Textbook of Addiction Treatment

Nady el-Guebaly
Giuseppe Carrà
Marc Galanter
Alexander M. Baldacchino
Editors

Textbook of Addiction Treatment

International Perspectives

Second Edition

Volume I

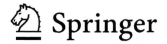
Springer

Editors
Nady el-Guebaly
Division of Addiction
Department of Psychiatry
University of Calgary
Calgary, AB
Canada

Marc Galanter
Division of Alcoholism and Drug Abuse
Department of Psychiatry
NYU School of Medicine
New York, NY
USA

Giuseppe Carrà
Mental Health Department
University of Milano-Bicocca
Monza
Italy

Alexander M. Baldacchino
Population and Behavioural Science
Division (Psychiatry and Addictions)
University of St Andrews
St.Andrews
UK

ISBN 978-3-030-36393-2   ISBN 978-3-030-36391-8   (eBook)
https://doi.org/10.1007/978-3-030-36391-8

This Springer imprint is published by the registered company Springer Nature Switzerland AG
The registered company address is: Gewerbestrasse 11, 6330 Cham, Switzerland

Preface: An International Perspective and Its Evolution

The International Society of Addiction Medicine (ISAM) was founded in Palm Springs, USA, in 1999. From the onset, the elements of its main mission were:

- *Advancement of the knowledge of addiction as a treatable disease*
- *Recognition that physicians worldwide have a major role to play in the management of addiction and associated disorders*
- *Enhancement of the credibility of the physician's role*
- *Emphasis of the importance of educational activities*
- *Establishment of consensus documents and practice guidelines*

To implement this mission, the Society organizes an annual global meeting and fundamental workshops. It also supports the International Certification in Addiction Medicine since 2005 with over 250 applicants from 17 countries sitting this internationally accredited exam.

In seeking reference texts to create the examination questions for the certification, it became evident that the two or three excellent multiauthored textbooks available in English are all originated from the USA, with an occasional contribution from an author from another country. These books are heavily centered on data arising from a US context and culture. ISAM decided that a textbook with a broader authorship representation was required as well as a search for data originating from across the world. We aimed to describe the multifaceted options available for culturally sensitive strategies prioritizing demand reduction.

The first edition in 2015 resulted from the collaborative efforts over 3 years of some 265 contributors from 30 countries. Based on the positive response of the first edition and also some constructive comments to make the second edition more accessible, it was decided to strive for more concise chapters aimed at highlighting the basics of the field and presented in an educationally sensitive format. Each chapter has key words and key points to anchor their main teaching insights. We endeavored to increase their clinical relevance and the authors provided sets of selective references.

The resulting second edition consists of ten sections, with some 222 contributors from 23 countries. It also presents an excellent opportunity to review the rapid evolution of our field over the course of a short 5 years.

Sociocultural, Neurological, and Genetic Foundations

The prevalence of drug intake is determined by not only individual stress factors but also regional and larger-scale cultural patterns of drug consumption, social role models, as well as legal requirements and prohibitions.

A common sequence is for the onset of substance abuse to be largely influenced by cultural factors; environmental and social factors are important in the transition to hazardous consumption, while neurobiological and other risk factors have become more salient in the transition to substance use disorder. The last 5 years have highlighted a number of new trends. While appropriate efforts were made since 2000 to legitimize addiction as a chronic disease, the public imagination has been captured by the acute aspects of the illness. Thousands upon thousands of overdoses with increasingly lethal compounds such as the opioid fentanyl have resulted in an unheard amount of media coverage and political discourse. Furthermore, a previously noted trend for the creation of laboratory manufactured chemicals just accelerated. Carfentanyl followed fentanyl in a matter of months. Traditional legal drugs such as nicotine, considered on the wane in western countries, made a resurgence using new delivery strategies, such as vaping. Medications are also benefitting from an expanding range of methods of delivery. A definite trend in basic sciences is the search for correlates between the prior scientific silos. Psychological symptoms have cerebral correlates. The genetic and now epigenetic components of the heritability of addiction also point to cross-population differences in risk susceptibility across large samples. This edition also includes a review of animal models of addictive behavior at the various stages of addiction. All these considerations consequently inform the spectrum of applied prevention strategies.

Differences in international perspectives and challenges in achieving a universal taxonomy remain. DSM-5 proposed the recent aggregation of the concept of dependence with that of substance use. This edition presents the nosology of the new ICD-11 (Diagnostic Definition, Criteria, and Classification of SUDs).

The Global Facets of Drug Use and the Current Trends in Biological Approaches

The differential availability of traditional drugs such as alcohol, tobacco, opioids, and cannabis along with newer drugs such as cocaine, amphetamines, hallucinogens, sedatives, and anabolic steroids is evident across the global stage and brings insights into the origins of abuse. Advances in neurosciences have so far yielded about a dozen drug-specific medications, and barriers to access to this small number by conservative national policies, economic constraints, and lack of clinicians' expertise are progressively eroding. A mounting evidence of efficacy arises from a number of diverse complementary options such as acupuncture, biologics, transcranial magnetic stimulation, nutrients, phytomedicines, and mind-body treatments. The evidence for these approaches originates from around the globe, where some of these techniques derive from a long-standing acculturation.

Behavioral Approaches and the Balance of Fidelity and Adaptation

Globally, behavioral approaches are a major element of treatment. Over the last 50 years, these therapies have evolved from generic advice-giving and confrontational strategies to more sophisticated, evidence-based techniques aimed at improving retention in treatment and positive reinforcement of change. Behavioral approaches are either directed at the individual or at groups, couples, families, and communities. Not all such approaches have been evaluated to the same extent, with the major effort directed at the investigation of motivational interviewing, cognitive behavioral therapy, and contingency management. Recent trends include the increased empirical evidence for the combination of behavioral approaches along with medication. More recent developing approaches have included mindfulness strategies, a multimodal approach to chronic pain, and the expansion of exercise components. These approaches are also benefitting from the new world of technology for improved access.

Challenges in the international dissemination of these approaches include the significant effort required for the transfer of knowledge and skills as well as the need to balance the evidence-based principles and methods of the approach with the adaptation needed to incorporate new cultural contexts and values in a translated language.

Screening and Major Components of a Systems Approach

While there is consensus about the benefits of screening and brief intervention strategies, the selection of optimal screening instruments, laboratory detection methods, and brief intervention techniques is the subject of an international effort to assess cross-cultural validity as well as investigate cost-effective laboratory tests and intervention strategies to accommodate the world's range of financial and practice resources.

A community treatment system requires a comprehensive network of different approaches, services, and participants. A public health perspective stresses connections among services. These services share concepts of different indications and rules for patient pathways through treatment phases following a stepped care model.

The network, in addition to formal therapeutic regimes, includes low-threshold approaches through outreach activities and harm reduction interventions. The resources and priorities will of course differ between developing and developed countries. A comprehensive network remains a work in progress with continuous adaptations. An overall drug policy document should reflect political support to provide adequate and sustainable resources.

Faced with the difficulties in abating, if not ending, the disease of addiction, a diverse group of socially grounded therapies have sprung worldwide. Approaches have included peer-led movements with no formal affiliation such as the 12-step programs which are spanning most of the globe. Other peer-led programs have evolved as institutions regulated by governments such as therapeutic communities. These approaches are not identical worldwide but have nevertheless many similarities. A major advantage of these approaches has been their cost-effectiveness rendering them accessible to a range of economic capabilities.

The second advantage has been their adaptability to social institutions as diverse as the workplace, the justice system, or the residential treatment programs. These approaches have gained widespread acceptance particularly in developing countries.

A system must include continuous monitoring and evaluation. The education and training of staff must be informed by the results of the evaluation. Stakeholders are to be involved in the priority setting as well as ethical and legal considerations.

Policies and Training in Addiction

There is increased recognition of the interplay between policy, legal, quality, and other governance standards in our field. A major trend accelerating over the last 5 years has been the increased recognition of addiction problems as public health rather than legal problems. This has led to prioritization of demand reduction strategies over supply reduction approaches. The social experiment over the last 5 years of the various aspects of legalization of cannabis is under scrutiny. Benefits and challenges are being reported.

The education, training, and sustenance of an appropriate workforce are critical to the survival of our field. A range of pioneering efforts is available. They are based on an increasingly consensual framework of identified competencies recognized by specialty associations as well as a number of universities through a master's degree.

Recognition of these competencies is facilitated through diverse pathways such as an American Board Examination, an International Certification (ISAM), and a number of diploma degrees. The knowledge base is accessible through a number of open access literature repositories or other educational activities. Fellowships in research training are available through NIDA, and a number of travel fellowships to conferences are offered.

Concerning the recognition of a specialty status, there is no "one-size-fits-all" model. This journey must adapt to local educational and licensing requirements that govern the national practices of medicine; options for recognition of competency may include certification by examination or completion of a comprehensive portfolio.

Beyond training, the recruitment of an adequate workforce must take into consideration the provision of attractive career paths countering stigma as well as adequate remuneration and working conditions.

What Constitutes a Behavioral Addiction?

Over the last 40 years, an increasing range of behaviors have been recognized as susceptible to develop from excessive engagement to a habitual or compulsive pattern. In addition to the investigation of common biological and psychological underpinnings, an international perspective highlights sociocultural differences. The same applies to the meeting of basic needs such as food, sex, or exercise and their evolution into compulsive behaviors. Ever-increasing access to services, products, and credit may accelerate this course.

Other insights are arising from the study of behavioral addictions as windows into human nature without the effects of substances. A model of addiction is emerging, depending less on "harm-based" negative consequences which are subject to ever-changing cultural values and judgment calls and more on the presence of concepts such as craving, loss of control, impulsivity, compulsion, mood dysregulation, and/or cognitive distortions.

Differences in treatment seeking patterns, treatment approaches, and settings as well as goals of treatment are highlighted in the international comparative analysis.

The major new additions in this Section are the updates on problematic Internet use and Internet gaming disorder. The new ICD-11 criteria as well as the DSM-5 appendix perspectives are discussed. Challenges about this concept and implications for the expansion of the range of potential correlated behaviors are outlined.

The Recognition of Medical Consequences and Comorbidities

The principles of assessment and management of the medical consequences of drug use ought not to be different around the world, and yet morbidity and mortality rates of drug users vary markedly due to differences in the general health status of the population, access to health care, and rates of treatment uptake and dropout. Almost every system is involved, including psychiatric, neurocognitive, cardiovascular, metabolic, and hepatic complications. An estimated one-third of the global population is living with one or more bacterial or viral infections. Nutrition is important, and nutritional disorders impact on recovery from other co-occurring illnesses. A new chapter on Oral Health has been added. The availability and acceptability of simple preventive measures like the use of a condom significantly affect the rate of sexually transmitted infections. The medical consequences of drug use interact in each country with the general level of hygiene as well as availability of preventive and treatment resources. While the management of acute disorders is the main focus of health resources in developing countries, chronic disorders including chronic pain become the major concern in developed countries, and substance use plays an important role in the course of both these acute and chronic disorders.

The Co-occurring Care of Substance Use and Psychiatric Disorders and System Change

While the recognition of medical comorbidities has not resulted in an overall health system change, reorganization is occurring in the addiction and mental health fields. Since the 1950s, the recognition of the co-occurrence of substance use and psychiatric disorders and its impact on the delivery of services has evolved. In most developed countries, the addiction field struggled to establish its own system of delivery of care based on the need to treat otherwise unrecognized or marginalized individuals with addictive disorders. In the United States, NIDA and NIAAA as separate research institutes led the building of a scientific knowledge foundation for our field. Worldwide, various degrees of separation remained in existence with many countries maintaining the addiction services under the umbrella of mental health.

For the last 30 years, increased recognition of the high prevalence of individuals with co-occurring disorders has resulted in replanning the coordination between addiction and other mental health services and in some cases integration of both systems. Based on improved empirical evidence in both fields, this renewed coordination is leading to enhanced attention to the neurobiological interface as well as pharmacological and psychotherapeutic combined options. It is also recognized that ethnic, racial, and cultural groups manifest their medical illnesses including psychiatric within the context of their heritage. The redesign of optimal systems of care as well as related workforce training is ongoing. Diagnostic-based approaches now integrate the treatment of substance use and other psychiatric disorders.

The Dilemmas of Special Populations

The challenge of prioritizing special groups for further recognition is a daunting one, and there is no international consensus. Our own selection included women, addressing half of humanity as well as the elderly soon to become a quarter of humanity. Two chapters describe the interactions between individuals abusing substances and the criminal justice system as well as the developing drug court network. Much attention has been directed at the care of physicians and other health care providers as an example of evidenced excellent outcome when well-defined workplace strategies are in place. Our last group involves the "displaced" populations either through conflicts or disasters; internationally, these groups are in the millions!

Perhaps a common feature of these groups is a sense that their fit within the general system of care may not be optimal, and there is demonstrated evidence that some of their needs may be better met wholly or partly in distinct pathways of care.

Meeting the Needs of Our Youth

Contrary to the previously listed groups, there is international consensus that the youth of the world deserve their own care. Much is to be gained by a focused system for young people who use drugs. They face the higher risk of initiating substance use. This initiation is determined by a multitude of risk factors in different developmental contexts, some of it originating from parental chronic substance use.

Adolescence is also a critical period where protective factors can also modify the pathways to substance use. The earlier the intervention during that period, the more chance there may be of a successful outcome including the prevention of chronicity and the reduction of the risk of suicide. Knowledge of the impact of both risk and protective factors can also optimize preventive strategies.

The engagement of a young person who is often vulnerable and even marginalized may require the involvement of multiple systems along with repeated assessments. Greater specificity in treatment choice that is developmentally appropriate such as CBT and MET along with family-based interventions has been demonstrated to provide the most consistent gains. Barriers to involvement such as stigma, safety, transportation, and family commitment must also be addressed.

In conclusion, as no country has so far been able to eradicate the misuse of substances or control excessive behaviors, pooling the international experience is warranted. A global scanning of the options allows us to forecast potentially promising approaches. Considering the world experience, we are also reminded of the dictum "Absence of evidence may not necessarily mean evidence of absence." It may just be that the evidence has yet not been unearthed and our current investigations are still not sensitive enough. The second edition is a testimony to the rapid evolution of our field, its challenges, and also its progress.

The COVID-19 pandemic started as we were concluding the final preparation of this edition. This pandemic brought home the critical need for global interconnectedness and the importance of comprehensive public health approaches. This pandemic superimposes itself on top of the many concerns reviewed in the rest of the textbook. An additional chapter has been added to the Section on Medical Disorders highlighting the conceptualization of syndemics and related strategies addressing the challenges of concurrent epidemics.

Calgary, AB, Canada   Nady el-Guebaly
Monza, Italy   Giuseppe Carrà
New York, NY, USA   Marc Galanter
St Andrews, UK   Alexander M. Baldacchino

Acknowledgments

From Nady el-Guebaly:

- To Joan, Jana, Lani, Nadia, Jalen, Nancy, and Robert, who sustained me through this second journey, and to the staff of the Addiction Centre, who over 20 years continue to allow my professional dreams.

From Giuseppe Carrá:

- To Caterina and Barbara

From Alex Baldacchino:

- To Sarah, my wife, and children Francesca and Stefan who support me throughout my sometime tortuous professional journey and who constantly reminded me of the essence of love and compassion. To NHS Fife Addiction Services which in the last 25 years provided the best of care to individuals and families experiencing substance-related problems.

The Editors also wish to acknowledge:

- The work of each and every one of our Section Editors and chapter authors, listed in the front. They defined for us the meaning of teamwork.
- The forbearance and dedication of our Administrative Assistant, Tracy Howden, and ISAM's Executive Administrator, Marilyn Dorozio, both of Calgary, Canada.
- The guidance and support of our Springer team: Donatella Rizza, Hemalatha Gunasekaran and Vasudevan Priyadarshini.
- The International Society of Addiction Medicine (ISAM) for sponsoring this textbook.
- ISAM Board of Directors 2016–2019:
  - Kathleen Brady, President [USA], Alex Baldacchino, President-Elect and Education [UK], Riaz Khan, Treasurer [Switzerland], Gregory Bunt, Past-President [USA], Hamad Al Ghaferi, International Liaison [UAE], Henrietta Bowden-Jones, Public Relations [UK], Sung-Gon Kim, Membership & Affiliates [South Korea], Nady el-Guebaly, Chief Examiner [Canada], Marc Galanter, Chief Editor [USA].

Contents

Part IV   Main Systems Components in Addictions Treatment
Ambros Uchtenhagen and Giuseppe Carrà

Contributors

Robert Ali University of Adelaide, Adelaide, SA, Australia

Joseph Althaus The National Problem Gambling Clinic, London, UK

The Barberry National Centre for Mental Health, Birmingham, UK

Stephen Amadala Alberta Health Services, Calgary, AB, Canada

Pedro J. Amor Department of Personality, Assessment and Psychological Treatment, National Distance Education University (UNED), Madrid, Spain

Garima Arora Dental Health Services Research Unit, University of Dundee, Dundee, UK

Sawitri Assanangkornchai Epidemiology Unit, Faculty of Medicine, Prince of Songkla University, Songkhla, Thailand

N. Avena University of Florida College of Medicine, Gainesville, FL, USA

Thomas F. Babor Department of Public Health Sciences, University of Connecticut School of Medicine, Farmington, CT, USA

Sudie E. Back Medical University of South Carolina, Charleston, SC, USA

Alexander M. Baldacchino Population and Behavioural Science Division (Psychiatry and Addictions), University of St Andrews and NHS Fife, St Andrews, UK

St Andrews Medical School, University of St Andrews, Scotland, UK

Jane Ballantyne University of Washington, Seattle, WA, USA

Manuel Barrera Jr Department of Psychology, Arizona State University, Tempe, AZ, USA

Pablo Barrio Addictions Unit, Department of Psychiatry, University of Catalonia, Barcelona, Spain

Francesco Bartoli Department of Medicine and Surgery, University of Milano-Bicocca, Milan, Italy

Department of Mental Health and Addiction, ASST Nord Milano, Milan, Italy

M. Teresa Bascarán INEUROPA-ISPA, Oviedo, Spain

CIBERSAM, Oviedo, Spain

David Best University of Derby, Derby, UK

Julio Bobes INEUROPA-ISPA, Oviedo, Spain

CIBERSAM, Oviedo, Spain

Department of Psychiatry, University of Oviedo, Oviedo, Spain

M. Teresa Bobes-Bascarán Servicio de Salud Del Principado de Asturias (SESPA), Oviedo, Spain

Department of Psychology, University of Oviedo, Oviedo, Spain

INEUROPA-ISPA, Oviedo, Spain

CIBERSAM, Oviedo, Spain

Kristopher Bough Division of Basic Neuroscience and Behavioral Research, National Institute on Drug Abuse, USA

Henrietta Bowden-Jones Honorary Professor, Division of Psychology and Language Science, University College London, London, UK

Honorary Senior Visiting Fellow, Cambridge University, London, UK

President of Psychiatry Section, Royal Society of Medicine, London, UK

The National Problem Gambling Clinic, London, UK

Kathleen T. Brady Department of Psychiatry and Behavioral Sciences, Clinical Neuroscience Division, Medical University of South Carolina, Charleston, SC, USA

Department of Psychiatry and Behavioral Sciences, Addiction Sciences Division, Medical University of South Carolina, Charleston, SC, USA

Distinguished University Professor, Vice President for Research, Medical University of South Carolina, Charleston, SC, USA

Jørgen G. Bramness Norwegian Competence Centre for Dual Diagnosis Innland Hospital Trust, Hamar, Norway

Norwegian Institute of Public Health, Oslo, Norway

Institute of Clinical Medicine, UiT, The Arctic University of Norway, Tromsø, Norway

María Dolores Braquehais Integral Care Program for Sick Health Professionals, Galatea Clinic, Galatea Foundation, Catalan Medical Association, Barcelona, Spain

Group of Psychiatry, Mental Health and Addictions, Vall Hebron Research Institute, Barcelona, Spain

Barbara Broers Unit for Dependencies, Division for Primary Care, Department for Community Medicine, Primary Care and Emergencies, Geneva University Hospitals, Geneva, Switzerland

Vivian B. Brown Prototypes: Centers for Innovation in Health, Mental Health, and Substance Use Disorders, Pittsboro, NC, USA

Eugeni Bruguera Integral Care Program for Sick Health Professionals, Galatea Clinic, Galatea Foundation, Catalan Medical Association, Barcelona, Spain

Group of Psychiatry, Mental Health and Addictions, Vall Hebron Research Institute, Barcelona, Spain

Department of Psychiatry and Legal Medicine, Hospital Universitari Vall d'Hebron, CIBERSAM, Universitat Autònoma de Barcelona, Barcelona, Spain

Alan J. Budney Center for Technology and Behavioral Health, Department of Psychiatry, Geisel School of Medicine at Dartmouth, Lebanon, NH, USA

Gregory Bunt Daytop Village, Inc., New York, NY, USA

Department of Psychiatry, NYU Langone Medical Center, New York, NY, USA

Gregor Burkhart EMCDDA, Lisbon, Portugal

Anja Busse United Nations Office on Drugs and Crime, Vienna, Austria

Giuseppe Carrà Mental Health Department, University of Milano-Bicocca, Milan, Italy

Department of Mental Health and Addiction, ASST Nord Milano, Milan, Italy

Division of Psychiatry, University College London, London, UK

Department of Medicine and Surgery, University of Milano-Bicocca, Milan, Italy

Daniele Carretta Department of Mental Health and Addiction, Azienda Socio Sanitaria Territoriale Papa Giovanni XXIII, Bergamo, Italy

Miquel Casas Department of Psychiatry and Legal Medicine, Hospital Universitari Vall d'Hebron, CIBERSAM, Universitat Autònoma de Barcelona, Barcelona, Spain

Richard Cash 360Edge, Melbourne, VIC, Australia

Felipe González Castro Edson College of Nursing and Health Innovation, Arizona State University, Phoenix, AZ, USA

Kai Yeng Chan Consultation Liaison and Addictions Psychiatry Medicine, Townsville Hospital, Douglas, QLD, Australia

Katrin Charlet Department of Psychiatry and Psychotherapy, CCM, Charité - Universitätsmedizin Berlin, Berlin, Germany

Guang Chen Drug Health, Western Sydney Local Health District, Westmead, NSW, Australia

Brian Conway Vancouver Infectious Diseases Centre, Vancouver, BC, Canada

Ryan Cotter Division of Cardiology, University of Colorado, Aurora, CO, USA

David Crockford Department of Psychiatry, University of Calgary, Calgary, AB, Canada

Ilana B. Crome Keele University, Staffordshire, UK

St George's, University of London, London, UK

Silvia L. Cruz Department of Pharmacobiology, CINVESTAV, Mexico City, Mexico

Naomi Dambreville The City College of New York, CUNY, New York, NY, USA

The Graduate Center, CUNY, New York, NY, USA

Leigh Dickerson Davidson David E. Smith, MD & Associates, San Francisco, CA, USA

Cornelis A. J. De Jong Radboud University, Nijmegen, The Netherlands

George De Leon BST at the School of Nursing, NYU, New York, NY, USA

Department of Psychiatry, NYU School of Medicine, New York, NY, USA

Zsolt Demetrovics Institute of Psychology, ELTE Eötvös Loránd University, Budapest, Hungary

John F. Dillon Gut Group, Division of Molecular and Clinical Medicine, School of Medicine, University of Dundee, Dundee, UK

Fernando Dinamarca Institut de Neuropsiquiatria i Addiccions, Hospital del Mar, Barcelona, Spain

IMIM (Institut Hospital del Mar d'Investigacions Mèdiques), Barcelona, Spain

Michael Dinh Royal Prince Alfred Hospital, The University of Sydney, Discipline of Emergency Medicine, Sydney, NSW, Australia

Hannah M. Dix Gastroenterology Department, NHS Tayside, Dundee, UK

Nicole Durham Addictions Division, Centre for Addiction and Mental Health (CAMH), Toronto, ON, Canada

Enrique Echeburúa Department of Clinical Psychology, University of the Basque Country UPV/EHU, San Sebastián, Spain

J. Guy Edwards Southampton University Hospitals, Southampton, UK

Department of Psychiatry and Epidemiology Unit, Faculty of Medicine, Prince of Songkla University, Hat Yai, Songkhla, Thailand

Hamed Ekhtiari Laureate Institute for Brain Research, Tulsa, OK, USA

Nady el-Guebaly Division of Addiction, Department of Psychiatry, University of Calgary, Calgary, AB, Canada

Ahmed Elkashef Division of Therapeutics and Medical Consequences, National Institute on Drug Abuse, National Institutes of Health, Bethesda, Maryland, USA

Nadine Ezard St Vincent's Hospital Sydney / UNSW, Sydney, Australia

L. Llamosas Falcón Centre for Addiction and Mental Health (CAMH), Toronto, ON, Canada

Preventive Medicine and Public Health, Hospital Universitario 12 de Octubre, Madrid, Spain

Magi Farré Universitat Autònoma de Barcelona, Barcelona, Spain

Hospital Universitari Germans Trias i Pujol (IGTP), Badalona, Spain

Thierry Favrod-Coune Unit for Dependencies, Division for Primary Care, Department for Primary Care Medicine, Geneva University Hospitals, Geneva, Switzerland

Marica Ferri EMCDDA, Lisbon, Portugal

Tatiana Zambrano Filomensky Impulse Control Disorders Outpatient Unit, University of São Paulo, São Paulo, Brazil

Francina Fonseca Institut de Neuropsiquiatria i Addiccions, Hospital del Mar, Barcelona, Spain

IMIM (Institut Hospital del Mar d'Investigacions Mèdiques), Barcelona, Spain

Universitat Autònoma de Barcelona, Barcelona, Spain

Ronald Fraser McGill University, Montreal, QC, Canada

Ruth Freeman Dental Health Services Research Unit, University of Dundee, NHS Tayside, Dundee, UK

Eva Friedel Charite - Universitätsmedizin Berlin, Berlin, Germany

Marc Galanter Division of Alcoholism and Drug Abuse, Department of Psychiatry, NYU School of Medicine, New York, NY, USA

Department of Psychiatry, NYU School of Medicine, New York, NY, USA

Hugh Garavan Department of Psychiatry, University of Vermont, Burlington, VT, USA

Maria Garbusow Department of Psychiatry and Psychotherapy, CCM, Charité - Universitätsmedizin Berlin, Berlin, Germany

M. Paz García-Portilla INEUROPA-ISPA, Oviedo, Spain

CIBERSAM, Oviedo, Spain

Department of Psychiatry, University of Oviedo, Oviedo, Spain

Eliot L. Gardner Neuropsychopharmacology Section, Molecular Targets and Medications Discovery Research Branch, Intramural Research Program, National Institute on Drug Abuse, US National Institutes of Health, Baltimore, MD, USA

Tony P. George Addictions Division, Centre for Addiction and Mental Health (CAMH), Toronto, ON, Canada

Department of Psychiatry, University of Toronto, Toronto, ON, Canada

Stephen Gilbert Anaesthesia and Pain Medicine, Townsville Hospital, Douglas, QLD, Australia

North Queensland Persistent Pain Management Service, Townsville Hospital, Townsville, QLD, Australia

Thomas Gilbertson Department of Neurology, Ninewells Hospital and Medical School, Dundee, UK

Division of Imaging Science and Technology, Medical School, University of Dundee, Dundee, UK

M. Gold Washington University, St. Louis, MO, USA

Hugo González National Institute of Psychiatry Ramón de la Fuente Muiz, Mexico City, Mexico

Christine M. Goodair Population Health Research Institute, St George's, University of London, London, UK

David A. Gorelick Department of Psychiatry, University of Maryland School of Medicine, Baltimore, MD, USA

Linda Gowing University of Adelaide, Adelaide, SA, Australia

Kevin M. Gray Department of Psychiatry and Behavioral Sciences, Medical University of South Carolina, Charleston, SC, USA

Paul Griffiths EMCDDA, Lisbon, Portugal

Antoni Gual Addictions Unit, Department of Psychiatry, University of Catalonia, Barcelona, Spain

Neurosciences Institute, Hospital Clínic, IDIBAPS, Barcelona, Spain

Steven W. Gust International Program, National Institute on Drug Abuse, National Institutes of Health, US Department of Health and Human Services, Washington, DC, USA

Anna Haber Western Sydney University School of Medicine, Sydney, Australia

Paul S. Haber Drug Health Services, Sydney Local Health District, The University of Sydney Central Clinical School, Sydney, NSW, Australia

University of Sydney and Drug Health Service, Royal Prince Alfred Hospital, Camperdown, NSW, Australia

Richard Hallinan Drug Health Services, Liverpool Hospital, South Western Sydney Local Health District, Liverpool, NSW, Australia

The Byrne Surgery, Redfern, NSW, Australia

Rebecca Hamer Sheffield Hallam University, Sheffield, UK

Jennifer Harland University of Adelaide, Adelaide, SA, Australia

Richard Hartnoll European Monitoring Centre for Drugs and Drug Addiction, Lisbon, Portugal (retired)

Deborah S. Hasin Department of Epidemiology, Columbia University Mailman School of Public Health, New York State Psychiatric Institute, New York, NY, USA

Dagmar Hedrich European Monitoring Centre for Drugs and Drug Addiction, Lisbon, Portugal

Andreas Heinz Department of Psychiatry and Psychotherapy, CCM, Charité - Universitätsmedizin Berlin, Berlin, Germany

Annemarie Hennessy Western Sydney University School of Medicine, Sydney, Australia

Susan Henry-Edwards University of Adelaide, Adelaide, SA, Australia

Mariely Hernandez The City College of New York, CUNY, New York, NY, USA

The Graduate Center, CUNY, New York, NY, USA

Meyen Hertzsprung M Hertzsprung Psychological Services, Calgary, AB, Canada

David C. Hodgins Department of Psychology, University of Calgary, Calgary, AB, Canada

Ben Houghton St George's University of London, London, UK

Lori Isaif McGill University Health Centre, Montreal, QC, Canada

Shelly Iskandar Psychiatric Department, Hasan Sadikin Hospital, Padjajaran University, Bandung, Indonesia

Alexandra Ivanciu Department of Psychiatry, University of Vermont, Burlington, VT, USA

Lauren M. Jansson The Johns Hopkins University School of Medicine, Baltimore, MD, USA

Chloe J. Jordan National Institute on Drug Abuse, Baltimore, MD, USA

Aloysius Joseph Daytop International, Inc., New York, NY, USA

Jakob Kaminski Charite - Universitätsmedizin Berlin, Berlin, Germany

Gen Kanayama Biological Psychiatry Laboratory, McLean Hospital, Belmont, MA, USA

Harvard Medical School, Boston, MA, USA

Linda K. Kaye Edge Hill University, Ormskirk, UK

Jag H. Khalsa Division of Therapeutics and Medical Consequences, National Institute on Drug Abuse, National Institutes of Health, Aldie, VA, USA

Division of Therapeutics and Medical Consequences, National Institute on Drug Abuse, National Institutes of Health, Bethesda, Maryland, USA

E. J. Khantzian Department of Psychiatry, Harvard Medical School, Boston, MA, USA

Jungjin Kim Division of Alcohol and Drug Abuse, McLean Hospital, Belmont, MA, USA

Department of Psychiatry, Harvard Medical School, Boston, MA, USA

Hyoun S. Kim Department of Psychology, University of Calgary, Calgary, AB, Canada

Orsolya Király Institute of Psychology, ELTE Eötvös Loránd University, Budapest, Hungary

Axel Klein Global Drug Policy Observatory, University of Swansea, Swansea, UK

Keith Klostermann Medaille College, Buffalo, NY, USA

Gail Koshorek Sleep Disorder & Research Center, Henry Ford Health System, Detroit, MI, USA

Christos Kouimtsidis Imperial College, London, UK

Mori J. Krantz Division of Cardiology, University of Colorado, Aurora, CO, USA

Denver Health Medical Center, Division of Cardiology, Denver, CO, USA

Daniel L. Krashin University of Washington, Seattle, WA, USA

Daria J. Kuss Nottingham Trent University, Nottingham, UK

Lise Laporte McGill University Health Centre, Montreal, QC, Canada

Noeline C. Latt Disciplines of Psychiatry and Addiction Medicine, Faculty of Medicine, University of Sydney, Camperdown, NSW, Australia

Formerly Northern Area Drug and Alcohol Service, Royal North Shore Hospital, St Leonards, NSW, Australia

Nicole K. Lee National Drug Research Institute (NDRI), Curtin University, Bentley, WA, Australia

360Edge, Melbourne, VIC, Australia

Robert F. Leeman Department of Health Education and Behavior, University of Florida, Gainesville, FL, USA

Department of Psychiatry, Yale University, New Haven, CT, USA

Bernard Le Foll Translational Addiction Research Laboratory, Centre for Addiction and Mental Health, University of Toronto, Toronto, ON, Canada

Alcohol Research and Treatment Clinic, Acute Care Program, Centre for Addiction and Mental Health, Toronto, ON, Canada

Campbell Family Mental Health Research Institute, Centre for Addiction and Mental Health, Toronto, ON, Canada

Department of Family and Community Medicine, University of Toronto, Toronto, ON, Canada

Department of Pharmacology and Toxicology, University of Toronto, Toronto, ON, Canada

Division of Brain and Therapeutics, Department of Psychiatry, University of Toronto, Toronto, ON, Canada

Institute of Medical Sciences, University of Toronto, Toronto, ON, Canada

Shea M. Lemley Geisel School of Medicine at Dartmouth, Lebanon, NH, USA

Frances Rudnick Levin Columbia University Medical Center, New York State Psychiatric Institute, New York, NY, USA

Luming Li Psychiatry, Yale University, New Haven, CT, USA

Jessica B. Lydiard University of Miami, Miami, FL, USA

Brian Mac Grory Brown University, Providence, RI, USA

Tianna Magel Vancouver Infectious Diseases Centre, Vancouver, BC, Canada

Hussein Manji United Nations Office on Drugs and Crime, Vienna, Austria

Marianne Marcus The University of Texas Health Science Center at Houston, Houston, TX, USA

Douglas B. Marlowe National Association of Drug Court Professionals, Chadds Ford, PA, USA

Lisa A. Marsch Geisel School of Medicine at Dartmouth, Lebanon, NH, USA

Flavio F. Marsiglia School of Social Work, Arizona State University, Phoenix, AZ, USA

Lisa Marzilli Dominion Diagnostics Lab, Narragansett, RI, USA

Jenna L. McCauley Medical University of South Carolina, Charleston, SC, USA

Andrew S. McClintock University of Wisconsin-Madison, Madison, WI, USA

Michael G. McDonell Washington State University, Spokane, WA, USA

R. Kathryn McHugh Division of Alcohol and Drug Abuse, McLean Hospital, Belmont, MA, USA
Department of Psychiatry, Harvard Medical School, Boston, MA, USA

S. McNamara Department of Respiratory & Sleep Medicine, Royal Prince Alfred Hospital, Camperdown, NSW, Australia

Sterling M. McPherson Washington State University, Spokane, WA, USA

Tim McSweeney Department of Psychology, University of Hertfordshire, Hatfield, UK

María Elena Medina-Mora Mental Health Global Research Center, National Institute of Psychiatry Ramón de la Fuente Muiz/UNAM, Mexico City, Mexico

Robert Milin Adolescent Day Treatment Unit, Royal Ottawa Mental Health Centre, Ottawa, ON, Canada
Department of Psychiatry University of Ottawa, Ottawa, ON, Canada

Michael Miller Department of Psychiatry, University of Wisconsin, Madison, WI, USA

Larissa J. Mooney Department of Psychiatry and Biobehavioral Sciences, University of California Los Angeles (UCLA), Los Angeles, CA, USA

VA Greater Los Angeles Healthcare System, Los Angeles, CA, USA

Christian A. Müller Department of Psychiatry and Psychotherapy, CCM, Charité - Universitätsmedizin Berlin, Berlin, Germany

Natalia Murinova University of Washington, Seattle, WA, USA

S. Murray Icahn School of Medicine, Mount Sinai, NY, USA

B. Nanayakkara Department of Respiratory & Sleep Medicine, Royal Prince Alfred Hospital, Camperdown, NSW, Australia

Edward V. Nunes Division on Substance Use Disorders, Department of Psychiatry, Columbia University Irving Medical Center, New York State Psychiatric Institute, New York, NY, USA

Michael Odenwald Department of Psychology, Konstanz University, Konstanz, Germany

Timothy J. O'Farrell Harvard Medical School, Brockton, NY, USA

Andrew T. Olagunju Department of Psychiatry and Behavioral Neurosciences McMaster University & St Joseph Healthcare Hamilton, Hamilton, ON, Canada

Department of Psychiatry, College of Medicine, University of Lagos, Lagos, Nigeria

Matthew Oliver Royal Prince Alfred Hospital, The University of Sydney, Discipline of Emergency Medicine, Sydney, NSW, Australia

Esther Papaseit Universitat Autònoma de Barcelona, Barcelona, Spain

Hospital Universitari Germans Trias i Pujol (IGTP), Badalona, Spain

Fernando B. Perfas Daytop International Training Academy, New York, NY, USA

Sara Park Perrins School of Environmental and Forest Sciences, University of Washington, Seattle, WA, USA

Harrison G. Pope Jr Biological Psychiatry Laboratory, McLean Hospital, Belmont, MA, USA

Harvard Medical School, Boston, MA, USA

Marc N. Potenza Department of Psychiatry, Yale University, New Haven, CT, USA

Departments of Child Study and Neurobiology, Yale University, New Haven, CT, USA

Ulrich W. Preuss Vitos Hospital for Psychiatry and Psychotherapy, Kassel, Germany

Department for Psychiatry, Psychotherapy and Psychosomatic Medicine, University of Halle, Halle, Germany

C. Probst Centre for Addiction and Mental Health (CAMH), Toronto, ON, Canada

Anna Quirk Department of Endocrinology, St Vincent's Hospital, Darlinghurst, NSW, Australia

Department of Endocrinology, Royal Prince Alfred Hospital, Camperdown, NSW, Australia

Rahul Rao Institute of Psychiatry, Psychology and Neuroscience, London, UK

Richard A. Rawson Vermont Center for Behavior and Health, University of Vermont, Burlington, VT, USA

Department of Psychiatry and Biobehavioral Sciences, University of California Los Angeles (UCLA), Los Angeles, CA, USA

Tania Real National Institute of Psychiatry Ramón de la Fuente Muiz, Mexico City, Mexico

J. Rehm Centre for Addiction and Mental Health (CAMH), Toronto, ON, Canada

Dalla Lana School of Public Health, University of Toronto, Toronto, ON, Canada

Institute of Medical Science, University of Toronto, Toronto, ON, Canada

Department of Psychiatry, University of Toronto, Toronto, ON, Canada

Institute of Clinical Psychology and Psychotherapy, Technische Universität Dresden, Dresden, Germany

Department of International Health Projects, Institute for Leadership and Health Management, I.M. Sechenov First Moscow State Medical University, Moscow, Russian Federation

Stephan Ripke Charite - Universitätsmedizin Berlin, Berlin, Germany

Emma M. Robinson Gut Group, Division of Molecular and Clinical Medicine, School of Medicine, University of Dundee, Dundee, UK

Rebeca Robles National Institute of Psychiatry Ramón de la Fuente Muiz, Mexico City, Mexico

Timothy Roehrs Sleep Disorder & Research Center, Henry Ford Health System, Detroit, MI, USA

Department of Psychiatry and Behavioral Neuroscience, Wayne State University, SOM, Detroit, MI, USA

John M. Roll Washington State University, Spokane, WA, USA

Evelien Rooke Department of Neurology, Ninewells Hospital and Medical School, Dundee, UK

Robin Room Centre for Alcohol Policy Research, La Trobe University, Bundoora, VIC, Australia

Centre for Social Research on Alcohol & Drugs, Department of Public Health Sciences, Stockholm University, Stockholm, Sweden

Hendrik G. Roozen University of New Mexico, Albuquerque, NM, USA

Paula Ross 360Edge, Melbourne, VIC, Australia

Thomas Roth Sleep Disorder & Research Center, Henry Ford Health System, Detroit, MI, USA

Department of Psychiatry and Behavioral Neuroscience, Wayne State University, SOM, Detroit, MI, USA

Hans-Jürgen Rumpf University of Lübeck, Lübeck, Germany

Brian Rush Centre for Addiction and Mental Health, Toronto, ON, Canada

Claudia Salazar Central North West London NHS Foundation Trust, London, UK

Siddharth Sarkar Department of Psychiatry and National Drug Dependence Treatment Center, All India Institute of Medical Sciences, New Delhi, India

Julia Sasiadek Addictions Division, Centre for Addiction and Mental Health (CAMH), Toronto, ON, Canada

John B. Saunders Centre for Youth Substance Abuse Research, University of Queensland, St Lucia, QLD, Australia

Disciplines of Psychiatry and Addiction Medicine, Faculty of Medicine, University of Sydney, Camperdown, NSW, Australia

Miriam Sebold Department of Psychiatry and Psychotherapy, CCM, Charité - Universitätsmedizin Berlin, Berlin, Germany

Bhags Sharma Addiction Services, NHS Fife, Scotland, UK

K. D. Shield Centre for Addiction and Mental Health (CAMH), Toronto, ON, Canada

Dalla Lana School of Public Health, University of Toronto, Toronto, ON, Canada

Dan Shlosberg Department of Psychological Medicine, Faculty of Medical and Health Sciences, University of Auckland, Auckland, New Zealand

Gal Shoval Geha Mental Health Center, Petah Tiqva, Israel

Sackler Faculty of Medicine, Tel Aviv University, Tel Aviv, Israel

Matisyahu Shulman Division on Substance Use Disorders, Department of Psychiatry, Columbia University Irving Medical Center, New York State Psychiatric Institute, New York, NY, USA

Roland Simon IFT Institute for Therapy Research, Munich, Germany

Jane Ellen Smith Department of Psychology, University of New Mexico, Albuquerque, NM, USA

David E. Smith David E. Smith, MD & Associates, San Francisco, CA, USA

Brendan Smyth Department of Renal Medicine, St. George Hospital, Sydney, Australia

Michael J. Sofis Center for Technology and Behavioral Health, Department of Psychiatry, Geisel School of Medicine at Dartmouth, Lebanon, NH, USA

Philip A. Spechler Department of Psychiatry, University of Vermont, Burlington, VT, USA

Douglas Steele Division of Imaging Science and Technology, Medical School, University of Dundee, Dundee, UK

Frederike Stöth Institute of Legal Forensic Medicine, University of Bern, Bern, Switzerland

Hermano Tavares Impulse Control Disorders Outpatient Unit, University of São Paulo, São Paulo, Brazil

Joe Tay Wee Teck University of Glasgow, Scotland, Glasgow, UK

Debora Teles Personality Disorder Program, McGill University Health Centre, Montreal, QC, Canada

Natasha Thon IDIBAPS Neurosciences Institute, Barcelona, Spain

Marta Torrens Institut de Neuropsiquiatria i Addiccions, Hospital del Mar, Barcelona, Spain

IMIM (Institut Hospital del Mar d'Investigacions Mèdiques), Barcelona, Spain

Universitat Autònoma de Barcelona, Barcelona, Spain

Christopher Tremonti Sydney Local Health District, Camperdown, NSW, Australia

Leanne Trick Translational Addiction Research Laboratory, Centre for Addiction and Mental Health, University of Toronto, Toronto, ON, Canada

Stephen Twigg Department of Endocrinology, Royal Prince Alfred Hospital, Camperdown, NSW, Australia

Sydney Medical School (Central), Faculty of Medicine and Health, The University of Sydney, Sydney, NSW, Australia

Ambros Uchtenhagen Swiss Research Foundation for Public Health and Addiction, Zurich University, Zurich, Switzerland

Annie Umbricht The Johns Hopkins University School of Medicine, Baltimore, MD, USA

Martha L. Velez The Johns Hopkins University School of Medicine, Baltimore, MD, USA

Antonio Verdejo-Garcia Turner Institute for Brain and Mental Health, Monash University, Melbourne, VIC, Australia

Jelena Verkler Sleep Disorder & Research Center, Henry Ford Health System, Detroit, MI, USA

Claudio Violato University of Minnesota Medical School, Minneapolis, MN, USA

Jonathan M. Wai Division on Substance Use Disorders, Department of Psychiatry, Columbia University Irving Medical Center, New York State Psychiatric Institute, New York, NY, USA

Nasir Warfa Maltepe University, Maltepe/İstanbul, Turkey

Wolfgang Weinmann Institute of Legal Forensic Medicine, University of Bern, Bern, Switzerland

Roger D. Weiss Division of Alcohol and Drug Abuse, McLean Hospital, Belmont, MA, USA

Department of Psychiatry, Harvard Medical School, Boston, MA, USA

Gabrielle Welle-Strand Norwegian Center of Addiction Research/Oslo University Hospital, Oslo, Norway

Blake Werner Yale University, New Haven, CT, USA

Jessica Wong Klinik am Homberg, Bad Wildungen, Germany

Kelli Wuerth Vancouver Infectious Diseases Centre, Vancouver, BC, Canada

Friedrich Martin Wurst Medical Faculty, University of Basel, Basel, Switzerland

Psychiatric University Hospital Basel, Basel, Switzerland

S. Yarnell-Mac Grory Yale School of Medicine – Department of Psychiatry, New Haven, CT, USA

Yvonne H. C. Yau Department of Neurology and Neurosurgery, McGill University, Montreal, QC, Canada

Michel Yegles Laboratoire National de Santé, Forensic Toxicology, Dudelange, Luxemburg

Mehran Zare-Bidoky Iranian National Center for Addiction Studies, Tehran University of Medical Sciences, Tehran, Iran

School of Medicine, Shahid Sadoughi University of Medical Sciences, Yazd, Iran

David Zendle University of York, York, UK

Part I

Basic Sciences and Clinical Foundations

Andreas Heinz and Nady el-Guebaly

Basic Sciences and Clinical Foundations: An Introduction

1

Andreas Heinz and Nady el-Guebaly

Content

Abstract

We here introduce the section "Basic Sciences and Clinical Foundations." In this section, we address the social, cultural, and regional as well as the neurobiological and genetic aspects of addiction. The foundational section of this international textbook on addiction treatment aims to provide a prologue to the topic. This section starts with chapters on neurobiology including a review of the neurotoxic and neuroadaptive consequences of chronic drug intake with a focus on alcohol. A chapter on genetics presents the heritability of addiction and its genetic and epigenetic components. The next chapter complements the focus on neurobiological correlates of addictive behavior with a discussion of animal models of addiction. The next chapter presents the international epidemiological aspects of addiction with a focus on the findings of the Global Burden of Disease Study. The role of socioenvironmental factors in diagnosis and treatment is addressed in the next chapter, which also describes their respective impact on the patient-clinician interpersonal dynamics as well as interactions in the family, intimate social networks, community at large, and policy makers. We thus emphasize how cultural factors, that is, shared beliefs, norms, and patterns of behavior, interact with drug consumption in different populations. The social patterning of psychoactive drug use differs as to whether it is medicinal, regular, intermittent, or addictive. The next chapter focuses on the prevention applications of the components discussed with a review of the international experience. These contributions underpin the evolution of diagnostic definitions and classifications reviewed in the subsequent chapter. In conclusion, this foundational section provides a focused scientific review of current knowledge. As this is the first section of this textbook, the aim is to demonstrate the basic sciences and clinical foundations and to reflect the commonalities and differences of broad global and international perspectives.

A. Heinz (✉)
Charité – Universitätsmedizin Berlin,
Berlin, Germany
e-mail: andreas.heinz@charite.de

N. el-Guebaly
Division of Addiction, Department of Psychiatry,
University of Calgary, Calgary, AB, Canada
e-mail: nady.el-guebaly@ahs.ca

Keywords

Basic science · Neurobiology · Genetics
Animal models · Global Burden of Disease
Diagnoses

Drug use and dependence are the leading causes of disability and suffering particularly among adolescence and younger adults [11]. Addictive disorders also contribute to a substantial percentage of interpersonal violence, partly due to the direct effect of drugs of abuse such as alcohol [13] and partly due to social consequences of illicit drug abuse [20, 21, 27]. In this section, we will discuss the social, cultural, and regional as well as the neurobiological and genetic aspects of addiction. The appreciation of this term has evolved. In 1976, Griffith Edwards suggested to focus on key aspects of drug dependence, namely, tolerance to drug effects developing with its chronic (ab)use and withdrawal symptoms appearing when chronic drug use is suddenly interrupted [4]. Edwards suggested replacing the term "addiction" as this more likely stigmatizes patients because it points to strong drug urges and the allegedly impaired ability to control such desires. He instead proposed to focus on the "somatic" aspects of the addictive disorders, most notably tolerance and withdrawal. However, tolerance also develops to nonaddictive drugs such as ß-blockers or antidepressive medication, and withdrawal symptoms emerge as a sign of impaired cerebral homoeostasis when drug consumption is suddenly stopped [15, 19]. Caffeine consumption can also cause withdrawal symptoms, which is relevant but not sufficient for diagnosing drug dependence. In accordance with these considerations, a "caffeine dependence" syndrome was described in ICD-10 but is no longer found in the current version of ICD-11, and DSM-5 lists "caffeine use disorder" only as a condition for further study [14]. Beyond tolerance development and withdrawal symptoms, current classification systems emphasize craving for the drug of abuse and the impaired ability to control the consumption of this drug in spite of its harmful effects as key aspects of addictive disorders [1].

Craving, loss of control, and consumption despite negative consequences have often been labeled as the "psychological" symptoms of an addictive disorder, while tolerance development and withdrawal symptoms have been called "somatic" signs of the disease; however, in our view, this distinction between psychological and somatic symptoms of addictive disorders should no longer be supported, as both withdrawal symptoms and craving for the drug of abuse have cerebral correlates. Tolerance development is associated with neuroadaptations within affected neurotransmitter systems, and withdrawal symptoms result from an imbalance between central excitatory and inhibitory neurotransmitters, causing an overshoot of autonomic nervous system responses [18]. Craving in turn might be attributable to dysfunctions of motivational systems including dopaminergic neurotransmission in the ventral striatum [8, 12]. Furthermore, current theories of addictive behavior emphasize a gradual shift from goal-directed, reward-seeking behavior toward automatic or even "compulsive" drug intake, a concept that has previously been promoted by Tiffany and Carter [26] with respect to nicotine dependence and that has currently gained a lot of behavioral as well as neurobiological support in animal experiments and human studies focusing on chronic drug intakes [6, 7]. These considerations show that far from being limited to either the psychological or somatic domain, all key aspects of addictive disorders such as tolerance development, withdrawal symptoms, drug craving, and impaired control of drug use are associated with central nervous system correlates and neuroadaptations.

Modern theories of psychiatric disorders integrate subjectively reported symptoms such as craving or urges to consume a drug with behavioral variables such as acute or habitual drug intake and their respective neurobiological correlates (e.g., activation of the ventral or dorsal striatum and the respectively associated frontocortical-striatal-thalamic loops [3, 10, 23]. Such neurobiological approaches are now complemented by computational approaches that compare different models of behavior for best fit and identify decisive computational steps (including reward prediction errors); the neurobiological correlates of such computations can then be identified, for example, with neuro-imaging [29].

Modern neurobiological research has often pointed to the intimate interaction between social stress effects and the development and maintenance of drug addiction [13, 17]. For example, exposure to developmentally early social isolation stress in nonhuman primates promotes excessive alcohol intake, and the degree to which such social effects impact on the neurobiological correlates of addiction is modulated by genetic variability [2, 9, 13, 16].

Beyond individual social stress factors, regional and large-scale cultural patterns of drug consumption, legal requirements, and prohibitions as well as complex social role models all contribute to the prevalence of drug intake [5, 24]. Also, modern cosmopolitan societies need to consider the effects of different explanatory models of addictive disorders. For example, we and others have observed that it may not suffice to translate information material to prevent the development of addictive disorders because the concept, the terms, and the general understanding of addictive behavior can vary substantially between persons and cultures, and misunderstandings can only be avoided if local and linguistic concepts of "normal" and "harmful" drug use are known [22, 28]. More recently, the stigmatizing effect of some of our current terminology has come under scrutiny [25].

Our textbook addresses all the above mentioned aspects of addiction. The foundational section of this international textbook on addiction treatment aims to provide an apt prologue to the topic. It consequently includes articles on the burden of disease, the cultural as well as genetic aspects of addictive disorders, and the neurobiology of addiction and also on the resulting strategies for prevention and treatment of drug use and dependence.

The second chapter on neurobiology by Dr. Sebold and coworkers is a review of the neurotoxic and neuroadaptive consequences of chronic drug intake with a focus on alcohol (Chap. 2). Dispositional factors are reviewed, and the neurobiological effects of alcohol consumption are outlined, followed by a discussion of some key animal and human studies underpinning the concept of a reward system and the important differentiation between the experiences of "liking" and "wanting." The chapter concludes with an analysis of the consequences for treatment options.

The third chapter on genetics by Dr. Friedel et al. presents a complementary perspective to the first one (Chap. 3). It reviews the heritability of addiction and its genetic and epigenetic components. It also highlights gene x environment interactions and explains how epigenetic mechanisms may mediate the impact of social stress factors on gene expression.

The fourth chapter by Dr. Gardner focuses on animal models of addictive behavior (Chap. 4). It shows how animal models of the various stages of addiction, from preexisting vulnerability to models of relapse, can be used to measure drug effects on the central nervous system and how these effects can modify drug-related behavior. It discusses key aspects of addictive behavior including the role of dopamine and further neurotransmitter systems on drug reinforcement.

The fifth chapter by Dr. Rehm et al. presents the international epidemiological aspects of addiction with a focus on the findings of the Global Burden of Disease Study (Chap. 5). Regional differences are compared. A sequence emerges whereby the onset of substance abuse is largely influenced by cultural factors; environmental and social factors are important in the transition to hazardous consumption, while neurobiological and other risk factors become more salient in the transition to substance use disorder. The public health impact of intravenous and polysubstance drug use and a resulting epidemic of infectious diseases are leading to a contemplation of much needed drug policy reforms.

An international textbook ought to pay particular attention to sociocultural dimensions. Consequently, the next chapter authored by Dr. Room focuses on the cultural factors, that is, the shared beliefs, norms, and patterns of behaviors (Chap. 6). The social patterning of psychoactive drug use differs as to whether it is medicinal, regular, intermittent, or addictive. The handling of alcohol and drug problems often changes over time, for example, from a judicial to a health problem. It thus complements the chapters on gene x environment interactions and explains how cultural diversity modifies patterns of drug consumption and respective norms. The chapter concludes with Alcoholics Anonymous as an example of core practices worldwide but also local cultural adaptations.

The next chapter focuses on the prevention applications of the components previously discussed with review of the international experience. This seventh chapter is authored by Drs. Simon and Burkhart and describes prevention strategies in different regional settings (Chap. 7). Drs. Burkhart and Simon from the European Monitoring Centre for Drugs and Drug Addiction first describe a logical frame for prevention and assessment of its effectiveness. The basics of several prevention strategies are then described including mass media campaigns and environmental prevention. The benefits and limitations of different targets of the preventative efforts range from the population at large to vulnerable groups to family-based prevention and indicated prevention for individuals. The authors then discuss important regional and cultural aspects of prevention. Societal values influence student and adolescent behaviors as well as parenting practices. Again, an international perspective is presented as to recent developments and trends in preventative measures. Examples of the previously described strategies in different regions of the world and their relative acceptance are presented along with resulting lessons about successful transfer and adaptation of the experience between continents and countries.

The last chapter (Chap. 8) by Drs. Saunders and Latt reviews the diagnostic evolution in the ICD and DSM systems.

In conclusion, we hope this foundational section provides an informative basic science review of current knowledge. The first section of this textbook aims to reflect the commonalities and differences of broad global and international perspectives as salient determinants of management strategies.

References

1. American Psychiatric Association and DSM-5 Task Force. Diagnostic and statistical manual of mental disorders: DSM-5. Arlington: American Psychiatric Association; 2013.
2. Barr CS, Newman TK, Becker ML, Champoux M, Lesch KP, Suomi SJ, Higley JD. Serotonin transporter gene variation is associated with alcohol sensitivity in rhesus macaques exposed to early-life stress. Alcohol Clin Exp Res. 2003;27(5):812–7.
3. Chen G, Cuzon Carlson VC, Wang J, Beck A, Heinz A, Ron D, Buck KJ. Striatal involvement in human alcoholism and alcohol consumption, and withdrawal in animal models. Alcohol Clin Exp Res. 2011;35(10):1739–48.
4. Edwards G, Gross MM. Alcohol dependence: provisional description of a clinical syndrome. Br Med J. 1976;1(6017):1058–61.
5. el-Guebaly N, Cathcart J, Currie S, Brown D, Gloster S. Public health and therapeutic aspects of smoking bans in mental health and addiction settings. Psychiatr Serv. 2002;53(12):1617–22.
6. Everitt BJ, Robbins TW. Neural systems of reinforcement for drug addiction: from actions to habits to compulsion. Nat Neurosci. 2005;8(11):1481–9.
7. Everitt BJ, Robbins TW. Drug addiction: updating actions to habits to compulsion. Ann Rev Psychol. 2016;67:23–50.
8. Everitt BJ, Belin D, Economidou D, Pelloux Y, Dalley JW, Robbins TW. Neural mechanisms underlying the vulnerability to develop compulsive drug-seeking habits and addiction. Philos Trans R Soc B Biol Sci. 2008;363(1507):3125–35.
9. Fahlke C, Lorenz JG, Long J, Champoux M, Suomi SJ, Higley JD. Rearing experiences and stress-induced plasma cortisol as early risk factors for excessive alcohol consumption in nonhuman primates. Alcohol Clin Exp Res. 2000;24(5):644–50.
10. Goldstein RZ, Volkow ND. Dysfunction of the prefrontal cortex in addiction: neuroimaging findings and clinical implications. Nat Rev Neurosci. 2011;12(11):652–69.
11. Gore FM, Bloem PJ, Patton GC, Ferguson J, Joseph V, Coffey C, Sawyer SM, Mathers CD. Global burden of disease in young people aged 10–24 years: a systematic analysis. Lancet. 2011;377(9783):2093–102.
12. Heinz A. Dopaminergic dysfunction in alcoholism and schizophrenia–psychopathological and behavioral correlates. Eur Psychiatry. 2002;17(1):9–16.
13. Heinz AJ, Beck A, Meyer-Lindenberg A, Sterzer P, Heinz A. Cognitive and neurobiological mechanisms of alcohol-related aggression. Nat Rev Neurosci. 2011;12(7):400–13.
14. Heinz A, Daedelow LS, Wackerhagen C, Di Chiara G. Addiction theory matters – why there is no dependence on caffeine or antidepressant medication. Addict Biol. 2019;25(2):e12735.
15. Henssler J, Heinz A, Brandt L, Bschor T. Antidepressant withdrawal and rebound phe-

nomena – a systematic review. Dt Arztebl Int. 2019;116(20):355–61.

16. Higley JD, Hasert MF, Suomi SJ, Linnoila M. Nonhuman primate model of alcohol abuse: effects of early experience, personality, and stress on alcohol consumption. Proc Natl Acad Sci. 1991;88(16):7261–5.

17. Hinckers AS, Laucht M, Schmidt MH, Mann KF, Schumann G, Schuckit MA, Heinz A. Low level of response to alcohol as associated with serotonin transporter genotype and high alcohol intake in adolescents. Biol Psychiatry. 2006;60(3):282–7.

18. Hughes JR. Alcohol withdrawal seizures. Epilepsy Behav. 2009;15(2):92–7.

19. Karachalios GN, Charalabopoulos A, Papalimneou V, Kiortsis D, Dimicco P, Kostoula OK, Charalabopoulos K. Withdrawal syndrome following cessation of antihypertensive drug therapy. Int J Clin Pract. 2005;59(5):562–70.

20. Macleod J, Oakes R, Copello A, Crome I, Egger M, Hickman M, Oppenkowski T, Stokes Lampard H, Smith GD. Psychological and social sequelae of cannabis and other illicit drug use by young people: a systematic review of longitudinal, general population studies. Lancet. 2004;363(9421):1579–88.

21. Nutt D, King LA, Saulsbury W, Blakemore C. Development of a rational scale to assess the harm of drugs of potential misuse. Lancet. 2007;369(9566):1047–53.

22. Penka S, Heimann H, Heinz A, Schouler-Ocak M. Explanatory models of addictive behaviour among native German, Russian-German, and Turkish youth. Eur Psychiatry. 2008;23(Suppl 1):36–42.

23. Peters J, Bromberg U, Schneider S, Brassen S, Menz M, Banaschewski T, et al. Lower ventral striatal activation during reward anticipation in adolescent smokers. Am J Psychiatry. 2011;168(5):540–9.

24. Rehm J, Rehn N, Room R, Monteiro M, Gmel G, Jernigan D, Frick U. The global distribution of average volume of alcohol consumption and patterns of drinking. Eur Addict Res. 2003;9(4):147–56.

25. Saitz R. Things that work, things that don't work, and things that matter: including words. J Addict Med. 2015;9:429–30.

26. Tiffany ST, Carter BL. Is craving the source of compulsive drug use? J Psychopharmacol. 1998;12(1):23–30.

27. Toumbourou J, Stockwell T, Neighbors C, Marlatt G, Sturge J, Rehm J. Interventions to reduce harm associated with adolescent substance use. Lancet. 2007;369(9570):1391–401.

28. Vardar A, Kluge U, Penka S. How to express mental health problems: Turkish immigrants in Berlin compared to native Germans in Berlin and Turks in Istanbul. Eur Psychiatry. 2012;27(Suppl 2):S50–5.

29. Voon V, Derbyshire K, Ruc C, Irvine MA, Worbe Y, Enander J, et al. Disorders of compulsivity: a common bias towards learning habits. Mol Psychiatry. 2015;20(3):345–52.

Neurobiology of Alcohol Dependence

2

Miriam Sebold, Christian A. Müller,
Maria Garbusow, Katrin Charlet,
and Andreas Heinz

Contents

Abstract

Chronic drug intake (including alcohol) has profound neurotoxic and neuroadaptive consequences on neurotransmitter systems and brain circuitries that are strongly involved in learning and memory. Neuroadaptive altera-
tions within these systems can contribute to addiction development and maintenance. Current brain imaging studies identified neural correlates of behavioral processes that play a key role in addiction, such as cue-induced craving or automatic action tendencies. In this chapter, we describe neurobiological theories of addiction development and maintenance with a focus on motivational alterations and their neurobiological correlates as revealed by current neuroimaging studies in alcohol dependence. We discuss findings that assess alterations in reward anticipation and processing and their respective effects on learning mechanisms implicated in alcohol dependence. A better understanding of neural pro-

M. Sebold · C. A. Müller · M. Garbusow · K. Charlet ·
A. Heinz (✉)
Department of Psychiatry and Psychotherapy, CCM,
Charité - Universitätsmedizin Berlin,
Berlin, Germany
e-mail: andreas.heinz@charite.de

© Springer Nature Switzerland AG 2021
N. el-Guebaly et al. (eds.), *Textbook of Addiction Treatment*,
https://doi.org/10.1007/978-3-030-36391-8_2

cesses directly associated with the development and maintenance of addiction can help to improve prevention programs as well as therapeutic and pharmacological interventions in the treatment of addicted patients.

2.1   Introduction

The dependence syndrome is characterized by cognitive and physiological phenomena after repeated substance intake including continuous drug intake despite the knowledge of its negative consequences. Further symptoms are drug craving and a high priority given to drug use, the development of tolerance towards the specific drug effects, and the inability to control drug intake (International Classification of Diseases, tenth Revision (ICD-10)). Alcohol is legal in most countries and therefore socially accepted and highly available, contributing to high consumption patterns worldwide. According to *the Global status report on alcohol and health*, the World Health Organization (WHO) described a prevalence of 4% of alcohol use disorders worldwide with more than 2.5 million people dying annually due to the consequences of hazardous alcohol intake, which as a causal factor exceeds global death rates caused by HIV/AIDS or tuberculosis. However, beyond somatic effects, alcohol dependence has profound social, economic, and psychological consequences. Since up to 85% of the patients with alcohol dependence relapse after detoxification, strong effort has been made to investigate the underlying pathophysiological mechanisms in the development and maintenance of substance use disorders. By using brain imaging techniques, neural correlates of processes have been identified that are assumed to be involved in relapse, such as cue-induced craving or dysfunctional decision-making. The goal of such studies is to shed light on the neurobiology of drug addiction as well as to provide new options for specific behavioral and pharmacological interventions. Neuroimaging studies that predict relapses in

detoxified patients have clinical implications, as programs treating addiction could use this information to assess patients with high risk of relapse and to refer them to higher levels of care. In this chapter, we will illustrate neurobiological theories of addiction development and maintenance. We focus on the neurobiology of alcohol dependence to illustrate key mechanisms of drug addiction and mostly refer to human studies. For other drugs of abuse and more reference to animal studies, please also see Koob and Volkow [28]. We will describe neuroadaptive effects of excessive chronic alcohol consumption and present studies that discovered alterations in neurotransmitter systems and neural activity.

2.2   Dispositional Factors for the Development of Alcohol Dependence

Several risk factors for the development of alcohol dependence have been reported in the literature including the influence of genes and environment. We will focus on key mechanisms identified in animal experiments and human studies.

2.2.1   Level of Response to Alcohol

One dispositional factor that has been discussed in the literature is the individual response to alcohol: individuals with a low level of response to alcohol, that is, those who need high amounts of alcohol to experience stimulating or sedative effects, tend to use alcohol excessively and seem therefore to be at a higher risk of developing alcohol dependence. Thus, low sensitivity toward the effects of ethanol predicts future heavy alcohol consumption and alcohol-related problems. This phenotype represents a genetically influenced trait with a heritability rate of 40–60% and can be observed more often in subjects with a positive versus negative family history of alcoholism, pointing to a close gene-environment association [43]. Concerning the neurobiological correlates of this trait, studies using functional magnetic resonance imaging (fMRI) reported that the neural processing of affective and cognitive stimuli [38] is affected by this trait. Subjects with low responses to alcohol show decreased activation towards these stimuli, which might contribute to their impaired ability to recognize modest levels of alcohol intoxication.

Early Social Deprivation

Another dispositional factor for the development of alcohol dependence is stress. Stress factors that can increase the risk to develop an addictive disorder include traumatic childhood experiences such as social deprivation early in life, isolation, or abandonment [32]. Experiencing social stress activates effector systems such as the hypothalamic-pituitary-adrenal (HPA) axis. As a result, this might alter the mesolimbic dopamine system, which is critically involved in the development of drug dependence (Chap. 3). In line with this, Morgan et al. [33] observed in a positron emission tomography (PET) study in nonhuman primates that low social status (which potentially induces stress) is associated with lower dopamine receptor availability (which has been associated with increased dopamine concentrations in the extracellular space [21] and increased cocaine intake).

Furthermore, primates experiencing early social deprivation showed serotonergic dysfunction associated with high levels of aggression and low levels of response to acute alcohol intoxication [16]. In accordance, young primates who were separated from their mother in early infancy displayed a lower level of serotonin turnover, a higher availability of serotonin transporters (5-HTT), and higher levels of alcohol intake [17]. Hinckers et al. [23] observed that subjects with a genetic disposition for a high availability of 5-HTT displayed lower levels of response to alcohol and higher alcohol consumption during adolescence. These findings suggest an important genetic role in the interaction between stress, serotonergic neurotransmission, and alcohol response.

2.3 Addiction and the Reward System

2.3.1 Disentangling "Liking" from "Wanting"

The above-described dispositional factors contribute to the development of substance dependence. However, it is not known in detail why some substances (e.g., alcohol, cocaine, nicotine) make individuals addicted whereas others (more natural and healthy substances) do not. There is accumulating evidence that this "addictive feature" critically relies on the dopaminergic transmission the substance induces.

All drugs of abuse have in common that their intake leads to increased dopaminergic neurotransmission in the ventral striatum and the nucleus accumbens (NAcc) [11]. As alternative reinforcers (like food, sex, money) also elicit dopaminergic release, it was initially suggested that dopamine mediates reward and causes hedonic feelings. Dopaminergic innervated regions of the mesocorticolimbic circuit have therefore commonly been termed as the "reward system." This system includes ascending dopaminergic pathways from the ventral tegmental area (VTA) and substantia nigra via the ventral (including the NAcc) and the dorsal striatum and the amygdala to frontal and limbic circuits (Fig. 2.1). However, the assumption that dopamine primarily causes hedonic feelings was challenged by studies demonstrating increased dopaminergic neurotransmission when reward occurs unexpectedly or when it is greater than expected (Sect. 3.2). Thus, instead of mediating pleasure, dopamine might play a crucial role in signaling salience and consequently motivating an individual to strive toward a certain reward. Further evidence for a role of dopamine in motivation comes from studies demonstrating symptoms of apathy instead of anhedonia in subjects who received pharmacological blockage of dopaminergic neurotransmission (e.g., via neuroleptics). Apathy is defined as the lack of interest, enthusiasm, or concern and can therefore be seen as the endpoint on a motivational continuum [40].

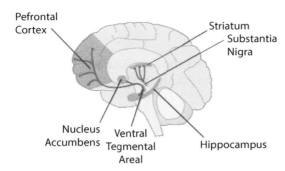

Fig. 2.1 The dopaminergic mesocorticolimbic circuit: the VTA; ventral striatum, including the nucleus accumbens (NAcc); dorsal striatum; amygdala; and frontal and limbic circuits. Key regions of the so-called neural reward system include the VTA and nucleus accumbens

Therefore, wanting (experience of desire and urge to strive for something) was suggested to be disentangled from liking (experience of pleasure, causes feelings of positive emotions and hedonism). Whereas the dopaminergic system is most commonly associated with "wanting" [4], the opioidergic is related to "liking." Evidence for the role of the opioidergic system in mediating hedonic effects of reward comes from animal studies using μ-opioid receptor (MOR) knockout mice, which show insensitivity toward the hedonic effects of morphine [31]. In accordance, nalmefene – a compound with antagonistic activity at MORs – decreases subjective pleasantness of palatable foods in humans [55]. Besides food reward, the opioid system further seems to mediate the affective value of drug reward, including alcohol consumption. Indeed, in vivo availability of MORs was elevated in alcohol-dependent patients [20], and naltrexone, a MOR antagonist that is administered for craving reduction in addiction treatment, is assumed to block the hedonic effects of alcohol, thus reducing relapse rates and alcohol intake in alcohol-dependent patients.

Beyond opioids, other neurotransmitters have been implicated in the mediation of "liking." For instance, stimulation of endocannabinoid and GABA-benzodiazepine sites in limbic structures increased pleasure of food rewards. Therefore, hedonic liking of the consumption of a fully predicted reward can be mediated through a variety of neurotransmitter systems.

2.3.2 Dopamine in Mediating Learning Effects

As described above, dopamine plays a major role in motivation. Schultz [44] was the first to demonstrate a shift in phasic dopaminergic activity from received reward to the reward-predicting cue, when subjects had learned the contingency between the reward and the stimulus. Moreover, Schultz and his colleagues observed a dip of dopaminergic transmission when the outcome was worse than expected, for instance, when the reward suddenly was omitted ([44]; see Fig. 2.2). These phasic dopaminergic signals serve as a teaching signal to adapt subsequent expectations and are then translated into actions. In other words, a dopaminergic signal makes us recognize that something important is about to happen; thus, it triggers motivation and encourages us to act either to achieve a reward or to avoid a punishment. It is important to bear in mind that there is a multifaceted role for dopamine in addiction. Beyond tonic dopamine release, phasic increases encode the magnitude of unexpected rewards and are also elicited by reward-associated cues, unless they are themselves predicted by preceding stimuli. Phasic dopamine release elicited by drugs of abuse is usually stronger than release evoked by natural reinforcers, thus biasing behavior toward drug intake [10].

2.3.3 Incentive Salience Theory of Addiction

The adaptation of phasic dopaminergic signals over the course of learning appears to reflect the assignment of value to cues (Fig. 2.2b). Thus, in addiction, environmental stimuli, which have repeatedly been paired with drugs, acquire incentive salience as a result of Pavlovian learning [40]. The attribution of incentive salience to drug-associated stimuli is closely linked to the observation that addicted subjects show significant responses to drug-related stimuli, a phenomenon referred to as cue reactivity [7]. In alcohol dependence, external stimuli of visual or olfac-

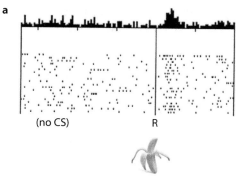

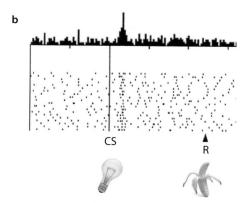

Occurence of unpredicted Reward
Dopaminergic release at reward onset

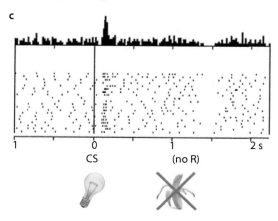

Occurence of predicted Reward
Dopaminergic Realease at CS onset

Absence of predicted Reward
Dip of dopaminergic firing at expected reward onset

Fig. 2.2 (**a**) Burst of dopaminergic firing in occurrence of an unpredicted reward (R) at reward onset (positive prediction error). (**b**) After Pavlovian conditioning: burst of dopaminergic firing not at reward but at conditioned stimulus (CS) onset. (**c**) No reward: dip of dopaminergic firing at expected reward onset (negative prediction error). (Adapted from Schultz [44])

tory modality, such as the sight of an alcohol bottle in the supermarket or the smell of a beer in a pub, might serve as such cues. Cue-induced responses in substance dependence exist on a variety of physiological levels including changes in heart rate, sweat gland activity, skin temperature, and functional brain activity [7]. Moreover, alcohol-dependent patients report increased craving whenever they are confronted with alcohol cues, which may help to explain the cue-reactivity phenomenon.

Experimentally, cue reactivity is most commonly operationalized by confronting subjects with substance-related cues (e.g., images) and neutral control images. fMRI studies have shown that substance-dependent subjects display increased activation of several core regions of the mesolimbic pathway, when confronted with substance-related stimuli. This finding has been reported in various substance dependencies, including heroin, cocaine, alcohol, cannabis, and nicotine dependence. Brain regions which have reliably been identified in different cue-reactivity fMRI studies include the anterior cingulate cortex (ACC), the medial prefrontal cortex (mPFC), the ventral and dorsal striatum and the orbitofrontal cortex (OFC), the dorsolateral prefrontal cortex (dlPFC), and the amygdala [42]. Crucially, physiological responses to substance-related cues supposedly reflect automatic conditioned responses that are not under conscious control (Sect. 3.4), as demonstrated by studies using drug cues that are presented below the threshold of consciousness.

Increased cue reactivity was also reported in relation to consciously experienced cues, as indicated by self-reported measurements that assess craving or the desire for a particular substance of abuse [45]. Importantly, subjective and physiological cue reactivity are sometimes dissociated. Indeed, physiological cue reactivity resembles responses elicited by positive stimuli, although these subjects deny conscious feelings of pleasure or even report aversive feelings to these drug cues [35]. Thus, one can conclude that physiological indicators of cue reactivity are more proximal to implicit associations compared to explicit self-reports and therefore may provide higher predictive validity.

One of the most important features about cue reactivity is that these stimuli can modulate behavior. Thus, cues that have acquired incentive salience attract attention and guide approach behavior and therefore act as "motivational magnets" [4]. Indeed, when drug administration is repeatedly paired with an external cue, rats approach the cue more likely and with increasing rapidity even when it no longer predicts drug administration. Likewise, alcohol-associated stimuli increase alcohol consumption in rats [8]. Besides alcohol cues, other reward-associated cues also play a role in substance dependence. For instance, cues that have been associated with monetary reward modulate subsequent behavior in alcohol dependence [14]. Thus, the extent to which reward-predicting cues acquire incentive salience can modulate subsequent behavior, and the resulting impact on neural responses may reflect the severity of substance dependence.

2.3.4 Habitual Drug Seeking

Whereas the incentive salience theory suggests that in addiction, drug-associated cues become motivationally highly attractive and therefore "wanted," Tiffany's theory of addiction suggests that drug consumption reflects a habitual responding that is controlled by automatically initiated action schemata [49]. Thus, in addiction, drug-associated stimuli might not elicit a positive affective or motivational state that results in drug-seeking behavior. Rather, according to Tiffany's theory, in addiction, drug consumption happens to occur in a habitual fashion. Theoretical arguments for habits were based on the observation that drug consumption in addiction seems to be initiated and completed without intention, difficult to impede in the presence of triggering stimuli, and conducted in the absence of awareness. Further evidence for habitual drug consumption comes from clinical observations of addicted patients: many relapses happen to occur without any preceding urges to consume drugs or conscious craving. According to their "transition to habit" theory, Everitt and Robbins [13] suggested that addiction reflects the end-point of a series of transitions: from initial drug

intake that causes hedonic feelings (liking) to a stage when substance use becomes habitual (wanting) and ultimately to loss of control, where drug consumption is compulsive and therefore disentangled from anticipatory drug effects. Evidence for this comes from animal studies: rats that have learned a specific response in order to self-administer drugs continue to perform this response even when drug delivery is suppressed [26]. Thus, actions of these rats were no longer guided by outcome expectancy (*lever press results in drug delivery and hedonic feelings*), but rather by external cues that elicit conditioned responses (*lever press whenever a cue is available*). This experiment manipulates the value of the cue-induced lever press, and such manipulations are typically used to test whether actions are goal-directed or habitual. In this procedure (devaluation design), the value of an action is suddenly decreased (by detaching it from the positive outcome or by associating it with a negative outcome). When actions are habitual, this devaluation does not alter choice behavior on that stimulus. Contrary to this, when actions are goal-directed, the devaluation of a stimulus decreases choice behavior of that stimulus. Studies demonstrated that unlimited access to alcohol fosters ethanol consumption in rats even when the alcohol is altered by bitter-tasting quinine [24]. Interestingly, responding for ethanol becomes insensitive to devaluation at a stage when responding for food reward still is sensitive to devaluation, indicating that the shift from goal- to stimulus-directed consumption is more rapid for alcohol than natural rewards [12].

On the neural level, "wanting" is probably mediated by the ventral striatum, while the state of habitual drug intake is modulated by the dorsal striatum. Thus, the development of an addiction is promoted by a transformation from goal-directed to stimulus-driven, automatic behavior, which is assumed to be accompanied by a shift of ventral to dorsal striatal activity. Animal studies seem to confirm this contention: once substance use becomes habitual, drug-associated stimuli foster release of dopamine in the dorsal striatum [9]. However, the translation of observations in animals excessively trained to perform lever presses for food or drugs to human behavior is controversial. In humans, studies investigating a shift from goal-directed to habitual control often use multistep paradigms. These tasks bear two important differences to the procedures commonly used in animals. First, they use non-drug-related rewards (e.g., monetary rewards). Secondly, they are rather complex and rely on cognitive abilities such as working memory. These limitations might have caused the inconsistent picture regarding habit formation in substance-dependent humans. Whereas some studies have demonstrated such a shift [47], others have shown no such link in alcohol dependence [46]. Based on these studies, the role of habitual versus goal-directed decision-making in human substance dependence remains to be further explored.

2.4 Consequences of Chronic Alcohol Consumption

2.4.1 Neuroadaptive Dopaminergic Changes

Chronic alcohol intake is associated with profound neuroadaptive and neurotoxic effects on dopaminergic, GABAergic, serotonergic, and glutamatergic neurotransmission. For instance, alcohol-dependent patients display low levels of dopamine synthesis and release as well as an decreased availability of D2 receptors (DRD2) in the ventral striatum [52]. The reduction of DRD2 is positively associated with lifetime alcohol intake, suggesting that excessive alcohol consumption causes DRD2 decreases. These dopaminergic changes can recover with prolonged abstinence. In early phases of abstinence, however, they can cause the individual to strive for particularly strong activators of the downregulated dopaminergic system (such as drugs or drug-associated stimuli). This is in line with the finding that the degree of striatal downregulation of DRD2 in alcohol dependence is associated with the extent of cue-induced neural activation and with the severity of alcohol craving [18]. The bias towards high dopaminergic stimulatory drugs can influence choices against

weaker primary and secondary reinforcers such as food, money, or social interactions. Thus, dopaminergic dysfunction may primarily interfere with learning of new conditional stimuli and contexts that predict non-drug reward. A study demonstrated impairments in learning from non-drug-related rewards in alcohol dependence [37], which correlated with craving for (well-learned non-explicit) alcohol intake. The shift of natural reward processing to preferential drug-related reward processing has been metaphorically described as a "hijacking of the reward system." In line with this, alcohol-dependent patients displayed a decrease in ventral striatum activity when confronted with monetary cues but an increased activation in the same region when confronted with drug cues [3], which further suggests an essential role for the ventral striatum in relapse prediction. In accordance with the assumption of a hijacked reward system, it was suggested that strong neural responses to rewarding and non-drug-related stimuli might serve as a potential protective brain mechanism against relapse. Indeed, increased ventral striatal responses to affectively positive pictures were related to more subsequent abstinent days and less prospective alcohol intake [22].

2.4.2 Neuroanatomical Alterations

Alcohol as a neurotoxic substance causes widespread neural alterations when chronically consumed: up to 70% of alcohol-dependent patients show alcohol-associated brain atrophy, that is, tissue loss of gray and white matter, ventricular enlargement, and sulci widening [6]. Morphometric studies investigating brain volume changes in alcohol dependence found that this atrophy mainly affects frontal, temporal, and parieto-occipital regions but also the hippocampus, the corpora mammillaria, and the cerebellum, with the most marked atrophic changes within the white and gray matter of the frontal lobe [34]. In particular, volume deficits of frontal and parieto-occipital regions appear to be clinically relevant, since these changes were reported to be predictive of higher risk of relapse [39].

These atrophic changes might lead to impairments of working memory and executive functioning, thus possibly reducing long-term action planning and inhibition of short-term reward-directed behavior (e.g., alcohol intake) [54]. However, the precise pathophysiological mechanism of alcohol-associated brain atrophy is not fully understood; possibly, a hyperglutamatergic state during alcohol withdrawal leads to a calcium influx via activation of glutamatergic NMDA receptors and thereby initiates cytotoxic cascades [50]. Furthermore, alcohol withdrawal was reported to activate the HPA axis, resulting in elevated cortisol concentrations. Cortisol concentrations in turn were associated with altered serotonergic neurotransmission, which also contributed to increased severity of depression in early abstinence [19]. Interestingly, these neuropathological changes seem to be partially reversible, because regenerations of brain volume during short-term and long-term alcohol abstinence were described in alcohol-dependent patients [56]

2.4.3   Alcohol Tolerance and Withdrawal

Chronic substance use results in different neuroadaptive changes in the brain, leading to tolerance towards the acute effects of the substance and causing withdrawal symptoms when substance use is reduced or stopped. Alcohol-related withdrawal symptoms are of psychological (e.g., anhedonia and anxiety) and physical (e.g., tachycardia, nausea, sweating, headaches, tremors) nature. Tolerance-related neuroadaptation seems to be essential for the maintenance of homeostasis between excitatory and inhibitory functions in the brain and counteracts the acute effects of the drug of abuse [27]. As a consequence of these alterations, a reduction or cessation of substance use may lead to a severe disturbance of homeostasis, which can clinically manifest as psychovegetative withdrawal symptoms, potentially including severe complications such as epileptic seizures or delirium. Both development of tolerance and withdrawal symptoms seem to be

related to alcohol's activation of GABAergic as well as inhibition of glutamatergic neurotransmission [29]. GABA represents the main inhibitory neurotransmitter in the human brain and is involved in rapid information processing in cortical and subcortical areas. While acute alcohol consumption induces activation of inhibitory GABA-A receptors, leading to sedation after intake of large amounts of ethanol, chronic alcohol consumption seems to result in an increased tolerance for acute alcohol effects due to a systematic downregulation of GABA-A receptors. Long-lasting GABA-A receptor changes have been found in alcohol-dependent patients after several weeks of alcohol abstinence and even may persist long during further abstinence [1]. Regarding psychovegetative withdrawal symptoms, neuroadaptive changes within the glutamatergic system appear to result from chronic alcohol-induced antagonism at glutamatergic NMDA receptors. Indeed, a compensatory upregulation of glutamatergic NMDA receptors as a consequence of chronic alcohol intake has been observed [53]. In case of reduction or cessation of alcohol consumption, the excitatory neurotransmitter glutamate then can activate an elevated number of NMDA receptors [15]. This process can also cause imbalances between inhibitory and excitatory functioning with a predominance of excitation, clinically resulting in withdrawal symptoms.

2.5   Pharmaco-fMRI: New Insights of Pharmacological Treatment

Albeit treatment of drug-associated harm with drug substitution has been proven to be a useful option in opioid addiction, in alcohol dependence, treatment with putative partially substitutive psychoactive compounds (such as γ-hydroxybutyric acid, GHB) is uncommon and can induce GHB dependence [51]. Instead, so-called anti-craving substances such as naltrexone, nalmefene, or acamprosate are temporarily applied for relapse prevention or reduction of alcohol consumption, respectively. Meta-analyses have demonstrated moderate effectiveness of naltrexone and acamprosate with regard to reduction of alcohol consumption or maintenance of abstinence, respectively [25]. The application of neuroimaging techniques in pharmacologically treated alcohol-dependent patients might potentially be useful in predicting which medication helps to prevent relapse. For example, elevated levels of MORs have been observed in the ventral striatum of some alcohol-dependent patients after withdrawal and are targeted by naltrexone, which blocks MORs [20].

A combination of fMRI and pharmacological treatment (pharmaco-fMRI) might allow to further elucidate how and where a specific compound acts on the central nervous system. For example, naltrexone treatment produced a significant reduction of cue-induced activity in the ventral striatum in alcohol-dependent subjects [36]. Notably, these changes in neural activity were additionally related to decreases in cue-induced craving, indicating a close link between pharmacological effects of naltrexone, striatal activation, and pharmacological craving modulation. Further studies were conducted to assess the effectiveness of acamprosate. Acamprosate is assumed to reduce neuronal hyperexcitability, which may be responsible for acute alcohol withdrawal on the level of both excitatory glutamate and inhibitory GABA neurotransmitter pathways. Findings of a preclinical study suggest a calcium-related mechanism in alcohol dependence [48], and acamprosate treatment resulted in a significant reduction of cue-induced activity in the striatum and the posterior cingulate in alcohol dependence [30].

Besides naltrexone and acamprosate, alternative pharmacological treatments have been suggested to reduce craving and relapse rates in alcohol-dependent patients. One example for a pharmacological treatment is baclofen, a GABA-B receptor agonist, which has raised attention since first clinical studies suggested its effectiveness in the treatment of alcohol-dependent patients. Recent meta-analyses reported inconsistent results with regard to its efficacy in alcohol dependence [5, 41]. In alcohol-dependent patients, a pharmaco-fMRI study found that patients receiving baclofen showed a stronger decrease, in cue-elicited brain activation in left orbitofrontal cortex, bilateral amygdala and left VTA than patients receiving a placebo treatment. Thus, baclofen might decrease cue-elicited brain activation in areas known to be involved in the processing of salient stimuli [2].

2.6 Conclusion

Altogether, neurochemical effects of acute alcohol intake can be experienced as rewarding and therefore reinforce drug intake via Pavlovian conditioning. These learning mechanisms appear to underlie a shift from occasional alcohol consumption to habitual intake. Neuroadaptive alterations (particularly regarding dopaminergic neurotransmission within the so-called reward system) are related to craving and increased processing of alcohol cues. Thus, neurobiological consequences of excessive alcohol intake are in accordance with the clinical observation that many alcohol-dependent patients find it particularly difficult to abstain from habitual consumption patterns and relapse after drug withdrawal, despite high individual motivation to remain abstinent. Neuroimaging studies might help to gain a better understanding of the neurobiological correlates of craving and motivation for alcohol intake. Furthermore, longitudinal and multimodal imaging studies might help to identify patients with a high relapse risk who could benefit from a higher intensity of treatment.

Acknowledgments This work was supported by the German Research Foundation (Deutsche Forschungsgemeinschaft, DFG, HE2597/14-1, HE2597/14-2, RA1047/2-1, RA1047/2-2, RO 5046/2-2, SCHA1971/1-2, SCHL 1969/2-2, SCHL 1969/4-1).

Glossary

Devaluation A psychological design for the assessment of stimulus-triggered (habitual) responding. Animals are trained to perform two responses, one for each of two different rewards. One reward is then devalued by associating it with bad taste (via quinine), sickness (lithium chloride), or satiety (via pre-feeding).

When given the opportunity to perform the instrumental responses again in extinction, the responses for the devalued reward should be selectively diminished, in case actions are controlled by outcome expectancy. Instead, when actions are stimulus-driven (thus habitual), actions for the devalued reward should not be altered.

Goal-directed actions Instrumental responses that are acquired through response-outcome associations. Goal-directed actions are performed with the intention of obtaining the goal. Goal-directed actions are sensitive to devaluation.

Habitual actions Instrumental responses that reflect the execution of stimulus-response associations. Habitual actions are enabled by particular stimulus configurations and thus insensitive to devaluation. Habitual behavior comprises features of automaticity such as speed, autonomy, lack of control, and absence of conscious awareness.

Incentive A stimulus that promotes approach to a reward as a result of predictive associations with this reward. Incentives serve as motivational devices, as they facilitate and energize behavior that has been associated with the reward. Incentives may acquire activational properties, which amplify the incentive properties of other stimuli that occur concurrently, but are not necessarily related to the reward.

Liking Emotional affective value of reward that has hedonic impact and causes feelings of pleasure. In addiction research, self-reported measure of hedonia has been used as a proxy for liking.

Pavlovian conditioning Associative learning, in which the conditioned stimulus (CS) comes to signal the occurrence of a second stimulus and the unconditioned stimulus (US) thus elicits conditioned responses following CS presentation.

Reinforcer A stimulus that increases the probability of a desired response. In contrast to incentives, reinforcers elicit responding on the basis of their contingency with actions (instrumental conditioning).

Reward A class of unconditioned motivational stimuli, which elicit pleasure and hedonic feelings that can act as positive reinforcers.

Wanting Motivational value of reward that has decision utility. In addiction research, craving for the positive effects of drugs has been used as a proxy for wanting.

References

1. Abi-Dargham A, et al. Alterations of benzodiazepine receptors in type II alcoholic subjects measured with SPECT and [123I]iomazenil. Am J Psychiatry. 1998;155:1550–5.
2. Beck A, et al. Effects of high-dose baclofen on cue reactivity in alcohol dependence: a randomized, placebo-controlled pharmaco-fMRI study. Eur Neuropsychopharmacol. 2018;28:1206–16. https://doi.org/10.1016/j.euroneuro.2018.08.507.
3. Beck A, et al. Ventral striatal activation during reward anticipation correlates with impulsivity in alcoholics. Biol Psychiatry. 2009;66:734–42. https://doi.org/10.1016/j.biopsych.2009.04.035.
4. Berridge KC. Wanting and liking: observations from the neuroscience and psychology laboratory. Inquiry. 2009;52:378. https://doi.org/10.1080/00201740903087359.
5. Bschor T, Henssler J, Muller M, Baethge C. Baclofen for alcohol use disorder-a systematic meta-analysis. Acta Psychiatr Scand. 2018;138:232–42. https://doi.org/10.1111/acps.12905.
6. Carlen PL, Wortzman G, Holgate RC, Wilkinson DA, Rankin JC. Reversible cerebral atrophy in recently abstinent chronic alcoholics measured by computed tomography scans. Science. 1978;200:1076–8.
7. Carter BL, Tiffany ST. Meta-analysis of cue-reactivity in addiction research. Addiction. 1999;94:327–40.
8. Corbit LH, Janak PH. Ethanol-associated cues produce general pavlovian-instrumental transfer. Alcohol Clin Exp Res. 2007;31:766–74. https://doi.org/10.1111/j.1530-0277.2007.00359.x.
9. Corbit LH, Nie H, Janak PH. Habitual alcohol seeking: time course and the contribution of subregions of the dorsal striatum. Biol Psychiatry. 2012;72:389–95. https://doi.org/10.1016/j.biopsych.2012.02.024.
10. Di Chiara G, Bassareo V. Reward system and addiction: what dopamine does and doesn't do. Curr Opin Pharmacol. 2007;7:69–76. https://doi.org/10.1016/j.coph.2006.11.003.
11. Di Chiara G, Imperato A. Drugs abused by humans preferentially increase synaptic dopamine concentrations in the mesolimbic system of freely moving rats. Proc Natl Acad Sci U S A. 1988;85:5274–8.
12. Dickinson A, Wood N, Smith JW. Alcohol seeking by rats: action or habit? Q J Exp Psychol B. 2002;55:331–48. https://doi.org/10.1080/0272499024400016.
13. Everitt BJ, Robbins TW. Neural systems of reinforcement for drug addiction: from actions to habits to compulsion. Nat Neurosci. 2005;8:1481–9. https://doi.org/10.1038/nn1579.

14. Garbusow M, et al. Pavlovian-to-instrumental transfer effects in the nucleus accumbens relate to relapse in alcohol dependence. Addict Biol. 2016;21:719–31. https://doi.org/10.1111/adb.12243.

15. Glue P, Nutt D. Overexcitement and disinhibition. Dynamic neurotransmitter interactions in alcohol withdrawal. Br J Psychiatry. 1990;157:491–9.

16. Heinz A, et al. In vivo association between alcohol intoxication, aggression, and serotonin transporter availability in nonhuman primates. Am J Psychiatry. 1998;155:1023–8.

17. Heinz A, Jones DW, Gorey JG, Bennet A, Suomi SJ, Weinberger DR, Higley JD. Serotonin transporter availability correlates with alcohol intake in nonhuman primates. Mol Psychiatry. 2003a;8:231–4. https://doi.org/10.1038/sj.mp.4001214.

18. Heinz A, et al. Correlation between dopamine D(2) receptors in the ventral striatum and central processing of alcohol cues and craving. Am J Psychiatry. 2004;161(10):1783–9.

19. Heinz A, et al. Relationship between cortisol and serotonin metabolites and transporters in alcoholism [correction of alcolholism]. Pharmacopsychiatry. 2002;35(4):127–34. https://doi.org/10.1055/s-2002-33197.

20. Heinz A, et al. Correlation of stable elevations in striatal mu-opioid receptor availability in detoxified alcoholic patients with alcohol craving: a positron emission tomography study using carbon 11-labeled carfentanil. Arch Gen Psychiatry. 2005;62:57–64. https://doi.org/10.1001/archpsyc.62.1.57.

21. Heinz A, Saunders RC, Kolachana BS, Jones DW, Gorey JG, Bachevalier J, Weinberger DR. Striatal dopamine receptors and transporters in monkeys with neonatal temporal limbic damage. Synapse. 1999;32:71–9. https://doi.org/10.1002/(SICI)1098-2396(199905)32:2<71::AID-SYN1>3.0.CO;2-Q.

22. Heinz A, et al. Brain activation elicited by affectively positive stimuli is associated with a lower risk of relapse in detoxified alcoholic subjects. Alcohol Clin Exp Res. 2007;31:1138–47. https://doi.org/10.1111/j.1530-0277.2007.00406.x.

23. Hinckers AS, Laucht M, Schmidt MH, Mann KF, Schumann G, Schuckit MA, Heinz A. Low level of response to alcohol as associated with serotonin transporter genotype and high alcohol intake in adolescents. Biol Psychiatry. 2006;60:282–7. https://doi.org/10.1016/j.biopsych.2005.12.009.

24. Hopf FW, Chang S-J, Sparta DR, Bowers MS, Bonci A. Motivation for alcohol becomes resistant to quinine adulteration after 3 to 4 months of intermittent alcohol self-administration. Alcohol Clin Exp Res. 2010;34:1565–73. https://doi.org/10.1111/j.1530-0277.2010.01241.x.

25. Jonas DE, et al. Pharmacotherapy for adults with alcohol use disorders in outpatient settings: a systematic review and meta-analysis. JAMA. 2014;311:1889–900. https://doi.org/10.1001/jama.2014.3628.

26. Katner SN, Weiss F. Ethanol-associated olfactory stimuli reinstate ethanol-seeking behavior after extinction and modify extracellular dopamine levels in the nucleus accumbens. Alcohol Clin Exp Res. 1999;23:1751–60.

27. Koob GF, Le Moal M. Drug abuse: hedonic homeostatic dysregulation. Science. 1997;278:52–8.

28. Koob GF, Volkow ND. Neurobiology of addiction: a neurocircuitry analysis. Lancet Psychiatry. 2016;3:760–73. https://doi.org/10.1016/S2215-0366(16)00104-8.

29. Krystal JH, et al. Gamma-aminobutyric acid type a receptors and alcoholism: intoxication, dependence, vulnerability, and treatment. Arch Gen Psychiatry. 2006;63:957–68.

30. Langosch JM, et al. The impact of acamprosate on cue reactivity in alcohol dependent individuals: a functional magnetic resonance imaging study. J Clin Psychopharmacol. 2012;32:661–5. https://doi.org/10.1097/JCP.0b013e318267b586.

31. Matthes HW, et al. Loss of morphine-induced analgesia, reward effect and withdrawal symptoms in mice lacking the mu-opioid-receptor gene. Nature. 1996;383:819–23. https://doi.org/10.1038/383819a0.

32. Meyer-Lindenberg A, Tost H. Neural mechanisms of social risk for psychiatric disorders. Nat Neurosci. 2012;15:663–8. https://doi.org/10.1038/nn.3083.

33. Morgan D, et al. Social dominance in monkeys: dopamine D2 receptors and cocaine self-administration. Nat Neurosci. 2002;5:169–74. https://doi.org/10.1038/nn798.

34. Moselhy HF, Georgiou G, Kahn A. Frontal lobe changes in alcoholism: a review of the literature. Alcohol Alcohol. 2001;36:357–68.

35. Mucha RF, Geier A, Stuhlinger M, Mundle G. Appetitive effects of drug cues modelled by pictures of the intake ritual: generality of cue-modulated startle examined with inpatient alcoholics. Psychopharmacology. 2000;151:428–32. https://doi.org/10.1007/s002130000508.

36. Myrick H, et al. Effect of naltrexone and ondansetron on alcohol cue–induced activation of the ventral striatum in alcohol-dependent people. Arch Gen Psychiatry. 2008;65:466–75. https://doi.org/10.1001/archpsyc.65.4.466.

37. Park SQ, Kahnt T, Beck A, Cohen MX, Dolan RJ, Wrase J, Heinz A. Prefrontal cortex fails to learn from reward prediction errors in alcohol dependence. J Neurosci. 2010;30:7749–53. https://doi.org/10.1523/JNEUROSCI.5587-09.2010.

38. Paulus MP, et al. High versus low level of response to alcohol: evidence of differential reactivity to emotional stimuli. Biol Psychiatry. 2012;72:848–55. https://doi.org/10.1016/j.biopsych.2012.04.016.

39. Rando K, Hong KI, Bhagwagar Z, Li CS, Bergquist K, Guarnaccia J, Sinha R. Association of frontal and posterior cortical gray matter volume with time to alcohol relapse: a prospective study. Am J Psychiatry. 2010;168(2):183–92.

40. Robinson TE, Berridge KC. The incentive sensitization theory of addiction: some current issues. Phil Trans R Soc B. 2008;363:3137–46. https://doi.org/10.1098/rstb.2008.0093.

41. Rose AK, Jones A. Baclofen: its effectiveness in reducing harmful drinking, craving, and negative mood. A meta-analysis. Addiction. 2018;113:1396–406. https://doi.org/10.1111/add.14191.

42. Schacht JP, Anton RF, Myrick H. Functional neuroimaging studies of alcohol cue reactivity: a quantitative meta-analysis and systematic review. Addict Biol. 2013a;18:121–33. https://doi.org/10.1111/j.1369-1600.2012.00464.x.

43. Schuckit MA, Risch SC, Gold EO. Alcohol consumption, ACTH level, and family history of alcoholism. Am J Psychiatry. 1988;145:1391–5. https://doi.org/10.1176/ajp.145.11.1391.

44. Schultz W. Predictive reward signal of dopamine neurons. J Neurophysiol. 1998;80:1–27.

45. Schulze D, Jones BT. Desire for alcohol and outcome expectancies as measures of alcohol cue-reactivity in social drinkers. Addiction. 2000;95:1015–20.

46. Sebold M, et al. When habits are dangerous: alcohol expectancies and habitual decision making predict relapse in alcohol dependence. Biol Psychiatry. 2017;82:847–56. https://doi.org/10.1016/j.biopsych.2017.04.019.

47. Sjoerds Z, de Wit S, van den Brink W, Robbins TW, Beekman AT, Penninx BW, Veltman DJ. Behavioral and neuroimaging evidence for overreliance on habit learning in alcohol-dependent patients. Transl Psychiatry. 2013;3:e337. https://doi.org/10.1038/tp.2013.107.

48. Spanagel R, et al. Acamprosate produces its anti-relapse effects via calcium. Neuropsychopharmacology. 2014;39:783–91. https://doi.org/10.1038/npp.2013.264.

49. Tiffany ST. A cognitive model of drug urges and drug-use behavior: role of automatic and nonautomatic processes. Psychol Rev. 1990;97:147–68.

50. Tsai G, Gastfriend DR, Coyle JT. The glutamatergic basis of human alcoholism. Am J Psychiatry. 1995;152:332–40.

51. van Noorden MS, Mol T, Wisselink J, Kuijpers W, BAG D. Treatment consumption and treatment re-enrollment in GHB-dependent patients in the Netherlands. Drug Alcohol Depend. 2017;176:96–101. https://doi.org/10.1016/j.drugalcdep.2017.02.026.

52. Volkow ND, et al. Decreases in dopamine receptors but not in dopamine transporters in alcoholics. Alcohol Clin Exp Res. 1996;20:1594–8.

53. Ward RJ, Lallemand F, de Witte P. Biochemical and neurotransmitter changes implicated in alcohol-induced brain damage in chronic or 'binge drinking' alcohol abuse. Alcohol Alcohol. 2009;44:128–35. https://doi.org/10.1093/alcalc/agn100.

54. Watanabe M. Reward expectancy in primate prefrontal neurons. Nature. 1996;382:629–32. https://doi.org/10.1038/382629a0.

55. Yeomans MR, Wright P. Lower pleasantness of palatable foods in nalmefene-treated human volunteers. Appetite. 1991;16:249–59.

56. Zou X, Durazzo TC, Meyerhoff DJ. Regional brain volume changes in alcohol-dependent individuals during short-term and long-term abstinence. Alcohol Clin Exp Res. 2018;42:1062–72. https://doi.org/10.1111/acer.13757.

Heritability of Alcohol Use Disorder: Evidence from Twin Studies and Genome-Wide Association Studies

3

Eva Friedel, Jakob Kaminski, and Stephan Ripke

Contents

Abstract

The genetics of addictions including alcohol dependence have been the focus of extensive research, albeit with variable and often conflicting results. Heritability estimations suggest that about 50% of the variance of addictive behavior is due to (epi)genetic effects, while associations between addictive behavior (such as amount of drinking and relapse) and specific genetic combinations are generally in a modest range. This chapter introduces the methods used to estimate heritability and specific genetic influences, such as twin and adoption studies, polygenic risk scores, and genome-wide association studies. Environmental influences on gene expression and possible pathways of epigenetic modifications will be addressed.

E. Friedel (✉) · J. Kaminski · S. Ripke
Charite - Universitätsmedizin Berlin,
Berlin, Germany
e-mail: eva.friedel@charite.de;
jakob.kaminski@charite.de;
stephan.ripke@charite.de

Keywords

Heritability · Single-nucleotide polymorphism (SNP) · Polygenetic risk score (PRS) · Epigenome · Genome-wide association studies (GWAS) · Linkage disequilibrium (LD)

© Springer Nature Switzerland AG 2021
N. el-Guebaly et al. (eds.), *Textbook of Addiction Treatment*,
https://doi.org/10.1007/978-3-030-36391-8_3

3.1   Introduction

Clinical observations indicate that alcohol use disorder (AUD) is more frequent among relatives. Discussion arises around the question whether alcohol use is genetically determined or rather a product of a shared environment. Although patients might experience alcohol use in their parents, there is no unavoidable road toward addiction when children of alcohol-dependent parents drink their first alcoholic beverage. This suggests that environmental factors interact with biological factors in a complex way. Moreover, in an adoption study, genetic and environmental factors were of similar magnitude [26].

3.2   What Is Heritability in Addiction?

In general, heritability is understood as a proportion of a given phenotypic variance that is due to genetic variability. There are different ways in order to estimate this genetic variability (see Box 3.1). Twin and adoption studies were the mainstay of investigations of how traits are inherited from parents to their offspring for decades. The fact that dizygotic twins share about half of their genes and monozygotic twins share all their genes allows to statistically model how much of a trait might be linked to additive genetic effects. Landmark studies investigating heritability of AUD include work by Heath et al. [17], who used tetrachoric correlation (a statistical test that exploits the abovementioned assumption of additive genetic effects) and found that 64% of the variance is explained by genetic risk factors. More recent estimates for heritability from meta-analysis of twin and adoption studies result in an approximation of 50% of the variance explained by genetic factors [47]. Interestingly, this study also found moderate shared environmental effects (e.g., 10% of the variance). The authors interpret that environmental factors contribute to the familial aggregation of AUD. As compared to the high estimates from twin studies, a smaller propor-

tion has been attributed to additive effects from common genetic variation, the so-called single-nucleotide polymorphism (SNP) heritability: 33% for AUD [34] and 18% [48] or 13% for average alcohol consumption [9]. Exploiting the aggregation of weighted counts of risk genes (single-nucleotide polymorphisms, SNPs) resulting in an individual polygenic risk score, up to 1% of the variance in AUD symptom scores has been explained [40]. Estimates from large genome-wide association studies (GWAS) and online surveys, treating alcohol use as continuous marker, find point estimates for heritability of 12% of the variance explained [39]. Interestingly, in their cohort, recruited via the online ancestry and health info service 23andMe, Inc., there was a positive association between educational attainment and AUDIT scores, suggesting a possible confound based on a selection bias.

In summary, there is a wide range in heritability estimates resulting from different kinds of methodological approaches (see Fig. 3.1). This phenomenon is frequently referred to as the case of the missing heritability. It is important to note that there is no easy answer when talking to patients about heritability of a complex trait that is highly polygenic and implies environmental factors. As a clinician, the best way to communicate disease risk is to underline the high probability of not passing on a genetic liability to the patients' offspring and to emphasize on environmental factors that are malleable in order to destigmatize and give hope for possible interventions.

3.3   Genome-Wide Association Studies

In the past 15 years, major advances in the field of human disease genetics have provided the path for novel research strategies such as GWAS to identify the genetic factors involved in various psychiatric traits and other genetically complex disorders. This progress started with the completion of the Human Genome Project in 2003. There, it became evident that the majority of

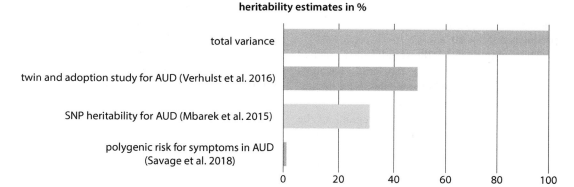

Fig. 3.1 Different heritability estimates from different methodologies. Heritability can be expressed as proportion of variance accounted for a certain phenotypic trait. Depending on the methodology, different estimates are obtained. Twin and adoption studies imply the whole genome; however, they might be biased toward an overestimation due to shared environment. SNP heritability evaluates the contribution of common variants by calculating the relatedness between apparently unrelated individuals and associating that measure to a certain phenotype. The explained variance with polygenic risk scores is expected to converge with the estimated SNP heritability with vastly increased sample size

bases do not differ, or are invariant, between two randomly chosen individuals in the world. Still, more than nine million unique SNPs exist in the genome of European individuals [45] with a minor allele frequency (MAF) of at least 1%. One important feature of the SNP genome was the haplotype block structure. This phenomenon is also called linkage disequilibrium (LD) and has important consequences for analysis methods like imputation and the development of SNP arrays that play a key role in GWAS.

Companies started to develop microarrays as SNP genotyping platforms to allow the simultaneous, rapid genotyping of hundreds of thousands of SNPs in an individual at affordable costs. The most commonly used approaches are allele discrimination by hybridization, as used by Affymetrix and the Infinium Assay of Illumina.

In a GWAS, a genome-wide set of SNPs is measured in a large number of cases (with disease) and controls (without disease) using commercially available high-throughput genotyping platforms (SNP microarrays). Currently, such genotyping platforms typically measure between 300,000 and 800,000 unique SNPs in each sample. Because many SNPs located in the same haplotype block are correlated via LD, it is computationally feasible to estimate the geno-

types of the remaining (not genotyped) ~8,500,000 SNPs with MAF >1% across the genome using a reference data set, such as that provided by the 1000 Genomes Project [45] or the Haplotype Reference Consortium. This method of estimating missing genotypes is called imputation and enables a more comprehensive analysis of the SNP variation present in the human genome as well as meta-analyses across multiple data sets that have used different genotyping platforms. This is an important step combining GWAS data from distinct sources, which is necessary to increase statistical power to detect novel genetic associations.

Since there is no requirement for prior biological knowledge of the trait undergoing investigation, a GWAS is an unbiased, genome-wide search for SNPs that are involved in the development of a disease. The costs of SNP microarrays have decreased substantially over time, so that it is now feasible to analyze tens of thousands of individuals. This is a crucial requirement to achieve the statistical power to detect the small genetic effects mediated by common risk variants. One limitation of GWAS is the large number of tested SNPs, posing a massive multiple testing problem. This is addressed by correction methods, and an SNP allele is assumed to be associated with the disease when the allele frequency difference between patients and controls produces $p < 5 \times 10^{-08}$.

This significance threshold, also named genome-wide significance threshold, accounts for testing one million independent SNPs, assuming a type 1 error rate of 5%.

Significant SNPs will point to regions of the genome that harbor potential causal variants. After the often inconsistent and frustrating results of the linkage and candidate gene era, the GWAS approach has led to a breakthrough and has discovered several thousands of genetic loci reliably associated with a range of complex phenotypes and diseases.[1] These findings not only provide novel biological insight into diseases but also have the potential to guide therapeutic development.

One limitation of GWAS is that it cannot identify the functionally causal variant(s) in an associated region. As a consequence of the LD between many variants within a haplotype block, the association signal typically covers a broad chromosomal region, sometimes spanning 500 kb or more and containing numerous genes. In practice, however, at least half of the associated regions encompass only one or two genes.

In other regions, pathway or gene set analyses or functional annotations may help prioritize candidate genes, but the identification of the responsible gene/functionally relevant variant remains a challenge.

3.4 Genome-Wide Association Studies in Psychiatric Disease

In 2006, the first GWAS of schizophrenia was published [33]. It comprised 320 patients and 325 controls, genotyped on 25,000 gene-based SNPs. No SNP was meeting today's threshold for genome-wide significance. The following published GWAS used the Affymetrix 500 K genotyping chip with much more comprehensive genomic coverage. However, by today's standards, sample sizes were still small: 178 cases and 144 controls in a study by Lencz et al. [30] and 738 cases and 733 controls in a sample by Sullivan et al. [44]. Again, none of the top hits met the criteria for genome-wide significance. The fourth published GWAS by O'Donovan et al. [10] could report the first reliable and consistent findings. Although the initial GWAS with 479 cases and 2937 controls did not yield genome-wide significant associations, there were a few findings that were very close to meet this significance threshold. A follow-up cohort with a sample size of 6666 cases and 9897 controls could confirm a lead SNP located in the transcription factor ZNF804A, considered by many in the field as the first, replicating finding in GWAS for schizophrenia. It became clear that the effect size of common risk genes for schizophrenia is generally lower than expected and that several hundreds of patients and controls did not suffice to detect genome-wide significant associations when appropriately correcting for multiple testing. Following this observation, researchers began to intensify collaborations and jointly analyzed GWAS data sets to substantiate the power of their analyses to trace variants with small genetic effects contributing to schizophrenia across the genome.

Large-scale collaborations like International Schizophrenia Consortium (ISC), SGENE, Molecular Genetics of Schizophrenia (MGS), the Bonn–Mannheim (BoMa) consortium, and, last but not the least, the Psychiatric Genomics Consortium (PGC) were founded and have substantially contributed to the success of GWAS for psychiatric traits in the past few years [43, 45]. A landmark paper from the ISC consortium could not only identify a handful of validated SNPs but also introduced the meanwhile widely applied polygenic risk score method into the field of psychiatric GWAS [24]. Since then, it has been shown in many different data sets that the polygenic risk score derived with an SNP set from an initial GWAS is capable of distinguishing schizophrenia patients from controls in independent data sets, albeit with low sensitivity and specificity. Notably, the predictive power of

---

[1] https://www.ebi.ac.uk/gwas/docs/diagram-downloads

the polygenic test improves (in terms of phenotypic variance explained) when SNPs with non-significant p-values are also included. This means that many schizophrenia-associated SNPs with small but true genetic effects still must be contained in this p-value range. The most important implication of that work was that further sample size increase would uncover many more yet unknown schizophrenia hits, while power of the polygenic risk score would become more powerful.

In 2011, Schizophrenia Working Group of the PGC published a GWAS study comprising 21,856 individuals (cases and controls) in combination with 29,939 individuals in a follow-up replication step, yielding to five novel gene loci [24]. This laid the foundation for a strongly accelerated collaboration. In 2014, the PGC published a second meta-analysis, including almost 37,000 individuals with schizophrenia, 302 investigators, 35 countries, and 4 continents [1]. One hundred twenty-eight statistically independent associations, implicating at least 108 schizophrenia-associated loci, were reported (Fig. 3.2).

Not only 83 of these loci were novel, but 25 previous findings could be confirmed supporting the use of large GWAS to create reproducible findings.

Genes from the reported 108 schizophrenia-associated loci were involved in the following functional categories: glutamatergic (and possibly dopaminergic) neurotransmission, neuronal calcium signaling, synaptic function and plasticity, neurodevelopment, and immune processes.

In the following years, GWAS of other psychiatric traits followed with a similar trajectory, most notably in major depression, identifying 102 independent variants.

This GWAS required a vastly increased sample size of 246,363 cases and 561,190 controls due to much smaller effect sizes of the underlying causal common variants.

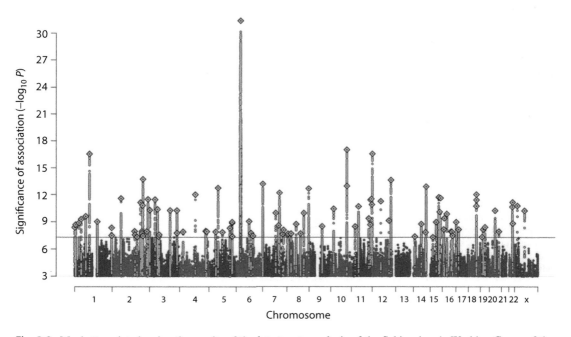

Fig. 3.2 Manhattan plot showing the results of the latest meta-analysis of the Schizophrenia Working Group of the PGC, implicating 108 independent schizophrenia-associated loci [1]

3.5 Future Directions of Psychiatric Genome-Wide Association Studies

When we illustrate number of schizophrenia-associated SNPs as a function of case sample size and compare them to two other genetically complex diseases/phenotypes, which showed great success in GWAS analyses (namely, Crohn's disease and human height), findings regarding schizophrenia are comparable to those for human height (Fig. 3.3).

It is apparent that, after a collective case number of roughly 15,000, we can observe an almost linear relationship between case number and the number of significantly associated genetic variants (~4 new hits per 1000 added cases). It is therefore reasonable to aim for further sample size increase to achieve a more sophisticated picture of the biology involved in psychiatric traits.

Two unpublished studies have been presented at various conferences: a GWAS of bipolar disorder, identifying more than 30 loci with 20,352 cases and 31,358 controls [42], and a GWAS of schizophrenia, with 65,205 cases and 87,919 controls, identifying 248 genome-wide significant regions (personal communication). These confirm the undamped effect of additional associations with further sample size increase.

GWAS in psychiatry is certainly a successful method for identifying common risk variants.

Even though these diagnoses harbor presumed high heterogeneity, the field succeeded in identifying far more than a handful genetic loci for various psychiatric traits.

Despite these successes, it is important to continue recruitment of new cohorts to further increase power and discover more risk variants to get a more distinguished picture of the biological processes involved in these disorders. Improved bioinformatics techniques, such as refined biological gene set analyses, and more comprehensive references of pre-annotated pathways will be helpful to even better exploit GWAS results. It should also be emphasized that psychiatric GWAS hits are characterized by a broad frequency spectrum of disease alleles.

In the future, extended analysis of polygenic risk scores will likely be useful in clinical settings, e.g., for improved phenotypic classifications or for guiding medication and therapy. It should be noted though that, to date, the field has not arrived at a broad clinical integration of polygenic risk scores.

Pathophysiological consequences of the many risk variants identified need to be investigated further. For example, it is unclear whether the schizophrenia-risk SNPs are the functionally relevant SNPs or just "proxies" in LD. Experimental approaches (molecular and cellular investigations) will be the key to understand the functional

Fig. 3.3 Number of genome-wide significant findings as a function of sample size, reflected as number of cases. Red, Crohn's disease; yellow, schizophrenia; black, bipolar disorder; green, adult height

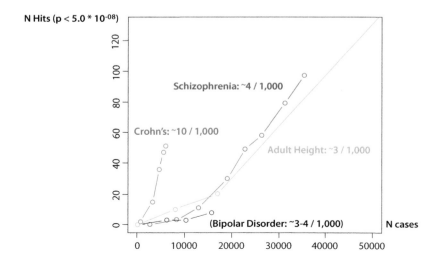

consequences of risk alleles and the underlying pathophysiological processes.

Some of the identified associations might already point to actionable therapeutic targets. Furthermore, we hope that with deeper insights into the biology of psychiatric disease, pharmacologic and non-pharmacologic therapy will become more beneficial to patients.

3.6   Potential Markers

The genetics of alcohol dependence is summarized in a comprehensive review by Rietschel and Treutlein [38]. Findings include 30 GWAS on AUD, alcohol consumption, and AUD-related traits. A more recent large GWAS for alcohol dependence of 16,087 subjects [13] report associations with genes relating to alcohol metabolism such as alcohol dehydrogenase and aldehyde dehydrogenase. Other studies identified several interesting candidate genes, for example, in the GATA4 gene that encodes a transcription factor of atrial natriuretic peptide [46] and XRCC5,

which is involved in sensitivity to alcohol in humans and animals [25]. Furthermore, Val66Met polymorphism might contribute to alcohol dependence vulnerability via lower executive function performance [3], and brain-derived neurotrophic factor (BDNF) serum levels have been linked to AUD [29]. Moreover, genotype of serotonin transporter has been shown to be correlated with alcohol intake in nonhuman primates [20] and response to alcohol in adolescents [23] pointing toward the importance of alcohol sensitivity as a possible trait variable associated with the development of AUD [41].

In summary, the abovementioned findings underline the polygenic character of inheritance involving several genetic variants. One has to consider that genetic risk factors for AUD may be part of a broad genetic burden for a range of disorders, including vulnerability to social isolation, stress, and adverse environments [19, 21, 27]. It has been discussed that genetic factors related to AUD may exert their influences on alcohol use via processes of reward learning and habituation [14].

Box 3.1 How Can We Estimate Heritability
Twin Studies
The fact that monozygotic twins share twice as many genes compared to monozygotic twins makes it rather straightforward to calculated heritability estimates using Falconer's formula $H^2 = 2(r_{(MZ)}-r_{(DZ)})$. H^2 signifies the heritability, which is calculated as the difference in correlation coefficients r for phenotypic variance in monozygotic and dizygotic twins. There are several relevant limitations in twin studies. Firstly, Falconer's formula assumes that all genetic effects are additive; however, most likely and biologically plausible, there are gene x gene interactions, which can create nonlinear effects. Moreover, genes in related subjects do not occur randomly but are inherited together, which may render the estimate of heritability too strong. Assortative mating (the tendency that similar people have

children together) might inflate heritability estimates from twin studies; eventually, it may overestimate dominant variance. And even in twin studies where the twins are raised apart, shared environment before separation and selective placement has to be considered [6].

Single-Nucleotide Polymorphism
Heritability
An almost reverse approach to twin studies is the estimation of SNP heritability. It makes use of tiny differences in the proportions of genome shared among seemingly unrelated individuals. Here, the heritability is derived from an estimate of relatedness between apparently unrelated individuals derived from SNP variation. That means it is calculated from the extent to which phenotypic variance for a trait can be explained by SNPs across the genome. A kinship matrix is calculated, which

represents the similarities between individuals that are unrelated. This matrix is then fitted to a vector of the phenotype in a mixed model in order to estimate heritability.

The unrelatedness of the subjects studied helps to disentangle possible effects of SNPs that are inherited together. In other words, SNP mutations that are associated with a phenotype are likely representing causal effects of this SNP, rather than being due to a different source of genetic variation, which is associated with a SNP that is inherited alongside with other SNPs.

However, SNP heritability is limited to additive effects from only a subset of common genetic variants that are investigated (sometimes referred to as the "chip heritability"), and SNP heritability does not identify specific SNP associations, meaning it is not made for the discovery of the underlying genetic variants.

Polygenic Scores

A polygenic score comprises thousands of SNPs that are associated with a specific trait. The aggregation of many associated SNPs provides a score that can be used as an individual estimate for individual differences. The SNPs are weighted by their correlation with the trait. Thus, polygenic scores give an estimate of the subjects genetic risk for a specific trait. One has to bear in mind that polygenic scores provide a probabilistic estimate for a certain trait. For research purposes, polygenic scores are a useful tool to investigate the extent to which a genetic estimate of a trait mediates effects on other variables of interest.

3.7   Environmental Influences on Heritability

3.7.1   Epigenetic Mechanisms

Epigenetics refer to molecular processes that alter gene expression without altering the deoxyribonucleic acid (DNA) sequence itself [35]. The most commonly accepted mechanisms coded as epigenetic mechanisms are DNA methylation, histone modifications, and noncoding RNAs (see Fig. 3.4). *DNA methylation* refers to the addition of a methyl group to DNA base pairs, primarily the cytosine base in cytosine-guanine (CG) dinucleotides. When CG dinucleotides occur in a high frequency (at least 200 base pairs), they form so-called CG islands. These islands play an important role in gene regulation, as they typically occur at or near the transcription start site (or the promoter region) of genes. *Histone modification* refers to the physical organization of DNA as part of the chromatin, as the DNA is wrapped around histones. This physical interaction (between DNA and histones) directly modifies the accessibility of the genome to transcription factors. There are numerous processes affecting this interaction, e.g., methylation, phosphorylation, acetylation, ubiquitylation, and sumoylation. Also, *noncoding RNAs* (microRNAs (miRNAs)) bind to mRNA, thus interfering with gene expression on a posttranslational level [50].

These mechanisms interact with chromatin, the protein complex that organizes DNA and thus can alter the extent to which genes are accessible to transcription factors. This chapter will focus on DNA methylation as the most commonly studied epigenetic mechanism in addiction.

Initial studies of aberrant DNA methylation patterns in AUD suggest that the "epigenetic" properties of ethanol may play an important role in the maintenance of alcohol consumption in AUD. Animal studies show that already before conception exposure to alcohol can cause alterations in DNA methylation in the brain of the offspring [15]. Ethanol induces methylation patterns in brain areas known to be involved in the development and maintenance of addictive behaviors are within the limbic system such as the ventral

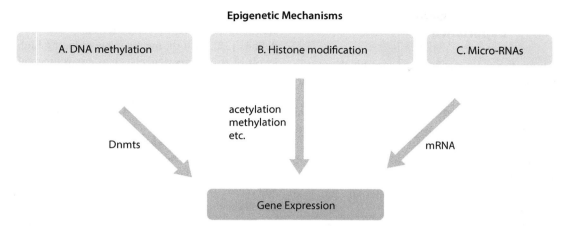

Fig. 3.4 Epigenetic mechanisms: A. DNA methylation is catalyzed by a family of DNA methyltransferases (Dnmts) that transfer a methyl group from *S*-adenyl methionine (SAM) to the fifth carbon of a cytosine residue to form 5mC. B. DNA is wrapped around histone proteins, which can be manipulated, e.g., through acetylation, methylation, phosphorylation and hence change accessibility to transcription factors without changing the DNA itself. C. MicroRNAs (miRNAs) are noncoding, single-stranded RNAs of 18–25 nucleotides. miRNAs affect gene expression through binding to mRNA. All processes are interrelated and affect gene expression (e.g., silencing or activation of target genes)

tegmental area (VTA), which is associated with reward dependent learning and memory and the hypothalamus, which contributes to stress and fear management [12]. Differences in methylations patterns induced by alcohol consumption have been shown to persist over generations [11] and can be reversed via specific chemical interventions [2].

Human postmortem brains show an overall decrease of methylation level after high alcohol exposure over life compared to healthy control brains [37]. In humans, the amount of alcohol exposure was directly linked to methylation patterns in genes highly relevant for addiction, including the γ-aminobutyric acid-A receptor (GABA) A and B gene [31]. Their differential methylation was associated with expression levels of a number of genes involved in immune function. Specifically, DNA methylation levels in promoter regions of genes implicated in addiction can be associated with AUD. These pathways include the dopaminergic system [5], the hypothalamus-pituitary-adrenal (HPA) stress axis [22], cell proliferation [18], and signaling

pathways [4]. Furthermore, changes in methylation level have been associated with behavioral patterns such as craving for alcohol and withdrawal symptoms [5, 22].

Assessing epigenetic modifications is an important step forward in closing the gap between high estimates of heritability in AUD on the one hand and moderate to low associations between gene expression and behavioral indicators of AUD (such as amount of drinking, time to relapse, and withdrawal symptoms) on the other hand.

Besides the epigenetic properties of alcohol itself, there are numerous other variables that have been identified as highly relevant in the induction of epigenetic modification, including, for example, (mal)nutrition, consumption of other drugs, and exposure to stressful life experience as early as preconception [15]. With respect to the development and maintenance of AUD, stress exposure has been identified as one of key mechanisms mediating environmental and epigenetic influences and will thus be discussed in further detail within this chapter [7, 28, 32].

3.8   Aversive or Stressful Life Experience

So far, the exact mechanisms causing changes in DNA methylation patterns have only been insufficiently understood. Environmental influences during critical periods of development can lead to changes in learning, perception, and behavior via epigenetic mechanisms and may increase the risk of AUD and other psychiatric disorders. Such environmental stressors can be chemical influences, malnutrition, lack of maternal care, and adverse life experiences [28].

Animal models give further insight into the molecular mechanisms by which environmental factors influence gene transcription and behavior regulation. Maternal (caring via licking and grooming) behavior in the first week after birth altered the offsprings' epigenome at a glucocorticoid receptor (GR) gene promoter in the hippocampus [49], a region highly relevant for learning and habitization processes. Animals with caring mothers showed higher glucocorticoid receptor levels and reduced corticosterone and were less anxious compared to the offspring of less-caring mothers. These changes in epigenetic programming can persist over generations; thus, heritability turns into a dynamic and time-sensitive process.

In humans, aversive and stressful life changes such as loss of a friend, change in occupation, or problems in love relationship have been identified as potential modulators of (epi)genetic processes with relevance for alcohol-related behavior. Peng et al. [36] recently identified two new gene loci for alcohol-related life events in humans performing genome-wide analyses. They report two rare variants: the potassium channel subfamily K member 2 (K2P channel gene KCNK2) and missense and splice-site variants in pro-inflammatory mediator gene phosphodiesterase 4C (PDE4C). These genes play an important role in cell signaling and immune modulation and have been identified as relevant for serotonergic neurotransmission and depressive symptoms [36]. In agreement with animal studies, stress exposure during pregnancy in humans leads to changes in the individuals' response to stress after birth at different ages and has been linked to behavioral changes such as inconsiderate behavior, sleep disturbance, and attention deficits [32]. In turn, mechanisms reducing high levels of stress experience such as environmental enrichment and physical exercise can partially reverse DNA methylation differences associated with drinking in human subjects at high risk for developing AUD [8].

Summing up, epigenetic mechanisms are numerous and can be caused by multiple factors, only a few of which have been directly linked to addictive behavior. The interplay between genetic, epigenetic, and environmental factors has an ongoing influence on brain development and the associated behavioral changes, thus causing resilience or vulnerability to mental disorders such as AUD.

A key challenge for future research in the field of epigenetics will be to disentangle how changes in gene transcription contribute to the development and maintenance of addictive behaviors. At present, to name only a few of the challenges, we have to rely on new technologies and a poor knowledge of the methylome. By focusing on the CPG-rich islands near promoter regions, relevant sites for addictive behavior might be missed. Methylation patterns change over time and tissue type; thus, it remains speculative to relate methylation patterns retrieved from peripheral blood cells to brain-based processes. Many studies have small sample sizes, and different tissues and cells are being used to identify molecular changes. Up to now, there is no validated and commonly accepted framework for the analysis of genome-wide epigenetic data, which makes it extremely difficult to replicate new findings [16]. Nevertheless, epigenetic changes are an interface between environmental and genetic factors and may help to close the "heritability gap."

References

1. Schizophrenia Working Group of the Psychiatric Genomics Consortium, Ripke S, Neale BM, Corvin A, Walters JTR, Farh K-H, et al. Biological insights from 108 schizophrenia-associated genetic loci. Nature. 2014;511:421–7. https://doi.org/10.1038/nature13595.

2. Bekdash RA, Zhang C, Sarkar DK. Gestational choline supplementation normalized fetal alcohol-induced alterations in histone modifications, DNA methylation, and proopiomelanocortin (POMC) gene expression in β-endorphin-producing POMC neurons of the hypothalamus. Alcohol Clin Exp Res. 2013;37(7):1133–42. https://doi.org/10.1111/acer.12082.

3. Benzerouk F, Gierski F, Gorwood P, Ramoz N, Stefaniak N, Hübsch B, et al. Brain-derived neurotrophic factor (BDNF) Val66Met polymorphism and its implication in executive functions in adult offspring of alcohol-dependent probands. Alcohol. 2013;47(4):271–4. https://doi.org/10.1016/j.alcohol.2013.03.001.

4. Biermann T, Reulbach U, Lenz B, Frieling H, Muschler M, Hillemacher T, et al. N-methyl-d-aspartate 2b receptor subtype (NR2B) promoter methylation in patients during alcohol withdrawal. J Neural Transm. 2009;116(5):615–22. https://doi.org/10.1007/s00702-009-0212-2.

5. Bönsch D, Greifenberg V, Bayerlein K, Biermann T, Reulbach U, Hillemacher T, et al. Alpha-synuclein protein levels are increased in alcoholic patients and are linked to craving. Alcohol Clin Exp Res. 2005;29(5):763–5. Retrieved from http://www.ncbi.nlm.nih.gov/pubmed/15897720

6. Boomsma D, Busjahn A, Peltonen L. Classical twin studies and beyond. Nat Rev Genet. 2002;3(11):872–82. https://doi.org/10.1038/nrg932.

7. Cecil CAM, Walton E, Viding E. Epigenetics of addiction: current knowledge, challenges, and future directions. J Stud Alcohol Drugs. 2016;77(5):688–91. https://doi.org/10.15288/jsad.2016.77.688.

8. Chen J, Hutchison KE, Bryan AD, Filbey FM, Calhoun VD, Claus ED, et al. Opposite epigenetic associations with alcohol use and exercise intervention. Front Psych. 2018;9:594. https://doi.org/10.3389/fpsyt.2018.00594.

9. Clarke TK, Adams MJ, Davies G, Howard DM, Hall LS, Padmanabhan S, et al. Genome-wide association study of alcohol consumption and genetic overlap with other health-related traits in UK biobank (N=112117). Mol Psychiatry. 2017;22(10):1376–84. https://doi.org/10.1038/mp.2017.153.

10. Donovan MCO, Craddock N, Norton N, Williams H, Peirce T, Moskvina V, et al. Identification of loci associated with schizophrenia by genome-wide association and follow-up. Nat Genet. 2008;40(9):1053–5. https://doi.org/10.1038/ng.201.

11. Finegersh A, Homanics GE. Paternal alcohol exposure reduces alcohol drinking and increases behavioral sensitivity to alcohol selectively in male offspring. PLoS One. 2014;9(6):e99078. https://doi.org/10.1371/journal.pone.0099078.

12. Gangisetty O, Bekdash R, Maglakelidze G, Sarkar DK. Fetal alcohol exposure alters proopiomelanocortin gene expression and hypothalamic-pituitary-adrenal Axis function via increasing MeCP2 expression in the hypothalamus. PLoS One. 2014;9(11):e113228. Retrieved from https://doi.org/10.1371/journal.pone.0113228

13. Gelernter J, Kranzler HR, Sherva R, Almasy L, Koesterer R, Smith AH, et al. Genome-wide association study of alcohol dependence:significant findings in African- and European-Americans including novel risk loci. Mol Psychiatry. 2014;19(1):41–9. https://doi.org/10.1038/mp.2013.145.

14. Goldman MS, Reich RR, Darkes J. Expectancy as unifying construct in alcohol-related cognition. In: Wiers RW, Stacy AW, editors. Handbook of implicit Congition and addiction. Thousand Oaks: Sage Publications; 2006. p. 105–15.

15. Govorko D, Bekdash RA, Zhang C, Sarkar DK. Male germline transmits fetal alcohol adverse effect on hypothalamic proopiomelanocortin gene across generations. Biol Psychiatry. 2012;72(5):378–88. https://doi.org/10.1016/j.biopsych.2012.04.006.

16. Harlaar N, Hutchison KE. Alcohol and the methylome: design and analysis considerations for research using human samples. Drug Alcohol Depend. 2013;133(2):305–16. https://doi.org/10.1016/j.drugalcdep.2013.07.026.

17. Heath AC, Bucholz KK, Madden PAF, Dinwiddie SH, Slutske WS, Bierut LJ, et al. Genetic and environmental contributions to alcohol dependence risk in a national twin sample: consistency of findings in women and men. Psychol Med. 1997;27(6):1381–96. https://doi.org/10.1017/S0033291797005643.

18. Heberlein A, Dürsteler-MacFarland KM, Frieling H, Gröschl M, Lenz B, Bönsch D, et al. Association of Nerve Growth Factor and Vascular Endothelial Growth Factor a with psychometric measurements of opiate dependence: results of a pilot study in patients participating in a structured Diamorphine maintenance program. Eur Addict Res. 2012;18(5):213–9. https://doi.org/10.1159/000337212.

19. Heinz A, Beck A, Meyer-Lindenberg A, Sterzer P, Heinz A. Cognitive and neurobiological mechanisms of alcohol-related aggression. *Nature Reviews*. Neuroscience. 2011;12(7):400–13. https://doi.org/10.1038/nrn3042.

20. Heinz A, Jones DW, Gorey JG, Bennet A, Suomi SJ, Weinberger DR, Higley JD. Serotonin transporter availability correlates with alcohol intake in non-human primates. Mol Psychiatry. 2003;8(2):231–4. https://doi.org/10.1038/sj.mp.4001214.

21. Hicks BM, Krueger RF, Iacono WG, McGue M, Patrick CJ. Family transmission and heritability of externalizing disorders: a twin-family study. Arch Gen Psychiatry. 2004;61(9):922–8. https://doi.org/10.1001/archpsyc.61.9.922.

22. Hillemacher T, Frieling H, Luber K, Yazici A, Muschler MAN, Lenz B, et al. Epigenetic regulation and gene expression of vasopressin and atrial natriuretic peptide in alcohol withdrawal. Psychoneuroendocrinology. 2009;34(4):555–60. https://doi.org/10.1016/j.psyneuen.2008.10.019.

23. Hinckers AS, Laucht M, Schmidt MH, Mann KF, Schumann G, Schuckit MA, Heinz A. Low level of

response to alcohol as associated with serotonin transporter genotype and high alcohol intake in adolescents. Biol Psychiatry. 2006;60(3):282–7. https://doi.org/10.1016/j.biopsych.2005.12.009.

24. International Schizophrenia Consortium, Purcell SM, Wray NR, Stone JL, Visscher PM, O'Donovan MC, et al. Common polygenic variation contributes to risk of schizophrenia and bipolar disorder. Nature. 2009;460(7256):748–52. https://doi.org/10.1038/nature08185.

25. Juraeva D, Treutlein J, Scholz H, Frank J, Degenhardt F, Cichon S, et al. XRCC5 as a risk gene for alcohol dependence: evidence from a genome-wide gene-set-based analysis and follow-up studies in drosophila and humans. Neuropsychopharmacology. 2015;40(2):361–71. https://doi.org/10.1038/npp.2014.178.

26. Kendler KS, Ji J, Edwards AC, Ohlsson H, Sundquist J, Sundquist K. An extended Swedish national adoption study of alcohol use disorder. JAMA Psychiat. 2015;72(3):211–8. https://doi.org/10.1001/jamapsychiatry.2014.2138.

27. Kendler KS, Myers JM, Keyes CLM. The relationship between the genetic and environmental influences on common externalizing psychopathology and mental wellbeing. Twin Research and Human Genetics: The Official Journal of the International Society for Twin Studies. 2011;14(6):516–23. https://doi.org/10.1161/ATVBAHA.114.303112.ApoA-I.

28. Kofink D, Boks MPM, Timmers HTM, Kas MJ. Epigenetic dynamics in psychiatric disorders: environmental programming of neurodevelopmental processes. Neurosci Biobehav Rev. 2013;37(5):831–45. https://doi.org/10.1016/j.neubiorev.2013.03.020.

29. Köhler S, Klimke S, Hellweg R, Lang UE. Serum brain-derived neurotrophic factor and nerve growth factor concentrations change after alcohol withdrawal: preliminary data of a case-control comparison. Eur Addict Res. 2013;19(2):98–104. https://doi.org/10.1159/000342334.

30. Lencz T, Morgan TV, Athanasiou M, Dain B, Reed CR, Kane JM, et al. Converging evidence for a pseudoautosomal cytokine receptor gene locus in schizophrenia. Mol Psychiatry. 2007;12(6):572–80. https://doi.org/10.1038/sj.mp.4001983.

31. Liu C, Marioni RE, Hedman ÅK, Pfeiffer L, Tsai P-C, Reynolds LM, et al. A DNA methylation biomarker of alcohol consumption. Mol Psychiatry. 2018;23(2):422–33. https://doi.org/10.1038/mp.2016.192.

32. Lupien SJ, McEwen BS, Gunnar MR, Heim C. Effects of stress throughout the lifespan on the brain, behaviour and cognition. Nat Rev Neurosci. 2009;10(6):434–45. https://doi.org/10.1038/nrn2639.

33. Mah S, Nelson MR, DeLisi LE, Reneland RH, Markward N, James MR, et al. Identification of the semaphorin receptor PLXNA2 as a candidate for susceptibility to schizophrenia. Mol Psychiatry. 2006;11(5):471–8. https://doi.org/10.1038/sj.mp.4001785.

34. Mbarek H, Milaneschi Y, Fedko IO, Hottenga J-J, de Moor MHM, Jansen R, et al. The genetics of alcohol dependence: twin and SNP-based heritability, and genome-wide association study based on AUDIT scores. Am J Med Genet. 2015;168(8):739–48. https://doi.org/10.1002/ajmg.b.32379.

35. Nestler EJ. Epigenetic mechanisms of drug addiction. Neuropharmacology. 2014;76:259–68. https://doi.org/10.1016/j.neuropharm.2013.04.004.

36. Peng Q, Bizon C, Gizer IR, Wilhelmsen KC, Ehlers CL. Genetic loci for alcohol-related life events and substance-induced affective symptoms: indexing the "dark side" of addiction. Transl Psychiatry. 2019;9(1):71. https://doi.org/10.1038/s41398-019-0397-6.

37. Ponomarev I, Wang S, Zhang L, Harris RA, Mayfield RD. Gene Coexpression networks in human brain identify epigenetic modifications in alcohol dependence. J Neurosci. 2012;32(5):1884–97. https://doi.org/10.1523/JNEUROSCI.3136-11.2012.

38. Rietschel M, Treutlein J. The genetics of alcohol dependence. Ann N Y Acad Sci. 2013;1282(1):39–70. https://doi.org/10.1111/j.1749-6632.2012.06794.x.

39. Sanchez-Roige S, Fontanillas P, Elson SL, Gray JC, de Wit H, Davis LK, et al. Genome-wide association study of alcohol use disorder identification test (AUDIT) scores in 20 328 research participants of European ancestry. Addict Biol. 2017:121–31. https://doi.org/10.1111/adb.12574.

40. Savage JE, Salvatore JE, Aliev F, Edwards AC, Hickman M, Kendler KS, et al. Polygenic risk score prediction of alcohol dependence symptoms across population-based and clinically ascertained samples. Alcohol Clin Exp Res. 2018;42(3):520–30. https://doi.org/10.1111/acer.13589.

41. Schuckit MA, Smith TL, Goncalves PD, Anthenelli R. Alcohol-related blackouts across 55 weeks of college: effects of European-American ethnicity, female sex, and low level of response to alcohol. Drug Alcohol Depend. 2016;169:163–70. https://doi.org/10.1016/j.drugalcdep.2016.10.026.

42. Stahl, E. A., Forstner, A. J., & Mcquillin, A. (2017). Genome-wide association study identifies 30 Loci Associated with Bipolar Disorder. ABSTRACT: Bipolar disorder is a highly heritable psychiatric disorder that features episodes of mania and. BioRxiv. doi: https://doi.org/10.1101/173062.

43. Stefansson H, Ophoff RA, Steinberg S, Andreassen OA, Cichon S, Rujescu D, et al. Common variants conferring risk of schizophrenia. Nature. 2009;460(7256):744–7. https://doi.org/10.1038/nature08186.

44. Sullivan PF, Lin D, Tzeng JY, Van Den Oord E, Perkins D, Stroup TS, et al. Genomewide association for schizophrenia in the CATIE study: results of stage 1. Mol Psychiatry. 2008;13(6):570–84. https://doi.org/10.1038/mp.2008.25.

45. The 1000 Genomes Project, McVean GA, Altshuler DM, Durbin RM, Abecasis GR, Bentley DR, et al. An integrated map of genetic variation from 1,092 human

genomes. Nature. 2012;491(7422):56–65. https://doi.org/10.1038/nature11632.

46. Treutlein J, Cichon S, Ridinger M, Wodarz N, Soyka M, Zill P, et al. Genome-wide association study of alcohol dependence. Arch Gen Psychiatry. 2009;66(7):773. https://doi.org/10.1001/archgenpsychiatry.2009.83.

47. Verhulst B, Neale MC, Kendler KS. The heritability of alcohol use disorders: a meta-analysis of twin and adoption studies. Psychol Med. 2015;45(5):1061–72. https://doi.org/10.1017/S0033291714002165.

48. Vrieze SI, McGue M, Miller MB, Hicks BM, Iacono WG. Three mutually informative ways to understand the genetic relationships among behavioral disinhibi-tion, alcohol use, drug use, nicotine use/dependence, and their co-occurrence: twin biometry, GCTA, and genome-wide scoring. Behav Genet. 2013;43(2):97–107. https://doi.org/10.1007/s10519-013-9584-z.

49. Weaver ICG, Cervoni N, Champagne FA, D'Alessio AC, Sharma S, Seckl JR, et al. Epigenetic pro-gramming by maternal behavior. Nat Neurosci. 2004;7(8):847–54. https://doi.org/10.1038/nn1276.

50. Wei JW, Huang K, Yang C, Kang CS. Non-coding RNAs as regulators in epigenetics (review). Oncol Rep. 2017;37(1):3–9. https://doi.org/10.3892/or.2016.5236.

Animal Models of Addiction

4

Eliot L. Gardner

Contents

Abstract

Addiction is a vastly complex disorder – with biological, psychological, social, and spiritual determinants. To a degree, the psychological, social, and spiritual determinants can be stud-

E. L. Gardner (✉)
Neuropsychopharmacology Section, Molecular Targets and Medications Discovery Research Branch, Intramural Research Program, National Institute on Drug Abuse, US National Institutes of Health, Baltimore, MD, USA
e-mail: egardner@intra.nida.nih.gov

ied at the human level. This is highly problematic for the biological determinants, as it would almost certainly involve probing and manipulating the living human brain – with its many neural circuits and systems subserving choice, impulsivity, compulsive behavior, positive affect, negative affect, drug-seeking, drug-taking, drug craving, and relapse. Therefore, animal models have been developed to model the various biological and, in parallel, behavioral aspects of drug-seeking, drug-taking, and relapse. These models possess both face validity and a significant degree

© Springer Nature Switzerland AG 2021
N. el-Guebaly et al. (eds.), *Textbook of Addiction Treatment*,
https://doi.org/10.1007/978-3-030-36391-8_4

of construct validity and predictive validity. Such models have yielded significant insights into the neurobiological substrates of addiction and have proven useful in the search for potentially effective anti-addiction, anti-craving, and anti-relapse medications to be used as adjuncts to other (e.g., cognitive, behavioral, psychosocial, group support) therapeutic modalities.

4.1 Introduction

Addiction is a complex disorder [44] involving dysfunction within vast regions of the central nervous system [49]. Given addiction's complexity, no single preclinical animal model can hope to satisfactorily capture the totality of its fundamental elements [62]. Rather, each animal model is an approximation that captures some but not all of the characteristics of the human condition. A major stumbling block in the development of animal models is that there is no generally accepted definition of addiction. Addiction is a term usually used to describe a self-administration habit involving an "addictive" substance, but there is no single criterion that distinguishes habits that qualify as addictions from habits that do not. People often talk glibly about being a "chocolate addict," but in the absence of a medical condition that makes sugar-rich chocolate consumption harmful to health (e.g., diabetes), it is hard to support the claim that indulging (even overindulging) in chocolate consumption qualifies as an addiction. Thus, there are many animal models, each of which reflects some real or presumed aspect of the habit-forming properties of addictive drugs. Although the models differ quite considerably, they each tend to identify the same major drugs, the same dose ranges, the same sites of action in the brain, and the same routes of administration as being associated with addiction liability [97]. The most strongly addictive substances are effective in each of the several models. Because each model seems, at least in terms of face validity, to reflect a different aspect

of the habit-forming actions of addictive drugs, the most balanced picture of the addictive liability of a given drug comes from an integrated consideration of the drug's actions across a full range of models. Nevertheless, preclinical laboratory models have made enormous contributions to our understanding of addiction, as animal models have the advantage of possessing both face validity and a significant degree of construct validity and predictive validity (vid., [18]). In addition, animal models can be used to probe the underlying neurobiology and neurocircuitry of addiction – to a far greater degree of precision than is currently allowed by human neuroimaging techniques (vid., [30]).

4.2 The Cycle of Addiction

Drug addiction can be conceptualized as a cyclical process [93]. It often begins with factors (biological, psychological, social) that predispose to initial drug use. This is then followed by actual first drug use – and the intoxication and drug-induced "high" that accompanies such initial use. This often progresses to moderate or relatively infrequent use ("chipping"). Although moderate and/or infrequent, even "chipping" of addictive substances can have serious legal, health, psychological, and/or social consequences (e.g., [36, 78]). Alternatively, addictive drug use can progress to extended, escalating, and/or "binge" use (e.g., [92]) – obviously more serious conditions with obviously more serious sequelae (e.g., compromised family, occupational, social, and/or recreational activities). Binge use is also problematic in that it often predicts subsequent severe drug addiction [11]. Drug use can then progress to "compulsive" use – often defined as continued addictive drug use in the face of obvious and serious drug-induced harmful consequences to the drug user. As addictive drug use continues, an "opponent process" trap [31, 61] opens, during which the drug-induced "high" diminishes and drug-induced dysphoria increases – leaving the addictive drug user with a net loss of subjective drug-induced positive affect. Another "opponent process" situation arises in the context of drug withdrawal and its concomitant negative affect

[47]. In both situations, the resultant negative affect or dysphoria can lead to stress and to preoccupation with further drug use [93]. This, in turn, often leads to relapse to drug-seeking and drug-taking behavior. Since the founding of the Alcoholics Anonymous organization in the 1930s and the publication of its so-called Big Book [2], it has been well recognized that relapse is *the* major problem in the successful clinical management of drug addiction. Further, it has been recognized that there are three primary triggers to drug craving and relapse to drug-seeking behavior in recovering drug addicts – re-exposure to drug, exposure to stress, and re-exposure to environmental cues and contexts previously associated with drinking or drugging. An especially pernicious clinical problem is "incubation of craving," in which – counterintuitively – vulnerability to relapse actually increases with the mere passage of time since cessation of drug use and initiation of abstinence [81, 82].

4.3 Animal Models of the Various Stages in the Cycle of Addiction

4.3.1 Preexisting Vulnerability to Addiction

A major preexisting vulnerability to addiction revolves around the concept of "reward deficiency" – decreased ability to derive pleasure and satisfaction from the normal events of daily life [7]. This concept has been amplified (e.g., [9]) and accepted into mainstream theory on the nature and underlying substrates of addiction (e.g., [26, 44, 90]). Importantly, it can be modeled at the preclinical laboratory animal level [29]. Just as excess reward (such as produced by addictive drugs) has been amply and unambiguously tied to excess levels of the neurotransmitter dopamine in the nucleus accumbens (vid., [30, 31, 92, 97]), "reward deficiency" has been tied to deficiencies of nucleus accumbens dopamine [31, 44]. Such deficiencies can be measured. One measurement technique that has been widely used is that of positron emission tomography (PET) scanning [87]. PET is a nuclear medicine imaging technique that detects pairs of gamma rays emitted by a positron-emitting radioligand that has been introduced into the body. Three-dimensional images of ligand concentration within the body are then constructed by computer analysis. Ligands specific for dopamine include [^{11}C]raclopride and [^{18}F]fallypride. Another widely used animal model for assessing nucleus accumbens dopamine levels is in vivo brain microdialysis (vid., [25]). In this procedure, a very small dialysis probe is constructed from stainless steel tubing and microdialysis tubing and then surgically implanted into the desired chemical sampling site in the brain (e.g., nucleus accumbens). Typically, the stainless steel tubing is concentric, with an exceedingly small piece of dialysis tubing connecting the tips of the two concentric stainless steel tubes deep in the brain. Artificial cerebral spinal fluid is perfused through the apparatus – the input tubing connected to a fluid pump and the output tubing connected to a chemical sampling device such as high-pressure liquid chromatography (HPLC). Within the chemical sampling site in the brain, molecules of neurotransmitters (or other chemicals) dialyze across the membrane and are carried to the chemical sampling device. In vivo brain microdialysis is a robust and reliable technique for measuring neurotransmitter levels within a small (1–2 mm) sampling domain within the brain and has proven itself very useful in studying the neurobiology of addiction, craving, and relapse (e.g., [51, 70]). Hypodopaminergic states within the nucleus accumbens have been tied to enhanced vulnerability to self-administer cocaine in laboratory rodents and in nonhuman laboratory primates [14, 60].

Another preexisting condition that confers vulnerability to addiction is impulsivity [71]. Impulsivity confers vulnerability to initial drug use, continued drug use, and relapse to drug use after periods of abstinence. Two types of impulsivity relevant to drug addiction have been identified – impulsive action and impulsive choice. Impulsive action refers to an inability to withhold a prepotent response. Impulsive choice refers to an inability to tolerate delayed rewards. These two types of impulsivity are likely modulated by different neural substrates [16]. Impulsive choice is most commonly measured using a reward delay discounting task in which the animal (or human) subject has a choice between an immediate small reward or a delayed large reward [1]. By altering the size of the reward and/or the delay for the larger reward, "reward delay discount" functions (i.e., the degree to which the test subject devalues a delayed reward) can be computed. Drug-abusing/dependent humans have high discount rates (i.e., they strongly prefer immediate rewards). This has been demonstrated for patients addicted to/dependent upon nicotine, ethanol, opioids, cocaine, and methamphetamine. Prior to becoming addicted to or dependent upon addictive substances, ordinary laboratory rats self-assort themselves into low-impulsive versus high-impulsive animals. For most laboratory rat strains, this self-assortment yields approximately 50% low-impulsive and 50% high-impulsive animals. High-impulsive laboratory rats are *extremely averse* to intermediate-to-long reward delays [33]. In low-impulsive rats, acute cocaine does not alter preexisting impulsivity. In high-impulsive rats, acute or chronic cocaine decreases impulsivity (arguably, a methylphenidate-like effect). In low-impulsive rats, chronic cocaine *dramatically increases* impulsivity [33]. Thus, in low-impulsive animals (less prone to drug-taking because of their preexisting low trait impulsivity), chronic cocaine increases impulsivity and therefore increases the tendency to drug-taking behavior [14]. One may therefore conclude that preexisting levels of trait impulsivity are of relevance to initial tendency to drug-taking behavior and also to the degree to which chronic drug exposure may alter a preexisting tendency to drug-taking behavior [33].

4.3.2 Addictive Drug Self-Administration

If one equates addiction with drug self-administration (an inaccurate homology, as the above-noted mention of "chipping" illustrates), the self-administration paradigm offers the most obvious animal model of addiction. Laboratory animals will self-administer several classes of addictive drugs by a wide variety of routes – oral, intragastric, intraperitoneal, intravenous, or intracranial. This is often done to the point of physiological dependence. Oral self-administration of ethanol and intravenous self-administration of heroin represent obvious analogues of human drug-seeking. In the strongest version of the model, the animal is required to work for access to the drug and not merely to ingest it. This is an instrumental conditioning paradigm, reflecting response learning, inasmuch as the drug is given in a response-contingent manner. In the case where the animal lever-presses for presentation of the drug, the lever-pressing is termed the instrumental response, and ingestion of the drug is termed the consummatory response.

Although the drug self-administration model is most often used with fixed-ratio reinforcement contingencies, an important variant is one in which progressive-ratio reinforcement is used [74]. In progressive-ratio drug self-administration, a progressively increasing workload is imposed upon the animal to receive a drug injection. For example, the workload may increase in a steeply incremental fashion: one lever press required for the first injection, two for the second injection, four for the third, eight for the fourth, and so on. Although typically the workload is not incremented so steeply, in every progressive-ratio drug self-administration session, a point is reached at which the animal's responding falls below some criterion level (often, an abrupt cessation of responding) – the progressive-ratio "break point." This "break point" is taken as a measure of reinforcing efficacy and "reward strength" of the self-administered substance [40]. Alternatively, some experts consider the progressive-ratio break point to reflect the degree of incentive motivation to self-administer drugs. Interestingly, psychostimulants yield different estimates of reward efficacy than do opioids in this animal model. Psychostimulants respond preferentially to incremental increases in response cost immediately following reinforcement, whereas opioids respond preferentially to incremental increases in response cost at the beginning of a discrete trial or daily test session. This has been taken to mean that motivation to self-administer psycho-stimulants versus opiates is qualitatively different [4]. Provocatively, progressive-ratio break point estimates of the rewarding efficacy of different classes of addictive drugs in animals parallel quite closely the verbal rank orderings of appetitiveness for different classes of addictive drugs given by experienced polydrug-abusing humans [28].

4.3.3 Intoxication and the Drug-Induced "High"

A striking feature of drug addiction is how few chemicals are subject to abuse. If all congeners of all chemicals are included, approximately 30,000,000 chemical substances are known [30]. Yet, only approximately 300 (including nicotine, ethanol, psychostimulants, opiates, barbiturates, benzodiazepines, and cannabinoids) are addictive, and this figure is likely an overestimate. Obviously, 300 is a stunningly small subset of 30,000,000. It poses the question: what makes those 300 chemicals addictive while the remaining 30,000,000 are not? There are, after all, few pharmacological similarities among addictive drugs. Some – including barbiturates, ethanol, opioids, and benzodiazepines – are sedatives, while others, including nicotine, cocaine, and the amphetamines, are stimulants. Some – including opiates and cannabinoids – are analgesic, while others, in the proper laboratory or clinical situation, augment pain perception. Some – such as ethanol and opioids – produce physical dependence, while others, such as cocaine, produce little if any physical dependence. However, a few commonalities are apparent and instructive. All addictive drugs are subjectively rewarding, reinforcing, and pleasurable [30]. Laboratory animals volitionally self-administer them [28], just as humans do. Furthermore, the rank order of appetitiveness in animals parallels the rank order of appetitiveness in humans [28, 62]. Most importantly, all addictive drugs (with the exception of the LSD-like and mescaline-like hallucinogens) activate the reward circuitry of the brain [27, 30], thereby producing the subjective "high" that the drug abuser seeks. Furthermore, the

degree of such activation of the brain's reward circuitry correlates well with the degree of the subjective "high."

4.3.3.1 The Brain's Reward Circuitry

The brain's reward circuitry was first discovered by Olds and Milner [63] at McGill University in Montreal. They found that animals would repeatedly return to an area of the laboratory in which they had received mild electrical stimulation of subcortical structures anatomically associated with the medial forebrain bundle. Subsequently, they found that animals would avidly perform tasks (e.g., depressing wall-mounted levers in their test chambers) in order to receive such brain stimulation. James Olds [64, 65] and his wife Marianne Olds [66, 67] subsequently extensively mapped the rodent brain, confirming that a large majority of the brain sites supporting brain stimulation reward are associated with the nuclei of origin, tracts, and terminal loci of the medial forebrain bundle. Other researchers (e.g., [77]) studied electrical brain stimulation reward in nonhuman primates and confirmed that the anatomic brain substrates supporting brain reward are homologous to those in rodents. Using sophisticated electrophysiological techniques, Gallistel et al. [23] determined that the primary neural substrate supporting electrical brain stimulation reward is the moderately fast-conducting, myelinated descending neural fiber system of the medial forebrain bundle. This system originates in the anterior bed nuclei of the medial forebrain bundle (an array of deep subcortical limbic loci anterior to the hypothalamus and preoptic area), descends to the ventral tegmental area of the midbrain via the medial forebrain bundle, and then ascends via the medial forebrain bundle to a select group of forebrain limbic loci including the nucleus accumbens, olfactory tubercle, and frontal cortex. Wise and Bozarth [98] were the first to realize that this assortment of brain loci and tracts constitutes a neural circuit containing three synaptically connected, in-series neuronal elements – a descending link running from the anterior bed nuclei of the medial forebrain bundle to the ventral tegmental area, an ascending link running from the ventral tegmental area to the nucleus accumbens, and a further link running from the nucleus accumbens to the ventral pallidum. The first link is a descending myelinated fiber tract of unknown neurotransmitter type. The second link is an ascending fiber tract from the ventral tegmental area to the nucleus accumbens, with dopamine as its neurotransmitter (see below). The third link is a projection from the nucleus accumbens to the ventral pallidum, using γ-aminobutyric acid (GABA), substance P, and enkephalin as conjoint neurotransmitters. This three-neuron, in-series circuit receives synaptic inputs from, and is functionally modulated by, a wide variety of other neural circuits using a wide variety of neurotransmitters.

Addictive drugs of different classes act on this three-neuron, in-series brain reward neural circuit at different points to activate the circuit and produce the euphoric drug-induced "high."

Importantly, this brain reward circuitry evolved over eons of evolution to subserve biologically essential normal rewarding behaviors such as feeding, drinking, sexual behavior, maternal and paternal behaviors, and social interactions. From an appreciation of the natural and biologically essential nature of these reward circuits comes the notion that addictive drugs "hijack" the brain's reward circuits, activating them more strongly than natural rewards and diverting the drug addict's life to pursuit of drug-induced pleasure at the expense of "getting off" on life's normal pleasures and rewards [34, 76].

4.3.3.2 The Intense Nature of Brain Stimulation Reward

Electrical brain stimulation reward is remarkable for the intensity of the reward and reinforcement produced [30]. When the stimulating electrode is properly on target within the ventral tegmental area, medial forebrain bundle, or nucleus accumbens, laboratory animals will volitionally self-stimulate those areas at maximal rates. They will, tellingly, ignore readily available food, water, toys, and sexually receptive animals of the opposite sex in order to self-deliver the brain stimulation reward. They will also volitionally accept aversive and painful consequences in order to self-deliver the brain stimulation reward (also see below under "Compulsive Use"). In awake humans, such electrical stimulation can evoke intense subjective feelings of pleasure [6, 38, 80], in some instances similar to descriptions of intense medieval religious ecstasies (Ward A. A. Jr., personal communication, 1967). As the most addictive drugs (e.g., cocaine, methamphetamine) evoke comparable levels of subjective reward, it is easy to understand their intensely addictive nature.

4.3.3.3 Dopamine: The Crucial Reward Neurotransmitter

Soon after the discovery of the electrical brain stimulation reward phenomenon (Olds and Milner, 1956) and subsequent mapping of the rodent and nonhuman primate brain for brain reward loci and neuronal tracts (e.g., [23, 65–67, 77]), many attempts were made to determine the neurotransmitter underlying the brain reward phenomenon. The first suggestion that dopamine was the crucial neurotransmitter was made in 1969 by Gardner, who selectively depleted neurotransmitters in the brains of rhesus monkeys working a complex operant task to receive electrical brain stimulation reward and then – crucially – repleted (in sequence) each neurotransmitter believed to have been pharmacologically depleted [24]. Working independently, and using a different research approach, Wise and colleagues in Montreal confirmed this suggestion in a brilliant series of published articles (e.g., [20, 96, 103]). By selective anatomic placement of intracerebral micro-catheters and intracranial micro-electrodes, both the Gardner group and the Wise group suggested that dopamine was the crucial brain reward neurotransmitter activated by addictive drugs, specifically in the "second-stage" ventral tegmental area to nucleus accumbens link in the brain's reward circuitry that had been anatomically identified by Wise and Bozarth [98, 99] and by Gallistel et al. [23]. That dopamine is indeed the crucial "reward" neurotransmitter in the brain has subsequently been confirmed by many investigators in laboratories worldwide and is based on many congruent findings. First, virtually all addictive drugs are functional dopamine agonists – some direct, some indirect, and some even transsynaptic (vid., [27, 30, 102]). With the exception of the LSD- and mescaline-like hallucinogens, functional dopamine agonism is the single pharmacological property that all addictive drugs share. Second, intracerebral microinjections of dopamine agonists produce conditioned place preference [86] and support volitional intracerebral self-administration [102]. Third, dopamine antagonists are negative reinforcers in animals (animals will work to avoid or escape their administration) and produce subjectively aversive effects in humans [30, 62]. Fourth, when dopamine antagonists are administered to animals volitionally self-administering addictive drugs, a compensatory increase in addictive drug intake occurs (to compensate for the decreased rewarding potency of the addictive drug), followed by extinction and cessation of the self-administration behavior (when the dopamine antagonism reaches a sufficient intensity so as to totally block the rewarding properties of the self-administered addictive drug) [62, 103]. Fifth, measures of real-time synaptic neurochemistry in the nucleus accumbens of test animals volitionally engaged in intravenous self-administration of addictive drugs show that following the first volitional self-administration of the test session, extracellular dopamine overflow in the nucleus accumbens displays a tonic increase of approximately 200%; thereafter, extracellular dopamine levels in the nucleus accumbens fluctuate phasically between approximately 200% and 100% over baseline; and the low point of each phasic dip in extracellular nucleus accumbens dopamine accurately predicts the next volitional intake of addictive drug by the test animal [100, 101]. Such data are extremely compelling, as they show that when animals self-administer heroin or cocaine (or other addictive drugs), they do so in order to, in turn, titrate blood lev-

els of addictive drug, brain levels of addictive drug, and – most importantly – nucleus accumbens levels of dopamine.

4.3.4 Moderate Addictive Drug Use Versus Extended Access, Augmented Incentive Motivation for Drug Use, and Enhanced Reward Value of Addictive Drugs

For purposes of economy in the use of animals, time, laboratory personnel, and laboratory budgets, most self-administration studies in laboratory animals have historically been limited to 2 or 3 hours of addictive drug access. This, of course, does not accurately model clinical reality. And, further, it raises the question: is addictive drug self-administration fundamentally different if animals (and, presumably, humans) are allowed extended drug access as opposed to limited drug access? This question has been systemically addressed in a series of elegant published articles by, among others, George Koob and colleagues (e.g., [46]). These researchers – and others – have found that giving laboratory animals extended access to addictive drug self-administration produces radically different behavioral and neurobiological sequelae. For example, Koob and colleagues have reported a series of findings in laboratory rats that are extremely provocative with respect to their analogy, and probably homology, to human opioid addiction [95]. First, under extended access conditions (as compared to limited access conditions), intravenous self-administration was maintained *and escalated* for heroin, oxycodone, and fentanyl, but not for buprenorphine. Rats that were allowed limited drug access showed low and stable lever-pressing for each of the four opioids, but not an escalation in drug intake. Following escalation of drug intake, a classic inverted U-shaped dose-effect function was demonstrated in the heroin, oxycodone, and fentanyl self-administering rats, suggesting that the animals were titrating their doses. These findings indicate that extended access to heroin, oxycodone, and fentanyl – but not buprenorphine – results in escalation of drug self-administration. Could this be an insight into buprenorphine's clinical efficacy but relative lack of addictive liability? This is an interesting question.

Second, extended access to drug self-administration was compared to limited access with respect to effects on self-administration break point under progressive-ratio reinforcement conditions. As noted above, shifts in progressive-ratio break points are believed to represent shifts in reward efficacy or motivational properties of the drug [40, 74]. Wade et al. [95] found increases in progressive-ratio break point (i.e., enhanced reward efficacy) for heroin, oxycodone, and fentanyl – but not for buprenorphine – under extended drug access conditions as compared to limited drug access conditions. Extended access rats showed increased motivation for intermediate doses of heroin, oxycodone, and fentanyl compared with limited access rats. No group differences for buprenorphine were found.

Additionally, it has been known for some time that increasing the dose of opioid, even in limited access conditions, can alter the reinforcing efficacy of the drug [48, 75]. The reason(s) for this may relate to differential binding affinities, efficacy, and opioid subtype preference. Heroin, oxycodone, fentanyl, and buprenorphine have few differences in time to onset when administered intravenously. However, each of these drugs shows differential binding affinities, efficacy, and opioid subtype preference. A comparison of the binding affinity for the mu opioid receptor may be an important factor in the reward value of these opioids. While heroin, oxycodone, and fentanyl have similar binding affinities [21, 94], buprenorphine has a much higher mu opioid receptor binding affinity – suggesting that time to offset from the receptor for buprenorphine may be longer than that for the other opioids [94]. Action at other receptors may also be relevant. Buprenorphine acts as a partial agonist at the mu opioid receptor, the nociceptin receptor (also known as the nociceptin/orphanin FQ receptor), and the kappa opioid receptor but also as an antagonist at the kappa opioid receptor [41]. Nociceptin

receptor activation produces opposite effects on mesolimbic dopamine receptors than does mu opioid receptor activation – by decreasing extracellular nucleus accumbens dopamine levels [54, 59]. Also, activation of kappa receptors directly inhibits dopaminergic neurons [54] – reducing brain reward. Thus, buprenorphine's relative lack of addictive liability may result from multiple actions at multiple brain sites – with the extended access animal drug self-administration model yielding important insights into some of these actions, as well as yielding insights into mechanisms underlying the increased drug reward and increased incentive motivation for drug self-administration observed with chronic opioid use.

4.3.5 Compulsive Drug Use

Loss of control over harmful drug-seeking and drug-taking is one of the most intractable aspects of addiction, as human substance abusers continue to pursue and use addictive drugs despite incurring massively negative consequences to themselves, their families, their jobs, and their health [3]. Many have made the cogent argument that drug-seeking and drug-taking do not adequately define addiction (see comments above relating to "chipping"). Therefore, considerable attention has been paid to developing animal models that incorporate harmful consequences to the animal either concomitant with or consequent to drug-seeking and drug-taking (e.g., [5, 15, 69, 88]).

Although there are many variants of this general approach, one will be sufficiently illustrative [15]. Deroche-Gamonet and colleagues measured persistence of responding for drug when drug delivery was associated with punishment. During these sessions with laboratory rats, nose-pokes under fixed-ratio 5 reinforcement (one drug infusion for every fifth nose-poke) resulted in delivery of both the drug and an electrical foot shock. The shock punishment was signaled by a new cue light that illuminated at the time of the first nose-poke and turned off after the delivery of the shock.

They then went on to analyze the relationship between drug-seeking in the face of harmful consequences and propensity to relapse to drug-seeking behavior. To study propensity to relapse, they used an animal relapse model ([73, 89]; see also discussion below) in which drug-seeking behavior is triggered – after a drug withdrawal period – by re-exposure to drug or re-exposure to conditioned cues (light, sound) previously associated with drug-taking. A 5-day and 30-day period of withdrawal following 3 months of drug self-administration were both studied. Responding during the relapse test was taken to measure vulnerability to relapse.

In the first experiment, rats were assigned to two groups on the basis of their relapse behavior. The high-relapse-prone animals differed profoundly from the low-relapse-prone animals. High-relapse-prone animals progressively increased their drug-seeking behavior during no-drug periods and also after punishment. They also had higher break points for drug self-administration under progressive-ratio reinforcement (i.e., displayed higher incentive motivation to self-administer; found the addictive drug to be more rewarding). Correlation analyses revealed that each addiction-like behavior (persistence of drug-seeking, resistance to punishment, motivation for drug) strongly predicted propensity to relapse.

In a second experiment, these researchers assessed whether addiction-like behaviors were also related to propensity to relapse after a longer period of withdrawal (30 days). Again, high propensity to relapse was positively correlated with persistence of drug-seeking, resistance to punishment, and motivation for drug.

These experiments show that after prolonged drug self-administration, addiction-like behaviors are found in rats. Importantly, addiction-like behaviors are not present after a short period of drug self-administration, but develop, as does addiction in humans, only after prolonged exposure to the drug. Furthermore, as do human addicts, rats showing an addiction-like behavior have a high propensity to relapse even after a long period of withdrawal. Finally, these findings indicate that the three addiction-like behaviors are measures of a single factor that reflects compulsive drug use.

4.3.6   The "Opponent Process" Trap

As noted, electrical brain stimulation reward is a powerful preclinical technique for measuring the reward value of addictive drugs (vid., [30]). In 1981, Gardner and colleagues decided to examine whether there were differences in morphine-enhanced brain reward depending upon the exact anatomic placement of the stimulating electrode in the ascending dopaminergic tract running from the ventral mesencephalon to the neostriatal forebrain [61]. These researchers found that when the brain stimulation reward electrode was in the medial portion of the tract, a single injection of morphine produced an *enhancement of brain reward* which waned as the morphine metabolized and dissipated during the hours following the injection. On subsequent days, the same pattern held, but *the degree of brain reward enhancement underwent tolerance (decreased) with each subsequent day*. When the brain stimulation reward electrode was in the lateral portion of the tract, a single injection of morphine produced *inhibition of brain reward* which waned as the morphine metabolized and dissipated during the hours following the injection. On subsequent days, *the degree of brain reward inhibition grew progressively on each subsequent day*. Further experiments, using in vivo voltammetry microelectrodes [25] to measure dopamine levels in different anatomic domains of the neostriatum revealed a similar picture [8]. Thus, the initial drug-enhanced reward dissipates, while the initial drug-induced inhibition of brain reward grows progressively stronger. It will be readily appreciated that this places the drug user in a nasty "trap" – the drug-induced euphoria undergoes tolerance, while the drug-induced dysphoria progressively grows. The opioid addict eventually comes to use opioids not to "get high," but rather to "get straight" (i.e., to try to push his/her diminished brain reward and, hence, subjective dysphoria back toward something approximating normal affect).

4.3.7 Drug Withdrawal and Negative Affect: Additional Drivers of Relapse to Drug-Seeking and Drug-Taking

George Koob, the director of the US National Institute on Alcohol Abuse and Alcoholism and one of the most creative and original thinkers in the field of addiction medicine, has pointed out that the negative affect and dysphoria produced by drug withdrawal are powerful drivers of relapse to drug-seeking and drug-taking behaviors [46–48]. As noted above, in addiction, healthful rewards lose their former motivational power. In a person with addiction, the reward and motivational systems become reoriented through conditioning to focus on the stronger release of dopamine produced by the drug and its cues. This is the concept behind the notion that addictive drugs "hijack" the normal reward mechanisms and processes of the brain.

For many years, it was believed that over time, persons with addiction would become more sensitive to the rewarding effects of drugs and that this increased sensitivity would be reflected in higher levels of dopamine in the circuits of their brains that process reward (including the nucleus accumbens and the dorsal striatum). However, we now know that this is incorrect. As noted above, in the presence of addiction, addictive drug consumption triggers *smaller* increases in dopamine levels [90, 91, 104]. This diminished dopamine release renders the brain's reward system much less sensitive to stimulation by both drug-related and non-drug-related rewards. Consequently, persons with addiction no longer experience the same degree of euphoria from a drug as they did when they first started using it. Thus, persons with addiction often become less motivated by everyday stimuli (e.g., relationships and activities) that they had previously found to be motivating and rewarding. It must be understood that these changes become deeply ingrained neurobiologically and cannot be quickly reversed through simple termination of drug use (e.g., detoxification). In fact, simple termination of drug use is so contraindicated by the underlying neurobiology of withdrawal and withdrawal-induced dysphoria that short-term detoxification programs can be considered to constitute medical malpractice. In addition to decreased nucleus accumbens dopamine tone, withdrawal actually recruits enhanced reactivity to stress and emergence of negative emotions – resulting in what has been termed a rebound "anti-reward" state [47]. This is different from the "opponent process trap" described above, in that the anti-reward state of Koob and Le Moal is a rebound phenomenon while the "opponent process trap" is the summation of opponent processes occurring simultaneously in anatomically different regions of the brain's reward circuitry. In Koob and Le Moal's "anti-reward" process, there is intense motivation to escape the discomfort associated with addictive drug withdrawal. As a result, the patient with addiction transitions from taking drugs simply to feel pleasure (to "get high") to taking them to obtain transient relief from dysphoria. In addition, stress responses in the brain are recruited [44, 45, 50, 85].

Persons with addiction frequently cannot understand why they continue to take the drug when it no longer yields pleasure. Many state that they continue to take the drug to escape the distress they feel when they are not intoxicated. Unfortunately, although the short-acting effects of increased dopamine levels triggered by drug administration temporarily relieve this distress, the result of repeated bingeing is to deepen the dysphoria during withdrawal, thus producing a vicious cycle.

4.3.8 Animal Models of Relapse

Relapse to drug-seeking and drug-taking is common and so pathognomonic of addiction that it is often used as a diagnostic criterion [3, 42]. As a result, many animal models of relapse have been developed and have added greatly to our knowledge of addiction and its underlying neurobiology (e.g., [12, 13, 73]). Fundamentally, animal models of relapse fall into two categories – those in which abstinence is achieved by experimenter-imposed behavioral extinction of the drug-taking habit and those in which drug relapse is assessed after either forced or voluntary abstinence. Arguably, it is the latter set of animal models that most closely resemble the human situation, as human abstinence is typically either forced (e.g., by incarceration or inpatient treatment in hospital or clinic settings) or voluntary due to either the negative consequences of chronic drug use or the availability of strong nondrug rewards in the drug user's environment [17, 43, 55].

4.3.8.1 Extinction-Based Relapse Models

There are two fundamental variants of this model – relapse based on extinction of an operant response (e.g., lever-pressing, nose-poking, running from a start box to a goal box) for drug self-administration and relapse based on extinction of a Pavlovian association of addictive drug intake and drug-receipt-associated unique environmental cues and/or contexts (e.g., conditioned place preference). Thus, the fundamental distinction is between models based on Skinner's [83] or Thorndike's [39] work and models based on Pavlov's work [57].

Relapse Based on Operant Response Extinction

In the operant self-administration variant of the model, laboratory animals are trained to self-administer a drug by emitting an operant response (e.g., lever-pressing, nose-poking, running from a start box to a goal box) to receive drug. During the extinction phase, the operant response is extinguished by omitting the drug reward. During the reinstatement (relapse) test, the ability of various acute stimuli (or "triggers") to reinstate the previous drug-seeking behavior is measured under extinction conditions. The amount of previous operant responding (now nonreinforced) is the operational measure of drug-seeking behavior [19, 56, 84]. The three classical relapse triggers in this model are the same as observed in human relapse – re-exposure to drug, stress, or re-exposure to conditioned cues or contexts previously associated with drug intake [2].

Relapse Based on Pavlovian Response Extinction

In the conditioned place preference variant of the model, laboratory animals are placed in an experimental device with two environmental cue-distinct chambers and allowed to freely explore. The distinct cues that identify the chambers are typically visual, tactile, and/or olfactory. The cues are arranged such that they are initially motivationally neutral (i.e., the animal prefers neither chamber over the other). A barrier is then placed between the two cue-distinct chambers. By placing the animal alternatively in one chamber and the other (usually a 3-hour exposure, with daily alternation between chambers), the animals are trained to associate one distinct set of environmental cues/contexts with drug injections and the second compartment with injections of vehicle. If the drug is appetitive, the animals develop a very distinct preference for the drug-associated chamber. Subsequently, rats are subjected to extinction training during which they are exposed – alternatingly – to both contexts in the absence of drug. Reinstatement of the preference for the drug-paired compartment is then determined after noncontingent exposure to such relapse "triggers" as re-exposure to drug or exposure to stress [58, 79].

4.3.8.2 Abstinence-Based Relapse Models

Forced Abstinence by Removal from the Drug-Taking Environment

This is essentially a withdrawal-based model analogous (perhaps even homologous) to human incarceration or placement in a secure hospital or treatment center. A typical forced abstinence study includes three phases: training, forced withdrawal from drug, and testing. During the training phase, laboratory animals are allowed to self-administer a drug by emitting standard operant responses (e.g., lever-pressing, nose-poking). This is typically paired with presentation of discrete environmental cue(s). During the withdrawal phase, the animals are housed in the animal facility for different periods of abstinence. During the test phase, the animals are returned to the drug self-administration environment/context, and the previous drug-yielding operant responses result in contingent presentation of the discrete cue(s) previously paired with drug infusions but not the drug itself [22, 72]. Nonreinforced lever-pressing in this single extinction session is the operational measure of "relapse to drug-seeking" and the main dependent measure.

Incubation of Craving

An exceptionally important variant of this model is the so-called "incubation of craving" model. In this model – otherwise identical to the "forced abstinence by removal from the drug-taking environment" model noted immediately above – groups of animals are subjected to different lengths of drug withdrawal before being tested for relapse [37]. Somewhat counterintuitively, it was found that (within limits) longer periods of drug withdrawal produced more intense relapse [37]. However, astute clinicians pointed out that this "counterintuitive" finding actually comported with clinical reality – Gawin and Kleber [35] having reported that cue-induced cocaine craving in human patients progressively increases over the first weeks of abstinence and remains high for a remarkably extended period. This "incubation of craving" model has been used extensively over the past 15 years in a large number of studies relating to the underlying neurobiology of drug reward, drug addiction, craving, and relapse.

Voluntary Abstinence Induced by Adverse Consequences of Drug Use

This, of course, comports nicely with observed clinical reality. In the preclinical model, laboratory animals are trained to self-administer a drug (usually paired with a discrete environmental cue). Then, drug-taking behavior is suppressed by aversive foot shock – either after the animal performs the operant response [68] or by introducing an electrical barrier in front of the drug-associated lever such as to deter the animal from making the operant response in the first place [10]. During the test phase, relapse to drug-seeking is precipitated by exposure to drug-priming injections or environmental cues. These models have recently been used to exceptional effect in identifying specific brain loci underlying relapse to drug-seeking behavior in the face of adverse consequences (e.g., [52, 53]).

4.4 Conclusion

Drug addiction at the human level is a biopsychosocial-spiritual disorder and is well-accepted in the field of addiction medicine. To a considerable extent, the psychological, social, and spiritual dimensions of this disorder can be studied – and even experimentally probed – at the human level. However, probing and manipulating the biological aspects of addiction are problematic, as they would – perforce – require probing and manipulating the living human brain. For this reason, animal models of addiction have been developed (and continue to be). The use of these models has yielded important insights into the biological aspects of addiction; has proven useful in identifying and testing potential anti-addiction, anti-craving, and anti-relapse medications that may prove useful at the human level; and has shed useful knowledge to inform the current debate on the possible medical utility of cannabis [28, 32].

References

1. Ainslie G. Specious reward: a behavioral theory of impulsiveness and impulse control. Psychol Bull. 1975;82(4):463–96.
2. Alcoholics Anonymous. Alcoholics anonymous big book. 1st ed. New York: Alcoholics Anonymous World Services; 1939.
3. American Psychiatric Association. Diagnostic and statistical manual of mental disorders, DSM-5. 5th ed. Washington, DC: American Psychiatric Association Publishing; 2013.
4. Arnold JM, Roberts DCS. A critique of fixed and progressive ratio schedules used to examine the neural substrates of drug reinforcement. Pharmacol Biochem Behav. 1997;57(3):441–7.
5. Belin D, Mar AC, Dalley JW, Robbins TW, Everitt BJ. High impulsivity predicts the switch to compulsive cocaine-taking. Science. 2008;320(5881):1352–5.
6. Bishop MP, Elder ST, Heath RG. Intracranial self-stimulation in man. Science. 1963;140(3565):394–6.
7. Blum K, Cull JG, Braverman ER, Comings DE. Reward deficiency syndrome. Am Sci. 1996;84:132–45.
8. Broderick PA, Gardner EL, van Praag HM. In vivo electrochemical and behavioral evidence for specific neural substrates modulated differentially by enkephalin in rat stimulant stereotypy and locomotion. Biol Psychiatry. 1984;19(1):45–54.

9. Comings DE, Blum K. Reward deficiency syndrome: genetic aspects of behavioral disorders. Prog Brain Res. 2000;126:325–41.

10. Cooper A, Barnea-Ygael N, Levy D, Shaham Y, Zangen A. A conflict rat model of cue-induced relapse to cocaine seeking. Psychopharmacology. 2007;194(1):117–25.

11. Courtney KE, Polich J. Binge drinking in young adults: data, definitions, and determinants. Psychol Bull. 2009;135(1):142–56.

12. Crombag HS, Bossert JM, Koya E, Shaham Y. Context-induced relapse to drug-seeking: a review. Phil Trans R Soc B. 2008;363(1507):3233–43.

13. Cruz FC, Babin KR, Leao RM, Goldart EM, Bossert JM, Shaham Y, Hope BT. Role of nucleus accumbens shell neuronal ensembles in context-induced reinstatement of cocaine-seeking. J Neurosci. 2014;34(22):7437–46.

14. Dalley JW, Fryer TD, Brichard L, Robinson ES, Theobold DE, Lääne K, Peña Y, Murphy ER, Shah Y, Probst K, Abakumova I, Aigbirhio FI, Richards HK, Hong Y, Baron JC, Everitt BJ, Robbins TW. Nucleus accumbens D2/D3 receptors predict trait impulsivity and cocaine reinforcement. Science. 2007;315(5816):1267–70.

15. Deroche-Gamonet V, Belin D, Piazza PV. Evidence for addiction-like behavior in the rat. Science. 2004;305(5686):1014–7.

16. Eagle DM, Baunez C. Is there an inhibitory-response-control system in the rat? Evidence from anatomical and pharmacological studies of behavioral inhibition. Neurosci Biobehav Rev. 2010;34(1):50–72.

17. Epstein DH, Preston KL. The reinstatement model and relapse prevention: a clinical perspective. Psychopharmacology. 2003;168(1–2):31–41.

18. Epstein DH, Preston KL, Stewart J, Shaham Y. Toward a model of drug relapse: an assessment of the validity of the reinstatement procedure. Psychopharmacology. 2006;189(1):1–16.

19. Ettenberg A. Haloperidol prevents the reinstatement of amphetamine-rewarded runway responding in rats. Pharmacol Biochem Behav. 1990;36(3):635–8.

20. Fouriezos G, Hansson P, Wise RA. Neuroleptic-induced attenuation of brain stimulation reward in rats. J Comp Physiol Psychol. 1978;92(4):661–71.

21. Frances B, Gout R, Monsarrat B, Cros J, Zajac JM. Further evidence that morphine-6 beta-glucuronide is a more potent opioid agonist than morphine. J Pharmacol Exp Ther. 1992;262(1):25–31.

22. Fuchs RA, Feltenstein MW, See RE. The role of the basolateral amygdala in stimulus-reward memory and extinction memory consolidation and in subsequent conditioned cued reinstatement of cocaine seeking. Eur J Neurosci. 2006;23(10):2809–13.

23. Gallistel CR, Shizgal P, Yeomans JS. A portrait of the substrate for self-stimulation. Psychol Rev. 1981;88(3):228–73.

24. Gardner EL. Pharmacological aspects of intracranial self-stimulation in rhesus monkeys. Paper presented at Winter Conference on Brain Research, Aspen, Colorado, January 1969. 1969.

25. Gardner EL, Chen J, Paredes W. Overview of chemical sampling techniques. J Neurosci Meth. 1993;48(3):173–97.

26. Gardner EL. Neurobiology and genetics of addiction: implications of "reward deficiency syndrome" for therapeutic strategies in chemical dependency. In: Elster J, editor. Addiction: entries and exits. New York: Russell Sage Foundation; 1999. p. 57–119.

27. Gardner EL, David J. The neurobiology of chemical addiction. In: Elster J, Skog OJ, editors. Getting hooked. rationality and the addictions. Cambridge: Cambridge University Press; 1999. p. 93–136.

28. Gardner EL. What we have learned about addiction from animal models of drug self-administration. Am J Addict. 2000;9(4):285–313.

29. Gardner EL. Reward behaviors as a function of hypodopaminergic activity: animal models of reward deficiency syndrome. Mol Psychiatry. 2001;6(Suppl 1):S4.

30. Gardner EL. Brain-reward mechanisms. In: Lowinson JH, Ruiz P, Millman RB, Langrod JG, editors. Substance abuse: a comprehensive textbook. 4th ed. Philadelphia: Lippincott Williams and Wilkins; 2005. p. 48–97.

31. Gardner EL. Addiction and brain reward and anti-reward pathways. Adv Psychosom Med. 2011;30:22–60.

32. Gardner EL. Cannabinoids and addiction. In: Pertwee RG, editor. Handbook of cannabis. Oxford: Oxford University Press; 2014. p. 173–88.

33. Gardner EL, Xi Z-X, Srivastava R. Laboratory rodent studies of cocaine's effects on impulsive choice: implications for the aetiology of psychostimulant drug abuse. Drug Alcohol Rev. 2018;37(Suppl 3):S32.

34. Garavan H, Pankiewicz J, Bloom A, Cho JK, Sperry L, Ross TJ, Salmeron BJ, Risinger R, Kelley D, Stein EA. Cue-induced cocaine craving: neuroanatomical specificity for drug users and drug stimuli. Am J Psychiatry. 2000;157(11):1789–98.

35. Gawin F, Kleber H. Pharmacologic treatments of cocaine abuse. Psychiatr Clin North Am. 1986;9(3):573–83.

36. Goldsmith RJ, Ries RK, Yuodelis-Flores C. Substance-induced mental disorders. In: Reis RK, Fiellin DA, Miller SA, Saitz R, editors. Principles of addiction medicine. 4th ed. Philadelphia: Lippincott Williams and Wilkins; 2009. p. 1139–50.

37. Grimm JW, Hope BT, Wise RA, Shaham Y. Incubation of cocaine craving after withdrawal. Nature. 2001;412(6843):141–2.

38. Heath RG. Electrical self-stimulation of the brain in man. Am J Psychiatry. 1963;120:571–7.

39. Herrnstein RJ. On the law of effect. J Exp Anal Behav. 1970;13(2):243–66.

40. Hodos W. Progressive ratio as a measure of reward strength. Science. 1961;134(3483):943–4.

41. Huang P, Kehner GB, Cowan A, Liu-Chen LY. Comparison of pharmacological activities of buprenorphine and norbuprenorphine: norbuprenorphine is a potent opioid agonist. J Pharmacol Exp Ther. 2001;297(2):688–95.

42. Hunt WA, Barnett LW, Branch LG. Relapse rates in addiction programs. J Clin Psychol. 1971;27(4):455–6.

43. Katz JL, Higgins ST. The validity of the reinstatement model of craving and relapse to drug use. Psychopharmacology. 2003;168(1–2):21–30.

44. Koob GF. Addiction is a reward deficit and stress surfeit disorder. Front Psychiatry. 2013;4:72. https://doi.org/10.3389/fpsyt.2013.00072. eCollection 2013.

45. Koob GF, Buck CL, Cohen A, Edwards S, Park PE, Schlosburg JE, Schmeichel B, Vendruscolo LF, Wade CL, Whitfield TW Jr, George O. Addiction as a stress surfeit disorder. Neuropharmacology. 2014;76(Pt B):370–82.

46. Koob GF, Ahmed SH, Boutrel B, Chen SA, Kenny PJ, Markou A, O'Dell LE, Parsons LH, Sanna PP. Neurobiological mechanisms in the transition from drug use to drug dependence. Neurosci Biobehav Rev. 2004;27(8):739–49.

47. Koob GF, Le Moal M. Plasticity of reward neurocircuitry and the "dark side" of drug addiction. Nat Neurosci. 2005;8(11):1442–4.

48. Koob GF, Le Moal M. Neurobiology of addiction. London: Academic Press; 2006.

49. Koob GF, Volkow ND. Neurobiology of addiction: a neurocircuitry analysis. Lancet Psychiatry. 2016;3(8):760–73.

50. Koob GF, Schulkin J. Addiction and stress: an allostatic view. Neurosci Biobehav Rev. 2019;106:245–62. https://doi.org/10.1016/j.neubiorev.2018.09.008.

51. Li X, Peng X-Q, Jordan CJ, Li J, Bi G-H, He Y, Yang H-J, Zhang H-Y, Gardner EL, Xi Z-X. mGluR5 antagonism inhibits cocaine reinforcement and relapse by elevation of extracellular glutamate in the nucleus accumbens via a CB1 receptor mechanism. Sci Rep. 2018;8(1):3686. https://doi.org/10.1038/s41598-018-22087-1.

52. Marchant NJ, Kaganovsky K. Effect of systemic and accumbens shell injections of the D1-family receptor antagonist on renewal of alcohol seeking after punishment-imposed abstinence. Behav Neurosci. 2015;129(3):281–91.

53. Marchant NJ, Rabei R, Kaganovsky K, Caprioli D, Bossert JM, Bonci A, Shaham Y. A critical role of lateral hypothalamus in context-induced relapse to alcohol seeking after punishment-imposed abstinence. J Neurosci. 2014;34(22):7447–57.

54. Margolis EB, Hjelmstad GO, Bonci A, Fields HL. Kappa opioid agonists directly inhibit midbrain dopaminergic neurons. J Neurosci. 2003;23(31):9981–6.

55. Marlatt AG. Models of relapse and relapse prevention: a commentary. Exp Clin Psychopharmacol. 1996;4(1):55–60.

56. McFarland K, Ettenberg A. Reinstatement of drug-seeking behavior produced by heroin-predictive environmental stimuli. Psychopharmacology. 1997;131(1):86–92.

57. McSweeney FK, Murphy ES. The Wiley Blackwell handbook of operant and classical conditioning. Malden: John Wiley & Sons; 2014.

58. Mueller D, Stewart J. Cocaine-induced conditioned place preference: reinstatement by priming injections of cocaine after extinction. Behav Brain Res. 2000;115:39–47.

59. Murphy NP, Ly HT, Maidment NT. Intracerebroventricular orphanin FQ/nociceptin suppresses dopamine release in the nucleus accumbens of anaesthetized rats. Neuroscience. 1996;75(1):1–4.

60. Nader MA, Morgan D, Gage HD, Nader SH, Calhoun TL, Buchheimer N, Ehrenkaufer R, Mach RH. PET imaging of dopamine D2 receptors during chronic cocaine self-administration in monkeys. Nat Neurosci. 2006;9(8):1050–6.

61. Nazzaro JM, Seeger TF, Gardner EL. Morphine differentially affects ventral tegmental and substantia nigra brain reward thresholds. Pharmacol Biochem Behav. 1981;14(3):325–31.

62. O'Brien C, Gardner EL. Critical assessment of how to study addiction and its treatment: human and non-human animal models. Pharmacol Ther. 2005;108(1):18–58.

63. Olds J, Milner P. Positive reinforcement produced by electrical stimulation of septal area and other regions of rat brain. J Comp Physiol Psychol. 1954;47(6):419–27.

64. Olds J. Pleasure centers in the brain. Sci Am. 1956;95:105–16.

65. Olds J. Hypothalamic substrates of reward. Physiol Rev. 1962;42:554–604.

66. Olds ME, Olds J. Approach-avoidance analysis of rat diencephalon. J Comp Neurol. 1963;120:259–95.

67. Olds ME, Olds J. Drives, rewards and the brain. In: Newcomb TM, editor. New directions in psychology. New York: Holt, Rinehart & Winston; 1965. p. 329–410.

68. Panlilio LV, Thorndike EB, Schindler CW. Reinstatement of punishment suppressed opioid self-administration in rats: an alternative model of relapse to drug abuse. Psychopharmacology. 2003;168(1–2):229–35.

69. Pelloux Y, Everitt BJ, Dickinson A. Compulsive drug seeking by rats under punishment: effects of drug taking history. Psychopharmacology. 2007;194(1):127–37.

70. Peng X-Q, Xi Z-X, Li X, Spiller K, Li J, Chun L, Wu K-M, Froimowitz M, Gardner EL. Is slow-onset long-acting monoamine transport blockade to cocaine as methadone is to heroin? Implication for anti-addiction medications. Neuropsychopharmacology. 2010;35(13):2564–78.

71. Perry JL, Carroll ME. The role of impulsive behavior in drug abuse. Psychopharmacology. 2008;200(1):1–26.

72. Reichel CM, Bevins RA. Forced abstinence model of relapse to study pharmacological treatments of substance use disorder. Curr Drug Abuse Rev. 2009;2(2):184–94.

73. Reiner DJ, Frederiksson I, Lofaro OM, Bossert JM, Shaham Y. Relapse to opioid seeking in rat models: behavior, pharmacology and circuits. Neuropsychopharmacology. 2018;44(3):465–77.

74. Richardson NR, Roberts DCS. Progressive ratio schedules in drug self-administration studies in rats: a method to evaluate reinforcing efficacy. J Neurosci Meth. 1996;66(1):1–11.

75. Roberts DCS, Loh EA, Vickers G. Self-administration of cocaine on a progressive ratio schedule in rats: dose-response relationship and effect of haloperidol pretreatment. Psychopharmacology. 1989;97(4):535–8.

76. Robbins TW, Everitt BJ. Drug addiction: bad habits add up. Nature. 1999;398(6728):567–70.

77. Routtenberg A, Gardner EL, Huang YH. Self-stimulation pathways in the monkey, *Macaca mulatta*. Exp Neurol. 1971;33(1):213–24.

78. Saitz R. Medical and surgical complications of addiction. In: Reis RK, Fiellin DA, Miller SA, Saitz R, editors. Principles of addiction medicine. 4th ed. Philadelphia: Lippincott Williams and Wilkins; 2009. p. 945–67.

79. Sanchez CJ, Sorg BA. Conditioned fear stimuli reinstate cocaine-induced conditioned place preference. Brain Res. 2001;908(1):86–92.

80. Sem-Jacobsen W, Torkildsen A. Depth recording and electrical stimulation in the human brain. In: Ramey ER, O'Doherty DS, editors. Electrical studies on the unanesthetized brain. New York: Harper (Hoeber Medical Division); 1960. p. 280–8.

81. Shaham Y, Shalev U, Lu L, de Wit H, Stewart J. The reinstatement model of drug relapse: history, methodology and major findings. Psychopharmacology. 2003;168(1–2):3–20.

82. Shalev U, Grimm JW, Shaham Y. Neurobiology of relapse to heroin and cocaine seeking: a review. Pharmacol Rev. 2002;54(1):1–42.

83. Skinner BF. The behavior of organisms: an experimental analysis. Cambridge, MA: B.F. Skinner Foundation; 1938.

84. Stewart J, de Wit H. Reinstatement of drug-taking behavior as a method of assessing incentive motivational properties of drugs. In: Bozarth MA, editor. Methods of assessing the reinforcing properties of abused drugs. New York: Springer-Verlag; 1987.

85. Tunstall BJ, Carmack SA, Koob GF, Vendruscolo LF. Dysregulation of brain stress systems mediates compulsive alcohol drinking. Curr Opin Behav Sci. 2017;13:85–90.

86. Tzschentke TM. Measuring reward with the conditioned place preference (CPP) paradigm: update of the last decade. Addict Biol. 2007;12(3–4):227–462.

87. Valk PE, Bailey DL, Townsend DW, Maisey MN, editors. Positron emission tomography: basic science and clinical practice. London: Springer-Verlag London Ltd.; 2003.

88. Vanderschuren LJ, Everitt BJ. Drug seeking becomes compulsive after prolonged cocaine self-administration. Science. 2004;305(5686):1017–9.

89. Venniro M, Caprioli D, Shaham Y. Animal models of drug relapse and craving: from drug priming-induced reinstatement to incubation of craving after voluntary abstinence. Prog Brain Res. 2016;224:25–52.

90. Volkow ND, Wang G-J, Fowler JS, Logan J, Gatley SJ, Hitzemann R, Chen AD, Dewey SL, Pappas N. Decreased striatal dopaminergic responsiveness in detoxified cocaine-dependent subjects. Nature. 1997;386(6627):830–3.

91. Volkow ND, Tomasi D, Wang GJ, Logan J, Alexoff DL, Jayne M, Fowler JS, Wong C, Yin P, Du C. Stimulant-induced dopamine increases are markedly blunted in active cocaine abusers. Mol Psychiatry. 2014;19(9):1037–43.

92. Volkow ND, Morales M. The brain on drugs: from reward to addiction. Cell. 2015;162(4):712–25.

93. Volkow ND, Koob GF, McLellan AT. Neurobiologic advances from the brain disease model of addiction. N Engl J Med. 2016;374(4):363–71.

94. Volpe DA, Tobin GAM, Mellon RD, Katki AG, Parker RJ, Colatsky T, Kropp TJ, Verbois SL. Uniform assessment and ranking of opioid mu receptor binding constants for selected opioid drugs. Regul Toxicol Pharmacol. 2011;59(3):385–90.

95. Wade CL, Vendruscolo LF, Schlosburg JE, Hernandez DO, Koob GF. Compulsive-like responding for opioid analgesics in rats with extended access. Neuropsychopharmacology. 2015;40(2):421–8.

96. Wise RA. Catecholamine theories of reward: a critical review. Brain Res. 1978;152(2):215–47.

97. Wise RA. The brain and reward. In: Liebman JM, Cooper SJ, editors. The neuropharmacological basis of reward. Oxford: Oxford University Press; 1989. p. 377–424.

98. Wise RA, Bozarth MA. Brain reward circuitry: four circuit elements "wired" in apparent series. Brain Res Bull. 1984;12(2):203–8.

99. Wise RA, Bozarth MA. Brain mechanisms of drug reward and euphoria. Psychiatr Med. 1985;3(4):445–60.

100. Wise RA, Leone P, Rivest R, Leeb K. Elevations of nucleus accumbens dopamine and DOPAC levels during intravenous heroin self-administration. Synapse. 1995a;21(2):140–8.

101. Wise RA, Newton P, Leeb K, Burnette B, Pocock D, Justice JB Jr. Fluctuations in nucleus accumbens dopamine concentration during intravenous cocaine self-administration in rats. Psychopharmacology. 1995b;120(1):10–20.

102. Wise RA, Gardner EL. Functional anatomy of substance-related disorders. In: D'Haenen H, den Boer JA, Willner P, editors. Biological psychiatry. New York: Wiley; 2002. p. 509–22.

103. Yokel RA, Wise RA. Increased lever pressing for amphetamine after pimozide in rats: implications for a dopamine theory of reward. Science. 1975;187(4176):547–9.

104. Zhang Y, Schlussman SD, Rabkin J, Butelman ER, Ho A, Kreek MJ. Chronic escalating cocaine exposure, abstinence/withdrawal, and chronic re-exposure: effects on striatal dopamine and opioid systems in C57BL/6J mice. Neuropharmacology. 2013;67:259–66.

Burden of Disease: The Epidemiological Aspects of Addiction

5

J. Rehm, C. Probst, L. Llamosas Falcón, and K. D. Shield

Contents

Abstract

This chapter describes epidemiological aspects of substance use disorders. It begins with a narrative review of the transition from substance use to a substance use disorder. A methodological introduction into global burden of disease estimates for substance use disorders follows, and finally, this chapter reports on regional differences on burden of disease.

J. Rehm (✉)
Centre for Addiction and Mental Health (CAMH), Toronto, ON, Canada

Dalla Lana School of Public Health, University of Toronto, Toronto, ON, Canada

Institute of Medical Science, University of Toronto, Toronto, ON, Canada

Department of Psychiatry, University of Toronto, Toronto, ON, Canada

Institute of Clinical Psychology and Psychotherapy, Technische Universität Dresden, Dresden, Germany

Department of International Health Projects, Institute for Leadership and Health Management, I.M. Sechenov First Moscow State Medical University, Moscow, Russian Federation

C. Probst
Centre for Addiction and Mental Health (CAMH), Toronto, ON, Canada

L. L. Falcón
Centre for Addiction and Mental Health (CAMH), Toronto, ON, Canada

Preventive Medicine and Public Health, Hospital Universitario 12 de Octubre, Madrid, Spain

K. D. Shield
Centre for Addiction and Mental Health (CAMH), Toronto, ON, Canada

Dalla Lana School of Public Health, University of Toronto, Toronto, ON, Canada

© Springer Nature Switzerland AG 2021
N. el-Guebaly et al. (eds.), *Textbook of Addiction Treatment*,
https://doi.org/10.1007/978-3-030-36391-8_5

The investigation of what influences the course of substance use from initiation to the development of a substance use disorder reveals a multiplicity of factors. The overall picture suggests that extra-individual, social factors such as the cultural background, or peer behavior, predominantly influence use initiation and the transition to hazardous patterns of use, whereas intraindividual factors such as personality traits and genes are more prominent in the development and potential chronification of substance use disorders.

1.4% and 0.9% of the global population were affected by alcohol use and by drug use disorders, respectively, according to estimates from the Global Burden of Disease (GBD) study, which only includes the more severe cases. For all substances, prevalence is higher in men than in women. These disorders cause substantial burden of disease: alcohol use disorders account for 0.7% of the global burden of disease, while drug use disorders account for 1.1%. While tobacco use disorders are defined in psychiatric classification systems, their prevalence and associated burden are not estimated by the GBD.

The burden of disease attributable to different substance use disorders varies strongly across countries and regions. Burden due to alcohol use disorders is highest in upper-middle-income countries, while burden due to drug use disorders is highest in high-income countries.

Keywords

Substance use disorders · Epidemiology Global burden of disease · Regional differences · Life course · Comorbidity

Addictions (substance use disorders), as currently defined in major classification systems, are highly prevalent and account for a considerable degree of the global burden of disease. This burden is typically defined as a summary health indicator, measured in disability-adjusted life years (DALYs) lost [45], which is composed of years of life lost due to premature mortality plus years of life lost to disability [18]. However, the burden of disease is not homogenous across substances, countries, and time. Furthermore, the transition from substance use to a substance use disorder is dependent on numerous factors. Accordingly, this chapter outlines these factors and describes the burden caused by substance use disorders as obtained from the [20].

5.1 The Transition into a Substance Use Disorder

There is a history of use initiation, and often an observable pattern of hazardous use, which precedes substance addiction. Generally, these observable trajectories can be approached from either a drug-centered or an individual-centered perspective [37]; we will focus on the main individual-centered aspects and will not deal with the differences between specific substances.

The initiation of substance use depends largely on social and environmental factors, such as the cultural context, advertising, or peer influence [19]. Worldwide per capita consumption and rates of abstention differ greatly between countries [14, 41, 49, 69]. For instance, lower abstention rates for alcohol consumption are observed in high-income countries, and higher abstention rates are observed in North African, Eastern Mediterranean, and South Asian countries [81, 82]; higher abstention rates are often associated with religion and with low economic wealth [41, 53, 68]. Substance use is often initiated in adolescence, but there are some economic, cultural, and substance-specific variations [13]; for instance, in India and in Thailand, the age of initiation has long been in or around the twenties [24, 46]. However, with economic and cultural changes, the age of initiation is dropping in some traditionally "dry" cultures. For example, in some states of India, the age of initiation has dropped by 5 years or more in recent years [26, 50].

Across substances and cultures, women are less likely to initiate substance use [12, 13]. Substance availability [39, 52, 67] and advertising [10, 25, 70] have been shown to influence the age of initiation. Beyond these influential cultural factors, the initiation of use is influenced by the individual's social network and immediate environment. Several studies have shown that social motives, peer or familial substance use, and normative beliefs of close peers influence the initiation of substance use across different substances [6, 17, 34, 48].

While most users maintain a low-risk pattern of use, some individuals will develop hazardous patterns of substance use [15, 73]. In particular, early onset of substance use has been shown to increase the risk of later hazardous substance use across substances [1, 2, 51, 55]. With respect to alcohol, research indicates that repeated intoxication at a young age is especially associated with later-in-life hazardous patterns of alcohol consumption [5, 36]. A review identifying the characteristics of people with hazardous alcohol consumption patterns in Europe [35] observed that hazardous drinking patterns were more prevalent in males, adolescents, and young adults. Furthermore, the review identified other social and environmental factors, such as the predominant drinking culture, peer influences [7, 42], parental monitoring [9], and concurrent use of other substances. Finally, the motivation for alcohol consumption seems to evolve from social motives and curiosity (predominantly controlled use) to hazardous consumption patterns motivated by self-enhancement and coping [32, 33].

The factors which influence the transition from hazardous use patterns to substance use disorders are less evident. Impulsivity-related personality traits, such as sensation seeking or the desire to be uninhibited, influence the transition from controlled use to hazardous use and from hazardous use to the development of a substance use disorder [31, 65, 71]. Intraindividual vulnerabilities, such as genetic factors [27, 37] and comorbid psychiatric or mental disorders [73], can be identified as characteristics of individuals who transition from substance use to a substance use disorder. In particular, high rates of incident substance use disorders have been observed, particularly for people with prior mood, anxiety, and personality disorders [72].

Almost three decades ago, Khantzian [30] developed the "self-medication hypothesis" in order to explain the development of addictive disorders where there was a prior background of mental illness or pain; this hypothesis is still discussed (e.g., [38]). Stress and stressful and traumatic life events are also important contributors to the development of substance use disorders [40]. Adolescents and young adults show an elevated prevalence of substance use disorders in several countries, with higher rates in males [29, 43, 44]. There are regions of the world, however, where middle-aged men (as opposed to adolescents and young adults) have the highest prevalence of substance use disorders (e.g., some countries in the European Union [59] and in Russia [47].

In summary, the onset of substance use is largely influenced by cultural factors and often begins at a young age. It may be assumed that hazardous use precedes the transition to a substance use disorder, but scientific evidence is limited in this regard. The majority of studies do not investigate the respective transitions separately, and longitudinal study designs risk missing the phase of hazardous use due to long study intervals. Furthermore, a large number of risk factors influence the transitions to hazardous use and then to substance use disorders. Environmental and social factors appear to be more important in the transition to hazardous consumption, whereas genetic risk factors and individual vulnerabilities appear to be more important in the transition from hazardous consumption to a substance use disorder [16, 28, 75]. Social factors also play a role in the transition from hazardous consumption to a substance use disorder. For example, during the Vietnam War, many American soldiers became dependent on heroin. After returning to the United States, the majority of these heroin addictions ceased [62, 63], but in the minority of cases where the addiction persisted, family history and genetically driven vulnerabilities are now considered to have played a major role. The risk factors and their differential influence on initiation and the hazardous progression of substance use are summarized in Fig. 5.1.

Fig. 5.1 Heuristic model of risk factors for the initiation of substance use, the transition to hazardous patterns of use, and then the transition to a substance use disorder

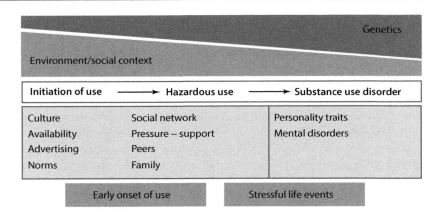

5.2 The Global Burden of Disease Associated with Substance Use Disorders

5.2.1 Methodology and Limitations of the Burden of Disease Estimations

To understand the burden of disease estimates and their potential limitations, it is necessary to understand how they are estimated. The definition of "substance use disorders" used in the GBD study [18] includes "substance dependence" as defined in the International Classification of Diseases Version 10 (ICD-10) [80] and "severe substance use disorders" as defined in the Diagnostic and Statistical Manual of Mental Disorders, Fifth Edition (DSM-5) [4] . Thus, the GBD studies do not include the burden of disease caused by "harmful use" as defined by the ICD-10 or "abuse" as defined in the DSM-IV [3]. As a result, the main burden reported in the GBD studies stems from alcohol dependence. In addition to dependence, the GBD category of alcohol use disorders includes alcohol poisonings and fetal alcohol spectrum disorder (FASD); however, the burden due to FASD is negligible in GBD study calculations.

The exclusion of "harmful use" or "abuse" (or the restriction to severe dependence) leads to an underestimation of the burden of substance use disorders, and the exclusion of these disorders impacts the relative burden of disease caused by

alcohol versus drug use disorders; for alcohol, contrary to drug use disorders, a large part of the disease burden is actually due to harmful use/abuse. While disability outcomes stemming from the abuse/harmful use of alcohol are lower than disability outcomes resulting from dependence [66], the rates of the former outcomes are not zero [22]. Further, the prevalence of harmful use/abuse globally is almost as high as the prevalence of dependence globally [82] and is markedly higher in some countries (such as the United States [22] and in regions such as Africa [82].

Thus, when comparing current estimates of the burden of disease attributable to alcohol use disorders to estimates from previous GBD studies [57, 58], where harmful use/abuse of alcohol was not excluded, or to estimates for the same year published in the World Health Organization's (WHO) Global Status Report on Alcohol and Health [82], we can conclude that the current GBD study substantially underestimates the global burden of alcohol use disorders.

On the other hand, for drug use disorders, other than cannabis use disorders, the difference between the burden of drug use disorders as a disease condition and as a risk factor is not nearly as large as it is for alcohol use disorders (see Table 5.1); 66% of the burden from illegal drugs as a risk factor for drug use disorders stems from drug dependence (compared to 16% for alcohol).

Tobacco use disorders are a late addition to the category of substance use disorders. Only 50 years ago the WHO still clearly separated the

Table 5.1 Burden of disease associated with substance use disorders and with substance consumption as a risk factor (GBD 2017)

Cause	DALYs lost (1000s)						Percentage (%) change (1990 to 2017)
	1990	95% CI	2010	95% CI	2017	95% CI	
Use disorders							
Tobacco							
Alcohol	11,588	(9305–14,376)	16,663	(13,470–20,561)	17,463	(14,084–21,627)	51.0
Drug	15,937	(12,268–19,835)	22,716	(17,521–28,355)	27,187	(21,120–33,583)	70.6
Opioid	11,609	(8590–14,841)	17,535	(13,230–22,288)	21,485	(16,256–27,143)	85.1
Cocaine	587	(411–804)	871	(649–1142)	992	(747–1291)	69.0
Amphetamine	1073	(633–1600)	1145	(723–1695)	1184	(757–1744)	10.3
Cannabis	400	(252–601)	501	(318–737)	518	(329–766)	29.5
Other drugs	2266	(1797–2887)	2663	(2223–3208)	3008	(2553–3537)	32.7
Risk factor							
Tobacco	198,928	(184,735–215,168)	202,534	(190,633–214,512)	213,385	(201,156–226,659)	7.3
Alcohol	74,493	(65,887–84,150)	105,425	(94,784–117,365)	107,971	(96,195–120,117)	44.9
Drug	22,984	(19,048–27,276)	36,358	(30,828–42,153)	41,658	(35,318–48,195)	81.2
All DALYs lost	2,562,010	(2,417,539-2,722,707)	2,543,062	(2,346,588–2,763,048)	2,499,292	(2,285,525–2,737,391)	−2.4

Source: Global Burden of Disease Collaborative Network [20]
CI Confidence Interval

legal, "habit-forming" drugs of alcohol and tobacco from the "addictive illegal drugs" [79]. It is now accepted that both alcohol and tobacco are addictive substances, as evidenced for tobacco by all the current classifications: in the ICD-10 as "Mental and behavioral disorders due to use of tobacco" [80], in the ICD-11 as "Disorders due to use of nicotine" [83], and in the DSM-5 as "Tobacco Use Disorders" [4].

However, in the case of tobacco, the psychiatric classification of tobacco use disorders has never entered mainstream epidemiology and burden of disease research. Thus, "tobacco use disorders" was not a disease category in the latest GBD study report [20], nor for other burden of disease calculations (e.g., [78]). While part of the burden of tobacco as a risk factor shown in Table 5.1 is due to tobacco use disorders, the exact proportion is unclear, but it is likely higher

than for either illegal drugs or alcohol (see also Table 5.1).

Another important aspect of the interpretation of the GBD study numbers concerns the underlying epidemiology. The methodology underlying the estimates of the prevalence of drug use disorders has been described in detail by Degenhardt and Hall [14]. With respect to alcohol use disorders, prevalence was based exclusively on a systematic review of high-quality general population surveys which measured alcohol dependence using standardized measures such as the Composite International Diagnostic Interview (CIDI; first version [64]; several versions are currently in use, most importantly the CIDI of the World Mental Health Survey [84], the Schedules for Clinical Assessment in Neuropsychiatry (SCAN; [77]), or the Alcohol Use Disorder and Associated Disabilities Interview Schedule

(AUDADIS) [23]. Studies in several countries under the aegis of the WHO have claimed that for alcohol dependence, as well as for illegal drug dependence, standardized instruments yield similar diagnoses; however, for the prevalence of "harmful use" and "abuse" and subsequently for alcohol use disorders within the DSM-5, marked differences in diagnoses have been reported [11, 54, 74].

Even when standardized instruments are used, prevalence may differ. For example, in the early years of the abovementioned CIDI being used for the World Mental Health Surveys, dependence-item questions were asked only if the respondent had at least one abuse symptom, thereby leading to a large underestimation of dependence prevalence [21]. Similarly, small changes in wording of these items seem to have been responsible for substantial changes in Dutch prevalence figures over the past decade (see [56] for comparisons and further considerations).

Finally, while the burden of substance use disorders is high (Table 5.1), the specific GBD framework hides the fact that the majority of the burden from substance use occurs in people with substance use disorders [60, 61]. For example, on average, individuals with alcohol use disorders in treatment in Nordic countries lost on average 24–28 years of their life [76]; however, alcohol use disorders or alcohol poisoning were not listed as underlying causes of death on death certificates, and thus, in burden of disease studies, these deaths were attributed to comorbidities such as injuries and other chronic diseases [8]. This approach provides similar results for other substance use disorders, and therefore, the overall impact of substance use disorders on global health tends to be underestimated.

5.2.2 Global Burden of Substance Use Disorders and Regional Differences

According to the GBD study in 2017, more than 107 million people in 2017 were classified as having an alcohol use disorder (107.4 million; 95% confidence interval (CI): 95.9–119.7 million); all prevalence data were obtained from [20]; about 75.1 million of these people were men (95% CI: 67.3–83.3 million), and 32.3 million were women (95% CI: 28.3–36.5 million). These numbers correspond to 1.4% of the world's population in that year (95% CI: 1.2%–1.6%), 2.0% of all men (95% CI: 1.8%–2.2%), and 0.8% of all women (95% CI: 0.7%–0.9%). All percentages and rates are age-standardized to be comparable across countries, regions, and time. For drug use disorders, the following prevalence estimates were provided: 71.2 million people (95% CI: 64.0–79.8 million), approximately 47 million men (47.4 million; 95% CI: 42.4–53.1 million), and 24 million women (23.8 million; 95% CI: 21.4–26.9 million). Thus, 0.9% of the world's population in that year suffered from a drug use disorder (95% CI: 0.8%–1.1%), 1.3% of all men (95% CI: 1.1%–1.4%), and 0.6% of all women (95% CI: 0.6%–0.7%).

In the 2017 GBD study, alcohol use disorders resulted in 17,463,000 DALYs lost, accounting for 0.7% of the global burden of disease (see Table 5.1). In addition to the global burden of disease from alcohol use disorders, there is a larger burden of disease from illegal drug use disorders (27,187,000 DALYs lost, accounting for 1.1% of the global burden of disease). Temporal trends from 1990 to 2017 indicate an increasing age-standardized burden of alcohol use disorders (an increase of 51.0%) and drug use disorders (an increase of 70.6%). The increase in the age-standardized burden of drug use disorders was greatest for opioids (85.1%), followed by cocaine (69.0%), other drugs (32.7%), cannabis (29.5%), and amphetamines (10.3%) (Table 5.2).

Globally, the burden of disease due to alcohol use disorders and drug use disorders varied greatly by geography. In 2017, alcohol use disorders were highest in Eastern Europe and in tropical Latin America, with 1016 (95% CI: 875–1201) and 424 (95% CI: 341–522) DALYs lost per 100,000 people, respectively (see Fig. 5.2). The lowest burden of alcohol use disorders was experienced in North Africa and the Middle East, with 74 (95% CI: 54–97) DALYs lost in 2017; clearly, religious beliefs (Islam is the main religion in most countries of this region) played an important role. The country that experienced the greatest burden of alcohol use disorders in 2017 was Belarus, with 1153 (95% CI: 959–1384) DALYs lost per 100,000 people. By comparison, the

Table 5.2 Age-standardized burden of disease associated with substance use disorders and with substance consumption as a risk factor (GBD 2017)

	Age-standardized DALYs lost per 100,000						
Cause	1990	95% CI	2010	95% CI	2017	95% CI	Percentage (%) change (1990 to 2017)
Use disorders							
Tobacco							
Alcohol	232	(187–285)	229	(186–282)	216	(174–268)	−6.6
Drug	296	(228–366)	310	(240–387)	343	(266–424)	15.9
Opioid	217	(161–277)	240	(181–305)	270	(204–342)	24.8
Cocaine	11	(8–15)	12	(9–16)	12	(9–16)	13.2
Amphetamine	19	(11–27)	15	(10–23)	15	(10–23)	−17.7
Cannabis	7	(4–11)	7	(4–10)	7	(4–10)	−5.8
Other drugs	43	(34–54)	37	(31–44)	38	(32–45)	−11
Risk factor							
Tobacco	4502	(4218–4803)	2996	(2821–3172)	2646	(2493–2811)	−41.2
Alcohol	1574	(1383–1785)	1482	(1330–1653)	1329	(1185–1482)	−15.6
Drug	441	(368–519)	501	(425–579)	521	(441–604)	18
All DALYs lost	48,595	(45,720–51,787)	37,379	(34,572–40,490)	32,797	(30,042–35,849)	−32.5

Source: Global Burden of Disease Collaborative Network [20]
CI Confidence Interval

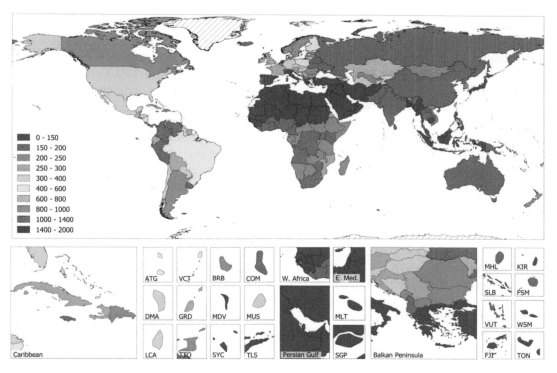

Fig. 5.2 Burden of disease in 2017 per 100,000 people resulting from alcohol use disorders (age-standardized, both sexes combined). (Source: https://vizhub.healthdata.org/gbd-compare/)

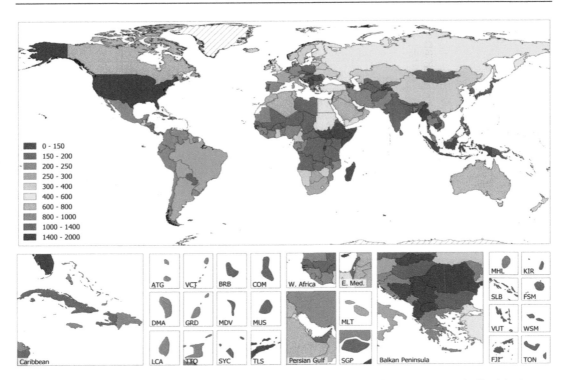

Fig. 5.3 Burden of disease in 2017 per 100,000 people resulting from drug use disorders (age-standardized, both sexes combined). (Source: https://vizhub.healthdata.org/gbd-compare/)

global burden of alcohol use disorders in 2017 was 216 (95% CI: 174–268) DALYs lost per 100,000 people.

In 2017, drug use disorders were highest in high-income North America, North Africa and the Middle East, and Australasia, with 1602 (95% CI: 1367–1843), 701 (95% CI: 514–902), and 566 (95% CI: 452–686) DALYs lost per 100,000 people, respectively (see Fig. 5.3). The largest country-level burden of drug use disorders was observed in the United States and the United Arab Emirates, with 1696 (95% CI: 1451–1947) and 1338 (95% CI: 1000–1706) DALYs lost per 100,000 people, respectively.

With respect to the burden of different categories of drug use disorders, opioid use disorders were highest in high-income North America, with 1155 (95% CI: 982–1340) DALYs lost per 100,000 people; cocaine use disorders were also highest in the same region, with 120 (95% CI: 93–154) DALYs lost per 100,000 people. Further, amphetamine use disorders were highest in Australasia, with 91 (95% CI: 60–131) DALYs lost per 100,000 people, and cannabis use disor-

ders were highest in high-income North America, with 24 (95% CI: 15–36) DALYs lost per 100,000 people. For comparison, the global burden of drug use disorders in 2017 was 343 (95% CI: 266–424) DALYs lost per 100,000 people: opioid use disorders were responsible for 270 (95% CI: 204–342) DALYs lost per 100,000 people, cocaine use disorders were responsible for 12 (95% CI: 9–16) DALYs lost per 100,000 people, amphetamine use disorders were responsible for 15 (95% CI: 10–23) DALYs lost per 100,000 people, cannabis use disorders were responsible for 7 (95% CI: 4–10) DALYs lost per 100,000 people, and other drug use disorders were responsible for 38 (95% CI: 32–45) DALYs lost per 100,000 people.

The age-standardized burden of alcohol use disorders was greatest in upper-middle-income countries (285 DALYs lost per 100,000 people), followed by high-income countries (272 DALYs lost per 100,000 people), lower-middle-income countries (181.7 DALYs lost per 100,000 people), and low-income countries (150.4 DALYs lost per 100,000 people) (see Table 5.3). The burden caused by drug use disorders in 2017 was

Table 5.3 Age-standardized burden of disease associated with substance use disorders and with substance consumption as a risk factor by World Bank region (GBD 2017)

Cause	Age-standardized DALYs lost per 100,000							
	Low-income countries	95% CI	Lower-middle-income countries	95% CI	Upper-middle-income countries	95% CI	High-income countries	95% CI
Use disorders								
Tobacco								
Alcohol	150	(112–198)	182	(145–225)	285	(230–351)	271.8	(224–331)
Drug	187	(138–244)	219	(163–282)	400	(298–504)	709.2	(596–823)
Opioid	162	(116–216)	185	(134–243)	326	(236–418)	500.0	(416–582)
Cocaine	2	(1–4)	2	(2–3)	12	(9–16)	50.2	(38–65)
Amphetamine	5	(3–7)	8	(5–13)	20	(12–31)	30.5	(21–42)
Cannabis	5	(3–7)	5	(3–8)	6	(4–9)	13.3	(8–20)
Other drugs	14	(11–19)	18	(15–23)	37	(29–45)	115.2	(99–133)
Risk factor								
Tobacco	1198	(1065–1345)	2294	(2128–2469)	3514	(3328–3720)	3370	(3130–3622)
Alcohol	1007	(847–1195)	1259	(1111–1417)	1730	(1491–1969)	1342	(1124–1599)
Drug	267	(214–326)	381	(319–451)	640	(532–748)	921	(801–1039)

Source: Global Burden of Disease Collaborative Network [20]
CI Confidence Interval

greatest in high-income countries (709 DALYs lost per 100,000 people), followed by upper-middle-income countries (400 DALYs lost per 100,000 people), lower-middle-income countries (219 DALYs lost per 100,000 people), and low-income countries (187 DALYS lost per 100,000 people). Thus, the burdens of disease for opioid, cocaine, amphetamine, cannabis, and other drug use disorders were all highest in high-income countries and lowest in low-income countries.

Examining the burden by risk factor, the tobacco- and alcohol-attributable burdens were highest in upper-middle-income countries (3514 and 1730 DALYs lost per 100,000 people, respectively) and lowest in low-income countries (1198 and 1007 DALYs lost per 100,000 people, respectively). The drug-attributable burden was highest in high-income countries (921 DALYs lost per 100,000 people) and lowest in low-income countries (267 DALYs lost per 100,000 people).

Appendix

Table 5.4 Definitions of scientific terms

Term	Definition
2017 global burden of Disease study	The largest systematic effort to describe the global distribution and causes of a wide array of major diseases, injuries, and health risk factors, with yearly updates
Age-standardized	Rates that have been adjusted to minimize the differences in age composition of populations (used when comparing rates from different populations)
Confidence interval	A range of values where there is a given probability (in this case, 95%) that the true value (in this case, disability-adjusted life years) is contained within this range of values
Delta	The percentage change in the value of a measure between two conditions (in this case, time)
Disability-adjusted life years	A measure of population health loss or burden of disease that takes into account years of life lost due to premature mortality and years of life lost due to disability

Table 5.4 (continued)

Term	Definition
Burden of disease	A measure of health loss from diseases, conditions, and injuries as measured by disability-adjusted life years
Incidence	The number of new cases of a disease, condition, or injury during a given period of time for a specified population
Mortality	Death
Prevalence	The number of people with a given disease, condition, or injury at any point during a given period of time (e.g., annual, lifetime, period, or point)
Systematic review	The application of search and evaluation strategies that limit bias in the assembly, critical appraisal, and synthesis of studies that are relevant to a topic
Years of life lost due to premature mortality	A measure of health loss due to premature mortality, which is calculated as an estimate of the number of years people would have lived if they had not died prematurely
Years of life lost due to disability	A measure of health loss due to disability, which was calculated in the 2010 Global Burden of Disease study as the point prevalence of a disease, condition, or injury multiplied by a corresponding disability weight (a measure of health loss caused by a disease condition compared to total health loss (i.e., death))

References

1. Adam A, Faouzi M, Gaume J, Gmel G, Daeppen JB, Bertholet N. Age of first alcohol intoxication: association with risky drinking and other substance use at the age of 20. Swiss Med Wkly. 2011;141:w13226.
2. Addolorato G, Vassallo GA, Antonelli G, Antonelli M, Tarli C, Mirijello A, Agyei-Nkansah A, Mentella MC, Ferrarese D, Mora V, Barbara M, Maida M, Camma C, Gasbarrini A, Alcohol Related Disease C. Binge drinking among adolescents is related to the development of alcohol use disorders: results from a cross-sectional study. Sci Rep. 2018;8:12624.
3. American Psychiatric Association. Diagnostic and statistical manual of mental disorders, 4th edition, primary care. Washington, DC: American Psychiatric Association; 2000.

4. American Psychiatric Association. Diagnostic and statistical manual of mental disorders: DSM-5. Arlington: American Psychiatric Association; 2013.
5. Asbridge M, Cartwright J, Wilson K, Langille D. Age at first drink, experiences of drunkenness, and alcohol-related problems in Canadian youth: is early onset bad if you are a moderate drinker? J Stud Alcohol Drugs. 2016;77:974–9.
6. Blanco EA, Duque LM, Rachamallu V, Yuen E, Kane JM, Gallego JA. Predictors of aggression in 3.322 patients with affective disorders and schizophrenia spectrum disorders evaluated in an emergency department setting. Schizophr Res. 2018;195: 136–41.
7. Borsari B, Carey KB. Peer influences on college drinking: a review of the research. J Subst Abus. 2001;13:391–424.
8. Charlson FJ, Baxter AJ, Dua T, Degenhardt L, Whiteford HA, Vos T. Excess mortality from mental, neurological, and substance use disorders in the global burden of disease study 2010. In: Patel V, Chisholm D, Dua T, Laxminarayan R, Medina-Mora ME, editors. Mental, neurological, and substance use disorders: disease control priorities, third edition (volume 4). Washington, DC: The International Bank for Reconstruction and Development/The World Bank; 2016.
9. Danielsson AK, Romelsjo A, Tengstrom A. Heavy episodic drinking in early adolescence: gender-specific risk and protective factors. Subst Use Misuse. 2011;46:633–43.
10. Davis JP, Pedersen ER, Tucker JS, Dunbar MS, Seelam R, Shih R, D'amico EJ. Long-term associations between substance use-Related media exposure, descriptive norms, and Alcohol use from adolescence to young adulthood. J Youth Adolesc. 2019;48:1311–26.
11. Degenhardt L, Bharat C, Bruno R, Glantz MD, Sampson NA, Lago L, Aguilar-Gaxiola S, Alonso J, Andrade LH, Bunting B, Caldas-de-Almeida JM, Cia AH, Gureje O, Karam EG, Khalaf M, McGrath JJ, Moskalewicz J, Lee S, Mneimneh Z, Navarro-Mateu F, Sasu CC, Scott K, Torres Y, Poznyak V, Chatterji S, Kessler RC, WHO World Mental Health Survey Collaborators. Concordance between the diagnostic guidelines for alcohol and cannabis use disorders in the draft ICD-11 and other classification systems: analysis of data from the WHO's World Mental Health Surveys. Addiction. 2019a;114:534–52.
12. Degenhardt L, Bharat C, Glantz MD, Sampson NA, Scott K, Lim CCW, Aguilar-Gaxiola S, Al-Hamzawi A, Alonso J, Andrade LH, Bromet EJ, Bruffaerts R, Bunting B, de Girolamo G, Gureje O, Haro JM, Harris MG, He Y, de Jonge P, Karam EG, Karam GE, Kiejna A, Lee S, Lepine JP, Levinson D, Makanjuola V, Medina-Mora ME, Mneimneh Z, Navarro-Mateu F, Posada-Villa J, Stein DJ, Tachimori H, Torres Y, Zarkov Z, Chatterji S, Kessler RC, WHO World Mental Health Survey Collaborators. The epidemiology of drug use disorders cross-nationally: findings from the WHO's World Mental Health Surveys. Int J Drug Policy. 2019b;71:103–12.
13. Degenhardt L, Chiu WT, Sampson N, Kessler RC, Anthony JC, Angermeyer M, Bruffaerts R, de Girolamo G, Gureje O, Huang Y, Karam A, Kostyuchenko S, Lepine JP, Mora MEM, Neumark Y, Ormel JH, Pinto-Meza A, Posada-Villa J, Stein DJ, Takeshima T, Wells JE. Toward a global view of alcohol, tobacco, cannabis, and cocaine use: findings from the who world mental health surveys. PLoS Med. 2008;5:1053–67.
14. Degenhardt L, Hall W. Extent of illicit drug use and dependence, and their contribution to the global burden of disease. Lancet. 2012;379:55–70.
15. Florez-Salamanca L, Secades-Villa R, Hasin DS, Cottler L, Wang S, Grant BF, Blanco C. Probability and predictors of transition from abuse to dependence on alcohol, cannabis, and cocaine: results from the National Epidemiologic Survey on Alcohol and Related Conditions. Am J Drug Alcohol Abuse. 2013;39:168–79.
16. Fowler T, Lifford K, Shelton K, Rice F, Thaper A, Neale MC, Mcbride A, van Den Bree MB. Exploring the relationship between genetic and environmental influences on initiation and progression of substance use. Addiction. 2007;102:413–22.
17. Galea S, Nandi A, Vlahov D. The social epidemiology of substance use. Epidemiol Rev. 2004;26:36–52.
18. GBD 2017 DALYs and HALE Collaborators. Global, regional, and national disability-adjusted life-years (DALYs) for 359 diseases and injuries and healthy life expectancy (HALE) for 195 countries and territories, 1990-2017: a systematic analysis for the Global Burden of Disease Study 2017. Lancet. 2018;392:1859–922.
19. Gell L, Bühringer G, Mcleod J, Forberger S, Holmes J, Lingford-Hughes A, Meier PS. What determines harm from addictive substances and behaviours? New York: Oxford University Press; 2016.
20. Global Burden of Disease Collaborative Network. Global Burden of Disease Study 2017 (GBD 2017) Results. [Online]. Seattle: Institute for Health Metrics and Evaluation. 2019. Available: http://ghdx.health-data.org/gbd-results-tool. Accessed 14 July 2019.
21. Grant BF, Compton WM, Crowley TJ, Hasin DS, Helzer JE, Li TK, Rounsaville BJ, Volkow ND, Woody GE. Errors in assessing DSM-IV substance use disorders. Arch Gen Psychiatry. 2007;64:379–80.
22. Grant BF, Goldstein RB, Saha TD, Chou SP, Jung J, Zhang H, Pickering RP, Ruan WJ, Smith SM, Huang B, Hasin DS. Epidemiology of DSM-5 alcohol use disorder: results from the national epidemiologic survey on alcohol and related conditions III. JAMA Psychiat. 2015;72:757–66.
23. Grant BF, Harford TC, Dawson DA, Chou PS, Pickering R. The ALCOHOL Use Disorder and Associated Disabilities Interview Schedule (AUDADIS): reliability of alcohol and drug modules in a general population sample. Drug Alcohol Depend. 1995;39:37–44.

24. Gururaj G, Pratima M, Girish N, Benegal V. Alcohol related harm: implications for public health and policy in India. Bangalore: National Institute of Mental Health and Neurosciences; 2011.

25. Hanewinkel R, Isensee B, Sargent JD, Morgenstern M. Cigarette advertising and teen smoking initiation. Pediatrics. 2011;127:E271–8.

26. Jaisoorya TS, Beena KV, Beena M, Ellangovan K, Jose DC, Thennarasu K, Benegal V. Prevalence and correlates of alcohol use among adolescents attending school in Kerala, India. Drug Alcohol Rev. 2016;35:523–9.

27. Kendler KS, Myers J, Prescott CA. Specificity of genetic and environmental risk factors for symptoms of cannabis, cocaine, alcohol, caffeine, and nicotine dependence. Arch Gen Psychiatry. 2007;64:1313–20.

28. Kendler KS, Prescott CA. Genes, environment, and psychopathology: understanding the causes of psychiatric and substance use disorders. Guilford Press. New York; 2006.

29. Khan SS, Secades-Villa R, Okuda M, Wang SC, Perez-Fuentes G, Kerridge BT, Blanco C. Gender differences in cannabis use disorders: results from the national epidemiologic survey of alcohol and related conditions. Drug Alcohol Depend. 2013;130:101–8.

30. Khantzian EJ. The self-medication hypothesis of addictive disorders: focus on heroin and cocaine dependence. Am J Psychiatry. 1985;142:1259–64.

31. Kotov R, Gamez W, Schmidt F, Watson D. Linking "big" personality traits to anxiety, depressive, and substance use disorders: a meta-analysis. Psychol Bull. 2010;136:768–821.

32. Kuntsche E, Gabhainn SN, Roberts C, Windlin B, Vieno A, Bendtsen P, Hublet A, Tynjala J, Valimaa R, Dankulincova Z, Aasvee K, Demetrovics Z, Farkas J, van Der Sluijs W, de Matos MG, Mazur J, Wicki M. Drinking motives and links to alcohol use in 13 European countries. J Stud Alcohol Drugs. 2014;75:428–37.

33. Kuntsche E, Knibbe R, Gmel G, Engels R. Why do young people drink? A review of drinking motives. Clin Psychol Rev. 2005;25:841–61.

34. Kuntsche E, Mueller S. Why do young people start drinking? Motives for first-time alcohol consumption and links to risky drinking in early adolescence. Eur Addict Res. 2012;18:34–9.

35. Kuntsche E, Rehm J, Gmel G. Characteristics of binge drinkers in Europe. Soc Sci Med. 2004;59:113–27.

36. Kuntsche E, Rossow E, Simons-Morton B, Ter Bogt T, Kokkevi A, Godeau E. Not early drinking but early drunkenness is a risk factor for problem behaviors among adolescents from 38 European and north American countries. Alcohol Clin Exp Res. 2013;37:308–14.

37. Le Moal M, Koob GF. Drug addiction: pathways to the disease and pathophysiological perspectives. Eur Neuropsychopharmacol. 2007;17:377–93.

38. Lembke A. Time to abandon the self-medication hypothesis in patients with psychiatric disorders. Am J Drug Alcohol Abuse. 2012;38:524–9.

39. Lipperman-Kreda S, Grube JW, Friend KB. Local tobacco policy and tobacco outlet density: associations with youth smoking. J Adolesc Health. 2012;50:547–52.

40. Logrip ML, Zorilla EP, Koob GF. Stress modulation of drug self-administration: implications for addiction comorbidity with post-traumatic stress disorder. Neuropharmacology. 2012;62:552–64.

41. Manthey J, Shield KD, Rylett M, Hasan OSM, Probst C, Rehm J. Global alcohol exposure between 1990 and 2017 and forecasts until 2030: a modelling study. Lancet. 2019;393:2493–502.

42. Mason WA, Toumbourou JW, Herrenkohl TI, Hemphill SA, Catalano RF, Patton GC. Early age alcohol use and later alcohol problems in adolescents: individual and peer mediators in a bi-national study. Psychol Addict Behav. 2011;25:625–33.

43. Mchugh RK, Votaw VR, Sugarman DE, Greenfield SF. Sex and gender differences in substance use disorders. Clin Psychol Rev. 2018;66:12–23.

44. Merikangas KR, Mcclair VL. Epidemiology of substance use disorders. Hum Genet. 2012;131:779–89.

45. Murray CJL. Rethinking DALYs. In: Murray CJL, Lopez A, editors. The global burden of disease: a comprehensive assessment of mortality and disability from diseases, injuries, and risk factors in 1990 and projected to 2020. Boston: Harvard School of Public Health; 1996.

46. National Statistics Office. Tobacco and alcohol consumption behaviors among Thai people in year 2004: Bangkok; National Statistical Office. 2005.

47. Neufeld M, Rehm J. Alcohol consumption and mortality in Russia since 2000 – are there any changes following the alcohol policy changes starting in 2006. Alcohol Alcohol. 2013;48:222–30.

48. Olds RS, Thombs DL, Tomasek JR. Relations between normative beliefs and initiation intentions toward cigarette, alcohol and marijuana. J Adolesc Health. 2005;37:75.

49. Peacock A, Leung J, Larney S, Colledge S, Hickman M, Rehm J, Giovino GA, West R, Hall W, Griffiths P, Ali R, Gowing L, Marsden J, Ferrari AJ, Grebely J, Farrell M, Degenhardt L. Global statistics on alcohol, tobacco and illicit drug use: 2017 status report. Addiction. 2018;113:1905–26.

50. Pillai A, Nayak MB, Greenfield TK, Bond JC, Hasin DS, Patel V. Adolescent drinking onset and its adult consequences among men: a population based study from India. J Epidemiol Community Health. 2014;68:922–7.

51. Pitkanen T, Lyyra AL, Pulkkinen L. Age of onset of drinking and the use of alcohol in adulthood: a follow-up study from age 8-42 for females and males. Addiction. 2005;100:652–61.

52. Popova S, Giesbrecht N, Bekmuradov D, Patra J. Hours and days of sale and density of alcohol outlets: impacts on alcohol consumption and damage: a systematic review. Alcohol Alcohol. 2009;44:500–16.

53. Probst C, Manthey J, Rehm J. Understanding the prevalence of lifetime abstinence from alcohol: an ecological study. Drug Alcohol Depend. 2017;178:126–9.
54. Pull CB, Saunders JB, Mavreas V, Cottler LB, Grant BF. Concordance between ICD-10 alcohol and drug use disorder criteria and diagnoses as measured by the AUDADIS-ADR, CIDI and SCAN: results of a cross-national study. Drug Alcohol Depend. 1997;47:207–16.
55. Qadeer RA, Georgiades K, Boyle MH, Ferro MA. An epidemiological study of substance use disorders among emerging and young adults. Can J Psychiatr. 2019;64:313–22.
56. Rehm J, Anderson P, Barry J, Dimitrov P, Elekes Z, Feijao F, Frick U, Gual A, Gmel G Jr, Kraus L, Marmet S, Raninen J, Rehm MX, Scafato E, Shield KD, Trapencieris M, Gmel G. Prevalence of and potential influencing factors for alcohol dependence in Europe. Eur Addict Res. 2015;21:6–18.
57. Rehm J, Mathers C, Popova S, Thavorncharoensap M, Teerawattananon Y, Patra J. Global burden of disease and injury and economic cost attributable to alcohol use and alcohol use disorders. Lancet. 2009;373:2223–33.
58. Rehm J, Room R, Monteiro M, Gmel G, Graham K, Rehn N, Sempos CT, Frick U, Jernigan D. Alcohol use. In: Ezzati M, Lopez AD, Rodgers A, Murray CJL, editors. Comparative quantification of health risks: global and regional burden of disease attributable to selected major risk factors. Geneva: World Health Organization; 2004.
59. Rehm J, Room R, Van Den Brink W, Jacobi F. Alcohol use disorders in EU countries and Norway: an overview of the epidemiology. Eur Neuropsychopharmacol. 2005;15:377–88.
60. Rehm J, Shield KD. Global burden of disease and the impact of mental and addictive disorders. Curr Psychiatry Rep. 2019;21:10.
61. Rehm J, Shield KD, Gmel G, Rehm MX, Frick U. Modeling the impact of alcohol dependence on mortality burden and the effect of available treatment interventions in the European Union. Eur Neuropsychopharmacol. 2013;23:89–97.
62. Robins LN. The sixth Thomas James Okey Memorial Lecture. Vietnam veterans' rapid recovery from heroin addiction: a fluke or normal expectation? Addiction. 1993;88:1041–54.
63. Robins LN, Slobodyan S. Post-Vietnam heroin use and injection by returning US veterans: clues to preventing injection today. Addiction. 2003;98:1053–60.
64. Robins LN, Wing J, Wittchen HU, Helzer JE, Babor TF, Burke J, Farmer A, Jablenski A, Pickens R, Regier DA, Sartorius N, Towle LH. The composite international diagnostic interview. An epidemiologic instrument suitable for use in conjunction with different diagnostic systems and in different cultures. Arch Gen Psychiatry. 1988;45:1069–77.
65. Romer Thomsen K, Callesen MB, Hesse M, Kvamme TL, Pedersen MM, Pedersen MU, Voon V. Impulsivity traits and addiction-related behaviors in youth. J Behav Addict. 2018;7:317–30.
66. Samokhvalov AV, Popova S, Room R, Ramonas M, Rehm J. Disability associated with alcohol abuse and dependence. Alcohol Clin Exp Res. 2010;34:1871–8.
67. Sherk A, Stockwell T, Chikritzhs T, Andreasson S, Angus C, Gripenberg J, Holder H, Holmes J, Makela P, Mills M, Norstrom T, Ramstedt M, Woods J. Alcohol consumption and the physical availability of take-away alcohol: systematic reviews and meta-analyses of the days and hours of Sale and outlet density. J Stud Alcohol Drugs. 2018;79:58–67.
68. Shield K, Rehm M, Patra J, Sornpaisarn B, Rehm J. Global and country specific adult per capita consumption of alcohol, 2008. Sucht. 2011;57:99–117.
69. Shield K, Rylett M, Gmel GS, Gmel G, Kehoe-Chan T, Rehm J. Global alcohol exposure estimates by country, territory and region for 2005 – a contribution to the Comparative Risk Assessment for the 2010 Global Burden of Disease Study. Addiction. 2013;108:912–22.
70. Smith LA, Foxcroft DR. The effect of alcohol advertising, marketing and portrayal on drinking behaviour in young people: systematic review of prospective cohort studies. BMC Public Health. 2009;9
71. Stautz K, Cooper A. Impulsivity-related personality traits and adolescent alcohol use: a meta-analytic review. Clin Psychol Rev. 2013;33:574–92.
72. Swendsen J, Conway KP, Degenhardt L, Glantz M, Jin R, Merikangas KR, Sampson N, Kessler RC. Mental disorders as risk factors for substance use, abuse and dependence: results from the 10-year follow-up of the National Comorbidity Survey. Addiction. 2010;105:1117–28.
73. Swendsen J, Le Moal M. Individual vulnerability to addiction. Ann N Y Acad Sci. 2011;1216:73.
74. Üstün BT, Compton W, Mager D, Babor T, Baiyewu O, Chatterji S, Cottler L, Gogus A, Mavreas V, Peters L, Pull C, Saunders J, Smeets R, Stipec M, Vrasti R, Hasin D, Room R, van Den Brink W, Regier D, Blaine J, Grant BF, Sartorius N. WHO study on the reliability and validity of the alcohol and drug use disorder instruments. Overview of methods and results. Drug Alcohol Depend. 1997;47:161–9.
75. Vink JM, Willemsen G, Boomsma DI. Heritability of smoking initiation and nicotine dependence. Behav Genet. 2005;35:397–406.
76. Westman J, Wahlbeck K, Laursen TM, Gissler M, Nordentoft M, Hallgren J, Arffman M, Osby U. Mortality and life expectancy of people with alcohol use disorder in Denmark, Finland and Sweden. Acta Psychiatr Scand. 2015;131:297–306.
77. Wing JK, Babor T, Brugha T, Burke J, Cooper JE, Giel R, Jablenski A, Regier D, Sartorius N. SCAN. Schedules for Clinical Assessment in Neuropsychiatry. Arch Gen Psychiatry. 1990;47:589–93.
78. Wittchen HU, Jacobi F, Rehm J, Gustavsson A, Svensson M, Jönsson B, Olesen J, Allgulander C, Alonso J, Faravelli C, Fratiglioni L, Jennum P,

Lieb R, Maercker A, van Os J, Preisig M, Salvador-Carulla L, Simon R, Steinhausen HC. The size and burden of mental disorders and other disorders of the brain in Europe 2010. Eur Neuropsychopharmacol. 2011;21:655–79.

79. World Health Organization. WHO expert committee on addiction-producing drugs, seventh report. Geneva; World Health Organization. 1957.

80. World Health Organization. ICD-10 classifications of mental and behavioural disorder: clinical descriptions and diagnostic guidelines. Geneva; World Health Organization. 1992.

81. World Health Organization. Global status report on alcohol and health. Geneva; World Health Organization. 2011.

82. World Health Organization. Global status report on alcohol and health 2018. 2018a. Available: https://www.who.int/substance_abuse/publications/global_alcohol_report/en/. Accessed 20 May 2019.

83. World Health Organization. ICD-11 International Classification of Diseases 11th Revision: The global standard for diagnostic health information. 2018b. Available: https://icd.who.int/en/. Accessed 12 July 2019.

84. World Health Organization. The world health organization world mental health composite international diagnostic interview (WHO WMH-CIDI). 2019. Available: https://www.hcp.med.harvard.edu/wmhcidi/download-the-who-wmh-cidi-instruments/. Accessed 11 July 2019.

Cultural Aspects and Responses to Addiction

6

Robin Room

Contents

Abstract

Use of psychoactive substances and our interpretations of the effects of the substances are affected by culture, defined broadly to include social worlds and subcultures as well as tribal, societal and linguistic groupings. Prototypical patternings of use include medicinal use, customary regular use and festival and other intermittent uses (where the psychoactivity is most attended to). A fourth pattern, addictive or dependent use, was a conceptualisation arising after the Enlightenment. Cultural norms may both encourage and discourage use and heavy use and may make the use more or less problematic. Cultural factors also shape responses to substance use, including the social handling of problematic situations and persons. Thus, there are characteristic differences between cultures in the institutional and professional location in the handling of substance use problems. In the modern world, there is substantial diffusion of practices and understandings between cultures, and in multicultural societies, drinking or drug use patterns often serve as markers of cultural distinctions. Despite all the diffusion, there are persisting cultural differences in thinking about, patterns of use of, and responses to psychoactive substance use.

R. Room (✉)
Centre for Alcohol Policy Research, La Trobe University, Bundoora, VIC, Australia

Centre for Social Research on Alcohol & Drugs, Department of Public Health Sciences, Stockholm University, Stockholm, Sweden
e-mail: r.room@latrobe.edu.au

Keywords

Norms on behaviour · Cultural practices
Social handling · Alcohol · Drugs · Concepts
of behaviour

6.1   Introduction

This chapter is concerned with cultural factors
in addiction. In discussing cultural aspects, we
are referring to shared beliefs, norms and patterns of behaviour, both about use of psychoactive substances and about how the use should
be interpreted and responded to. "Cultural"
here pertains to a variety of kinds and levels of
collectivity. This can range from a small tribal
group, for instance, the traditional inhabitants
of Easter Island in the Pacific, to a large multinational aggregation, as in a discussion of how
English speakers understand addiction, in contrast, say, to French speakers.

Often in discussing cultural factors, we are
dealing with multicultural situations, with a
diversity of cultures or subcultures. In such situations, the particular norms and behaviours of a
group may serve as markers differentiating
between groups; where most people drink alcohol, for instance, abstaining from alcohol may
become a mark of difference for Muslims or
Mormons [33].

We also use "cultural" here to refer to "social
worlds" [37, 39] within a society in which
understandings, norms and behaviours are
shared but in which the cultural boundaries are
less marked. For instance, one can speak of a
social world of heavy drinkers who know what
is expected behaviour at the bar in a tavern in a
particular society [10]. Are male drinkers
expected to buy drinks for each other, or does
each always pay just for himself? What signals
are being sent between a man and a woman
when he buys a drink for her and she accepts?
Among young adults in Oslo, Norway, for
instance, "when men buy drinks for women, this
may be interpreted as a negotiation for further
intimacy" [38]. Answers to such questions will

be obvious to those within the social world, but
may not be to outsiders.

6.2   Cultural Expectations About and Definitions of Psychoactive Substances and Their Effects

By definition, psychoactive substances change
our mental state. But how we interpret that
change, and how we behave under the influence, is strongly influenced by "set and setting"
[43] – including our expectancies about the
effects, which in turn are influenced by cultural
factors as well as previous experience. Although
the psychoactive effect of tobacco may not register in the consciousness of a habituated cigarette smoker, in other circumstances, the effect
of tobacco use may be so strong that the user is
rendered unconscious, as early Spanish observ-
ers reported in describing tobacco use among
native South Americans [26]. How those under
the influence of a given dose of alcohol behave
differs widely between cultures, as MacAndrew
and Edgerton [22] argued in their landmark
work on *Drunken Comportment*. Whether or
not someone taking LSD experienced a "bad
trip" in the United States in the 1960s and
1970s, Bunce [9] argued, was strongly influenced not only by subcultural expectations but
also by the extent of sociopolitical controversy
at that particular historical moment concerning
the drug.

Three social patternings of psychoactive drug
use can be distinguished as prototypical: medicinal use, customary regular use and intermittent
use. In many traditional societies, some drugs or
formulations have been confined to medicinal
use, that is, use under the supervision of a healer
to alleviate mental or physical illness or distress.
For several centuries after the technique for dis-
tilling alcoholic spirits had diffused from the
Arab world to Europe, for instance, spirits-based
drinks were regarded primarily as medicines
[40]. This way of framing drug use has been rou-
tinised and made subject to official control in the
modern state through a prescription system, with

physicians writing the prescriptions and pharmacists filling them. However, alongside this allopathic system in many societies, there is also legal provision for what are termed herbal, alternative or complementary medicines [12], some of which have psychoactive properties [6] – even apart from cannabis, which in the late 2010s is de facto becoming an herbal medicine in parts of North America. Drugs included in the prescription system usually are forbidden for nonmedicinal use [1], although the modern international drug control system has been fighting a losing battle to enforce this rule.

When a drug becomes a regular accompaniment of everyday life, its psychoactivity often is muted and even unnoticed, as is often the case for a habitual cigarette smoker. Similarly, in Southern European wine cultures, wine is often differentiated from intoxicating "alcohol"; wine drinkers are expected to maintain their original comportment after drinking. This may be called a pattern of *banalised use*: a potentially powerful psychoactive agent is domesticated into a mundane article of daily life that is available relatively freely in the consumer market.

Intermittent use – for instance, on sacred occasions, at festivals or only on weekends – minimises the build-up of tolerance to a drug. It is in the context of such patterns that the greatest attention is likely to be paid to a drug's psychoactive properties. The drug may be understood by both the user and others as having taken control of the user's behaviour and thus explain otherwise unexpected behaviour, whether bad or good [31]. As in Robert Louis Stevenson's fable of Jekyll and Hyde, normal self-control is expected to return when the effects of the drug wear off. In light of the power this framing attributes to the substance, access to it may be limited – in traditional societies by sumptuary rules keyed to social differentiations and in industrial societies by other forms of market restriction, including outright prohibition.

In modern societies, a fourth pattern of use is commonly recognised: addicted or dependent use that is marked by regular use, often of large doses. Where such use for the particular substance is not defined in the society as banalised,

addiction tends to be defined as an individual failing rather than a social pattern. Conceptualising repeated heavy use in terms of addiction means that the categorisation becomes an explanation – an explanation of why the pattern of use continues, despite problems resulting from the use for the individual and often for others. The concept thus focuses not on the pattern of use in itself, but rather on an apparent inability to control or refrain from use despite adverse consequences.

The addiction concept became established for alcohol in general understandings of European societies in the period after the Enlightenment. Particularly as temperance movements sprang up in response to the waves of very heavy alcohol consumption that accompanied the Industrial Revolution, the addiction idea came into common use as an explanation of why backsliding was common among temperance members who had pledged to give up drinking [21, 32]. In the late nineteenth century, the concept was extended by doctors to cover other psychoactive substances, and more recently, popular and professional discourse has commonly applied it also to other behaviours such as gambling [25, 36], though not without dispute [16]. However, as terminology for psychoactive substances has shifted in the International Classification of Diseases from "alcoholism" and "addiction" to "dependence" [29], in ICD's 11th revision, ironically, a term derived from "addiction" comes up only with respect to "addictive behaviours" such as gambling, now classified alongside substance use disorders [2]. But though the addiction concept has diffused into many cultures and is applied to a range of behaviours extending beyond substance use, there are substantial differences in cultural understandings of what the concept characterises and implies [34].

6.3   Norms Concerning Use and Related Behaviour

The use of psychoactive substances in any society or cultural group is structured by norms concerning use and behaviour while and after using. Laws and regulations on these matters, such as laws forbidding sales to or use by those under a certain age or prohibiting driving after use or regulations such as a church denomination's rubric specifying how leftover consecrated wine from a communion service is to be handled (that it is to be "reverently" consumed; [5]:198), may be described as formal norms. At least as important in structuring use are informal norms concerning use, which are often highly differentiated according to the social context [13] and to the user's demographic and social position. Bruun's division between controls at the phases of use, pattern and consequences [8] – whether use at all is disallowed or there are controls on the pattern of use or controls aiming to insulate the use from adverse consequences – describes the main strategies of both formal and informal norms in limiting the damage from substance use.

It is important to note that norms may encourage use – and indeed heavy use – as well as discourage it and may make the use riskier or more problematic. Heavy drinking or drug use is not always a matter of individual choice, but in particular social contexts may be a strong expectation. Taking alcohol as an example, in cultures where buying rounds is customary, once the round has been established, a man drinking with a group of friends will face a strong expectation to stay and drink as many drinks as there are men in the group. In a Mongolian cultural group in China, competitive drinking is a norm: "a refusal to drink signifies a refusal to engage the other on equal and respectful terms. Drinking partners take turns challenging each other to drain the cup, and the cups are inverted immediately afterward to prove the liquor is gone" [41]. Among young adult Italians, as also elsewhere in Europe, drinking games, enforced as a group ritual, serve the function of "becoming drunk quickly so as to amplify the effects of drinking: less shyness and disinhibition" [4]. Cultural expectations may thus facilitate heavy drinking and even enforce it, so that in some circumstances, addiction or dependence might better be described as located at collective levels rather than in the individual's mind or body [27]. This idea is carried by the French term *alcoolisation*, used concerning a society such as France when alcohol consumption was at its highest there in the 1950s [17].

6.4 Cultural Factors in Responses to Substance Use

Intoxication and habitual use of psychoactive substances can be problematic in many ways for those around the user, and societies and cultures respond in many ways in efforts to limit or prevent the problems. Informal responses by those around the drinker, smoker or drug user are very common (e.g. [14, 15]) – at levels ranging from a spouse's raised eyebrow to strenuous retribution.

Societies also respond to alcohol and drug problems at more formal levels. In the modern world, there is considerable uniformity across societies in the general roster of agencies and professions with responsibility for the social handling of problematic situations and persons. In most societies, there are hospitals and other health services and medical professionals, courts and police and judges, welfare institutions and social workers and churches and other faith institutions and clergy. But none of these sets of agencies and professions have clear and unchanging custody of alcohol and drug problems. Typically, all of them handle some part of drug and alcohol problems, but drug and alcohol problems are not central to the jurisdiction of any one of them [35]. The result is a diversity of competing models of how alcohol and drug problems should be handled [7]. As an eminent addiction doctor, Norman Kerr, put it already in the late nineteenth century, "in drunkenness of all degrees of every variety, the Church sees only the sin; the World the vice; the State the crime. On the other hand the medical profession uncovers a state of disease" [18].

There are characteristic cultural differences in the location of the handling of alcohol and drug problems. For alcohol problems, for instance, the welfare system has been the traditional central location in several Nordic countries; liver clinics within the medical system have played a major role in France and Italy; psychiatry has had a principal role in Switzerland and Austria [3, 19, 20]. But it is also true that, in a given society, the handling of alcohol and drug problems has often changed over time – particularly because these are "wicked problems" [42] where whatever solution is in effect will seem inadequate. As

Bruun [7] remarked about the Finnish history of the social handling of alcohol problems, "the consistent frustrations concerning the relative lack of success in fighting alcoholism made [Finland] move compulsively from one model [of response] to another."

The responses to alcohol and drug problems, both informal and formal, are thus just as subject to cultural definitions and norms as are the substance use and related behaviours. The responses are influenced both by the cultural definitions and norms concerning the substance use and by cultural beliefs and practices concerning appropriate responses. For the formal responses, general cultural and societal understandings and practices concerning the social handling of social and health problems also come into play.

6.5   Intercultural Influences and Diffusion

Almost no cultural group in the modern world is completely on its own. A particular solution to a set of problems that worked out in the cultural conditions of one society may travel far. Thus, for example, there is much about the ideas and organisation of Alcoholics Anonymous (AA) that reflects cultural understandings and practices in a particular society, the United States [24, 28]. But AA has diffused widely across the world, into cultures with considerable differences from US society. Even so, it is clear that the patterns of diffusion of AA show some regularities in terms of which societies it has flourished in, and these regularities tell us something both about core characteristics of AA and about patterns of culture [23]. And to some extent, AA practices have been adapted to the local culture [11]. Furthermore, even where AA was seen as culturally alien in some way, the news of its existence stimulated adaptations seen as more culturally congenial, and often the outcome has been AA and the adaptation coexisting side by side [30].

We have already mentioned above the tendency of cultural groups in multicultural societies to define themselves in distinction from each other, with drinking or drug use practices fairly often used as markers of the distinctions. On the other hand, it is clear that there is also some assimilation: immigrant groups take on practices from the receiving society, often forming a new cultural bricolage [33]. Influences and diffusion are also common between societies and cultures. Such influences are carried by four major forces: mass media, producers and other economic actors, intergovernmental bodies and agreements and the professions. News reports, television and film entertainment, and now also internet channels, convey information and images between cultural groups, perhaps particularly between youth cultures in different societies. In an increasingly globalised world with diminishing trade barriers, global corporations and other economic actors (and their equivalents for illicit drug markets) actively and tirelessly try out promotion methods and materials which have worked elsewhere in new cultural settings. Dissemination and influence also flow through the international drug and tobacco treaties and the agencies which implement them, as well as increasingly through other agencies such as international non-governmental organisations in a cross-national policy community. And doctors, police and other professionals, through professional societies, journals, newsletters and meetings, diffuse ideas, evidence and practices internationally.

Despite all the dissemination, cultural differences persist. In terms of cultural differentiations in psychoactive substance use and problems, and in the societal and cultural responses, it is possible to point to trends both of change and of stasis and both of convergence and of divergence, depending on where one looks. In thinking and acting across cultures concerning alcohol and other drugs, it is wise to take into account that even matters that are taken for granted in a given society or culture, or that are assumed to be universally valid in a profession's thinking, are often understood differently in different cultural traditions.

References

1. Babor T, Caulkins J, Fischer B, Foxcroft D, Humphreys K, Medina-Mora ME, Obot I, Rehm J, Reuter P, Room R, Rossow I, Strang J. Drug policy and the public good. 2nd ed. Oxford: Oxford University Press; 2018.

2. Basu D, Ghosh A. Substance use and other addictive disorders in International Classification of Diseases-11, and their relationship with DSM-5 and ICD-10. Indian J Soc Psychiatry. 2018;34(Suppl S1):54–62. http://www.indjsp.org/text.asp?2018/34/5/54/245838.

3. Baumohl J, Room R. Inebriety, doctors and the state: alcoholism treatment institutions before 1940. In: Galanter M, editor. Recent developments in alcoholism, vol. 5. New York: Plenum; 1987. p. 135–74.

4. Beccaria F, Guidoni OV. Young people in a wet culture: functions and patterns of drinking. Contemp Drug Probl. 2002;29:305–34.

5. Blunt JJ. The annotated book of common prayer. 5th ed. London: Rivingtons; 1871.

6. Bostock ECS, Kirkby KC, Garry MI, Taylor BV, Hawrelak JA. Mania associated with herbal medicines, other than cannabis: a systematic review and quality assessment of case reports. Front Psychol. 2018;9:280. https://doi.org/10.3389/fpsyt.2018.00280.

7. Bruun K. Finland – the non-medical case. In: Kiloh LG, Bell DS, editors. 29th international congress on alcoholism and drug dependence. Sydney, Australia, February, 1970. Australia: Butterworths, 1971; p. 545–559.

8. Bruun K. Implications of legislation relating to alcoholism and drug dependence: government policies. In: Kiloh LG, Bell DS, editors. 29th international congress on alcoholism and drug dependence. Sydney, Australia, February, 1970. Australia: Butterworths, 1971. p. 173–181.

9. Bunce R. Social and political sources of drug effects: the case of bad trips on psychedelics. J Drug Issues. 1979;9(2):213–33.

10. Cavan S. Liquor license: an ethnography of bar behavior. Chicago: Aldine; 1966.

11. Eisenbach-Stangl I, Rosenqvist P, editors. Diversity in unity: studies of Alcoholics Anonymous in eight societies. NAD Publication No. 33. Helsinki: Nordic Council for Alcohol & Drug Research; 1998.

12. Enioutina EY, Salis ER, Job KM, Gubarev MI, Krepkova LV, Sherwin CM. Herbal medicines: challenges in the modern world. Part 5. status and current directions of complementary and alternative herbal medicine worldwide. Expert Rev Clin Pharmacol. 2017;10(3):327–38.

13. Greenfield T, Room R. Situational norms for drinking and drunkenness: trends in the U.S. adult population, 1979-1990. Addiction. 1997;92:33–47.

14. Hemström Ö. Informal alcohol control in six EU countries. Contemp Drug Probl. 2002;29:577–604.

15. Hradilova Selin K, Holmila M, Knibbe R. Informal social control of drinking in intimate relationships – a comparative analysis. Contemp Drug Probl. 2009;36:31–59.

16. Jaffe J. Trivializing dependence. Br J Addict. 1990;85:1425–7.

17. Jellinek EM. International experience with the problem of alcoholism. Prepared for the joint meeting of expert committee on mental health and on alcohol, Geneva, 27 September – 2 October 1954. Geneva: World Health Organization, WHO/MENT/58 & WHO/APD/ALC/12, 2 June 1954.

18. Kerr N. Inebriety, or narcomania: its etiology, pathology, treatment and jurisprudence. 3rd ed. New York: J. Selwin Tait and Sons; 1888.

19. Klingemann H, Hunt G, editors. Drug treatment systems in an international perspective: drugs, demons and delinquents. Thousand Oaks: Sage; 1998.

20. Klingemann H, Takala J-P, Hunt G, editors. Cure, care or control: alcoholism treatment in fourteen countries. Albany: State University of New York Press; 1992.

21. Levine HG. The discovery of addiction: changing concepts of habitual drunkenness in American history. J Stud Alcohol. 1978;39:143–74.

22. MacAndrew C, Edgerton R. Drunken comportment: a social explanation. Chicago: Aldine; 1969.

23. Mäkelä K. Social and cultural preconditions of Alcoholics Anonymous (AA) and factors associated with the strength of AA. Br J Addict. 1991;86(11):1405–13.

24. Mäkelä K, Arminen I, Bloomfield K, Eisenbach-Stangl I, Helmersson Bergmark K, Kurube N, Mariolini N, Ólafsdóttir H, Peterson JH, Phillips M, Rehm J, Room R, Rosenqvist P, Rosovsky H, Stenius K, Świątkiewicz G, Woronowicz B, Zieliński A. Alcoholics Anonymous as a mutual-help movement: a study in eight societies. Madison and London: University of Wisconsin Press; 1996.

25. Marks I. Behavioural (non-chemical) addictions. Br J Addict. 1990;85:1389–94.

26. Robicsek F. The smoking gods: tobacco in Maya art, history and religion. Norman: University of Oklahoma Press; 1978.

27. Room R. Social psychology of drug dependence. In: The epidemiology of drug dependence: report on a conference: London 25–29 Sept 1972. Copenhagen: Regional Office for Europe, World Health Organization; 1973. p. 69–75.

28. Room R. Alcoholics Anonymous as a social movement. In: McCrady BS, Miller WR, editors. Research on Alcoholics Anonymous: opportunities and alternatives. New Brunswick: Rutgers Center of Alcohol Studies; 1993. p. 167–87.

29. Room R. Alcohol and drug disorders in the International Classification of Diseases: a shifting kaleidoscope. Drug Alcohol Rev. 1998;17:305–17.

30. Room R. Mutual help movements for alcohol problems in an international perspective. Addict Res. 1998;6:131–45.

31. Room R. Intoxication and bad behaviour: understanding cultural differences in the link. Soc Sci Med. 2001;53:189–98.

32. Room R. The cultural framing of addiction. Janus Head. 2003;6:221–34.

33. Room R. Multicultural contexts and alcohol and drug use as symbolic behaviour. Addict Res Theory. 2005;13:321–31.

34. Room R. Taking account of cultural and societal influences on substance use diagnoses and criteria. Addiction. 2006;101(Suppl. 1):31–9.

35. Room R, Hall W. Frameworks for understanding drug use and societal responses. In: Ritter A, King T, Hamilton M, editors. Drug use in Australian society. 2nd ed. Sydney: Oxford University Press; 2017. p. 69–83.
36. Saïet M. Les Addictions [The addictions]. Que-sais-je? Series no. 3911. Paris: Presses Universitaires de France; 2011.
37. Shibutani T. Reference groups as perspectives. Am J Sociol. 1955;60:562–9.
38. Træen B, Hovland A. Games people play: sex, alcohol and condom use among urban Norwegians. Contemp Drug Probl. 1998;25:3–48.
39. Unruh DR. The nature of social worlds. Pac Sociol Rev. 1980;23(3):271–96.
40. Wasson RG. Distilled alcohol dissemination. Drinking Drug Practices Surveyor. 1984;19:6.
41. Williams DM. Alcohol indulgence in a Mongolian community of China. Bull Concern Asian Sch. 1998;30:13–22.
42. Rittel HWJ, Webber MW. Dilemmas in a general theory of planning. Policy Sci. 1973;4:155–69.
43. Zinberg N. Drug, set, and setting: the basis for controlled intoxicant use. New Haven: Yale University Press; 1986.

Prevention Strategies

Roland Simon and Gregor Burkhart

Contents

Abstract

Prevention has the potential to positively affect problem substance use and related behaviors such as delinquency, violence, and sexual behavior. Science-based prevention interventions and strategies focus on the key determinants of successful socialization, such as nurturing and safe environments, social norms, parental skills and monitoring, executive and social skills, and impulse control. Information provision is necessary but as such contributes little to changing behavior.

Thus, universal prevention addresses the population at large and targets the development of skills and values, norm perception, and interaction with peers and social life; selective prevention addresses vulnerable

R. Simon (✉)
IFT Institute for Therapy Research,
Munich, Germany

G. Burkhart
EMCDDA, Lisbon, Portugal
e-mail: Gregor.Burkhart@emcdda.europa.eu

© Springer Nature Switzerland AG 2021
N. el-Guebaly et al. (eds.), *Textbook of Addiction Treatment*,
https://doi.org/10.1007/978-3-030-36391-8_7

groups and focuses on improving their opportunities in difficult living and social conditions; and indicated prevention addresses vulnerable individuals and helps them to deal and cope with the individual personality traits that make them more vulnerable to escalating drug use. Environmental prevention can complementarily and effectively change human behavior by modifying its regulatory, physical, and economic context. This means to subtly alter social and other environmental cues and social norms and their perception. Effective examples range from intervening at society level through market regulations of substances and changing the physical environment of nightlife and neighborhoods, to more rule-setting and monitoring within families.

The challenge for drug prevention lies therefore in helping people to adjust their behavior, capacities, and well-being in fields of multiple influences — such as behavioral opportunities and incentives, perceived norms, interaction with others, and their own personality traits — in order to reduce risk behaviors related to substances. The key challenge for this century, however, is to bridge the gap between the advances made in prevention science and the implementation of effective programs and local policies in prevention practice.

Keywords

Environmental prevention · Universal prevention · Selective prevention Family-based prevention · Indicated prevention Norms

7.1   Introduction

Drug prevention is traditionally conceived of as interventions or policies to avoid or delay the initiation into substance use by adolescents. It is a key element of national and international drug policies. Prevention is thought to act on the demand reduction side of drug interventions,

helping people to contain their use (or problem use) of psychoactive substances and their negative consequences. This understanding of prevention is complementary to treatment (which targets recovery and cure) and harm reduction (which helps people avoid the secondary negative effects of the use or problem use of addictive substances).

7.1.1   Factors for the Development of Problem Drug Use

Neuroscience has considerably contributed to prevention by providing an explanation why and how the developing brains of adolescents are particularly vulnerable to the noxious effects of alcohol, tobacco, and illicit drugs and to environmental factors. Prevention work can use findings from neuroscience to tailor interventions to the peculiarities in the functioning of adolescents.

Neuroscience has also (re)introduced concepts such as personality traits and temperament as risk factors, giving a longer-term perspective to prevention, which starts in early childhood. Many prevention professionals still focus on substance use, which should in their understanding be prevented altogether or early detected and treated. However, other variables may be of crucial importance in the transition from experimental use to substance use disorder (SUD). The same variables that predict initial acute drug effects and early use may significantly contribute to continued use, escalation, and dependence [12]. Recent research has introduced the common liability model, which suggests that early-manifesting traits such as neurobehavioral (i.e., cognitive, affective, and behavioral) disinhibition predict both early initiation of substance use and rapid escalation into problem use. Shared genetic and environmental influences and early externalizing behavior may lead to later substance use problems. Other personality traits, such as high levels of sensation seeking and low levels of shyness and avoidance, have shown to increase the risk of progressing from smoking to cannabis use. Hopelessness and sensation seeking were predictive for using alcohol, tobacco, and marijuana. Sloboda et al. [41] provide an exhaustive revision of the risk factor models relevant for prevention, which include many developmental factors in early childhood. Instead of detecting and addressing drug users, these findings point to a need to early target individual vulnerability traits.

Findings in the field of neuropsychology have shed light on why information provision does not deter young people from drug use and other problem behaviors: at their age, behavior is determined more by social context than by individual choice, and neurobiological imbalances may result in impaired judgment of risk. More crucially, though, adolescents respond more intensely to emotional and social stimuli and have increased awareness of others' opinions. Reward seeking is increased in the presence of their peers when the brain's socio-emotional system is stimulated. The interplay of these processes explains why adolescents take risks like substance use more often in peer group environments. Therefore, it seems to be normative, biologically driven, and to a certain degree inevitable and evolutionary function that adolescents are prone to risk-taking explorations during adolescence. Mature judgment needs time to develop, and therefore, cognitive–informative strategies seem unlikely to make adolescents wiser, less impulsive, or less short-sighted.

7.1.2 An Overarching Model for Prevention

The last section has described a number of factors influencing the risk of developing problematic patterns of substance use. The following section aims to show that the challenge of prevention is more than just avoiding or delaying substance use. Instead, it should help youth to positively develop from childhood to adulthood and to adjust their behavior, capacities, and well-being to their own personality traits influenced by, among others, living conditions, social norms, interaction with peers and parents, and opportu-

nities. Prevention could therefore be defined as evidence-based socialization where the primary focus is sustaining healthier behaviors. It includes preventing or delaying substance use initiation or related behaviors, reducing their intensification, or preventing the escalation of use into problem use.

The three classical forms of prevention defined by the Institute of Medicine [35] are based on people's vulnerability, which was found more practical for substance use prevention than the medical paradigm of primary, secondary, and tertiary prevention. While the latter works fine for the natural course of, for example, cancer and infectious diseases, it seems less adequate to describe human behavior.

The four forms of prevention described below address the most relevant spheres of behavior influence: opportunities, incentives, and behavioral norms are targeted by environmental strategies; interaction with peers and social life by universal prevention; social conditions and exclusion by selective prevention; and personality traits by indicated prevention. This simplified classification provides us with an overview of the different preventive approaches taken. Prevention can in addition be segmented according to the level of environment on which it is acting, into macro, meso, and micro level [3]. As the majority of prevention activities focus in practice on substance use and problem behavior in general, they mostly do not differentiate between alcohol, tobacco, and illicit drugs.

7.1.3 Considerations for Practice

The considerations above have manifold implications and underpin the following considerations for practice:

- Adolescent impulsivity and risk taking have an important evolutionary function. Prevention, though, can provide skills and nurturing environments in order to reduce the potential harm of these specific adolescent characteristics.

- Information provision has little impact on behavior, particularly of adolescents and in "hot" situations.
- Cultural values, descriptive norms, and the social acceptability of use influence people's initiation into substance use and problem behavior directly as well as indirectly through parenting practices.
- An increase of normative beliefs, that is, giving the implicit impression that most or many people do engage in a given problem behavior, is an important harmful effect of sub-optimal public messaging, for example, in mass media campaigns that were not perfectly pretested and evaluated.
- Publicly visible sanctions and reinforcement of social norms, for example, in schools and nightlife venues, have important potentials for changing and sustaining behavior, while legislation, which prosecutes individuals, often fails to dissuade adolescents from continuing to use substances.
- Informal social control and social sanctions (from family and peers) may have more of an impact than the certainty and severity of formal legal sanctions [37].

7.2 Prevention Strategies: Definitions and Effects

A large proportion of the general public and substantial numbers of policy makers have, for some time, seen drug prevention as purely informing or warning young people about the effects or dangers of drugs. Quite logically then, mass media campaigns (see Sect. 7.2.1) were often the first choice of prevention intervention. Environmental prevention strategies aim to alter the immediate regulatory, cultural, social, physical, and economic environments in which people make their choices about substance use (see Sect. 7.2.2).

Prevention approaches are classified according to differences in the vulnerability (and risk) of the target group. For universal prevention (see Sect. 7.2.3), all members of the population are assumed to share the same general risk for substance use problems, although the risk may vary greatly between individuals. Selective prevention

(see Sect. 7.2.4) applies social and demographic indicators that roughly indicate increased levels of vulnerability among some groups. In indicated prevention (see Sect. 7.2.5), vulnerable individuals are screened and have to be defined on the basis of properly diagnosed risk conditions, such as attention deficit disorder or conduct disorders.

7.2.1 Mass Media Campaigns

Mass media campaigns can reach large and heterogeneous audiences and have shown to be beneficial in promoting health behaviors like healthier nutrition, physical activity, and participation in screening for breast and cervical cancer [50]. However, they seem to be much less successful in discouraging problem behaviors, which have a strong impulsive component. While some positive effects on tobacco smoking have been found, there is actually no evidence that simply informing adolescents about the effect of drugs has a beneficial impact on their illicit drug use, as a Cochrane Review [2] confirms. Mass media campaigns seem to be more effective in tackling adolescent use of legal drugs and when they target parents instead of young people [10]. Perceptions of normality seem to play an essential role in their success and failure, which can also lead to detrimental effects: intention to use cannabis seemed to have increased in certain subgroups with greater exposure to a US warning campaign – most likely due to misperceived high popularity and prevalence of marijuana use.

It is an important ethical concern that mass media campaigns may have iatrogenic effects by changing normative beliefs, resulting in higher intentions to use. This is even more problematic, as the target population has typically not requested this (potentially harmful) kind of social intervention.

Against this background, the lack of adequate evaluations of media campaigns is a concern. In Europe, only the Netherlands and the UK have assessed the effects of these campaigns on behavior or intentions, while the large majority of reported campaigns have not been evaluated at all or only assessed how the campaign was perceived or affected knowledge alone.

7.2.2 Environmental Prevention

This approach takes into account that potential substance users are influenced by a complex set of factors in their environment, including social norms, defining what is considered normal, expected, or accepted in their reference group; the rules, regulations, and taxes of their state; the commercial advertisements to which they are exposed; and the availability of alcohol, tobacco, and illicit drugs. Many human behaviors performed everyday are automatic and are generally reactions to common and familiar stimuli. This demonstrates the importance of environmental and social cues and automatic processes in influencing behavior. It may explain the limited success of prevention approaches that focus solely on individual responsibility for decision-making and self-control.

The purpose of environmental prevention policies and interventions is to limit the availability of opportunities for unhealthy or risky behavior and/or promote the availability of healthy ones. This approach differs from traditional behavioral prevention approaches as it targets the automatic system of behavior (one that doesn't require deliberate cognition). Thus, it requires lower individual "agency": individual personal resources such as conscious decision-making, motivation, and intent are less important in these types of intervention.

Environmental prevention strategies often entail changes at the macro level (legislation or society), such as market control using taxes and publicity bans or coercive measures including age controls and tobacco bans, which are effective but often resisted in parts of the population. Regulations and market interventions are currently considered as the only evidence-based mechanisms to prevent the harm caused by commodity industries [34]. Efforts to create protective and positive school and family climates also belong to environmental prevention.

7.2.2.1 Environmental Influences in Schools and Communities

There is evidence that the school climate and the nature of the school environment substantially influence substance use and violence in school.

Students' perceptions of school safety, teacher support, and whether they are treated fairly are also related to substance use. Interventions that increase student participation, improve relationships, and promote a positive school ethos appear to reduce substance use.

Other strategies at the meso level include municipal strategies to reduce public nuisance, drug "policies" in schools, targeted policing, conditional venue and event licensing, fines and venue design guidelines, and community action strategies such as neighborhood watch schemes.

7.2.2.2 Environmental Influences in Nightlife

The known environmental determinants of alcohol abuse and violence also apply to nightlife settings: dirty conditions, poor ventilation, high levels of noise and music, low comfort, high density of patrons, predominant male patronage, high numbers of intoxicated patrons, and high boredom [33]. A European review [23] found that important environmental contributions to alcohol-related problems include a permissive environment, discounted drinks promotions, poor cleanliness, crowding, loud music, and poor staff practice. Environmental approaches addressing these factors to reduce drug use and other risky behaviors may be more profitable for a business, improve its image, reduce the risk of city and police interference, and limit problems in its neighborhood.

Reviews of prevention interventions in nightlife settings conclude that they can effectively reduce high-risk alcohol consumption, alcohol-related injury, violent crimes, access to alcohol by underage youth, and provision of alcohol to intoxicated people. Providing information and pill testing were not considered evidence based. Interventions such as "responsible beverage services" or "designated driver programs," often backed by the industry, are less effective, especially if they are not enforced. The most effective strategies were those that combined training, cooperation, and enforcement with "classical" environmental measures such as taxation, reduced blood alcohol concentration (BAC) limits for driving, and reinforced minimum legal purchasing age.

7.2.2.3 Environmental Influences within Families

The climate of norms, parental modeling and behavior, and the associated exposure to sensorial and visible cues such as substances, screens, and food are microenvironments that subtly shape adolescent behavior and attitudes. Later in this chapter, we will describe family-based programs that aim to improve the behavior of children and young people through better parenting. In this section, we address some aspects of families that are not necessarily related to direct parent–child interaction but reflect micro-level environmental influences on the socialization of youth.

One aspect is the amount of pocket money, which has been found to be associated with increased prevalence of risky alcohol use and higher odds of smoking, getting drunk, using cannabis, and using ecstasy, even after controlling for socioeconomic status and other aspects. The role of families' socioeconomic situation in this respect is still unclear. How parents tell their own substance use history may also play a role. A more recent study found an association between parents admitting their own past drug use in detail and teenagers having a more positive attitude to substances [24].

Parental ingenuousness about their offspring's substance use can have a protective function in the sense of a Pygmalion effect. In a longitudinal study [28], adolescent users whose parents indicated that their children used marijuana at baseline were more than twice as likely to continue use, compared to children of parents who assumed that their children had not initiated marijuana use, even if this assumption might have been wrong. Obviously, monitoring and family rules play major roles in creating protective environments, but since such elements imply an active role by parents, we discuss those in the section dedicated to family-based prevention.

7.2.2.4 Environment, Social Norms, and Substance Use

Even if environmental prevention targets predominantly legal drugs and antisocial behavior, its approaches are important for the whole prevention field because early, widespread, and accepted use of alcohol and tobacco is associated with illicit drug use in many countries. Alcohol has a key role in the initiation of illicit drug use, especially among adolescents. European School Survey Project on Alcohol and Other Drugs [13] data for 22 countries showed that 86% of the 15- to 16-year-old students who had used ecstasy during the last month had also consumed five or more alcoholic drinks on one occasion. Similar relationships were found for alcohol with cannabis and cocaine. In prospective longitudinal studies, tobacco smoking has been shown to mediate the initiation into cannabis and predict an earlier initiation [1]. It seems that the social and physical contexts of consumption are also influencing the level of alcohol, tobacco, and illicit drug use in the same way. Environmental prevention focuses on these contexts.

The effectiveness of environmental prevention is well established in the alcohol and tobacco fields. At the macro level, taxation and regulations have been found to be effective, reducing alcohol use and related problems [49]. At the meso level, a study showed that adolescents living in areas with lower outlet density and proximity were drinking less. In a US study [38], a legal age of below 21 years for buying alcohol was associated with an increased risk of binge drinking later in life. Additionally, drinkers who lived in states with lower minimum drinking ages were more likely to drink alcohol heavily, but not to consume more overall or to drink more frequently.

Guidelines for the creation of better environments in recreational settings, such as the "safer dancing" guidelines, were developed since the end of the 1990s. They include access to free drinking water, rules on glassware and noise, monitoring of interior space in respect of risky sexual or aggressive behavior and drugs, training staff for medical emergencies and handling drug-related problems, and excluding "problem" patrons (drug dealers, drug users, persons carrying weapons).

Besides the perceived availability of substances, environmental aspects such as cultural values, descriptive norms, and the social acceptance of use seem to influence initiation into substance use.

Close contact with substance-using peers is strongly related to individual substance use. Establishing an overarching environment of disapproval may be an effective means of preventing cannabis use by adolescents. Overall, normative beliefs are also important factors in the success or failure of interventions. While several studies confirm that behavioral change is mediated by descriptive norms, the social norms approach has to be used with caution as social groups may also develop minority norms that deliberately deviate from the healthy injunctive norm that is being promoted [9].

It is unlikely that environmental prevention will have much of an impact on the behavior of highly vulnerable individuals. However, the prevention paradox postulates that the majority of alcohol-related problems in a population are associated with low to moderate drinkers simply because they are much more numerous than heavy drinkers. A study in 23 European countries [11] confirmed this for adolescent boys' and girls' annual consumption and heavy episodic drinking; similar results were found in Brazil. Still, there are limitations to this concept. A minority of people with frequent heavy episodic drinking accounted for a large proportion of all problems in one study [11], and most illicit drug use was found in the high-risk group (15% of the sample) in a different study.

The practical consequence of the prevention paradox is that all available approaches should be used: environmental and universal prevention strategies should aim to reduce initiation and overall levels of substance use, and targeted strategies should address particularly vulnerable subgroups and individuals, addressing harm related to early-age drug use or frequent cannabis use.

7.2.3 Universal Prevention: Intervening with Populations

Universal prevention addresses the population at large, regardless of differing vulnerabilities of individuals or subgroups. It aims to reduce substance-related risk behavior by providing necessary competences to avoid or delay initiation into substance use, acting like a "behavioral vaccine." In Europe, at least, universal prevention predominantly takes place in schools, as they facilitate access to the large share of the youth populations.

The overall effectiveness of school-based universal prevention has been repeatedly questioned, but there is abundant evidence from reviews (e.g., [5, 16, 32, 43]) that programs based on the social influence approach have consistently been more effective than programs based on any other approaches. The approach consists of components such as social skills training (listening, making compliments, empathy, and communication), strengthening personal skills (goal setting, coping, identifying feelings), and correcting normative beliefs (i.e., on the level of acceptance and use of substances among peers). It has to be delivered in an interactive way that engages young people. While life skills components of such programs are well known and have been well researched, the role of social norms (see Sect. 7.2.2) has gained the attention of researchers only more recently. Evidence from trials suggests that this approach might be an additional pathway for reducing substance-use-related harm [29, 30].

Even if the effects of school-based prevention at the intervention level are often small, social influence programs can be an important mechanism for transmitting societal norms on substance use to young people. They can help them to further develop their skills to make and implement safer decisions about substance use or in situations where others are using. They also offer the potential of creating a more sympathetic environment for complementary systemic strategies, such as restrictions on advertising for legal psychotropic substances [32]. In this field, we find some "manualized" programs which provide detailed material and guidance for teachers and pupils.

"Unplugged" is the only multisite randomized controlled trial (RCT) of a school-based prevention program in Europe to date. This comprehensive social influence program consists of twelve 1-h interactive sessions delivered by class teachers. It has proven its effectiveness with respect to drunkenness and cannabis use and problematic drug and alcohol use among boys, but not among girls [47]. Participation in the program was also associated with positive effects among adolescents from a low socioeconomic level. The program was implemented in several additional countries, in Eastern Europe, South America, and Asia, replicating in some cases the initial promising outcomes.

The "Good Behavior Game" (GBG) is a way of managing whole primary school classes during regular lessons and socializing children to be self-controlled, emphasizing the role of significant others (teachers and peers) in children's social adjustment in school. Children systematically learn over a period of one school year to respect basic class rules. RCTs reported a beneficial impact up to the middle school years and even young adulthood including reductions in alcohol and drug dependency disorders and a reduction in many other behavioral problems. Substances and substance use are not explicit themes in GBG but targeted through a focus on socialization. "Unplugged" and GBG can be accessed at the Xchange registry[1] of the EMCDDA.

7.2.4 Selective Prevention: Intervening with (Vulnerable) Groups

Selective prevention intervenes with specific groups, families, or communities that may be more likely to develop drug use or progress into dependency. Often, this higher vulnerability to problem drug use stems from social exclusion, lack of opportunities, and less nurturing family or community environments. For example, European countries most frequently report about young (drug law) offenders, youth in deprived neighborhoods, ethnic minorities and immigrant groups, school dropouts, students who are failing academically, and vulnerable families as target groups of this type of intervention. This means that – different from universal prevention – the

[1] http://www.emcdda.europa.eu/best-practice/xchange_en

situation and vulnerability pattern of a given target group has to be studied before starting the invention. Since this vulnerability assessment relies on the group level, individual risk cannot be assessed. Evidence for the effectiveness of selective prevention is currently limited because evaluations are difficult and scarce.

The effective components in selective prevention seem to be virtually the same as in universal prevention. Interventions that do not solely address drug use, adapt to young people's experiences, and avoid rigid abstinence-oriented messages have proven to be more effective. They address social needs connected to drug use, rather than drug use behavior as such which in these populations are considered as just one of several expressions of behavioral maladjustment.

In summary, prevention that targets vulnerable people may moderate the effect of an early developmental disadvantage, its translation into social marginalization, and progression into substance abuse. Interventions delivered during the early school years that aimed to improve educational environments and reduce social exclusion also had a moderating effect on later substance use [45], without specifically targeting youth who experiment with drugs. Such prevention programs can also be beneficial in behavioral domains beyond substance use, such as violence, delinquency, academic failure, teenage pregnancies, and unprotected sex. Smoking, drinking, safe sex, and healthy nutrition among adolescents share common factors: beliefs about immediate gratification and social advantages, peer norms, peer and parental modelling, and refusal self-efficacy.

While in Europe the concept of selective prevention has been accepted quite well, several researchers have raised concerns regarding possible iatrogenic effects when vulnerable young people are grouped together in selective interventions. Problem behavior may get worse when members of this selective group model to each other's problem behavior ("deviance modelling"), thereby corroborating their belief that their deviant behavior is "normal" while the surrounding social environment is not ("norm narrowing"). Such iatrogenic effects are unlikely to occur in universal prevention, where some program evaluations in school and family settings [26] found that the more vulnerable subgroups within the target population benefited more from the intervention, possibly because they adjusted their behavior to that of the "conventional" majority.

Increasingly in the EU, vulnerable groups have been primary targets for prevention interventions. In most cases, these were young offenders and pupils with academic and social problems, who share many risk factors with problem drug users. While young offenders as a group are easy to identify, interventions provided are often not appropriate for them. The manualized program for young offenders (FreD) takes a more specific approach. Developed at the national level in Germany, it has been expanded to and adapted by one-third of all EU member states. Some countries have reacted specifically to the increased vulnerability to drug use found among pupils in vocational schools, for example, with tailored programs to generally improve literacy and numeracy levels among disadvantaged students. At the community level, municipalities in Northern Europe and in Italy aim to combine drug and alcohol policies, action plans, and youth work through binding cooperation agreements between local authorities and nongovernmental organizations.

Early intervention approaches provide social, emotional, and learning support to children in the early years of life. They can delay or prevent future problems including substance misuse more effectively and economically than intervening only when problems appear. Parenting programs at a local level can be an essential part of early intervention, but proactive parental work and training is still an exception.

As the prevention of different problem behaviors belongs to segregated political portfolios in most countries, a common, cohesive, coherent, and efficient approach to adolescent vulnerability is often lacking. In those few countries where such policy responses to multiple risk behaviors have emerged, there is increasing evidence for the effectiveness of such approaches [21].

7.2.5 Family-Based Prevention: Universal and Selective

Many parents in the Western world tend to assume that a close, warm, and open relationship with their children is protective against SUD, by providing them with a space to test their own boundaries. Recent research has provided considerable support for the idea that not only parental support but also monitoring are strong determinants of lower prevalence levels of adolescent risk behavior. Research indicates that the "authoritative style" (strict and warm) is the most protective against substance use, while the "neglectful style" (lenient and distant) increases the risk of drug use. Research however is as yet inconclusive as factors beyond parenting style, such as parents' drug use, emotional support and warmth, family structure, and influence of culture have to be considered as well [7, 19].

Monitoring and warmth together appear to predict adolescents' social and interpersonal perceptions of drug use and their actual drug use. A recent study in the Netherlands suggests that clear parental rule-setting is more strongly related to lower levels of risk behaviors in adolescents than are more general parenting practices. The findings give additional etiological underpinning to an intervention study that tested the Swedish Örebro program in the Netherlands. The program combines parent and student interventions and establishes simple drinking rules, coordinated between home and school ([25]). It can be accessed at the Xchange registry[1] of the EMCDDA.

Strict family rules about drinking were also tested against a (harm minimization) model according to which alcohol use is a part of normal adolescent development while parents should supervise their children's use to encourage responsible drinking. McMorris et al. [31] compared adolescent alcohol use and related harms among adolescents in Washington State, USA, and Victoria, Australia, two states that have, respectively, adopted zero tolerance and harm minimization policies. Despite those differences, family context was related to alcohol use and harmful use in a very similar way, but adult-supervised alcohol use resulted in higher levels of harmful alcohol consequences. Both Mediterranean drinking cultures and Danish drinking parties where parents organize and supervise alcohol consumption among their teenage offspring are based on this rationale of adult-supervised alcohol use.

The need to break intergenerational cycles of poor parenting practices was addressed by Hill et al. [22], who examined the extent to which interactions between behavioral disinhibition and family management during adolescence (from age 10) predict alcohol abuse and alcohol dependence at age 27. Young people who were high in behavioral disinhibition were at increased risk of later alcohol abuse and dependence but only in consistently poorly managed family environments, while in consistently well-managed families, high levels of behavioral disinhibition did not increase the risk of later alcohol abuse or dependence.

Most of the effective family-based programs contain elements of monitoring, rule-setting, and contingency management. A systematic review [4] of programs for substance-affected families found interventions to be effective when their duration was longer than 10 weeks and when they involved components of parenting and children and family skills training. Proximal outcomes (e.g., knowledge, coping skills, and family relations) were stronger than more distal outcomes (e.g., self-worth and substance use initiation). Apart from a few studies, the long-term effects on young people's substance use, delinquency, mental health, physical health, and school performance have rarely been assessed in the evaluations. Several of these programs can be accessed at the Xchange registry[1] of the EMCDDA.

Overall, across universal and selective interventions, Cochrane Reviews found good evidence that family-based prevention interventions are effective in reducing young people's alcohol, tobacco, and drug use [18].

7.2.6 Indicated Prevention: Intervening with (Vulnerable) Individuals

Indicated prevention aims to identify individuals with behavioral or psychological problems that may be predictive of developing problem substance use later in life and to target them individually with special interventions. Indicators of increased risk can be dissocial behavior and early aggression as well as alienation from parents, school, and peer groups. The aim of indicated prevention is not necessarily to prevent substance use but to prevent or at least delay development of a dependence or to prevent more risky patterns of use. Problematic substance use is seen as just one among the behavioral or mental health problems that lead to SUD, which can be diagnosed at the individual level. This is highly relevant for practice and policy because vulnerabilities at the social (demographic) level, those at the individual (mental health) level, and those at the environmental level affect the pathways to substance use disorder in quite distinct ways and phases of life [41]. The focus of the respective prevention strategies should match the kind of vulnerability found at the target populations.

There are no systematic reviews or meta-analyses assessing the effectiveness of interventions that target individuals with behavioral or psychological problems independent of substance use. Nevertheless, the few available single intervention studies in Europe tend to be better designed and to provide stronger outcomes than those in selective prevention.

For example, the school-based program "Preventure" targets adolescents (aged 13–14 years) with specific personality risk factors for early-onset substance use disorder and other risky behaviors in only two sessions. Even when implemented by nonspecialists, participants showed a lower likelihood of later onset of drinking or a less steep increase in consumption and binge drinking. Effects beyond substance use included reduced scores in depression, panic attacks, truancy, and shoplifting [36]. SKOLL (www.skoll.de), a 10-week program of training in self-control for young people with risky substance use, was implemented nationwide in Germany at schools and in other settings. Results showed reductions in drug use and risky behaviors over the course of several months, more self-confidence, alternatives to risky behavior, and social contacts. Those young people who were more vulnerable benefited the most.

Brief interventions (BI) consist of one-to-one counselling sessions, sometimes including follow-up sessions, which are delivered by trained health and social workers to people at risk. BI were found to be effective for alcohol-related problems when delivered in the primary healthcare system and colleges. This approach is increasingly used also to target young people and their cannabis use. Putting these one-to-one personal interventions to scale continues to be a challenge, and their overall effectiveness is under debate [8, 17, 20, 44]. They are increasingly delivered via interactive counselling websites or m-health technologies [15], which might attract substance users who would not approach any regular assessment or counselling service. BI often makes use of the technique of motivational interviewing (MI), which in a Cochrane Review [42] showed significant effects in short- to midterm follow-ups in comparison to nonintervention. For club-goers, Kurtz et al. [27] suggest that even simple assessment and feedback interviews can reduce substance use.

As young alcohol or drug users mostly have no self-perception of problems, screening and assessing them for possible problems is a particular challenge. In Europe, drug tests are very rarely used for assessing drug-related problems in pupils (under suspicion), and in most countries, testing is not allowed since they are judged as ethically questionable and ineffective [14], In the USA, by contrast, even random drug tests seem to be common.

Overall, indicated prevention could reduce the negative impact of neurobehavioral problems, such as early aggression on later substance use, and other problem behavior from childhood on.

7.2.7 Considerations for Practice

The considerations above underpin a number of considerations for practice:

- The use of mass media campaigns should be considered with highest caution, since warning campaigns can backfire. They are useful if targeted at parents, if they correct erroneous normative beliefs, or if they support environmental strategies by explaining their rationales (e.g., "protect our youth from industry influences").
- The underused potentials of environmental prevention are gaining more attention. Public (often local) policies modifying the regulatory, economic, and physical environments, which inconspicuously shape human behavior, can achieve positive changes in substance use behaviors and sustain them. An intrinsic dilemma for policy makers might be that such strategies are either invisible or unpopular: contrary to mass media campaigns, they don't deliver political capital.
- Universal prevention in schools should focus both on conveying social and personal behavioral skills by means of evidence-based programs and on guaranteeing safe and positive school climate.
- Selective prevention is in Europe often delivered through prevention services rather than by programs. There is much potential for improvement of intervention content (skills and competence training instead of information and counseling). Concerns exist about their safety because of the small number of evaluations and the particular risk of grouping young people with problem behaviors together.
- Indicated prevention offers an important potential of targeting early temperamental and behavioral issues, which might increase the propensity for SUD later in life. Few promising programs are available, but coverage is very low, and the most frequently found intervention type targets regular substance users

with brief interventions. New e-health methods might reduce the obstacles in scaling up their delivery.

- Families are an important but underused resource in helping adolescents in adjusting their behavior to environmental and social influences. Evidence-based approaches range from environmental (rules and monitoring) to universal and selective (parenting techniques). However, reaching and engaging parents and promoting parental monitoring is a major challenge for implementation. For this purpose, mass media campaigns can be helpful.

After careful development and evaluation of effects, prevention strategies and programs need proper implementation to affect a relevant part of the population.

- Despite the limited evidence, it is possible that mass media campaigns still have a wider role to play in comprehensive social marketing strategies, such as those trying to support environmental strategies.
- A practical problem for different strategies is that many parents cannot be reached using the classic instruments such as parents' evenings or invitations for a talk during office hours.
- Some universal programs might predominantly attract the well-off, low-risk families; however, effective (often selective) programs tackle this imbalance by offering transportation, childcare, and food at the venues – elements that might be essential for families in need.
- Addressing all families using a universal prevention approach might allow more vulnerable families to adopt educational, normative, and behavior models from the more conventional families in the same group, and more vulnerable families may profit the most.
- As developing prevention programs is expensive, transfer of well-established programs should be a very interesting approach. Despite some difficulties and hesitations [40], a number of manualized prevention programs from North America have been successfully transferred to European environments.

More details on these programs, results of their effectiveness in European evaluation studies, and the experiences of practitioners in implementing them can be found at the EMCDDA Xchange registry[1].

7.2.8 Transfer of Prevention Technologies

Prevention research in North America is generally more developed than in Europe. This is related to structural differences in social policies and prevention practice as well as to research funding. In the European Union, however, services such as health and social care and education are generally of higher quality and are widely available, which is not the case in most other regions of the world. As a consequence, in these regions outside of Europe, prevention programs are developed or used to promptly address a range of emerging social problems; this approach might hence be a consequence of a lower availability of universal social, youth, and health services.

The evidence for the effectiveness of substance use disorder prevention comes almost exclusively from evaluations of sophisticated manualized programs (e.g., [18, 46]). Their implementation is more likely to be manualized to assure accuracy and reach of implementation. Such programs are also more likely to have been pretested, to have been checked for unintentional (iatrogenic) effects, and to prove positive behavioral outcomes. Overall, such interventions could be considered "high-tech prevention." In medicine, most people would naturally expect such a level of "technology assessment", especially of medications, before they can be distributed to the population. In Europe, such high-tech programs are rare, especially outside classrooms. Prevention strategies consist in most cases of varying combinations of policies for vulnerable populations; activities for school-aged youth to raise their awareness, self-competence, social skills, and/or autonomy; and events and advice for parents and in some countries in local environmental prevention policies. Such approaches make use of the existing infrastructure, and they allow for innovation and adaption to local needs and perceptions. However, they are sometimes based on little more than common sense and, except for the environmental approaches, often lack evidence of effectiveness and have possible iatrogenic effects. In broad terms, it seems that the relative lack of prevention infrastructure in the USA has led to more prevention research and program development. Europe, on the other hand, relies on a more elaborate infrastructure but spends much less energy on ensuring the quality, effectiveness, and safety of interventions.

Well-developed programs from North America have been culturally adapted to suit other parts of the world. Using an existing program means that the resources, manuals, and methodologies are ready for immediate use, facilitating implementation. However, in Europe, there has been an aversion to the standardization inherent in manualized interventions and a belief that cultural and organizational differences between North America and Europe would make the adaptation problematic. Countries in Latin America and in Asia do not appear to have such problems in adopting and adapting evidence-based programs from other parts of the world.

Despite the difficulties and hesitations described above, in the past decade, a number of manualized substance use prevention programs from North America have been successfully transferred and adapted to European environments. They and their effectiveness ratings can be accessed at http://www.emcdda.europa.eu/best-practice/xchange_en alongside the experiences of the implementers in Europe that adaptation and implementation are both feasible and effective (where outcomes are available). While a considerable amount of time and effort was necessary to adjust the programs to culture and context, in most cases, it was preferable to adapt an available effective program than to develop a new one from scratch. Yet, several American flagship programs appear to yield less convincing results when implemented in Europe, either due to better services provided to the control conditions, questions of fidelity, or the noninvolvement of the developers in the evaluations.

7.3   Conclusion

7.3.1   Prevention, Treatment, and Harm Reduction

Prevention has made considerable progress in recent years, but there is still much room for improvement. Despite considerable support also through findings from neurosciences, evidence is still limited, which might hinder a broader use of prevention. However, the number of options available to tackle substance-related problems is limited. Harm reduction interventions are important but limited in scope, and treatment often comes late after problem substance use has started and reaches only a part of people in need. So we have to use all tools at hand to work on the drug problem, and prevention is absolutely core in this respect despite its limitations and shortcomings.

Reflecting on the criticism that prevention is only abstinence oriented, the term "risk reduction" has been coined as a viable alternative for vulnerable or drug-using youth. In fact, the evidence, intervention examples, and theoretical frameworks discussed here show that "risk reduction" is intrinsically included in all prevention measures, and most prevention interventions in fact try to achieve generally better behavioral control and adequate socialization or to avoid rapid escalation from experimental use to SUD or even addiction, hence reducing risk and harms.

Especially for selective and indicated prevention, we do see a considerable overlap with treatment where low treatment rates and considerable delays before treatment initiation have led to a more generic debate on the role of treatment itself. Putting more emphasis on outcomes targeting "healthy lifestyle" instead of "avoidance of addiction" and "low-risk use" instead of "abstinence," the conceptual gap between treatment and prevention is shrinking [6]. The vicinity between these concepts becomes obvious when we look at websites for cannabis users, which offer information and self-tests on one side and access to treatment in case of need on the other side.

7.3.2 Conceptual Developments

Findings from country-level ecological analyses on the health of young people [48] show that the strongest determinants of adolescent health worldwide are structural factors such as national wealth, income inequality, and access to education. As a consequence, nurturing environments, with safe and supportive families and schools, together with positive and supportive peers, are crucial in addressing risk and building protective factors in the course of child and adolescent development.

Social norms and other environmental cues have a strong influence on behavior, suggesting that the effect of informal social control and social sanctions (from family and peers) may be more important than the certainty and severity of formal sanctions. This illustrates that comprehensive prevention policies ought not only to address individual vulnerabilities and illicit drug use. Informal social norms have a major but largely underestimated influence on initiation and level of substance use and related behaviors.

Also based on neuropsychological findings, prevention has become more unified at conceptual level, and a number of problematic behaviors, including antisocial and violent behavior, substance use, and pathological use of computer and the Internet, today are targeted often with the same interventions. The need for a strong evidence base, critical reflection of practice, and adequate training of the staff involved remains central to all these approaches.

In terms of gender differences, a number of program evaluations found, overall, less or no effects for girls. One possible explanation might be a lower vulnerability at baseline, which could also reflect the fact that neurobehavioral disinhibition is found more frequently in boys. Alternative hypotheses are that these interventions are less appealing to girls or that the timing of delivery with regard to their cognitive, social, and emotional development is less appropriate, since girls mature earlier. So girls who, overall, use psychoactive substances less and have fewer problems might also gain less from existing prevention programs.

7.3.3 Implementation

Overall, the field still seems to be dominated by interventions that might attract more public attention than be effective in changing and sustaining consumption behavior. Policy interest in selective prevention has increased, but this has not translated into better interventions for vulnerable youth or more evaluation research. There has been some recent interest in indicated prevention in Europe, and well-designed evaluation studies have taken place, but the intervention coverage as such is still limited to a few countries. Too many prevention interventions continue to appeal to cognitive processes only, namely, information provision, regardless of the lacking evidence. Policy makers and professionals have only reluctantly begun to acknowledge that social norms and their perception (environmental prevention) as well as impulse control (indicated prevention) are powerful determinants of adolescent behavior. The potential for addressing emotional and unconscious processes in prevention is virtually unacknowledged.

But on the implementation side also, promising developments can be found:

- There is a (limited) number of prevention programs with well-proven evidence of effectiveness that are relatively easy to implement through manuals and other supporting materials. Better use could be made of these interventions.
- A further potential lies in the complementary approach of developing environmental prevention strategies at local level, which provide safe and nurturing environments within and around schools (no outlets nearby), at nightlife venues, and during leisure time. These are, for example, the key component of the so-called Icelandic approach [39].
- Web-based offers are already widespread and should be developed further. BI and MI can serve as tools. While prevention has been traditionally linked to school curricula, and TV, today, Internet and social media approaches play an important role which should be further developed.

- Standards can help to better implement new programs and interventions. Since the publication of the international standards for prevention by UNODC and the European drug prevention quality standards (EDPQS), a steadily increasing number of countries are introducing such quality standards in their own strategies.
- A unified prevention training syllabus for relevant professionals has the potential to improve prevention systems by developing skills and competences in evidence-based prevention. The Universal Prevention Curriculum (UPC)[2] is a first step into this direction. Based on the UNODC standards of evidence and the EDPQS it transmits key competences such as needs and resource assessment, selection and implementation of interventions and/or policies, and monitoring and evaluation. A much shortened European version is now available the EUPC https://www.emcdda.europa.eu/best-practice/european-prevention-curriculum.
- Very heterogeneous professional cultures, beliefs, and assumptions are a challenge for transferring the progress made in prevention science into routine practice. In order to achieve this, further training and development of the prevention workforce is crucial.
- A focus on informational and educational approaches is still common in many countries despite the known limited evidence to their effectiveness.
- Despite often necessary adjustments to national culture and conditions, the transfer of well-developed prevention programs mainly from Northern America has shown to provide a considerable chance to improve the quality of services also in other parts of the world.

Taking all these elements together, we do see prevention as highly promising tools to work on substance-related behaviors and problems. There has been a considerable number of developments in recent years, and more investment in research, training of professionals, and especially implementation of findings from preventions science would seem a good investment.

---

[2]https://www.issup.net/training/universal-prevention-curriculum

References

1. Agrawal A, Madden PAF, Martin NG, Lynskey MT. Do early experiences with cannabis vary in cigarette smokers? Drug Alcohol Depend. 2013;128(3):255–9. https://doi.org/10.1016/j.drugalcdep.2012.09.002.
2. Allara E, Ferri M, Bo A, Gasparrini A, Faggiano F. Are mass-media campaigns effective in preventing drug use? A Cochrane systematic review and meta-analysis. BMJ Open. 2015;5(9):e007449. https://doi.org/10.1136/bmjopen-2014-007449.
3. Bronfenbrenner U. The ecology of human development: experiments by nature and design. Cambridge, MA: Harvard University Press; 1979.
4. Bröning S, Kumpfer K, Kruse K, Sack PM, Schaunig-Busch I, Ruths S, et al. Selective prevention programs for children from substance-affected families: a comprehensive systematic review. Subst Abuse Treat Prev Policy. 2012;7(1):23. https://doi.org/10.1186/1747-597X-7-23.
5. Bühler A, Thrul J (2015) Prevention of addictive behaviours. Updated and extended version of Prevention of Substance Abuse. Luxembourg. doi: https://doi.org/10.2810/742866.
6. Bühringer G, Rumpf HJ. Future of addiction treatment: Plea for a paradigmatic change. Sucht. 2018;64(3):125–8.
7. Calafat A, García F, Juan M, Becoña E, Fernández-Hermida JR. Which parenting style is more protective against adolescent substance use? Evidence within the European context. Drug Alcohol Depend. 2014;138:185. https://doi.org/10.1016/j.drugalcdep.2014.02.705.
8. Carney T, Myers BJ, Louw J, Okwundu CI. Brief school-based interventions and behavioural outcomes for substance-using adolescents. In: Carney T, editor. Cochrane database of systematic reviews. Chichester: John Wiley and Sons, Ltd.; 2014. https://doi.org/10.1002/14651858.CD008969.pub2.
9. Comello MLG. Characterizing drug non-users as distinctive in prevention messages: implications of optimal distinctiveness theory. Health Commun. 2011;26(4):313–22. https://doi.org/10.1080/10410236.2010.550022.
10. Crano WD. Applying established theories of persuasion to problems that matter: on becoming susceptible to our own knowledge. In: Forgas JP, Cooper J, Crano WD, editors. The psychology of attitudes and attitude change. New York: Psychology Press; 2010.
11. Danielsson AK, Wennberg P, Hibell B, Romelsjö A. Alcohol use, heavy episodic drinking and subsequent problems among adolescents in 23 European countries: does the prevention paradox apply? Addiction. 2012;107(1):71–80. https://doi.org/10.1111/j.1360-0443.2011.03537.x.
12. de Wit H, Phillips TJ. Do initial responses to drugs predict future use or abuse? Neurosci Biobehav Rev. 2012;36(6):1565–76. https://doi.org/10.1016/j.neubiorev.2012.04.005.

13. EMCDDA. Responding to drug use and related problems in recreational settings. Luxembourg: Publications Office of the European Union; 2012.

14. EMCDDA. Drug testing in schools. Luxembourg: Publications Office of the European Union; 2017a. Retrieved from http://www.emcdda.europa.eu/system/files/publications/6575/tdau17003enn.pdf.

15. EMCDDA. m-Health applications for responding to drug use and associated harms. Luxembourg: Publications Office of the European Union; 2018. https://doi.org/10.2810/379921.

16. Faggiano F, Minozzi S, Versino E, Buscemi D. Universal school-based prevention for illicit drug use. In: Faggiano F, editor. Cochrane database of systematic reviews. Chichester: John Wiley and Sons; 2014. https://doi.org/10.1002/14651858.CD003020.

17. Foxcroft DR, Coombes L, Wood S, Allen D, Almeida Santimano NML, Moreira MT. Motivational interviewing for the prevention of alcohol misuse in young adults. In: Foxcroft DR, editor. Cochrane database of systematic reviews, vol. 7. Chichester: John Wiley and Sons; 2016. https://doi.org/10.1002/14651858.CD007025.

18. Foxcroft DR, Tsertsvadze A. Universal family-based prevention programs for alcohol misuse in young people. Cochrane Database Sys Rev. 1469–493X (Electronic). 2011:CD009308.

19. García OF, Serra E, Zacarés JJ, García F. Parenting styles and short- and long-term socialization outcomes: a study among Spanish adolescents and older adults. Psychosoc Interv. 2018;27(3):153–61. https://doi.org/10.5093/pi2018a21.

20. Glass JE, Hamilton AM, Powell BJ, Perron BE, Brown RT, Ilgen MA. Revisiting our review of Screening, Brief Intervention and Referral to Treatment (SBIRT): meta-analytical results still point to no efficacy in increasing the use of substance use disorder services. Addiction. 2016;111(1):181–3. https://doi.org/10.1111/add.13146.

21. Hale DR, Viner RM. Policy responses to multiple risk behaviours in adolescents. J Public Health. 2012;34(Suppl 1):i11–9. https://doi.org/10.1093/pubmed/fdr112.

22. Hill KG, Hawkins JD, Bailey JA, Catalano RF, Abbott RD, Shapiro VB. Person-environment interaction in the prediction of alcohol abuse and alcohol dependence in adulthood. Drug Alcohol Depend. 2010;110(1–2):62–9. https://doi.org/10.1016/j.drugalcdep.2010.02.005.

23. Hughes K, Quigg Z, Eckley L, Bellis M, Jones L, Calafat A, et al. Environmental factors in drinking venues and alcohol-related harm: the evidence base for European intervention. Addiction. 2011;106(Suppl 1):37–46. https://doi.org/10.1111/j.1360-0443.2010.03316.x.

24. Kam JA, Middleton AV. The associations between parents' references to their own past substance use and youth's substance-use beliefs and behaviors: a comparison of Latino and European American youth.

Hum Commun Res. 2013;39(2):208–29. https://doi.org/10.1111/hcre.12001.

25. Koning IM, Maric M, MacKinnon D, Vollebergh WAM. Effects of a combined parent-student alcohol prevention program on intermediate factors and adolescents' drinking behavior: a sequential mediation model. J Consult Clin Psychol. 2015;83(4):719–27. https://doi.org/10.1037/a0039197.

26. Koning IM, Verdurmen JEE, Engels RCME, Van den Eijnden RJJM, Vollebergh WAM. Differential impact of a Dutch alcohol prevention program targeting adolescents and parents separately and simultaneously: low self-control and lenient parenting at baseline predict effectiveness. Prev Sci. 2012;13(3):278–87. https://doi.org/10.1007/s11121-011-0267-9.

27. Kurtz SP, Surratt HL, Buttram ME, Levi-Minzi M, Chen M. Interview as intervention: the case of young adult multidrug users in the club scene. J Subst Abus Treat. 2013;44(3):301–8. https://doi.org/10.1016/j.jsat.2012.08.004.

28. Lamb CS, Crano WD. Parents' beliefs and children's marijuana use: evidence for a self-fulfilling prophecy effect. Addict Behav. 2014;39(1):127–32. https://doi.org/10.1016/j.addbeh.2013.09.009.

29. Livingstone AG, McCafferty S. Explaining reactions to normative information about alcohol consumption: a test of an extended social identity model. Int J Drug Policy. 2015;26(4):388–95. https://doi.org/10.1016/j.drugpo.2014.10.005.

30. McAlaney J, Bewick B, Hughes C. The international development of the "Social Norms" approach to drug education and prevention. Drug Educ Prev Polic. 2011;18(2):81–9. https://doi.org/10.3109/09687631003610977.

31. McMorris BJ, Catalano RF, Kim MJ, Toumbourou JW, Hemphill SA. Influence of family factors and supervised alcohol use on adolescent alcohol use and harms: similarities between youth in different alcohol policy contexts. J Stud Alcohol Drugs. 2011;72(3):418–28. Retrieved from http://www.ncbi.nlm.nih.gov/pmc/articles/PMC3084357/.

32. Midford R. Drug prevention programmes for young people: where have we been and where should we be going? Addiction. 2010;105(10):1688–95.

33. Miller BA, Holder HD, Voas RB. Environmental strategies for prevention of drug use and risks in clubs. J Subst Abus. 2009;14(1):19–38. https://doi.org/10.1080/14659890802305887.

34. Moodie R, Stuckler D, Monteiro C, Sheron N, Neal B, Thamarangsi T, et al. Profits and pandemics: prevention of harmful effects of tobacco, alcohol, and ultra-processed food and drink industries. Lancet. 2013;381(9867):670–9. https://doi.org/10.1016/S0140-6736(12)62089-3.

35. Mrazek PJ, Haggerty RJ. Reducing risks for mental disorders: frontiers for preventive intervention research. Washington, DC: National Academy Press; 1994.

36. O'Leary-Barrett M, Castellanos-Ryan N, Pihl RO, Conrod PJ. Mechanisms of personality-targeted intervention effects on adolescent alcohol misuse, internalizing and externalizing symptoms. J Consult Clin Psychol. 2016;84(5):438–52. https://doi.org/10.1037/ccp0000082.

37. Paternoster R. The deterrent effect of the perceived certainty and severity of punishment: a review of the evidence and issues. Justice Q. 1987;4(2):173–217. Retrieved from http://libra.msra.cn/Publication/42492252/the-deterrent-effect-of-the-perceived-certainty-and-severity-of-punishment-a-review-of-the.

38. Plunk AD, Cavazaos-Rehg P, Bierut LJ, Grucza RA. The persistent effects of minimum legal drinking age laws on drinking patterns later in life. Alcohol Clin Exp Res. 2013;37(3):463–9. https://doi.org/10.1111/j.1530-0277.2012.01945.x.

39. Sigfúsdóttir ID, Thorlindsson T, Kristjánsson ÁL, Roe KM, Allegrante JP, Kristjánsson AL, et al. Substance use prevention for adolescents: the Icelandic Model. Health Promot Int. 2009;24(1):16–25. https://doi.org/10.1093/heapro/dan038.

40. Simon R, Burkhart G. Regional and cultural aspects of prevention. In: El-Guebaly N, Carrà G, Galanter M, editors. Textbook of addiction treatment: international perspectives. Milano: Springer Milan; 2015. https://doi.org/10.1007/978-88-470-5322-9_134.

41. Sloboda Z, Glantz MD, Tarter RE. Revisiting the concepts of risk and protective factors for understanding the etiology and development of substance use and substance use disorders: implications for prevention. Subs Use Misuse. 2012;47(8–9):944–62. https://doi.org/10.3109/10826084.2012.663280.

42. Smedslund G, Berg RC, Hammerstrøm KT, Steiro A, Leiknes KA, Dahl HM, Karlsen K. Motivational interviewing for substance abuse. Cochrane Database of Systematic Reviews Online. John Wiley and Sons; 2011. doi: https://doi.org/10.1002/14651858.CD008063.

43. Tanner-Smith EE, Durlak JA, Marx RA. Empirically based mean effect size distributions for universal prevention programs targeting school-aged youth: a review of meta-analyses. Prev Sci. 2018;19(8):1091–101. https://doi.org/10.1007/s11121-018-0942-1.

44. Tanner-Smith EE, Lipsey MW. Brief alcohol interventions for adolescents and young adults: a systematic review and meta-analysis. J Subst Abus

Treat. 2015;51:1–18. https://doi.org/10.1016/j.jsat.2014.09.001.

45. Toumbourou JW, Stockwell T, Neighbors C, Marlatt GA, Sturge J. Interventions to reduce harm associated with adolescent substance use. Lancet. 2007;369(9570):1391–401.

46. UNODC. International standards on drug use prevention. 2nd ed. Vienna: United Nations; 2018. Retrieved from http://www.unodc.org/documents/prevention/prevention_standards.pdf.

47. Vigna-Taglianti FD, Galanti MR, Burkhart G, Caria MP, Vadrucci S, Faggiano F. "Unplugged," a European school-based program for substance use prevention among adolescents: overview of results from the EU-Dap trial. New Dir Youth Dev. 2014;2014(141):67–82, 11–12. https://doi.org/10.1002/yd.20087.

48. Viner RM, Ozer EM, Denny S, Marmot M, Resnick M, Fatusi A, Currie C. Adolescence and the social determinants of health. Lancet. 2012;379(9826):1641–52. https://doi.org/10.1016/S0140-6736(12)60149-4.

49. Wagenaar AC, Tobler AL, Komro KA. Effects of alcohol tax and price policies on morbidity and mortality: a systematic review. Am J Public Health. 2010;100(11):2270–8. https://doi.org/10.2105/AJPH.2009.186007.

50. Wakefield MA, Loken B, Hornik RC. Use of mass media campaigns to change health behaviour. Lancet. 2010;376(9748):1261–71. https://doi.org/10.1016/S0140-6736(10)60809-4.

Further Reading

EMCDDA. European drug prevention quality standards: a manual for prevention professionals. Luxembourg: Publications Office of the European Union; 2011.

EMCDDA. Health and social responses to drug problems. A European guide. Luxembourg: Publications of the European Union; 2017.

Oncioiu SI, Burkhart G, Calafat A, Duch M, Perman-Howe P, Foxcroft DR. Environmental substance use prevention interventions in Europe. EMCDDA: Lisbon; 2018.

Strang J, Babor T, Caulkins J, Fischer B, Foxcroft D, Humphreys K. Drug policy and the public good: evidence for effective interventions. Lancet. 2012;379(9810):71–83.

Diagnostic Definitions and Classification of Substance Use Disorders

8

John B. Saunders and Noeline C. Latt

Contents

Abstract

Diagnostic terms exist to identify forms of substance use which are causing clinical impairment or risk and to distinguish them from normality. Both repetitive substance use and single-occasion use exist along a gradation of severity. Repetitive substance use which confers the risk of harmful consequences is termed Hazardous Substance Use,

J. B. Saunders (✉)
Centre for Youth Substance Abuse Research, University of Queensland, St Lucia, QLD, Australia

Disciplines of Psychiatry and Addiction Medicine, Faculty of Medicine, University of Sydney, Camperdown, NSW, Australia
e-mail: mail@jbsaunders.net

N. C. Latt
Disciplines of Psychiatry and Addiction Medicine, Faculty of Medicine, University of Sydney, Camperdown, NSW, Australia

Formerly Northern Area Drug and Alcohol Service, Royal North Shore Hospital, St Leonards, NSW, Australia
e-mail: Unknown_6574809@Meteor.com

© Springer Nature Switzerland AG 2021
N. el-Guebaly et al. (eds.), *Textbook of Addiction Treatment*,
https://doi.org/10.1007/978-3-030-36391-8_8

which is a new diagnostic term in the latest (eleventh) revision of the International Classification of Diseases (ICD-11). Harmful Substance Use in ICD-10 and ICD-11 denotes repetitive substance use which has caused physical or mental harm but where the guidelines for the diagnosis of Substance Dependence have not been met. At the top of this hierarchy in ICD-10 and ICD-11 is Substance Dependence. This is defined as a psychobiological syndrome that is a disorder of regulation of substance use. It comprises impaired control over substance use, continued use of the substance despite harmful consequences and often increased tolerance and withdrawal symptoms. It is underpinned by enduring neurobiological changes in brain reward, stress, salience and control systems, which result in an "internal driving force" to use and continue to use a substance (or group of substances) in a self-perpetuating way. The most recent (fifth) edition of the Diagnostic and Statistical Manual of Mental Disorders (DSM-5) changed the diagnostic landscape with its deletion of its forerunner, DSM-IV's diagnoses of Substance Dependence and Substance Abuse (which denoted a maladaptive and repetitive pattern of substance use causing social problems), and replacing them with a broader condition of "substance use disorder" that can exist in varying degrees of severity (mild, moderate or severe) depending on the number of criteria fulfilled. In addition to these forms of repetitive substance use, single-occasion use may lead to substance intoxication (in both ICD and DSM), and episode of Harmful Substance Use (ICD-11). Where substance use is curtailed in substance-dependent individuals, substance withdrawal can occur, this being a cluster of symptoms and features specific to the substance taken. In general, the features of substance withdrawal are opposite to those of the pharmacological effects of the substance concerned. There are also numerous mental and neurocognitive sequelae which occur in both the ICD and DSM systems, some with rather different diagnostic names and definitions. They

include substance-induced mental disorders, such as substance-induced mood disorder, and similarly termed anxiety disorder, psychotic disorder, sleep-wake disorder, sexual dysfunction, obsessive-compulsive disorders, and substance-induced delirium. Neurocognitive disorders include substance-induced amnestic syndrome and substance-induced dementia. The ICD system also has comprehensive coverage of all physical disorders induced by psychoactive substance use. DSM-5 does not include the medical/physical complications of substance use and has abandoned the multiaxial system, which included (as Axis III) associated physical conditions. For all these disorders, diagnosis is based on a set of specific diagnostic guidelines (ICD) or criteria (DSM), which reflect the substance used, the pattern of use and the specific features of the disorder.

8.1 Introduction and Background

8.1.1 Introduction

Psychoactive substance use exists as a continuum and substance use disorders as a hierarchy. Some forms of substance use in small amounts, for example, alcohol, are not harmful, or at least low risk. Other psychoactive substances such as prescribed opioids or benzodiazepines are medically necessary and appropriate in many situations. Illicit drugs, such as cannabis (marijuana), may have functional value to some people, and there may be a threshold of use for some beneath which little harm occurs. The line between substances which are medically prescribed and those which are medically inappropriate (and typically illegal) is becoming increasingly blurred, with the more widespread use of psychostimulants for various disorders and the availability of medicinal cannabinoids (and in some countries legally available cannabis (marijuana) and the prescribing, albeit uncommonly, of oxybate (gamma-hydroxybutyric acid) as a treatment for alcohol dependence. A fundamental property of all the substances covered by this chapter is their inherent capacity to cause intoxicating effects and reinforcement of use and to induce neurobiological processes that lead to Substance Dependence/Addiction, withdrawal syndromes (in most cases) and a range of physical, neurocognitive, psychological and social harms.

Diagnoses are made to facilitate communication between different healthcare providers and to provide a basis for an intervention. Diagnosis is an intellectual discipline characteristic of medicine that seeks to define the patient's symptoms, behaviours and clinical features and match them against an array of human disorders such that the disorder that most satisfactorily covers what the patient experiences is selected. The intellectual process underlying diagnosis also serves to distinguish the patient's condition from normality. Some diagnoses indicate forms of substance use that confer the risk of harmful consequences in the future, others a syndromal disorder and others a complicating disorder or impairment. A coherent system of diagnosis and classification provides a vital structure for the practice of addiction medicine.

The present time is a period of considerable change in diagnostic concepts and terms. The latest edition (the fifth) of one of the principal diagnostic systems, the Diagnostic and Statistical Manual of Mental Disorders (DSM-5), was published by the American Psychiatric Association (APA) in 2013 [4]. In mid-2019, the latest revision (the eleventh) of the International Classification of Diseases, which is the international basis for disease, morbidity and mortality diagnosis and coding, was approved by the World Health Organization (WHO) [72]. Whereas there was considerable similarity between the major substance use diagnoses in their forerunners DSM-IV and ICD-10, there is a divergence in the central disorders of repetitive substance use in DSM-5 and ICD-11. Specifically, ICD-11 has retained the central ICD-10 [70] diagnoses of Substance Dependence and Harmful Substance Use, with some modifications, whereas DSM-5 has combined the DSM-IV diagnoses of Substance Dependence and Substance Abuse [3]

into an umbrella diagnosis of substance use disorder [4]. Many addiction medicine specialists in North America and elsewhere adopt the diagnostic concepts and criteria developed by the American Society of Addiction Medicine (ASAM) and the International Society of Addiction Medicine (ISAM) [5, 25]. The conceptual understanding of substance disorders is rather different in these formulations, and the diagnostic criteria have only passing resemblance to those employed in the DSM and ICD systems. A further contrast is provided by the emphasis in the fields of epidemiology and public health on quantification of substance use and not to define specific behavioural or psychophysiological disorders.

It will be apparent from the foregoing comments that a synthesis of diagnostic concepts in the current classification systems is not possible. In this chapter, we shall present a history of common concepts of substance use disorders and then review the key diagnoses in the current international diagnostic systems. Before this, we shall briefly review the range of addictive (dependence-inducing) and potentially harmful psychoactive substances and also the patterns of substance use that need to be captured by a diagnostic classification system.

8.1.2 The Range of Addictive Substances

There are many thousands of naturally occurring and synthetic substances that have the capacity to induce addiction, and new ones are continually being synthesised. Substances with addictive potential tend to have acute psychological effects which consumers find pleasant, at least initially and in the majority of cases. They tend to cause euphoria and, in many cases, a sense of relaxation. Certain substances are valued because they relieve pain or sickness and therefore are described as having a medicinal effect as opposed to a primary hedonic one. The pharmacokinetic properties of the substance influence its addictive potential, with the rapidity of absorption (and therefore action), ease of penetrating the blood/

brain barrier and duration of action influencing the likelihood of recurrent self-administration and therefore addiction. Addictive potential is also influenced by the mode of administration, with the smoking and intravenous injecting routes inducing more rapid addiction than oral ingestion. Addictive substances tend to have a biphasic action, whereby the hedonic effect is typically followed by negative symptoms consequent on declining blood and tissue levels of the substance. The neurobiological changes which occur in this phase could be regarded as "restorative", with the aim of returning neuronal systems to their normal functioning state.

The propensity of psychoactive substances to induce addiction therefore ranges considerably depending on the mode of administration, the substance's pharmacodynamic and pharmacokinetic properties, individual vulnerability and also the social setting in which the substance is taken. Caffeine as occurs in coffee, tea and certain soft drinks and once considered a minor stimulant at the lowest end of the addiction spectrum is listed in DSM-5, ICD-10 and ICD-11. Certain other substances have psychoactive properties and are harmful but are not or only rarely addictive. These include most of the hallucinogens, where the acute psychoactive effects (often of a psychedelic or psychotomimetic nature) commonly result in clinical presentations but where addiction/dependence is uncommon. Other substances such as sugar and certain commercial soft drinks exist in a borderline area where addiction is described but is not typical and is often rare. Substances in this last domain will not be further considered in the present chapter.

Many prescribed and proprietary ("over the counter") medications have addictive potential. Because of the therapeutic benefits (and commercial value) of these medications, there has been controversy as to whether they should be termed addictive substances as opposed to their inducing physiological dependence. The DSM system has an exclusion for tolerance and withdrawal as diagnostic criteria where the drug has been prescribed medically. There is a divergence of opinion between those who would exclude medication

use when it is being prescribed by a medical practitioner and those authorities who regard the occurrence of a desire for repeated administration of such medications and the occurrence of withdrawal symptoms to indicate that addictive processes are present in the individual. This debate has entered the public domain with the huge and increasing number of deaths in the USA and many other countries from prescribed opioids, the risks of overdose and clear evidence of their addictive capacity.

Both the ICD and DSM systems aim to encompass the range of psychoactive substances used recreationally and medically. Substances may be used individually, but increasingly, they are used in combinations, each of which has its own psychiatric and physical morbidities [15]. ICD-11 has an expanded listing of psychoactive substance groups in its primary structure. This reflects the emergence in many parts of the world of new psychoactive substances such as synthetic cannabinoids, synthetic psychostimulants and hallucinogens [40]. Table 8.1 compares and contrasts those substances covered in DSM-IV, DSM-5, ICD-10 and ICD-11.

8.1.3 Mechanisms Underlying Repetitive Substance Use

There are numerous psychological and social influences which determine whether a substance with psychoactive properties is actually used, periodically or repeatedly, and may potentially lead to harmful consequences and addiction. An important determinant is the availability of a particular substance in a society, and this in turn may be determined by whether it is of plant origin and requires particular climatic conditions or level of rainfall to grow. Other substances are chemically synthesised and require a corresponding level of knowledge and technical equipment to produce.

Psychological mechanisms are involved in substance use becoming repetitive use, and classical conditioning theory, operant conditioning theory and social learning theory [8] all contribute to our understanding of how this eventuates.

Table 8.1 Coverage of psychoactive substance groups in DSM-IV and DSM-5 and ICD-10 and ICD-11

Class	DSM-IV	DSM-5	ICD-10	ICD-11	Comments
CNS depressants	Alcohol	Alcohol	Alcohol	Alcohol	
	Cannabis	Cannabis	Cannabinoids	Cannabis	
				Synthetic cannabinoids	
	Inhalants	Inhalants	Volatile solvents	Volatile inhalants	
	Opioids[a]	Opioids[a]	Opioids[a]	Opioids[a]	
	Sedatives, hypnotics or anxiolytics	Sedatives, hypnotics or anxiolytics	Sedative-hypnotics	Sedatives, hypnotics or anxiolytics	
	Nicotine	Tobacco	Tobacco	Nicotine	
CNS stimulants	Caffeine	Caffeine	Other stimulants including caffeine	Caffeine	
	Amphetamines	Stimulants		Stimulants including amphetamines, methamphetamine or methcathinone	The stimulants category in DSM-5 includes amphetamine-type substances, cocaine and other or unspecified stimulants. For some diagnoses, the type of substance can be specified
				Synthetic cathinones	
	Cocaine		Cocaine	Cocaine	
Hallucinogens, Empathogens and dissociative drugs	Hallucinogens	Hallucinogens	Hallucinogens	Dissociative drugs including ketamine and phencyclidine	In DSM-5, there are separate descriptions for phencyclidine and for other hallucinogens. MDMA is classified under other hallucinogens
	Phencyclidine			Hallucinogens	
				MDMA and related drugs including MDA	
Polysubstance use	Polysubstance		Multiple drug use and use of other psychoactive substances		The category polysubstance use does not appear in DSM-5 or ICD 11
Other and unknown substances	Other substances	Other or unknown substances		Other specified psychoactive substances	There is no category for unknown or unspecified substances in DSM-IV
				Unknown or unspecified psychoactive substances	

[a]Includes prescription opioids

The reader is referred to suitable reviews for further reference.

Neurobiological mechanisms come into play in particular when a pattern of repetitive substance use has developed and result in that repetitive use tending to become more stereotyped and self-perpetuating, being driven by internal cues rather than external circumstances. The essential result of the neurobiological mechanisms of addiction is the generation of an internal driving force, which is enduring and which promotes further substance use even in the absence of external cues and continues to do so even when circumstances are inappropriate for substance use and the person may actually be experiencing harm as a result of that use. The driving force of what is termed Substance Dependence or Addiction results in substance use occupying a more and more central role in the person's life, with other interests, enjoyments, activities and responsibilities being relegated to the periphery. Much has been learnt about the neurobiological processes, and it appears there are interlinked neurocircuits which are "reset" in a person with addiction. These subserve reward, alertness (excitation) and salience on behavioural control.

In summary, in the early period of psychoactive substance use, that use is influenced strongly by external circumstances and also by the person's mood state. As repeated use continues and dependence develops, the repetitive use reflects more the internal neurobiological mechanisms that have developed. It is these mechanisms that result in repetitive substance use becoming more and more syndromal and to produce the clinical disorders we recognise as addiction.

8.2 Concepts of Substance Use Disorders

8.2.1 Personality Disorder

In the first edition of DSM, published in 1952, substance misuse was included in the personality disorders [1]. Drug addiction was not specifically defined, but there was a statement that it was usually symptomatic of a personality disorder. The second edition, published in 1968 [2], had substance use disorders classified within the personality disorders. There were no specific definitions or criteria and little description of the conditions. The diagnosis of drug dependence required "evidence of habitual use or a clear sense of a need for the drug" [2].

8.2.2 The Disease Concept

Many groups view substance use disorders as reflecting a disease process, which is biologically determined and results in the individual having an individualistic reaction to a psychoactive substance and a relatively predictable natural history. This conceptualisation influenced and was subsequently embraced by the self-help movements, such as Alcoholic Anonymous. Jellinek developed the concept of the disease of alcoholism in the 1940s and 1950s [26], although in his later work he increasingly recognised the role of environmental influences. During the 1960s and 1970s, the concept that substance misuse might represent a disease process was dismissed by most scientists and professionals. Likewise, the role of genetic predisposition was thought to be inconsequential, with the familial aggregation of substance misuse explained by cultural influences, role modelling or malfunction within families. With the increasing understanding of neurobiological changes underpinning Substance Dependence/Addiction, the concept of their being a primary disease entity has become more popular with statements such as "addiction is a brain disease" [35]. The question is more whether addiction is a primary disease or an acquired one, with most recent neurobiological data indicating the latter. This is discussed further below.

8.2.3 Epidemiological and Sociological Formulations

A third tradition may be described as the epidemiological and sociological one. Put simply, substance misuse and problems arise fundamentally because of the overall level of use of that particular substance in society. In the 1950s, Ledermann [32] proposed a relationship between the level of alcohol consumption in a community and the prevalence of alcoholism. The level of use is, in turn, influenced by the availability of alcohol, its manufacture and distribution, its price (importantly) and cultural traditions and sanctions. Inherent in these conceptualisations is that individual pathology is considered of secondary importance. The social constructionist school views substance use problems as disaggregated, with no special relationship among them. This school of thought was concerned about the stigma attributable to diagnostic labels and the potential of treatment as a form of social control [48].

8.2.4 Learnt Behaviour

The 1970s saw the rise of social cognitive theory [8] as an influential paradigm to explain the development and resolution of alcohol and drug problems. This school of thought teaches that the (many) influences that determined behaviour in general apply to the uptake of substance use and the development of disordered use. Positive consequences encourage repeated use, negative ones the opposite. Patterns of substance use behaviour could become established in this way, but equally, repetitive substance use could be "unlearnt". This led to the development of a range of cognitive behavioural therapies, some of which aimed at moderated or "controlled" substance use.

8.2.5 Clinical Syndrome

The need for an understanding of substance misuse which spanned these various discipline-bound conceptualisations and terms was largely met by the formulation of the concept of a "substance dependence syndrome" originally proposed with regard to alcohol dependence by Edwards and Gross in 1976 [19]. The basis of the dependence syndrome was a clinical description of key clinical features in a way that was essentially theoretical and was not based on any aetiological understanding of the disorder, be it biological, behavioural or sociological. Rather, certain experiences, behaviours and symptoms related to repetitive alcohol use were identified as tending to cluster in time and to occur repeatedly. The advantage of a descriptive account of dependence is that it can accommodate aetiological models but not be beholden to them.

The concept of the dependence syndrome applies to many other psychoactive substances that have the potential for reinforcement of use, including benzodiazepines, illicit and prescribed opioids, cannabis, inhalants, psychostimulants such as cocaine and the amphetamines, nicotine, caffeine and anabolic steroids [21, 39, 51, 65]. It may also apply to repetitive behaviours that do not involve self-administration of a psychoactive substance. These include pathological gambling and compulsive shopping and exercise [34, 42]. "Disordered gambling" has now been added to DSM-5 [4].

The dependence syndrome has been at the heart of the classification systems of psychoactive substance use disorders since the 1980s [57]. It is the principal substance use disorder in DSM-IV [3], ICD-10 [70] and ICD-11 [72]. However, in DSM-5, the dependence syndrome is subsumed under substance use disorder [4].

8.2.6 Neurobiological Disorder

Neurobiological mechanisms come into play particularly when a pattern of repeated use has become established. They induce a driving force to use the substance in preference to other human activities or interests and do so in a continuing and seemingly compulsive way. They cause reinforcement and indeed self-perpetuation of psychoactive substance use. Increases in tolerance favour consumption of larger and larger doses of the substance. The three key neurobiological changes in dependence are as follows:

(i) Activation and then inhibition of brain reward systems, particularly involving dopaminergic transmission and opioidergic transmission. These have the effect of resetting the reward systems such that larger amounts of the substance are needed to produce the desired effect and natural rewards are not as reinforcing [67, 68].

(ii) Recruitment of brain stress systems, including those subserved by glutamate neurotransmission and corticotrophin-releasing factor (CRF) [29] and suppression or uncoupling of antistress systems [49].

(iii) Impairment of inhibitory control pathways from the prefrontal cortex to the mesolimbic systems, resulting in impaired decision-making capacity [73].

(iv) Resetting of the salience circuitry arising from the cingulate gyrus of the frontal lobe and changing the importance of substance use relative to other interest, activities and responsibilities [28].

A publication on the neuroscience of addiction by the World Health Organization summarises the key developments in biomedical research over this period [71].

8.2.7 Genetic Influences

Investigations into possible genetic influences have accompanied this research on neural circuitry. Biometric genetic studies have shown that children born of parents with Substance Dependence are more likely to have Substance Dependence themselves [56] and that this is largely explained by genetic transmission rather than environmental factors [16, 17, 33, 56]. Genomic analysis in human and laboratory animals has identified several areas of the genome where mutations are associated with increased risk of substance use disorders [16, 17, 20].

8.3 Diagnoses Applied to Use of Psychoactive Substances in DSM-IV, DSM-5, ICD-10 and ICD-11

8.3.1 Overview

The current versions of the DSM and ICD systems are DSM-5 [4] and ICD-10 [70], respectively. In May 2019, ICD-11 was formally published by the World Health Organization (WHO). Accordingly, the diagnoses listed and discussed in this section will include those in DSM-5, ICD-10 and ICD-11. In addition, certain DSM-IV diagnoses [3] will be described as they are well known and much of the empirical basis for modern treatment draws upon them as the basis for recruitment into both pharmacological and psychological therapies. DSM-IV and ICD-10 diagnoses were developed almost simul-

taneously and were underpinned by the US National Institute of Health Joint Project on Diagnosis and Classification [55].

The DSM and ICD systems differ in their emphasis. The DSM system focuses on the needs of clinicians and researchers and encompasses the range of mental, behavioural and addictive diagnoses. Diagnostic criteria are provided for each diagnosis and these are quite specific.

The ICD system, which is overseen by the WHO, is a compendium of all human disorders including physical and psychiatric disorders, external causes such as trauma and also health risk factors. In addition to being a resource for clinicians and researchers, it is also the basis for the systematic recording, compilation and analysis of morbidity and mortality statistics worldwide. The ICD listing includes definitions of all the disorders. For mental, behavioural and addictive disorders, there is a more detailed version also containing diagnostic guidelines and explanatory material which is termed the ICD Clinical Descriptions and Diagnostic Guidelines (CDDG). The term "diagnostic guidelines" is employed in the ICD in preference to the term diagnostic criteria to emphasise the more flexible nature of the guidance provided, which is intended to allow scope for clinical judgement and cultural variations. It attempts to avoid strict cut-offs in duration or symptom count, unless these have been widely accepted and specifically validated [22]. The ICD-11 has also been developed with an explicit public health framework [45], and this is evident from the spectrum of repetitive substance use ranging from hazardous use, harmful use and Substance Dependence that it incorporates (Fig. 8.1). It comprises diagnoses which reflect a single occasion of use (substance intoxication and episode of Harmful Substance Use) and those which reflect a pattern of repeated use.

8.3.1.1 Substance Intoxication (ICD-10, ICD-11, DSM-IV, DSM-5)
(See Table 8.2)
Substance intoxication is an episode of excessive use, producing clinically significant pharmaco-

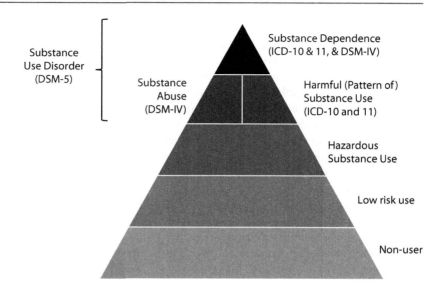

Fig. 8.1 Pyramid ICD-10, ICD-11, DSM-IV, DSM-5

Table 8.2 Diagnostic guidelines for substance intoxication (DSM-5, ICD-10, ICD-11)

	DSM-5	ICD-10	ICD-11
Primary definition	Acute intoxication is a transient condition following administration of a psychoactive substance resulting in disturbance of level of consciousness, cognition, perception, affect or behaviour or other psycho-physiological functions and responses. Symptoms of intoxication are substance specific and may produce different types of effect at different levels	A transient condition following the administration of alcohol or other psychoactive substances, resulting in disturbances in level of consciousness, cognition, perception, affect or behaviour, or other psycho-physiological functions and responses	Substance intoxication is a clinically significant transient condition that develops during or shortly after the consumption of a substance that is characterized by disturbances in consciousness, cognition, perception, affect, behaviour or coordination. These disturbances are caused by the known pharmacological effects of the substance, and their intensity is closely related to the amount of substance consumed. They are time limited and abate as the substance is cleared from the body
Additional guidelines and text	Acute intoxication is closely related to dose levels. Exceptions occur with certain underlying organic conditions such as renal or hepatic insufficiency where smaller doses may produce an intoxicating effect	Acute intoxication is a transient condition. Intensity of intoxication lessens with time and effects eventually disappear in the absence of further use of the substance. Recovery is therefore complete except where tissue damage or another complication has arisen Acute intoxication is usually closely related to dose levels. Exceptions may occur in individuals with certain underlying organic conditions. Disinhibition due to social context should also be taken into account	Further guidelines describe it as a reversible substance-specific syndrome with requirements of: A. Recent ingestion of a substance B. Clinically significant problematic behavioural or psychological changes that develop during or shortly after use C. The signs and symptoms are not attributable to another medical condition and are not better explained by another mental disorder, including intoxication with another substance. Substance intoxication is common in those with a substance use disorder but may occur in individuals without a substance use disorder
Explanatory notes	*Note that substance-specific features of intoxication are listed under the primary criteria*		*Note that substance-specific features of intoxication are listed under the primary definitions*

logical effects but which may in severe cases be termed poisoning or overdose. Substance intoxication is defined in DSM-5 as a reversible substance-specific syndrome due to recent ingestion of a substance, together with clinically significant problematic behavioural or psychological changes that develop during, or shortly after, use of the substance, and the signs and symptoms are not attributable to another medical condition and are not better explained by another mental disorder, including intoxication with another substance [4]. ICD-10 and ICD-11 define substance intoxication quite similarly, namely, a clinically significant transient condition that develops during or shortly after the consumption of a substance that is characterised by disturbances in consciousness, cognition, perception, affect, behaviour and coordination. There is a further statement that these disturbances are caused by the known pharmacological effects of the substance, their intensity is closely related to the amount of substance consumed and the disturbances are time-limited and abate as the substance is cleared from the body [70, 72].

Substance intoxication can be life threatening particularly in non-tolerant individuals. Patients may present with coma following intoxication with CNS depressants like alcohol, benzodiazepines or opiates; the risk is compounded when a mixture of these drugs is taken, as is often the case. In addition to neuropsychiatric complications such as paranoia and psychosis, intoxication with psychostimulants (MDMA, amphetamines, cocaine) may lead to a variety of cardiovascular, central nervous system, musculoskeletal, electrolyte and renal complications [61].

8.3.1.2 Episode of Harmful Use of a Substance

This is a new diagnosis in ICD-11 [72] and is designed to capture harm which is considered to be due to substance use but where there is no or insufficient evidence that the person either had an episode of substance intoxication or had a repetitive pattern of substance use where Harmful Substance Use or Substance Dependence could be diagnosed. This diagnosis has proven useful in early studies of the ICD-11 system in capturing

persons attending emergency departments who had an alcohol-related injury but no available information about a prior pattern of alcohol consumption [9].

8.3.1.3 Repetitive Substance Use which Does Not Fulfil Dependence Criteria

Repetitive substance use which does not fulfil the criteria for the dependence syndrome is still of clinical significance. It is handled differently in the two systems. In ICD-10 and ICD-11, the term Harmful Substance Use applies to repetitive use of a psychoactive substance which has caused physical or mental harm to that person [70, 72]. In DSM-IV, the term Substance Abuse refers to repetitive use of a psychoactive substance which essentially is causing social harm or problems [3]. There is no equivalent term in the ICD system; indeed, the ICD eschews the notion of a disorder that is defined by social criteria. In addition, ICD-11 has defined an entity of Hazardous Substance Use which is a health risk factor and is at the mid-range of the hierarchy of substance use and misuse (Fig. 8.1).

Hazardous Substance Use (ICD-11)

Hazardous Substance Use (Fig. 8.1) is listed in a separate chapter "Factors Influencing Health Status" and not included with substance use disorders [72]. Hazardous Substance Use is defined as a pattern of psychoactive substance use that appreciably increases the risk of harmful physical or mental health consequences to the user or to others to an extent that warrants attention and advice from health professionals. The risk may be related to the short-term effects of the substance or to longer-term cumulative effects on physical or mental health or functioning. Hazardous Substance Use has not yet reached the level of having caused harm to the physical or mental health of the user or others around the user.

In support of including hazardous use in a diagnostic system is the evidence that it can be defined and it responds to therapy, the evidence base for the effectiveness of interventions for hazardous alcohol consumption being particularly strong [27].

Hazardous alcohol use is also termed "risky", "high-risk" use, or "unhealthy" use [10, 36, 37]. Hazardous use defines men and women drinking in excess of national low-risk guidelines.

In the USA, the National Institute on Alcohol Abuse and Alcoholism defines risky drinking as men under 65 years drinking more than 14 standard drinks per week on average or more than four standard drinks on any day and women and adults 65 years and older consuming more than seven standard drinks per week on average or more than three standard drinks on any day where one standard drink is defined as 12 grams of ethanol, 5 ounces of wine, 12 ounces of beer or 1.5 ounces of 80 proof spirits [53, 54]. Heavy episodic drinking, defined as repeated heavy drinking episodes of more than five standard drinks (65 g alcohol) by men and more than four US standard drinks (50 g alcohol) by women, confers a risk of alcohol use disorders, acute and chronic illnesses and injuries [37, 52].

In Australia, hazardous or risky consumption is now defined as daily consumption by men and women of more than two standard drinks (20 g alcohol) for some years [36]. In the UK, drinking in excess of 14 units of alcohol per week on a regular basis is considered risky drinking. For people regularly drinking more than 14 units per week, it is recommended to spread drinking evenly over three or more days [66, 69].

Data from the National Epidemiologic Survey on Alcohol and Related Conditions (NESARC) indicate that hazardous alcohol consumption (defined as the US 5+/4+ standard drink criterion) exists within the continuum of abuse and dependence criteria. As the frequency of this level of consumption increases, this experience moves along the severity continuum to overlap with abuse and dependence criteria [52].

Unhealthy alcohol use is an umbrella term encompassing a whole range of alcohol use disorders and a practical means of grouping all the diagnoses [53].

Harmful Substance Use (ICD-10) or Harmful Pattern of Substance Use (ICD-11)

Harmful Substance Use (Fig. 8.1) is an ICD term which denotes a repetitive pattern of sub-stance use, which does not fulfil the criteria for Substance Dependence but has caused damage to a person's physical or mental health or (in ICD-11) has resulted in behaviour leading to harm to the health of others [72]. The pattern of substance use is evident over a period of at least 12 months if substance use is episodic or at least one-month use is continuous, i.e. daily or almost daily [70, 72]. The harmful effects may be acute or chronic. Examples of acute complications include fractures and other forms of trauma, acute gastritis and acute psychotic symptoms following substance use. Chronic medical complications encompass liver disease, (e.g. alcoholic liver disease or hepatitis C-induced liver disease following injecting drug use), cardiovascular diseases, respiratory diseases, various neurological sequelae and many others. Examples of mental complications are depressive episodes secondary to heavy alcohol intake and substance-induced psychosis. In clear distinction to DSM-IV, social complications per se are insufficient to justify a diagnosis of Harmful Substance Use in the ICD [70, 72].

Substance Abuse (DSM-IV)

Substance Abuse in DSM-IV was defined as repetitive substance use which has resulted in one or more social or occupational problems. Substance Abuse was envisaged as one axis of a biaxial conceptualisation of substance use disorders, which separates the core syndrome of dependence from the consequences. However, there is blurring of this conceptualisation because of its hierarchical relationship with dependence, i.e. as a less severe disorder. DSM-5 does not have a separate diagnosis of Substance Abuse, as this has been subsumed within DSM-5 substance use disorder.

8.3.1.4 Substance Dependence (DSM-IV and ICD-10; ICD-11)

Substance Dependence was the central substance use diagnosis in DSM-IV and ICD-10 and remains so in ICD-11 [3, 70, 72]. Essentially, it is a syndrome where there is an "internal drive" to continued and self-perpetuating use [57, 59, 61, 63].

Substance Dependence is defined similarly in DSM-IV, ICD-10 and ICD-11 (Table 8.3). Essentially, Substance Dependence is a syndromal cluster of behavioural, cognitive and physiological phenomena that develop after repeated substance use. In ICD-11, two or more of the three diagnostic guidelines set out below need to be present within a 12-month period or continuous for at least 1 month [43, 44, 58, 63, 72]. The diagnostic guidelines are the following:

1. *Impaired control* over substance use – in terms of the onset, level, circumstances or termination of use, often but not necessarily accompa-

nied by a subjective sensation of urge or craving to use the substance.
2. Substance use becomes an increasing *priority in life* in such that it takes precedence over other interests or enjoyments, daily activities, responsibilities or health or personal care. Substance use takes an increasingly central role in the parson's life and relegates other areas of life to the periphery. Substance use often continues despite the occurrence of problems.
3. *Physiological features* (indicative of neuroadaptation to the substance) as manifested by i) tolerance, ii) withdrawal symptoms following

Table 8.3 Diagnostic criteria for substance dependence and substance use disorder in DSM-IV and DSM-5 and ICD-10 and ICD-11

	DSM-IV dependence	DSM-5 substance use disorder	ICD-10 substance dependence	ICD-11 substance dependence
Stem	A maladaptive pattern of substance use, leading to clinically significant impairment or distress, as manifested by three or more of the following occurring at any time in the same 12-month period	A problematic pattern of substance use leading to clinically significant impairment or distress, as manifested by at least two of the following occurring within a 12-month period	A cluster of physiological, behavioural and cognitive phenomena in which the use of alcohol takes on a much higher priority for a given individual than other behaviours that once had greater value. Three or more of the following (six) manifestations should have occurred together for at least 1 month or occurred together repeatedly within a 12-month period	A disorder of regulation of alcohol use arising from repeated or continuous use of alcohol. The characteristic feature is a strong internal drive to use alcohol. The diagnosis requires two or more of the three central features to be present in the individual at the same time and to occur repeatedly over a period of at least 12 months or continuously over a period of at least 1 month
1	No equivalent criterion – Mentioned in text	Craving or a strong desire or urge to use the substance	A strong desire or sense of compulsion to take the psychoactive substance (craving or compulsion)	1. Impaired control over substance use – In terms of the onset, level, circumstances or termination of use and often, but not necessarily, accompanied by a subjective sensation of urge or craving to use the substance
2	There is persistent desire or unsuccessful attempts to cut down or control substance use	There is persistent desire or unsuccessful efforts to cut down or control substance use	No equivalent criterion but text states that the subjective awareness of compulsion is most commonly seen during attempts to stop or control substance use	
3	The substance is often taken in larger amounts or over a longer period of time than was intended	The substance is often taken in larger amounts or over a longer period than was intended	Difficulties in controlling substance-taking behaviour in terms of its onset, termination or levels of use *(loss of control)*	

Table 8.3 (continued)

	DSM-IV dependence	DSM-5 substance use disorder	ICD-10 substance dependence	ICD-11 substance dependence
4	Important social, occupational or recreational activities are given up or reduced because of drinking or psychoactive substance use	Recurrent substance use resulting in a failure to fulfil major role obligations at work, school or home	Progressive neglect of alternative pleasures and responsibilities because of psychoactive substance use or increased amount of time necessary to obtain or take the substance or to recover from its effects	2. Substance use becomes an increasing priority in life such that its use takes precedence over other interests or enjoyments, daily activities, responsibilities or health or personal care. It takes an increasingly central role in the person's life and relegates other areas of life to the periphery. Substance use often continues despite the occurrence of problems
5	A great deal of time is spent in activities necessary to obtain the substance, use the substance or recover from its effects	A great deal of time is spent in activities necessary to obtain the substance, use the substance or recover from its effects	Subsumed in the above criterion	
6.	The substance use is continued despite knowledge of having a persistent or recurrent physical or psychological problem that is likely to have been caused or exacerbated by the substance	Substance use is continued despite knowledge of having a persistent or recurrent physical or psychological problem that is likely to have been caused or exacerbated by that substance	Persisting with substance use despite clear evidence of overtly harmful consequences	
7.	Tolerance: As defined by either (a) a need for markedly increased amounts of the substance to achieve the desired effects or (b) markedly diminished effect with continued use of the same amount of the substance	Tolerance is defined by either of the following: a) a need for markedly increased amounts of the substance to achieve intoxication or desired effect or b) a markedly diminished effect with continued use of the same amount of the substance	Tolerance: Such that increased doses of the psychoactive substances are required in order to achieve effects originally produced by lower doses	3. Physiological features (indicative of neuroadaptation to the substance) as manifested by (i) tolerance, (ii) withdrawal symptoms following cessation or reduction in use of that substance or (iii) repeated use of the substance (or pharmacologically similar substance) to prevent or alleviate withdrawal symptoms. Withdrawal symptoms must be characteristic for the withdrawal syndrome for that substance and must not simply reflect a hangover effect
8.	Withdrawal as manifested by either (a) the characteristic withdrawal syndrome for the substance or (b) the same (or a closely related) substance is taken to relieve or avoid withdrawal symptoms	Withdrawal is manifested by either of the following: a) the characteristic withdrawal syndrome for the substance or b) the substance (or a closely related substance) is taken to relieve or avoid withdrawal symptoms	A physiological withdrawal state when substance use has ceased or been reduced, as evidenced by the characteristic withdrawal syndrome for the substance, or use of the same (or a closely related substance) with the intention of relieving or avoiding withdrawal symptoms	

(continued)

Table 8.3 (continued)

	DSM-IV dependence	DSM-5 substance use disorder	ICD-10 substance dependence	ICD-11 substance dependence
9.Former DSM-IV abuse	Continued substance use despite having persistent or recurrent social or interpersonal problems caused or exacerbated by the effects of the substance (e.g. arguments with spouse about consequences of intoxication, physical fights)	Continued substance use despite having persistent or recurrent social or interpersonal problems caused or exacerbated by the effects of the substance	To some extent subsumed in criterion no. 4	To some extent subsumed in criterion no. 2
10. Former DSM-IV abuse	Recurrent substance use in situations in which it is typically hazardous (drink driving)	Recurrent use in situations in which it is physically hazardous	No equivalent criterion	No equivalent criterion
11. Former DSM-IV abuse	Recurrent substance use which results in failure to fulfil major obligations at work, school or home	Important social, occupational or recreational activities are given up or reduced because of substance use	To some extent subsumed in criterion no. 4	To some extent subsumed in criterion no. 2
Former DSM-IV abuse, now omitted	Recurrent substance-related legal problems (e.g. driving an automobile or operating a machine when impaired by substance use)			

In DSM-5, the diagnosis of substance use disorder is further classified according to severity: presence of 2–3 symptoms, mild; presence of 4–5 symptoms, moderate; and presence of 6 or more symptoms, severe

cessation or reduction in use of that substance and iii) repeated use of the substance (or pharmacologically similar substance) to prevent or alleviate withdrawal symptoms. Withdrawal symptoms must be characteristic for the withdrawal syndrome for that substance and must not simply reflect a hangover effect.

The concordance of the ICD-11 Substance Dependence diagnostic guidelines with their counterparts in ICD-10 and the criteria in DSM-IV have been found to be in almost perfect agreement for alcohol dependence, cannabis dependence and prescribed opioid dependence with the ICD-10 and DSM-IV classifications of dependence [12, 13, 30]. However, there is much less agreement with DSM-5 substance use disorder for alcohol or cannabis [12, 30].

Substance Dependence typically occurs in people who use large amounts of psychoactive substances, for example, people consuming alcohol in excess of 120 g/day (men) or 80 g/day (women). The diagnosis of Substance Dependence is not, however, made primarily on the level of consumption.

8.3.1.5 Substance Use Disorder (DSM-5)

DSM-5 has radically restructured the conceptualisation and classification of substance-related disorders [4]. Substance Dependence and Abuse have been replaced by the broader concept of substance use disorder. Substance use disorder is now the central diagnosis and represents essentially a combination of the diagnostic features of DSM-IV Substance Dependence and Substance Abuse (Table 8.3), with one Substance Abuse criterion omitted and the ICD-10 criterion of craving added. This offers a simplified diagnostic system.

In DSM-5, substance use disorder is defined as a problematic pattern of substance use leading to clinically significant impairment or distress, manifested by at least two of the following 11 criteria occurring within a 12-month period:

1. The substance is often taken in larger amounts over a longer period than was intended.
2. There is persistent desire or unsuccessful efforts to cut down or control substance use.
3. A great deal of time is spent in activities necessary to obtain the substance, use the substance or recover from its effects.
4. Craving or a strong desire or urge to use the substance.
5. Recurrent substance use resulting in a failure to fulfil major role obligations at work, school or home.
6. Continued substance use despite having persistent or recurrent social or interpersonal problems caused or exacerbated by the effects of the substance.
7. Important social, occupational or recreational activities are given up or reduced because of substance use.
8. Recurrent substance use in situations in which it is physically hazardous.
9. Continued substance use despite knowledge of having a persistent or recurrent physical or psychological problem that is likely to have been caused or exacerbated by that substance.
10. Tolerance as defined by either of the following: (a) a need to markedly increase amounts of substance to achieve intoxication or desired effect or (b) a markedly diminished effect with continued use of the same amount of substance.
11. Withdrawal as manifested by either of the following: (a) the characteristic withdrawal

syndrome for the substance or (b) the substance (or a closely related substance) is taken to relieve or avoid withdrawal symptoms.

The severity is graded on the number of criteria met, namely, mild, 2–3; moderate, 4–5; and severe, 6 or more (Table 8.3). Moderate to severe substance use disorder in DSM-5 is roughly equivalent to Substance Dependence in ICD-10 and ICD-11 [24, 72].

DSM-5 substance use disorder is a very broad and heterogeneous condition, and there is a risk that its extended scope means that it is less useful for determining treatment than the concept of Substance Dependence. The change occurred despite Substance Dependence being a psychometrically robust syndrome [11, 23, 38, 57, 64]. An example of this is the requirement for dependence on heroin or other opioids for there to be justification in prescribing opioid agonist maintenance therapy with methadone or buprenorphine.

8.3.1.6 Other Definitions of Dependence or Addiction

The two systems that have most impact internationally are the ICD and the DSM, under the auspices of the World Health Organization and the American Psychiatric Association (APA), respectively. Several professional organisations have developed definitions for use by their own members/fellows (the APA is a national professional organisation. But the DSM has such international reach that it is more appropriately classified as an international system). Foremost of these other organisations is the American Society of Addiction Medicine (ASAM). It employs the term "addiction" rather dependence or "use disorders". The ASAM definition of "addiction" [5] is as follows:

> Addiction is a primary, chronic disease of brain reward, motivation, memory and related circuitry. Dysfunction in these circuits leads to characteristic biological, psychological, social and spiritual manifestations. This is reflected in an individual pathologically pursuing reward and/or relief by substance use and other behaviours.

Addiction is characterized by inability to consistently abstain, impairment in behavioural control, craving, diminished recognition of significant problems with one's behaviours and interpersonal relationships, and a dysfunctional emotional response. Like other chronic diseases, addiction often involves cycles of relapse and remission. Without treatment or engagement in recovery activities, addiction is progressive and can result in disability or premature death.

This is a fundamentally different concept to those of dependence in the ICD and DSM systems and even more distant to the DSM-5 understanding of substance use disorders. The main points of distinction are as follows:

1. The disorder is described as "primary" and suggests a fundamental (presumably) biological difference between those who are addicted and those who are not, rather than the notion of an acquired syndrome which is the nature of the dependence syndrome.
2. The disorder is described as "progressive" in an unqualified way, which is different to the concept that dependence can undergo "natural" remission (i.e. without treatment).
3. There is no sense of a spectrum of disorder.

There are five central features of addiction in this conceptualisation, which are the following:

(a) Inability to consistently abstain
(b) Impairment in behavioural control
(c) Craving or increased "hunger" for drugs or rewarding experiences
(d) Diminished recognition of significant problems with one's behaviours and interpersonal relationships
(e) A dysfunctional emotional response

These features might be considered diagnostic criteria for addiction, although it is not clear how many are required for the diagnosis and in what combination. The psychometric performance of the criteria is unknown. Despite these shortcomings, the ASAM definition well summarises the experience of patients at the severe end of the spectrum of substance use disorders. It has an intuitive appeal to many clinicians, particularly those working in in-patient treatment programmes and residential recovery programmes. The definition has been adopted, on a temporary basis, by the International Society of Addiction Medicine and the Canadian Society of Addiction Medicine.

8.3.1.7 Substance Withdrawal (DSM-IV, DSM-5, ICD-10 and ICD-11)

Substance withdrawal refers to a state which may occur when substance use is curtailed in persons with Substance Dependence or a physiological dependence on a psychoactive substance even though the diagnosis of Substance Dependence may not apply. Substance withdrawal is also likely to occur in DSM-5 substance use disorder of the moderate or severe subtypes. It is an important manifestation of the neurobiological changes that underpin dependence. In general, the features of the withdrawal syndrome are opposite to those of the acute pharmacological effects of the substance. In contrast to dependence, the withdrawal syndrome varies appreciably according to the substance. Psychostimulant withdrawal is very different to withdrawal from sedative-hypnotics. Substance withdrawal is often listed as a "substance-induced disorder"; however, given its intimate relationship with dependence, it is discussed at this point.

Substance withdrawal is generally stated to be a clinically significant cluster of symptoms specific to the known withdrawal state of that substance. The ICD system specifies that there has been repeated and usually prolonged and/or high-dose use of that substance. The withdrawal syndrome develops in a period from hours to a few days (or more rarely longer) after cessation or reduction in use. There is variable severity and duration of symptoms. The DSM system requires that the signs or symptoms cause clinically significant distress or impairment in social, occupational or other areas of functioning. The specific criteria in DSM-5, ICD-10 and ICD-11 are listed in Table 8.4. The onset and course of the withdrawal state are time-limited and are related to the type of substance and the dose being used immediately before abstinence. Three types of

Table 8.4 Diagnostic guidelines for substance withdrawal (DSM-5, ICD-10, ICD-11)

	DSM-5	ICD-10	ICD-11
Primary definitions and criteria	A. Characteristic withdrawal syndrome that develops within hours or a few days after the cessation of (or reduction in) heavy and prolonged substance use B. The development of two or more signs/symptoms specific to the substance, developing within hours to a few days after cessation or reduction in use C. The signs or symptoms cause clinically significant distress or impairment in social, occupational or other areas of functioning	A group of symptoms of variable clustering and severity occurring on absolute or relative withdrawal of a substance For diagnosis of withdrawal syndrome, there should be clear evidence of recent cessation or reduction of substance use after repeated and usually prolonged and/or high dose use of that substance. A withdrawal state is one of the main indicators of the dependence syndrome	A clinically significant cluster of symptoms, behaviours and/or physiological features, varying in degree of severity and duration that occurs upon cessation or reduction of use of a substance in individuals who have developed substance dependence or have used the substance for a prolonged period or in large amounts
Additional guidelines		Symptoms and signs compatible with the known features of a withdrawal state from the particular substance or substances. Physical symptoms vary according to the substance being used. Psychological disturbances (e.g. anxiety, depression, sleep disorders) are also common features of withdrawal. Typically, the patient reports that withdrawal symptoms are relieved by further substance use. The features are not accounted for by a medical disorder unrelated to the substance use, and not better accounted for by another mental or behavioural disorder	Physical symptoms vary according to the substance being used. Psychological disturbances (e.g. anxiety, depression, sleep disorders) also are common features of withdrawal. Typically, the patient reports that withdrawal symptoms are relieved by further substance use Onset and course of the withdrawal state are time limited and are related to the type of substance and the dose being used immediately before abstinence. Less commonly, the withdrawal state is complicated by seizures. Substance-induced delirium includes withdrawal states which are complicated by delirium
Explanatory notes	*Note that substance-specific features of withdrawal are listed under the primary criteria*		*Note that substance-specific features of withdrawal are listed under the primary definitions*

withdrawal are recognised in DSM-5 and ICD-10, but in ICD-11, withdrawal with delirium is subsumed in the diagnosis of substance-induced delirium [72]. More broadly, substance withdrawal may vary from mild to very severe. For example, alcohol withdrawal may vary from mild features of autonomic hyperactivity to delirium tremens (DTs) [62]. Convulsions generally herald the onset of delirium tremens which has a mortality rate of about 15%. The acute alcohol withdrawal syndrome needs to be differentiated from Wernicke's encephalopathy [31]. Benzodiazepine withdrawal has a similar picture but may persist for weeks or months [41]. Opioid withdrawal resembles a flulike illness [61] with aches, pains, rhinorrhoea, nausea, vomiting, sweating, features of autonomic hyperactivity, irritability, agitation, insomnia and strong cravings for opioids. Dilatation of the pupils is a characteristic physical sign. Cannabis withdrawal

[61] includes irritability, restlessness, anxiety, insomnia and mood changes. Cannabis withdrawal was not recognised in DSM-IV, although it is now included in DSM-5 [4]. Withdrawal from psychostimulants [61] is an exaggeration of the "crash" and is characterised by craving, low mood, irritability, sleep disturbance, anxiety, dysphoria, depression and increased risk of suicide.

8.3.1.8 Substance-Induced Disorders

Substance-induced or substance-related problems or disabilities encompass the multiple physical disorders, mental health disorders, neurocognitive impairments and social, personal, occupational and legal problems. The World Health Organization Committee conceptualised substance-related problems or disabilities as the *consequences* of repetitive substance use [18, 19, 57, 59].

Substance-Induced Mental and Neurocognitive Disorders (DSM-IV, DSM-5, ICD-10 and ICD-11)

In DSM-IV and ICD-10, there are several substance-related mental disorders. These include substance-induced depression, substance-induced anxiety disorder, substance-induced bipolar disorder and substance-induced psychotic disorder. In DSM-5, the same disorders are present, but they are located in the chapters describing the respective generic mental disorder. For example, substance-induced anxiety disorder is grouped within the anxiety disorders section.

In addition, there are neurocognitive consequences of substance use disorders. Here, we shall briefly describe one of the former – psychotic disorder – and two of the latter, delirium and amnesic syndrome. In DSM-IV, DSM-5, ICD-10 and ICD-11, there are several substance-related mental disorders of variable in severity and duration. They are usually temporary but may persist over weeks or more rarely months [61, 72]. They include substance-induced mood disorders, anxiety disorder, sleep-wake disorder, sexual dysfunction and for psychostimulants substance-induced obsessive-compulsive disorder. Different syndromes are caused by different substances. Here, we shall discuss just three of

them: delirium, psychotic disorder and amnesic syndrome.

(i) *Substance-Induced Delirium (DSM-IV, DSM-5 and ICD-11)*

Delirium is an uncommon feature of substance misuse, although sometimes the diagnosis is made in persons with acute intoxication. Substance intoxication with delirium is an accepted diagnosis in DSM-IV and DSM-5 [3, 4] but not in ICD-10 [70], but it is included in ICD-11 [72]. Most commonly, it is seen in those with a severe withdrawal syndrome from alcohol or sedative drugs [62].

The classical disorder is delirium tremens (DTs) [62], which is a short-lived but occasionally life-threatening toxic confusional state with accompanying somatic disturbances. It is usually a consequence of absolute or relative cessation of alcohol in severely dependent drinkers with a long history of use. Its onset may be preceded by features of simple withdrawal and/or by withdrawal convulsions. A similar withdrawal delirium is seen after cessation of benzodiazepines and other sedative hypnotics although with less tremor. In DSM-5, substance intoxication delirium is differentiated from substance withdrawal delirium in the chapter on neurocognitive disorders [4].

(ii) *Substance-Induced Psychotic Disorder (DSM-IV, DSM-5, ICD-10 and ICD-11)*

Psychosis or psychotic symptoms occur in many people with substance use disorders. In some, the psychosis is a consequence of drug use. In others, it reflects an underlying independent disorder such as schizophrenia. Sometimes the aetiology and mechanisms are unclear.

Substance-induced psychotic disorder is presented as an example of a mental disorder induced by substance use. It features in both the DSM and ICD systems. Substance-induced psychotic disorder is a phenomenon that occurs during or soon after (usually within 48 hours) intoxication with, or withdrawal from, a psychoactive substance. It is characterised by psychotic symptoms, e.g.

delusions, vivid hallucinations (typically auditory but often in more than one sensory modality), disorganised thinking, grossly disorganised behaviour, misidentifications, psychomotor disturbances (excitement or stupor), and an abnormal affect, which may range from intense fear to ecstasy. The disorder typically resolves within 1 month and fully within 6 months. The sensorium is usually clear, but some degree of clouding of consciousness, though not severe confusion, may be present. The disorder typically resolves at least partially within 1 month and fully within 6 months. The diagnosis is excluded if the psychotic state is a manifestation of substance withdrawal syndrome. The ICD-11 definition emphasises that the amount and duration of substance use must be capable of producing psychotic symptoms and that the symptoms are not better explained by a primary mental disorder, for example, if they preceded the onset of substance use or persisted for a substantial period of time after cessation of substance use or if there is a pre-existing primary mental disorder with psychotic symptoms.

In DSM-5, substance/medication-induced psychotic disorders are mentioned in the chapter on schizophrenia spectrum and other psychotic disorders with the psychotic disorder associated with alcohol, cannabis, phencyclidine, other hallucinogens, inhalants, sedative/hypnotic/anxiolytic, amphetamine (or other stimulant), cocaine and other unknown substance. The psychotic symptoms are thought to be a physiological consequence of a drug of abuse (medication or toxin) and cease after removal of the agent. The diagnostic criteria in DSM-5 are the following:

A. The presence of one or both of the following symptoms: (a) delusions and (b) hallucinations.
B. Evidence that the symptoms developed during or soon after substance intoxication or withdrawal and the substance is capable of producing the symptoms.
C. The disturbance is not better explained by an independent psychotic disorder (not substance-induced), as evidenced by the fol-

lowing: (a) the symptoms preceded the onset of substance use, (b) the symptoms persist for a substantial period of time (e.g. about 1 month) after cessation of acute withdrawal or intoxication, and (c) there is no evidence of non-substance-induced disorder (e.g. history of recurrent non-substance-related episodes).
D. The disturbance does not occur exclusively during the course of a delirium.
E. The disturbance causes clinically significant distress or impairment in social, occupational or other important areas of functioning [4].

For psychostimulants such as amphetamines and cocaine, there is a dose-response relationship, with psychosis occurring especially in those who have been using high doses and/or using the drug over a lengthy period. According to ICD-10, a diagnosis of psychotic disorder should not be made merely on the basis of perceptual distortions or hallucinatory experiences when substances having primary hallucinogenic effects (e.g. lysergic acid, mescaline and cannabis in high doses) have been taken. In such cases, and also for confusional states, a possible diagnosis of substance intoxication should be considered.

(iii) *Substance-Induced Amnesic Syndrome (DSM-IV, DSM-5, ICD-10 and ICD-11)*

Amnesic (amnestic) syndrome is an example of a substance-related disorder where there is anatomical brain damage, caused in this case by the combined effects of thiamine deficiency and toxicity of the substance, typically alcohol [7, 61]. The most common chronic form is characterised by impairment of recent memory, with relative preservation of remote memory and with normal immediate recall. Disturbances of time sense and ordering of events are usually evident, as are difficulties in learning new material. Confabulation may be marked but is not invariably present and should not be regarded as a prerequisite for diagnosis. Importantly, other cognitive functions are usually relatively well preserved; the amnesic defects are, therefore, out of proportion to other disturbances. Personality changes, often with apparent apathy and loss of initiative, and tendency towards self-neglect may be present but are not necessary for the diagnosis.

Substance-induced amnesic syndrome is classified in DSM-5 within the neurocognitive disorders and not as a substance-induced mental disorder. The diagnostic criteria are those of substance/medication-induced neurocognitive disorder, and although an amnesic-type disorder seen with alcohol is noted, no specific criteria are included. In ICD-10, substance-induced amnesic syndrome is included in the substance disorders chapter, with a specific definition and diagnostic guidelines. However, in ICD-11, it is included in the neurocognitive disorders chapter within the section of amnestic disorders (and therefore distinct from the dementias) and under the heading of "Amnestic Disorder Due to Psychoactive Substances Including Medications".

Substance-Induced or Substance-Related Physical Disorders

Complications arising from repetitive substance use stem not only from the pharmacological properties of a particular substance but also from unknown potency and purity and sterility from contaminants and adulterants with which the substance is prepared, unsafe injecting practices and the associated lifestyle of the user. The spread of bacterial infections and viral infections, such as hepatitis C and HIV and to a lesser extent hepatitis B, is important in this regard [61]. The disinhibiting effect of alcohol and substance use also places users at risk of sexually transmitted diseases.

In DSM-III, DSM-IIIR and DSM-IV, relevant physical disorders were noted in Axis III of the multiaxial system. DSM-5 has abandoned this multiaxial system, and comorbid physical disorders receive little attention. ICD-10 by contrast lists an array of these disorders, in keeping with its objective of encompassing all human disorders irrespective of aetiology.

Alcohol consumption can cause disease in virtually every organ system in the body and is also associated with a range of malignancies. Cannabis and tobacco use commonly induce respiratory disorders with the latter being a major cause of bronchial cancer [46, 47, 50, 61].

In the ICD system, substance-induced physical disorders are not included with the main grouping of disorders due to substance use but are classified in the respective organ and body systems sections. For example, alcoholic cirrhosis of the liver is included as one of several forms of alcoholic liver disease in the section on diseases of the liver within the chapter "Diseases of the Digestive System". It should be noted that alcohol and certain other substances are risk factors for many physical disorders in addition to those for which they are a principal causal agent. At the same time, to examine relationships between use patterns and consequences without considering whether a diagnosable substance use disorder is present, as is usual in epidemiological studies, is limiting. In support of including hazardous use in a diagnostic system is the evidence that it can be defined and it responds to therapy, the evidence base for the effectiveness of interventions for hazardous alcohol consumption being particularly strong [6, 14, 60, 61, 69]. Thus, in a comprehensive diagnostic system, there are grounds for having a dependence category, a nondependence disorder that is of clinical consequence and a "subthreshold" disorder that indicates risk to individuals and populations.

Substance-Related Social Problems

The adverse consequences of a substance use disorder are legion. Some will be the presenting problem(s) and will be uppermost in the patient's (or relative's) mind. Examples of social problems are the following:

- Relationship problems
- Interpersonal difficulties
- Financial problems
- Work-related problems/unemployment/prostitution
- Legal/forensic problems such as drunk driving

Acknowledgement We thank Corinne Lim for her expert contribution to the literature and cross-checking of the citations to the literature.

References

1. American Psychiatric Association (APA). Diagnostic and statistical manual for mental disorders. American Psychiatric Association, Washington, DC, USA; 1952.
2. American Psychiatric Association (APA). The diagnostic and statistical manual of mental disorders, Second Edition (DSM-II). American Psychiatric Association, Washington, DC, USA; 1968.
3. American Psychiatric Association (APA). The diagnostic and statistical manual of mental disorders, Fourth Edition (DSM-IV). American Psychiatric Association, Washington, DC, USA; 1994.
4. American Psychiatric Association (APA). The diagnostic and statistical manual of mental disorders, Fifth Edition (DSM-5). American Psychiatric Association, Washington, DC, USA; 2013.
5. American Society of Addiction Medicine (ASAM). Public policy statement: definition of addiction. American Society of Addiction Medicine, Chevy Chase; 2011. Retrieved from https://www.asam.org/resources/definition-of-addiction.
6. Babor TF, Higgins-Biddle JC, Saunders JB, et al. The alcohol use disorders identification test- guidelines for use in primary care. 2nd ed. Geneva: World Health Organization (WHO); 2001. Department of Mental Health and Substance Dependence 2001. Retrieved from http://whqilbdoc.who.int/hq/2001/WHO_MSD_MSB_01.6a.pdf.
7. Baigent M. Physical complications of substance abuse: what the psychiatrist needs to know. Curr Opin Psychiatry. 2003;16:291–6.
8. Bandura A. Social learning theory. Englewood Cliffs: Prentice-Hall; 1977.
9. Cherpitel CJ, Ye Y, Poznyak V. Single episode of alcohol use resulting in injury: a cross-sectional study in 21 countries. Bull World Health Organ. 2018;96:335–42.
10. Commonwealth Department of Health and Ageing. Australian alcohol guidelines: health risks and benefits. Commonwealth of Australia. 2012. Retrieved from http://www.alcohol.gov.au/internet/alcohol/publishing.nsf/Content/guide-adult.
11. Cottler LB, Grant BF, Blaine J, et al. Concordance of DSM-IV alcohol and drug use disorder criteria and diagnoses as measured by AUDADIS-ADR, CIDI and SCAN. Drug Alcohol Depend. 1997;47:195–205.
12. Degenhardt L, Bharat C, Bruno R, Glantz MD, Sampson NA, Lago L, Aguilar-Gaxiola S, Alonso J, Andrade LH, Bunting B, Caldas-de-Almeida JM, Cia AH, Gureje O, Karam EG, Khalaf M, McGrath JJ, Moskalewicz J, Lee S, Mneimneh Z, Navarro-Mateu F, Sasu CC, Scott K, Torres Y, Poznyak V, Chatterji S, Kessler RC, on behalf of the WHO World Mental Health Survey Collaborators. Concordance between the diagnostic guidelines for alcohol and cannabis use disorders in the draft ICD-11 and other classification systems: analysis of data from the WHO's world mental health surveys. Addiction. 2019;114:534–52.
13. Degenhardt L, Bruno R, Lintzeris N, et al. Agreement between definitions of pharmaceutical opioid use disorders and dependence in people talking opioids for chronic non-cancer (POINT) study. Lancet Psychiatry. 2015;2:314–22.
14. Degenhardt L, Hall W. Extent of illicit drug use and dependence, and their contribution to the global burden of disease. Lancet. 2012;379:55–70.
15. Degenhardt L, Hall W, Lynskey M. Alcohol, cannabis and tobacco use among Australians: a comparison of their associations with other drug use and use disorders, affective and anxiety disorders, and psychosis. Addiction. 2001;96:1603–14.
16. Ducci F, Goldman D. The genetic basis of addictive disorders. Psychiatr Clin North Am. 2012;35:495–519.
17. Edenberg HJ, Foroud T. Genetics and alcoholism. Nat Rev Gastroenterol Hepatol. 2013;10:487–94.
18. Edwards G, Arif A, Hodgson R. Nomenclature and classification of drug and alcohol-related problems: a WHO memorandum. Bull World Health Org. 1981;59:225–42.
19. Edwards G, Gross MM. Alcohol dependence: provisional description of a clinical syndrome. Br Med J. 1976;1:1058–61.
20. Ehlers CL, Walter NAR, Dick DM, Buck KJ, Crabbe JC. A comparison of selected quantitative trait loci associated with alcohol use phenotypes in humans and mouse models. Addict Biol. 2010;15: 185–99.
21. Feingold A, Rounsaville B. Construct validity of the dependence syndrome as measured by DSM-IV for different psychoactive substances. Addiction. 1995;90:1661–9.
22. First MB, Reed GM, Saxena S, Hyman SE. The development of the ICD-11 clinical descriptions and diagnostic guidelines for mental and behavioural disorders. World Psychiatry. 2015;14:82–90.
23. Hasin D, Hatzenbuehler ML, Keyes K, Ogburn E. Substance use disorders: diagnostic and statistical manual of mental disorders, fourth edition (DSM-IV) and international classification of diseases, tenth edition (ICD-10). Addiction. 2006;101(1):59–75.
24. Hasin DS, O'Brien CP, Auriacombe M, Borges G, Bucholz K, Budney A, Compton WM, Crowley T, Ling W, Petry NM, Schuckit M, Grant BF. DSM-5 criteria for substance use disorders: recommendations and rationale. Am J Psychiatry. 2013;170: 834–51.
25. International Society of Addiction Medicine (ISAM). Definition of addiction. Calgary/Alberta: International Society of Addiction Medicine; 2013.
26. Jellinek EM. The disease concept of alcoholism. New Brunswick/New Jersey: Hillhouse Press; 1960.
27. Kaner EFS, Beyer FR, Muirhead C, Campbell F, et al. Effectiveness of brief alcohol interventions in primary care populations. Cochrane Database Syst Rev. 2018;2:CD004148.
28. Koob GF, Le Moal M. Plasticity of reward neurocircuitry and the dark side of drug addiction. Nat Rev Neurosci. 2005;8:1442–4.

29. Koob GF, Volkow NB. Neurobiology of addiction: a neurocircuitry analysis. Lancet Psychiatry. 2016;3:760–73.

30. Lago L, Bruno R, Degenhardt L. Concordance of ICD-11 and DSM-5 definitions of alcohol and cannabis use disorders: a population survey. Lancet Psychiatry. 2016;3:673–84.

31. Latt N, Dore G. Thiamine in the treatment of Wernicke encephalopathy in patients with alcohol use disorders. Intern Med J. 2014;44:911–5.

32. Ledermann, S. Alcool, alcoolism, alcoolisation: données scientifiques de caractère physiologique, économique et social. Presses Universitaires de France, Institut National d'Etudes Demographiques, Paris; 1960.

33. Lessov CN, Martin NG, Statham DJ, Todorov AA, Slutske WS, Bucholz KK, Heath AC, Madden PAF. Defining nicotine dependence for genetic research: evidence from Australian twins. Psychol Med. 2004;34:865–79.

34. Lejoyeux M, McLoughlin M, Ades J. Epidemiology of behavioural dependence: literature review and results of original studies. Eur Psychiatry. 2000;15:129–34.

35. Leshner A. Addiction is a brain disease. Issues Sci Technol. 2001;17:75–80.

36. National Health and Medical Research Council (NHMRC). Australian guidelines to reduce health risks from drinking alcohol 2009. 2009. Retrieved from https://www.nhmrc.gov.au/health-advice/alcohol.

37. National Institute on Alcohol Abuse and Alcoholism (NIAAA). Helping patients who drink too much: a clinician's guide. Rockville: National Institute on Alcohol Abuse and Alcoholism; 2005.

38. Nelson CB, Rehm J, Üstün TB, Grant B, Chatterji S. Factor structures for DSM-IV substance disorders criteria endorsed by alcohol, cannabis, cocaine and opiate users: results from the WHO reliability and validity study. Addiction. 1999;94:843–55.

39. Owen RT, Tyrer P. Benzodiazepine dependence: a review of the evidence. Drugs. 1983;25:385–98.

40. Papaseit E, Farré N, Schifano F, Torrens M. Emerging drugs in Europe. Curr Opin Psychiatry. 2014;27:243–50.

41. Park, T.W. Benzodiazepine use disorder: epidemiology, pathogenesis, clinical manifestations, course and diagnosis. UpToDate, Waltham, MA, USA: UpToDate Inc; 2018. Retrieved from https://www.uptodate.com/home/content.

42. Potenza MN. Should addictive disorders include non-substance related conditions? Addiction. 2006;101(s1):142–51.

43. Poznyak, V. Alcohol use disorders: their status in the draft ICD-11. Presented at the Joint Congress of the Research Society on Alcoholism and the International Society for Biomedical Research on Alcoholism, Seattle, USA, June 2014.

44. Poznyak, V. Background to the development of the section on disorders due to substance use and related conditions in the draft ICD-11. Presented at the World Congress of the World Psychiatric Association, Madrid, Spain, September 2014. Available through the Department of Mental Health and Substance Abuse, World Health Organization, Geneva, Switzerland; 2014.

45. Poznyak V, Reed GM, Medina-Mora ME. Aligning the ICD-11 classification of disorders due to substance use with global service needs. Epidemiol Psychiatr Sci. 2018;27:212–8.

46. Rehm J, Baliunas D, Borges GLG, Graham K, Irving H, Kehoe T, Parry CD, Patra J, Popova S, Poznyak V, Roerecke M, Room R, Samokhvalov AV, Taylor B. The relation between different dimensions of alcohol consumption and burden of disease: an overview. Addiction. 2010;105:817–43.

47. Roerecke N, Rehm J. Alcohol use disorders and mortality: a systematic review and meta-analysis. Addiction. 2013;108:1562–78.

48. Room R. Drugs, consciousness and self-control: popular and medical conceptions. Int Rev Psychiatry. 1989;1:63–70.

49. Roy A, Pandey SC. The decreased cellular expression of neuropeptide Y protein in rat brain structures during ethanol withdrawal after chronic ethanol exposure. Alcohol Clin Exp Res. 2002;26:796–803.

50. Russell M, Light JM, Gruenewald PJ. Alcohol consumption and problems: the relevance of drinking patterns. Alcohol Clin Exp Res. 2004;28:921–30.

51. Saha TD, Chou PS, Grant BF. Toward an alcohol use disorder continuum using item response theory: results from the national epidemiologic survey on alcohol and related conditions. Psychol Med. 2006;36:931–41.

52. Saha TD, Stinson FS, Grant BF. The role of alcohol consumption in future classification of alcohol use disorders. Drug Alcohol Depend. 2007;89:82–92.

53. Saitz R. Unhealthy alcohol use. N Engl J Med. 2005;352:596–607.

54. Saitz, R. Screening for unhealthy use of alcohol and other drugs in primary care. UpToDate, Waltham, MA, USA: UpToDate Inc; 2019. Retrieved from https://www.uptodate.com/home/content.

55. Sartorius N, Kaelber CT, Cooper JE, Roper NT, Rae DS, Gulbinat W, Üstün TB, Regier DA. Progress toward achieving a common language in psychiatry: the clinical guidelines accompanying the WHO classification of mental and behavioural disorders in ICD-10. Arch Gen Psychiatr. 1993;50:115–24.

56. Saunders JB. Alcoholism: new evidence for a genetic contribution. Br Med J. 1982;284:1137–8.

57. Saunders JB. Substance dependence and non-dependence in the diagnostic and statistical manual of mental disorders (DSM) and the international classification of diseases (ICD): can an identical conceptualization be achieved? Addiction. 2006;101(s1):49–59.

58. Saunders, J.B. Rationale for changes in the clinical descriptions and diagnostic guidelines of disorders due to substance use and related conditions in the

draft ICD-11. Presented at the World Congress of the World Psychiatric Association, Madrid, Spain, September 2014; 2014.

59. Saunders JB. Substance use and addictive disorders in DSM-5 and ICD-10 and the draft ICD-11. Curr Opin Psychiatry. 2017;30:227–37.

60. Saunders JB, Aasland OG, Babor TF, et al. Development of the alcohol use disorders identification test (AUDIT): WHO collaborative project on early detection of persons with harmful alcohol consumption II. Addiction. 1993;88:791–804.

61. Saunders JB, Conigrave KM, Latt NC, Nutt DJ, Marshall EJ, Ling W, Higuchi S. Addiction medicine. 2nd ed. Oxford: Oxford University Press; 2016. ISBN:978-0-19-871475-0.

62. Saunders JB, Janca A. Delirium tremens: its aetiology, natural history and treatment. Curr Opin Psychiatr. 2000;13:629–33.

63. Saunders JB, Peacock A, Degenhardt L. Alcohol use disorders in the draft ICD-11, and how they compare with DSM-5. Curr Addict Rep. 2018;5:257–64.

64. Saunders JB, Schuckit MA. The development of a research agenda for substance use disorders diagnosis in the diagnostic and statistical manual of mental disorders, fifth edition (DSM-V). Addiction. 2006;101(1):1–5.

65. Teesson M, Lynskey M, Manor B, Baillie A. The structure of cannabis dependence in the community. Drug Alcohol Depend. 2002;68:255–62.

66. UK chief medical officers' low risk drinking guidelines. 2016. Retrieved from https://www.gov.uk/government/publications/alcohol-consumption-advice-on-low-risk-drinking.

67. Volkow ND, Fowler JS, Wang GJ. The addicted brain viewed in the light of imaging studies: brain circuits and treatment strategies. Neuropharmacology. 2004;47(s1):3–13.

68. Volkow ND, Koob GF, McLellan T. Neurobiologic advances from the brain disease model of addiction. N Engl J Med. 2016;374:363–71.

69. Wood AM, Kaptoge S, Butterworth AS, Wallet P, et al. Risk thresholds for alcohol consumption: combined analysis of individual-participant data for 599 912 current drinkers in 83 prospective studies. Lancet. 2018;391:1513–23.

70. World Health Organization (WHO). The ICD-10 classification of mental and behavioural disorders: clinical descriptions and diagnostic guidelines. Geneva: World Health Organization; 1992.

71. World Health Organization (WHO). Neuroscience of psychoactive substance use and dependence. Geneva: World Health Organization; 2004.

72. World Health Organization (WHO). International classification of diseases 11th revision (ICD-11). Geneva: World Health Organization; 2019. Retrieved from via https://icd.who.int/en/.

73. Yücel M, Lubman DI. Neurocognitive and neuroimaging evidence of behavioural dysregulation in human drug addiction: implications for diagnosis, treatment and prevention. Drug Alcohol Rev. 2007;26:33–9.

Part II

Drugs of Abuse and Pharmacotherapies for Substance Disorders

Jag Khalsa and Kristopher Bough

Drugs of Abuse and Pharmacotherapies for Substance Use Disorders: Introduction

9

Jag H. Khalsa

Contents

Abstract

Substance use/abuse remains a major problem in the world. The use of both *legal* (alcohol, tobacco, caffeine) and *illegal* drugs (androgenic anabolic steroids, amphetamines, benzodiazepines, cannabis, cocaine, heroin/opiates, hallucinogens, inhalants, khat, and prescribed/misused drugs) is associated with serious morbidity (health consequences) and mortality. Several chapters in this section discuss epidemiology, pharmacology, and various therapeutic interventions available for clinical management of health consequences of various substance use disorders. It should be noted that even though the treatment of substance use disorders with a wide range of clinical symptoms is complex, effective clinical management is achievable with integrated programs of health care. It is anticipated that the reader at the global level will benefit from the current knowledge on clinical management of health effects of drugs of abuse presented in this section.

Keywords

Drug abuse · Pharmacotherapies · SUDS

9.1 Introduction

Substance abuse and associated addiction/dependence continue to remain some of the major problems in the world. According to the 2018 WHO Drug Report [1], an estimated 275 million people worldwide, which is roughly *5.6 percent of the global population* aged 15–64 years, used drugs at least once during 2016. Some 31 million people who use drugs

J. H. Khalsa (✉)
Division of Therapeutics and Medical Consequences, National Institute on Drug Abuse, National Institutes of Health, Aldie, VA, USA
e-mail: jag.khalsa@nih.gov

© Springer Nature Switzerland AG 2021
N. el-Guebaly et al. (eds.), *Textbook of Addiction Treatment*,
https://doi.org/10.1007/978-3-030-36391-8_9

suffer from drug use disorders, meaning that their drug use is harmful to the point where they may need treatment. Roughly 450,000 people died as a result of drug use in 2015. Of those deaths, 167,750 were directly associated with drug use disorders (mainly overdoses). Opioids continued to cause the most harm, accounting for 76 percent of deaths where drug use disorders were implicated. In the USA, an estimated 19.7 million American adults (aged 12 and older) battled a substance use disorder in 2017 [2]. Almost 74% of adults suffering from a substance use disorder in 2017 struggled with an alcohol use disorder. There were 70,000 deaths from opiate overdoses. In addition, the total economic cost to the USA alone was $740 billion (tobacco, $300B; alcohol, $249B; illicit drugs, $193B; prescription drugs, $78.5B); the health-related costs were estimated to be $168B, $27B, $11B, and $26B for tobacco, alcohol, illicit drugs, and prescription drugs, respectively.

Regardless of the incidence and prevalence of legal and illegal drug use/abuse, we must recognize that we will never be able to completely eradicate drug abuse. But we *must* be able to recognize and characterize the wide range of serious health and medical consequences of both legal and illegal drugs and reduce their impact on society by using the best and effective intervention (prevention and treatment) strategies. The health consequences of legal substances (e.g., caffeine, tobacco, and alcohol), prescription drugs (e.g., benzodiazepines, opioid pain medications, and androgenic anabolic steroids), and illegal substances (e.g., amphetamines, cocaine, opiates, hallucinogens, and marijuana) involve almost every biochemical and physiological system, and these may include psychiatric, cardiovascular, metabolic, and hepatic complications and infectious diseases.

In the first edition of the textbook on drug treatment, all the important aspects of medical consequences of substance abuse were discussed. This section of the second edition of the text book will have updated chapters discussing the currently available interventions (prevention and treatment) for reducing the impact of health consequences of substance abuse.

A typical patient with a substance use disorder (SUD) has multiple problems rather than single pathology, yet it is not generally feasible for multiple specialists to become involved. In addition, it is also not adequately covered in medical school training. Consequently, the addiction medicine specialist needs a broad range of clinical skills to adequately manage patients with complex health problems including pain. Alcohol and other drugs particularly affect the neurological systems but may also involve other physiological and biochemical systems including gastrointestinal, cardiovascular, hepatic, and metabolic systems as well. The medical comorbidities may include psychiatric, cardiovascular, co-occurring infections, or other physiological system involvement; this section will briefly address specific non-infectious drug-related consequences and their clinical management.

9.2 Use/Abuse of Legal Substances

The two most toxic substances of use, alcohol and tobacco, are legal and are associated with significant morbidity and mortality. In Chap. 10 on *alcohol* use disorder (*AUD*), Trick and LeFoll discuss several pharmacological combined with behavioral and psychosocial interventions that are effective for treating AUD. In addition to the already approved medications such as disulfiram, naltrexone, acamprosate, and nalmefene, some "off-label" medications are also under investigation for treating AUD. Research is underway to better understand predictors of treatment response which may ultimately lead to improved treatment outcomes in the future.

In Chap. 15 on *tobacco* use and its treatment, Sasiadek, Durham, and George point out that even though the rates of tobacco use and tobacco use disorder have reduced substantially over the past 40 years, an estimated 1.1 billion people worldwide and 34 million people in the USA still smoke tobacco. A substantial number of these people develop tobacco use disorder (*TUD*) with significant morbidity and commonly, cancer-related mortality. An estimated 10% are successful in quitting smoking (CDC [3]). The chapter presents the available research on clinical assessment; various psychosocial and pharmacological treatments, including the FDA-approved pharmacotherapies: nicotine replacement therapies (NRTs), sustained-release bupropion, and varenicline; and finally the integration of tobacco use disorder treatment into mental health settings. There are future challenges such as developing safer and more effective therapies for smoking cessation and making these therapies available to all smokers who want to quit.

Finally, in the chapter on *caffeine* (Chap. 16), Favrod-Coune and Broers report on a substance that is used by >90% of the world's population. They provide insight into health consequences of caffeine and other xanthines, especially focusing on coffee, tea, or energy drinks. They recommend the distribution of more and better information to the population about the risk of acute intoxication of caffeine, the nutritional and metabolic risks of energy drinks, and the problems of mixing these with alcohol. They recommend placing warning messages on caffeine-containing food or drinks as well as a legal limitation of the content of caffeine. In addition, they discuss possible treatment modalities for their excessive use and abuse.

9.3 Illegal or Medically Prescribed but Misused Drugs

With regard to addiction to *amphetamine*-type stimulants (*ATS*, Chap. 14), Elkashef and Khalsa discuss the consequences of and pharmacotherapies for treating addiction to amphetamine-type stimulants. They suggest that treatment to ATS addiction should begin early, be comprehensive and integrated, and should be long term and that treatment modalities such as psychotherapeutic interventions, medications including agonists like d-amphetamine and methylphenidate and other medications like bupropion, modafinil, naltrexone, and topiramate have been found to be promising for treating addiction to ATS.

In the chapter on *anabolic androgenic steroids* (Chap. 21), Kanayama and Pope report that AAS

use was common among athletes in the past, but now their use has spread widely in the general population with an estimated 2.9 to 4.0 million users in the USA. The AAS use is associated with significant morbidity resulting in cardiovascular, psychiatric, endocrine, and musculoskeletal complications and dependence in AAS users. Though there are no known specific anti-AAS medications available to treat AAS consequences, medications have been used to treat specific consequences of AAS such as endocrine effects and muscle dysmorphic syndrome.

The use of *benzodiazepine and benzodiazepine-like drugs (z-type)* such as sedatives, hypnotics, antiepileptics, and muscle relaxants continues to be a major problem in the world. Umbricht and Valez (Chap. 11) report that the use of these drugs, particularly among adolescents, women, elderly, and polydrug abusers, is associated with significant morbidity and mortality. In the USA alone, 12.5% of adults aged 65 years old are prescribed BZDs or Z-drugs in spite of a clear increase in mortality in this age group. An estimated 3–41% of patients with alcohol use disorder also misuse BZDs. Opioids are also involved in about 75–86% of benzodiazepine deaths. Nearly 30% of fatal opioid overdoses in the USA also involve benzodiazepines. The authors present an excellent discussion on adverse consequences of BZD in various populations and currently available prevention and non-pharmacologic interventions for benzodiazepine users.

As mentioned above, *cannabis* remains the most illicit drug used in the world, and its associated cannabis use disorder (*CUD*) poses a major public health problem. In a chapter on CUD (Chap. 12), Budney, Sofis, and Borodovsky discuss cannabis use, the associated social and health problems, and intervention therapeutic (tested and novel), pharmacologic, and behavioral (MET/CBT/CM) modalities for treating CUD and relapse. They also discuss novel approaches of modulating the endocannabinoid system; alternative dosing with CB1 agonists, and combinations of medications targeting withdrawal and co-occurring symptoms and disorders that may interfere with cannabis reduction or prompt relapse.

Cocaine use is also associated with significant morbidity and mortality. Currently, there are no specific FDA-approved medications for treating cocaine use disorder (*CUD*). However, in a chapter on cocaine (Chap. 13), Gorelick reports that treatment strategies such as "off-label" medications including disulfiram, tricyclic antidepressants such as desipramine and imipramine, the anticonvulsant topiramate, and behavioral modalities are being used for treating CUD. He suggests that by understanding neurobiology of cocaine addiction, one could develop innovative treatment modalities for treating CUD. Importantly, clinicians should keep in mind the distinctions between efficacy and effectiveness and between a statistically significant and clinically meaningful treatment effect.

According to Odenwald, Kline, and Warfa (Chap. 17), although the epidemiology of *khat* use is not very clear, its use is associated with neurocognitive deficit and other health problems similar to those produced by other CNS stimulants. The authors highlight that not much is known about any effective treatments for khat addiction. Thus, Odenwald suggests the following measures: there is a strong need to (a) develop reliable and cross-culturally valid diagnostic instruments, (b) develop effective and adequate treatment strategies applicable in traditional khat use countries and among immigrant communities elsewhere in the world, (c) support strong empirical research designs to guide national and international politics, and (d) support the development of law and public health strategies, both in the "khat belt" and among the diaspora.

In the chapter on *hallucinogens* (Chap. 19), Farre and her colleagues describe a heterogeneous group of substances that act via 5-HT2A, NMDA, and opioid-kappa receptors, producing primarily perception but also substance use disorder with acute tolerance but without withdrawal syndrome. For treating hallucinogen use disorder, there are no specific therapeutic modalities available, but the aim would be to reduce consumption and achieve abstinence. According to the authors, hallucinogens like LSD, psilocybin, ayahuasca, and the designer drug MDMA are being evaluated for the treatment of different mental disorders. With regard to *inhalant* use,

Real and her colleagues discuss (Chap. 20) the epidemiology, policy issues, pharmacology, short- and long-term health effects, and prevention and treatment interventions, with particular attention to special and vulnerable populations including children, adolescents, students, indigenous groups like workers exposed to solvents, and anesthesiologists, affected by inhalant use.

Opiate abuse and resulting epidemic have become a major problem in the world. In Chap. 18 on opioid use disorder (*OUD*) and its treatment, Torrens and colleagues have discussed pharmacology of different opioid drugs and currently available pharmacotherapies including methadone and buprenorphine, combined with psychosocial interventions to treat opioid use disorder and associated complications including overdose or naltrexone depot formulations for preventing relapse. They also discuss the possibility of using alternative pharmacotherapeutics such as slow-release morphine and diacetylmorphine for treating opiate use disorder.

Finally, the use of *prescription* drugs including sedatives, stimulants, hypnotics, and analgesics has recently caused havoc in the USA and elsewhere. The use of these drugs is associated with serious morbidity (adverse health consequences) and mortality as discussed by Bramness. Chapter 22 discusses a number of important aspects of prescription drugs, differences between various class of prescription drugs, their pharmacokinetics, assessment of adverse effects, and various prevention and treatment strategies available to the treating clinician.

In summary, this section describes the morbidity and mortality that can result from substance use/abuse. Although treatment of drug addiction and associated medical and health consequences is complex, effective clinical management is achievable with integrated programs of health care. Societally, it will begin with providing the population with an accurate description of consequences of substance use/abuse and highlighting options for treatment. And, medically, the information contained herein will also provide care providers a better understanding of the disorders and outline possible options for treatment and future research. It is anticipated that the reader at the global level will benefit from the current knowledge on clinical management of health effects of drugs of abuse presented in this section.

Acknowledgments The author is grateful to the National Institute on Drug Abuse, NIH, for an opportunity to continue to serve as a special volunteer to be able to collaborate with NIH and other national and international colleagues. The author is also grateful to his NIDA colleague, Dr. Kris Bough, program director, Division of Basic Neuroscience and Behavior Research, for valuable suggestions in the preparation of this chapter and the section as the co-editor.

Disclosures The opinions in this chapter are of the author and do not reflect those of the National Institute on Drug Abuse, National Institutes of Health, USA.

References

1. Center for Behavioral Health Statistics and Quality. 2017 national survey on drug use and health: detailed tables. Substance abuse and mental health services administration, Rockville, MD; 2018. https://www.samhsa.gov/.../NSDUHDetailedTabs2017/NSDUHDetailedTabs2017.pdf; https://www.samhsa.gov/sites/default/files/nsduh-ppt-09-2018.pptx. Accessed 14 July 2019.
2. Centers for Disease Control and Prevention. Quitting smoking among adults—United States, 2000–2015. Morb Mortal Wkly Rep. 2017;65(52):1457–64. https://www.cdc.gov/mmwr/volumes/65/wr/mm6552a1.htm. Accessed 14 July 2019.
3. World Drug Report. United Nations publication, Sales No. E.18.XI.9; 2018. https://www.unodc.org/wdr2018. Accessed 14 July 2019.

Pharmacological Treatment of Alcohol Use Disorder

10

Leanne Trick and Bernard Le Foll

Contents

L. Trick
Translational Addiction Research Laboratory, Centre for Addiction and Mental Health, University of Toronto, Toronto, ON, Canada
e-mail: Leanne.Trick@camh.ca

B. Le Foll (✉)
Translational Addiction Research Laboratory, Centre for Addiction and Mental Health, University of Toronto, Toronto, ON, Canada

Alcohol Research and Treatment Clinic, Acute Care Program, Centre for Addiction and Mental Health, Toronto, ON, Canada

Campbell Family Mental Health Research Institute, Centre for Addiction and Mental Health, Toronto, ON, Canada

Department of Family and Community Medicine, University of Toronto, Toronto, ON, Canada

Department of Pharmacology and Toxicology, University of Toronto, Toronto, ON, Canada

Division of Brain and Therapeutics, Department of Psychiatry, University of Toronto, Toronto, ON, Canada

Institute of Medical Sciences, University of Toronto, Toronto, ON, Canada
e-mail: Bernard.LeFoll@camh.ca

© Springer Nature Switzerland AG 2021
N. el-Guebaly et al. (eds.), *Textbook of Addiction Treatment*,
https://doi.org/10.1007/978-3-030-36391-8_10

Abstract

Alcohol use disorder (AUD) is a severe condition associated with negative health, social and economic consequences, yet it often remains untreated. Pharmacological treatments for AUD are effective, especially in combination with other behavioural or psychosocial interventions. Disulfiram, naltrexone, acamprosate and nalmefene are approved pharmacological treatments for AUD. In addition, medications for other health conditions can be prescribed 'off-label', and further potentially useful drugs are under investigation. Current research is seeking to better understand predictors of treatment response which may ultimately lead to improved treatment outcomes in the future. This chapter provides a summary of approved pharmacological treatments and other medications that may prove useful in the treatment of AUD.

Keywords

Alcohol use disorder · Pharmacological treatment · Pharmacotherapy · Medication Abstinence · Relapse

10.1   Introduction

Alcohol use disorder (AUD) is a chronic relapsing condition characterized by compulsive alcohol use and loss of control over drinking, accompanied by clinically important impairment or distress. Current diagnostic criteria (DSM-5; *American Psychiatric Association*) require the presence of at least 2 out of 11 symptoms, with severity intensifying as the number of symptoms increase. In the USA estimates of 12-month and lifetime prevalence of AUD in adults are 13.9% and 29.1%, respectively [1]. According to a 2018 report by the *World Health Organization* [2], the harmful use of alcohol results in three million deaths each year, and 5.1% of all disease burden worldwide is related to alcohol use. AUD is asso-

ciated with a variety of other physical and mental health conditions including neurological impairments, cardiovascular disease, liver disease, cancer, mood and anxiety disorders and foetal alcohol syndrome, along with other adverse outcomes such as risk of injury [3]. Furthermore AUD imposes a huge economic burden, for example, in the USA alone AUD has been estimated to cost $223.5 billion annually [4].

Despite the prevalence of AUD and increased morbidity, mortality and economic costs associated with it, many people with AUD remain untreated. A large US survey suggests that only 14.6% of those with a diagnosis of AUD receive treatment [5]. Thus, a large proportion of people with AUD do not receive treatment despite the availability of effective interventions (e.g. studies show that treatments for AUD are associated with reductions in risk for relapse and AUD-associated mortality [6, 7]).

Available treatments for AUD include pharmacotherapy, behavioural or psychosocial therapies involving professional counselling and mutual support groups such as *Alcoholics Anonymous*. These treatments are complementary; each addresses a different aspect of alcohol dependence, while they share the common goal of maintaining abstinence. Pharmacological treatments for AUD are recommended in conjunction with other behavioural or psychosocial approaches, and such combinations have proven to be successful [8, 9]. The US *National Institute on Alcohol Abuse and Alcoholism* recommends pharmacological treatment particularly where patients who have recently stopped drinking are experiencing problems with craving or 'slips', or in cases where behavioural or psychosocial treatments alone have previously failed.

Existing pharmacological treatments work to eliminate or reduce drinking and prevent relapse by causing unpleasant side effects if alcohol is consumed, by blocking the rewarding effects of alcohol or by suppressing craving for alcohol. Several of these medicines have been approved for the treatment of AUD by regulatory agencies (e.g. the US *Food and Drug Administration*; FDA), although approval status varies by country. Additionally, medications developed and licensed for the treatment of other health conditions, but which have shown utility in the management of AUD, can be used 'off-label', and other new medications are under investigation which may provide treatment alternatives in the near future.

This chapter provides an overview of approved pharmacological treatments for AUD, along with other medications that appear to be useful in the treatment of AUD. Factors influencing the choice of pharmacotherapy and predictors of treatment response are briefly discussed. Other medicines used in the early stages of treatment to assist with safely managing symptoms of withdrawal from alcohol (e.g. benzodiazepines) will not be considered since this chapter focuses on pharmacological treatments intended to reduce alcohol consumption and prevent relapse. The information presented here is based on a synthesis of evidence from any country where relevant research has been conducted. In general, where reviews or meta-analyses exist (especially systematic or Cochrane reviews), these are presented in favour of the results of individual studies.

10.2 Approved Pharmacological Treatments

Four pharmacological treatments are widely approved for the treatment of AUD: disulfiram, naltrexone, acamprosate and nalmefene. This section summarizes available information about the mechanism of action, efficacy and administration of each medication in turn, followed by a head-to-head comparison of the four drugs.

10.2.1 Disulfiram

Disulfiram (marketed under the trade name Antabuse®) is licensed in many countries for the treatment of AUD including the USA, Canada and in Europe and has been in use since the 1940s.

The potential of disulfiram as a treatment for AUD was discovered by chance in the 1930s after factory workers in the rubber industry reported feeling sick when they drank alcohol, following exposure to a by-product of rubber manufacturing – disulfiram. It was later learned that disulfiram interferes with the metabolism of alcohol and discourages alcohol consumption by causing unpleasant effects such as nausea, vomiting, flushing and palpitations if alcohol is consumed. Early attempts to utilize disulfiram as a treatment for alcoholism were based on a paradigm of aversion conditioning using high doses, although this led to a number of serious adverse side effects and even deaths. Subsequently the dose was lowered, and the focus of treatment shifted to supporting abstinence by strengthening the patient's motivation to avoid alcohol.

The use of disulfiram is indicated, following initial withdrawal, for complete cessation of alcohol consumption in highly motivated patients.

10.2.1.1 Mechanism of Action

The effect of disulfiram is thought to be mainly due to its interference with the metabolism of alcohol. The majority of alcohol taken into the body is metabolized by the liver. First, the enzyme alcohol dehydrogenase (ADH) converts alcohol molecules into acetaldehyde, a toxic chemical compound. Then acetaldehyde is converted by another enzyme, aldehyde dehydrogenase (ALDH), into acetic acid. Finally, acetic acid can be broken down into water and carbon dioxide and eliminated from the body. Disulfiram blocks the natural degradation of alcohol by inhibiting the liver enzyme ALDH, which results in an accumulation of acetaldehyde. This accumulation of toxic acetaldehyde causes symptoms such as nausea, vomiting, headache, flushing, diarrhoea and hypotension. Given a sufficiently high dose of alcohol, the interaction with disulfiram can cause serious adverse events and even death. Several genetic polymorphisms exist in the genes that encode the liver enzymes ADH and ALDH, and these can have implications for drinking behaviour, responses to alcohol, risk for dependence and potentially also the treatment of AUD. For example, ALDH2 is one of two main genes responsible for encoding ALDH, and variants of this gene have been identified that are either 'active' or 'inactive' in the elimination of acetaldehyde. The inactive form of ALDH2 (the ALDH2*2 allele) is found among approximately 50% of the Asian population and is responsible for the 'flushing' response seen after alcohol consumption, thought to be due to the accumulation of acetaldehyde (since the inactive variant of the gene inhibits breakdown of acetaldehyde). This allele is also associated with lower risk for alcohol dependence and slower development of symptoms of alcohol dependence. Polymorphisms of both ALDH2 and other genes that encode ADH (e.g. ADH1A) have also been associated with increased risk of cancer and other physical illnesses such as liver disease and diabetes in heavy drinkers, and it is proposed that this is due not only to differences in levels of alcohol consumption but also to the way alcohol is metabolized.

Disulfiram also acts as a dopamine beta-hydroxylase inhibitor [10, 11]. This inhibition creates a decrease of norepinephrine and an increase of dopamine levels in the brain. Such an imbalance may have therapeutic properties for the treatment of substance use disorders and could explain why disulfiram can affect behavioural responses related to addiction (even in animals never exposed to alcohol).

Finally, some consider disulfiram a form of psychological treatment, since the anticipation of adverse effects (if alcohol is consumed) is a key element of successful treatment. For example, randomized controlled studies have shown that disulfiram is only effective at reducing alcohol consumption when it is administered in open-label (i.e. unblinded) conditions and where patients receive clear and repeated information about the adverse effects produced by the disulfiram-alcohol interaction [12].

10.2.1.2 Efficacy

Evidence of the effectiveness of disulfiram for the treatment of AUD is limited. Several reviews report mixed findings, with a reduction in the amount of alcohol consumed and/or a reduction in the number of drinking days in disulfiram-treated patients compared to placebo in some studies but no improvements in relapse rates. Concerns have also been raised about heterogeneity among existing trials and weak study quality [13–16].

A recent meta-analysis of 22 randomized controlled trials (cumulative total $N = 2414$) highlighted several methodological inconsistencies among existing studies [12]. Importantly, this review also demonstrated the impact of study design on appraisals of effectiveness. Two-thirds of the studies included in the meta-analysis used an open-label design, and the remainder used a blinded design. Results showed that disulfiram was effective only in open-label trials. While the 'gold standard' for trials of this type would usually dictate blinded treatment administration, the findings here are in fact consistent with disulfiram's mechanism of action; since the expectation of unpleasant effects due to the disulfiram-alcohol interaction is thought to motivate abstinence, it follows that the certain knowledge of having received active treatment is a necessary condition for its success.

Treatment supervision has been identified as another important variable that appears to impact on efficacy. For example, in one small review, the only study that showed a positive effect of disulfiram compared to placebo was also the only study to use supervised administration. The authors reported a further comparison of five studies using supervised versus unsupervised treatment and concluded that best outcomes were achieved where disulfiram administration was supervised by a healthcare provider [17]. Some existing studies have been criticized because of poor treatment compliance and low retention rates (e.g. 46% of patients dropped out before the end of one study), and this has been particularly problematic in studies where treatment was unsupervised [15]. This suggests that enhanced compliance may be one mechanism by which treatment supervision might improve outcomes.

The optimal duration of disulfiram treatment is currently unclear. A review comparing short- and long-term treatments found improvements in days until relapse and number of drinking days with short-term disulfiram treatment compared to placebo, but only limited positive effects of disulfiram with longer-term (12 months) treatment [18]. On the other hand, in a single study of patients with severe AUD in long-term treatment, an abstinence rate of more than 50% was observed using guided administration of disulfiram over 9 years follow-up. This suggests that extended treatment with disulfiram might be useful but only in the context of comprehensive outpatient treatment with adequate supervision [19].

Studies showing reduced craving and increased consecutive days of abstinence in alcoholics with co-morbid psychiatric diagnoses [20] and reductions in alcohol consumption in poly-substance users [21] following disulfiram treatment suggest that disulfiram may have value in patients with other psychiatric and substance use co-morbidities.

10.2.1.3 Administration

Dose and Regimen

An oral dose of disulfiram should be taken once daily, tapered up over 1–2 weeks to an average maintenance dose of 250 mg daily (maximum dose 500 mg). Patients should receive a thorough explanation of the rationale and effects of disulfiram treatment, including information about the disulfiram-alcohol interaction, strong cautions about drinking while taking disulfiram and warnings about ingestion of products that may not obviously contain alcohol (e.g. sauces, cough mixtures, liniments, sanitizing gels, etc.). It is not necessary to 'test' the disulfiram-alcohol interaction (i.e. to induce an aversive reaction by administering alcohol under supervision) since this does not improve efficacy as long as adequate education is provided [19].

Non-compliance is one of the biggest problems with disulfiram use. It is therefore important that patients are committed to treatment and it is administered under supervision. Ideally, the clinician should arrange for the pill to be taken under supervision by a family member to ensure better adherence to treatment. Treatment may last for months or years, and after initial treatment has been discontinued patients may choose to restart disulfiram in anticipation of exposure to high-risk situations or during periods of acute stress that may challenge their resolve to remain abstinent.

Contraindications

Patients must be detoxified (ideally for a few days), free of alcohol for at least the past 12 hours and free of withdrawal symptoms before treatment with disulfiram can commence. It should be noted that a disulfiram-alcohol reaction can occur for up to 2 weeks after disulfiram has been discontinued.

Disulfiram is contraindicated in patients with psychosis, severe myocardial disease and coronary occlusion and in pregnant or nursing mothers. Caution is recommended in patients with cardiac disease, diabetes mellitus, hypothyroidism, epilepsy, cerebral damage, kidney disease, cirrhosis of the liver, liver failure and hepatitis C. Caution is also recommended in children, adolescents and older adults (dose reductions should be considered in adults aged over 60 years). Prescribers should be aware of interactions with other drugs including benzodiazepines, isoniazid, monoamine oxidase inhibitors, tricyclic antidepressants, warfarin, metronidazole, theophylline, phenytoin and lithium. Dose adjustments and careful monitoring may be necessary to ensure patient safety.

Side Effects

If alcohol is not consumed, side effects associated with disulfiram are generally mild and appear within the first 1–2 weeks of treatment. Tiredness is the main side effect. Other common side effects include headache, metallic taste in the mouth, skin rash, impotence in men and a swollen or sore tongue. Less common but serious side effects include optic neuritis, peripheral neuropathy, hepatitis, liver failure and psychosis.

A meta-analysis of randomized controlled trials investigating the efficacy of disulfiram also collated information relating to adverse effects. While more adverse events were reported in disulfiram-treated groups overall compared to controls, there was no difference in the number of deaths or serious adverse events requiring hospitalization suggesting that disulfiram is safe in carefully screened groups, such as those included in clinical trials [12].

10.2.2 Naltrexone

Naltrexone is approved for use in the treatment of AUD in over 30 countries worldwide [22]. The FDA approved an oral formulation in 1994, followed in 2006 by an extended-release injectable formulation that was developed to improve treatment retention and adherence. Oral naltrexone is marketed under trade names including ReVia®, Natrel® and Depade® and extended-release as Vivitrol®.

In the treatment of AUD, naltrexone may be useful in preventing relapse by blocking the pleasurable rewarding effects of alcohol. It is indicated in detoxified patients who are not currently using, or who have not recently used, opioids.

10.2.2.1 Mechanism of Action

Naltrexone is an opioid receptor antagonist with high affinity for the μ-receptor and weaker affinity at δ- and κ-receptors. The mechanism by which naltrexone reduces alcohol consumption is not fully understood, although it is thought to be mediated by the endogenous opioid and dopamine systems. In the brain, acute alcohol consumption triggers the release of the endogenous opioid β-endorphin, which in turn stimulates dopamine release in the nucleus accumbens and other areas of the mesolimbic-dopamine pathway involved in the processing of reward and thought to be responsible for the positive reinforcing effects of alcohol. Due to its antagonist properties at the μ-opioid receptor, naltrexone may suppress alcohol consumption by blockade of the receptor (therefore also blocking dopamine release), thus disrupting the pleasurable positive reinforcing effects of alcohol and reducing alcohol craving. This hypothesis is supported by animal studies showing that mice without the μ-opioid receptor do not self-administer alcohol, presumably due to lack of positive reinforcement [23].

10.2.2.2 Efficacy

Interest in naltrexone for the treatment of AUD was stimulated by two early clinical trials which showed that among alcohol-dependent patients 12 weeks of treatment with naltrexone as an adjunct to psychosocial interventions improved drinking outcomes including abstinence, relapse rates, number of drinking days, severity of alcohol-related problems and craving. Both studies suggested that naltrexone was particularly effective in preventing relapse to dependence following alcohol exposure [24, 25]. Approval of naltrexone by the FDA soon followed, along with a raft of controlled and randomized controlled trials.

Several meta-analyses have supported the early positive findings, with modest improvements in a variety of drinking outcomes, most commonly relapse to heavy drinking [16, 26–31]. The most recent Cochrane review of opioid antagonists for the treatment of alcohol dependence identified 47 randomized controlled trials involving naltrexone as an adjunct to psychosocial interventions [32]. Oral naltrexone significantly reduced two of three primary outcomes, return to heavy drinking (number needed to treat (NNT) = 10, i.e., ten patients require treatment to prevent one patient returning to heavy drinking) and the number of drinking days (NNT = 25), but had no effect on return to any drinking. All secondary outcomes were improved by naltrexone including a 3% reduction in number of heavy-drinking days and an almost 11 g reduction in alcohol consumption on drinking days. In the majority of studies, a standard 50 mg daily dose was used, and treatment typically lasted for 3 months. A small subset of studies that included post-treatment follow-ups indicated that the benefits of treatment fade after discontinuation, although naltrexone-treated patients had a 14% lower risk of return to heavy drinking compared to placebo at up to 12 months follow-up. Extended-release naltrexone was not associated with significant improvements, although few studies were available for review.

A small number of studies have not shown any positive effects of oral naltrexone, although these studies have tended to be limited by small sample sizes or poor treatment compliance or have used samples with other psychiatric or substance use co-morbidities (e.g. severe depression, eating disorders).

Of all the approved treatments for AUD, naltrexone has the largest evidence base regarding efficacy. However, previous reviews have highlighted several issues with the existing evidence, including the following:

(a) Heterogeneity in study design which has limited the generalizability of findings of individual studies.
(b) A large number of outcome measures have been used, and there is inconsistency among studies in the measure for which largest or most consistent effects have been observed.
(c) In many studies treatment duration was short, and so it is still unclear how long treatment effects will last and what the appropriate length of treatment may be.
(d) Currently there is limited evidence of the efficacy of injectable naltrexone, although existing studies suggest specific subgroups may see benefit with this formulation, e.g. males and individuals with lead-in abstinence [33, 34].

On the other hand, consistent positive observations are that (a) many individual studies are of moderate to high quality; (b) time to relapse is the most consistently improved outcome variable, suggesting that naltrexone is particularly effective for relapse prevention; and (c) naltrexone should be given in combination with psychosocial therapy.

Research is increasingly turning its attention to predictors of treatment response. This may help to explain inconsistencies in treatment effects but also suggests the possibility of optimizing efficacy in the future by tailoring treatments. Pharmacogenetic studies, for example, have initially suggested that variants of the OPRM1 gene that encodes the μ-opioid receptor may affect naltrexone treatment response in AUD patients [35, 36]. However, this result was not replicated in a prospective cohort study [37], and so at this point pharmacogenetic tailoring is not yet ready to be implemented in routine clinical care until more robust findings emerge from further studies.

10.2.2.3 Administration

Dose and Regimen
The standard dose of oral naltrexone is 50 mg once daily, taken for 3–6 months (although it can be continued for up to 24 months if required). The optimal duration of treatment is unclear, although some studies suggest that after initial treatment has been discontinued a regimen of targeted use at 'high-risk' times may maintain treatment effects [38, 39].

Extended-release naltrexone is available as a 380 mg dose, given by intramuscular injection approximately every 4 weeks.

Contraindications
Patients should not be drinking at treatment initiation, and naltrexone should not be used in patients with current, recent (past 7 days) or anticipated use of opioid medication since naltrexone can precipitate severe opioid withdrawal.

Naltrexone is contraindicated in patients with acute hepatitis or liver failure. Caution is advised in patients with active liver disease, kidney disease and pregnant or nursing mothers.

Side Effects
Naltrexone is generally well tolerated, with mainly mild side effects. The most common side effects include nausea, vomiting, headache, tiredness, anxiety and insomnia. Less common side effects include gastrointestinal complaints (e.g. diarrhoea, abdominal pain, constipation), joint/muscle aches, rash, dizziness, increased or decreased energy, ringing in the ears, sweating, mild depression and delayed ejaculation. Uncommon but serious side effects include liver toxicity and failure (usually at higher than standard doses, so naltrexone can typically be initiated even in patients with mild liver problems, i.e. AST or ALT levels below 3 times normal), suicidal thoughts, hallucinations, blurred vision, swelling of the face, feet or legs and shortness of breath.

A meta-analysis of efficacy studies found no significant difference between naltrexone versus placebo in the number of patients who experienced at least one adverse event or in the number of patients who discontinued due to an adverse event, suggesting that side effects do not impact upon naltrexone compliance or discontinuation [30].

10.2.3 Acamprosate

Acamprosate (also known by the trade name Campral®) was first approved for the treatment of AUD in Europe in 1989. It is currently approved worldwide including in the USA, Canada, South America, Australia and parts of Asia and Africa.

It is indicated for the prevention of relapse in patients with established abstinence. Unlike naltrexone, acamprosate can be used in patients receiving opioid treatment, e.g. for chronic pain conditions.

10.2.3.1 Mechanism of Action

While its exact mechanism of action is unknown, it is believed that acamprosate may work by modulating activity of the glutamatergic neurotransmitter system. Chronic excessive alcohol use is thought to cause neuroadaptive changes that result in an imbalance between the excitatory glutamatergic and inhibitory GABAergic neurotransmitter systems. In turn this is thought to be involved in the development of tolerance to alcohol and symptoms of alcohol withdrawal (such as craving). It has been proposed that acamprosate may normalize pathological glutamatergic hyperactivity by modulating activity at NMDA and mGLu5 glutamate receptors, thereby restoring the balance between glutamatergic and GABAergic systems and blunting the negative effects of alcohol withdrawal thought to trigger relapse [40, 41].

10.2.3.2 Efficacy

Many randomized controlled trials have been conducted to compare the efficacy of acamprosate with placebo for the treatment of AUD. The majority of these trials have shown moderate improvements with acamprosate treatment on outcomes including continuous abstinence rates,

cumulative number of abstinent days, return to any drinking and percentage of patients remaining in treatment [16, 27, 31, 42]. One review reported a 7–13% improvement in outcomes with acamprosate compared to placebo [31]. Beneficial effects of treatment may persist after treatment is discontinued, with improvements in abstinence rates (but not number of drinking days) having been reported at 6–12 months post-treatment [43].

A Cochrane review identified 24 randomized controlled trials investigating the effectiveness of acamprosate (cumulative total N = 6915). Treatment typically commenced after patients had achieved 3–7 days of abstinence and was administered for 6 months as an adjunct to psychosocial interventions. The most commonly used outcome measure was return to any drinking (or the opposite; continuous abstinence). Analysis of pooled data showed that acamprosate reduced the risk of return to drinking to 86% of that in the placebo group (NNT = 9) and increased cumulative abstinence duration by 11%. However, there was no significant positive effect of acamprosate treatment on the secondary outcomes return to heavy drinking or gamma-glutamyl transferase (a biochemical marker of heavy alcohol use) [44].

A small number of studies have shown no improvement in drinking outcomes following acamprosate treatment. Aspects of study design such as small sample sizes, short treatment duration and a long lead-in abstinence period may have contributed to the failure to find treatment benefit in these studies. However, two large well-designed trials (the US COMBINE study [45] and the PREDICT study conducted in Germany [46]) have also reported no improvement in drinking outcomes following 3 months (PREDICT) or 4 months (COMBINE) of treatment. It is not immediately clear why these trials should have found no positive effect of acamprosate. The authors suggest that differences in patient characteristics and treatment settings may explain the contrary findings. The details of psychosocial interventions are not well described in many reports, but it is also possible that more comprehensive psychosocial interventions employed in COMBINE and PREDICT may have masked any beneficial effects of acamprosate.

A strength of the existing evidence base is that individual studies have generally been of adequate quality and are reasonably comparable. These studies demonstrate that as an adjunct to psychosocial interventions acamprosate appears to be helpful in maintaining abstinence in AUD patients who have recently stopped drinking. On the other hand, acamprosate does not seem to be as effective in preventing return to heavy drinking [16], and it is unclear whether the type of psychosocial intervention impacts on efficacy.

Several potential predictors of treatment response have been identified. For example, sex, psychiatric and substance use co-morbidities (including anxiety), family history of alcoholism or late age of AUD onset may be factors that modify treatment response [47]. In the COMBINE study, where no overall positive treatment effects were found, a subgroup analysis showed that acamprosate improved abstinence from heavy drinking in patients with shorter duration of abstinence at treatment initiation, those who had received prior treatment or those with a goal of total abstinence. This may suggest that individuals with more severe AUD respond better to acamprosate (e.g. since they have greater upregulation of the glutamatergic system, the supposed target of acamprosate treatment [48]) and that motivation to abstain is an important factor in the success of acamprosate treatment. Finally, pharmacogenetic studies have identified potential genetic markers of treatment response including variants of the GATA binding protein 4 [49], GABARA6 and GABARA2 [40] genes.

10.2.3.3 Administration

Dose and Regimen
Treatment with acamprosate is generally initiated after 5 days of alcohol abstinence, although it is safe to begin treatment prior to cessation of drinking or during alcohol withdrawal. Acamprosate is available in 333 mg tablets, and an oral dose of 666 mg should be taken three times per day. A lower dose (333 mg three times per day) may be used for some patients including those with impaired kidney function. Treatment should be administered as an adjunct to behav-

ioural or psychosocial interventions and should persist even if the patient relapses.

Contraindications
Since acamprosate is excreted primarily by the kidneys, it is contraindicated in patients with severe renal impairment. Caution is advised in patients with moderate renal impairment, children, adolescents, older adults (65 years and older) and pregnant or nursing mothers.

Side Effects
Side effects of acamprosate are generally mild and transient. The most common side effect is diarrhoea. Other less common side effects include gastrointestinal complaints (cramps, flatulence), headache, change in libido, insomnia, anxiety, muscle weakness, nausea, itchiness and dizziness. Suicidal ideation is a rare but serious side effect.

10.2.4 Nalmefene

Nalmefene is the most recently approved pharmacological treatment for AUD and is currently available within Europe and a small number of other countries (including Australia and Hong Kong). It was approved by the *European Medicines Agency* in 2012 and has been marketed since April 2013 under the brand name Selincro®.

The use of nalmefene is indicated for reducing the number of heavy-drinking days as part of a harm reduction strategy. In the UK the *National Institute for Health and Care Excellence* (NICE) recommends the use of nalmefene for patients with high drinking levels (greater than 60 g alcohol daily for men and greater than 40 g alcohol daily for women) who do not have physical withdrawal symptoms and who do not require immediate detoxification.

10.2.4.1 Mechanism of Action
Nalmefene is a selective opioid antagonist, structurally similar to naltrexone, with high affinity to μ-receptors and medium affinity to δ-receptors, although unlike naltrexone it is also a partial ago-

nist at κ-receptors. The therapeutic action of nalmefene in the treatment of AUD is thought to be due mainly to its antagonist effect at μ-receptors, which blocks the positive reinforcing effects of acute alcohol consumption. However animal studies suggest that in addition to μ-receptor-mediated blockade of positive reinforcing effects of alcohol, the activity of nalmefene at κ-receptors may also play an important role in its mechanism of action by blocking negative reinforcing effects of alcohol.

10.2.4.2 Efficacy

Few trials of nalmefene efficacy have been conducted to date, although the majority of existing studies have shown small positive effects, with fewer heavy-drinking days and a reduction in total alcohol consumption among AUD patients and heavy drinkers [50]. Improvements in drinking outcomes have been found following daily dosing as well as targeted (i.e. 'as needed') administration of nalmefene [51, 52]. Studies indicate that nalmefene is effective in reducing heavy drinking even among AUD patients who are unable to abstain from drinking [53]; indeed it may be most effective in subgroups of AUD patients who do not abstain from drinking prior to treatment initiation [52]. To date the best effects of nalmefene have been found in the first 4 weeks of treatment although evidence supports treatment durations of 6–12 months.

One relatively small multisite study found that 12 weeks of nalmefene treatment combined with motivational enhancement therapy had no effect on heavy drinking, craving, time to first heavy-drinking day or biochemical markers of alcohol use compared with placebo [54]. Variation between study sites and the relatively small sample size may explain the failure to find a positive effect in this study however.

Moving forward, more careful specification of the populations included in studies of nalmefene treatment is required. There is currently little or no evidence of safety or efficacy in adolescents, older adults and patients with other medical or psychiatric co-morbidities. It is also unclear whether the type or intensity of psychosocial intervention that patients engage with may impact on the efficacy of nalmefene, since in the majority of existing studies these were either unstandardized or poorly described.

Little work has investigated potential predictors of nalmefene treatment response. Preclinical research suggests the possibility that nalmefene may be more effective in severe alcohol dependence, although this remains to be confirmed in humans [55]. In addition, while pharmacogenetic studies suggest a role for the OPRM1 gene in predicting naltrexone treatment response, no moderating effects of OPRM1 genotypes on drinking outcomes following nalmefene treatment were found [56].

10.2.4.3 Administration

Dose and Regimen

An oral dose of 20 mg nalmefene can be taken daily, or 'as needed', 1–2 hours before drinking alcohol. It is recommended that nalmefene is used in conjunction with psychosocial support.

Contraindications

Since nalmefene can cause severe opioid withdrawal, it should not be used in patients with recent, current or anticipated opioid use. It is also contraindicated in patients with severe liver or renal impairment or recent acute alcohol withdrawal syndrome.

Although there are no dose-dependent effects of nalmefene on liver toxicity, caution is advised in patients with mild or moderate liver dysfunction. Caution is also advised in patients with mild or moderate renal dysfunction, a history of seizures (including alcohol withdrawal seizures), conditions that interfere with the absorption of lactose and concurrent use of potent UGT2B7 inhibitors, older adults (aged over 65 years) and pregnant or nursing mothers. Glucoronyl transfe UDP rasi

Side Effects

Nalmefene is reasonably well tolerated at daily doses of 20–40 mg [50]. The most common side effects are mild to moderate nausea, dizziness, insomnia and headache. Other side effects that have been reported include loss of appetite, confusion, restlessness, reduced libido, drowsiness,

Codeine, morphine, Oxycodone metabolized

tachycardia, dry mouth, diarrhoea, excessive sweating, muscle spasms, weakness, hallucinations, dissociation, itching, rash and swelling in the face, lips or tongue.

10.2.5 Comparison of Approved Treatments

Few head-to-head comparisons of disulfiram with other approved medications exist. However, studies suggest that disulfiram is superior to acamprosate in patients with a long duration of alcohol dependence [57], that disulfiram is more effective than naltrexone at reducing alcohol consumption but not craving in alcohol-dependent men [58] and that disulfiram in combination with a brief cognitive behavioural intervention is more effective than both naltrexone and acamprosate at reducing alcohol consumption and number of heavy-drinking days, extending time to first drink and increasing total number of abstinent days [59].

Of the four approved medications, acamprosate and naltrexone have the best evidence to support their use, showing they are both effective adjunct treatments. However, trials directly comparing acamprosate with naltrexone have not established significant differences between them in treatment outcomes. The most recent Cochrane review reported that the evidence base comparing them was too small to draw conclusions [33] and another that drug choice may be more usefully guided by other factors such as ease of administration, adverse effects and availability [16]. On the other hand, it has been suggested that acamprosate and naltrexone may impact on different facets of alcohol dependence, with studies showing that acamprosate may be more useful for eliminating drinking while naltrexone is better for achieving controlled consumption [60]. Limitations in the design of some of these studies make it unclear whether this observation is reliable.

Nalmefene is structurally similar to naltrexone but with potential pharmacological and clinical advantages including more effective binding at opioid receptors, higher bioavailability and lack of dose-dependent liver toxicity [61].

However, there is limited evidence directly comparing these drugs. A laboratory study in non-treatment seeking alcohol-dependent patients showed that both nalmefene and naltrexone reduced alcohol consumption, although more side effects were noted in the nalmefene condition [62].

10.3 'Off-Label' Pharmacological Treatments

A number of medications approved for treating other health conditions, but not currently AUD, have been suggested for 'off-label' use. This includes drugs from a variety of classes including anticonvulsants, serotonergic agents and GABAergic agents. This section briefly summarizes the most promising 'off-label' treatments for AUD.

10.3.1 Topiramate

Topiramate is approved for the treatment of epilepsy and migraine. It is thought that it may reduce the positive reinforcing effects of alcohol and alcohol craving due to suppression of dopamine release via a dual process of glutamatergic blockade and GABAergic facilitation. Through this mechanism it is also likely to be able to prevent/attenuate withdrawal symptoms, which are an important contributor of drinking, notably at the beginning of treatment. It should be noted that in the seminal trials performed by Johnson et al. [63, 64], topiramate is typically started when the patient is still drinking and the dose is gradually titrated up over 2 months. Usually patients will gradually decrease their alcohol intake and ultimately abstain from alcohol during the same period, an effect likely produced through the direct impact of topiramate on withdrawal symptoms and possibly also on the reinforcing effects of alcohol.

Few studies evaluating the efficacy of topiramate in AUD have been conducted to date. The first randomized controlled trials showed that, compared to placebo, a daily oral dose of up to

300 mg topiramate combined with a brief psychosocial intervention improved drinking outcomes including percentage of heavy-drinking days, percentage of days abstinent, drinks per day, craving for alcohol and biochemical markers of heavy alcohol use [63, 64]. Other studies have showed improvements in outcomes related to relapse. For example lower relapse rates in topiramate treated patients compared to placebo (67% vs. 86% [65]), although in one study relapse rate was superior after 4 weeks of treatment but not at 8 or 12 weeks so it is unclear how long treatment benefits are maintained [66]. A minority of studies have found no effect of topiramate although these have tended to be limited by weak study design (e.g. unblinded design or lack of placebo control), and one was unusual in using a sample of inpatients and an intense psychosocial intervention which may have masked topiramate effects [67, 68]. Interestingly, preliminary evidence suggests that a gene involved in encoding a subunit of the glutamate receptor (GRIK1) may moderate topiramate treatment effects [69].

Several side effects of topiramate have been reported including headache, numbness, taste abnormalities, cognitive impairments, anorexia and, more rarely, serious visual problems including glaucoma. There is a teratogenic risk, so pregnancy testing should be conducted in women of child-bearing age, and women should be informed of this risk and ideally use contraceptive measures. Gradual dose titration is important due to the adverse side effect profile, although the optimal dose and duration of treatment for AUD is still unclear. The fact that topiramate is started while patients are still drinking makes it quite useful for situations in which individuals are not ready to detoxify or in which there is no medical infrastructure to oversee detoxification (in which case topiramate treatment can be initiated on an ambulatory basis with close monitoring).

10.3.2 Gabapentin

Gabapentin is another anticonvulsant medication, also used for the treatment of neuropathic pain. Animal models suggest its mechanism in

the treatment of AUD may be due to indirect modulation of GABAergic neurotransmission. Laboratory and clinical studies support the safety and efficacy of gabapentin for the treatment of AUD, although the evidence base is currently small. A recent review identified six small randomized controlled trials that reported drinking outcomes among alcohol dependent patients. Five of the studies demonstrated positive effects of 4–12 weeks of treatment with gabapentin (daily doses 600–1800 mg), combined with behavioural support. Several outcomes related to drinking quantity and frequency were improved. Gabapentin also delayed onset of relapse to heavy drinking, reduced craving and improved sleep quality [70]. Positive effects were particularly evident at higher doses and where patients were already abstinent at commencement of treatment. Side effects are generally mild but can include headache, insomnia, fatigue, muscle aches and gastrointestinal complaints. Abrupt withdrawal has precipitated seizures and so dose titration is necessary. Reports of abuse have been documented in high-risk populations, and so these patients should be monitored for potential gabapentin misuse.

10.3.3 Baclofen

Baclofen is a $GABA_b$ receptor agonist, approved for the treatment of muscle spasticity. $GABA_b$ receptors are thought to be involved in emotion regulation, and a role for baclofen in treating AUD in patients with co-morbid mood and anxiety disorders has been proposed [71]. A recent narrative review found beneficial effects of baclofen on a number of drinking-related outcomes in some studies (e.g. case studies, open-label studies), although in studies with more rigorous design (i.e. randomized controlled trials) findings have been mixed despite the fact it is widely used as an off-label treatment for AUD [72]. Randomized controlled trials have used baclofen doses of 30–180 mg per day, given over 3–26 weeks, and have demonstrated that it is well tolerated with few side effects in AUD patients, even among patients with cirrhosis. However, these studies have typically excluded patients with psychiatric co-morbidities, and inconsistent effects of baseline anxiety or depression levels on treatment response have been found. At this point in time, the use of baclofen seems appropriate for patients that have AUD associated with liver cirrhosis. It should still be considered experimental otherwise.

10.4 Other Pharmacological Agents Under Investigation

While research has shown that existing pharmacological treatments can be efficacious, effect sizes are typically only small to moderate, and relapse rates are often high [73]. Thus, there is a need to develop more effective treatments. As our understanding of the neurobiology of alcohol addiction grows, new treatment targets are emerging (for a review see [74]). Covering the different drug targets is beyond the scope of the present chapter. Instead, this section describes only varenicline, a partial agonist at $\alpha4\beta2*$ acetylcholine nicotinic receptors, that is approved for smoking cessation.

In animal models varenicline has been shown to reduce alcohol self-administration and cue-induced relapse. In humans, it attenuates alcohol intake and craving for alcohol among non-dependent heavy drinkers [75], and neuroimaging studies show that in heavy-drinking smokers it decreases cue-elicited activation in areas related to reward (e.g. anterior cingulate cortex, nucleus accumbens and orbitofrontal cortex).

A recent review identified four randomized controlled trials of the safety and efficacy of varenicline in alcohol dependent patients [76]. One of these was a large multisite trial that found moderate positive effects of varenicline: after 13 weeks varenicline-treated patients had fewer heavy-drinking days per week (38% vs. 48%) and fewer drinks per day (4.4 vs. 5.3) compared to a placebo group. The varenicline group also reported less craving than the placebo group, although drinking outcomes related to abstinence were not different [77]. Two smaller trials also showed beneficial effects of varenicline treatment, with decreased

craving being the most consistent finding. The evidence for outcomes related to alcohol consumption and abstinence was more mixed. Subgroup analyses suggest that varenicline may be most effective at reducing heavy drinking among alcohol-dependent patients who are also smokers, smokers who also reduce their tobacco consumption and individuals with less severe alcohol dependence [77, 78]. Varenicline may therefore be especially effective in reducing alcohol craving and consumption among AUD patients who are highly motivated to decrease both alcohol use and smoking. The subgroups for whom varenicline is most effective, and for which outcomes, remain to be confirmed. Existing studies have all used relatively short treatment durations, and so it is also unclear what the optimal length of varenicline treatment should be.

Regarding safety, the majority of studies have found that varenicline is generally well tolerated, with mild nausea being the most frequently reported adverse effect. Therefore, varenicline represents a good option for individuals with AUD who are smokers. It could also be tested for patients that are non-smokers; however it is still experimental for this group.

10.5 Choice of Pharmacotherapy

The choice of pharmacological treatment for any given AUD patient is likely to depend on multiple factors, e.g. other medical, psychiatric or substance use co-morbidities, concurrent medication, patient preference and motivation, the goal of treatment (complete abstinence vs. reduction of alcohol consumption) and specific challenges the patient may face, whether the patient is already abstinent, ease of administration, side effects and adherence. Sequential use is common and may be necessary where the treatment initially selected is not successful, although there is no evidence to suggest a 'best order'.

It is unclear if combinations are more effective than single drug therapy. Alcohol dependence is a complex disorder involving multiple neurotransmitter and other systems, suggesting that a combination of drugs acting at different sites may provide the most comprehensive treatment strategy. However, studies comparing combination treatments with monotherapy have provided no or mixed evidence of enhanced treatment effects [45, 79, 80]. Combination therapy may be warranted if initial monotherapy is not successful.

10.6 Predictors of Treatment Response

Inconsistent treatment effects have been observed for some pharmacotherapies. Research is increasingly investigating predictors of treatment response to make sense of these mixed findings. Better understanding the characteristics of populations for whom treatments are most effective could also provide a strategy for maximizing treatment benefits by facilitating the development of personalized treatments.

One such avenue is pharmacogenetics. Research is currently investigating genetic heterogeneity in multiple systems in the body involved in both the positive and negative reinforcing effects of alcohol including the opioid system (the OPRM1 gene that encodes the μ-opioid receptor), GABAergic system (the GABRA2 and GABRG3 genes that encode the $GABA_A$ receptor), serotonergic system (the short versus long allele of the serotonin transporter gene) and corticotrophin-releasing factor system (the CRFR1 gene).

10.7 Conclusion

This chapter reviewed available information about approved and other pharmacological treatments for AUD. Key points are summarized below:

- Few treatments with clear evidence of safety and efficacy are available, and effect sizes tend to be modest.
- Disulfiram, naltrexone, acamprosate and nalmefene are the only currently approved medications for AUD.
- Disulfiram may be appropriate under certain conditions (especially with open-label, super-

vised administration where treatment compliance is good) but the existing evidence base is limited.
- There is reasonable evidence to support the use of acamprosate and naltrexone as adjunct treatments, although it is unclear which produces best effects.
- Nalmefene is approved for the reduction of alcohol consumption, but its use is relatively recent, and it is not available yet in North America.
- Topiramate, gabapentin and varenicline appear to be promising agents, although further research is required.
- Baclofen may also be worth considering, particularly in patients with liver disease, although evidence of efficacy is mixed and more research is required.
- Pharmacological treatments are recommended as an adjunct to psychosocial interventions, although the impact of the type of psychosocial intervention is unclear.
- There is currently limited evidence of efficacy in special populations, such as those with other medical, psychiatric or substance use co-morbidities, adolescents, older adults and minority groups.
- Optimal duration of treatment with pharmacological agents is unclear. Guidelines recommend continuing treatment for at least 3 months, although acamprosate is the only agent for which long-term efficacy and safety have been established.
- Better understanding predictors of treatment response may lead to improvements in treatment, including use of personalized treatment approaches.

References

1. Grant BF, et al. Epidemiology of DSM-5 alcohol use disorder: results from the National Epidemiologic Survey on Alcohol and Related Conditions III. JAMA Psychiat. 2015;72(8):757–66.
2. WHO. Global status report on alcohol and health 2018. Geneva: World Health Organization; 2018.
3. Cargiulo T. Understanding the health impact of alcohol dependence. Am J Health Syst Pharm. 2007;64(5_Supplement_3):S5–S11.

4. Bouchery EE, et al. Economic costs of excessive alcohol consumption in the U.S., 2006. Am J Prev Med. 2011;41(5):516–24.

5. Cohen E, et al. Alcohol treatment utilization: findings from the national epidemiologic survey on alcohol and related conditions. Drug Alcohol Depend. 2007;86(2):214–21.

6. Dawson DA, et al. Estimating the effect of help-seeking on achieving recovery from alcohol dependence. Addiction. 2006;101(6):824–34.

7. Timko C, et al. Predictors of 16-year mortality among individuals initiating help-seeking for an alcoholic use disorder. Alcohol Clin Exp Res. 2006;30(10):1711–20.

8. O'Malley SS, O'Connor PG. Medications for unhealthy alcohol use: across the spectrum. Alcohol Res Health. 2011;33(4):300–12.

9. Huebner RB, Kantor LW. Advances in alcoholism treatment. Alcohol Res Health. 2011;33(4):295–9.

10. Bourdelat-Parks BN, et al. Effects of dopamine beta-hydroxylase genotype and disulfiram inhibition on catecholamine homeostasis in mice. Psychopharmacology. 2005;183(1):72–80.

11. Di Ciano P, et al. Effects of disulfiram on choice behavior in a rodent gambling task: association with catecholamine levels. Psychopharmacology. 2018;235(1):23–35.

12. Skinner MD, et al. Disulfiram efficacy in the treatment of alcohol dependence: a meta-analysis. PLoS One. 2014;9(2):e87366.

13. Agosti V. The efficacy of treatments in reducing alcohol consumption: a meta-analysis. Int J Addict. 1995;30(8):1067–77.

14. Hughes JC, Cook CC. The efficacy of disulfiram: a review of outcome studies. Addiction. 1997;92(4):381–95.

15. Williams SH. Medications for treating alcohol dependence. Am Fam Physician. 2005;72(9):1775–80.

16. Jonas DE, et al. Pharmacotherapy for adults with alcohol use disorders in outpatient settings: a systematic review and meta-analysis. JAMA. 2014;311(18):1889–900.

17. Berglund M, et al. Treatment of alcohol abuse: an evidence-based review. Alcohol Clin Exp Res. 2003;27(10):1645–56.

18. Jorgensen CH, Pedersen B, Tonnesen H. The efficacy of disulfiram for the treatment of alcohol use disorder. Alcohol Clin Exp Res. 2011;35(10):1749–58.

19. Krampe H, et al. Follow-up of 180 alcoholic patients for up to 7 years after outpatient treatment: impact of alcohol deterrents on outcome. Alcohol Clin Exp Res. 2006;30(1):86–95.

20. Petrakis IL, et al. Naltrexone and disulfiram in patients with alcohol dependence and comorbid post-traumatic stress disorder. Biol Psychiatry. 2006;60(7):777–83.

21. Carroll KM, et al. Treatment of cocaine and alcohol dependence with psychotherapy and disulfiram. Addiction. 1998;93(5):713–27.

22. Litten RZ, Allen JP. Advances in development of medications for alcoholism treatment. Psychopharmacology. 1998;139(1–2):20–33.

23. Roberts AJ, et al. Mu-opioid receptor knockout mice do not self-administer alcohol. J Pharmacol Exp Ther. 2000;293(3):1002–8.

24. O'malley SS, et al. Naltrexone and coping skills therapy for alcohol dependence: a controlled study. Arch Gen Psychiatry. 1992;49(11):881–7.

25. Volpicelli JR, et al. Naltrexone in the treatment of alcohol dependence. Arch Gen Psychiatry. 1992;49(11):876–80.

26. Srisurapanont M, Jarusuraisin N. Naltrexone for the treatment of alcoholism: a meta-analysis of randomized controlled trials. Int J Neuropsychopharmacol. 2005;8(2):267–80.

27. Bouza C, et al. Efficacy and safety of naltrexone and acamprosate in the treatment of alcohol dependence: a systematic review. Addiction. 2004;99(7):811–28.

28. Snyder JL, Bowers TG. The efficacy of acamprosate and naltrexone in the treatment of alcohol dependence: a relative benefits analysis of randomized controlled trials. Am J Drug Alcohol Abuse. 2008;34(4):449–61.

29. Jarosz J, et al. Naltrexone (50 mg) plus psychotherapy in alcohol-dependent patients: a meta-analysis of randomized controlled trials. Am J Drug Alcohol Abuse. 2013;39(3):144–60.

30. Streeton C, Whelan G. Naltrexone, a relapse prevention maintenance treatment of alcohol dependence: a meta-analysis of randomized controlled trials. Alcohol Alcohol. 2001;36(6):544–52.

31. Kranzler HR, Van Kirk J. Efficacy of naltrexone and acamprosate for alcoholism treatment: a meta-analysis. Alcohol Clin Exp Res. 2001;25(9):1335–41.

32. Rosner S, et al. Opioid antagonists for alcohol dependence. Cochrane Database Syst Rev. 2010;12:CD001867.

33. Garbutt JC, et al. Efficacy and tolerability of long-acting injectable naltrexone for alcohol dependence: a randomized controlled trial. JAMA. 2005;293(13):1617–25.

34. O'Malley SS, et al. Efficacy of extended-release naltrexone in alcohol-dependent patients who are abstinent before treatment. J Clin Psychopharmacol. 2007;27(5):507–12.

35. Thorsell A. The μ-opioid receptor and treatment response to naltrexone. Alcohol Alcohol. 2013;48(4):402–8.

36. Krishnan-Sarin S, O'Malley S, Krystal JH. Treatment implications: using neuroscience to guide the development of new pharmacotherapies for alcoholism. Alcohol Res Health. 2008;31(4):400–7.

37. Gelernter J, et al. Opioid receptor gene (OPRM1, OPRK1, and OPRD1) variants and response to naltrexone treatment for alcohol dependence: results from the VA Cooperative Study. Alcohol Clin Exp Res. 2007;31(4):555–63.

38. Heinala P, et al. Targeted use of naltrexone without prior detoxification in the treatment of alcohol dependence: a factorial double-blind, placebo-controlled trial. J Clin Psychopharmacol. 2001;21(3):287–92.

39. Niciu MJ, Arias AJ. Targeted opioid receptor antagonists in the treatment of alcohol use disorders. CNS Drugs. 2013;27(10):777–87.

40. Mason BJ, Heyser CJ. Acamprosate: a prototypic neuromodulator in the treatment of alcohol dependence. CNS Neurol Disord Drug Targets. 2010;9(1):23–32.

41. De Witte P, et al. Neuroprotective and abstinence-promoting effects of acamprosate: elucidating the mechanism of action. CNS Drugs. 2005;19(6):517–37.

42. Mann K, Lehert P, Morgan MY. The efficacy of acamprosate in the maintenance of abstinence in alcohol-dependent individuals: results of a meta-analysis. Alcohol Clin Exp Res. 2004;28(1):51–63.

43. Garbutt JC, et al. Pharmacological treatment of alcohol dependence: a review of the evidence. JAMA. 1999;281(14):1318–25.

44. Rosner S, et al. Acamprosate for alcohol dependence. Cochrane Database Syst Rev. 2010;9:CD004332.

45. Anton RF, et al. Combined pharmacotherapies and behavioral interventions for alcohol dependence: the COMBINE study: a randomized controlled trial. JAMA. 2006;295(17):2003–17.

46. Mann K, et al. Results of a double-blind, placebo-controlled pharmacotherapy trial in alcoholism conducted in Germany and comparison with the US COMBINE study. Addict Biol. 2013;18(6):937–46.

47. Verheul R, et al. Predictors of acamprosate efficacy: results from a pooled analysis of seven European trials including 1485 alcohol-dependent patients. Psychopharmacology. 2005;178(2–3):167–73.

48. Spanagel R, Kiefer F. Drugs for relapse prevention of alcoholism: ten years of progress. Trends Pharmacol Sci. 2008;29(3):109–15.

49. Kiefer F, et al. Involvement of the atrial natriuretic peptide transcription factor GATA4 in alcohol dependence, relapse risk and treatment response to acamprosate. Pharmacogenomics J. 2011;11(5):368–74.

50. Mann K, et al. Nalmefene for the management of alcohol dependence: review on its pharmacology, mechanism of action and meta-analysis on its clinical efficacy. Eur Neuropsychopharmacol. 2016;26(12):1941–9.

51. Mann K, et al. Extending the treatment options in alcohol dependence: a randomized controlled study of as-needed nalmefene. Biol Psychiatry. 2013;73(8):706–13.

52. Gual A, et al. A randomised, double-blind, placebo-controlled, efficacy study of nalmefene, as-needed use, in patients with alcohol dependence. Eur Neuropsychopharmacol. 2013;23(11):1432–42.

53. Mason BJ, et al. A double-blind, placebo-controlled study of oral nalmefene for alcohol dependence. Arch Gen Psychiatry. 1999;56(8):719–24.

54. Anton RF, et al. A multi-site dose ranging study of nalmefene in the treatment of alcohol dependence. J Clin Psychopharmacol. 2004;24(4):421–8.

55. Walker BM, Zorrilla EP, Koob GF. Systemic κ-opioid receptor antagonism by nor-binaltorphimine reduces dependence-induced excessive alcohol self-administration in rats. Addict Biol. 2011;16(1):116–9.

56. Arias AJ, et al. Effects of opioid receptor gene variation on targeted nalmefene treatment in heavy drinkers. Alcohol Clin Exp Res. 2008;32(7):1159–66.

57. Diehl A, et al. Why is disulfiram superior to acamprosate in the routine clinical setting? A retrospective long-term study in 353 alcohol-dependent patients. Alcohol Alcohol. 2010;45(3):271–7.

58. De Sousa A, De Sousa A. A one-year pragmatic trial of naltrexone vs disulfiram in the treatment of alcohol dependence. Alcohol Alcohol. 2004;39(6):528–31.

59. Laaksonen E, et al. A randomized, multicentre, open-label, comparative trial of disulfiram, naltrexone and acamprosate in the treatment of alcohol dependence. Alcohol Alcohol. 2008;43(1):53–61.

60. Maisel NC, et al. Meta-analysis of naltrexone and acamprosate for treating alcohol use disorders: when are these medications most helpful? Addiction. 2013;108(2):275–93.

61. Soyka M. Nalmefene for the treatment of alcohol dependence: a current update. Int J Neuropsychopharmacol. 2014;17(4):675–84.

62. Drobes DJ, et al. A clinical laboratory paradigm for evaluating medication effects on alcohol consumption: naltrexone and nalmefene. Neuropsychopharmacology. 2003;28(4):755–64.

63. Johnson BA, et al. Oral topiramate for treatment of alcohol dependence: a randomised controlled trial. Lancet. 2003;361(9370):1677–85.

64. Johnson BA, et al. Topiramate for treating alcohol dependence: a randomized controlled trial. JAMA. 2007;298(14):1641–51.

65. Paparrigopoulos T, et al. Treatment of alcohol dependence with low-dose topiramate: an open-label controlled study. BMC Psychiatry. 2011;11:41.

66. Baltieri DA, et al. Comparing topiramate with naltrexone in the treatment of alcohol dependence. Addiction. 2008;103(12):2035–44.

67. Likhitsathian S, et al. Topiramate treatment for alcoholic outpatients recently receiving residential treatment programs: a 12-week, randomized, placebo-controlled trial. Drug Alcohol Depend. 2013;133(2):440–6.

68. Florez G, et al. Using topiramate or naltrexone for the treatment of alcohol-dependent patients. Alcohol Clin Exp Res. 2008;32(7):1251–9.

69. Kranzler HR, et al. Topiramate treatment for heavy drinkers: moderation by a GRIK1 polymorphism. Am J Psychiatry. 2014;171(4):445–52.

70. Mason BJ, Quello S, Shadan F. Gabapentin for the treatment of alcohol use disorder. Expert Opin Investig Drugs. 2018;27(1):113–24.

71. Brennan JL, et al. Clinical effectiveness of baclofen for the treatment of alcohol dependence: a review. Clin Pharmacol. 2013;5:99–107.

72. Agabio R, Leggio L. Baclofen in the treatment of patients with alcohol use disorder and other mental health disorders. Front Psych. 2018;9:464.

73. Charney DA, Zikos E, Gill KJ. Early recovery from alcohol dependence: factors that promote or impede abstinence. J Subst Abus Treat. 2010;38(1):42–50.

74. Litten RZ, et al. Development of medications for alcohol use disorders: recent advances and ongoing challenges. Expert Opin Emerg Drugs. 2005;10(2):323–43.

75. McKee SA, et al. Varenicline reduces alcohol self-administration in heavy-drinking smokers. Biol Psychiatry. 2009;66(2):185–90.

76. Erwin BL, Slaton RM. Varenicline in the treatment of alcohol use disorders. Ann Pharmacother. 2014;48(11):1445–55.

77. Litten RZ, et al. A double-blind, placebo-controlled trial assessing the efficacy of varenicline tartrate for alcohol dependence. J Addict Med. 2013;7(4):277–86.

78. Plebani JG, et al. Results from a pilot clinical trial of varenicline for the treatment of alcohol dependence. Drug Alcohol Depend. 2013;133(2):754–8.

79. Pettinati HM, Anton RF, Willenbring ML. The COMBINE study: an overview of the largest pharmacotherapy study to date for treating alcohol dependence. Psychiatry (Edgmont). 2006;3(10):36–9.

80. Scott LJ, et al. Acamprosate: a review of its use in the maintenance of abstinence in patients with alcohol dependence. CNS Drugs. 2005;19(5):445–64.

Benzodiazepine and Nonbenzodiazepine Hypnotics (Z-Drugs): The Other Epidemic

11

Annie Umbricht and Martha L. Velez

Contents

A. Umbricht · M. L. Velez (✉)
The Johns Hopkins University School of Medicine,
Baltimore, MD, USA
e-mail: mvelez@jhmi.edu

© Springer Nature Switzerland AG 2021
N. el-Guebaly et al. (eds.), *Textbook of Addiction Treatment*,
https://doi.org/10.1007/978-3-030-36391-8_11

Abstract

Benzodiazepines (BZDs) are CNS depressant drugs with sedative, hypnotic, anticonvulsant, and muscle relaxant properties. BZDs replaced barbiturates and other hypnotics in the late 1950s and became the most prescribed medications in 1977. Generally considered effective and safe for short-term use, long-term BZD use beyond 6 weeks is controversial due to loss of efficacy and cognitive adverse outcomes. Side effects include alteration of sleep architecture, nightmares, agitation, amnesia, cognitive impairment, confusion, depression, and dementia. BZD-induced psychomotor impairments lead to increased risks of falls and motor vehicle accidents. Abrupt BZD discontinuation may lead to rebound of the symptoms for which they were prescribed and withdrawal symptoms. The mortality risk of BZD use disorder is of special concern in vulnerable populations given the current opioid overdose epidemic, as BZDs use by patients with opioid use disorders (OUD) contributes significantly to an increase in opioid-related death. In the early 1990s, nonbenzodiazepine $GABA_A$ receptor agonists at the BZD receptor site, the Z-drugs (zaleplon, zolpidem, zopiclone, and eszopiclone), were introduced for treatment of insomnia. Z-drugs have been promoted as safer than traditional BZDs and rapidly gained wide acceptance with the public and practitioners. However, given their similar mechanism of action, their risks and side effects are similar. Given the risks, prescription of sedatives should be avoided or, if necessary, should be limited to short-term use for acute issues. Studies demonstrate that BZD discontinuation after long-term use is associated with improved quality of life once the withdrawal syndrome has been overcome.

Keywords

Benzodiazepines · Sedative use disorder
Nonbenzodiazepine hypnotics
Benzodiazepine withdrawal · Z-drugs

11.1 Scope of the Problem

From 1996 to 2013, the proportion of the population prescribed benzodiazepines (BZDs) doubled from 3% to 6.2% and the quantity prescribed tripled from 1.1 to 3.6 kg of lorazepam equivalent per 100,000 population [27]. Chlordiazepoxide sedative activity was serendipitously discovered by Sternbach in 1955, and it was approved in 1960 for the treatment of anxiety and insomnia, followed by diazepam in 1963. Given a lower toxicity, BZDs soon replaced barbiturates and other hypnotic drugs and became the most prescribed medications in 1977. Generally considered effective and safe for short-term use, the long-term use of BZDs is much more controversial due to a loss of efficacy (tolerance) and their association with adverse outcomes. Nevertheless, BZDs are frequently prescribed for long time despite recommendations to use evidence-based behavioral therapies first, such as relaxation techniques, sleep hygiene, or psychotherapy, or prescribe antidepressants [36]. In the USA, 12.5% of adults aged 65 and older are prescribed BZD or Z-drugs in spite of a clear increase in mortality in this age group [5, 29, 36].

Although the abuse liability of BZDs has been disputed in the general population, the risk of BZD use disorder including physical dependence is undisputed in vulnerable populations, contributing to the lethality of the current opioid overdose epidemic of the twenty-first century. Public health problems associated with BZDs are due to chronic prescriptions for legitimate symptoms, diversion to other persons than the patients for whom the prescription was initially ordered, and broader illegal trade for recreational use. Diversion of prescription drugs has soared in the last decades, and, after marijuana, prescription drug misuse is the most common type of nonmedical drug use. Data from the 2015–2016 National Surveys on Drug Use and Health estimate that in the past year 12.5% adults used BZDS, 2.1% misused BZDs at least once, and 0.2% had BZD use disorder. Among BZD users, 17.1% misused them, and 1.5% had BZD use disorder [7].

The illegal trade on the dark web of counterfeited tranquilizer, mostly alprazolam, is increasing, targeting teens and young adults. These pills may be adulterated with fentanyl or fentanyl analogues, making them deadly [3]. BZD use is associated with emergency room visits, suicidal ideation, use of other substances, and psychiatric disorders [7]. Treatment programs for substance use disorders (SUDs) and emergency departments' data indicate that 95% of patients with BZD use disorders are polysubstance users, with 82% reporting primary abuse of another substance and 12.9% reporting primary abuse of BZD [40]. An estimated 3–41% of patients with alcohol use disorders also misuse BZDs.

Between 1998 and 2008, the proportion of admissions to addiction treatment for BZD use disorder tripled in the USA compared to an 11% overall increase in substance abuse admissions. The number of annual admissions for combined abuse of benzodiazepine and narcotic pain reliever increased 570% from 2000 to 2010. After opioids, BZDs are the second most common medication class linked with overdose deaths, the rate of which grew more than fourfold from 1996 to 2013 [5]. Despite the increased risk of overdose in patients taking BZDs with other substances such as alcohol or opioids, rates of co-prescription of benzodiazepines and opioids nearly doubled between 2001 and 2013, including among patients receiving medication for opioid use disorder. Emergency department (ED) visits involving combined use of opioids and BZDs (19.1%) were higher than that for ED visits involving opioids without benzodiazepines (12.6%) and for ED visits involving benzodiazepines without opioids (11.4%). Opioids are involved in between 75 and 86% of benzodiazepine deaths. Nearly 30% of fatal "opioid" overdoses in the USA also involve benzodiazepines, suggesting that some of the increase in opioid-related deaths might be caused by increases in cocurrent benzodiazepine/opioid use over time [41].

In the early 1990s, a new group of nonbenzodiazepine $GABA_A$ receptor ($GABA_AR$) agonists at the benzodiazepine receptor site, the Z-drugs (zaleplon, zolpidem, zopiclone, and eszopiclone), was introduced for the treatment of insomnia. Chemically distinct from the BZDs, Z-drugs have been promoted as safer than traditional BZDs and rapidly gained wide acceptance with the public and practitioners. However, given their similar mechanism of action at the benzodiazepine site of the $GABA_AR$, their side effects are similar. The FDA, on May 14, 2013, released a safety announcement recommending a dose reduction for zolpidem extended release as well as a warning not to operate a vehicle or machinery requiring mental alertness on the day following the use of zolpidem due to residual psychomotor impairment. Next day sedation, cognitive and psychomotor impairment, and physical dependence and withdrawal are observed in patients receiving Z-drugs. Abuse of Z-drugs is on the increase, and studies suggest that Z-drugs may also increase the risk of depression. The extent of their participation to untoward effects of public health importance is minimized due to the fact that common toxicology screens do not include detection of these Z-drugs. The use of Z-drugs such as zolpidem and eszopiclone alone or in combination with opioids is also associated with increased mortality although the documentation is lacking as toxicology screen may fail to detect Z-drugs. For simplification, in this chapter, the use of the word benzodiazepine also covers Z-drugs.

BZD misuse disproportionately impacts vulnerable populations, including the elderly, adolescents, young adults, pregnant women, victims of sexual assaults, and those with a history of SUD or other psychiatric disorders. BZD misuse is among the most widespread forms of adolescent prescription drug misuse. The 2017 Monitoring the Future reported annual prevalence rates of prescription BZD use of 2.0%, 4.1%, and 4.7% in grades 8, 10, and 12, respectively. A longitudinal study showed that by age 18, the lifetime medical or nonmedical use of BZD was 20.1% and was a predictor of SUD at age 35. Given their risks, prescription of sedatives especially in pediatric populations is best avoided and, if necessary, should be limited to short-term use for acute issues.

Although difficult, studies demonstrate that BZD discontinuation after long-term use is associated with improved quality of life once the withdrawal syndrome has been overcome. This chapter will describe specific patient populations at risk for BZD use disorders, how to identify them, as well as best management practices, including interventions for BZD taper.

11.2 Pharmacology of Benzodiazepines and Other BZD-Site Agonists

Gamma-aminobutyric acid (GABA) is the primary inhibitory neurotransmitter, and its actions are mediated by receptors that are widely distributed throughout the CNS. BZD, Z-drugs, barbiturates, and ethanol are positive modulators of the gamma-aminobutyric A receptor (GABA$_A$R) functions (i.e., their binding induces a neuronal response only in the presence of the actual agonist GABA). The GABA$_A$Rs are ligand-gated ion channels allowing influx of chloride (Cl-), causing hyperpolarization of the neuronal membrane, thus inhibiting the firing of new action potentials. The GABA$_A$R is a transmembrane receptor made of five subunits (2 a, 2 b, and 1 g) binding GABA on the extracellular side of the receptor. Two GABA molecules are needed to open the chloride channel. BZDs and Z-drugs act as GABA potentiators by increasing the frequency with which the chlorine channel opens when two GABA molecules bind to GABA$_A$R. The increase in intracellular chloride concentration hyperpolarizes the neuron, reducing its excitability [20, 43].

It is through their ability to increase the GABA$_A$R's affinity for GABA that BZDs and Z-drugs produce a transient subjective relaxation effect for patients with anxiety or insomnia disorders. In addition to symptom relief, data from animal models indicate that BZDs, by modulating GABA$_A$Rs, increase firing of dopaminergic neurons in the ventral tegmental area, in effect stimulating the mesolimbic reward system and setting the stage for further drug seeking and explaining further the addictive properties of BZDs [44]. The shorter the onset of action after drug taking, the

more efficient is the learning of the rewarding effect associated to the drug. When using BZDs with short onset of action (30 minutes), the individual learns that relaxation, stress relief, or sleep is obtained by taking a pill rather than by learning effective practices of stress reduction and healthy sleep habits (or sleep hygiene). Repeated use induces alterations of the GABA$_A$Rs with the development of tolerance, requiring increases in doses and frequency of dosing to maintain the effects. Attempts to discontinue medications after several (≥ 4) weeks of regular intake lead to resurgence or rebound of the primary symptom of anxiety or insomnia, triggering further drug seeking and leading to automatic and compulsive drug-taking behaviors or initiating the cycle of addiction [17]. Like with ethanol, abrupt benzodiazepine discontinuation unmasks the "downregulated" state of inhibitory transmission leading to the characteristic hyperexcitable state or withdrawal symptoms of anxiety, panic, insomnia, irritability, autonomic hyperactivity, sweats, increased sensorium, and possibly seizures.

Given their specific binding and allosteric modulation of GABA$_A$R, Z-drugs have similar long-term negative effects to BZDs including adverse cognitive (amnesia) and psychomotor effects, compromise in balance, unsteadiness, night falls, and driving impairments. Due to their heterogeneous chemical classes, routine toxicology screens for drugs of abuse do not include the Z-drug hypnotics, so the extent of their impact on emergency room visits and other societal costs remains underreported. In clinical trials, these sedative hypnotics were found to more than double the risk of depression compared to the groups taking placebo. Consequently, the long-term use of sedative hypnotic drugs increases the suicide risk as well as overall mortality risk. The Z-drugs have similar risks of rebound and withdrawal as BZDs.

11.3 Pharmacokinetic

Pharmacokinetic differences between BZDs relate to their respective time to peak effect (onset of action) and duration of action, as well as whether metabolites are psychoactive. BZDs are rapidly absorbed by the gastrointestinal tract after oral administration with onset of action within 30 minutes (diazepam) to 2 hours (chlordiazepoxide). A shorter onset of action leads to higher abuse liability. BZDs are metabolized by the liver via two pathways: glucuronide conjugation by the cytochrome P450 system and/or microsomal oxidation (demethylation and hydroxylation). Some metabolites are psychoactive and undergo further metabolism, thus prolonging the drug duration of action. Intravenous administration of BZDs has quasi immediate onset of action due to fast delivery to the CNS and is reserved for use in emergency (grand mal seizures) or hospital setting (pre-anesthesia). Most BZDs cannot be administered intramuscularly due to erratic absorption, except for midazolam.

Upon discontinuation, BZD pharmacokinetic characteristics predict the time of onset, duration, and severity of the BZD withdrawal syndrome: BZD with shorter half-life and no active metabolites, like alprazolam, is more likely to cause withdrawal symptoms even between scheduled doses. This tends to increase its abuse liability. Long-acting BZDs or those with long-acting metabolites (diazepam, chlordiazepoxide, and active metabolite desmethyldiazepam among others) tend to have an insidious onset of withdrawal starting about 24 hours, with peak intensity 7–14 days after the last dose. Other drugs inhibiting or activating the cytochrome P450 system may change BZD duration of action, causing increase in impairment or withdrawal. The long half-life of some BZDs and metabolites mean that the terminal elimination time can last for up to 4 weeks, even after one dose, longer after chronic dosing since BZD accumulates in fat.

11.4 Clinical Indications for BZDs and Z-Drugs

In this section, we are first reviewing accepted indications for BZDs, reminding the reader that BZDs and other BZD-site agonists are only indicated for incidental or short-term use (less than 4–6 weeks) and at the lowest effective dose, as physical dependence can develop after just 1 month of continuous BZD use. Indications for this type of use include phobias preventing specific functions or procedures (e.g., flying in an airplane, undergoing an MRI for patients with claustrophobia). They are also indicated for short-term management (7–10 days) of reactive anxiety (e.g., sudden stressor such as grief); short-term management of insomnia, including insomnia associated with alcohol withdrawal; and management of withdrawal from alcohol or sedatives with short half-lives. Another indication is the intravenous emergency intervention for grand mal seizures. BZDs have been shown to reduce mortality in acute cocaine toxicity, or in the treatment of acute delirium tremens, a severe complication of alcohol withdrawal. BZD can be used in short-term intervention of psychiatric emergencies accompanied by psychosis or mania, before the onset of action of lithium or other antipsychotic medications (neuroleptics). BZDs are indicated for premedication in anesthesia and for sedation in intensive care (to facilitate mechanical ventilation and/or sedate patients in distress). Note that this indication is coming into question as the use of BZD in this setting has been associated with intensive care delirium and longer ICU length of stay.

11.5 Problems Related to the Long-Term Use of BZDs

The long-term clinical use of BZDs is controversial given the increased morbidity and mortality associated with sedatives. Advocates of long-term management with BZDs claim the patients' acceptability and widespread belief of safety and efficacy. However, several academic and public health policies strongly advise against long-term use of BZDs for PTSD, generalized anxiety disorder (GAD), insomnia, depression, and panic attacks due to the lack of evidence of demonstrated long-term efficacy and their problematic side effects (Table 11.1). Sedatives adversely affect cognitive (memory, attention) and psycho-

Table 11.1 Potential problems related to the use of BZDs

Side effects of BZDs
Sedation, psychomotor impairment impacting driving and operating machinery
Cerebellar dysfunction: unsteadiness (falls), nystagmus, poor coordination, slurred speech, disorientation (space)
Cognitive impairment of memory, attention, disorientation (time), amnesia, decreased learning efficiency, and consolidation
Decreased self-awareness (metacognition) and self-regulation
Increased impulsivity associated with disinhibition and poor working memory
Potentiation of respiratory depression in combination with other substances (alcohol and opioids, including buprenorphine) or in chronic lung disease and obstructive sleep apnea
Reinforcement of avoidance, inflexibility prevents coping/learning of adaptive response
In elderly, TBI and other CNS disorders: acceleration of cognitive decline or dementia
Behavioral problems with forensic implications: increase in motor vehicle accidents (60–80% more accidents in drivers on BZDs or Z-drugs)
Problems of disinhibition in persons with borderline personality disorders or impulse disorders, with paradoxical increase in anxiety and agitation, with consequent aggressive or even violent actions; due to anterograde amnesia (black-out), the person may not have any recollection of the incident (fugue states)

motor functions impacting daily activities and performance. BZD-associated impairments in reaction time, attention, and visuospatial skills increase vulnerability for motor vehicle accidents. Emerging research indicates that BZD use in older adults may increase the risk of developing dementia [19], risk of falls, fractures, and traffic accidents [18]. Similarly, psychomotor impairment, falls, and hip fractures are more likely to occur with Z-drugs that have longer half-lives.

Among war veterans with PTSD, BZD prescriptions are not effective and may increase the risk of misuse and worsening outcome in the setting of SUD. BZD-induced disinhibition has been described in patients with traumatic brain injury (TBI), an important issue, given the frequent comorbid (often underdiagnosed) conditions of TBI and PTSD among veterans returning from war zones. The use of BZDs in this population is also increasing their risk of suicide.

Given the fact that physical dependence may develop after just 30 days of daily BZD use, prescriptions should be for 14 days, with warning about the risk of developing physical dependence and strong resistance for renewing the prescription. If a patient is already under psychiatric care, a general or emergency room practitioner should not prescribe BZD as it will undermine the therapeutic alliance and encourage doctor shopping.

11.6   BZD Use Disorders

Most people prescribed with sedatives take them responsibly and may benefit from their use, if they are taken for short term (less than 4–6 weeks). Longer duration or high doses of benzodiazepine, however, increase the odds of developing BZD use disorders including dependence [23]. BZD should be avoided in those who have preexisting cognitive impairment (elderly, TBI) and patients with panic disorders, suicidal ideations, and underlying SUD due to their elevated odds of developing dependence on benzodiazepines [46].

Overuse of psychoactive medications may also stem from an erosion of quality health-care service. Health-care providers may inadvertently play a role in misuse behaviors by failing to recognize a patient's vulnerability for developing a SUD, missing depression diagnoses when evaluating insomnia or anxiety complaints, overprescribing medications, or just due to time pressure: it takes more time to refuse a patient's request and teach alternative behavioral strategies for anxiety or insomnia than to agree and write the requested prescription. Of patients started on BZD, 36% will still be taking them at 3 months and 15% at 1 year. Very worrisome is the fact that 46–71% of OUD patients on medication-assisted treatment (methadone, buprenorphine) are also prescribed BZDs in spite the overwhelming risk of overdose and untoward treatment outcome. Similarly worrisome is the concurrent chronic prescription of opiates and sedatives for chronic pain, given the increased potential for respiratory depression and cardiac arrest especially with comorbid diagnoses of chronic obstructive pulmonary disease (COPD) or obstructive sleep apnea (OSA). The fact that these drugs are considered "medication" and are endorsed by physicians may give a false sense of safety. Some people intentionally seek to use sedatives for their direct rewarding psychoactive properties (e.g., to get euphoric feelings similar to those induced by alcohol or other illegal drugs; [48]) but also to alleviate negative emotions, such as to lessen anxiety and decrease inhibitions, thus facilitating social encounters or other situations. Recreational BZD users purchase them from legal or illegal sources, from acquaintances, or from family members who have prescriptions. Other sources include illicit sales of diverted supplies and/or the Internet where counterfeited drugs are sold without any quality assurance or regulations [15].

While "doctor shoppers," nonethical physician behaviors, and the Internet receive much media attention regarding diversion, data suggest that numerous active street markets involving patients, pharmacies, distributors, and pharmaceutical corporations are involved in fraudulent practices as well [21].

11.7 BZD Withdrawal Syndrome

Onset of BZD physical dependence can occur after as little as 4 weeks of daily BZD use and occurs in about half of the patients after 4 months or more of daily use [13]. Withdrawal symptoms as well as the resurgence, or even rebound (increase in intensity), of the initial symptoms for which the drug was prescribed are to be expected when BZDs are voluntarily or involuntarily reduced or stopped after more than a month of regular use.

Onset and duration of BZD withdrawal symptoms are function of their pharmacokinetics, duration of use, underlying diagnoses, and individual personality. Onset of BZD withdrawal may start within hours of the last dose for short-acting BZD or within 1–10 days after long-acting BZD. Withdrawal symptoms may linger for 6–8 weeks or even months after discontinuation.

However, many patients report more restorative sleep and improved quality of life due to improved cognitive and psychomotor functioning after resolution of withdrawal symptoms. Therefore, it is worth encouraging and supporting patients during these efforts.

The onset of withdrawal symptoms can be insidious, producing a subjective "need" or craving for BZDs in spite the realization that they are no longer effective and are causing adverse effects [4]. BZD withdrawal corresponds to CNS hyperexcitability and autonomic hyperarousal. Symptoms can be divided into physical, autonomic, sensory, and psychological clusters [39].

Physical and neurological symptoms include muscle tension, weakness, twitching or spasms, tremor, unsteadiness, and grand mal seizures.

Autonomic symptoms include flu-like illness, sweats, shivering, decreased appetite, nausea, tachycardia (palpitations), increased blood pressure, and dry mouth.

Sensory symptoms include pain, myalgia, paresthesia, blurred vision, hyperacusis, tinnitus, headaches, photophobia, dysesthesia, allodynia, hypersensitivity to touch, hyperosmia, altered taste, and eye soreness.

Psychological symptoms include anxiety, panic attack, restlessness, agitation, depression, mood swings, decreased concentration, fatigue made worse due to inability to fall asleep, lethargy, light-headedness, faintness, depersonalization, derealization, hallucination, and delirium.

Kindling, a neurologic sensitization phenomenon, leads to increased withdrawal intensity upon repeat and successive withdrawal episodes, including increased propensity to seizures.

11.8 BZD Use in Specific Populations

The growing problems related to prescription drug affect individuals of both genders and of all ages, starting in middle school-aged children (ages 12–16) worldwide. The high prevalence of BZD use and BZD use disorder among specific populations reflects the presence of underlying conditions that explain in part the known relationship between sedatives and morbidity/mortality. For example, the presence of underlying psychiatric conditions, such as anxiety, ADHD, and bipolar disorders, explains partially the prevalence of use among these at-risk populations. In addition, other preexisting conditions such as obesity or respiratory insufficiency mediate the known relationship between sedative use and increased morbidity/mortality. For example, sedatives increase the risk of sudden death in obesity-related OSA or in COPD. This creates a vicious cycle since respiratory insufficiency and chronic sleep disruption are both anxiogenic.

11.8.1 Adolescents and Young Adults

The lifetime prevalence of anxiety ranges between 15% and 20%, and the median age of onset is 11 years of age, constituting one of the most common and earliest type of psychopathology among children and adolescents [32]. Anxiety disorders are found in 5–19% of all children and adolescents. Sleep disorders are also very common in pediatric populations, with as many as 17% of adolescents having unrestorative sleep. Sleep problems among children often go unrecognized, in part because of parents underreporting them. Awareness of the importance and potential consequences of sleep problems on academic performance, neurocognitive function, and daytime behavioral problems must be emphasized. Children and adolescents are frequently sleeping less than 9 hours at night, the required minimum amount of sleep for this age group. Intrinsic contributors to inadequate sleep patterns in children and adolescents include developmental changes causing a shift in circadian rhythm during puberty, delayed sleep-phase syndrome (7% of adolescents), sleep-disordered breathing, and insomnia-type symptoms found in up to 34% of adolescents. Extrinsic factors include early school start time and poor sleep habits such as use of electronic devices near or during bedtime and caffeine consumption, especially problematic when undisclosed in soda or other foods [42].

Anxiety, poor academic performance, behavioral problems, and sleep problems have been recognized as risk factors for later SUDs, and the nonprescribed use of sedatives among adolescents and young adults is a cause of concern in many countries. Fast brain development during this life stage, especially the development of executive function and learning acquisition, implies that exposure to amnesia-inducing drugs may stunt development and result in neurobiological changes and behavioral consequences such as academic problems, increased impulsivity (inversely correlated with short-term memory), and school dropouts. Young people report using sedatives to relieve anxiety symptoms and insomnia, and a high percentage of teenagers and some parents believe that prescription drugs, even taken nonmedically, are safer than illegal drugs. Due to dramatic societal changes, children and adolescents are increasingly exposed to direct-to-consumer advertisement of medications, rushed medical visits promoting fixing of problems via prescription while decreasing patient-clinician interaction, increased media distractions, and increased time competition for numerous activities all potentially resulting in increased anxiety. Parents must closely monitor the children who have been prescribed these drugs, making sure they are safely stored and not diverted.

11.8.2 Elderly

Published guidelines advise against the prescribing of benzodiazepines or Z-hypnotics (BZD-Z) to patients over 65 years old [2]. However, inappropriate use of BZDs and Z-drugs among this age group is widespread despite a risk-benefit ratio that is clearly greater than 1, as BZDs are proven to increase mortality. As sleep disruption and insomnia increase with age affecting more than 30% of older people, studies report that a third to half of seniors in North America and the UK are prescribed either a Z-drug or BZD for sleep disturbance [16, 35]. Given the high illness burden and accompanying polypharmacy in older adults and their decreased drug metabolism, their susceptibility to toxic effects due to drug interactions and cumulation is increased. BZDs may also interact with over-the-counter medications and dietary supplements, which are consumed in significant quantities by seniors. Cognitive adverse events (memory loss, confusion, disorientation, dementia), psychomotor-type adverse events (dizziness, loss of balance, falls), and morning impairment (residual morning sedation) can lead to accidents, including when operating vehicles. In addition, patients over 65, being less flexible, are significantly less likely to stop BZDs than younger patients, and drug dependence is often unrecognized among older adults. Nevertheless, when successful, BZD taper and change to more appropriate medications such as antidepressants result in improved quality of life for both patients and their caregivers.

11.8.3 Women

Women are more likely than men to suffer from depression, anxiety, and victimization, all of which are associated with SUD. Frequently women report starting drug use in an attempt to cope with stressful situations or traumatic memories. Women are significantly more likely than men to engage in "doctor shopping" and to be prescribed medications with high abuse liability for long periods of time or in combination.

It is estimated that between 1% and 4% of pregnant women use benzodiazepines and/or Z-hypnotics [28]. BZDs cross the placenta and have the potential to accumulate in the embryo/ fetus. Although the general consensus is that BZDs have low teratogenic potential, studies of their safety in pregnancy have been neglected, compared to other psychotropic substances. There has been inconsistent reporting on the relative risk of orofacial clefts among infants exposed to benzodiazepines during the first trimester. Risks of congenital malformations may increase with exposure to more than one psychotropic: higher risks of congenital heart defects were found in children born to pregnant women taking SSRIs and BZDs. Studies evaluating the neurodevelopmental effects on children prenatally exposed to BZD or Z-drugs have yielded mixed

results, with some reporting gross motor and communication impairments in toddlers [28]. During pregnancy, it is best to taper BZDs, or if absolutely indicated, BZDs should be prescribed at the lowest effective dose and for the shortest possible duration, avoiding use in the first trimester and avoiding polypharmacy [12].

It is known that BZD use in poly-SUD is a poor prognostic indicator of recovery, and the same holds true during pregnancy. A portion of pregnant women with BZD use disorder are unable to discontinue BZDs despite the knowledge of their associated risk on the developing brain. Pregnant women and women of childbearing age in general with BZD SUD (which usually includes polysubstance use disorder) tend to be very impaired and emotionally challenged with high impulsivity, frequent relapses, and trust issues, including nonadherence with treatment recommendations. BZDs should never be prescribed to pregnant women with SUD as they promote impulsivity, by decreasing inhibition and memory, thus preventing learning more adaptive coping skills. In addition, behaviors associated with BZD use increase risks of assaults and victimization further complicating the pregnancy and risks of harm to mother and fetus. When BZDs are continued into the late pregnancy, sedative neonatal abstinence syndrome (NAS) may occur. In the experience of one of the authors (MV) BZD NAS can be prolonged and protracted, with the newborn displaying major physiological and behavioral difficulties including high sensitivity to internal and external stimuli. The newborn cries easily, has difficulty with feeding, and has major difficulties tolerating regular touch, sounds, movement, visual stimuli, or internal stressors. Indeed, the child's uncontrollable crying and irritability may complicate the care and the mother/infant interaction, given the preexisting emotional vulnerabilities of the mother, as she may internalize the child's behaviors as rejection or overwhelmingly stressful. Given the high developmental stakes, alternative approaches to treating anxiety, anxiety sensitivity, stress, and distress intolerance during pregnancy are desperately needed. Funding should target efforts to validate the effectiveness of integrative interventions to improve self-regulation and reduce stress during pregnancy. If successful, such interventions would have positive intergenerational impacts.

11.8.4 Polysubstance Users

The prevalence of BZD use reaches up to 50% individuals with OUD, including those on medication treatment (methadone, buprenorphine). BZD use in opioid-dependent populations is a predictor of overdose, lethality, and poor treatment outcome including cocaine and other drug use, self-harm behaviors, and poor psychosocial functioning. Methadone fatalities include BZDs in 75% of cases as do almost all buprenorphine fatalities. Benzodiazepines are frequently abused in combination with alcohol or other drugs (mainly opiates) to enhance the subjective reward of the primary substance, offset their adverse effects (e.g., irritability induced by stimulants), or alleviate withdrawal symptoms including insomnia. The risk of overdose death is greater when opioids and benzodiazepines are used in combination with alcohol due to the sedating and respiratory depression properties of all three substances.

The rehabilitation of patients who abuse BZDs in combination to other drugs is very challenging as they represent a treatment-resistant population. This phenomenon could have several explanations: the concurrent dependence on BZDs and opioids could lead to more severe withdrawal symptoms than opioid withdrawal alone, resulting in higher treatment attrition rates. Comorbid anxiety disorders are associated with avoidant behaviors, fears of discomfort, anxiety sensitivity resulting in lack of openness and flexibility, and resistance to alternative treatment modalities. The negative impact of BZDs on memory and cognition prevents learning more effective coping strategies that are indispensable to achieve abstinence.

11.8.5 Drug-Facilitated Sexual Assault (DFSA)

DFSA is a term used to describe sexual crimes that involve the surreptitious administration of psychoactive substances to compromise an unsuspecting individual's ability to consent to sexual activity. Although alcohol remains the most frequent substance used by perpetrators of sexual assault crimes, sedative drugs such as flunitrazepam (Rohypnol®), a fast-acting BZD, and other BZDs, ketamine, and gamma-hydroxybutyrate (GHB) are known to be slipped in a victim's beverage. Perpetrators choose these drugs because they act rapidly, produce disinhibition followed by deep sedation and relaxation of voluntary muscles, and cause the victim to have lasting anterograde amnesia for events that occurred under the influence of the drug. Many drugs associated with rape are given via alcohol to potentiate the drug effects [22]. The victim is left with a profound sense of betrayal, devastating powerlessness, and shame, in addition to the disorientation caused by the amnesia. The destructive emotions resulting from these assaults may derail a person's life goals and create vulnerabilities to resort to substance use to manage the emotional and physical pain.

11.9 Treatment of BZD Use Disorders

The management of patients with BZD use disorders includes several concurrent aspects: (1) management of the acute withdrawal phase, (2) treatment of underlying condition(s), (3) relapse prevention, and (4) crisis management, if needed. Clinicians need to work closely with patients showing empathy in helping managing distress, while providing choices of integrative or supportive therapies. Educational materials and tips regarding insomnia (sleep hygiene, sleep diary) and anxiety (CBT programs, self-help materials, referrals to mindfulness resources, breathing retraining) should be provided.

11.9.1 Intervention and BZD Detoxification

For some long-term BZD user patients, minimal interventions such as brief consultation or a letter with information about risks of long-term use of BZDs and the recommendation for their discontinuation can be effective and do not produce adverse effects [34].

The management of BZD withdrawal includes, either independently or in combination, (1) gradual tapering of the BZD, (2) switching to an equivalent dose of a long half-life BZD before gradual tapering of the latter, (3) the use of adjuvant medications, (4) treatment of the underlying conditions (e.g., SSRIs for anxiety) prior to detoxification and continuing these medications after BZD discontinuation, and (5) non-pharmacologic treatments of underlying conditions [25, 24]).

Although the rate of BZD taper needs to be individualized, there are some common recommendations as a function of the pattern of BZD use. A common recommendation is a reduction by 10–15% every 1–2 weeks, leaving some decision power to the patient. There is evidence that most patients will be able to complete a taper in 6–10 weeks.

For patients dependent on the more potent BZDs or those with higher abuse liability due to their short onset of action (lorazepam, clonazepam) or on those with short duration of action (alprazolam, triazolam, zaleplon, zolpidem), it is recommended to switch to a diazepam equivalent (https://clincalc.com/Benzodiazepine/default.aspx) for a few days and then rapidly taper off diazepam by 25% weekly over 4 weeks. This ensures a smooth detoxification as the drug long half-life and active metabolites will continue to taper itself for another 3–4 weeks after discontinuation. For heavy BZD-dependent polysubstance abusers, the availability of BZD from illegal sources may jeopardize outpatient detoxification, and residential treatment may be necessary to complete the detoxification.

11.9.2 Adjuvant Medications for BZD Withdrawal Treatment

Antiepileptic medications such as carbamazepine, its safer metabolite oxcarbazepine [11], and valproic acid are useful adjunct medications for attenuating BZD withdrawal symptoms especially for those coming off higher BZD doses, exceeding 20 mg diazepam equivalent daily. The newer antiepileptic zonisamide, which acts as both GABA enhancer and glutamate inhibitor, should also be investigated as it was found superior to diazepam on symptoms of craving, withdrawal, and depression for alcohol withdrawal [37].

Other GABA medications, such as pregabalin [8] and gabapentin, have been evaluated for BZD detoxification, but their benefits have not been confirmed [47]. Antiepileptic medications should not be considered for long-term BZD substitution because of their negative effects on cognition and potential risk of abuse (gabapentin).

11.9.3 Pharmacologic Treatment of Underlying Conditions

It is important to treat underlying condition(s) before, during, and after BZD withdrawal treatment. SSRIs and other antidepressant with low stimulating potential (sertraline, paroxetine, citalopram, escitalopram, mirtazapine, trazodone) are recommended for underlying anxiety disorders, especially with concurrent depressive symptomatology. Melatonin is recommended for insomnia, concurrently to adequate sleep hygiene. The recently approved orexin receptor antagonist, suvorexant, which was FDA approved in 2014 for the treatment of insomnia, should be evaluated for its potential in treating rebound insomnia in the setting of BZD and Z-drug withdrawal.

11.9.4 Non-pharmacologic Treatment of BZD Use Disorders

Maximizing the use of non-pharmacologic interventions is critically important, and a multidisciplinary approach is recommended. Although the review of non-pharmacologic interventions for anxiety and sleep disorders is beyond the scope of this chapter, clinicians will benefit their patients in developing familiarity with self-empowering strategies aimed at improving vagal tone and self-regulation as these practices lead to improved quality of life and better health by reducing stress reactivity, while minimizing risks associated with polypharmacy. Effective target-oriented short-term psychotherapy, cognitive behavioral therapy (CBT), exposure therapy, and mindfulness-based stress reduction are but a few examples.

Several promising therapies target anxiety: Creating Opportunities for Personal Empowerment (COPE) is a brief group CBT-based intervention that can be delivered to teens in school settings. Adolescents who received this therapy scored significantly lower in depression and anxiety on the Beck Youth Inventories and showed increases in self-reported confidence in managing negative emotions. Evaluations showed that the COPE intervention was well received by the teens [30].

A 12-session program of mindfulness-based stress reduction (MBSR) in seventh and eighth graders at a small school for low-income urban boys resulted in less anxiety, improved coping, and a trend to attenuation of cortisol response to academic stress, when compared with health education participants [38].

Pathological worry is considered a central symptom of GAD but can be seen in other types of anxiety (e.g., excessive worry over future panic attacks). A meta-analysis found that CBT for GAD is highly effective treatment for reducing pathological worry, including younger adults and geriatric patients, and the improvement was sustained at long term [10]. Tolin demonstrated that a 4-week breathing training aimed to correct hypo-

capnia in three anxiety clinics resulted in reduction of at least 40% of symptoms among 85% of completers and remission in 56% [45]. Battery-powered transcranial brain stimulation has been shown to stimulate vagal tone and found in uncontrolled trials to help with anxiety and insomnia. Recordings of imagery for insomnia or anxiety can help with sleep initiation and symptom reductions. The regular use of the recordings nudges the listener via metaphors to change usual ruminations toward more hopeful and restorative inner dialogues and is a cost-effective tool for change that one of us (AU) has found to be very well received by patients and effective. A collection of such recordings by B. Naparsteck and others can be found at https://www.healthjourneys.com/.

Avoidance of the discomfort of the withdrawal or rebound reactions during BZD tapering is a major difficulty in interrupting the vicious cycle of BZDs use to combat painful subjective states during the recovery from BZD misuse and dependence. To break this cycle, it is essential for individuals with co-occurring disorders to learn strategies to self-regulate anxiety symptoms as well as alternative coping strategies. Psychological support is required during and after BZD withdrawal as patients remain extremely vulnerable for several months after discontinuation. CBTs are among the most efficacious psychosocial interventions to treat individuals with co-occurring disorders and SUDs. The CB model of relapse is based on linear progression of responses in high-risk situations. Increase in self-efficacy leads to increased coping with anxiety and stress and less substance use. Combination of CBT with contingency management and relapse prevention combined with pharmacotherapy are among the most successful treatments [14].

Acceptance commitment therapy (ACT) [6] is a third-wave CBT intervention focusing on methods such as acceptance, mindfulness, cognitive defusion, decentering, and metaphors meant to reduce the impact of negative thoughts and feelings. ACT has also found wide acceptance as effective treatment for avoidance and anxiety disorders.

Physical exercise may enhance sleep and contribute to an increased quality of life in older adults [33], and increased physical activity also helps with insomnia [26]. CBT for insomnia is as effective for improving sleep quality, while decreasing depression and improving mental health.

11.10 Prevention of BZD UD

11.10.1 Awareness of Professional Guidelines

Countries have created guidelines aimed at curbing the chronic use of BZD to prevent the risks of misuse and abuse. Several health organizations (American Psychiatric Association (APA), the National Institute for Health and Care Excellence (NICE), The Royal Australian and New Zealand College of Psychiatrists (RANZCP), the UK Committee on Safety of Medicines (1988)) and governmental agencies (US Department of Veterans Affairs (VA) and the US Department of Defense (DoD), the UK Department of Health via the Chief Medical Officer (2004)) have created evidence-based guidelines describing indications and recommended length of time for BZD use. Most of these guidelines emphasize selective serotonin reuptake inhibitors (SSRI) as first-line treatment for GAD, panic attacks, and post-traumatic stress disorder and generally discourage the use of BZDs. However, primary and mental health-care providers frequently continue prescribing BZDs outside indications included in the guidelines [1]. Clinicians should avoid prescribing sedatives to children, as studies have documented that adolescents who received a medical prescription for sedatives are more likely to use nonprescribed medications of this type. Receiving a prescription reinforces the belief among adolescents that sedatives are "low risk" and that medications are the answers to life's challenges or unpleasant emotions.

11.10.2 Screening

Due to the strong association between anxiety disorders and SUDs, it is imperative to include screening questions regarding alcohol, smoking, and substance use histories when evaluating patients presenting with anxiety or insomnia complaints. A history of chronic lung disease or obstructive sleep apnea is relative contraindication to BZDs due to increased lethality. Identifying and counseling at-risk individuals, promoting alternative treatments where appropriate, and education on the safe and effective use of BZDs or Z-drugs may all decrease BZD diversion and misuse [31]. If in the last resort BZDs or Z-drug treatment is considered, it should be done with clear expectation of short duration and with education. To this effect, developing an explicit treatment contract with the patient and obtaining patient's signature to limit and monitor the duration of therapy for 2–6 weeks maximum are other ways of preventing BZD-related problems.

11.10.3 Patient Education

Education needs to highlight:

1. The side effects of BZDs, including their potential for physical dependence, symptom rebound upon discontinuation, and adverse effects on memory, cognition, and mood, including increased risk of dementia and increased risk of falls and accidents when operating vehicles or machinery within 24 hours of taking the medication
2. Risks of diversion, including ensuring safe keeping of medication in locked cabinets or boxes in order to prevent use of the medication by other persons living in the household
3. Safe handling of leftover medications which should be disposed appropriately by returning them to the pharmacist for environmentally safe disposal

More education is needed regarding the importance of sleep requirements, especially in children and adolescents, and the timely recognition of poor sleep habits and/or sleep problems. Observing regular sleep hygiene behaviors is universally beneficial in improving sleep quality and for optimal mental health. Combination of sleep hygiene intervention, CBT, and stress reduction has been used to improve sleep and decrease the risk of relapse among adolescents with substance abuse problems [9].

11.10.4 Monitoring Patients Receiving BZD Prescriptions

An office policy should be in place to prevent BZD or Z-drug medication refill beyond 4–6 weeks. Depression should be addressed with antidepressant medications indicated for mood disorders, or patients should be referred to mental health providers. Inform patients in writing of the risks of BZDs if prescriptions for BZDs exceed 3 months, requesting patient signature acknowledging reception of the information, via certified letter if needed.

Pharmacies should be engaged in patient monitoring, informing practitioners when prescriptions are obtained from multiple providers and preventing duplication.

Programs treating OUD, such as opiate detoxification, need to screen for concurrent benzodiazepine dependence and modify the detoxification protocol accordingly and assess underlying psychiatric issues given their high prevalence in this population.

11.11 Conclusions

– While the true extent of BZD and Z-drug use/misuse and diversion is unknown, it is well known that they are among the most frequently prescribed medications and that they are prescribed chronically for insomnia, anxiety, and as muscle relaxants, which is against professional guidelines.
– BZD-related problems are found in all ages from adolescence to seniors and widely different populations such as war veterans and women.

– Due to their adverse effects on memory and cognition, BZDs impact daily activities such as driving or taking care of children.
– BZD use disorder is a common and costly comorbidity in patients with anxiety disorders or other SUDs complicating treatment outcome. In the last two decades, BZD use increase has contributed to the current epidemic of lethal drug overdose in the USA.
– BDZ discontinuation is a challenging process and needs to be closely monitored with compassion and encouragement given the severe discomfort and underlying distress, while knowing that improved quality of life lies ahead.
– Non-pharmacologic therapies, sleep hygiene, exercise, outdoor activities, CBT, mindfulness-based stress reduction, yoga, breathing retraining, or other relaxation interventions have been shown to be more efficacious than BZDs for insomnia and anxiety. These interventions have the benefits of long-term stress reduction, improvement of cognition and life satisfaction, and decrease in disease burden.
– Health-care providers and society in general need to be aware of BZD intrinsic abuse liability but also of individual vulnerabilities in risk for misuse and diversion.

References

1. Abrams TE, Lund BC, Bernardy NC, Friedman MJ. Aligning clinical practice to PTSD treatment guidelines: medication prescribing by provider type. Psychiatr Serv. 2013;64(2):142–8.
2. American Geriatrics Society Beers Criteria Update Expert Panel. American Geriatrics Society updated Beers Criteria for potentially inappropriate medication use in older adults. J Am Geriatr Soc. 2012;60(4):616–31. https://doi.org/10.1111/j.1532-5415.2012.03923.x.
3. Arens AM, van Wijk XM, Vo KT, Lynch KL, Wu AH, Smollin CG. Adverse effects from counterfeit alprazolam tablets. JAMA Intern Med. 2016;176(10):1554–5.
4. Ashton H. The diagnosis and management of benzodiazepine dependence. Curr Opin Psychiatry. 2005;18:249–55.
5. Bachhuber MA, Hennessy S, Cunningham CO, Starrels JL. Increasing benzodiazepine prescriptions and overdose mortality in the United States, 1996-2013. Am J Public Health. 2016;106:686–8.

6. Blackledge JT, Hayes SC. Emotion regulation in acceptance and commitment therapy. J Clin Psychol. 2001;57(2):243–55, review.

7. Blanco C, Han B, Jones CM, Johnson K, Compton WM. Prevalence and correlates of benzodiazepine use, misuse and use disorders among adults in the United States. J Clin Psychiatry. 2018;79(6):18m12174.

8. Bobes J, Rubio G, Terán A, Cervera G, López-Gómez V, Vilardaga I, Pérez M. Pregabalin for the discontinuation of long-term benzodiazepines use: an assessment of its effectiveness in daily clinical practice. Eur Psychiatry. 2012;27(4):301–7.

9. Bootzin RR, Stevens SJ. Adolescents, substance abuse, and the treatment of insomnia and daytime sleepiness. Clin Psychol Rev. 2005;25:629–44.

10. Covin R, Ouimet AJ, Seeds PM, DJA D. A meta-analysis of CBT for pathological worry among clients with GED. J Anxiety Disord. 2008;22:108–16.

11. Croissant B, Grosshans M, Diehl A, Mann K. Oxcarbazepine in rapid benzodiazepine detoxification. Am J Drug Alcohol Abuse. 2008;34(5):534–40.

12. Dell'osso B, Lader M. Do benzodiazepines still deserve a major role in the treatment of psychiatric disorders? A critical reappraisal. Eur Psychiatry. 2013;28(1):7–20.

13. El-Guebaly N, Sareen J, Stein MB. Are there guidelines for the responsible prescription of benzodiazepines? Can J Psychiatr. 2010;55(11):709–14.

14. Epstein DH, Hawkins WE, Covi L, Umbricht A, Preston KL. Cognitive-behavioral therapy plus contingency management for cocaine use: findings during treatment and across 12-month follow-up. Psychol Addict Behav. 2003;17(1):73–82.

15. Forman RF, Marlowe DB, McLellan AT. The internet as a source of drug of abuse. Curr Psychiatry Rep. 2006;8:377–82.

16. Glass J, Lanctot KL, Herrmann N, et al. Sedative hypnotics in older people with insomnia: meta-analysis of risks and benefits. BMJ. 2005;331(7526):1169.

17. Gravielle MC. Activation-induced regulation of GABAA receptors: is there a link with the molecular basis of benzodiazepine tolerance? Pharmacol Res. 2016;109:92–100.

18. Gunja N. In the ZZZ zone: the effects of Z-drugs on human performance and driving. J Med Toxicol. 2013;9(2):163–71.

19. He Q, Chen X, Wu T, Li L, Fei X. Risk of dementia in long-term benzodiazepine users: evidence from a meta-analysis of observational studies. J Clin Neurol. 2019;15(1):9–19.

20. Heikkinen AE, Moykkynen TP, Korpi ER. Long-lasting modulation of glutamatergic transmission in VTA dopamine neurons after a single dose of benzodiazepine agonists. Neuropsychopharmacology. 2009;34:290–8.

21. Inciardi JA, Surratt HL, Kurtz SP, Cicero TJ. Mechanisms of prescription drug diversion among drug-involved club- and street-based populations. Pain Med. 2007;2(8):171–83.

22. Isorna Folgar M, Souto Taboada C, Rial Boubeta A, Alias A, McCartan K. Drug-facilitated sexual assault and chemical submission. Psychol Soc Educ. 2017;9(2):263–82.

23. Kan CC, Hilberink SR, Breteler MH. Determination of the main risk factors for benzodiazepine dependence using a multivariate and multidimensional approach. Compr Psychiatry. 2004;45(2):88–94.

24. Kennedy KM, O'Riordan J. Prescribing benzodiazepines in general practice. Br J Gen Pract. 2019;69:152–3.

25. Lader M, Tylee A, Donoghue J. Withdrawing benzodiazepines in primary care. CNS Drugs. 2009;23(1):19–34. doi:10.2165/0023210-200923010-00002.

26. Lang C, Brand S, Feldmeth AK, Holsboer-Trachsler E, Pühse U, Gerber M. Increased self reported and objectively assessed physical activity predict sleep quality among adolescents. Physiol Behav. 2013;120:46–53.

27. Lembke A, Papac J, Humphreys K. Our other prescription drug problem. N Engl J Med. 2018;378:693–5.

28. Lupattelli A, Chambers CD, Bandoli G, Handal M, Skurtveit S, Nordeng H. Association of maternal use of benzodiazepines and z-hypnotics during pregnancy with motor and communication skills and attention-deficit/hyperactivity disorder symptoms in preschoolers. JAMA Netw Open. 2019;2(4):e191435. https://doi.org/10.1001/jamanetworkopen.2019.1435.

29. Maust DT, Blow FC, Wiechers IR, et al. National trends in antidepressant, benzodiazepine, and other sedative-hypnotic treatment of older adults in psychiatric and primary care. J Clin Psychiatry. 2017;78:e363–71.

30. Mazurek Melnyk B, Kelly S, Lusk P. Outcomes and feasibility of a manualized cognitive behavioral skills building intervention: group COPE for depressed and anxious adolescents in school settings. J Child Adolesc Psychiatr Nurs. 2013;27:1073–6077.

31. McLarnon M, Monaghan T, Stewart S, Barrett SP. Drugs misuse and diversion in adults prescribed anxiolytics and sedatives. Pharmacotherapy. 2011;31(3):262–72. www.ncbi.nlm.nih.gov/pubmed/21361736.

32. Mohr C, Schneider S. Anxiety disorders. Eur Child Adolesc Psychiatry. 2013;22(Suppl 1):S17–22.

33. Montgomery P, Dennis J. Physical exercise for sleep problems in adults aged 60+. Cochrane Database Syst Rev. 2002;4:CD003404.

34. Mugunthan K, McGuire T, Glasziou P. Minimal interventions to decrease long-term use of benzodiazepines in primary care: a systematic review and meta-analysis. Br J Gen Pract. 2011;61(590):e542–3. https://doi.org/10.3399/bjgp11X593857.

35. Nubukpo P, Clement JP. Medical drug abuse and aging. Geriatr Psychol Neuropsychiatr Vieil. 2013;11(3):305–15.

36. Olfson M, King M, Schoenbaum M. Benzodiazepine use in the United States. JAMA Psychiatry. 2015;72:136–42.

37. Rubio G, López-Muñoz F, Ponce G, Pascual JM, Martínez-Gras I, Ferre F, Jiménez-Arriero MA, Alamo C. Zonisamide versus diazepam in the treatment of alcohol withdrawal syndrome. Pharmacopsychiatry. 2010;43(7):257–62.

38. Sibinga EM, Perry-Parrish C, Chung SE, Johnson SB, Smith M, Ellen JM. School-based mindfulness instruction for urban male youth: a small randomized controlled trial. Prev Med. 2013;57:799–801.

39. Soyka M. Treatment of benzodiazepine dependence. N Engl J Med. 2017;376(24):2399–400.

40. Substance Abuse and Mental Health Services Administration. Treatment episode data set (TEDS): 2011. Discharges from substance abuse treatment services. BHSIS series S-70, HHS publication no. (SMA) 14-4846. Rockville: Substance Abuse and Mental Health Services Administration; 2014.

41. Sun EC, Dixit A, Humphreys K, et al. Association between concurrent use of prescription opioids and benzodiazepines and overdose: retrospective analysis. BMJ. 2017;356:j760.

42. Tan E, Healey D, Gray AR, Galland BC. Sleep hygiene intervention for youth aged 10 to 18 years with problematic sleep: a before-after pilot study. BMC Pediatr. 2012;12:189. Published 2012 Dec 7. doi:10.1186/1471-2431-12-189.

43. Tan KR, Brown M, Labouèbe G, et al. Neural bases for addictive properties of benzodiazepines. Nature. 2010;463(7282):769–74.

44. Tan KR, Rudolph U, Luscher C. Hooked on benzodiazepines: GABA-a receptor subtypes and addiction. Trends Neurosci. 2011;34(4):188–97.

45. Tolin DF, Billingsley AL, Hallion LS, Diefenbach GJ. Low pre-treatment end-tidal CO_2 predicts dropout from cognitive-behavioral therapy for anxiety and related disorders. Behav Res Ther. 2017;90:32–40.

46. Voyer P, Preville M, Roussel ME, Berbiche D, Beland SG. Factors associated with benzodiazepine dependence among community-dwelling seniors. J Community Health Nurs. 2009;26(3):101–13.

47. Welsh JW, Tretyak V, McHugh RK, Weis RD, Bogunovic O. Review: adjunctive pharmacologic approaches for benzodiazepine tapers. Drug Alcohol Depend. 2018;189:96–107.

48. Yu HY. The prescription drug abuse epidemic. Clin Lab Med. 2012;32:361–77.

Cannabis Use Disorder and Its Treatment

12

Alan J. Budney and Michael J. Sofis

Contents

Abstract

Scientific advances and clinical epidemiology provide clear evidence of cannabis' potential for addiction and adverse psychosocial and health consequences, yet skepticism about its addictive potential remains, and perceived risk of its potential for harm continues to decrease. Indeed, treatment seeking for cannabis use disorder (CUD) comprises a substantial proportion of all substance use treatment admissions. This chapter is focused on cannabis' potential for misuse and addiction and reviews what is known about behavioral and pharmacological interventions for cannabis use reduction or cessation. Behavioral treatments, brief interventions, and digital health interventions have demonstrated efficacy, although there remains much room for continued improvement in outcomes. Unfortunately, a growing body of research has yet to identify an effective pharmacotherapy, and no medications are currently approved by the FDA for treating CUD. Continued efforts to identify and increase access to effective interventions for misuse and CUD are imperative to the public health considering the loosening of cannabis laws for both therapeutic and recreational use, the burgeoning of cannabis industry, and societal and cultural trends toward acceptance of cannabis use. The field will continue to benefit

A. J. Budney (✉) · M. J. Sofis
Center for Technology and Behavioral Health,
Department of Psychiatry, Geisel School of Medicine
at Dartmouth, Lebanon, NH, USA
e-mail: alan.j.budney@dartmouth.edu

© Springer Nature Switzerland AG 2021
N. el-Guebaly et al. (eds.), *Textbook of Addiction Treatment*,
https://doi.org/10.1007/978-3-030-36391-8_12

from efforts to develop innovative treatments that leverage scientific and technological advances and that better tailor interventions to individuals or subgroups of cannabis users.

Keywords

Cannabis · Cannabis use disorder · Marijuana Treatment · Medication

12.1 Introduction

Cannabis remains one of the most widely used regulated psychoactive substances in the United States and other developed countries, and the prevalence of cannabis use continues to rise. Debate about its addictive potential, health consequences, legal status, and therapeutic use has troubled governments, scientists, and the general public for more than a century. Advances in clinical and basic science have provided clear evidence of cannabis' potential for addiction and adverse psychosocial and health consequences, yet skepticism remains, and perceived risk of its potential for harm continues to decrease.

The discovery of the endogenous cannabinoid system in the late 1980s triggered a plethora of scientific investigation exploring the biological underpinnings of cannabis use and its effects and the potential mechanisms by which it impacts physical health and psychiatric disorders. Clear similarities were observed in the neurobiological processes involved in cannabis use and the development of cannabis use disorder (CUD) and those involved with other types of substance use and addictions. A withdrawal syndrome was identified, and increased concern about CUD and its treatment began to pervade the scientific literature. Clinical epidemiological studies and clinical studies of behavioral and pharmacotherapy interventions for CUD increased in numbers and unfortunately demonstrated that CUD was relatively common and, like other substance use disorders, not easy to treat [14].

The growing awareness of these clinical concerns related to cannabis misuse has been paralleled by an escalation of attention on the potential therapeutic use of cannabis and its constituent compounds, the acceleration of legalization of cannabis possession and use, and a flourishing cannabis industry, all of which contribute to a cultural context of reduced concern about the personal risks and public health consequences of cannabis use. Notably, lower perceived risk of harm in the general population corresponds with increases in prevalence. Such cultural changes raise concern about increased risk for CUD and the risk of harm related to cannabis misuse.

This chapter will focus solely on cannabis use and its potential for misuse and addiction and on what is known about interventions for helping those who develop problems with cannabis. Because we will not be focusing on therapeutic use of cannabis, it is important to clarify what we are referring to when we use the word "cannabis" in this chapter. Cannabis will refer only to cannabis plant material or extracts from the cannabis plant *that contain substantial amounts of delta-9-tetrahydrocannabinol (THC). THC* is the compound that produces the euphoric-like effects or the high experienced when cannabis is consumed [32]. Hence it is the THC in cannabis that relates most closely to its addictive potential. In this chapter, "cannabis" will *not* be referring to cannabidiol (CBD) products that contain no or only trace amounts of THC. CBD is the compound in the cannabis plant that has garnered much attention for its potential therapeutic effects, but CBD does not produce a high when ingested [25]. Given the current cultural climate, discussions of treatment for CUD or cannabis misuse need to distinguish between use of substances with THC and those with primarily CBD and little to no THC. Below, we provide a brief overview of the pharmacology, phenomenology, and epidemiology of cannabis and CUD, followed by an update and review of the current evidence base for effective treatments for those seeking to reduce or quit cannabis use.

12.2 Pharmacology and Phenomenology

12.2.1 Cannabis Use

Cannabis is the generic and most appropriate scientific term for the psychoactive compounds that comprise *Cannabis sativa* or *indica* plants that have been used by humans to alter consciousness or to enhance physical and mental well-being for thousands of years. The cannabis plant contains well over 100 compounds; however, the compound of most relevance to the development of problematic use or addiction is delta-9-tetrahydrocannabinol (hereafter referred to as THC). Ingestion of THC is the primary mediator of the *positive reinforcing effects of cannabis use* (i.e., pleasurable feelings or sensations) via its interaction with the endogenous cannabinoid system and, in particular, activation of CB1 cannabinoid receptors located in abundance throughout the brain [26]. The common positive effects of cannabis use include euphoria or "high"; sense of relaxation, calm, or stress reduction; increased propensity for laughter; a slowed time perception; and increased creativity and appreciation for music or other art mediums. Common adverse or negative effects of cannabis use include feelings of paranoia, anxiety, and mild to moderate impairment in attention, memory, learning, and judgment. Of note, the contribution of cannabinoids (other than THC) and other compounds in the cannabis plant in producing these positive and negative effects and putative therapeutic effects is not clear but continues to be an important focus of current research [55].

12.2.2 Cannabis Use Disorder

The accumulated body of neurobiological, behavioral, clinical, epidemiological, and health services data collected over the past 30 years should render the debate over cannabis' addictive potential obsolete [12]. Nonetheless skepticism remains; hence, here we provide a brief overview of this body of work and the clinical epidemiological data that illustrate the significant public health issues that arise related to cannabis misuse and CUD.

Neurobiological and behavioral research As alluded to above, preclinical nonhuman and human laboratory research has characterized the endogenous cannabinoid system and identified how exogenous cannabinoids, like THC, interact with CB1 receptors, stimulate dopamine production in the brain's reward pathways, and produce the psychoactive and reinforcing effects of cannabis, which are the common neurobiological features of mostly all substances with addictive potential [78]. Human laboratory studies have demonstrated positive subjective reinforcing effects of THC, with higher doses preferred over lower doses among current cannabis users, and a preference for THC over placebo [32].

Withdrawal Experimental research has demonstrated another key marker of cannabis' addictive potential, a withdrawal syndrome that can occur when regular cannabis use is discontinued, i.e., a person is deprived of THC. Human and animal research has clearly demonstrated how THC deprivation can precipitate withdrawal, CB1 agonists such as THC can relieve such withdrawal (pharmacological specificity), and CB1 antagonists can precipitate withdrawal in animals that have been regularly administered CB1 agonists. Numerous human clinical studies have now identified the common signs and symptoms of a cannabis withdrawal syndrome: irritability/anger/aggression, restlessness, anxiety, sleep difficulty, strange dreams, decreased appetite, weight loss, and depressed mood [11]. Physical symptoms are reported less frequently but include chills, headaches, physical tension, sweating, and stomach pain. The time course of this withdrawal syndrome is like most other types of substance withdrawal with onset within the first 24–48 hours of cessation, peaking within the first week, with a duration of approximately 1–2 weeks [11, 13].

Cannabis withdrawal is now included as a substance withdrawal disorder and a CUD criterion item in the DSM-5 and the ICD-11 (see below for CUD definitions). The syndrome can play a part in the development and maintenance CUD by contributing to the continuation of problematic cannabis use patterns and by precipitating relapse (i.e., negative reinforcement processes). Of note, this withdrawal syndrome [3], although clinically important, does not typically precipitate serious medical or psychiatric risk [3]. In summary, the behavioral and neural processes observed related to cannabis administration and withdrawal parallel those of most substances that carry risk for development of an addiction.

Genetics As would be expected, genetic contributions to the development of CUD have been observed. Heritable risk factor studies suggest that genetic risk comprises 30–80% of the total variance in risk of developing a CUD, and genetic linkage studies strongly suggest a genetic link to CUD [1]. Cannabis-specific genes, i.e., those that impact vulnerability to the addictive potential of cannabis; genes that are related to a general vulnerability to mostly all SUDs, i.e., those that increase or decrease vulnerability to externalizing behavior problems; and genes that impact reactivity to environmental variables such as stress, have all been linked to cannabis use, misuse, and CUD.

Diagnosis and definition The *Diagnostic and Statistical Manual of Mental Disorders* (DSM-5) [3] and the *International Statistical Classification of Diseases and Related Health Problems (ICD-10 or 11)* provide clear operational definitions of *CUD*. Both classification systems describe a syndrome that develops from excessive use of cannabis and which includes all the same generic criteria for diagnosis as for most other substance use disorders [77]. The DSM-5 criteria denote 11 criteria that relate to impaired control over one's consumption, social impairment, risky use, and physical dependence, i.e., tolerance or withdrawal. Severity can range from mild (2–3 criteria), to moderate (4–6 criteria), to severe (7 or more criteria). The ICD operationalizes CUD somewhat differently by including two distinct disorders: *harmful use* and a *dependence syndrome* (which are highly similar to previous DSM versions of abuse and dependence diagnoses). *Harmful use* entails a pattern of psychoactive substance use causing damage to physical or mental health. The *dependence syndrome* entails

a cluster of physiological, behavioral, and cognitive phenomena, which operationalize patterns of substance use that reflect increasing value of such use over other prosocial behaviors that previously had greater value. The *dependence syndrome* requires 3 of 6 specified criteria. Inclusion of CUD in the DSM and ICD taxonomies imparts the clear message that medical experts and scientists deem CUD to be a valid and clinically important substance use disorder that is not rare and is experienced in much the same way as other substance use disorders [3, 12].

Prevalence Cannabis remains the most commonly used psychoactive and regulated substance in the world after alcohol and tobacco. Globally, prevalence of its *use* has trended slightly upward since 2009, stabilizing over the past few years at approximately 4% (~190,000,000) of the adult and adolescent population who report using cannabis in the past year [69]. Greater increases over the past decade have been observed in the United States and Canada. Of note, in the United States, self-reported past-month cannabis use among pregnant women was approximately 7% in 2017, which reflects an increase from 3.4% in 2002. Reports of daily use among pregnant women also increased from 0.9% to 3.4% [72]. In Canada, a recent report also indicated an increase in cannabis use among pregnant women but at an overall lower prevalence rate (1.2–1.8% from 2012 to 2017) and reported a much higher rate of use (>6%) among younger women (15–24 years) [18]. Cannabis use during pregnancy, particularly during the first two trimesters, has been associated with effects on fetal growth and later childhood outcomes.

Global estimates of CUD indicate that over 13 million individuals meet criteria for a current diagnosis (~0.2% of the population or ~6% of those who use cannabis) [22]. In the United States, prevalence of current CUD appears substantially higher (1.5–3%) based on estimates provided by two general population surveys from the United States [37, 56]. Other high-income countries have also reported relatively high prevalence of CUD compared with the global population (e.g., Germany, 0.5%;

Australia, 1%). Conditional prevalence, or the percentage of those who use cannabis who develop CUD, has been estimated at 11.6% and 30% for past-year cannabis users across two US population studies [31, 36]. Of relevance to assessing the "addictive potential" of cannabis use, the conditional prevalence of CUD (30%) among past-year users observed in the US NESARC study appears higher than for alcohol (17.5%) but lower than for tobacco (80%) [17]. Like with other SUDs, the most prominent demographic risk factors associated with CUD are male gender and younger age (i.e., 18–25 or 18–29) [37, 59]. The relative risk of CUD among younger individuals is unique to CUD compared with other SUDs [59]. Overall, it is evident that CUD is not a rare disorder, and its prevalence appears to be increasing, leading the WHO to conclude that CUD is a clear public health problem, particularly among higher-income nations [74].

Phenomenology The estimated distribution of lifetime severity levels of CUD in the United States using DSM criteria is approximately 2.85% mild, 1.42% moderate, and 2.0% severe [37]. Severity level shows robust positive relationship with other mental health and substance use problems and a negative relationship to social, emotional, and cognitive functioning. Hence, like other SUDs, the more severe the CUD diagnosis, the greater the increase in the risk of physical and psychological symptoms that can negatively impact one's life. Those with CUD report greater disability [37] and are more likely to report inpatient and emergency room visits than those without CUD [16]. Additional consequences that have been associated with CUD relate to the pharmacological effects of cannabis intoxication and chronic use (e.g., driving accidents, risky sex behavior).

Treatment-seeking adults and adolescents identify multiple problems associated with their cannabis misuse. For adults these include procrastination/low productivity, memory issues, low energy, financial or employment difficulties, guilt about use, cannabis withdrawal, low self-confidence/self-esteem, insomnia, and distressed personal relationships [66]; and for adolescents these include neglected responsibilities, inability to do homework or study, missed school or work, went to school high, missed out on things because they spent too much money on cannabis, arguments with family, continued using despite promising oneself not to, and noticing unpleasant changes in personality [43].

Additionally, approximately 35% of those 12 years and older who are seeking treatment for CUD also report at least one additional psychiatric disorder [58]. Moreover, estimates from a general population study suggest that those with past-year CUD are more likely than those without CUD to have one or more additional SUDs (OR = 9.3) and to suffer from anxiety (OR = 2.8), personality (OR = 4.8), mood (OR = 3.8), and post-traumatic stress disorders (OR = 4.3) [37]. Importantly, those with CUD and another psychiatric disorder or another SUD demonstrate worse cannabis cessation outcomes and worse outcomes related to specific psychiatric conditions [6]. Given the notable prevalence of co-occurring CUD and psychiatric disorders, such findings indicate a clear need for services that provide integrated treatments.

Treatment seeking Across most parts of the globe, treatment admissions for CUD substantially increased in proportion to treatment for all SUDs from 2003 to 2016 (e.g., 8–15% in Eastern/Southeastern Europe, 19–30% in Western/Central Europe, 9–16% in Asia, 28–33% in North America) [68]. In the United States, treatment admissions for SUDs in general declined 18.6% from 2002 to 2015, with CUD admissions declining at an even higher rate (26%) perhaps related to escalating legalization policies [58]. Nonetheless, the number of CUD admissions remains substantial. In the United States, admissions for CUD make up approximately 13% of all SUD admissions, behind only alcohol and opioid use disorders as the primary substances reported by those entering treatment [57]. For those aged 15–17 years, the proportion of all SUD admissions for primary CUD is exponentially higher, comprising about 73% all admissions for these youth [57]. Notably, the percentage of admissions of cases for CUD decreases by age: 12–17 years, 77%; 18–19 years, 44%; 20–24 years, 22.5%; and 25–34 years, 12%.

Although substantial numbers of those with CUD seek treatment, just as with all other SUDs, the great majority does not utilize treatment services. Estimates from the United States suggest that only 7–8% of those with CUD engage in treatment related to their cannabis use during the past year [37], which is even lower than the estimated 13.5% of those with any past-year SUD who sought treatment [5]. Postulated reasons for this lack of utilization include perception that treatment is not necessary, lack of problem awareness, stigma, and self-reliance [27, 70]. Overall these statistics suggest a strong need for effective treatment services for CUD, increased treatment access, and interventions that motivate treatment seeking.

12.3   Treatment for Cannabis Misuse and CUD

The CUD treatment research literature parallels that of most other SUDs. Pharmacotherapy laboratory studies and clinical trials testing a wide range of medications have proliferated over the past 10–15 years. Psychosocial treatment studies have primarily focused on evaluating motivational enhancement, cognitive-behavioral or coping skills, and contingency management interventions and their combinations. Research on treatments for adolescents with CUD or cannabis misuse comprises multiple types of family-based interventions in addition to similar approaches to those used with adults. Most recently, multiple studies have focused on the development of digital or mHealth approaches that can increase access to effective CUD interventions and perhaps enhance outcomes when integrated with standard treatments. Below we provide a brief overview of this clinical literature highlighting promising approaches, current trends, and future directions.

Behavioral/psychosocial treatments Multiple reviews and book chapters summarizing the CUD treatment literature have appeared over the past decade (e.g., [14, 28, 62]). The most frequently evaluated interventions and those that have been deemed efficacious have been motivational enhancement therapy (MET), cognitive behavioral therapy (CBT), and contingency management (CM).

MET, the briefest (1–4 sessions) of the interventions, focuses on the individual's ambivalence toward quitting or reducing use, as well as targeting increased motivation and commitment to change. Counseling skills, such as empathy, reflective listening, summarizing, and affirmation, to engender motivation and action toward change are strategically employed. CBT is a skills training-based approach focused on enhancing cannabis abstinence/reduction, coping, and relapse prevention skills. Skills training is taught and practiced in session and assigned for practice in-between sessions. Group and individual delivery of CBT of varying length session (6–14 sessions) has been evaluated. Typical CM interventions systematically arrange a program of reinforcement (rewards or incentives) to elicit behavior change related to therapeutic targets, which in most cases is cannabis abstinence but also can be attendance at sessions, completion of homework, or engagement in prosocial activities. In most cases, CM has been evaluated as part of an intervention that includes MET or CBT.

The published reviews of the CUD treatment literature generally converge on several key conclusions [14, 28]. For adults, CBT, MET, combined MET/CBT, and combined MET/CBT/CM have each demonstrated efficacy for reducing cannabis use and decreasing CUD severity. CBT or the combination of MET and CBT appears to engender greater effects on cannabis use than MET alone. The integration of abstinence-based CM with MET, CBT, or MET/CBT optimizes short-term treatment abstinence outcomes, and frequency of cannabis use, abstinence, and severity of dependence are enhanced out to 12 months posttreatment. Overall, longer behavioral treatments (4 or more sessions) have shown more robust outcomes than brief MET motivational approaches, although threshold or optimal durations of treatment have not been identified.

As observed with controlled outpatient clinical trials of behavioral treatments for other substance use disorders, the outcomes observed in these CUD trials leave much room for improvement. The majority of participants does not achieve abstinence or substantial reduction in cannabis use indicative of significant clinical improvement. Moreover, of those who do achieve a positive response, a substantial number relapse either during outpatient treatment or shortly posttreatment.

Behavioral interventions for adolescents Although many clinical trials evaluating interventions for adolescents with SUDs include youth who use and misuse various substances, cannabis is typically the primary substance used by the adolescents and CUD the primary SUD diagnosis. Multiple reviews of this literature have appeared in the last 10 years (e.g., [39, 64, 67, 76]).

The largest clinical trial for youth with CUD, the Cannabis Youth Treatment (CYT), was a multi-site study ($N = 600$) comparing five outpatient treatments: individual MET/CBT, individual adolescent community reinforcement approach, group MET/CBT, the MET/CBT with family support network, and multidimensional family therapy [23]. Results indicated that the efficacy of these five approaches was not significantly different. That is, adolescents across conditions evidenced significant improvement in days of abstinence and recovery rates at the 1-year follow-up, and no one treatment outperformed the other. Most youth, however, did not achieve abstinence, with the great majority relapsing during treatment or during the 12-month follow-up period.

Most reviews have concluded that several family-based therapies, including functional family therapy, multidimensional family therapy,

and brief strategic family therapy, have clear support for their efficacy, as do individual- and group-delivered CBT. The evidence-based family approaches likely have significantly larger effects on substance use than MET and CBT interventions. As concluded for adult CUD treatments, integrated models that increase the scope and intensity of treatments by combining evidence-based approaches can enhance outcomes [39]. A notable example of successful integration is the combination of CM with MET/CBT and behavioral parent training [65]. The youth CM program included abstinence-based rewards delivered by both the clinic and guardians. This integrative model optimized during treatment cannabis reduction and abstinence, but unfortunately longer-term effects for youth with CUD remain elusive. The most favorable combinations, duration, and CM reward parameters have yet to be identified, and alternative approaches are clearly needed to enhance maintenance of treatment effects.

12.4 Digital Health Interventions

Digital health interventions (DHIs) hold substantial promise to extend reach and enhance outcomes for those with cannabis-related problems and CUD [7]. DHIs can increase access to evidence-based CUD interventions by reducing the need for highly trained personnel, lessening burden associated with attending the treatment clinic, allowing treatment to be provided in nonspecialty clinics, and reducing provider and patient costs. Some DHIs may improve treatment outcomes by making therapeutic tools available 24/7 via smartphone apps or web-based programs [7]. Moreover, new mobile technologies can potentially monitor risk factors for substance use in real time and provide individualized and automated approaches to dealing with high-risk situations. Readily available therapeutic tools (e.g., self-monitoring programs, skills training modules, social support platforms) hold promise for enhancing engagement with these evidence-based clinical interventions and maximizing outcomes and long-term maintenance of change.

DHIs for adults with CUD have been tested in multiple, controlled clinical trials. The early DHIs for CUD adapted face-to-face evidence-based MET/CBT interventions for delivery in community clinics using a computer or mobile devices. Initial controlled trials indicated a positive impact on treatment outcomes comparable to or exceeding therapist-delivered interventions, and some data suggest that these outcomes were achieved at lower cost and that community clinicians are open to using these DHIs [15, 41, 42, 48].

DHIs targeting cannabis use and related problems have also been applied and evaluated outside traditional healthcare settings. A meta-analysis of four controlled trials ($n = 1928$) conducted in three different countries assessed the effectiveness of online-delivered DHIs that combined MET/CBT for reducing problematic cannabis use and showed evidence of positive small effects at 3-month follow-up [38]. Another trial from Switzerland evaluated an eight-session web-based MET/CBT self-help program for the general population of cannabis users and tested it with vs. without 1–2 internet-delivered "chat" counseling sessions [60]. Program retention and completion were not high, but those who received the program with the chat counseling reported greater cannabis reduction outcomes than those who received only the web-based program or those assigned to a waitlist control group. Other DHIs for cannabis use have focused on college students. For example, a one-session web-based MET-personalized feedback intervention for cannabis-using students transitioning to college did not show treatment effects, but positive effects were observed among those with higher motivation to change and those with family histories of substance use problems [44].

A more recent systematic review and meta-analysis of diverse DHIs for reducing cannabis use identified 20 controlled treatment studies and concluded that these types of interventions significantly reduced cannabis use, but the posttreatment effects tended not to maintain during the year following these interventions [7]. As with in-person interventions, combination approaches appear to provide increased efficacy.

DHIs for youth have received less attention and have primarily been assessed with youth who are using cannabis but who are not seeking or enrolled in treatment [47]. One innovative study integrated ecological momentary assessments (EMA) via mobile phones with MET with cannabis-using youth [63]. After two in-person MET sessions, youth reported triggers, cravings, and cannabis use via their mobile phone for 2 weeks. Youth also received text messages to help them cope with the identified triggers. The use of this program reduced frequency of cannabis use and was acceptable to youth. Another small trial with youth entering an SUD treatment program replaced in-person sessions with CBT-based digitally delivered modules and achieved similar reductions in substance use and mental health outcomes compared with the therapist-delivered intervention; youth rated the DHI as highly acceptable [47]. Last, a pilot study targeting enhanced recovery support tested the use of daily collection of risk factors via an EMA mobile program and 24/7 availability of automated ecological momentary interventions (i.e., automated coping skills interventions) for youth recently discharged from residential treatment [24]. Youth readily used the intervention, particularly those at high risk, and the use of the EMIs was associated with less substance use; note that a large randomized trial of this DHI for youth is in progress.

In summary, digital interventions have the potential to reduce problematic cannabis use when used as part of in-person interventions in traditional treatment settings, as primary interventions in non-healthcare settings, and as stand-alone, online interventions for the general population. Although having at least minimal in-person contact appears to increase the efficacy of DHIs, significant effects can be achieved even with no clinical contact. Future technological innovations will most certainly increase the possibilities for DHI provision, which will have substantial impact on reducing barriers to treatment, increasing access for at-risk cannabis users, and hopefully increasing the potency of interventions for CUD.

12.5 Brief Interventions

Another treatment modality for CUD and cannabis misuse is the brief intervention (BI). BIs for CUD usually comprise 1–2 sessions and primarily utilize interviewing and counseling strategies drawn from the MET literature. These have been tested in specialty and non-specialty treatment settings and demonstrated small to moderate effects [53]. As with DHIs, the availability of BIs can increase access to treatment and decrease burden, which can help reach a larger proportion of those with CUD or cannabis-related problems who might benefit from the intervention.

Opportunistic settings such as schools or medical settings offer the ability to identify and reach more persons experiencing problems related to their use of cannabis. Several brief interventions aimed at youth have been developed to facilitate intervention efforts in these settings. Two brief interventions for youth were developed for use in primary care or the emergency department, one with a focus on substance abuse generally [19] and the other for cannabis specifically [4]. Both used MET counseling principles and delivered the intervention via a 15–20-minute session plus a 10-minute booster phone call and reported significant reductions in cannabis use indicating that primary care and emergency room settings can be utilized effectively to identify and intervene on cannabis use.

Schools, both high school and college, provide advantageous environments for reaching youth who misuse cannabis. Several BI studies have recruited and delivered the intervention in school settings and shown positive effects. Two sessions of an MET-based BI reduced cannabis use and CUD symptoms assessed at a 1-year follow-up [75]. Findings from two studies comprised of only one session of MET showed significant reductions in cigarettes, alcohol, and cannabis in one trial, but not in a second trial [51].

The most well-established school-based intervention is the *Teen Marijuana Check-Up (TMCU* [73]). This alternative school-based approach focuses on recruiting teens who are not necessarily interested or willing to go to treatment, those who may have questions about their cannabis use but do not identify as having a problem, and even those who are not thinking about changing their use. The TMCU is advertised in schools as a confidential meeting with a healthcare counselor and is not labeled as treatment. Three trials have shown that teens with cannabis use frequency levels comparable to that observed in outpatient treatment studies readily volunteer for the TMCU and show reliably greater decreases in cannabis use relative to teens in control conditions [73]. Of note, the TMCU has also been adapted and evaluated in Australia [49] and the Netherlands [21]. An ongoing implementation trial will evaluate different strategies for effectively translating the TMCU to community school systems [35].

Overall, BIs provide an important intervention modality that can reach cannabis users who are not likely to seek treatment. Initial evidence suggests that these interventions have significant positive impact on cannabis use, but this effect is not large.

12.6 Pharmacotherapies for CUD

The development of medications to use as adjuncts to behavioral interventions or as stand-alone treatment has the potential to enhance outcomes for those seeking to reduce or stop using cannabis. Increased understanding of the neurobiology of cannabis and the complexities of the endogenous cannabinoid system, together with a clearer characterization of the cannabis withdrawal syndrome, has led to an escalating number of human laboratory and clinical trials exploring the effects of a diverse cadre of medications. Reviews of this literature, including a most recent Cochrane review, have unfortunately yet to identify an effective pharmacotherapy (e.g., [9, 52, 62]), and no medications are currently approved by the FDA for treating CUD nor are there sufficient data to justify clear clinical recommendations. Below, we briefly summarize findings from the reviews and highlight a few more recently published studies.

Pharmacotherapy approaches explored to date include the following:

(a) Targeting of the withdrawal syndrome, either by use of CB1 agonists or intervening on specific withdrawal symptoms

(b) Use of CB1 receptor antagonists or inverse agonists to block the effects of THC and reduce the reinforcing effects of cannabis

(c) Targeting of mood, stress, or craving with diverse medications

(d) Opioid antagonists that block opioid receptors, which putatively contribute to the reinforcing effects of THC via interactions with the cannabinoid system

(e) Novel medications that directly target the endogenous cannabinoid system and directly manipulate brain levels of specific endocannabinoids, i.e., FAAH inhibitors

(f) Medications that target comorbid psychiatric conditions (e.g., depression, anxiety)

Agonist therapies such as dronabinol and nabilone have demonstrated clear efficacy for reducing cannabis withdrawal symptoms and self-administration in human laboratory studies when delivered alone and in combination with other medications; however, CUD outpatient treatment studies have failed to demonstrate the efficacy of dronabinol or a combination of lofexidine (an alpha-2 agonist) and dronabinol, although some data suggest that perhaps higher doses of dronabinol should be evaluated [46, 61]. Nabilone has yet to be tested in a clinical trial. Similarly, nabiximols (i.e., Sativex) an oramucosal preparation of THC combined with cannabidiol (CBD) reduced cannabis withdrawal symptoms but did not show an effect on cannabis use or abstinence [2]. An antagonist-like medication, i.e., rimonabant, a CB1 receptor inverse agonist, effectively blocked the intoxicating effects of smoked cannabis in a human study [40] but has not been tested in clinical trials because it was withdrawn from the European market because of psychiatric side effects. Unfortunately, no other antagonists or inverse agonists have received systematic study in humans. Zolpidem, a nonbenzodiazepine GABA-A receptor agonist used for the treatment of insomnia, reduced cannabis-withdrawal-related disruptions in sleep [71], and results from a clinical efficacy trial are pending. Guanfacine, an alpha-2a-adrenergic

agonist, has also shown positive effects on multiple symptoms of cannabis withdrawal [33].

Multiple laboratory studies and clinical trials have evaluated medications targeting mood, stress, or craving and have undergone tests in the laboratory and research clinics (e.g., baclofen, buspirone, bupropion, divalproex, fluoxetine, lithium, mirtazapine, nefazodone, oxytocin, quetiapine, topiramate, venlafaxine; [9]). Results of these studies have generally been unremarkable in that no robust evidence for potential efficacy has been observed. A few initial small clinical studies have reported positive findings. For example, the GABAergic medication, gabapentin, showed reductions in withdrawal symptoms and days and amount of cannabis use and improved sleep [50], but replication of these outcomes has not appeared in the literature. A trial of the naturally occurring amino acid, N-acetylcysteine (NAC), showed positive effects in reducing cannabis use in treatment-seeking youth [29], but a subsequent multi-site trial targeting CUD in adults did not observe positive effects on cannabis use [30].

Naltrexone, an opioid antagonist, has been considered as medication for CUD because of the bidirectional modulatory effects of the endogenous cannabinoid and opioid systems and the potential for opioid receptor blockade to decrease the positive effects of cannabis. Laboratory studies indicate that chronic dosing can decrease the reinforcing effects of cannabis smoking and may impact use patterns in the home environment [34]; however, no CUD clinical trials have been reported.

A recent novel approach to CUD medication development is to directly manipulate brain levels of specific endocannabinoid, for example, potentiating signaling by inhibiting fatty acid amide hydrolase (FAAH), the enzyme that degrades the endocannabinoid, anandamide. A small initial controlled trial of a FAAH inhibitor supported the safety of the FAAH inhibitor, and findings indicated positive effects on cannabis withdrawal symptoms during the initial 5-day inpatient stay and indicators of reduced cannabis use during a short 3-week outpatient period [20]. A larger controlled trial of this FAAH inhibitor is in progress.

Because the majority of those with CUD also has a psychiatric disorder, there has been some interest in testing medications for these co-occurring disorders. A large multi-site trial evaluated methylphenidate for teens with attention deficit hyperactivity disorder (ADHD) and an SUD (over 90% had CUD) [54]. Medication effects on ADHD were minimal, and no difference was observed on days of substance use. A small significant effect was reported on abstinence verified by urine toxicology. Prior studies that evaluated atomoxetine for ADHD and CUD and venlafaxine or fluoxetine for depression and CUD reported similarly weak results. Observational studies have reported that clozapine reduced cannabis use in those with schizophrenia and CUD, and a small, controlled trial supported this observation, observing a small effect on reductions in cannabis use [10].

12.7 Conclusions and Future Directions

Cannabis use and CUD, like other psychoactive substances and substance use disorders, pose an important public health problem impacting a substantial number of individuals across the globe. The changing landscape of cannabis legalization and the parallel burgeoning of a multibillion cannabis industry strongly suggest that problems related to the misuse of cannabis and the development of CUD will continue and likely escalate. Existing evidence-based behavioral treatments for CUD produce positive outcomes, with combination interventions such as MET/CBT/CM showing the largest effects. However, at least half of those who seek treatment for CUD do not show a positive response to these interventions, and many relapse. The majority of those with CUD does not seek or receive treatment. Digital health approaches delivered online or via mobile technologies such as smartphones hold promise for both increasing access to efficacious interventions and enhancing treatment potency and outcome. Integration of in-person and digital treatment approaches warrants further investigation.

Identifying of pharmacotherapies for CUD remains an important goal and one that could greatly enhance intervention options and enhance efficacy for those seeking to reduce or quit cannabis use. Finding an efficacious medication continues to be elusive. Novel approaches that warrant continued study include modulation of the endocannabinoid system, alternative dosing with CB1 agonists, and combinations of medications targeting withdrawal and co-occurring symptoms and disorders that may interfere with cannabis reduction or prompt relapse.

Methodological variability, particularly the lack of uniform outcome measures across CUD intervention studies, causes difficulties not only in comparing treatment efficacy but also in determining clinically meaningful outcomes [45]. To date, most studies have focused on cannabis abstinence to assess treatment efficacy, but substantial reductions in cannabis are also likely to result in improvement in psychosocial functioning [8]. In lieu of the current loosening of cannabis laws for both therapeutic and recreational use and societal and cultural trends toward acceptance of such use, broadening the range of outcomes used to evaluate CUD and cannabis use interventions is rationale and in line with the goals of those interested in addressing perceived problems associated with patterns of use that vary on frequency and amount of consumption. Persons who misuse cannabis and develop a CUD are a diverse group, with various patterns of cannabis use (frequency and quantity), differing symptom profiles, a wide range of severity levels, and assorted co-occurring problems. Behavioral and pharmacological treatment approaches that tailor interventions and outcome goals to specific subgroups may prove beneficial for enhancing their efficacy and can help better identify effective treatments for those struggling with cannabis use-related problems.

References

1. Agrawal A, Lynskey MT. Candidate genes for cannabis use disorders: findings, challenges and directions. Addiction. 2009;104(4):518–32. doi: ADD2504 [pii] https://doi.org/10.1111/j.1360-0443.2009.02504.x.
2. Allsop DJ, Copeland J, Lintzeris N, Dunlop AJ, Montebello M, Sadler C, et al. Nabiximols as an agonist replacement therapy during cannabis with-

drawal: a randomized clinical trial. JAMA Psychiatry. 2014;71(3):281–91. https://doi.org/10.1001/jamapsychiatry.2013.3947.

3. APA. Diagnostic and statistical manual of mental disorders. Arlington: American Psychiatric Association; 2013.

4. Bernstein E, Edwards E, Dorfman D, Heeren T, Bliss C, Bernstein J. Screening and brief intervention to reduce marijuana use among youth and young adults in a pediatric emergency department. Acad Emerg Med. 2009;16(11):1174–85. https://doi.org/10.1111/j.1553-2712.2009.00490.x.

5. Blanco C, Iza M, Rodríguez-Fernández JM, Baca-García E, Wang S, Olfson M. Probability and predictors of treatment-seeking for substance use disorders in the U.S. Drug Alcohol Depend. 2015;149:136–44.

6. Borodovsky JT, Budney AJ. Cannabis regulatory science: risk–benefit considerations for mental disorders. Int Rev Psychiatry. 2018;30:1–20. https://doi.org/10.1080/09540261.2018.1454406.

7. Boumparis N, Loheide-Niesmann L, Blankers M, Ebert DD, Korf D, Schaub MP, et al. Short- and long-term effects of digital prevention and treatment interventions for cannabis use reduction: a systematic review and meta-analysis. Drug Alcohol Depend. 2019;200:82–94. https://doi.org/10.1016/j.drugalcdep.2019.03.016.

8. Brezing CA, Choi CJ, Pavlicova M, Brooks D, Mahony AL, Mariani JJ, Levin FR. **Abstinence and reduced frequency of use are associated with improvements in quality of life among treatment-seekers with cannabis use disorder. Am J Addict. 2018;27(2):101–7. https://doi.org/10.1111/ajad.12660.

9. Brezing CA, Levin FR. The current state of pharmacological treatments for cannabis use disorder and withdrawal. Neuropsychopharmacology. 2018;43(1):173–94. https://doi.org/10.1038/npp.2017.212.

10. Brunette MF, Dawson R, O'Keefe CD, Narasimhan M, Noordsy DL, Wojcik J, Green AI. A randomized trial of clozapine vs. other antipsychotics for cannabis use disorder in patients with schizophrenia. J Dual Diagn. 2011;7(1–2):50–63.

11. Budney AJ, Hughes JR, Moore BA, Vandrey RG. A review of the validity and significance of the cannabis withdrawal syndrome. Am J Psychiatry. 2004;161(11):1967–77.

12. Budney AJ, Lile JA. Moving beyond the cannabis controversy into the world of the cannabinoids. Int Rev Psychiatry. 2009;21(2):91–5. doi: 910429540 [pii] https://doi.org/10.1080/09540260902782729.

13. Budney AJ, Moore BA, Vandrey RG, Hughes JR. The time course and significance of cannabis withdrawal. J Abnorm Psychol. 2003;112(3):393–402.

14. Budney AJ, Roffman R, Stephens RS, Walker D. Marijuana dependence and its treatment. Addict Sci Clin Pract. 2007;4(1):4–16.

15. Budney AJ, Stanger C, Tilford JM, Scherer EB, Brown PC, Li Z, et al. Computer-assisted behavioral therapy and contingency management for cannabis

16. Campbell CI, Bahorik AL, Kline-Simon AH, Satre DD. The role of marijuana use disorder in predicting emergency department and inpatient encounters: a retrospective cohort study. Drug Alcohol Depend. 2017;178:170–5.

17. Chou SP, Goldstein RB, Smith SM, Huang B, Ruan WJ, Zhang H, et al. The epidemiology of DSM-5 nicotine use disorder: results from the National Epidemiologic Survey on Alcohol and Related Conditions-III. J Clin Psychiatry. 2016;77(10):1404–12. https://doi.org/10.4088/JCP.15m10114.

18. Corsi DJ, Hsu H, Weiss D, Fell DB, Walker M. Trends and correlates of cannabis use in pregnancy: a population-based study in Ontario, Canada from 2012 to 2017. Can J Public Health. 2019;110(1):76–84. https://doi.org/10.17269/s41997-018-0148-0.

19. D'Amico EJ, Miles JN, Stern SA, Meredith LS. Brief motivational interviewing for teens at risk of substance use consequences: a randomized pilot study in a primary care clinic. J Subst Abus Treat. 2008;35(1):53–61. https://doi.org/10.1016/j.jsat.2007.08.008.

20. D'Souza DC, Cortes-Briones J, Creatura G, Bluez G, Thurnauer H, Deaso E, et al. Efficacy and safety of a fatty acid amide hydrolase inhibitor (PF-04457845) in the treatment of cannabis withdrawal and dependence in men: a double-blind, placebo-controlled, parallel group, phase 2a single-site randomised controlled trial. Lancet Psychiatry. 2019;6(1):35–45. https://doi.org/10.1016/S2215-0366(18)30427-9.

21. de Gee EA, Verdurmen JE, Bransen E, de Jonge JM, Schippers GM. A randomized controlled trial of a brief motivational enhancement for non-treatment-seeking adolescent cannabis users. J Subst Abus Treat. 2014;47(3):181–8. https://doi.org/10.1016/j.jsat.2014.05.001.

22. Degenhardt L, Ferrari AJ, Calabria B, Hall W, Norman RE, McGrath J, et al. The global epidemiology and contribution of cannabis use and dependence to the global burden of disease: results from the GBD 2010 study. PLoS One. 2013;8(10):e76635. https://doi.org/10.1371/journal.pone.0076635.

23. Dennis ML, Godley SH, Diamond G, Tims FM, Babor T, Donaldson J, et al. The cannabis youth treatment (CYT) study: main findings from two randomized trials. J Subst Abus Treat. 2004;27:197–213. https://doi.org/10.1016/j.jsat.2003.09.005.

24. Dennis ML, Scott CK, Funk RR, Nicholson L. A pilot study to examine the feasibility and potential effectiveness of using smartphones to provide recovery support for adolescents. Subst Abus. 2015;36(4):486–92. https://doi.org/10.1080/08897077.2014.970323.

25. ElSohly. Chemical constituents of marijuana: the complex mixture of natural cannabinoids. Life Sci. 2005;78:539–48.

26. Gardner EL. Endocannabinoid signaling system and brain reward: emphasis on dopamine. Pharmacol Biochem Behav. 2005;81:263–84.

27. Gates P, Copeland J, Swift W, Martin G. Barriers and facilitators to cannabis treatment. Drug Alcohol Rev. 2012;31(3):311–9. https://doi.org/10.1111/j.1465-3362.2011.00313.x.

28. Gates PJ, Sabioni P, Copeland J, Le Foll B, Gowing L. Psychosocial interventions for cannabis use disorder. Cochrane Database Syst Rev. 2016;(5). https://doi.org/10.1002/14651858.CD005336.pub4.

29. Gray KM, Carpenter MJ, Baker NL, DeSantis SM, Kryway E, Hartwell KJ, et al. A double-blind randomized controlled trial of N-acetylcysteine in cannabis-dependent adolescents. Am J Psychiatry. 2012;169(8):805–12. https://doi.org/10.1176/appi.ajp.2012.12010055.

30. Gray KM, Sonne SC, McClure EA, Ghitza UE, Matthews AG, McRae-Clark AL, et al. A randomized placebo-controlled trial of N-acetylcysteine for cannabis use disorder in adults. Drug Alcohol Depend. 2017;177:249–57. https://doi.org/10.1016/j.drugalcdep.2017.04.020.

31. Grucza RA, Agrawal A, Krauss MJ, Cavazos-Rehg PA, Bierut LJ. Recent trends in the prevalence of marijuana use and associated disorders in the United States. JAMA Psychiatry. 2016;73(3):300–1. https://doi.org/10.1001/jamapsychiatry.2015.3111.

32. Haney M, Comer SD, Ward AS, Foltin RW, Fischman MW. Factors influencing marijuana self-administration by humans. Behav Pharmacol. 1997;8:101–12.

33. Haney M, Cooper ZD, Bedi G, Herrmann E, Comer SD, Reed SC, et al. Guanfacine decreases symptoms of cannabis withdrawal in daily cannabis smokers. Addict Biol. 2019;24(4):707–16. https://doi.org/10.1111/adb.12621.

34. Haney M, Ramesh D, Glass A, Pavlicova M, Bedi G, Cooper ZD. Naltrexone maintenance decreases cannabis self-administration and subjective effects in daily cannabis smokers. Neuropsychopharmacology. 2015;40(11):2489–98. https://doi.org/10.1038/npp.2015.108.

35. Hartzler B, Lyon AR, Walker DD, Matthews L, King KM, McCollister KE. Implementing the teen marijuana check-up in schools—a study protocol. Implement Sci. 2017;12(1):103. https://doi.org/10.1186/s13012-017-0633-5.

36. Hasin D, Saha T, Kerridge B, Goldstein R, Chou P, Zhang H, et al. Prevalence of marijuana use disorders in the United States between 2001-2002 and 2012-2013. JAMA Psychiatry. 2015;72(12):1235–42. https://doi.org/10.1001/jamapsychiatry.2015.1858.

37. Hasin DS, Kerridge BT, Saha TD, Huang B, Pickering R, Smith SM, et al. Prevalence and correlates of DSM-5 cannabis use disorder, 2012-2013: findings from the National Epidemiologic Survey on Alcohol and Related Conditions-III. Am J Psychiatry. 2016;173(6):588–99. https://doi.org/10.1176/appi.ajp.2015.15070907.

38. Hoch E, Preuss UW, Ferri M, Simon R. Digital interventions for problematic cannabis users in non-clinical settings: findings from a systematic review and meta-analysis. Eur Addict Res. 2016;22(5):233–42. https://doi.org/10.1159/000445716.

39. Hogue A, Henderson CE, Ozechowski TJ, Robbins MS. Evidence base on outpatient behavioral treatments for adolescent substance use: updates and recommendations 2007-2013. J Clin Child Adolesc Psychol. 2014;43(5):695–720. https://doi.org/10.1080/15374416.2014.915550.

40. Huestis MA, Gorelick DA, Heishman SJ, Preston KL, Nelson RA, Moolchan ET, Frank RA. Blockade of effects of smoked marijuana by the CB1-sective cannabinoid receptor antagonist SR141716. Arch Gen Psychiatry. 2001;58:322–8.

41. Kay-Lambkin FJ, Baker AL, Kelly B, Lewin TJ. Clinician-assisted computerised versus therapist-delivered treatment for depressive and addictive disorders: a randomised controlled trial. Med J Aust. 2011;195(3):S44–50.

42. Kay-Lambkin FJ, Simpson AL, Bowman J, Childs S. Dissemination of a computer-based psychological treatment in a drug and alcohol clinical service: an observational study. Addict Sci Clin Pract. 2014;9:15. https://doi.org/10.1186/1940-0640-9-15.

43. Knapp AA, Babbin SF, Budney AJ, Walker DD, Stephens RS, Scherer EA, Stanger C. Psychometric assessment of the marijuana adolescent problem inventory. Addict Behav. 2018;79(4):113–9.

44. Lee CM, Neighbors C, Kilmer JR, Larimer ME. A brief, web-based personalized feedback selective intervention for college student marijuana use: a randomized clinical trial. Psychol Addict Behav. 2010;24(2):265–73. https://doi.org/10.1037/a0018859.

45. Lee DC, Schlienz NJ, Peters EN, Dworkin RH, Turk DC, Strain EC, Vandrey R. Systematic review of outcome domains and measures used in psychosocial and pharmacological treatment trials for cannabis use disorder. Drug Alcohol Depend. 2019;194:500–17. https://doi.org/10.1016/j.drugalcdep.2018.10.020.

46. Levin FR, Mariani JJ, Pavlicova M, Brooks D, Glass A, Mahony A, et al. Dronabinol and lofexidine for cannabis use disorder: a randomized, double-blind, placebo-controlled trial. Drug Alcohol Depend. 2016;159:53–60. https://doi.org/10.1016/j.drugalcdep.2015.11.025.

47. Marsch LA, Borodovsky JT. Technology-based interventions for preventing and treating substance use among youth. Child Adolesc Psychiatry Clin N Am. 2016;25(4):755–68. https://doi.org/10.1016/j.chc.2016.06.005.

48. Marsch LA, Carroll KM, Kiluk BD. Technology-based interventions for the treatment and recovery management of substance use disorders: a JSAT special issue. J Subst Abus Treat. 2014;46(1):1–4. https://doi.org/10.1016/j.jsat.2013.08.010.

49. Martin G, Copeland J. The adolescent cannabis check-up: randomized trial of a brief intervention for young cannabis users. J Subst Abus Treat. 2008;34(4):407–

14. doi: S0740-5472(07)00190-0 [pii] https://doi.org/10.1016/j.jsat.2007.07.004.

50. Mason BJ, Crean R, Goodell V, Light JM, Quello S, Shadan F, et al. A proof-of-concept randomized controlled study of gabapentin: effects on cannabis use, withdrawal and executive function deficits in cannabis-dependent adults. Neuropsychopharmacology. 2012;37(7):1689–98. https://doi.org/10.1038/npp.2012.14.

51. McCambridge J, Slym RL, Strang J. Randomized controlled trial of motivational interviewing compared with drug information and advice for early intervention among young cannabis users. Addiction. 2008;103(11):1809–18. https://doi.org/10.1111/j.1360-0443.2008.02331.x.

52. Nielsen S, Gowing L, Sabioni P, Le Foll B. Pharmacotherapies for cannabis dependence. Cochrane Database Syst Rev. 2019;(1):CD008940. https://doi.org/10.1002/14651858.CD008940.pub3.

53. Parmar A, Sarkar S. Brief interventions for cannabis use disorders: a review. Addict Disord Treat. 2017;16(2):80–93. https://doi.org/10.1097/ADT.0000000000000100.

54. Riggs PD, Winhusen T, Davies RD, Leimberger JD, Mikulich-Gilbertson S, Klein C, et al. Randomized controlled trial of osmotic-release methylphenidate with cognitive-behavioral therapy in adolescents with attention-deficit/hyperactivity disorder and substance use disorders. J Am Acad Child Adolesc Psychiatry. 2011;50(9):903–14. https://doi.org/10.1016/j.jaac.2011.06.010.

55. Russo EB. The case for the entourage effect and conventional breeding of clinical cannabis: no "strain," no gain. Front Plant Sci. 2019;9:1969. https://doi.org/10.3389/fpls.2018.01969.

56. SAMHSA. Results from the 2016 National Survey on Drug Use and Health: summary of national findings. Rockville: Substance Abuse and Mental Health Services Administration, Center for Behavioral Health Statistics and Quality; 2017.

57. SAMHSA. Treatment episode data set. In 2015 SPSS Data. 2017. Retrieved from https://wwwdasis.samhsa.gov/dasis2/teds.htm.

58. SAMHSA. Treatment episode data set (TEDS): 2005-2015. National admissions to substance abuse treatment services. BHSIS series S-91, HHS publication no. (SMA) 17-5037 (BHSIS series S-71, HHS publication no. (SMA) 14-4850). Rockville: Substance Abuse and Mental Health Services Administration, Center for Behavioral Health Statistics and Quality; 2017. Website: http://www.samhsa.gov/data/sites/default/files/TEDS2012N_Web.pdf.

59. SAMHSA. Results from the 2017 National Survey on Drug Use and Health: detailed tables. Rockville: Substance Abuse and Mental Health Services Administration, Center for Behavioral Health Statistics and Quality; 2018.

60. Schaub MP, Wenger A, Berg O, Beck T, Stark L, Buehler E, Haug S. A web-based self-help intervention with and without chat counseling to reduce cannabis use in problematic cannabis users: three-arm randomized controlled trial. J Med Internet Res. 2015;17(10):e232. https://doi.org/10.2196/jmir.4860.

61. Schlienz NJ, Lee DC, Stitzer ML, Vandrey R. The effect of high-dose dronabinol (oral THC) maintenance on cannabis self-administration. Drug Alcohol Depend. 2018;187:254–60. https://doi.org/10.1016/j.drugalcdep.2018.02.022.

62. Sherman BJ, McRae-Clark AL. Treatment of cannabis use disorder: current science and future outlook. Pharmacotherapy. 2016;36(5):511–35. https://doi.org/10.1002/phar.1747.

63. Shrier LA, Rhoads A, Burke P, Walls C, Blood EA. Real-time, contextual intervention using mobile technology to reduce marijuana use among youth: a pilot study. Addict Behav. 2014;39(1):173–80. https://doi.org/10.1016/j.addbeh.2013.09.028.

64. Stanger C, Lansing AH, Budney AJ. Advances in research on contingency management for adolescent substance use. Child Adolesc Psychiatry Clin N Am. 2016;25(4):645–59. https://doi.org/10.1016/j.chc.2016.05.002.

65. Stanger C, Ryan SR, Scherer EA, Norton GE, Budney AJ. Clinic- and home-based contingency management plus parent training for adolescent cannabis use disorders. J Am Acad Child Adolesc Psychiatry. 2015;54(6):445–53. e442. https://doi.org/10.1016/j.jaac.2015.02.009.

66. Stephens RS, Babor TF, Kadden R, Miller M. The marijuana treatment project: rationale, design, and participant characteristics. Addiction. 2002;97(S1):109–24.

67. Tanner-Smith EE, Wilson SJ, Lipsey MW. The comparative effectiveness of outpatient treatment for adolescent substance abuse: a meta-analysis. J Subst Abus Treat. 2013;44(2):145–58. https://doi.org/10.1016/j.jsat.2012.05.006.

68. UNODC. World drug report: pre-briefing to the member states. Vienna: United Nations Office on Drugs and Crime; 2018.

69. UNODC. World drug report 2019. Vienna: United Nations Office on Drugs and Crime; 2019.

70. van der Pol P, Liebregts N, de Graaf R, Korf DJ, van den Brink W, van Laar M. Facilitators and barriers in treatment seeking for cannabis dependence. Drug Alcohol Depend. 2013;133(2):776–80. https://doi.org/10.1016/j.drugalcdep.2013.08.011.

71. Vandrey R, Smith MT, McCann UD, Budney AJ, Curran EM. Sleep disturbance and the effects of extended-release zolpidem during cannabis withdrawal. Drug Alcohol Depend. 2011;117(1):38–44. https://doi.org/10.1016/j.drugalcdep.2011.01.003.

72. Volkow ND, Han B, Compton WM, McCance-Katz EF. Self-reported medical and nonmedical cannabis use among pregnant women in the United States medical and nonmedical cannabis use among pregnant women in the United States letters. JAMA. 2019;322(2):167–9. https://doi.org/10.1001/jama.2019.7982.

73. Walker DD, Stephens RS, Blevins CE, Banes KE, Matthews L, Roffman RA. Augmenting brief interventions for adolescent marijuana users: the impact of motivational check-ins. J Consult Clin Psychol. 2016;84(11):983–92. https://doi.org/10.1037/ccp0000094.

74. WHO. The health and social effects of nonmedical cannabis use. Geneva: World Health Organization; 2016.

75. Winters KC, Lee S, Botzet A, Fahnhorst T, Nicholson A. One-year outcomes and mediators of a brief intervention for drug abusing adolescents. Psychol Addict Behav. 2014;28(2):464–74. https://doi.org/10.1037/a0035041.

76. Winters KC, Tanner-Smith EE, Bresani E, Meyers K. Current advances in the treatment of adolescent drug use. Adolesc Health Med Ther. 2014;5:199–210. https://doi.org/10.2147/AHMT.S48053.

77. World Health Organization. The ICD-10 classification of mental and behavioural disorders: clinical descriptions and diagnostic guidelines. Geneva: World Health Organization; 1992.

78. Zehra A, Burns J, Kure Liu C, Manza P, Wiers C, Volkow N, Wang G. Cannabis addiction and the brain: a review. J Neuroimmune Pharmacol. 2018;13:1–15. https://doi.org/10.1007/s11481-018-9782-9.

Cocaine Addiction and Treatment

13

David A. Gorelick

Contents

D. A. Gorelick (✉)
Department of Psychiatry, University of Maryland
School of Medicine, Baltimore, MD, USA
e-mail: dgorelick@som.umaryland.edu

© Springer Nature Switzerland AG 2021
N. el-Guebaly et al. (eds.), *Textbook of Addiction Treatment*,
https://doi.org/10.1007/978-3-030-36391-8_13

Abstract

Cocaine use disorder represents a substantial clinical and public health burden in many countries, yet there are no well-proven and broadly effective pharmacological treatments available and no medication approved for this indication by any national regulatory authority. Medications with efficacy in more than one controlled clinical trial include disulfiram, oral stimulants in sustained-release formulation, bupropion, and the anticonvulsant topiramate. Cocaine-metabolizing enzyme, an anti-cocaine vaccine, and repetitive transcranial magnetic stimulation (rTMS) have each shown promise in small clinical trials. In the absence of proven, broadly effective medications, the mainstay of treatment remains psychosocial interventions, such as contingency management and cognitive-behavioral therapy.

Keywords

Cocaine · Pharmacological treatment · Disulfiram · Agonist maintenance · Topiramate · rTMS · Anti-cocaine vaccine

13.1 Introduction

Cocaine is a plant alkaloid found in leaves of the coca bush, *Erythroxylon coca*, which grows in the Andes Mountains region of South America. Its psychoactive properties make cocaine one of the most widely used and abused illicit drugs in the world. There were an estimated 18 million cocaine users worldwide in 2014, representing 0.4% of the 15- to 64-year-old population [96]. Cocaine use is associated with a variety of psychological and physical health problems, resulting in a substantial clinical and public health burden in countries where use is prevalent. About one in six cocaine users (via the intravenous or smoked routes of administration) develop addiction (moderate-severe cocaine use disorder in DSM-5 terms) to the drug, with subsequent psychological and socioeconomic problems [14]. In 2010, cocaine use disorder was associated globally with an estimated 1.09 million years lived with disability (rate of 16 per 100,000 persons) [97], 1.1 million disability-adjusted life years (16 per 100,000 persons) [67], and 500 deaths (<0.05 per 100,000 persons) [54]. Data from longitudinal studies in five different countries (Brazil, Canada, Denmark, France, and Italy) suggest that addicted cocaine users have death rates four- to eightfold higher than those of the same age and sex in the general population [13].

Notwithstanding this substantial health burden, there are no widely used, broadly effective treatments for cocaine use disorder. No medication is approved for this indication by any national regulatory authority because no medication has met the scientifically rigorous standard of consistent, statistically significant efficacy in adequately powered, replicated, controlled clinical trials. The mainstay of treatment is psychosocial, with good-quality evidence from controlled clinical trials for the efficacy of contingency management, which may have enhanced effectiveness when used in conjunction with pharmacological treatment [87] and cognitive-behavioral therapy [44, 76]. This chapter reviews the current state of pharmacological treatment for cocaine use disorder.

13.2 Overview of Pharmacological Treatment

The goals of pharmacological treatment of cocaine use disorder are to reduce or eliminate the desire (craving) to take cocaine, reduce or eliminate the acute positive reinforcement (euphoria, "high") from taking cocaine, and reduce or eliminate the negative reinforcement from cocaine withdrawal. To achieve these goals in clinical practice, medication should be used in conjunction with some psychosocial treatment component, if only to enhance medication adherence. There are few data to guide the choice of optimum psychosocial treatment to combine with pharmacotherapy [6]. As no medication currently has national regulatory authority approval for treatment of cocaine use disorder, psychosocial modalities should be the mainstay of treatment [18].

Four pharmacologic approaches are potentially useful to achieve these treatment goals [28]: (1) substitution treatment with a cross-tolerant stimulant (analogous to methadone maintenance treatment of opioid use disorder), (2) treatment with an antagonist medication that blocks the binding of cocaine at its site of action (true pharmacologic antagonism, analogous to naltrexone treatment of opioid use disorder), (3) treatment with a medication that functionally antagonizes the effects of cocaine (as by reducing the reinforcing effects of or craving for cocaine), and (4) alteration of cocaine pharmacokinetics so that less drug reaches or remains at its site(s) of action in the brain.

Most current clinical and research attention focuses on the second and third approaches. The first approach has been evaluated in a small number of clinical trials, with mixed results. The fourth approach has shown promise in animal studies and early phase II clinical trials [27].

Cocaine has two major neuropharmacological actions: blockade of presynaptic neurotransmitter transporters (reuptake pumps), thereby inhibiting the uptake of previously released monoamine neurotransmitters and resulting in psychomotor stimulant effects, and blockade of sodium ion channels in nerve membranes, resulting in local anesthetic effects [29].

Cocaine's positively reinforcing effects derive from its blockade of the dopamine reuptake pump, causing presynaptically released dopamine to remain in the synapse and enhancing dopaminergic neurotransmission [36]. Cocaine's local anesthetic effects are believed to contribute to cocaine-induced kindling, the phenomenon by which previous exposure to cocaine sensitizes the individual so that later exposure to low doses produces an enhanced response.

13.3 Medication Options

13.3.1 Antidepressants

Antidepressants are the most studied class of medication for the treatment of cocaine use disorder, but evidence for their efficacy is weak. A meta-analysis of 28 published clinical trials that involved 2547 participants found that antidepressants as a class (including tricyclics, selective serotonin reuptake inhibitors, serotonin-norepinephrine uptake inhibitors, and the MAO inhibitor selegiline) were no more effective than placebo in terms of dropout from treatment (relative risk 1.03, 95% CI 0.92–1.16) or number of weeks of continuous abstinence (8 studies, 942 participants, mean difference 0.08, 95% CI −0.17 to 0.32) [73].

There is variation across types of antidepressants, with some evidence of efficacy in controlled clinical trials for desipramine and bupropion. A meta-analysis of 16 published clinical trials with desipramine (plus one trial using imipramine) that involved 1293 participants found a significant benefit from desipramine in proportion of participants achieving at least 3 weeks of continuous abstinence (relative risk 1.55, 95% CI 1.10–2.17), but no benefit in treatment retention (relative risk 1.00, 95% CI 0.85–1.18) [73]. However, the abstinence benefit was limited to participants with mild cocaine use disorder. There is weak evidence that patients with steady-state desipramine plasma concentrations above 200 ng/mL have poorer outcomes [43], with better outcomes at concentrations around 125 ng/mL [47]. A meta-analysis of two published controlled clinical trials that involved 176 participants found bupropion significantly better than placebo in promoting at least 3 weeks of sustained abstinence in participants with moderate-severe cocaine use disorder (risk ratio 1.63, 95% CI 1.03, 2.59) [8].

Several other antidepressants have shown efficacy in small, open-label trials, including reboxetine, maprotiline, and mirtazapine [28].

Heterocyclic antidepressants have not been associated with unexpected or medically serious side effects. While theoretically possible, there is no evidence that patients who relapse to cocaine use while still on medication are at increased risk of cardiovascular side effects [68].

Selective serotonin reuptake inhibitors (SSRIs), such as fluoxetine, paroxetine, and sertraline, have not been effective in controlled clinical trials [73, 98]. A meta-analysis of 8 published clinical trials involving 662 participants found no significant advantage over placebo in dropout rate (relative risk 0.99, 95% CI 0.70–1.41) or craving for cocaine (standardized mean difference −0.22, 95% CI −0.52 to 0.54) [73]. One clinical trial found citalopram (20 mg/day) significantly better than placebo [63]. That study, unlike previous studies, used contingency management, in addition to cognitive-behavioral therapy, as the concomitant psychosocial treatment, suggesting the importance influence of psychosocial treatment on medication efficacy.

13.3.2 Dopamine Agonists (Antiparkinson Agents)

Direct and indirect dopamine agonist medications have not generally been found effective for the treatment of cocaine use disorder. A meta-analysis of 24 published clinical trials involving 2147 participants that evaluated both direct dopamine receptor agonists (bromocriptine, pergolide, pramipexole, cabergoline, hydergine) and indirect agonists (amantadine and the amino acid dopamine precursor L-dopa [sometimes combined with the peripheral dopa decarboxylase inhibitor carbidopa]) together as a class found no evidence of efficacy compared to placebo [61].

13.3.3 Disulfiram

Disulfiram increases dopamine concentrations by blocking the conversion of dopamine to norepinephrine by the enzyme dopamine-β-hydroxylase, so it can be considered a functional dopamine agonist [21]. A systematic review of seven published clinical trials involving 492 participants identified several trials in which disulfiram (250 mg daily) was significantly better than placebo in reducing dropout rate or cocaine use [72]. The trials could not be combined for meta-analysis because of high heterogeneity and differences in outcome measures. Only one [48] of five larger controlled clinical trials not included in the earlier review [28] found significant efficacy for disulfiram compared to placebo.

Some of the heterogeneity in treatment response to disulfiram may be due to genetic fac-

tors and gender. Three recent clinical trials found significant efficacy for disulfiram in genetically defined subgroup of patients: with dopamine-β-hydroxylase gene alleles associated with higher enzyme activity [48], with functional variants in the ankyrin repeat and kinase domain-containing 1 (*ANKK1*) and dopamine D_2 receptor (*DRD2*) genes [95], and in the α_{1A}-adrenoreceptor (*ADRA1A*) gene [91]. A review of five published controlled clinical trials involving 434 participants found that disulfiram was less effective in reducing cocaine use in women than in men [15]. There was no such gender difference in response to behavioral treatments. These findings suggest that disulfiram may be a promising treatment for cocaine use disorder in some subgroups of patients.

Although disulfiram is generally well tolerated in clinical trials, where subjects are carefully screened and closely monitored, it may be less safe in routine clinical practice [56].

13.3.4 Stimulants

Stimulant medications might be useful for the treatment of cocaine use disorder as a form of agonist maintenance treatment, conceptually similar to methadone maintenance treatment of opioid use disorder or nicotine replacement treatment of tobacco use disorder. The evidence to date is very promising, but not conclusive. A meta-analysis of 14 published clinical trials involving 1549 participants found that stimulants as a class (including dexamphetamine, mixed amphetamine salts, methamphetamine, lisdexamfetamine, methylphenidate, modafinil, and mazindol) were significantly better than placebo in promoting at least 3 weeks of sustained abstinence (risk ratio 1.36, 95% CI 1.05–1.77), but did not increase proportion of cocaine-free urine samples among those who did not achieve sustained abstinence (standardized mean difference 0.16, 95% CI −0.02 to 0.33) nor improve study retention (risk ratio 1.00, 95% CI 0.93–1.06) [8]. Among specific stimulants, only dexamphetamine (risk ratio 1.98, 95% CI 1.12–3.52) and mixed amphetamine salts (risk ratio 3.63,

95% CI 1.15–11.48) were significantly better than placebo in promoting at least 3 weeks of sustained abstinence. A recent 12-week, controlled clinical trial, not included in the earlier meta-analysis, found that sustained-release dexamphetamine significantly reduced frequency of cocaine use among 73 participants with cocaine use disorder who were also receiving heroin treatment for opioid use disorder (mean difference of 16.7 [95% CI 3.1–28.4] fewer days of cocaine use) compared to placebo [70]. None of these studies reported significant adverse effects, suggesting that stimulant substitution treatment might be safe in cocaine-using patients.

Cocaine itself could be used for agonist maintenance treatment in a slow-onset formulation or route of administration [26], conceptually similar to the use of slow-onset formulations of nicotine (transdermal or transbuccal) for the treatment of tobacco (nicotine) use disorder. Oral formulations of cocaine (cocaine salt capsules and coca leaf tea) substantially reduced coca paste smoking in two large case series of adult patients in Lima, Peru (where oral cocaine products are legal) [53]. Among a case series of 50 coca paste smokers in La Paz, Bolivia, coca leaf chewing (100–200 g of coca leaf per week for a mean of 2 years) substantially improved the mental health of one-third and improved the socioeconomic functioning of almost half (data on cocaine smoking were not reported) [37].

13.3.5 Antipsychotics

Neither the older so-called first-generation (typical) antipsychotics nor the newer second-generation (atypical) antipsychotics have shown consistent efficacy in the treatment of cocaine use disorder in patients without a comorbid psychotic disorder. A meta-analysis of 14 published clinical trials involving 719 participants found that antipsychotics as a class (aripiprazole, olanzapine, quetiapine, risperidone, and one study each with haloperidol or reserpine) reduced study dropout (risk ratio 0.75, 95% CI 0.57–0.97), but did not significantly reduce proportion of subjects achieving at least 3 weeks of continuous absti-

nence (risk ratio 1.30, 95% CI 0.73–2.32) or proportion of participants using cocaine during treatment (risk ratio 1.02, 95% CI 0.65–1.62) [38]. A recent controlled clinical trial of aripiprazole, not included in the earlier meta-analysis, in individuals who had achieved 2 weeks of continuous cocaine abstinence with contingency management, found no significant reduction in lapse or relapse rates, but a significant increase in cocaine craving [66].

Any antipsychotic should be prescribed with caution to cocaine users because of their potential vulnerability to the neuroleptic malignant syndrome [1]. Cocaine users may also be at elevated risk of antipsychotic-induced movement disorders [17, 34].

13.3.6 Anticonvulsants

Anticonvulsants might be effective in the treatment of cocaine use disorder because they increase inhibitory GABA activity and/or decrease excitatory glutamate activity in the brain, both actions that decrease the response to cocaine in the dopaminergic cortico-mesolimbic brain reward circuit [4]. However, controlled clinical trials show little or no effectiveness for anticonvulsants, except for topiramate. A meta-analysis of 20 published clinical trials involving 2068 participants found that anticonvulsants as a class (carbamazepine, gabapentin, lamotrigine, phenytoin, tiagabine, topiramate, and vigabatrin) had no significant effect on dropout rate (risk ratio 0.95, 95% CI 0.86–1.05), cocaine use (risk ratio 0.92, 95% CI 0.84–1.02), or cocaine craving (standardized mean difference −0.25, 95% CI −0.59 to 0.09) nor did any individual anticonvulsant show any significant benefit over placebo [62]. A separate meta-analysis of two topiramate trials involving 210 participants found a significant difference in the proportion of participants achieving sustained cocaine abstinence for at least 3 weeks (relative risk 2.43, 95% CI 1.31–4.53) [93]. A more recent controlled clinical trial involving 59 participants (not included in the meta-analyses) found topiramate significantly better than placebo in increasing cocaine-negative urine samples (odds ratio 8.69, p <0.001) and reducing self-reported cocaine use (mean reduction −3.1 g [p <0.001] for amount; mean reduction −0.78 times per week [p <0.005] for frequency), but only during the first 4 weeks of the 12-week trial [2].

13.3.7 Serotonergic Medications

Serotonergic medications such as buspirone and gepirone, used to treat generalized anxiety disorder, and ritanserin, developed as an antidepressant, showed no efficacy in controlled clinical trials [28]. Ondansetron, approved for the treatment of nausea and vomiting, significantly reduced cocaine use in a small controlled clinical trial, but only at the highest dose (4 mg twice daily) [39].

13.3.8 Cholinergic Medications

Several cholinergic medications have shown mixed results in controlled clinical trials. Varenicline, a partial agonist at $\alpha 4\beta 2$ nicotinic acetylcholine receptors approved for smoking cessation, significantly reduced cocaine use in one small controlled clinical trial [80]. Biperiden (2 mg tid), a muscarinic cholinergic receptor antagonist used to treat movement disorders, significantly reduced cocaine use in a small controlled clinical trial [16]. In contrast, mecamylamine, a nicotinic cholinergic receptor antagonist, and donepezil or galantamine, which nonspecifically increase brain cholinergic activity by inhibiting acetylcholinesterase activity, did not reduce cocaine use in small controlled clinical trials [28].

13.3.9 Opioid Medications

Mu-opiate receptor (mOR) antagonists have been evaluated as treatment for cocaine use disorder because of the role of brain mORs in cocaine use [22]. Three small controlled clinical trials (two placebo-controlled) found that naltrexone (50 mg daily) significantly reduced cocaine use compared to placebo [88, 90] or to cognitive-behavioral therapy without medication [31]. Buprenorphine (4 mg or 16 mg sl), a partial mOR agonist/kappa opioid antagonist used to treat opioid use disorder, combined with naloxone, was not effective in a controlled clinical trial of outpatients with moderate-severe cocaine use disorder [52].

13.3.10 Other Medications

A wide variety of other medications have been evaluated for the treatment of cocaine use disorder, often on the basis of promising case reports or animal studies suggesting that they reduce the reinforcing effects of cocaine. None of these medications has shown effectiveness in a large controlled clinical trial [28].

Doxazosin, an α_1-adrenergic receptor antagonist approved for treatment of hypertension, when rapidly titrated over 4 weeks to a daily dosage of 8 mg, significantly reduced cocaine use in one small, controlled clinical trial [92].

13.3.11 Medication Combinations

Concurrent use of two different medications, which might enhance efficacy while minimizing side effects, has been effective in several small clinical trials. Concurrent use of pergolide (a dopamine D_1/D_2 receptor agonist) and haloperidol (a dopamine D_2 receptor antagonist) and of amantadine (indirect dopamine agonist) and propranolol (beta-adrenergic antagonist) both showed efficacy in small clinical trials [41, 55]. The combination of extended-release mixed amphetamine salts and topiramate was significantly better than placebo in achieving three consecutive weeks of cocaine abstinence [57].

13.3.12 Nutritional Supplements and Herbal Products

The use of nutritional supplements (e.g., amino acids, vitamins, minerals) and herbal products is attractive because of their relative freedom from regulatory oversight and perceived safety and absence of side effects, but there is no support for efficacy from controlled clinical trials [28]. Trials of tyrosine (amino acid precursor of L-DOPA) and tryptophan (amino acid precursor of serotonin) (1 gram of each daily), L-tryptophan coupled with contingency management treatment, L-carnitine (500 mg/d) plus coenzyme Q10 (200 mg/d), and magnesium L-aspartate (732 mg daily), an easily absorbed form of magnesium, found them no better than placebo in reducing cocaine craving or use.

One herbal product that has received substantial publicity, but not yet rigorous clinical evaluation, is ibogaine, an indole alkaloid found in the root bark of the West African shrub *Tabernanthe iboga*. This compound maintained cocaine abstinence for a median of 8 months in 70% of 66 patients with moderate-severe substance use disorder (83% cocaine) after abstinence was initiated in a residential treatment program [86]. However, clinical research with ibogaine has been suspended in the USA because of the risk of life-threatening cardiac arrhythmia [45]. *Ginkgo biloba* (120 mg/d for 8 weeks) was no better than placebo in a controlled clinical trial [40].

13.3.13 Other Physical Treatments

Acupuncture is an ancient Chinese treatment that involves mechanical (with needles), thermal (moxibustion), or electrical (electroacupuncture) stimulation of specific points on the body surface. The mechanism of action is unknown; speculation has included stimulation of endogenous opioid systems. Meta-analyses of nine published studies did not find a significant benefit of active acupuncture over sham treatment [20, 60].

Transcranial magnetic stimulation (TMS) involves activation of brain neurons by fluctuating magnetic fields generated by electromagnetic coils placed on the scalp. Single and multiple sessions of repetitive TMS (rTMS) applied to the prefrontal cortex reduced cocaine craving and reduced cocaine use in a small, open-label pilot study [3]. Controlled clinical trials are currently underway.

13.4 Special Treatment Situations

13.4.1 Mixed Addictions

Concurrent opioid use, including comorbid substance use disorder, is a common clinical problem among individuals with cocaine use disorder. Some individuals use cocaine and opioids simultaneously (as in the so-called speedball) to enhance the drugs' subjective effects. Up to 20% or more of patients with opioid use disorder in methadone maintenance treatment also use cocaine [50]. Three different pharmacologic approaches have been used for the treatment of dual cocaine and opioid use disorders: (1) adjustment of methadone dose, (2) maintenance with another opioid medication, and (3) addition of medication targeting the cocaine use disorder.

Higher daily methadone doses (60 mg or more) generally are associated with less opioid use by patients in methadone maintenance. This relationship also holds in general for cocaine use among patients in methadone maintenance [75], although exceptions have been reported. Increasing the methadone dose as a contingency in response to cocaine use can be effective in reducing such use (and more so than decreasing the methadone dose).

Buprenorphine is a partial opioid agonist (μ-receptor agonist/κ-receptor antagonist) used for the agonist substitution treatment of opioid dependence [58]. Some (but not all) studies in patients with concurrent opioid and cocaine use disorders suggest that cocaine use (as well as opioid use) is reduced at higher buprenorphine doses (16–32 mg sl daily) [65].

Non-opioid medications for the treatment of cocaine use disorder frequently are evaluated in methadone- or buprenorphine-maintained outpatients with concomitant opioid use disorder because the opioid agonist maintenance component substantially enhances treatment adherence, improving the internal validity of the trial. There is no evidence that such agonist maintenance treatment significantly influences medication efficacy, but no studies have directly addressed this issue.

Alcohol use disorder is a common problem among individuals with cocaine use disorder, both in the community and in treatment settings, with rates of comorbidity as high as 90% [24]. Two medications used in the treatment of alcohol use disorder are also effective in the treatment of outpatients with concurrent cocaine and alcohol use disorders. Disulfiram substantially decreased both cocaine and alcohol use in two clinical trials and a small case series, but not in a third clinical trial [28]. Naltrexone, a μ-opioid receptor antagonist approved for the treatment of both alcohol and opioid use disorders, substantially decreased both cocaine and alcohol use at 150 mg po daily, but not at 50 mg daily or 100 mg daily or when given as a monthly long-acting injection [79]. Combined treatment with both disulfiram (250 mg daily) and naltrexone (100 mg daily) significantly improved abstinence from cocaine and alcohol [77].

A controlled clinical trial found no significant effect of topiramate compared to placebo in reducing cocaine or alcohol use in outpatients with comorbid cocaine and alcohol use disorders [42].

13.4.2 Psychiatric Comorbidity

Treatment-seeking individuals with cocaine use disorder have high rates of psychiatric diagnoses other than substance use disorder, with rates as high as 65% for lifetime disorders and 50% for current disorders. The commonest comorbid disorders tend to be major depression, bipolar spectrum, phobias, and post-traumatic stress disorder [12]. Personality disorders are also common, with rates as high as 69%. The commonest is antisocial personality disorder [11].

Antidepressants vary in their efficacy for reducing cocaine use among patients with comorbid major depression, although there are few direct comparisons or controlled clinical trials [71, 83]. Desipramine, imipramine, and bupropion have usually, but not always, been found effective, whereas SSRIs and mirtazapine are usually not effective. Venlafaxine (150–300 mg daily) and nefazodone (200 mg twice daily) showed some efficacy in small clinical trials [28].

Both anticonvulsant "mood stabilizers" and antipsychotics are used to treat comorbid bipolar disorder and cocaine use disorder. Case series and small clinical trials suggest that anticonvulsants such as valproate and lamotrigine and antipsychotics such as quetiapine and risperidone have some efficacy in reducing cocaine use in dually diagnosed patients [10]. Combining lithium with an anticonvulsant may be helpful in treatment-resistant patients.

Up to one-fourth of adults with cocaine use disorder have either adult attention-deficit hyperactivity disorder (ADHD) or a history of childhood ADHD [46]. Stimulant and dopaminergic medications are the mainstay of treatment for ADHD, suggesting that some of these patients may be self-medicating their ADHD with cocaine. Case series and clinical trials generally find that such medications successfully treat ADHD symptoms and reduce cocaine use in adults: dextroamphetamine, methamphetamine, extended-release mixed amphetamine salts, and bupropion, but not methylphenidate and bupropion [28].

Schizophrenia is not a common comorbid psychiatric disorder among patients in treatment for cocaine use disorder (about 1% prevalence) [51], but cocaine use disorder is commoner among treatment-seeking patients with schizophrenia (8–10% prevalence) [85]. Clinical experience suggests that first-generation antipsychotics, at doses that are effective in the treatment of schizophrenia, do not significantly alter cocaine craving or use.

Several case series and open-label trials suggest that the second-generation antipsychotics, including clozapine, olanzapine, quetiapine, risperidone, and aripiprazole, may be more effective than older (first-generation) antipsychotics in reducing cocaine and other drug use among patients with schizophrenia [84]. However, three head-to-head controlled clinical trials found no difference between olanzapine and haloperidol or risperidone in reducing cocaine use, with each medication reducing cocaine craving in one of the trials [28].

The use of cocaine can exacerbate or provoke antipsychotic-induced movement disorders [17, 34] and increase vulnerability to the neuroleptic malignant syndrome [1].

13.4.3 Medical Comorbidity

Few data are available to guide the pharmacotherapy of cocaine use disorder in medically ill patients, making this an important issue for future clinical research. Prudent clinical practice requires a careful medical evaluation of any patient before starting medication, with special attention to medical conditions common in individuals with cocaine use disorder. Such conditions would include viral hepatitis and alcoholic liver disease, which might alter the metabolism of prescribed medications, and HIV infection. The presence of the latter necessitates caution in prescribing medications with a known potential for inhibiting immune function. Clinical experience suggests that buprenorphine [5] and bupropion can be used safely in HIV-positive patients, although antiretroviral medications may decrease bupropion plasma concentrations [35].

13.4.4 Gender-Specific Issues

Women tend to be excluded from or underrepresented in many clinical trials of cocaine use disorder pharmacotherapy [30], in part because of concern over risk to the fetus and neonate should a female subject become pregnant. Thus, there is a substantial lack of information about gender-specific issues of pharmacotherapy in general and the pharmacotherapy of cocaine use disorder in particular [33]. Meanwhile, clinicians must deal on an *ad hoc* basis with the treatment implications of possible gender differences in medication pharmacokinetics (such as those resulting from differences in body mass and composition) and in pharmacodynamics (such as those related to the menstrual cycle or exogenous hormones such as oral contraceptives).

In the absence of directly relevant and systematically collected data, caution should be used when prescribing medications to pregnant women with cocaine use disorder and to those with pregnancy potential, keeping in mind both the risks of medication and the risks of continued cocaine use. Some medications proposed for the treatment of cocaine use disorder (such as tricyclic antidepressants, bupropion, and buprenorphine) have little potential for morphologic teratogenicity or disruption of pregnancy, although there are few or no data on behavioral teratogenicity [28]. Some medications do pose at least slight risk, such as amantadine (associated with pregnancy complications), lithium (associated with cardiac malformations and neonatal toxicity), anticonvulsants (associated with increased risk of congenital malformations), and antipsychotics (associated with nonspecific congenital anomalies and neonatal withdrawal).

Some medications (e.g., disulfiram, naltrexone) may generate different treatment responses in men versus women [7, 78]. The reasons for such gender differences are poorly understood but may include differences in medication pharmacokinetics, hormonal interactions, or subjects' psychological or socioeconomic status.

13.4.5 Age

Although adolescents make up a substantial minority of heavy cocaine users, they have been largely excluded from clinical trials of cocaine pharmacotherapies because of legal and informed consent considerations. On the basis of the scarcity of published case reports, it is likely that medication is not often used in the treatment of adolescent cocaine use disorder.

Similarly, we are not aware of any published studies on the pharmacological treatment of cocaine use disorder in elderly patients.

13.5 International Perspectives

The prevalence of cocaine use varies substantially by geographic region, based in part on the relative availability of cocaine [96]. In addition, national differences in modes of cocaine use result in variation in cocaine use disorder and related problems. The acute psychological effects of cocaine, and therefore its abuse liability, depend greatly on the rate at which drug reaches the brain. The more rapid the onset of the effect, the more intense the psychological effect [69]. This is the so-called rate hypothesis of psychoactive drug effect [26]. Routes of administration that produce rapid onset of effect, such as intravenous and smoked, are associated with greater abuse liability than those with slower onset, such as intranasal and oral [9, 25]. Thus, the Andean countries in which oral cocaine ingestion is legal and common (e.g., by chewing the leaves, drinking coca tea) tend to have lower prevalence of cocaine use disorder than might be expected from their prevalence of cocaine use [64].

Treatment of cocaine addiction is generally comparable worldwide, with the exception of the Andean countries. The legal availability of oral forms of cocaine in those countries makes possible the agonist substitution approach using cocaine itself [37, 53]. However, such treatment has never been evaluated in controlled clinical trials.

13.6 Future Prospects

Future progress in pharmacologic treatment for cocaine use disorder is likely to come from development of new medications with novel or more selective mechanisms of action and from development of pharmacokinetic approaches and new physical treatments such as TMS (see Sect. 13.3.13 above). New medications should evolve from an improved understanding of the neuropharmacology of cocaine use disorder and animal studies of the interactions of cocaine with novel compounds.

Preclinical studies with compounds that bind to the same presynaptic dopamine transporter site as does cocaine (thereby keeping cocaine from acting), but which do not themselves produce robust reinforcing effects (because of slow onset of effect and tight, long-lasting binding), suggest that such compounds may be useful as functional cocaine "antagonists" [82]. Manipulation of brain dopamine activity with selective dopamine

receptor ligands, especially for the D_3 type, attenuated the rewarding effects of cocaine in several animal studies [32] and awaits the development of compounds suitable for clinical trials. Medications that presynaptically release both dopamine and serotonin also show promise in animal studies [81].

Cocaine administration, like stress, activates the hypothalamic-pituitary-adrenal (HPA) axis, and stress may play a role in relapse to cocaine use after abstinence. These observations stimulated interest in corticotrophin-releasing factor receptor antagonists, some of which reduce cocaine self-administration in animals [94].

The endogenous cannabinoid (endocannabinoid) brain neurotransmitter system modulates the dopaminergic reward system [74], and blockade of cannabinoid CB_1 receptors inhibits relapse to cocaine self-administration after abstinence in animals [99]. Therefore, CB_1 receptor antagonists (or inverse agonists) and cannabinoids such as cannabidiol (which does not produce a subjective "high") [19] have promising therapeutic potential. The failure of existing medications to show consistent efficacy in the treatment of cocaine use disorder has prompted growing interest in pharmacokinetic approaches, that is, preventing ingested cocaine from entering the brain and/or enhancing its elimination from the body [27]. The former approach could be implemented by active or passive immunization to generate binding antibodies that keep cocaine from crossing the blood-brain barrier. The latter approach could be implemented by administration of an enzyme (e.g., butyrylcholinesterase [BChE]) that catalyzes cocaine hydrolysis or by passive or active immunization with a catalytic antibody. A 12-week controlled clinical trial found that weekly intramuscular injections of a mutated BChE with enhanced catalytic efficiency significantly increased the proportion of cocaine-negative urine samples (14.6% vs. 4.7%), although there was no significant difference in the proportion of participants achieving abstinence [23]. In a phase II controlled clinical trial, an anti-cocaine vaccine (i.e., active immunization to generate cocaine-binding antibodies) significantly reduced cocaine use among the one-third of participants who mounted a substantial antibody response, but only during the first 8 weeks of treatment [49]. Further work is needed to increase the consistency of the antibody response and lengthen the duration that antibody concentrations remain high enough to block cocaine use.

13.7 Conclusion

The absence of any medication that meets national regulatory standards for efficacy and safety leaves physicians with little clear-cut guidance for pharmacologic treatment of cocaine use disorder. Among existing medications marketed for other indications, none has yet shown consistent efficacy in replicated controlled clinical trials. Disulfiram appears the most promising, especially for patients with comorbid alcohol use disorder. Tricyclic antidepressants such as desipramine and imipramine (but not SSRIs) may be of use in patients with mild cocaine use disorder or with comorbid depression. The anticonvulsant topiramate has shown promise in controlled clinical trials and warrants further evaluation. The stimulant maintenance approach also warrants further evaluation using medications with low abuse potential (e.g., sustained-release amphetamine) or perhaps even a slow-onset (e.g., oral or transdermal) form of cocaine itself.

More sophisticated patient-treatment matching could enhance the efficacy of current medications by taking into account both patient characteristics that can influence treatment response (e.g., severity, withdrawal status, psychiatric comorbidity, or concomitant medications) and characteristics of the psychosocial treatment accompanying the medication. For example, a few studies suggest that some medications (e.g., L-DOPA, SSRIs) that are not effective when used with drug abuse counseling or cognitive-behavioral therapy may be effective when combined with contingency management treatment [63, 89].

Improved understanding of the neurobiology of cocaine use disorder should lead to new and more effective medications in the future, possibly by manipulation of the glutamate or endocannabinoid systems or HPA axis or by a pharmacokinetic mechanism. Regardless of which medications show promise in the future, their adoption into clinical practice should be guided by acceptable scientific proof of efficacy and safety, based on data from replicated, well-designed, adequately powered controlled clinical trials. Clinicians should also keep in mind the distinctions between efficacy (treatment works in a research setting in a selected research population getting close attention) and effectiveness (treatment works in a heterogeneous population in a realistic clinical environment) and between a statistically significant and clinically meaningful treatment effect [59].

Acknowledgments Dr. Gorelick receives royalties from UpToDate for writing articles about cocaine.

References

1. Akpaffiong MJ, Ruiz P. Neuroleptic malignant syndrome: a complication of neuroleptics and cocaine abuse. Psychiatry Q. 1991;62:299–309.
2. Baldacara L, Cogo-Moreira H, Parreira BL, et al. Efficacy of topiramate in the treatment of crack cocaine dependence: a double-blind, randomized, placebo-controlled trial. J Clin Psychiatry. 2016;77:398–406.
3. Balloni C, Badas P, Corona G, et al. Transcranial magnetic stimulation for the treatment of cocaine addiction: evidence to date. Subst Abuse Rehabil. 2018;9:11–21.
4. Brown RM, Kupchik YM, Kalivas PW. The story of glutamate in drug addiction and of N-acetylcysteine as a potential pharmacotherapy. JAMA Psychiat. 2013;70:895–7.
5. Carrieri MP, Vlahov D, Dellamonica P, et al. Use of buprenorphine in HIV-infected injection drug users: negligible impact on virologic response to HAART. The Manif-2000 Study Group. Drug Alcohol Depend. 2000;60:51–4.
6. Carroll KM, Rounsaville BJ. A perfect platform: combining contingency management with medications for drug abuse. Am J Drug Alcohol Abuse. 2007;33:343–65.
7. Carroll KM, Nich C, Shi JM, et al. Efficacy of disulfiram and Twelve Step Facilitation in cocaine-dependent individuals maintained on methadone: a randomized placebo-controlled trial. Drug Alcohol Depend. 2012;126:224–31.

8. Castells X, Cunill R, Pérez-Mañá C, et al. Psychostimulant drugs for cocaine dependence. Cochrane Database Syst Rev. 2016;9:CD007380.

9. Chen C-Y, Anthony JC. Epidemiological estimates of risk n the process of becoming dependent upon cocaine: cocaine hydrochloride powder versus crack cocaine. Psychopharmacologia. 2004;172:78–86.

10. Coles AS, Sadiadek J, George TP. Pharmacotherapies for co-occurring substance use disorder and bipolar disorders: a systematic review. Bipolar Disord. 2019;21:595.

11. Compton WM, Conway KP, Stinson FS, Colliver JD, Grant BF. Prevalence, correlates, and comorbidity of DSM-IV antisocial personality syndromes and alcohol and specific drug use disorders in the United States: results from the National Epidemiologic Survey on Alcohol and Related Conditions. J Clin Psychiatry. 2005;66:677–85.

12. Conway KP, Compton W, Stinson FS, Grant BF. Lifetime comorbidity of DSM-IV mood and anxiety disorders and specific drug use disorders: results from the National Epidemiologic Survey on Alcohol and Related Conditions. J Clin Psychiatry. 2006;67:247–57.

13. Degenhardt L, Singleton J, Calabria B, McLaren J, Kerr T, Mehta S, Kirk G, Hall WD. Mortality among cocaine users: a systematic review of cohort studies. Drug Alcohol Depend. 2011;113:88–95.

14. Degenhardt L, Hall WD. Extent of illicit drug use and dependence, and their contribution to the global burden of disease. Lancet. 2012;379:55–70.

15. DeVito EE, Babuscio TA, Nich C, et al. Gender differences in clinical outcomes for cocaine dependence: randomized clinical trials of behavioral therapy and disulfiram. Drug Alcohol Depend. 2014;145:156–67.

16. Dieckmann LH, Ramos AC, Silva EA, et al. Effects of biperiden on the treatment of cocaine/crack addiction: a randomised, double-blind, placebo-controlled trial. Eur Neuropsychopharmacol. 2014;24:1196–202.

17. Duggal HS. Cocaine use as a risk factor for ziprasidone-induced acute dystonia. Gen Hosp Psychiatry. 2007;29:278–9.

18. Fischer B, Blanken P, Da Silveira D, et al. Effectiveness of secondary prevention and treatment interventions for crack-cocaine abuse: a comprehensive narrative overview of English-language studies. Int J Drug Policy. 2015a;26:352–63.

19. Fischer B, Kuganesan S, Gallassi A, et al. Addressing the stimulant treatment gap: a call to investigate the therapeutic potential of cannabinoids for crack-cocaine use. Int J Drug Policy. 2015b;26:1177–82.

20. Gates S, Smith LA, Foxcroft DR. Auricular acupuncture for cocaine dependence. Cochrane Database Syst Rev. 2006;(1):CD005192.

21. Gaval-Cruz M, Weinshenker D. Mechanisms of disulfiram-induced cocaine abstinence: Antabuse and cocaine relapse. Mol Interv. 2009;9:175–87.

22. Ghitza UE, Preston KL, Epstein DH, et al. Brain mu-opioid receptor binding predicts treatment outcome in cocaine-abusing outpatients. Biol Psychiatry. 2010;68:697–703.

23. Gilgun-Sherki Y, Eliaz RE, McCann DJ, et al. Placebo-controlled evaluation of a bioengineered, cocaine-metabolizing fusion protein, TV-1380 (AlbuBChE), in the treatment of cocaine dependence. Drug Alcohol Depend. 2016;166:13–20.

24. Gorelick DA. Alcohol and cocaine: clinical and pharmacological interactions. Recent Dev Alcohol. 1992a;11:37–56.

25. Gorelick DA. Progression of dependence in male cocaine addicts. Am J Drug Alcohol Abuse. 1992b;18:13–9.

26. Gorelick DA. The rate hypothesis and agonist substitution approaches to cocaine abuse treatment. Adv Pharmacol. 1998;42:995–7.

27. Gorelick DA. Pharmacokinetic strategies for treatment of drug overdose and addiction. Future Med Chem. 2012;4:227–43.

28. Gorelick DA. Pharmacological treatment of stimulant use disorders. In: Miller SC, Fiellin DA, Rosenthal RN, Saitz R, editors. Principles of addiction medicine. 6th ed. Philadelphia: Wolters Kluwer; 2019. p. 847–62.

29. Gorelick DA, Baumann MH. The pharmacology of stimulants. In: Miller SC, Fiellin DA, Rosenthal RN, Saitz R, editors. Principles of addiction medicine. 6th ed. Philadelphia: Wolters Kluwer; 2019. p. 150–75.

30. Gorelick DA, Montoya ID, Johnson EO. Sociodemographic representation in published studies of cocaine abuse pharmacotherapy. Drug Alcohol Depend. 1998;49:89–93.

31. Grassi MC, Cioce AM, Guidici FD, et al. Short-term efficacy of disulfiram or naltrexone in reducing positive urinalysis for both cocaine and cocaethylene in cocaine abusers: a pilot study. Pharmacol Res. 2007;55:117–21.

32. Heidbreder CA, Newman AH. Current perspectives on selective dopamine D_3 receptor antagonists as pharmacotherapies for addictions and related disorders. Ann N Y Acad Sci. 2010;1187:4–34.

33. Helmbrecht GD, Thiagarajah S. Management of addiction disorders in pregnancy. J Addict Med. 2008;2(1):1–16.

34. Henderson JB, Labbate L, Worley M. A case of acute dystonia after single dose of aripiprazole in a man with cocaine dependence. Am J Addict. 2007;16:244.

35. Hogeland GW, Swindells S, McNabb JC, et al. Lopinavir/ritonavir reduces bupropion plasma concentrations in healthy subjects. Clin Pharmacol Ther. 2007;81:69–75.

36. Howell LL, Kimmel HL. Monoamine transporters and psychostimulant addiction. Biochem Pharmacol. 2008;75:196–217.

37. Hurtado-Gumucio J. Coca leaf chewing as therapy for cocaine maintenance. Ann Med Interne. 2000;151(Suppl B):B44–8.

38. Indave BI, Minozzi S, Pani PP, et al. Antipsychotic medications for cocaine dependence. Cochrane Database Syst Rev. 2016;(3):CD006306.

39. Johnson BA, Roache JD, Daoud N, et al. A preliminary randomized, double-blind, placebo-controlled study of the safety and efficacy of ondansetron in

the treatment of cocaine dependence. Drug Alcohol Depend. 2006;84:256–63.

40. Kampman KM, Majewska MD, Tourian K, et al. A pilot trial of piracetam and ginkgo biloba for the treatment of cocaine dependence. Addict Behav. 2003;28:437–48.

41. Kampman KM, Dackis C, Lynch KG, et al. A double-blind, placebo-controlled trial of amantadine, propranolol, and their combination for the treatment of cocaine dependence in patients with severe cocaine withdrawal. Drug Alcohol Depend. 2006;85:129–37.

42. Kampman KM, Pettinati HM, Lynch KG, et al. A double-blind, placebo-controlled trial of topiramate for the treatment of comorbid cocaine and alcohol dependence. Drug Alcohol Depend. 2013;133:94–9.

43. Khalsa ME, Gawin FH, Rawson R, et al. A desipramine ceiling in cocaine abusers. Problems of drug dependence, 1992 (NIDA research monograph 132). National Institute on Drug Abuse: Rockville; 1993. p. 18.

44. Knapp WP, Soares BG, Farrel M, Lima MS. Psychosocial interventions for cocaine and psychostimulant amphetamines related disorders. Cochrane Database Syst Rev. 2011;(3):CD003023.

45. Koenig X, Hilber K. The anti-addiction drug ibogaine and the heart: a delicate balance. Molecules. 2015;20:2208–28.

46. Kollins SH. A qualitative review of issues arising in the use of psychostimulant medications in patients with ADHD and co-morbid substance use disorders. Curr Med Res Opin. 2008;24:1345–57.

47. Kosten T, Oliveto A, Feingold A, et al. Desipramine and contingency management for cocaine and opioid dependence in buprenorphine maintained patients. Drug Alcohol Depend. 2003;70:315–25.

48. Kosten TR, Wu G, Huang W, et al. Pharmacogenetic randomized trial for cocaine abuse: disulfiram and dopamine-β-hydroxylase. Biol Psychiatry. 2013;73:219–24.

49. Kossten TR, Domingo CB, Shorter D, et al. Vaccine for cocaine dependence: a randomized double-blind placebo-controlled efficacy trial. Drug Alcohol Depend. 2014;140:42–7.

50. Leri F, Bruneau J, Stewart J. Understanding polydrug use: review of heroin and cocaine co-use. Addiction. 2003;98:7–22.

51. Libuy N, de Angel V, Ibanez C, et al. The relative prevalence of schizophrenia among cannabis and cocaine users attending addiction services. Schizophr Res. 2018;194:13–7.

52. Ling W, Hillhouse MP, Saxon AJ, et al. Buprenorphine + naloxone plus naltrexone for the treatment of cocaine dependence: the Cocaine Use Reduction with Buprenorphine (CURB) study. Addiction. 2016;111:1416–27.

53. Llosa T. Smoking coca paste and crack-tobacco must be treated as double addiction. Subst Abus. 2009;30:81.

54. Lozano R, Naghavi M, Foreman K, et al. Global and regional mortality from 235 causes of death for 20 age groups in 1990 and 2010: a systematic analysis for the Global Burden of Disease Study 2010. Lancet. 2012;380:2095–128.

55. Malcolm RM, Moore JA, Brady KT, et al. Pergolide/haloperidol for the treatment of cocaine dependence. College on Problems of Drug Dependence 1999. Rockville: National Institute on Drug Abuse; 1999. p. 165.

56. Malcolm R, Olive MF, Lechner W. The safety of disulfiram for the treatment of alcohol and cocaine dependence in randomized clinical trials: guidance for clinical practice. Expert Opin Drug Saf. 2008;7:459–72.

57. Mariani JJ, Pavlicova M, Bisaga A, et al. Extended-release mixed amphetamine salts and topiramate for cocaine dependence: a randomized controlled trial. Biol Psychiatry. 2012;72:950–6.

58. Mattick RP, Breen C, Kimber J, et al. Buprenorphine maintenance versus placebo or methadone maintenance for opioid dependence. Cochrane Database Syst Rev. 2014;(2):CD002207.

59. Miller WR, Manuel JK. How large must a treatment effect be before it matters to practitioners? An estimation method and demonstration. Drug Alcohol Rev. 2008;27:524–8.

60. Mills EJ, Wu P, Gagnier J, Ebbert JO. Efficacy of acupuncture for cocaine dependence: a systematic review & meta-analysis. Harm Reduct J. 2005;2:4.

61. Minozzi S, Amato L, Pani PP, et al. Dopamine agonists for the treatment of cocaine dependence. Cochrane Database Syst Rev. 2015;(5):CD003352.

62. Minozzi S, Cinquini M, Amato L, et al. Anticonvulsants for cocaine dependence. Cochrane Database Syst Rev. 2015;(4):CD006754.

63. Moeller FG, Schmitz JM, Steinberg JL, et al. Citalopram combined with behavioral therapy reduces cocaine use: a double-blind, placebo-controlled trial. Am J Drug Alcohol Abuse. 2007;33:367–78.

64. Montoya ID, Chilcoat HD. Epidemiology of coca derivatives use in the Andean Region: a tale of five countries. Subst Use Misuse. 1996;31:1227–40.

65. Montoya ID, Gorelick DA, Preston KL, et al. Randomized trial of buprenorphine for treatment of concurrent opiate and cocaine dependence. Clin Pharmacol Ther. 2004;75:34–48.

66. Moran LM, Phillips KA, Kowalczyk WJ, et al. Aripiprazole for cocaine abstinence: a randomized-controlled trial with ecological momentary assessment. Behav Pharmacol. 2017;28:63–73.

67. Murray CJL, Vos T, Lozano R, et al. Disability-adjusted life years (DALYs) for 291 diseases and injuries in 21 regions, 1990–2010: a systematic analysis for the Global Burden of Disease Study 2010. Lancet. 2012;380:2197–223.

68. Nelson RA, Gorelick DA, Keenan RM, et al. Cardiovascular interactions of desipramine, fluoxetine, and cocaine in cocaine-dependent outpatients. Am J Addict. 1996;5:321–6.

69. Nelson RA, Boyd SJ, Ziegelstein RC, et al. Effect of rate of administration on subjective and physiological effects of intravenous cocaine in humans. Drug Alcohol Depend. 2006;82:19–24.

70. Nuijten M, Blanken P, van de Wetering B, et al. Sustained-release dexamfetamine in the treatment of chronic cocaine-dependent patients on heroin-assisted treatment: a randomised, double-blind, placebo-controlled trial. Lancet. 2016;2387:2226–34.

71. Nunes EV, Levin FR. Treatment of depression in patients with alcohol or other drug dependence: a meta-analysis. JAMA. 2004;291:1887–96.

72. Pani PP, Trogu E, Vacca R, et al. Disulfiram for the treatment of cocaine dependence. Cochrane Database Syst Rev. 2010;(1):CD007024.

73. Pani PP, Trogu E, Vecchi S, Amato L. Antidepressants for cocaine dependence and problematic cocaine use. Cochrane Database Syst Rev. 2011;(12):CD002950.

74. Parolaro D, Rubino T. The role of the endogenous cannabinoid system in drug addiction. Drug News Perspect. 2008;21:149–57.

75. Peles E, Kreek MJ, Kellogg S, Adelson M. High methadone dose significantly reduces cocaine use in methadone maintenance treatment (MMT) patients. J Addict Dis. 2006;25:43–50.

76. Penberthy JK, Ait-Daoud N, Vaughan M, Fanning T. Review of treatment for cocaine dependence. Curr Drug Abuse Rev. 2010;3:49–62.

77. Pettinati HM, Kampman KM, Lynch KG, et al. A double blind, placebo-controlled trial that combines disulfiram and naltrexone for treating co-occurring cocaine and alcohol dependence. Addict Behav. 2008a;33:651–67.

78. Pettinati HM, Kampman KM, Lynch KG, et al. Gender differences with high-dose naltrexone in patients with co-occurring cocaine and alcohol dependence. J Subst Abuse Treat. 2008b;34:378–90.

79. Pettinati HM, Kampman KM, Lynch KG, et al. A pilot trial of injectable, extended-release naltrexone for the treatment of co-occurring cocaine and alcohol dependence. Am J Addict. 2014;23:591–7.

80. Plebani JG, Lynch KG, Yu Q, et al. Results of an initial clinical trial of varenicline for the treatment of cocaine dependence. Drug Alcohol Depend. 2012;121:163–6.

81. Rothman RB, Blough BE, Baumann MH. Dual dopamine/serotonin releasers as potential medications for stimulant and alcohol addictions. AAPS J. 2007;9:E1–E10.

82. Rothman RB, Baumann MH, Prisinzano TE, Newman AH. Dopamine transport inhibitors based on GBR12909 and benztropine as potential medications to treat cocaine addiction. Biochem Pharmacol. 2008;75:2–16.

83. Rounsaville BJ. Treatment of cocaine dependence and depression. Biol Psychiatry. 2004;56:803–9.

84. San L, Arranz B, Martinez-Raga J. Antipsychotic drug treatment of schizophrenic patients with substance abuse disorders. Eur Addict Res. 2007;13:230–43.

85. Sara GE, Large MM, Matheson SL, et al. Stimulant use disorders in people with psychosis: a meta-analysis of rate and factors affecting variation. Australia NZ J Psychiatry. 2015;49:106–17.

86. Schenberg EE, de Castro Comis MA, Chaves BR, et al. Treating drug dependence with the aid of ibogaine: a retrospective study. J Psychopharmacol. 2014;28:993–1000.

87. Schierenberg A, van Amsterdam J, van den Brink W, Goudriaan AE. Efficacy of contingency management for cocaine dependence treatment: a review of the evidence. Curr Drug Abuse Rev. 2012;5:320–31.

88. Schmitz JM, Stotts AL, Rhoades HM, et al. Naltrexone and relapse prevention treatment for cocaine-dependent patients. Addict Behav. 2001;26:167–80.

89. Schmitz JM, Mooney ME, Moeller FG, et al. Levodopa pharmacotherapy for cocaine dependence: choosing the optimal behavioral therapy platform. Drug Alcohol Depend. 2008;94:142–50.

90. Schmitz JM, Green CE, Stotts AL, et al. A two-phased screening paradigm for evaluating candidate medications for cocaine cessation or relapse prevention: modafinil, levodopa-carbidopa, naltrexone. Drug Alcohol Depend. 2014;136:100–7.

91. Shorter D, Nielsen DA, Huang W, et al. Pharmacogenetic randomized trial for cocaine abuse: disulfiram and α_{1A}-adrenoreceptor gene variation. Eur Neuropsychopharmacol. 2013a;23:1401–7.

92. Shorter D, Lindsay JA, Kosten TR. The alpha-1 adrenergic antagonist doxazosin for treatment of cocaine dependence: a pilot study. Drug Alcohol Depend. 2013b;131:66–70.

93. Singh M, Keer D, Klimas J, et al. Topiramate for cocaine dependence: a systematic review and meta-analysis of randomized controlled trials. Addiction. 2016;111:1337–46.

94. Specio SE, Wee S, O'Dell LE, et al. CRF(1) receptor antagonists attenuate escalated cocaine self-administration in rats. Psychopharmacology (Berl). 2008;196:473–82.

95. Spellicy CJ, Kosten TR, Hamon SC, et al. ANKK1 and DRD2 pharmacogenetics of disulfiram treatment for cocaine abuse. Pharmacogenet Genomics. 2013;23:333–40.

96. United Nations Office on Drugs and Crime. World drug report 2016. United Nations publication E.16.XI.7. Vienna: United Nations Office on Drugs and Crime; 2016.

97. Vos T, Flaxman AD, Naghavi M, et al. Years lived with disability (YLDs) for 1160 sequelae of 289 diseases and injuries 1990–2010: a systematic analysis for the Global Burden of Disease Study 2010. Lancet. 2012;380:2163–96.

98. Winstanley EL, et al. A randomized controlled trial of fluoxetine in the treatment of cocaine dependence among methadone-maintained patients. J Subst Abuse Treat. 2011;40:255–64.

99. Wiskerke J, Pattij T, Schoffelmeer ANM, De Vries TJ. The role of CB1 receptors in psychostimulant addiction. Addict Biol. 2008;13:225–38.

Pharmacotherapy of Addiction to Amphetamine-Type Stimulants

14

Ahmed Elkashef and Jag H. Khalsa

Contents

Abstract

Amphetamine-like stimulants (ATS) use is second to marijuana as the most widely used illicit substances worldwide with an estimated 59 million people using these at least once a year. Their use is associated with significant morbidity including cardiovascular complications, psychosis, and mortality. A wide range of modalities including psychotherapeutic and pharmacologic interventions are available for the treatment of dependence to amphetamine-type stimulants. Although many clinical trials are currently in progress for treating addiction to ATS, there is no FDA-approved medication for the indication. In the meantime, it is highly recommended that the available treatment should be started early and should be comprehensive, integrated, and long term.

Keywords

Amphetamine · Methamphetamine · Treatment · Medication

A. Elkashef · J. H. Khalsa (✉)
Division of Therapeutics and Medical Consequences,
National Institute on Drug Abuse, National Institutes
of Health, Bethesda, Maryland, USA

14.1   Introduction

Amphetamine-like stimulants (ATS) include a group of other synthetic stimulants like amphetamine, methamphetamine, 3,4-methylenedioxym ethamphetamine (MDMA), and related

© Springer Nature Switzerland AG 2021
N. el-Guebaly et al. (eds.), *Textbook of Addiction Treatment*,
https://doi.org/10.1007/978-3-030-36391-8_14

substances. These are highly addictive, and their chronic use may result in a series of mental and physical symptoms including anxiety, confusion, insomnia, mood disturbances, cognitive impairments, paranoia, hallucinations, and delusion. Though there is no specific FDA-approved drug to treat addiction to any of the amphetamines, there are behavioral and other pharmacotherapeutic modalities and agents that have used to treat ATS dependence. Currently, according to the 2017 World Drug Report [57], amphetamine-type stimulants use is second only to marijuana as the most widely used illicit substance worldwide. In 2015, an estimated 59 million people, aged 15–64 years, used amphetamines, prescription amphetamines, and 3,4-methylenedioxymethama phetamine (MDMA, ecstasy) at least once in the last year. Regions with highest prevalence are Oceania and North and Central America. Increases in seizure of methamphetamine are also being reported in East, Southeast, and Central Asia and Transcaucasia [57]. Incidentally, in the USA, in 2016, there were 20,203 methamphetamine-associated ER admissions [46]; and between 2003 and 2015, there were 1,292,300 weighted amphetamine-related hospitalizations with annual hospital costs increasing from $436 million in 2003 to $2.17 billion by 2015 [60].

14.2 Pharmacology

Methamphetamine and amphetamine have very similar pharmacodynamic effects; either can be metabolized to the other [2, 21, 43]. METH was first synthesized in the late 1800s by a Japanese pharmacologist [9], while amphetamine was originally synthesized by the German chemist Lazăr Edeleanu in 1887. Both were used during war to reduce fatigue and were available over the counter in Japan as *Philopon* and *Sedrin*.

Both amphetamine and methamphetamine are highly addictive stimulants that can be easily manufactured in clandestine labs. Common street names vary from country to country, e.g., "speed," "meth," "ice," "crystal," "crank," "glass," "Yaba," and "Ceptagon" just to name few.

ATS are potent dopamine uptake as well as vesicular monoamine transporter (VMAT2) blockers. The latter action is unique to ATS and not shared by other addictive stimulants like cocaine. VMAT2 blockers inhibit the incorporation of synthesized monoamines into the neuronal vesicles which lead to high concentrations of dopamine and other amines in the presynaptic terminal. This leads to higher levels of dopamine release which can cause oxidative stress and damage to the presynaptic terminals.

14.3 Health Consequences

Amphetamine and methamphetamine are approved in the USA and other countries worldwide for the treatment of attention deficit hyperactivity disorder, narcolepsy, and obesity. The weak isomer L-methamphetamine is used in the over the counter Vicks inhaler. ATS are powerful stimulants, with short-term effects that include euphoria, alertness, wakefulness, increased energy, and loss of appetite. Methamphetamine use is significantly associated with cardiovascular and cerebrovascular events [25]; some of the cardiovascular effects include irregular heartbeat, increased heart rate and blood pressure, aortic dissection, acute coronary syndrome, pulmonary arterial hypertension, and methamphetamine-associated cardiomyopathy [40]. Hyperthermia, convulsions, and stroke have also been reported with ATS overdose and can result in death if not treated.

Long-term ATS abuse can lead to weight loss, paranoia, chronic sleep disturbance, addiction, dependence, and psychosis almost indistinguishable from schizophrenia. Other psychiatric symptoms may include chronic anxiety, confusion, insomnia, mood disturbances, and violent behavior. PET studies have shown significant changes in striatal dopamine in chronic methamphetamine users in the form of downregulation or degeneration; these changes were associated with cognitive impairment. Some of the effects of chronic methamphetamine abuse appear to be, at least partially, reversible. A recent neuroimaging study showed recovery in some brain regions following prolonged abstinence (2 years, but not 6 months). This was associated with improved performance on motor and verbal memory tests. However, function in other brain regions did not display recovery even after 2 years of abstinence, indicating that some methamphetamine-induced changes are long-lasting [59]. Withdrawal symptoms have been reported in patients attempting to stop or entering treatment and include depression, anxiety, fatigue, and an increased craving for the drug. Other serious long-term effect of methamphetamine is tooth decay known as "meth mouth" [39].

Injection drug use and risky sexual behavior among methamphetamine users have been associated with increase in HIV, especially among men who have sex with men (MSMs) [54]. Methamphetamine abuse may also worsen the progression of HIV and its consequences including greater neuronal injury and cognitive impairment compared with nondrug abusers [33, 41].

Prenatal exposure to methamphetamine can lead to premature delivery, placental abruption, fetal growth retardation, and heart and brain abnormalities [14, 15, 30, 48, 61]. Ongoing research is continuing to study developmental outcomes such as cognition, social relationships, motor skills, and medical status of children exposed to methamphetamine before birth. However, the use of other substances or alcohol and maternal poor nutrition and health make the interpretation of these results difficult.

14.3.1 Treatment of Addiction to ATS

The treatment of addiction to amphetamines can be challenging because of the changes in brain structure that occur with chronic use of amphetamines. Research has shown that the treatment of ATS addiction, as any other addiction, should by integrated, comprehensive, individualized, and long term. Psychotherapeutic interventions like contingency management, cognitive behavioral therapy, relapse prevention, matrix, and 12-step-based therapy, which have shown effectiveness in the treatment of other addictions, have also shown efficacy in treating ATS addictions. These are detailed elsewhere in this book. Combining medications and psychotherapy like CM has been shown to have synergistic effect and should be the rule in any treatment plan depending on the treatment setting. Early intervention will also guarantee better outcomes as most addictions

start in adolescence. To guarantee best care, treatment should be integrated to address the multiple comorbid mental and physical problems that ATS addicts usually suffer.

In this chapter we will focus on pharmacological interventions that have been tried so far in the treatment of addiction to ATS.

14.3.2 Agonist Medications

Methylphenidate A dopaminergic stimulant approved for the treatment of ADHD was tried in methamphetamine dependence. An initial report of efficacy of SR methylphenidate (54 mg) against placebo and aripiprazole for intravenous amphetamine dependence in a 20-week randomized trial was not replicated in the larger double-blind study of 79 patients [56, 35].

Dextroamphetamine Another dopaminergic stimulant approved for weight loss, narcolepsy, and ADHD was tried in two double-blind studies in meth-dependent patients. The first trial used 110 mg of sustained release d-amphetamine daily for 12 weeks with gradual reduction over an additional 4 weeks. Medications were administered daily under supervision. The primary outcome was meth concentration in hair samples at baseline compared to follow-up using hair analysis. Although there was no significant effect for the primary outcomes, there was significantly greater reduction in meth withdrawal symptoms and craving compared to placebo [32]. Another double-blind study [19] of 60 mg sustained release d-amphetamine for 8 weeks showed no effect for the primary outcome of reducing meth use as evidenced by negative urines. Similar to the first study, this study also reported significant effect on craving and meth withdrawal symptoms for the d-amphetamine group.

Bupropion The safety of co-administering bupropion and methamphetamine was assessed in a clinical pharmacology study with no evidence of cardiovascular adverse events of PK interaction [38]. Three double-blind controlled outpatient studies investigated the effects of bupropion SR 150 mg BID in methamphetamine-dependent patients. Significantly a positive effect in reducing meth use was reported in light users. The effect was not seen in heavy users defined as >18 days of use in a month or more than two positive urine samples per week on screening [18, 53]. Another study [24] did not report an effect for bupropion as measured by abstinence in the last 2 weeks of the trial; however the group that showed compliance with medication as measured by plasma showed a significant effect highlighting the very important issue of medication adherence as a factor in many failed addiction medication trials.

Modafinil Modafinil is a weak stimulant approved for the treatment of narcolepsy and obstructive sleep apnea. It is proposed to exert its action on the glutamate and hypocretin system. However, recent PET study suggests that it may also bind to the dopamine transporter. Clinical trials in cocaine suggest that it may have a role in treating addiction to other stimulants [39–41]. Modafinil at a dose of 200 mg/day was tested in a double-blind, placebo-controlled trial for 10 weeks in 80 methamphetamine-dependent patients. The trial outcomes were negative except for a trend of reducing methamphetamine use in those who were medication compliant and attended counseling sessions [49]. In another single-blind study, modafinil combined with cognitive behavioral therapy (CBT) was tested in 13 HIV+ gay men with methamphetamine dependence. Six of the 10 patients completed the study with reduction of their methamphetamine use by over 50% [34]. In a more recent multisite trial [1, 23], 71 methamphetamine-dependent treatment seeking patients were randomized to placebo or 400 mg of daily modafinil for 12 weeks. The primary outcome was weeks of negative methamphetamine in their urine. The patients provided three urine samples weekly. The trial was negative; however, a post hoc analysis showed a significant effect on duration of abstinence (23 days vs. 10 days) favoring modafinil among compliant patients.

A recent meta-analysis of the use of prescription amphetamines for the treatment of stimulant use disorders (SUD) reported that prescription psychostimulants increased the rates of sustained abstinence in SUD, specifically for cocaine use disorders ([55], CPDD 2019, poster presentation).

14.3.3 Antagonist Medications

Aripiprazole A partial agonist second-generation antipsychotic was studied in two human laboratory studies with significant effects on attenuation of subjective effects of orally administered d-amphetamine [50]. However, outpatient studies with aripiprazole have been negative. One double-blind randomized study of 15 mg daily had to be stopped prematurely because of high dropout rate and increased amphetamine use [56]. Another double-blind study of aripiprazole in 90 patients for 12 weeks failed to show significant results [10].

14.3.4 Other Medications

GABA agonists Baclofen 60 mg and gabapentin 2400 mg daily were tried in a double-blind study of 25 meth-dependent patients in a 3-arm study for 16 weeks. Neither medication had an effect on reducing meth use compared to placebo. A post hoc analysis suggests a positive effect in patients who took higher doses of baclofen [22]. Topiramate interaction with meth and effect on its subjective effects were studied in a human lab double-blind study which showed that topiramate enhanced some of the positive effects of methamphetamine. This was attributed to possible PK interaction on meth metabolism [27]. A multisite outpatient trial of topiramate 200 mg for reducing meth use was negative for the primary outcome. However, there was a positive effect in the subgroup of patients that had negative urines at randomization suggesting a role in relapse prevention [17]. Vigabatrin was tried in an open-label study of 30 patients for 9 weeks. 18/30 subjects completed the study, and 16/18 tested negative for methamphetamine and cocaine during the last 6 weeks of the trial [8]. A safety clinical pharmacology interaction study was conducted in nontreatment-seeking methamphetamine-dependent patients given 15 and 30 mg i.v. doses of methamphetamine and doses of GVG up to 5 mg [13]. There were no reports of cardiovascular interactions and no effects of GVG on methamphetamine subjective effects. No published reports currently exist of follow-up outpatient trials of GVG for the treatment of addition to methamphetamine.

Antidepressants Mirtazapine was tried in a double-blind controlled study in 60 methamphetamine-dependent patients for 12 weeks with significant effect in reducing methamphetamine-positive urines [11]. The SSRIs, fluoxetine, paroxetine, and sertraline were tried in double-blind controlled studies [3, 4, 42, 44, 52] with no effect on methamphetamine use.

Calcium channel blockers Two calcium channel blockers, isradipine and amlodipine, were tried in human laboratory studies [26, 6] and reported to reduce the subjective and physiological responses to methamphetamine. However, a controlled outpatient clinical trial of amlodipine failed to show any efficacy in reducing methamphetamine use [5].

Ondansetron A serotonin 5-HT3 receptor antagonist was postulated to reduce dopaminergic activity in the striatum. A double-blind multisite, randomized, trial of three doses of ondansetron (0.25, 1, or 4 mg twice daily) for 8 weeks combined with CBT failed to show an effect over placebo at decreasing methamphetamine use [28].

Naltrexone Naltrexone moderates the predictive relationship between cue-induced craving and positive subjective effects of methamphetamine [45], 49]. In a preliminary randomized clinical trial, using functional MRI, naltrexone significantly reduced methamphetamine use and striatal resting-state functional connectivity between the ventral striatum, amygdala, hippocampus, and midbrain in people with methamphetamine use disorder [29]. In a human lab study of abstinent meth-dependent patients, naltrexone 50 mg significantly reduced the subjective effects of d-amphetamine. In a double-blind placebo-controlled outpatient study, naltrexone 50 mg was effective in reducing amphetamine use [31].

Rivastigmine Acetyl cholinesterase inhibitors have been shown in animal studies to reduce methamphetamine-seeking behavior. Rivastigmine was tried in a 2-week double-blind placebo-controlled human laboratory study, to study its interactions with methamphetamine 30 mg given i.v. Rivastigmine reduced the cardiovascular and subjective effects of methamphetamine. The 3 mg dosage significantly reduced methamphetamine-induced increases in diastolic blood pressure and self-reports of craving and anxiety. In another controlled study, the same dosage reduced the positive subjective effects of intravenous meth self-administered in human volunteers [12]. Outpatient trials are underway to test its efficacy in reducing meth use.

Varenicline In a double-blind randomized phase II clinical trial, varenicline at 1 mg, bid, combined with cognitive behavioral therapy, was ineffective in treating methamphetamine dependence in methamphetamine-dependent subjects [7].

Combination therapy (1) Midazolam-droperidol combination versus droperidol alone or midazolam-droperidol versus olanzapine was tested in a multicenter, randomized, double-blind, controlled, clinical trial in 92 methamphetamine-affected subjects. The primary outcome was the proportion of patients sedated adequately at 10 min. Results showed that a midazolam-droperidol combination provided more rapid sedation of patients with methamphetamine-related acute agitation than droperidol or olanzapine alone [58]. (2) Another combination therapy with naltrexone and N-acetyl-cysteine failed to show a significant effect on methamphetamine use in methamphetamine users [20]. (3) Two combinations trails of naltrexone and bupropion are published; the first is a human lab study [51] of 50 mg naltrexone and 300 mg of bupropion alone and in combination that failed to show an effect for the combination in reducing subjective effects of methamphetamine. An outpatient study of depot naltrexone monthly injection and 300 mg of bupropion SR daily showed a higher response in the medication group vs. placebo as defined by at least 6 negative urine tests out of 8 collected in the last 4 weeks of the trial [36].

14.4 Future Medication Options

VMAT2-inhibitors are being developed as methamphetamine antagonists to block its action on the VMAT receptors. Lobeline, a nicotinic alkaloid, has been shown in animal studies to decrease self-administration of methamphetamine and block meth-induced dopamine release [16, 37]. Tetrabenazine, another VMAT2 inhibitor recently approved in the USA for the treatment of Huntington's disease and other hyperkinetic disorders, is being studied in animal models of addiction. Research is also ongoing for more selective VMAT2 compounds.

CRF-1 antagonists have been shown in preclinical data to block stress-induced relapse to alcohol, cocaine, and heroin. The search for a safe CRF-1 antagonist to advance to clinical trials is underway.

D3 antagonists have been shown to block priming, cues, and stress-induced self-administration of nicotine, cocaine, and heroin, suggesting a role in relapse prevention in humans.

Cannabinoid-1 (CB-1) receptor antagonists have been reported to reduce or block self-administration and conditioned cue relapses in preclinical models of THC, nicotine, cocaine, MA, opiates, and ethanol.

Other compounds of interest are group I and group II metabotropic glutamate receptors.

mGluR5 antagonists and AMPA receptor antagonists have been shown to block cue-induced relapse to cocaine and heroin.

The CRF-1antagonists, dopamine D3receptor antagonists, cannabinoid CB1 antagonists, and glutamate site modulators, data in animal models of addiction, show nonselectivity. Further development of these compounds in man will have far-reaching application in treating substance use disorders particularly polysubstance use.

Cognitive enhancers like D-1agonists, 5-HT 6 antagonists, and D-cycloserine may have a role in strengthening the frontal lobe's inhibitory controls on impulsive behavior. They are also expected to improve cognition in methamphetamine-addicted patients.

Other area of therapeutic development for addiction is *immunotherapy*. Vaccines and monoclonal antibodies are in early development for nicotine, cocaine, methamphetamine, and heroin, details of which are highlighted in another chapter.

Global impact ATS is a global public health problem with severe comorbidities and economic burdens that are in the billions of dollars. The global trends of use seem unchanged since the last decade according to the WHO drug reports. This is indicative of ineffective, inefficient, or insufficient application of prevention and treatment approaches across the globe. It is time for an international task force on the issue lead by the WHO, involving all countries affected. Effective approaches need to be shared across countries, e.g., contingency management coupled with medications, with consideration of unique and cultural issues for each. Programs like training the trainers and cross-training are vital for proper application of treatment programs especially ones that focus on vulnerable populations, e.g., adolescents and pregnant women. The cost of implementing such a global intervention should be figured out and shared among the members if they are serious about tackling the problem. Programs that proved successful in other areas of addiction, e.g., screening, brief intervention, and referral to treatment (SBIRT) and drug courts, should be adapted to ATS.

14.5   In Summary

- ATS addiction ranks second to cannabis globally and contributes greatly to the total burden of the disease of addiction.
- ATS addiction is associated with multiple health problems like HIV and psychiatric diseases like psychosis.
- ATS addiction treatment like other addiction treatment should be started early and should be comprehensive, integrated, and long term.
- Psychotherapeutic interventions like CM, MI, CBT, matrix, RP, and 12 steps are equally effective for the treatment of ATS addiction and should be utilized as appropriate.
- Agonist medications like d-amphetamine and methylphenidate may have a role in treating ATS withdrawal symptoms and craving, particularly in patients with comorbid ADHD/ADD.
- Other medications that may be helpful are bupropion and modafinil for low to moderate users.
- Naltrexone and topiramate are also promising especially for ATS addicts who are also addicted to other substances like nicotine, alcohol, or opiates.
- There are many trials that are currently in progress for treating addiction to ATS. It is highly recommended that clinicians search the literature periodically for updates prior to initiating medication treatment for their patients.

References

1. Anderson AL, Li SH, et al. Modafinil for the treatment of methamphetamine dependence. Drug Alcohol Depend. 2011;120:135.
2. Anglin MD, et al. History of the methamphetamine problem. J Psychoactive Drugs. 2000;32(2):137–41.
3. Batki SL, Moon J, et al. Methamphetamine dependence. A controlled trial: a preliminary analysis. In: CPDD 61st Annual Scientific Meeting. Acapulco; 1999. p. 235.
4. Batki SL, Moon J, et al. Methamphetamine quantitative urine concentrations during a controlled trial of fluoxetine treatment. Preliminary analysis. Ann N Y Acad Sci. 2000;909:260–3.
5. Batki SL, Moon J, et al. Amlodipine treatment of methamphetamine dependence, a controlled out-patient trial: preliminary analysis. Drug Alcohol Depend. 2001;63(Suppl. 1):12.
6. Batki SL, Bui L, et al. Methamphetamine-amlodipine interactions: preliminary analysis (abstract). Drug Alcohol Depend. 2002;66:S12.
7. Briones M, Shoptaw S, Cooke R, et al. Varenicline treatment for methamphetamine dependence: a randomized, double-blind phase II clinical trial. Drug Alcohol Depend. 2018;189:30–6.
8. Brodie JD, Figueroa E, et al. Safety and efficacy of gamma-vinyl GABA(GVG) for the treatment of methamphetamine and/or cocaine addiction. Synapse. 2005;55(2):122–5.
9. Cho AK, Segal DS. Amphetamine and its analogs: psychopharmacology, toxicology, and abuse. 1st ed. San Diego: Academic Press; 1994.
10. Coffin PO, Santos GM, et al. Aripiprazole for the treatment of methamphetamine dependence: a randomized, double-blind, placebo-controlled trial. Addiction. 2012;108:751. https://doi.org/10.1111/add.12073.
11. Colfax GN, Santos GM, et al. Mirtazapine to reduce methamphetamine use: a randomized clinical trial. Arch Gen Psychiatry. 2011;68(11):1168–75.
12. De La Garza R, Maohoney JJ, et al. The acetylcholinesterase inhibitor rivastigmine does not alter total choices for methamphetamine, but may reduce positive subjective effects, in a laboratory model of intravenous self-administration in human volunteers. Pharmacol Biochem Behav. 2008;89:200–8.
13. De La Garza IIR, Zorick T, et al. The cardiovascular and subjective effects of methamphetamine combined with γ-vinyl-γ-aminobutyric acid (GVG) in non-treatment seeking methamphetamine-dependent volunteers. Pharmacol Biochem Behav. 2009;94(1):186–93.
14. Diaz SD, Smith LM, LaGasse LL, et al. Effects of prenatal methamphetamine exposure on behavioral and cognitive findings at 7.5 years of age. J Pediatr. 2014;164(6):1333–8.
15. Dinger J, Hinner P, Reichert J, Rüdiger M. Methamphetamine consumption during pregnancy - effects on child health. Pharmacopsychiatry. 2017;50(3):107–13.
16. Dwoskin LP, Crooks PA, et al. A novel mechanism of action and potential use for lobeline as a treatment for psychostimulant abuse. Biochem Pharmacol. 2002;63:89–98.
17. Elkashef A, Kahn R, et al. Topiramate for the treatment of methamphetamine addiction: a multi-center placebo-controlled trial. Addiction. 2012;107(7):1297–306.
18. Elkashef AM, Rawson RA, et al. Bupropion for the treatment of methamphetamine dependence. Neuropsychopharmacology. 2008;33:1162–70.
19. Galloway GO, Buscemi R, et al. A randomized, placebo-controlled trial of sustained-release dextroamphetamine for treatment of methamphetamine addiction. Clin Pharmacol Ther. 2011;89(2):276–82.

20. Grant JE, Odlaug BL, Kim SW. A double-blind, placebo-controlled study of N-acetyl cysteine plus naltrexone for methamphetamine dependence. Eur Neuropsychopharmacol. 2010;20(11):823–8.
21. Haile CN. Neurochemical and neurobehavioral consequences of methamphetamine abuse. In: Karch SB, editor. Drug abuse handbook. 2nd ed. Boca Raton: CRC Press; 2007. p. 478–503.
22. Heinzerling KG, Shoplaw S, et al. Randomized, placebo-controlled trial of baclofen and gabapentin for the treatment of methamphetamine dependence. Drug Alcohol Depend. 2006;85:177–84.
23. Heinzerling KG, Swanson AN, et al. Randomized, double-blind, placebo-controlled trial of modafinil for the treatment of methamphetamine. Drug Alcohol Depend. 2010;109(1–3):20–9.
24. Heinzerling KG, Swanson AN, et al. Randomized, double-blind, placebo-controlled trial of bupropion in methamphetamine-dependent patients with less than daily methamphetamine use. Addiction. 2014;109(11):1878–86.
25. Huang MC, Yang SY, Lin SK, Chen KY, et al. Risk of cardiovascular disease and stroke events in methamphetamine users: a 10-year follow-up study. J Clin Psychiatry. 2016;77(10):1396–403.
26. Johnson B, Roache J, et al. Isradipine, a dihydropyridine-class calcium channel antagonist, attenuates some of d-methamphetamine's positive subjective effects: a preliminary study. Psychopharmacology. 1999;144:295–300.
27. Johnson BA, Roache JD, et al. Effects of acute topiramate dosing on methamphetamine induced subjective mood. Int J Neuropsychopharmacol. 2007;10: 85–98.
28. Johnson BA, Ait-Daoud N, et al. A preliminary randomized double-blind, placebo-controlled study of the safety and efficacy of ondansetron in the treatment of methamphetamine dependence. Int J Neuropsychopharmacol. 2008;11:1–14.
29. Kohno M, Dennis LE, McCready H, Schwartz DL, et al. A preliminary randomized clinical trial of naltrexone reduces striatal resting state functional connectivity in people with methamphetamine use disorder. Drug Alcohol Depend. 2018;192:186–92.
30. Kwiatkowski MA, Roos A, Stein DJ, et al. Effects of prenatal methamphetamine exposure: a review of cognitive and neuroimaging studies. Metab Brain Dis. 2014;29(2):245–54.
31. Lindstrom NJ, Konstenius M, et al. Naltrexone attenuates the subjective effects of amphetamine in patients with amphetamine dependence. Neuropyschopharmacology. 2008;33:1856–63.
32. Longo M, Wickes W, et al. Randomized controlled trial of dexamphetamine maintenance for the treatment of methamphetamine dependence. Addiction. 2010;105(1):146–54.
33. Mediouni S, Marcondes MC, Miller C, et al. The cross-talk of HIV-1 Tat and methamphetamine in HIV-associated neurocognitive disorders. Front Microbiol. 2015;6(1164):1–24.
34. McElhiney MC, Rabkin JG, et al. Provigil (modafinil) plus cognitive behavioral therapy for methamphetamine use in HIV+ gay men: a pilot study. Am J Drug Alcohol Abuse. 2009;35(1):34–7.
35. Miles SW, Sheridan J, et al. Extended release methylphenidate for treatment of amphetamine/methamphetamine dependence: a randomized, double blind, placebo controlled trial. Addiction. 2013;108:1279. https://doi.org/10.1111/add.12109.
36. Mooney LJ, Hillhouse MP, Thomas C, et al. Utilizing a two-stage design to investigate the safety and potential efficacy of monthly naltrexone plus once-daily bupropion as a treatment for methamphetamine use disorder. Addiction. 2016;10(4):236–43.
37. Neugebauer NM, Harrod SB, et al. Lobeline decreases methamphetamine self-administration in rats. Eur J Pharmacol. 2007;571:33–8.
38. Newton TF, Roche JD, et al. Safety of intravenous methamphetamine administration during treatment with bupropion. Psychopharmacology. 2005;182:426–35.
39. Pabst A, Castillo-Duque JC, Mayer A, et al. Meth mouth-a growing epidemic in dentistry? Dent J (Basel). 2017;5(4):E29. https://doi.org/10.3390/dj5040029.
40. Paratz ED, Cunningham NJ, MacIsaac AI. The cardiac complications of methamphetamine. Heart Lung Circ. 2016;25(4):325–32.
41. Passaro RC, Pandhare J, Qian HZ, Dash C. The complex interaction between methamphetamine abuse and HIV-1 pathogenesis. J Neuroimmune Pharmacol. 2015;10(3):477–86.
42. Piasecki MP, Steinagel GM, et al. An exploratory study: the use of paroxetine for methamphetamine cravings. J Psychoactive Drugs. 2002;34:301–4.
43. Rasmussen N. America's first amphetamine epidemic 1929-1971: a quantitative and qualitative retrospective with implications for the present. Am J Public Health. 2008;98(6):974–85.
44. Rawson RA, Marinelli-Casey P, et al. A multi-site comparison of psychosocial approaches for the treatment of methamphetamine dependence. Addiction. 2004;99:708–14.
45. Ray LA, Bujarski S, Courtney KE, Moallem NR, et al. The effects of naltrexone on subjective response to methamphetamine in a clinical sample: a double-blind, placebo-controlled laboratory study. Neuropsychopharmacology. 2015;40(10):2347–56.
46. Richards JR, Hamidi S, Grant CD, Wang CG, et al. Methamphetamine use and emergency department utilization: 20 years later. J Addict. 2017;2017:4050932. https://doi.org/10.1155/2017/4050932. Epub 17 Aug 2017.
47. Roche DJ, Worley MJ, Courtney KE, et al. Naltrexone moderates the relationship between cue-induced craving and subjective response to methamphetamine in individuals with methamphetamine use disorder. Phychopharmacology (Berl). 2017;234(13):1997–2007.

48. Roos A, Jones G, Howells FM, et al. Structural brain changes in prenatal methamphetamine-exposed children. Metab Brain Dis. 2014;29(2):341–9.
49. Shearer J, Darke S, et al. A double-blind, placebo-controlled trial of modafinil 200mg/day for methamphetamine dependence. Addiction. 2009;104(2):224–33.
50. Stoops WW, Lile JA, Glaser PE, et al. A low dose of aripiprazole attenuates the subject-rated effects of d-amphetamine. Exp Clin Psychopharmacol. 2006;14:413–21.
51. Stoops WW, Pike E, Hays LR, et al. Naltrexone and bupropion, alone or combined, do not alter the reinforcing effects of intranasal methamphetamine. Pharmacol Biochem Behav. 2015;129:45–50.
52. Shoptaw S, Huber A, Peck J, et al. Randomized, placebo-controlled trial of sertraline and contingency management for the treatment of methamphetamine dependence. Drug Alcohol Depend. 2006;85:12–8.
53. Shoptaw S, Heinzerling KG, Rotheram-Fuller E, et al. Randomized, placebo-controlled trial of bupropion for the treatment of methamphetamine dependence. Drug Alcohol Depend. 2008;96:222–32.
54. Shoptaw S, Reback CJ. Methamphetamine use and infectious disease-related behaviors in men who have sex with men: implications for interventions. Addiction. 2007;102(Suppl 1):130–5.
55. Tardelli VS, Lago MPPD, Mendez M, Bisaga A et al. Contingency management with pharmacologic treatment for stimulant use disorder: A review. Behav Res Ther 2018;111:57–63.
56. Tiihonen J, Kuoppasalmi K, et al. A comparison of aripiprazole, methylphenidate and placebo for amphetamine dependence. Am J Psychiatry. 2007;164:160–2.
57. United Nations Office on Drugs and Crime. World drug report 2017 (ISBN: 978-92-1-148291-1, eISBN: 978-92-1-060623-3, United Nations publication, Sales No. E.17.XI.6).
58. Yap CY, Taylor DM, Knott JC, et al. Intravenous midazolam-droperidol combination, droperidol or olanzapine monotherapy for methamphetamine-related agitation: subgroup analysis of a randomized controlled trial. Addiction. 2017;112(7):1262–9.
59. Wang GJ, Volkow ND, Chang L, et al. Partial recovery of brain metabolism in methamphetamine abusers after protracted abstinence. Am J Psychiatry. 2004;161(2):242–8.
60. Winkelman TNA, Admon LK, Jennings L, et al. Evaluation of amphetamine-related hospitalizations and associated clinical outcomes and costs in the United States. JAMA Netw Open. 2018;1(6):e183758. https://doi.org/10.1001/jamanetworkopen.2018.3758.
61. Wright TE, Schuetter R, Tellei J, Sauvage L. Methamphetamines and pregnancy outcomes. J Addict Med. 2015;9(2):111–7.

Nicotine and Tobacco

15

Julia Sasiadek, Nicole Durham, and Tony P. George

Contents

Abstract

Although rates of tobacco use and tobacco use disorder have reduced substantially over the past 40 years, one in (six) Americans continue to smoke. The prevalence of smoking appears to be substantially higher in persons with psychiatric and substance use disorders and has remained unchanged, as these smokers have less success in quitting smoking. The epidemiology of tobacco use disorder and the pharmacological effects of nicotine and tobacco are reviewed followed by a discussion of the clinical assessment of tobacco users. The increasingly popular electronic cigarette will be examined as a possible form of treatment for tobacco use disorder. We then review psychosocial and pharmacological treatments, including the FDA-approved pharmacotherapies:

J. Sasiadek · N. Durham
Addictions Division, Centre for Addiction and Mental Health (CAMH), Toronto, ON, Canada

T. P. George (✉)
Addictions Division, Centre for Addiction and Mental Health (CAMH), Toronto, ON, Canada

Department of Psychiatry, University of Toronto, Toronto, ON, Canada
e-mail: tony.george@camh.ca

© Springer Nature Switzerland AG 2021
N. el-Guebaly et al. (eds.), *Textbook of Addiction Treatment*,
https://doi.org/10.1007/978-3-030-36391-8_15

nicotine replacement therapies (NRTs), sustained-release bupropion, and varenicline. Finally, integration of tobacco use disorder treatment into mental health settings is discussed with the view that tobacco use disorder is a chronic medical disorder and that more effective treatment of this comorbidity in psychiatric disorders may require targeted treatments based on a better understanding of the pathophysiology of individual psychiatric disorders.

15.1 Introduction: Epidemiology of Tobacco Use

Tobacco smoking is the leading preventable cause of morbidity and mortality in the Western world [5]. In the USA, approximately 14% of the population are currently tobacco users, which translates to roughly 34 million people. Worldwide, approximately 1.1 billion people use tobacco on a regular basis [17]. Around 33% of those who try cigarettes will become addicted, and 70% of those people will go on to want to quit completely. Most smokers who begin smoking in adolescence have difficulty quitting, with almost 2% of current 12th graders using cigarettes daily and, increasingly, 20% of 12th graders vaping nicotine [48, 81]. Since the release of the Surgeon General's report in 1965, however, smoking prevalence has been steadily declining, but this reduction appears to have slowed in recent years. Cigarette smoking remains the most common (>90%) method of tobacco use. In addition to cigarette smoking, pipe tobacco, cigars, hookah, and smokeless tobacco (e.g., chewing tobacco, snuff) are also common forms of tobacco use. Each year, approximately 480,000 people in the USA die as a result of smoking-attributable medical illnesses such as lung cancer, chronic obstructive pulmonary disease (COPD), cardiovascular disease, and stroke, including 41,000 people dying as a result of secondhand smoke. Additionally, roughly eight million people are sick or disabled because of their cigarette use, and smoking has been estimated to cost the USA $170 billion in smoking-related medical expenses, as well as $156 billion in lost

productivity annually [5]. Smoking is now increasing rapidly throughout the developing world, and it is estimated that current cigarette smoking will cause about 450 million deaths worldwide in the next 50 years. Reducing current smoking by 50% would prevent 20–30 million premature deaths in the first quarter of this century and 150 million in the second quarter. For most smokers, quitting is the single most important thing they can do to improve their health, and the results of epidemiological studies in Norway suggest that even with sustained reductions (>50%) in smoking consumption, there is little if any reduction in cardiovascular disease and lung or other smoking-related cancer risk [79]. However, reducing the amount of cigarettes smoked for individuals who have no intention to quit smoking did increase the probability of a quit attempt [41]. Although reductions in smoking consumption may not reduce risks of morbidity in the short term, it will more likely lead to self-quitting in the future.

15.2 Biology of Nicotinic Receptors

Nicotine is the main psychoactive ingredient in tobacco smoke. When tobacco is smoked, the primary site of action of nicotine is the $\alpha4\beta2$ nicotinic acetylcholine receptor (nAChR), which is also activated by the endogenous neurotransmitter acetylcholine. nAChRs in the CNS are pentameric ion channel complexes [11] comprised of two α and three β subunits. The seven α subunits are designated $\alpha2–\alpha9$ and the three β subunits are designated $\beta2–\beta4$. Due to this, there is considerable diversity in subunit combinations, which may explain some of the region-specific and functional selectivity of nicotinic effects throughout the CNS. These pentameric receptors are either homomerically or heteromerically arranged (e.g., $(\alpha4)_3(\beta2)_2$ or $(\alpha7)_5$). Activation of nAChRs leads to Na^+/Ca^{2+} ion channel fluxes and neuronal firing, and chronic exposure to nicotine results in desensitization of the receptors. nAChRs are situated presynaptically on several different neurotransmitter secreting neuron types due to their wide dispersement throughout the CNS. Of importance for nicotine addiction are the nAChRs situated on mesolimbic dopamine (DA) neurons that project from the ventral tegmental area (VTA) to the nucleus accumbens (NAc). Activation of nAChRs on mesolimbic DA neurons leads to DA release in the NAc, which helps to facilitate the addictive process involved in chronic tobacco use.

At low concentrations of nicotine, $\alpha4\beta2$ nAChR stimulation of afferent GABAergic projections onto mesoaccumbal DA neurons predominates, leading to reduced mesolimbic DA neuron firing and DA release. At higher nicotine concentrations, $\alpha4\beta2$ nAChRs desensitize, and activation of $\alpha7$ nAChRs on glutamatergic projections predominates, leading to increased mesolimbic DA neuron firing and DA secretion. Subsequently, nAChRs desensitize within several millisecond of activation by nicotine; nAChRs then resensitize after overnight abstinence, which presumably explains why most smokers report that the first cigarette in the morning is the most satisfying. Interestingly, the nAChR saturation levels reached after smoking to satiety are similar to the saturation levels seen after smoking just a few puffs. Therefore, while binding to central nAChRs is an important first step in the effects of nicotine, it is not a complete explanation for continued smoking behaviors.

15.3 Clinical Effects of Nicotine and Tobacco

The majority of tobacco users (>90%) smoke cigarettes. Most of these individuals smoke daily and have some degree of physiological dependence [60]. However, smoking patterns have lowered in recent years, and non-daily smokers now constitute 14% of all adult smokers in the USA [5]. While these non-daily smokers seem dependence-resistant, they still show the same difficulty with quitting as daily smokers do [77]. Smokers typically describe a "rush" and feelings of alertness and relaxation when smoking, and it is well known that nicotine has both stimulating and anxiolytic effects depending on basal level of arousal. Stimulation of the airway is an aspect of smoking that many individuals will report as reinforcing, and additives such as menthol

enhance the experience by increasing the taste and reducing the harshness of smoked tobacco. A diagnosis of tobacco use disorder is accomplished clinically by following the criteria outlined in the *Diagnostic and Statistical Manual of Mental Disorders 5* (DSM-5). These include increased tobacco use for longer periods of time, tobacco cravings, evidence of tolerance (e.g., increased amounts of tobacco needed to achieve the desired effect), and the presence of symptoms of tobacco withdrawal upon smoking cessation. Withdrawal symptoms, which begin within 24 hours of cessation, peak at 2–3 days, and usually subside within 2–3 weeks, include irritability, anxiety, decreased heart rate, insomnia, increased appetite, difficulty concentrating, and restlessness. Additionally, most dependent smokers state that they smoke their first cigarette of the day within 30 minutes of awakening, smoke daily, and increase their use of cigarettes per day. Timeline follow-back procedures [71] and smoking diaries have been used successfully to monitor smoking consumption over time. Scales such as the Fagerstrom Test for Nicotine Dependence (FTND) [28] allow assessment of the level of nicotine dependence with scores of ≥4 on a scale of 0–10 consistent with physiological dependence to nicotine. Nicotine craving and withdrawal can be reliably monitored using validated scales such as the Tiffany Questionnaire for Smoking Urges [76] and the Minnesota Nicotine Withdrawal Scale [31].

Besides positive reinforcement, withdrawal, and craving, there are several secondary effects of nicotine and tobacco use that may contribute to both maintenance of smoking and to smoking relapse including mood modulation (e.g., reduction of negative affect), stress reduction, and weight control. In addition, conditioned cues can elicit the urge to smoke even after prolonged periods of abstinence [2]. Specific effects might be most relevant to individuals high on dietary restraint (weight reduction) and psychiatric disorders (mood modulation, cognitive enhancement, stress reduction). These secondary effects may present additional targets for pharmacological intervention in certain subgroups of smokers (e.g., smokers with schizophrenia, depression, or obesity; [17]).

15.4 Electronic Cigarettes

Electronic nicotine delivery systems (ENDS), also known as e-cigarettes, are an alternative and increasingly common method of consuming nicotine. From 2010 to 2013, e-cigarette use in the adult population has drastically risen from approximately 1.8% to 13.0% in the USA [50]. The rise of electronic cigarettes has also been increasingly popular specifically among the adolescent population. In fact, data from the National Youth Tobacco Survey reported that the number of high-school children reporting use of e-cigarettes rose from 11.7% to 20.8% and 3.3% to 4.9% in middle-school children between 2017 and 2018. This increase in children was likely a result of peer pressure, high impulsivity, and interest in the device as a nicotine delivery system. Individuals with mental disorders and particularly substance use disorders are another subpopulation with twice the prevalence rate compared to those without mental health conditions [10, 46, 57].

Unlike traditional cigarettes, e-cigarettes contain no tobacco and do not require a flame. E-cigarettes contain a cartridge that houses the liquid (e-liquid), a heating element, and a battery. The liquid is a solution comprised of additives such as propylene glycol or glycerol, nicotine, flavoring, distilled water, etc. A lithium battery that powers the e-cigarette is connected to a vaporization chamber which is a tube containing electronic controls and an atomizer. When the e-liquid solution is rapidly heated and then cooled, it vaporizes into an aerosol mist that allows for inhalation or "vaping" of the liquid through a mouthpiece. Inhalation activates the atomizer to heat the liquid in the cartridge, converting the liquid to vapor, delivering nicotine to the lungs. Simple inhalation or manual initiation of a switch/button can activate the vaporizer inside [16].

There are approximately 460 brands sold in the market with a variety of e-liquid flavors, concentrations of nicotine (ranging from 0 to 24 mg/mL to max of 36 mg/mL), and pH levels. The typical concentration of e-cigarettes is 18 mg/mL, which is higher in comparison to the traditional cigarette (6–13 mg). However, the concentration levels of nicotine that is delivered to the bloodstream is still lower in comparison to the tobacco-smoked cigarette. E-cigarettes are also being used for other purposes. For example, cannabis, a popular substance choice, has been vaporized due to its decreased amount of smoke and odor. However, cannabis consumption via e-cigarette poses a risk since THC levels can exceed combustion mechanisms by 4- to 30-fold [52].

Despite risk factors associated with their use, e-cigarettes have also been suggested to be beneficial. Advocates welcome e-cigarettes as a gateway to smoking cessation or reduction of tobacco use [90]. Nicotine in an aerosol contains fewer tobacco toxicants compared to tobacco smoke and are thus considered less harmful and a less addictive alternative to tobacco cigarettes [12]. E-cigarettes have become the topic of a public health dispute as their popularity increased. The most significant barrier to e-cigarette regulation is the current lack of experimental evidence regarding their use. Although the evidence is limited and contested, some studies suggest that the majority of e-cigarette users treat them as cessation aides and report that they have been key to quitting smoking. For example, e-cigarettes compared favorably to nicotine replacement therapies (NRTs) in terms of the likelihood of having returned to smoking 6 months after a cessation attempt and have been perceived to be more efficacious than NRTs overall [12, 16, 69].

15.5 Psychosocial Treatments (See Table 15.1)

Several non-pharmacological interventions for smoking cessation are available. These include telephone quit lines, group and individual counseling, and self-help techniques ranging from the community to the individual domain. Behavioral treatments for tobacco use disorder can facilitate motivation to quit, provide an emphasis on the social and contextual aspects of smoking, and enhance overall success at smoking cessation [55]. Six-month quit rates with behavior thera-

Table 15.1 Pharmacological and behavioral treatments for tobacco use disorder

Treatment (*FDA-approved)	Mechanism of action	Rating
*Nicotine replacement therapies**		
Gum (OTC)	Slow nicotine absorption gradually reduces nicotine craving and withdrawal	1
Transdermal nicotine patch (OTC)	Slow nicotine absorption gradually reduces nicotine craving and withdrawal	1
Lozenge (OTC)	Slow nicotine absorption gradually reduces nicotine craving and withdrawal	1
Vapor inhaler (prescription)	Fast nicotine absorption leads to stimulation of nAChR which rapidly reduces nicotine craving and withdrawal	1
Nasal spray (prescription)	Fast nicotine absorption leads to stimulation of nAChR which reduces craving and withdrawal	1
Non-nicotine pharmacotherapies		
Bupropion SR*	Blocks reuptake of DA and NA; high-affinity, noncompetitive nAChR antagonism reduces nicotine reinforcement, withdrawal, and craving	1
Varenicline*	Acts as a partial agonist of $\alpha_4\beta_2$ nAChRs	1
Nortriptyline	Blocks reuptake of NA and 5-HT; probably reduces withdrawal symptoms and comorbid depressive symptoms; side effects limit utility	1–2
Clonidine	α_2-Adrenoreceptor agonist reduces nicotine withdrawal symptoms	2
Mecamylamine Cytisine	Noncompetitive, high-affinity nAChR antagonist combined with TNP reduces nicotine reinforcement, craving, and withdrawal. Acts as a partial agonist of $\alpha_4\beta_2$ nAChRs but might have limited efficacy at dose necessary for cessation	2 2
Naltrexone	Endogenous μ-opioid peptide receptor antagonist reduces nicotine craving and withdrawal in combination with TNP, may reduce alcohol use, and obviate cessation-induced weight gain	3
Nicotine vaccine	Limited evidence of efficacy for smoking cessation in early human trials and may also have utility in relapse prevention	2
Psychosocial treatments		
Brief interventions	Increase motivation to quit and impart cessation skills (e.g., community support, telephone counseling, self-help materials)	2
Cognitive-behavioral therapy	Behavioral strategies are developed to manage triggers; cognitive coping strategies target maladaptive thoughts to prevent relapse	1
Motivational interventions	Promotes patient's self-motivational statements, and in turn, patient gains greater awareness of the problems with smoking; increases intention for smoking cessation	2
Relapse prevention	A specified cognitive-behavioral approach that focuses on relapse prevention skills (e.g., recognizing high-risk situations and coping with lapses)	1
Contingency management	Uses positive reinforcement through tangible rewards to increase positive behaviors such as abstinence	2
Exposure therapy	Behavioral technique used to expose smokers to situational cues that induce cravings	2
Internet-based intervention	Strategies used via internet- or mobile-based platforms targeting adolescents, young adults, and adults	1

Effectiveness rating 1 strong evidence to support efficacy. *2* moderate evidence to support efficacy, *3* little evidence to support efficacy
*Indicates FDA-approved medications for tobacco use disorder

pies are 20–25%, and behavior therapy typically increases quit rates up to twofold over control groups. Additionally, providing behavioral support in addition to pharmacotherapy can increase the chance of a successful quit attempt by approx-imately 10–25% [73]. The primary goals of behavioral therapies in treatment of tobacco use disorder include (1) providing necessary skills to smokers to aid them to initiate smoking cessation and (2) teaching skills to avoid smoking in high-risk situations and smoking-related cues. Overall, studies have shown how more intensive counseling intervention approaches for smoking cessation have been more effective than less intensive interventions [45]. Although there is no sufficient evidence that suggests groups are more effective compared to individual interventions, group therapy seems to be a more effective intervention compared to self-help and less intensive interventions [72].

(a) *Brief interventions.* Brief advice has been found to increase the rate of smoking cessation (USPHS Guidelines, [14]); therefore it is recommended that doctors use the 5 A's with all patients (*ask* patients if they smoke, *advise* patients to quit, *assess* patients' motivation level for quitting, *assist* with quit attempts, and *arrange* follow-up contacts). Similar forms of smoking education in school settings have shown to reduce tobacco use as well as increase quit attempts in adolescent smokers [65]. Providing self-help material is a form of brief intervention used to increase motivation to quit and impart smoking cessation skills. Several studies have documented that minimal behavioral interventions such as community support groups, telephone counseling, and computer-generated tailored self-help materials can augment smoking cessation rates in controlled settings [73]. Additionally, the greatest quitting success rates may be seen when adding some support (at least 4 therapy sessions) compared to no support at all [73].

(b) *Motivational interventions.* The goal of motivational interviewing (MI) interventions is to elicit change through addressing ambivalence, increasing intrinsic motivation for change, and creating an atmosphere of acceptance in which patients take responsibility for making changes happen. Brief MI interventions have been developed for smoking cessation, and there is some evidence for increased smoking cessation using MI techniques [4]. MI interventions can also be especially effective for adolescents [29], possibly making MI useful for preventative efforts. Rollnick and colleagues [61] reported that clinicians found MI interventions to be feasible and acceptable due to the brief nature of the intervention and the focus on patient responsibility and enhancement of the clinician-patient relationship.

(c) *Cognitive-behavioral therapies.* In CBT (cognitive-behavioral therapy), patients learn strategies to anticipate and cope with situations in which they are likely to relapse to smoking. Some degree of efficacy of cognitive-behavioral therapies in smokers with and without psychiatric and substance use disorders has been observed for both individual [45] and group [72] counseling formats. Additionally, work by Brody et al. [3] has shown that reduced smoking with CBT (without pharmacotherapies) can reduce nAChR densities to normal receptor levels.

(d) *Relapse prevention.* A large number of smokers relapse within 6 months of quitting, with the majority of smokers relapsing within the first week after a quit attempt [32]. Focusing on relapse prevention skills including recognizing high-risk situations and coping with lapses can be included in initial smoking cessation treatment or following a quit attempt. However, some studies have not found an overall benefit for including relapse prevention with smokers after a quit attempt and suggest that more work is needed in this area of treatment research [44].

(e) *Contingency management.* CM (contingency management) is a type of behavioral therapy in which external reinforcers are used to change behavior. By using tangible rewards, smokers are conditioned to reinforce positive behaviors such as abstinence or a negative CO screen. Voucher-based reinforcement therapy (VBRT) uses vouchers or other monetary incentives, whereas prize incentive CM uses chances to win cash prizes to reinforce positive behaviors. These methods have been increasingly proven to be one of the more effective ways to minimize tobacco use and strengthen motivation to quit [75]. Studies have evaluated the strong positive correlation

CM has on tobacco abstinence in adolescent smokers, although treatment adherence and posttreatment efficacy seem to be poor [42]. Additionally, more recent studies have shown increasing reductions in smoking when incorporating delay discounting into a contingency management approach [26].

(f) *Exposure therapy.* Most cravings smokers experience are induced by situational cues. Cue-exposure treatment addresses cue-induced cravings and coping responses to avoid relapse [13]. This method has been shown to decrease cue-related cravings in individuals, especially those who have displayed initial cue reactivity [80]. Virtual reality has been an increasingly common type of cue-exposure therapy method along with photographs, video, auditory, and in vivo and imagery scripts. Evidence has shown that VR is a great way to produce strong cue-reactivity effects and cue-induced craving in real-world settings, however, may increase risks of relapse [56]. Overall, exposure therapy has been more promising when used to enhance other support interventions such as CBT [9].

(g) *Internet-based interventions.* Increasingly, methods such as mobile applications (MapMySmoke), social media platforms, and mobile text messages are being used, especially among adolescents. Website-delivered programs, such as 1-2-3 Smokefree, have shown to help maintain smoking abstinence in the short term. Wangberg et al. [82] have reported that tailored interventions delivered on a website and via email have shown to be almost twice as effective than nontailored internet interventions only in the short term. Both web-based and mobile-based approaches had shown to increase smoking cessation over a short term, suggesting this method would not be sufficient to aid in long-term tobacco abstinence.

(h) By using both a psychosocial and pharmacological approach, both biological and psychological dependence can be addressed. Providing behavioral support in addition to pharmacotherapy can increase the chance of a successful quit attempt by approximately

10–25%, with more intensive behavioral support increasing abstinence.

15.6 Pharmacological Treatments (See Table 15.1)

There are three FDA-approved classes of smoking cessation pharmacotherapies – nicotine replacement therapies (NRTs), sustained-release bupropion, and varenicline. According to the 2008 update to the Public Health Service *Treating Tobacco Use and Dependence Clinical Practice Guideline* [14], five NRTs, as well as bupropion SR and varenicline, all reliably increase cessation rates in comparison to placebo. Several other off-label and novel medications are also discussed in this section.

15.6.1 Nicotine Replacement Therapies

The goal of nicotine replacement therapy (NRT) is to relieve tobacco withdrawal, by providing nicotine without the harmful effects of cigarette additives, which allows smokers to focus on habit and conditioning factors when attempting cessation. After the acute withdrawal period, nicotine replacement therapy is gradually reduced so that little withdrawal should occur. NRTs rely on systemic venous absorption and so do not produce the rapid high levels of arterial nicotine achieved when cigarette smoke is inhaled. All commercially available forms of NRT are effective and increase quit rates by approximately 1.5–2.5-fold compared to placebo [68]. The transdermal patch, gum, and lozenge are over the counter (OTC), while the nasal spray and inhaler are by prescription.

(a) *Nicotine gum:* Nicotine ingested orally is extensively metabolized on first pass through the liver. Nicotine polacrilex gum avoids this problem via buccal absorption. Nicotine gum contains 2 or 4 mg of nicotine that can be released from a resin by chewing. The original recommended duration of treatment was

3 months though many experts believe longer treatment is more effective. Nicotine absorption from the gum peaks 30 minutes after beginning to use the gum. Venous nicotine levels from 2 and 4 mg gum are about one-thirds and two-thirds, respectively, of the steady-state (i.e., between cigarettes) levels of nicotine achieved with cigarette smoking. Nicotine via cigarettes is absorbed directly into the arterial circulation; thus, arterial levels from smoking are 5–10 times higher than those from the 2 and 4 mg gums.

Several placebo-controlled trials established the safety and efficacy of nicotine gum for smoking cessation [68]. There appears to be some evidence to support using higher doses of nicotine gum (4 mg pieces) in more highly dependent cigarette smokers (≥25 cpd), which supports the idea of matching nicotine gum dose to dependence level of the smoker [74].

Side effects from nicotine gum are rare and are mostly limited to those of mechanical origin (e.g., difficulty chewing, sore jaw) or of local pharmacological origin (e.g., burning in mouth, throat irritation) and most minimize over the course of 1 week.

(b) *Nicotine polacrilex lozenges.* Nicotine lozenges deliver nicotine (2 and 4 mg preparations) by buccal absorption. A 6-week double-blind, placebo-controlled RCT of 2 and 4 mg nicotine lozenges has shown their superiority to placebo lozenge [66], with significant reduction in nicotine craving and withdrawal. Furthermore, high doses of lozenge may be more efficacious in heavily dependent smokers suggesting that lozenge dose can be matched with dependence level. Just as with nicotine gum, mild throat and mouth irritation have been reported in preliminary trials [66].

(c) *Nicotine transdermal patch.* The four transdermal nicotine formulations take advantage of ready absorption of nicotine across the skin. Three of the patches are for 24-hour use and one is for 16-hour use. Starting doses are 21–22 mg/24-hour patch and 15 mg/16-hour patch. Nicotine via patches is slowly absorbed so that on the first day venous nicotine levels peak 6–10 hours after administration. Thereafter, nicotine levels remain fairly steady with a decline from peak to trough of 25% to 40% with 24-hour patches. Nicotine levels obtained with the use of patches are typically half those obtained by smoking. After 4–6 weeks on high-dose patch (21 or 22 mg/24 h, and 15 mg/16 h), smokers are tapered to a middle dose (e.g., 14 mg/24 hours or 10 mg/16 hours) and then to the lowest dose after 2–4 more weeks (7 mg/24 hours or 5 mg/16 hours). Most studies suggest that abrupt cessation of the use of patches often causes no significant withdrawal; thus, tapering does not appear to be necessary [68]. The recommended total duration of treatment is usually 6–12 weeks.

The overall efficacy of the nicotine transdermal patch (NTP) for smoking cessation has been well documented [68]. A meta-analysis of 17 RCTs in 1994 [15] reported end of treatment abstinence rates for NTP of 27% versus 13% for placebo patch (OR 2.6) and 22% vs. 9% at 6-month follow-up (OR 3.0). The effects of active NTP were independent of patch type, treatment duration, tapering procedures, and behavioral therapy format or intensity, though it should be noted that behavioral treatment enhanced outcomes with patch compared to patch alone. Additionally, combining the patch with nicotine lozenge has been shown to produce the greatest benefit for smoking cessation relative to placebo (above that of lozenge alone, patch alone, bupropion SR, and bupropion + nicotine lozenge relative to placebo) [58].

Significant adverse events with nicotine patches have not been found, with the most common minor side effects being skin reactions (50%), insomnia and increased or vivid dreams (15% with 24-hour patches), and nausea (5–10%). Tolerance to these side effects usually develops within a week of use. There appears to be little dependence liability associated with patch use as only 2% of patch users continue to use this product for an extended period after a cessation trial

[84], and this continued abstinence may be due to the desire to maintain abstinence.

(d) *Nicotine nasal spray.* Nicotine nasal spray is a prescribed NRT that is formulated as a nicotine solution in a nasal spray bottle similar to those used with saline sprays. Nasal spray delivers droplets that average about 1 mg per administration and is administered (10 mg/ml) to each nostril every 4–6 hours. The nicotine spray produces a more rapid rise in nicotine levels than that of nicotine gum but falls below the levels achieved by cigarettes. Peak nicotine levels occur within 10 minutes, and venous nicotine levels are about two-thirds those of between-cigarette levels. Smokers may use the nasal spray ad-lib up to 30 times/day for 12 weeks, including a tapering period.

Randomized, double-blind, placebo-controlled trials of nasal spray versus placebo spray [68] have established the safety and efficacy of the nasal spray for smoking cessation. Both trials employed treatment for 3–6 months, and active nasal spray led to a doubling of quit rates during active use relative to placebo use. Differences were reduced or absent with extended follow-up suggesting the need for maintenance use of this agent.

The major side effects associated with the use of nicotine nasal spray are nasal and throat irritation, rhinitis, sneezing, coughing, and watering eyes. Nicotine nasal spray may have some dependence liability; in a controlled study by West et al. [85], prolonged use of nasal spray was determined to be the case in 10% of smokers using the nasal spray, so follow-up of smokers using nasal spray is recommended.

(e) *Nicotine vapor inhalers (NVI).* NVI are cartridges (plugs) of nicotine (containing about 1 mg of nicotine each) placed inside hollow cigarette-like plastic rods. When warm air is passed through the cartridges, a nicotine vapor is produced, which is then inhaled. Absorption from nicotine inhaler is primarily buccal rather than respiratory. More recent versions of inhalers produce a rise in venous nicotine levels more rapidly than with nicotine gum but less rapidly than with nicotine nasal spray, with nicotine blood levels of about one-third that of between-cigarette levels. Smokers are instructed to puff continuously on the inhaler (0.013 mg/puff) during the day, and recommended dosing is 6–16 cartridges daily. The inhaler is to be used ad-lib for about 12 weeks.

No serious medical side effects have been reported with nicotine inhalers. Fifty percent of subjects report throat irritation or coughing. Double-blind, placebo-controlled RCTs [68] have demonstrated the superiority of NVI to placebo inhalers for smoking cessation. Results revealed a two- to threefold increase in quit rates (17–26%) at trial endpoint compared to placebo inhalers and smaller differences at follow-up periods of 1-year or longer. These data support the short-term efficacy of NVI in cigarette smokers, but longer-term trials with the inhaler are needed, and there is some modest concern about abuse liability, due to long-term use of the product in less than 10% of smokers [85].

15.6.2 Sustained-Release Bupropion

The phenylaminoketone, atypical antidepressant agent bupropion, in the sustained-release (SR) formulation (Zyban®), is a non-nicotine first-line pharmacological treatment for nicotine-dependent smokers who want to quit smoking. The mechanism of action of this antidepressant agent in the treatment of nicotine use disorder likely involves dopamine and norepinephrine reuptake blockade [1], as well as antagonism of high-affinity nAChRs [70]. The exact mechanism for bupropion's anti-smoking effects is unclear. The goals of bupropion therapy are (1) smoking cessation, (2) reduction of nicotine craving and withdrawal symptoms, and (3) prevention of cessation-induced weight gain.

The target dose of this agent in nicotine use disorder is 300 mg daily (150 mg bid), and it is typically started 7 days prior to the target quit date (TQD) at 150 mg daily, then increased to

150 mg bid after 3–4 days. Unlike the NRTs, there is no absolute requirement that smokers completely cease smoking by the TQD, though many smokers report a significant reduction in urges to smoke and craving, which facilitates cessation at the time of the TQD when drug levels reach steady-state plasma levels. Some smokers gradually reduce their cigarette smoking over several weeks prior to quitting. Smokers who are faster metabolizers of nicotine (as determined by genetic variation at the CYP2A6 allele) may benefit more from bupropion therapy, as opposed to NRT or counseling [59].

A pivotal multicenter study by Hurt and colleagues [34] established the efficacy and safety of sustained-release (SR) bupropion for treatment of nicotine use disorder which led to its FDA approval in the USA in 1998. In a 7-week double-blind, placebo-controlled multicenter trial, three doses of bupropion SR (100, 150, and 300 mg/day in BID dosing), in combination with weekly individual cessation counseling, were given to 615 cigarette smokers using at least 15 cigarettes per day. The end of trial 7-day point prevalence cessation rates for each of the bupropion doses, placebo, 100 mg/day, 150 mg/day, and 300 mg/day, were 19.0%, 28.8%, 38.6%, and 44.2%, respectively. At 1-year follow-up, cessation rates were 12.4%, 19.6%, 22.9%, and 23.1%, respectively. Bupropion treatment also dose-dependently reduced weight gain associated with smoking cessation and significantly reduced nicotine withdrawal symptoms at the 150 and 300 mg/day doses.

The primary side effects reported with bupropion administration in cigarette smokers are headache, nausea and vomiting, dry mouth, insomnia, and activation. Many of these side effects are observed in the first week of treatment. The main contraindication for the use of bupropion is a past history of seizures of any etiology. The rates of de novo seizures are low with this agent (<0.5%) at doses of 300 mg daily or less but have been observed when daily dosing exceeds 450 mg/day.

The combination of bupropion SR with nicotine transdermal patch (NTP) was evaluated in a double-blind, placebo-controlled, random-ized multicenter trial [36]. A total of 893 cigarette smokers, using at least 15 cigarettes per day (cpd), were randomized to one of four experimental groups: (1) placebo bupropion (0 mg/day) + placebo patch; (2) bupropion (300 mg/day) + placebo patch; (3) placebo bupropion + nicotine patch (21 mg/day for 4 weeks, with 2 weeks of 14 mg/day and 2 weeks of 7 mg/day); and (4) bupropion + patch. Bupropion was administered 1 week prior to the target quit date (Day 15) at which time patch treatment was initiated for a total of 8 weeks. All subjects received weekly individual smoking cessation counseling. Cessation rates at the 1-year follow-up assessment were 15.6% for placebo, 16.4% for active NTP alone, 30.3% for bupropion alone, and 35.5% for the combination of patch and bupropion. Both bupropion + patch and bupropion alone groups were significantly better than the placebo and patch alone conditions, but the combination was not significantly better than bupropion alone. Weight suppression after cessation was most robust in the combination therapy group. Side effects were consistent with the profiles of patch and bupropion, and the combination was well tolerated. However, a higher than expected rate of treatment-emergent hypertension (4–5%) was noted with the combination of bupropion and patch [36]. Of note, patch alone treatment was significantly different from placebo at the end of the trial, but not at the follow-up assessments.

Hays et al. [27] examined the effects of bupropion versus placebo on the prevention of smoking relapse in 784 cigarette smokers who achieved smoking abstinence after a 7-week open-label trial of bupropion (300 mg/day). Abstinent smokers were then randomized to bupropion (300 mg/day) or placebo for a total of 45 weeks. Fifty-nine percent of smokers enrolled in the open-label phase of the trial quit smoking. Significantly more smokers were abstinent at the end of the 52-week treatment period in bupropion vs. placebo groups (55.1 vs. 42.3%, $p < 0.01$), but not at the 1-year follow-up assessment. In addition, days to smoking relapse were higher in the bupropion vs. placebo group (156 vs. 65 days, $p < 0.05$).

Weight gain was significantly less in the bupropion group at both the end of treatment and 1-year follow-up. The results of this study suggest the efficacy of bupropion in preventing smoking relapse. Data regarding the optimal duration of bupropion therapy for maintenance treatment requires further study.

15.6.3 Varenicline

Varenicline tartrate (Chantix® in the USA, Champix® in Europe and Canada), an $\alpha_4\beta_2$ nAChR partial agonist and weak $\alpha7$ agonist, was approved as a first-line smoking cessation agent by the US FDA in 2006. The results of two independent but identical 12-week phase III trials comparing varenicline (1 mg bid) to bupropion SR (150 mg bid) and placebo have been published [21, 35]. The quit rate for both studies were similar for continuous abstinence over the last 4 weeks (weeks 9–12) of the study: study 1 [35], varenicline 43.9%, bupropion SR 29.8%, and placebo 17.6%; study 2 [21], varenicline 44.0%, bupropion SR 29.5%, and placebo 17.7%. Quit rates were significantly higher for participants taking varenicline compared to bupropion SR (ps <0.0001), and both drugs resulted in significantly higher quit rates than placebo. Continuous abstinence over the follow-up period (week 9 to 52) was lower, and participants taking varenicline continued to show a higher rate of abstinence (study 1, 22.1%; study 2, 23.0%) than participants taking bupropion (study 1, 16.4%, p <0.001 compared to varenicline; study 2, 15.0%, $p = 0.064$ compared to varenicline) and placebo (study 1, 8.4%; study 2, 10.3%). A third study examining the efficacy of the drug on smoking relapse prevention used a 12-week open-label varenicline phase followed by randomization to12 weeks of varenicline or placebo [78]. These investigators found that participants taking varenicline versus placebo were more likely to be continuously abstinent during weeks 13–24 (70.5% vs. 49.6%, p <0.001) and weeks 13–52 (43.6% vs. 36.9%, $p = 0.02$). Varenicline was found to reduce cravings and smoking satisfaction and to be safe and well tolerated. There were similar discontinuation rates for varenicline and bupropion, and the most common adverse event reported by the varenicline group was nausea (study 1, 28.1%; study 2, 29.4%).

There have been significant concerns about treatment emergent neuropsychiatric adverse events such as suicidal and homicidal ideation, psychosis, mania, and aggression with the use of varenicline for smoking cessation. However, evidence from controlled smoking cessation clinical trials in psychiatric populations such as schizophrenia [87] and bipolar disorder [89] suggest the safety of this agent for smoking cessation including in high-risk psychiatric populations. Further research on the safety and utility of these agents in psychiatric and addicted populations is clearly warranted.

15.6.4 Off-Label Medications

(a) *Cytisine.* Cytisine (Tabex® in Europe) is a nicotinic partial agonist that binds with high affinity to the $\alpha4\beta_2$ nicotinic acetylcholine receptor. West et al. [86] assessed the safety and efficacy of cytisine in the first randomized, placebo-controlled trial for the drug and found that it was significantly more effective for smoking cessation than placebo.

(b) *Nortriptyline.* Nortriptyline is a tricyclic antidepressant which has been shown in several double-blind, placebo-controlled trials to be superior to placebo [24] and to have comparable efficacy to bupropion [23]. Higher-intensity behavioral therapies may help to improve its efficacy. The mechanism of action is thought to relate to norepinephrine and serotonin reuptake blockade. Side effects include dry mouth, blurred vision, constipation, and orthostatic hypotension. It appears to have some utility in smokers with past histories of major depression, but its potential for fatal overdose has likely limited its utilization in smokers. However, nortriptyline can be recommended as a second-line agent after nicotine replacement therapies and bupropion, though more study of this agent is necessary.

(c) *Clonidine.* Clonidine is a presynaptic alpha-2 receptor agonist that dampens sympathetic activity originating at the locus coeruleus. It appears to have efficacy for treating opioid withdrawal and thus was tested with nicotine withdrawal during smoking cessation trials. The most common side effects of clonidine are dry mouth, sedation, and constipation. Postural hypotension, rebound hypertension, and depression are rare with smoking cessation treatment. Several clinical trials tested oral or transdermal clonidine in doses of 0.1–0.4 mg/day for 2–6 weeks with and without behavior therapy and have suggested clonidine is more effective in women than in men. In general, the effects of clonidine have not proven to be as robust as NRTs. A meta-analysis by Covey and Glassman [7] of 9 placebo-controlled studies and 813 patients found short-term quit rates of 39% on clonidine versus 21% on placebo (OR 2.4, 1.7–32.8) and suggested that clonidine was effective in the transdermal preparation and more helpful in female smokers. A subsequent meta-analysis by Gourlay and Benowitz [22] found long-term follow-up quit rates in 4 subsequent studies of 31% on clonidine and 17% on placebo (OR 2.0, 1.3–3.0). It appears to be useful in reducing nicotine withdrawal symptoms acutely and may have a role in smokers who have high levels of anxiety during early cessation [53]. This agent should be considered as a second-line therapy for smokers failing initial treatment with NRTs or bupropion.

(d) *Mecamylamine.* Mecamylamine (MEC) is a noncompetitive blocker at the ion channel site of both high-affinity central nervous system and peripheral nAChRs. When MEC is given to smokers who are not trying to stop smoking, they initially increase their smoking in an attempt to overcome the blockade produced by this drug. MEC does not precipitate withdrawal in humans perhaps because it is a noncompetitive nAChR antagonist. Common side effects included abdominal cramps, constipation, dry mouth,

and headaches. Based on a theory that combined blockade and agonist therapy at the nAChR might be beneficial, similar to the nAChR partial agonist profile of varenicline, two randomized trials compared MEC in combination with nicotine patch to placebo and nicotine patch, with the rationale that MEC would reduce the rewarding effects of nicotine and patch would reduce nicotine withdrawal symptoms [62, 63]. In the first trial [63], MEC (up to 10 mg/day; 5 mg bid for 5 weeks) or placebo was given in combination with nicotine patch (21 mg/day) for up to 8 weeks, and cessation rates were significantly higher in the combination group than the patch alone group (12/24 [50.0%] vs. 4/24 [16.7%], p <0.05). Mecamylamine was reported to reduce cigarette craving and negative effect and appetite increases associated with tobacco withdrawal. In a subsequent study of 80 cigarette smokers [62], MEC at doses of up to 10 mg/day was given as a pre-treatment for 4 weeks prior to nicotine patch initiation at the TQD, and the combination of MEC and patch was continued for 6 weeks. Similar to the first study, the combination of MEC with NTP increased continuous abstinence rates after the TQD compared to NTP alone (19/40 [47.5%] vs. 11/40 [27.5%], p <0.05). These data suggest the efficacy of the combination of MEC with NTP, and this combination should be considered a second-line therapy.

(e) *Naltrexone.* Naltrexone is a long-acting congener of the μ-opioid receptor antagonist naloxone. The rationale for using naltrexone for smoking cessation is that the performance-enhancing and other positive effects of nicotine may be opioid-mediated. Early studies observed that naltrexone monotherapy increases smoking, presumably an attempt to overcome blockade; however, a study of naltrexone in heavy smoking alcoholics found that cigarette smoking was decreased modestly [64]. Adverse events include elevated liver enzymes, nausea, and vomiting. A trial by Covey and colleagues [8] in 68 cigarette smokers using at least 20 cpd and highly motivated to quit compared naltrexone (up to 75 mg/day) initiated 3 days prior to the TQD to placebo for a total of 4 weeks. Cessation rates in the naltrexone group were nonsignificantly higher than placebo (46.7% vs. 26.3%, p <0.10), and at 6-month follow-up, there were no group differences.

Additional promising data with naltrexone was observed with the combination of naltrexone and NRT. A preliminary study by Krishnan-Sarin et al. [43] suggested that the combination of naltrexone and NTP is superior to NTP alone when NTP administration precedes that of naltrexone (presumably to decrease naltrexone-related withdrawal). In a larger trial of the combination of nicotine patch (21 mg/day) with four active doses of naltrexone (0, 25, 50, and 100 mg/day), it was shown that the highest dose of naltrexone with patch significantly improves continuous smoking abstinence rates compared to placebo [54], but these effects appeared to be confined to the first weeks of treatment. Further studies of naltrexone either alone or in combination with the patch are needed, including in patients with concurrent alcohol misuse.

(f) *Nicotine vaccines.* Nicotine vaccines are being developed by a number of companies, but they are not currently available for public use. A systematic review of smoking cessation trials conducted by pharmaceutical companies as part of the drug development process showed that nicotine vaccines, while well tolerated, did not enhance long-term cessation rates [25], and recent phase III trials of one nicotine vaccine preparation suggested that these agents did not increase rates of smoking cessation in nicotine-dependent smokers. However, the nicotine vaccine may have promise for the prevention of smoking relapse or initiation of smoking. Side effects include soreness at the injection site and hypersensitivity reactions to vaccine components.

15.7 Integration of Tobacco Use Disorder Treatment into Mental Healthcare Settings

High rates of tobacco use disorder and low rates of smoking cessation are becoming increasingly appreciated in psychiatric and addicted populations [38]. Individuals with substance use issues such as alcohol are two to four times more likely to be dependent on tobacco compared to the general population. It is increasingly evident that mental health and addiction clinics have done little to address the tobacco culture that permeates these institutional environments. However, smoking bans are becoming increasingly common in psychiatric hospitals and addiction treatment programs and appear to be successfully implemented in the majority of reported cases, but these developments have shown little uptake and application in community settings [47].

The utilization of standard tobacco use disorder treatments such as behavioral therapies, NRT, bupropion, and varenicline has been increasingly reported in psychiatric and substance-abusing smokers. For example, various formulations of NRT including nicotine patch [20] and nasal spray [88] and sustained-release bupropion [19] and varenicline [87] have been reported to be well-tolerated and efficacious in increasing rates of both smoking reduction and cessation in patients with schizophrenia, when combined with cognitive-behavioral and motivational enhancement therapies. Both NRTs and bupropion have also been studied in smokers with major depression [6, 39], post-traumatic stress disorder [30], and alcohol [33, 37] and opioid [67] use disorder and have been found to be well tolerated and effective; small trials with bupropion SR [83] and varenicline [89] have suggested their safety and effectiveness in smokers with bipolar illness. Interestingly, most effective treatments for polysubstance users are combinations of counseling and NRT or non-NRT. Moreover, interventions addressing all drugs for polysubstance users can be a more effective strategy for smoking cessation with concurrent cessation or sequentially. Furthermore, studies which compared integration of behavioral and pharmacological treatments in a mental health setting for smokers with PTSD found enhanced quit rates compared to nonintegrated smoking cessation therapies [49], suggesting that provision of integrated mental health and tobacco treatment produces enhanced cessation outcomes.

Finally, a better understanding of the pathophysiology of mental disorders may lead to improved treatments for this population. There is increasing evidence that available pharmacological and behavioral treatments, modified for those with mental disorders, can be used safely and effectively in these populations [47]. For example, schizophrenia is associated with a broad range of cognitive deficits particularly those related to prefrontal lobe dysfunction, and atypical antipsychotic drugs (e.g., clozapine, olanzapine), which improve certain cognitive deficits associated with schizophrenia, may facilitate reduction of smoking [18] or smoking cessation with standard pharmacotherapies such as nicotine patch [20] or bupropion SR [19]. The development of novel medications which target the underlying pathophysiology of psychiatric or substance use disorders may well lead to important advances in the management of tobacco use disorder in these special populations of smokers.

15.8   Conclusions

Tobacco use disorder remains one of the leading preventable causes of morbidity and mortality in the Western world. Nonetheless, smoking cessation therapies are among the most cost-effective and proven therapies in psychiatry and medicine. Yet, most healthcare providers do not identify tobacco use in their patients. In fact, a survey of psychiatric practices found that only 9.1% of smokers under the care of psychiatrists received treatment for nicotine use disorder [51]. Nonetheless, the American Psychiatric Association has recently published an update of its clinical practice guidelines for nicotine dependence [40] which should provide standards for the field of psychiatry in the assessment and treatment of tobacco use disorder. Furthermore,

while medication and behavioral treatments have documented efficacy in treating tobacco use disorder, it is important that these therapies be used in combination to achieve the best overall results and ensure adequate skill acquisition and treatment adherence. Future challenges include developing safer and more effective smoking cessation therapies and making these therapies available to all smokers who want to quit.

Key Points
- Rates of tobacco use disorder have decreased substantially, but many of the remaining smokers appear to have comorbidities that reduce their chance of quitting such as psychiatric and substance use disorders.
- Identification of smokers in clinical settings is of critical importance to the treatment of tobacco use disorder.
- There are effective pharmacological and behavioral therapies for tobacco use disorder, which work best when used in combination.
- E-cigarettes are an increasingly common smoking cessation aid, although may be misused by adolescents.
- A better understanding of the pathophysiology of mental health and addictive disorders may lead to improved treatment approaches for tobacco use disorder in these smoking populations.
- Smokers with psychiatric and substance use comorbidity may be best treated in settings which integrate smoking cessation treatments with mental health and addiction treatment.

References

1. Ascher JA, Cole JO, Colin JN, Feighner JP, Ferris RM, Fibiger HC, Golden RN, Martin P, Potter WZ, Richelson E. Bupropion: a review of its mechanism of antidepressant activity. J Clin Psychiatry. 1995;56:395–401.
2. Bedi G, Preston KL, Epstein DH, Heishman SJ, Marrone GF, Shaham Y, de Wit H. Incubation of cue-

induced cigarette craving during abstinence in human smokers. Biol Psychiatry. 2011;69:708–11.

3. Brody AL, Mukhin AG, Shulenberger S, Mamoun MS, Kozman M, Phoung J, Neary M, Luu T, Mandelkern MA. Treatment for tobacco dependence: effect on brain nicotinic acetylcholine receptor density. Neuropsychopharmacology. 2013; https://doi.org/10.1038/hpp.2013.53.

4. Carpenter MJ, Hughes JR, Solomon LJ, Callas PW. Both smoking reduction with nicotine replacement therapy and motivation advice increase future cessation among smokers unmotivated to quit. J Consult Clin Psychol. 2004;72:371–81.

5. CDC. Current cigarette smoking among adults – United States, 2016. MMWR Morb Mortal Wkly Rep. 2018;67(2):53.

6. Chengappa KN, Kambhampati RK, Perkins K, Nigam R, Anderson T, Brar JS, Vemulapalli HK, Atzert R, Key P, Kang JS, Levine J. Bupropion sustained-release as a smoking cessation treatment in remitted depressed patients maintained on treatment with selective serotonin reuptake inhibitors. J Clin Psychiatry. 2001;62:503–8.

7. Covey LS, Glassman AH. A meta-analysis of double-blind placebo-controlled trials of clonidine for smoking cessation. Br J Addict. 1991;86:991–8.

8. Covey LS, Glassman AH, Stetner F. Naltrexone effects on short-term and long-term smoking cessation. J Addict Dis. 1999;18:31–40.

9. Culberston CS, Schulenberger S, De La Garza R, Newton TF, Brody AL. Virtual reality cue exposure therapy for the treatment of tobacco dependence. J Cyber Ther Rehabil. 2012;5(1):57–64.

10. Cummins SE, Shu-Hong Z, Tedeschi GJ, Gamst AC, Myers MG. Use of e-cigarettes by individuals with mental health conditions. Tobacco Control. 2014; https://doi.org/10.1136/tobaccocontrol-2013-051511.

11. Dani JA, Jenson D, Broussard JI, De Biasi M. Neurophysiology of nicotine addiction. J Addict Res Ther. 2011;20(Suppl 1):001.

12. Etter JF, Bullen C. Electronic cigarette: users utilization, satisfaction and perceived efficacy. Addiction. 2011;106(11):2017–28.

13. Ferguson SG, Shiffman S. The relevance and treatment of cue-induced cravings in tobacco dependence. J Subst Abuse. 2009;36(3):235–43.

14. Fiore MC, Jaen CR, Baker TB, et al. Treating tobacco use and dependence: 2008 update US Public Health Service Clinical Practice Guideline executive summary. Respir Care. 2008;53:1217–22.

15. Fiore MC, Smith SS, Jorenby DE, Baker TB. The effectiveness of the nicotine patch for smoking cessation: a meta-analysis. JAMA. 1994;271:1940–7.

16. Foulds J, Veldheer S, Berg A. Electronic cigarettes (e-cigs): views of aficionados and clinical/public health perspectives. Int J Clin Pract. 2011;65(10):1037–42.

17. George TP, O'Malley SS. Current pharmacological treatments for nicotine dependence. Trends Pharmacol Sci. 2004;25:42–8.

18. George TP, Sernyak MJ, Ziedonis DM, Woods SW. Effects of clozapine on smoking in chronic schizophrenic outpatients. J Clin Psychiatry. 1995;56:344–6.

19. George TP, Vessicchio JC, Termine A, Bregartner TA, Feingold A, Rounsaville BJ, Kosten TR. A placebo-controlled study of bupropion for smoking cessation in schizophrenia. Biol Psychiatry. 2002;52:53–61.

20. George TP, Zeidonis DM, Feingold A, Pepper WT, Satterburg CA, Winkel J, Rounsaville BJ, Kosten TR. Nicotine transdermal patch and atypical antipsychotic medications for smoking cessation in schizophrenia. Am J Psychiatry. 2000;157:1835–42.

21. Gonzales D, Rennard SI, Nides M, Oncken C, Azoulay S, Billing CB, Watsky EJ, Gong J, Williams KE, Reeves KR. for the Varenicline Phase 3 Study Group. Varenicline, an alpha4 beta2 nicotinic acetylcholine receptor partial agonist, vs. sustained release bupropion and placebo for smoking cessation. JAMA. 2006;296:47–55.

22. Gourlay SG, Benowitz N. Is clonidine an effective smoking cessation therapy? Drugs. 1995;50:197–207.

23. Hall SM, Humfleet GL, Reus VI, Munoz RF, Hartz DT, Maude-Griffin R. Psychological intervention and antidepressant treatment in smoking cessation. Arch Gen Psychiatry. 2002;59:930–6.

24. Hall SM, Reus VI, Munoz RF, Sees KL, Humfleet G, Hartz DT, Frederick S, Triffleman E. Nortriptyline and cognitive-behavioral therapy in the treatment of cigarette smoking. Arch Gen Psychiatry. 1998;55:683–90.

25. Hartmann-Boyce J, Cahill K, Hatsukami D, Cornuz J. Nicotine vaccines for smoking cessation. Cochrane Database Syst Rev. 2012;(8):CD007072.

26. Harvanko AM, Strickland JC, Slone SA, Shelton BJ, Reynolds BA. Dimensions of impulsive behavior: predicting contingency management treatment outcomes for adolescent smokers. Addict Behav. 2019;90:334–40.

27. Hays JT, Hurt RD, Rigotti NA, Niaura R, Gonzales D, Durcan MJ, Sachs DP, Wolter TD, Buist AS, Johnston JA, White JD. Sustained-release bupropion for pharmacologic relapse-prevention after smoking cessation: a randomized, controlled trial. Ann Int Med. 2001;135:423–33.

28. Heatherton TF, Kozlowski LT, Frecker RC, Fagerstrom KO. The Fagerstrom test for nicotine dependence: a revision of the Fagerstrom tolerance questionnaire. Br J Addict. 1991;86:1119–27.

29. Heckman CJ, Egleston BL, Hofmann MT. Efficacy of motivational interviewing for smoking cessation: a systematic review and meta-analysis. Tob Control. 2010;19:410–6.

30. Hertzberg MA, Moore SD, Feldman ME, Beckham JC. A preliminary study of bupropion sustained-release for smoking cessation in patients with chronic posttraumatic stress disorder. J Clin Psychopharmacol. 2001;21:94–8.

31. Hughes JR, Hatsukami DK. Signs and symptoms of tobacco withdrawal. Arch Gen Psychiatry. 1986;43:289–94.

32. Hughes JR, Keely J, Naud S. Shape of the relapse curve and long-term abstinence among untreated smokers. Addiction. 2004;99:29–38.

33. Hurt RD, Dale LC, Offord KP, Croghan IT, Hays JT, Gomez-Dahl L. Nicotine patch therapy for smoking cessation in recovering alcoholics. Addiction. 1995;90:1541–6.

34. Hurt RD, Sachs DPL, Glover ED, Offord KP, Johnston JA, Dale LC, Khayrallah MA, Schroeder DR, Glover PN, Sullivan CR, Croghan IT, Sullivan PM. A comparison of sustained-release bupropion and placebo for smoking cessation. N Engl J Med. 1997;337:1195–202.

35. Jorenby DE, Hays JT, Rigotti NA, Azoulay S, Watsky EJ, Williams KE, Billing CB, Gong J, Reeves KR. for the Varenicline Phase 3 Study Group. Efficacy of varenicline, an alpha4 beta2 nicotinic acetylcholine receptor partial agonist, vs. placebo or sustained release bupropion for smoking cessation. JAMA. 2006;296:56–63.

36. Jorenby DE, Leischow SJ, Nides MA, Rennard SI, Johnston JA, Hughes AR, Smith SS, Muramato ML, Daughton DM, Doan K, Fiore MC, Baker TB. A controlled trial of sustained-release bupropion, a nicotine patch, or both for smoking cessation. N Engl J Med. 1999;340:685–91.

37. Kalman D, Kahler C, Tirch D, Penk W, Kaschib C, Monti PM. Twelve-week outcomes from an investigation of high dose nicotine patch therapy for heavy smokers with a past history of alcohol dependence. Psychol Addict Behav. 2004;18:78–82.

38. Kalman D, Morrisette SB, George TP. Co-morbidity of smoking with psychiatric and substance use disorders. Am J Addict. 2005;14:106–23.

39. Kinnunen T, Doherty K, Militello FS, Garvey AJ. Depression and smoking cessation: characteristics of depressed smokers and effects of nicotine replacement. J Consult Clin Psychol. 1996;64:791–8.

40. Kleber HD, Weiss RD, Anton RF Jr, George TP, Greenfield SF, Kosten TR, O'Brien CP, Rounsaville BJ, Strain EC, Ziedonis DM, Hennessey G, Connery H. American Psychiatric Association. Clinical practice guidelines for the treatment of patients with substance use disorders, 2nd edition. Am J Psychiatry. 2006;163:5–82.

41. Klemperer EM, Hughes JR, Naud S. Reduction in cigarettes per day prospectively predicts making a quit attempt: a fine-grained secondary analysis of a natural history study. Nicotine Tob Res. 2019;21(5):648–54.

42. Krishnan-Sarin S, Cavallo DA, Cooney JL, Schepis TS, Kong G, Liss TB, Liss AK, McMahon TJ, Nich C, Babuscio T, Rounsaville BJ, Carroll KM. An exploratory randomized controlled trial of a novel high-school based smoking cessation intervention for adolescent smokers using abstinence-contingent incentives and cognitive behavioral therapy. Drug Alcohol Depend. 2013;132(1–2):346–51.

43. Krishnan-Sarin S, Meandjiza B, O'Malley SS. Nicotine patch and naltrexone for smoking cessation: a preliminary study. Nicotine Tob Res. 2003;5:851–7.

44. Lancaster T, Hajek P, Stead LF. Prevention of relapse after quitting smoking: a systematic review of trials. Arch Intern Med. 2006;166(8):828–35.

45. Lancaster T, Stead LF. Individual behavioural counselling for smoking cessation. Cochrane Database Syst Rev. 2017;(3):CD001292.

46. Leventhal AM, Strong DR, Sussman S, Kirkpatrick MG, Unger JB, Barrington-Trimis JL, Audrain-McGovern J. Psychiatric comorbidity in adolescent electronic and conventional cigarette use. J Psychiatr Res. 2016;73:71–8.

47. Mackowick KM, Lynch M-J, Weinberger AH, George TP. Treatment of tobacco dependence in people with mental health and addictive disorders. Curr Psychiatr Rep. 2012;14:478–85.

48. Miech R, Johnston L, O'Malley PM, Bachman JG, Patrick ME. Adolescent vaping and nicotine use in 2017–2018 – U.S. National Estimates. N Engl J Med. 2019;380(2):192–3.

49. McFall M, Atkins DC, Yoshimoto D, Thompson CE, Kanter E, Malte CA, Saxon AJ. Integrating tobacco cessation treatment into mental health care for patients with posttraumatic stress disorder. Am J Addict. 2006;15:336–44.

50. McMillen RC, Gottlieb MA, Shaefer RM, Winckoff JP, Klein JD. Trends in electronic cigarette use among US adults: use is increasing in both smokers and non-smokers. Nicotine Tob Res. 2015;17(10):1195–202.

51. Montoya ID, Herbeck DM, Sviks DS, Pincus HA. Identification and treatment of patients with nicotine problems in routine clinical psychiatry practice. Am J Addict. 2005;14:441–54.

52. Morean ME, Kong G, Camenga DR, Cavallo DA, Krishnan-Sarin S. High school students' use of electronic cigarettes to vaporize cannabis. Pediatrics. 2015;136(4):611–6.

53. Niaura R, Brown RA, Goldstein MG, Murphy JK, Abrams DB. Transdermal clonidine for smoking cessation: a double-blind randomized dose-response study. Exp Clin Psychopharmacol. 1996;4:285–91.

54. O'Malley SS, Cooney JL, Krishnan-Sarin S, Dubin JA, McKee SA, Cooney NL, Blakeslee A, Meandzija B, Romano-Dahlgard D, Wu R, Makuch R, Jatlow P. A controlled trial of naltrexone augmentation of nicotine replacement therapy for smoking cessation. Arch Int Med. 2006;166:667–74.

55. Patten CA, Brockman TA. Combining medications with behavioral treatment. In: George TP, editor. Medication treatments for nicotine dependence. Boca Raton, Florida: Taylor Francis; 2006. p. 225–44.

56. Pericot-Valverde I, Secades-Villa R, Guterrez-Maldonado J. A randomized clinical trial of cue exposure treatment through virtual reality for smoking cessation. J Subst Abuse Treat. 2019;96:26–32.

57. Peters EN, Harrell PT, Hendricks PS, O'Grady KE, Pickworth WB, Vocci FJ. Electronic cigarettes in adults in outpatient substance use treatment: aware-

ness, perceptions, use and reasons for use. Am J Addict. 2015;24(3):233–9.

58. Piper ME, Smith SS, Schlam TR, Fiore MC, Jorenby DE, Fraser D, Baker TB. A randomized placebo-controlled clinical trial of five smoking cessation pharmacotherapies. Arch Gen Psychiatry. 2009;66:1253–62.

59. Ray R, Tyndale RF, Lerman C. Nicotine dependence pharmacogenetics: role of genetic variation in nicotine-metabolizing enzymes. J Neurogenet. 2009;23:252–61.

60. Rigotti NA. Clinical practice: treatment of tobacco use and dependence. N Engl J Med. 2002;346:506–12.

61. Rollnick S, Butler CC, Stott N. Helping smokers make decisions: the enhancement of breif intervention for general medical practice. Patient Educ Counsel. 1997;31:191–203.

62. Rose JE, Behm FM, Westman EC. Nicotine-mecamylamine treatment for smoking cessation: the role of pre-cessation therapy. Exp Clin Psychopharmacol. 1998;6:331–43.

63. Rose JE, Behm FM, Westman EC, Levin ED, Stein RM, Ripka GV. Mecamylamine combined with nicotine skin patch facilitates smoking cessation beyond nicotine patch treatment alone. Clin Pharmacol Ther. 1994;56:86–99.

64. Rosenhow DJ, Monti PM, Colby SM, Guillver SB, Swift RM, Abrams DB. Naltrexone treatment fort alcoholics: effect on cigarette smoking rates. Nicotine Tob Res. 2003;5:231–6.

65. Shakleton N, Jamal F, Viner RM, Dickson K, Patton G, Bonell C. School-based interventions going beyond health education to promote adolescent health: systematic review of reviews. J Adolesc Health. 2016;58(4):382–96.

66. Shiffman S, Dresler CM, Hajek P, Bilburt SJ, Targett DA, Strahs KR. Efficacy of a nicotine lozenge for smoking cessation. Arch Int Med. 2002;162:1267–76.

67. Shoptaw S, Rotheram-Fuller E, Yang X, Frosch D, Nahom D, Jarvik ME, Rawson RA, Ling W. Smoking cessation in methadone maintenance. Addiction. 2002;97:1317–28.

68. Silagy C, Lancaster T, Stead L, Mant D, Fowler G. Nicotine replacement therapies for smoking cessation. Cochrane Database Syst Rev. 2004;(3):CD000146.

69. Siegel MB, Tanwar KL, Wood KS. Electronic cigarettes as a smoking-cessation: tool results from an online survey. Am J Prev Med. 2011;40(4):472–5.

70. Slemmer JE, Martin BR, Damaj MI. Bupropion is a nicotinic antagonist. J Pharmacol Exp Therap. 2000;295:321–7.

71. Sobell LC, Sobell MB, Leo GI, Cancilla A. Reliability of a timeline method: assessing normal drinkers' reports of recent drinking and a comparative evaluation across several populations. Brit J Addict. 1988;83:393–402.

72. Stead LF, Carroll AJ, Lancaster T. Group therapy programmes for smoking cessation. Cochrane Database Syst Rev. 2017;(3):CD001007.

73. Stead LF, Lancaster T. Combined pharmacotherapy and behavioural interventions for smoking cessation. Cochrane Database Syst Rev. 2012;(10):CD008286.

74. Stead LF, Perera R, Bullen C, Mant D, Hartmann-Boyce J, Cahill K, Lancaster T. Nicotine replacement therapy for smoking cessation. Cochrane Database Syst Rev. 2012;(11):CD000146.

75. Tevyaw TO'L, Colby SM, Jennifer WT, Kahler CW, Rohsenow DJ, Barnett NP, Gwaltney CJ, Monti PM. Contingency management and motivational enhancement: a randomized clinical trial for college student smokers. Nicotine Tob Res. 2009;11(6):739–49.

76. Tiffany ST, Drobes DJ. The development and initial validation of a questionnaire on smoking urges. Addiction. 1991;86:1467–76.

77. Tindle HA, Shiffman S. Smoking cessation behavior among intermittent smokers versus daily smokers. Am J Public Health. 2011;101:e1–3.

78. Tonstad S, Tonnesen P, Hajek P, Williams KE, Billing CB, Reeves KR. for the Varenicline Phase 3 Study Group . Effect of maintenance therapy with varenicline on smoking cessation. JAMA. 2006;296:64–71.

79. Tverdal A, Bjartveit K. Health consumption of reduced daily cigarette consumption. Tob Control. 2006;15:472–80.

80. Unrod M, Drobes DJ, Stasiewicz PR, Ditre JW, Heckman B, Miller RR, Sutton SK. Decline in Cue-provoked craving during Cue exposure therapy for smoking cessation. Nicotine Tob Res. 2014;16(3):306–15.

81. Walker JF, Loprinzi PD. Longitudinal examination of predictors of smoking cessation in a national sample of U.S. adolescent and young adult smokers. Nicotine Tob Res. 2014;16(6):830–27.

82. Wangberg SC, Nilsen O, Antypas K, Gram IT. Effect of tailoring in an internet-based intervention for smoking cessation: randomized controlled trial. J Med Internet Res. 2011;13(4):e121.

83. Weinberger AH, Vessicchio JC, Sacco KC, Creeden CL, Chengappa KN, George TP. A preliminary study of sustained-release bupropion for smoking cessation in bipolar disorder. J Clin Psychopharmacol. 2008;28:584–7.

84. West R, Hajek P, Foulds J, Nilsson F, May S, Meadows A. A comparison of the abuse liability and dependence potential of nicotine patch, gum, spray, and inhaler. Psychopharmacology. 2000;149:198–202.

85. West R, Hajek P, Nilsson F, Foulds J, May S, Meadows A. Individual differences in preferences for and responses to four nicotine replacement products. Psychopharmacology. 2001;153:225–30.

86. West R, Zatonski W, Cedzynska M, Lewandowska D, Pazik J, Aveyard P, Stapleton J. Placebo-controlled trial of cytisine for smoking cessation. N Engl J Med. 2011;365:1193–200.

87. Williams JM, Anthenelli RM, Morris C, Tredow J, Thompson JR, Yunis C, George TP. A double-blind, placebo-controlled study evaluating the safety and efficacy of varenicline tartrate for smoking cessation

in schizophrenia and schizoaffective disorder. J Clin Psychiatry. 2012;73:654–60.

88. Williams JM, Ziedonis DM, Foulds J. A case series of nicotine nasal spray in the treatment of tobacco dependence among patients with schizophrenia. Psychiatr Serv. 2004;55:1064–6.

89. Wu BS, Weinberger AH, Mancuso E, Wing VC, Haji-Khamenh B, Levinson AJ, George TP. A preliminary feasibility study of varenicline for smoking cessation in bipolar disorder. J Dual Diagn. 2012;8:131–2.

90. Zawertailo L, Pavlov D, Ivanova A, Ng G, Baliunas D, Selby P. Concurrent E-cigarette use during tobacco dependence treatment in primary care settings: association with smoking cessation at three and six months. Nicotine Tob Res. 2017;19(2):183–9.

Addiction to Caffeine and Other Xanthines

16

Thierry Favrod-Coune and Barbara Broers

Contents

Abstract

Xanthine (3,7-dihydro-purine-2,6-dione) is a purine base that can naturally be found in human body tissues and fluids as well as in plants and other organisms. Methylated xanthines (methylxanthines) are phosphodiesterase inhibitors and adenosine receptor antagonists. Methylxanthines have thus different effects: reduce inflammation and immunity, reduce sleepiness, and increase alertness, but also stimulate the heart rate and contraction and dilate the bronchi. The most well-known methylxanthines are caffeine, methylbromine, and theophylline. Large observational studies suggest that caffeine may have long-term health benefits. Coffee and caffeine withdrawal symptoms exist and

T. Favrod-Coune (✉) · B. Broers
Unit for Dependencies, Division for Primary Care,
Department for Primary Care Medicine, Geneva
University Hospitals, Geneva, Switzerland
e-mail: thierry.favrod-coune@hcuge.ch;
barbara.broers@hcuge.ch

are often not recognized, especially in treatment settings, where caffeine withdrawal can be confounded with other symptoms. Caffeine intoxication and withdrawal are recognized clinical entities, but caffeine dependence is currently not. Caffeine withdrawal symptoms occur in half of regular coffee drinkers, even at moderate caffeine intake. The most common symptoms are headache, fatigue, and difficulty to concentrate. Health professionals and patients should be better informed about these symptoms and the risk of occurrence of caffeine withdrawal. There is little research on treatments for clinical problems associated with xanthine use or abuse.

16.1 Introduction

For professionals in the addiction field, discussing the issue of caffeine, in a private or professional context, is a pleasure. Finally there is a domain that allows us to have a sort of positive message: "drink your coffee, it's probably good for you, it's probably good for your patients."

Our image of "controllers" telling in general frightening stories about the risks of smoking, drinking, sniffing, or injecting different psychoactive substances can be slightly improved if we can enchant the benefits of a few cups of espresso in the morning. And it is even better if we can carefully formulate the recommendation not to forget the daily bit of dark chocolate, full of theobromine, another member of the methylxanthine group.

But is this really so? Are we sure there are no acute or long-term risks related to caffeine use? Is there a safe level of use? Should we talk about coffee or caffeine use? Are there subgroups of patients that should avoid xanthine use? And what about caffeine addiction or dependence, is it a clinical entity or a popular but misused term?

In this chapter we will focus mostly on caffeine and marginally on other methylxanthines. The objective of this chapter is to describe the effects, risks, and benefits of use of caffeine; dis-cuss "caffeinism and chocoholism"; and provide some clinical recommendations.

16.2 Caffeine and Methylxanthines

Xanthine (3,7-dihydro-purine-2,6-dione) is a purine base that can naturally be found in human body tissues and fluids as well as in plants and other organisms. Methylated xanthines (methylxanthines; *see* Fig. 16.1 *for chemical structure*) are phosphodiesterase inhibitors (increasing intracellular cAMP, activating protein kinase A, inhibiting the synthesis of tumor necrosis factor (TNF)-alpha and leukotriene) and adenosine receptor antagonists (inhibiting sleepiness-inducing adenosine). Methylxanthines have thus different effects: reduce inflammation and immunity, reduce sleepiness, and increase alertness, but also stimulate the heart rate and contraction and dilate the bronchi. The most well-known methylxanthines are caffeine, methylbromine, and theophylline.

Caffeine can be found naturally in coffee beans but also in tea leaves, guarana, and mate plants or kola nuts. Theobromine and theophylline are found in cacao beans and mate plants; tea leaves contain some theophylline. Caffeine and other methylxan-

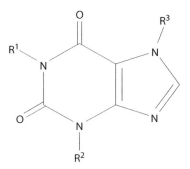

Caffeine: R1 = R2 = R3 = CH3

Theobromine: R1 = H, R2 = R3 = CH3

Theophylline: R1 = R2 = CH3, R3 = H

Fig. 16.1 Chemical structure of methylxanthines. (Source: https://en.wikipedia.org/wiki/Xanthine#/media/File:Methylxanthin_(R1,_R2,_R3).svg)

thines can be manufactured. Theophylline is a well-known asthma medication.

Caffeine is absorbed rapidly and completely through the gastrointestinal tract. After oral consumption the plasma peak is after 30–45 min, and the half-time elimination is around 3.5–6 h [16] with high variability related to age, hormones, use of nicotine or medications, etc. Metabolization takes essentially place in the liver through the cytochrome P450 pathway, especially through the cytochrome CYP1A2. The deficiency of CYP1A2 enzymes has been shown to impair caffeine metabolism and prolong caffeine half-life [9], as can certain medications, such as disulfiram [2] or quinolones, through CYL1A2 inhibition. Also during pregnancy, the half-life of caffeine increases, with one study suggesting that in the last month of pregnancy, half-life increases to 10.5 h on average [27]. Smokers seem to metabolize caffeine more quickly through acceleration of demethylation steps, with normalization of the enzyme-inducing effects of nicotine occurring after 4 days of abstinence [6].

Caffeine is metabolized in the liver into 10% theobromine, 4% theophylline, and 80% paraxanthine (Cornish and Christman 1957), so this means that theobromine can be found in the human body even without intake of chocolate.

Only 3% of non-metabolized caffeine is excreted through the urine.

16.3 Caffeine, Coffee, Tea, and Energy Drinks

Caffeine (1,3,7-trimethylxanthine) taken in coffee and tea can be considered the world's most widely consumed psychostimulant. About 90% of the adult population takes these beverages daily, with important regional differences [16]. Coffee is preferred to tea in most developed countries (except in England and Ireland) where 71.5% of the total amount of coffee is consumed. Tea is (until now) preferred in the developing countries, particularly in Asia, Argentina, Chile, Paraguay, and Uruguay. These countries count

for over three quarters of the tea consumption in the world. The total quantity of tea consumed is much higher than coffee, and tea is thus the second beverage consumed after water.

The use of the so-called energy drinks seems to be on the rise especially among young people in the developed world [37, 43] and in the sports population, with between 50% and 70% of elite athletes taking these drinks [11]. In the USA the sale of energy drinks increased from 100 to 600 million dollars between 2002 and 2006 [37], with prevalence of use increasing significantly in adolescents and middle-aged adults between 2003 and 2016 [42].

It should be kept in mind that coffee and tea contain several other components that can be responsible for potential beneficial and adverse health effects, such as antioxidants (e.g., polyphenols, catechins, flavonoids). Also, the way the beverages are prepared (filtered or unfiltered coffee) and what is added (sugar, milk, creamer, flavors) will have a potential impact on health. Caffeine (mostly artificial) is also added in different soft and energy drinks, as well as in prescribed and over-the-counter medications.

In Europe, the typical dose of caffeine for a cup a coffee is around 60–70 mg; for a cup of tea, 35 mg; for a glass of Coca-Cola, 46 mg; and for an energy drink, about 80 mg [13].

In the USA, the average consumption of caffeine is 280 mg per day, which is the equivalent of two cups of filtered coffee per day. Soft drinks contain variable amounts of caffeine, but official FDA limits are 71 mg per drink of 12 oz. (355 mL). The so-called energy drinks can contain up to 300 mg of caffeine per drink of 250 mL and up to 500 mg for a bottle [37] (*see* Table 16.1 *for caffeine content of selected foods, beverages, and drugs*).

Individuals taking six or more cups of coffee per day (over 600–1000 mg of caffeine daily) are considered to be heavy coffee users [5]. In adults, caffeine consumption is considered to be safe at a dose up to 400 mg per day and for adolescents and children up to 2.5 mg/kg per day [10, 36].

With regard to chocolate consumption, inhabitants of Central Europe are considered the champions with over 5 kg of chocolate taken per year,

Table 16.1 Caffeine content in selected food, beverages, and drugs

Product	Serving size	Caffeine per serving (mg)	Caffeine (mg/L)
Percolated coffee	207 mL (7 US fl oz)	80–135	386–652
Drip coffee	207 mL (7 US fl oz)	115–175	555–845
Coffee, decaffeinated	207 mL (7 US fl oz)	5–15	24–72
Coffee, espresso	44–60 mL (1.5–2.0 US fl oz	100	1691–2254
Tea – black, green, and other types – steeped for 3 min	177 mL (6 US fl oz)	22–74	124–416
Guayakí yerba mate (loose leaf)	6 g (200 US fl oz)	85	Approx. 358
Hot cocoa	207 mL (7 US fl oz)	3–13	14–62
Hershey's special dark chocolate (45% cacao content)	1 bar (43 g or 1.5 oz)	31	–
Hershey's milk chocolate (11% cacao content)	1 bar (43 g or 1.5 oz)	10	–
Coca-Cola classic or diet	355 mL (12 US fl oz)	34	96
Mountain dew	355 mL (12 US fl oz)	54	154
Guaraná Antarctica	355 mL (12 US fl oz	30	100
Red bull	250 mL (8.5 US fl oz)	80	320
Cocaine energy drink	250 mL (8.5 US fl oz)	288	1152
Caffeine tablet (regular strength)	1 tablet	100	–
Caffeine tablet (extra strength)	1 tablet	200	–
Excedrin tablet	1 tablet	65	–

References: Bordeaux 2019 and http://en.wikipedia.org/wiki/Caffeine with different validated sources

with Swiss citizens as champions with 8.8 kg/year in 2017, whereas in most Asian countries the average citizen takes less than 200 g of chocolate per year (https://www.statista.com/statistics/819288/worldwide-chocolate-consumption-by-country/). According to the International Cocoa Organization (www.icco.org), the world per capita consumption of cocoa has increased over the last 10 years, from 0.54 kg in 2002/2003 to 0.61 kg in 2010/2011. No updated data are available, but the world cocoa production in 2016 was globally stable compared to 2010/2011.

16.4 Main Effects of Caffeine

Caffeine is mostly taken for its psychostimulating properties: it increases alertness, energy, and ability to concentrate, predominantly in sleep-deprived individuals and also in those working in night shifts and suffering from jet lags [24].

A normal portion of chocolate has also this "arousing" effect, probably through the combined effect of caffeine and theobromine [40]. The counter side of the stimulating effect of caffeine is the occurrence of sleeping difficulties, with little or no tolerance developing for this effect, and the risk of anxiety symptoms including panic attacks in sensitive individuals (Wikoff et al. 2017). Part of these symptoms, occurring after (in general high dose of) coffee intake, can be related to both the psychostimulating effect and tachycardia induced by caffeine [5].

Caffeine increases physical performance, with different studies suggesting that even at 1–2 mg of caffeine per kg of body weight (around one 250 mL serving of an energy drink), reaction time, alertness, and aerobic and anaerobic performance are improved. At higher dose (3 mg caffeine/kg body weight), the ability to repeatedly sprint and the distance covered at high intensity improve, and the jump height increases [11].

The cardiovascular effects of caffeine include mainly the acceleration of heart rate and increase of force of contraction, with heavy caffeine use potentially triggering tachycardia and arrhythmia in susceptible persons. With regard to gastrointestinal effects, caffeine will increase gastric secretion and gastric acidity, possibly influencing absorption of different nutritional and pharmacological elements (e.g., iron), but most studies have been inconclusive. Caffeine stimulates the smooth muscles, thus impacting on bowel function and decreasing constipation [5].

Caffeine probably has a diuretic effect, an effect that is rapid and strong [4], but that has not been found in other study [1]. Probably both gastric and urinary discomforts contribute to spontaneous cessation of coffee intake in the elderly [16].

16.5 Risks of Caffeine Use

Acute Risks
Caffeine has a low-risk profile, but after intake of quantities over 250 mg, especially in non-tolerant subjects, an overstimulation of the central nervous and the cardiovascular system can occur, resulting in what is called a "caffeine intoxication." This clinical entity is mentioned in both the *Diagnostic and Statistical Manual of Mental Disorders* (DSM) and *International Classification of Diseases* (ICD).

In DSM-IV, the caffeine-related disorders were as follows:

- 292.89 – induced anxiety disorder
- 292.89 – induced sleep disorder
- 305.90 – intoxication
- 292.9 – related disorder NOS

The fifth edition of the DSM (DSM-V) includes the following diagnoses related to caffeine: caffeine intoxication, caffeine withdrawal, other caffeine-induced disorders (e.g., anxiety and sleep disorders), and unspecified caffeine-related disorder.

"Caffeine use disorder" is not included in DSM-V, but is included in Sect. III (Emerging measures and models) in order to encourage further research on the issue (www.dsm5.org).

For the ICD-10 criteria of caffeine intoxication, please see Table 16.2.

The incidence of caffeine intoxication seems to be increasing; it occurs mainly in young patients, mainly due to the use of caffeine-containing medications or energy drinks (not due to coffee intake), and when hospitalization is necessary, there is in general co-occurring use of other psychoactive substances or pharmaceutical products [32]. Death from caffeine overdose has been described [19], but it is not clear if in these cases patients have taken medications or have genetic cytochrome abnormalities inhibiting caffeine metabolism. Based on animal studies, the median lethal dose was estimated to be 192 mg/kg; when extrapolating to humans, this should correspond to an intake of around 10 g of caffeine, corresponding to 80–100 cups of coffee [34], making the occurrence of overdose with regular coffee not very probable.

16.6 Chronic Risks of Caffeine Use

Caffeine Dependence and Addiction
"Caffeine dependence" and "caffeine abuse" were not included in the DSM-IV, even if these terms are frequently used in the lay and medical literature. In general, there are not sufficient criteria to establish the diagnosis of caffeine dependence, even if 50% of regular caffeine users will present with withdrawal symptoms in case of acute abstinence. In the DSM-V "caffeine use disorder" has been added as a research diagnosis only (see above).

As caffeine intoxication, the caffeine withdrawal syndrome is included in both DSM and ICD classifications. The ICD-10 criteria for the caffeine withdrawal state (F15.3) are found in Table 16.2. ICD-11, to be introduced in the coming years, also covers caffeine withdrawal (and different other caffeine-related symptoms) but not caffeine use disorder (https://icd.who.int/browse11/l-m/en).

The caffeine withdrawal syndrome is probably largely underdiagnosed. It can occur after sudden abstinence from regular caffeine even at rather low intake of 100 mg daily [21]. The most frequent symptoms are headache, fatigue, decreased energy/activeness, decreased alertness, drowsiness, decreased contentedness, depressed mood, difficulty concentrating, irritability, and being foggy/not clearheaded. Symptoms occur after 12–24 h of abstinence and last for several days. The severity and duration of symptoms are related to the amount of regular caffeine intake. Juliano and Griffiths (2004) suggest that expectancies are not a prime determinant of caffeine withdrawal and that avoidance of withdrawal symptoms plays a central role in habitual caffeine consumption.

Patients who are hospitalized and depending on their state or inpatient regulations (decaffeinated coffee only in psychiatric settings) can find themselves in caffeine withdrawal with symptoms that can be misinterpreted or unrecognized. For instance, for a patient suffering from head trauma and not receiving his daily coffee, the severity of the headache can very well be influenced by the lack of caffeine.

The same misinterpretation can occur during expeditions at high altitude. For practical reasons or fear of increasing sleeplessness and risk of dehydration, caffeine intake is often stopped in this context. Several symptoms of altitude sickness and caffeine withdrawal are common, such as headache, fatigue, and lassitude [17]. Hackett suggests that during expeditions caffeine likely will have more beneficial than negative effects, especially in regular coffee drinkers.

Table 16.2 ICD 10 criteria for intoxication and withdrawal state of caffeine and other stimulants (other than cocaine, F 14.0)

F15.0 Acute intoxication due to use of other stimulants, including caffeine

A. The general criteria for acute intoxication (F1x.0) must be met

B. There must be dysfunctional behavior or perceptual abnormalities, as evidenced by at least one of the following:

  1. Euphoria and sensation of increased energy

  2. Hypervigilance

  3. Grandiose beliefs or actions

  4. Abusiveness or aggression

  5. Argumentativeness

  6. Lability of mood

  7. Repetitive stereotyped behaviors

  8. Auditory, visual, or tactile illusions

  9. Hallucinations, usually with intact orientation

  10. Paranoid ideation

  11. Interference with personal functioning

C. At least two of the following signs must be present

  1. Tachycardia (sometimes bradycardia)

  2. Cardiac arrhythmias

  3. Hypertension (sometimes hypotension)

  4. Sweating and chills

  5. Nausea and vomiting

  6. Evidence of weight loss

  7. Pupillary dilatation

  8. Psychomotor agitation (sometimes retardation)

  9. Muscular weakness

  10. Chest pain

  11. Convulsions

F15.3 Withdrawal state from other stimulants, including caffeine

A. The general criteria for withdrawal state (F1x.3) must be met

B. There is dysphoric mood (for instance, sadness or anhedonia)

C. Any two of the following signs must be present

  1. Lethargy and fatigue

  2. Psychomotor retardation or agitation

  3. Craving for stimulant drugs

  4. Increased appetite

  5. Insomnia or hypersomnia

  6. Bizarre or unpleasant dreams

From ICD-10 [20]

16.6.1 Other Chronic Risks

Heavy caffeine use is often associated with increased risk for other substance use or addictive disorders and mental health disorders such as adult hyperactivity syndrome. This correlation does absolutely not mean causality, but different studies suggest a two- to threefold increase of prevalence of tobacco dependence or problematic alcohol use for those consuming more than six to seven cups of coffee per day compared to those taking one to two cups [5, 16]. The combined (and increasing) use of energy drinks with alcohol in adolescents and young adults deserves specific attention.

Caffeine can induce panic attacks in some individuals, but seems not be correlated to the occurrence of negative outcomes of chronic psychiatric problems. A link between heavy caffeine use and schizophrenic relapse has been suggested but not confirmed [16]. Generally speaking, no association between psychiatric disorders and caffeine has been found after controlling for genetic and environmental factors [23].

Several studies suggest a correlation between high caffeine intake (>5 cups of coffee daily) and risk of lower bone density and increased risk of fracture, especially in lean elderly women and/or those having low calcium intake, but with tea intake correlated to higher bone density [5, 28].

The use of unfiltered coffee has been associated with increased level of cholesterol, a major risk factor for cardiovascular disease [38]. Still, the effect of filtered and unfiltered coffee on other risk factors is not fully clear, and even if caffeine can induce tachycardia and arrhythmia, the available literature suggests that caffeine has more benefits than risks for cardiovascular disease. A recent study suggests that while energy drink consumption up to a dose of 200 mg is safe, some cardiovascular adverse effect (including QT prolongation) is possible at more than 320 mg [12].

The same seems to be true for the oncology field (see below).

16.7 Benefits of Methylxanthine

16.7.1 Caffeine

As said before, when considering the benefits of caffeine, we remind that there is a difference between the benefits of caffeine itself and the benefits of coffee or other caffeine-containing drinks. Coffee contains hundreds of other com-

pounds that are antioxidants (polyphenols, flavonoids, catechins, melanoidins, etc.) that pass through coffee filters.

Moreover, it is globally difficult to speak only of caffeine because only few publications are about caffeine itself. Most scientific evidence is related to studies on coffee and do not consider the biologic effect of caffeine. In energy drinks, the consequences of caffeine are difficult to isolate from those due to the high content of sugar and other components like vitamins or the amino acid taurine.

First of all, there are strong suggestions that taking caffeine from coffee is associated with a diminution of the risk of total or specific mortality [14]. This study is based on the follow-up of more than 229,000 men and 173,000 women for 13 years. At inclusion, participants' age varied between 50 and 71 years. After adjustment for tobacco-smoking status and other possible biases, the risk of death was inversely correlated to coffee consumption. The benefit became significant at one cup of coffee per day for men (hazard ratio 0.94, 95% confidence interval 0.86–0.93) and at two or three cups of coffee for women (hazard ratio 0.87, 95% confidence interval 0.83–0.92). The benefit tended to rise with the amount of coffee taken, with a statistical inverse correlation between caffeine and mortality. An inverse correlation was also observed for death from respiratory disease, injuries, diabetes, and infection. No association was found between caffeine and cancer-related mortality. These results were confirmed in subgroups, including people in very good health at inclusion. In this study, the inverse correlation for heart disease and stroke was at the limit of statistical significance. An umbrella review of meta-analyses [36] comes to the same conclusions, with an optimal risk reduction for overall mortality at three to four cups of coffee per day. A recent meta-analysis, covering 40 studies and almost four million subjects [25], confirmed these findings and concluded that, compared to no coffee consumption, moderate coffee consumption (defined as two to four cups/day) was associated with reduced all-cause and cause-specific mortality. This inverse association between coffee and all-cause mortality was consistent by potential modifiers (age, overweight, alcohol and tobacco use), except region. The lowest relative risks were 3.5 cups per day for all-cause mortality, 2.5 cups for cardiovascular mortality, and 2 cups for cancer-related mortality.

When searching specific potential benefits of coffee for specific diseases, the most impressive observed effect is on liver disease. A large cohort study [26] (more than 129,000 subjects) was conducted over 20 years, from the 1980s in the USA. A strong inverse correlation was found between cirrhosis and coffee drinking especially when the origin of the cirrhosis was alcohol. In this case, there was a 40% risk reduction in 16-year cirrhosis incidence when people drank one to three cups of coffee (relative risk 0.6, 95% confidence interval 0.4–0.8) and an 80% risk reduction for four or more cups (relative risk 0.2, 95% confidence interval 0.1–0.4). For nonalcoholic cirrhosis, there was no significant risk reduction of caffeine on mortality and a non-significant 30% risk reduction for people drinking four or more cups (relative risk 0.7, 95% confidence interval 0.4–1.3). This relation was not observed for tea drinkers. Other cohort and case-control studies found strong reduction in the risk of liver cancer in coffee drinkers, with an increase in consumption of two cups of coffee per day being associated with a 43% reduced risk of liver cancer (relative risk 0.57, 95% confidence interval 0.49–0.67) (Larsson and Wolk 2007).

Coffee use is also inversely correlated to progression of fibrosis in hepatitis C liver disease (Freedman et al. 2009). The relative risk of two-point increase in fibrosis was 0.70 (0.48–1.02) for one or two cups of coffee a day and 0.47 (0.27–0.85) for three or more cups per day (significant trend). Although these are observational data (for evident ethical reasons, randomized studies will be difficult to realize), it is probable that people suffering from chronic hepatitis C are partially protected from fibrosis progression if they drink coffee on a regular basis.

Furthermore, the same authors found later that drinking coffee was a predictor to improved response to hepatitis C treatment with pegylated interferon and ribavirin (Freedman et al. 2011). The probability to achieve sustained virological response was almost twice for coffee drinkers of three or more cups of coffee daily (odds ratio 1.8, 95% confidence interval 0.8–3.9).

Patients suffering from substance use disorders (legal or illegal) have a higher prevalence cardiovascular risk factors and disease than the general population. Tobacco smoking is more common in this population; one study suggests there is not a lower physical activity or unbalanced diet (Berg and Høstmark 1996), but this study included few and young participants (22-year-olds). Interventions promoting cardiovascular and heart health are important in the addicted population.

For the general population, caffeine consumption was considered to have a negative impact on the cardiovascular system until the 1990s. More recent studies suggest that coffee has no effect on the incidence of cardiovascular events and even suggest a small benefit for people without preexisting cardiac disease.

While people drinking coffee had a trend (at the limit of statistical significance) for beneficial cardiovascular effect in the first study discussed in this section [14], other studies show an inverse relation was mortality [25], and others detected no association concerning men and a reduction in the cardiovascular mortality for women (relative risk of death 0.83, confidence interval 0.73–0.95) [30]. For stroke, a 20% reduction of relative risk has been found in a cohort study of women (Larsson et al. 2011); this was consistent with the results of another study concerning men (Larsson et al. 2008).

The effect of caffeine on insulin resistance is controversial and probably depends on the source of caffeine and the duration of exposition. At short term, caffeine has been shown to diminish insulin sensitivity (Beaudoin and Graham 2011). In a randomized controlled study, a dosage from 400 mg caffeine per day for a week showed a decrease of 35% (95% confidence interval 7–62%) of insulin sensitivity [31]. In another study, sweet caffeinated beverages tended to increase type 2 diabetes (Malik et al. 2010). Still, it was not possible to separate the effect of sugar or caffeine. The long-term effect of pure caffeine from other sources than tea or coffee seems to have the opposite effect in animal models, ameliorating the insulin sensitivity and neutralizing the negative metabolic of sucrose in rats [33], but this study was conducted not in humans but in type I diabetic rats. In humans, the regular consumption of coffee has been clearly linked to decrease the incidence of type 2 diabetes (Huxley et al. 2009). In this study, the relative risk was diminished by 7% for any additional cup of coffee or tea absorbed. This effect was not associated with certainty to caffeine as it was also observed with decaffeinated coffee.

Caffeine also influences the metabolism of uric acid and occurrence of gout [8]. In this large observational study, more than 50,000 men without former episode of gout were followed for 12 years. The relative risk of incidental gout was reduced by almost 60% (relative risk 0.41, 95% confidence interval 0.19–0.88) for the group consuming a large amount of coffee (six cups a day or more). The smallest efficient dose for gout protection was four to five cups of coffee a day with a 40% risk reduction (relative risk 0.60, 95% confidence interval 0.41–0.87). This was clearly linked to coffee and not caffeine, as this protective effect was not observed with tea or other sources of caffeine.

Tea and coffee (at a dosage of 300 mg caffeine per day) have been shown to protect against Parkinson's disease, with a risk reduction of 25% (relative risk 0.75, 95% confidence interval 0.68–0.82) (Costa et al. 2010), excluding women taking hormonal replacement after menopause.

A neuroprotective effect of coffee on Alzheimer's disease has been suggested, but this assumption is based on a small number of observational studies (Barranco Quintana 2007). The risk reduction could be 30% (relative risk 0.7, 95% confidence interval 0.55–0.9). Still, a more recent meta-analysis [29] suggested there was no link between caffeine intake and Alzheimer's disease or other forms of dementia.

A case-control study in Australia confirmed the potential benefit of caffeine to prevent road accidents (Sharwood et al. 2013). More than 500 professional drivers involved in crash accidents were compared to controls. After adjustment for confounding factors, drivers who consumed caffeine (from coffee, tea, energy drinks, or tablets) had a risk reduction of 63% of being involved in an accident (odds ratio 0.37, 95% confidence interval 0.27–0.50). This is probably due to the psychostimulant properties of caffeine (increase alertness, lessen fatigue, promote memory, prevent errors to people who are tired or working on night shift) [24]. Also in light drinkers, the accident reduction was found; this is an argument against that it was only an effect of the reversal of withdrawal (Childs and de Wit 2006).

Another well-established positive effect from caffeine is the enhancement of physical capacities [7]. The most effective dosage for this purpose seems to be around 3 mg caffeine per kilogram of weight. Positive impact was found on intermittent effort sports (e.g., soccer), continued effort sports lasting until 1 h (e.g., swimming), or endurance sports (e.g., running). The enhancing effect of caffeine is so significant that for a long time, caffeine was considered a doping substance controlled by the World Anti-Doping Agency (WADA). In 2004 caffeine was removed from the list (www.wada-ama.org).

The potential analgesic properties of caffeine are subject of debate. Caffeine is successfully used in the treatment of headache or migraine [15] and is a frequent component of combined analgesics or other medication (e.g., when mixed with paracetamol or salicylates or antihistamines). On the other hand, it can be the cause of headache [3] as caffeine withdrawal symptom.

Coffee and tea also seem to present benefit for mental health based on a data of a large cohort from the Nurses' Health Study. More than 50,000 women not suffering from depression at baseline were followed between 1996 and 2006 and stratified by their consumption of caffeine (Lucas et al. 2011). During the follow-up, women consuming four cups or more of coffee per day had a 0.80 relative risk of developing depression when compared to the group consuming one cup per week or less (95% confidence interval 0.68–0.95). This effect seems related to caffeine itself as it was not observed for women drinking decaffeinated coffee. These results are coherent with data from other studies showing an inverse correlation between coffee, depression, and suicide [22].

16.7.2 Theophylline

Theophylline, another methylxanthine (1,3-dimethyl-xanthine), is found in medication and in small quantity in tea, coffee, chocolate, mate, and guarana. Its principal indications are related to its bronchodilatative properties and immunomodulatory effects [41]. It is known to restore the sensitivity to corticosteroids in asthma. Consequently, theophylline is used in asthma and chronic obstructive pulmonary disease. It seems that it could also be useful for the prevention of acute kidney injury caused by radiologic contrast product (Dai et al. 2012). It is not as psychoactive as caffeine and not known to be a substance of abuse.

16.7.3 Theobromine

There is a popular belief that theobromine, a third methylxanthine, found principally in guarana, cacao, and chocolate, has a euphoric effect, but no studies can confirm this. The appetite for chocolate would be more linked to other methylxanthine such as caffeine and taste or cultural influences. So up to know, there are no proven benefits for theobromine [39].

16.7.4 Caffeine Abuse Treatment

In case of acute intoxication (Yew 2018), which necessitates more than 70 mg/kg of caffeine intake, (Bronstein et al. 2010), clinical management should be "supportive." The first action is to give standard protocols for cardiac life or other support (ABCs) [35], then give oxygen to the patient, and check the blood glucose. In case of extreme anxiety, agitation, or seizure and lack of effect of non-pharmacological interventions, give short-acting benzodiazepines (e.g., lorazepam orally when possible or intravenously/intramuscularly).

Activated charcoal is effective in reducing the absorption of methylxanthine and recommended early in the treatment. If needed, the patient should be transferred to an emergency unit where the care will also be supportive. Cardiovascular or neurologic toxicities are the most frequent. Sinus tachycardia occurs but does, in general, not require any intervention, but arrhythmia does. In case of extremely high caffeine levels, a dialysis or hemofiltration may be necessary.

Gastric lavage is rarely done because of aspiration risk. Caffeine is rapidly absorbed, and gastric lavage should not be considered unless in less than one hour after intake.

In case of withdrawal, no specific treatment or intervention was found in scientific publications. Anyway, caffeine withdrawal is not dangerous and self-limited, so no intervention is needed and a wait-and-see approach privileged. Nevertheless, the main problems during caffeine withdrawal are fatigue, lack of concentration, or headache. We can recommend general interventions such as rest, physical activity, and good fluid and electrolyte supply. In case of severe headaches, simple analgesia (e.g., paracetamol) could be used. If the time to go through withdrawal is really not adequate, for example, in case of professional or familial obligations, caffeine (in a limited dose) could be taken in the form of coffee, a caffeine-containing drink, or a tablet, and complete and slow withdrawal conducted later. For regular caffeine users who will be exposed to a period of caffeine abstinence (e.g., planned medical intervention), a decrease of daily caffeine intake days before is recommended [13]. Currently, no effective interventions to reduce excessive energy drink consumption exist [42].

16.8 International Perspectives

Currently, coffee, tea, and other caffeine-containing drinks are legally available in all countries and not subjected to regulation. Based on our review of benefits and risks of methylxanthines, we believe that there is no rationale to change this. This seems neither necessary nor useful in a public health or cultural perspective, as prohibition certainly will have a number of unwanted side effects. Nevertheless, information and warning (on package of food or drinks) are probably warranted, indicating the risk of high doses of caffeine and when mixed with alcohol and when relevant the risk of sugar, calories, or other compounds.

The FDA has warned four companies about adding caffeine to alcoholic beverages in 2010 [18] and stated that a further action, including the seizure of products, is possible under federal law. The FDA stated that caffeine is an "unsafe food additive" when mixed with alcohol.

Another international measure that we consider useful would be a limitation of the amount of caffeine in energy drinks. It seems difficult to reach toxic levels of caffeine when a drink contains 50–100 mg of caffeine. Nevertheless, content of 500 mg caffeine in one drink can represent a real danger, especially for children or teenagers, given their lower body weight and the propensity to like those drinks.

16.9 Conclusion

Safe caffeine use is possible and moderate coffee use (200–400 mg of caffeine per day) probably has more physical and psychological benefits than risks. Relative contraindications for caffeine intake are uncompensated heart disease, anxiety, and sleeping problems. Since most studies on caffeine use are observational, we can of course not recommend the use of caffeine or other methylxanthines for medical reasons to those who do not drink. The studies are merely based on cohorts of individuals drinking coffee and tea, so the use of these beverages should be privileged and not of energy drinks. Energy drinks lack several compounds found in coffee or tea (antioxidants) and contain others that possibly have a negative impact on health (sugar). In case of liver disease, especially if related to alcohol and HCV, a daily intake of at least five cups of coffee can be reasonably rec-

ommended to diminish the progression of the disease.

Coffee and caffeine withdrawal symptoms exist and are often not recognized, especially in treatment settings, where caffeine withdrawal can be confounded with other symptoms. Caffeine withdrawal occurs in half of regular coffee drinkers, even at moderate caffeine intake. The most common symptoms are headache, fatigue, and difficulty to concentrate. Health professionals and patients should be better informed about these symptoms and the risk of occurrence of caffeine withdrawal.

Caffeine intoxication and withdrawal are recognized clinical entities, but caffeine dependence, nor caffeine use disorder, is currently not. Some individuals can meet difficulties in controlling their caffeine intake and present withdrawal symptoms in case of abstinence, but most often other criteria of dependence are lacking. In some cases, such behavior seems close to an obsessive-compulsive or eating disorder.

In psychiatric inpatient settings, often only decaffeinated coffee is available. We recommend, for the reasons mentioned above, and a probable positive effect of caffeine in depressive symptoms, that both caffeinated and decaffeinated coffee be at the disposition of the patients, with restriction for those who suffer from anxiety or insomnia. Caffeine taken from coffee seems to be without risk for most psychiatric patients. Personalized recommendations (maximum daily quantity of caffeine, time limit) are probably more appropriate than constraining all patients to abstain from coffee consumption.

Finally, we highly recommend more and better information to the population about the risk of acute intoxication of caffeine, the nutritional and metabolic risks of energy drinks, and the problems of mixing these with alcohol. Warning messages on caffeine-containing food or drinks as well as a legal limitation of the content of caffeine (e.g., maximum 200 mg per unit) are certainly justified. They should be promoted in all countries.

References

1. Armstrong LE, Pumerantz AC, Roti MW, Judelson DA, Watson G, Dias JC, Sokmen B, Casa DJ, Maresh CM, Lieberman H, Kellogg M. Fluid, electrolyte, and renal indices of hydration during 11 days of controlled caffeine consumption. Int J Sport Nutr Exerc Metab. 2005;15:252.
2. Beach CA, Mays DC, Guiler RC, Jacober CH, Gerber N. Clinical inhibition of elimination of caffeine by disulfiram in normal subjects and recovering alcoholics. Pharmacol Ther. 1986;39:265–70.
3. Bigal ME, Sheftell FD, Rapoport AM, Tepper SJ, Lipton RB. Chronic daily headache: identification of factors associated with induction and transformation. Headache. 2002;42:575–81.
4. Bird ET, Parker BD, Kim HS, Coffield KS. Caffeine ingestion and lower urinary tract symptoms in healthy volunteers. Neurourol Urodyn. 2005;24:611.
5. Bordeaux B, Lieberman HR. Benefits and risks of caffeine and caffeinated beverages. 2019. UpToDate. http://www.uptodate.com. Accessed 7 July 2019.
6. Brown CR, Jacob P 3rd, Wilson M, Benowitz NL. Changes in rate and pattern of caffeine metabolism after cigarette abstinence. Clin Pharmacol Ther. 1988;43(5):488–91.
7. Burke LM. Caffeine and sports performance. Appl Physiol Nutr Metab 2008; 33:1319.
8. Choi HK, Willett W, Curhan G. Coffee consumption and risk of incident gout in men: a prospective study. Arthritis Rheum. 2007;56:2049.
9. Cornelis MC, El-Sohemy A, Kabagambe EK, Campos H. Coffee, CYP1A2 genotype, and risk of myocardial infarction. JAMA. 2006;295(10):1135–41.
10. Cornelis MC. The impact of caffeine and coffee on human health. Nutrients. 2019;11(2):416.
11. Del Coso J, Muñoz-Fernández VE, Muñoz G, Fernández-Elías VE, Ortega JF, Hamouti N, Barbero JC, Muñoz-Guerra J. Effects of a caffeine-containing energy drink on simulated soccer performance. PLoS One. 2012;7(2):e31380.
12. Ehlers A, Marakis G, Lampen A, Hirsch-Ernst KI. Risk assessment of energy drinks with focus on cardiovascular parameters and energy drink consumption in Europe. Food Chem Toxicol. 2019;130: 109–21.
13. Favrod-Coune F, Broers B. The health effect of psychostimulants: a literature review. Pharmaceuticals. 2010;3:2333–61.
14. Freedman ND, Park Y, Abnet CC, Hollenbeck AR, Sinha R. Association of coffee drinking with total and cause-specific mortality. N Engl J Med. 2012;366(20):1891–904.
15. Goldstein J, Silberstein SD, Saper JR, Ryan RE Jr, Lipton RB. Acetaminophen, aspirin, and caffeine in combination versus ibuprofen for acute migraine: results from a multicenter, double-blind, randomized, parallel-group, single-dose, placebo-controlled study. Headache. 2006;46:444–53.
16. Greden JF, Walters A. Caffeine. In: Lowinson JH, et al., editors. Substance abuse, a comprehensive textbook. 2nd ed. Baltimore: Williams & Wilkins; 1992. p. 356–70.
17. Hackett PH. Caffeine at high altitude: java at base-cAMP. High Alt Med Biol. 2010;11(1):13–7.
18. Herndon M. FDA warning letters issued to four makers of caffeinated alcoholic beverages. This beverages present a public health concern. U.S. Food and Drugs Administration. 2010. http://www.fda.gov/NewsEvents/Newsroom/PressAnnouncements/ucm234109.htm. Accessed 2 May 2013.
19. Holmgren P, Nordén-Pettersson L, Ahlner J. Caffeine fatalities—four case reports. Forensic Sci Int. 2004;139(1):71–73.
20. ICD-10 classification of mental and behavioural disorders: diagnostic criteria for research. WHO http://www.who.int/substance_abuse/terminology/icd_10/en/index.html. Accessed 7 July 2019.
21. Juliano LM, Griffiths RR. A critical review of caffeine withdrawal: empirical validation of symptoms and signs, incidence, severity, and associated features. Psychopharmacology (Berl) 2004;176:1.
22. Kawachi I, Willett WC, Colditz GA, Stampfer MJ, Speizer FE. A prospective study of coffee drinking and suicide in women. Arch Intern Med. 1996;156(5):521–5.
23. Kendler KS, Myers J, O Gardner C. Caffeine intake, toxicity and dependence and lifetime risk for psychiatric and substance use disorders: an epidemiologic and co-twin control analysis. Psychol Med. 2006;36:1717.
24. Ker K, Edwards PJ, Felix LM, Blackhall K, Roberts I. Caffeine for the prevention of injuries and errors in shift workers. Cochrane Database Syst Rev. 2010;(5):CD008508.
25. Kim Y, Je Y, Giovannucci E. Coffee consumption and all-cause and cause-specific mortality: a meta-analysis by potential modifiers. Eur J Epidemiol. 2019;34:731. https://doi.org/10.1007/s10654-019-00524-3. [Epub ahead of print].
26. Klastky AL, Morton C, Udaltsova N, Friedman GD. Coffee, cirrhosis and transaminases enzymes. Arch Int Med. 2006;166:1190–5.
27. Knutti R, Rothweiler H, Schlatter C. The effect of pregnancy on the pharmacokinetics of caffeine. Arch Toxicol. 1982;5:187–92.
28. Korpelainen R, Korpelainen J, Heikkinen J, et al. Lifestyle factors are associated with osteoporosis in lean women but not in normal and overweight women: a population-based cohort study of 1222 women. Osteoporos Int. 2003;14:34.
29. Larsson CL, Orsini N. Coffee consumption and risk of dementia and Alzheimer's disease: a dose-response meta-analysis of prospective studies. Nutrients. 2018;10(10):1501. https://doi.org/10.3390/nu10101501.
30. Lopez-Garcia E, van Dam RM, Li TY, Rodriguez-Artalejo F, Hu FB. The relationship of coffee consumption with mortality. Ann Intern Med. 2008;148:904–14.

31. MacKenzie T, Comi R, Sluss P, Keisari R, Manwar S, Kim J, Larson R, Baron JA. Metabolic and hormonal effects of caffeine: randomized, double-blind, placebo-controlled crossover trial. Metabolism. 2007;56:1694–8.

32. McCarthy DM, Mycyk MB, DesLauriers CA. Hospitalization for caffeine abuse is associated with abuse of other pharmaceutical products. Am J Emerg Med. 2008;26:799.

33. Park S, Jang JS, Hong SM. Long-term consumption of caffeine improves glucose homeostasis by enhancing insulinotropic action through islet insulin/insulin-like growth factor 1 signaling in diabetic rats. Metabolism. 2007;56(5):599–607.

34. Peters JM. Factors affecting caffeine toxicity: a review of the literature. J Clin Pharmacol and J New Drugs. 1967;7:131–41.

35. Pohler H. Caffeine intoxication and addiction. The Journal for Nurse Practicioners 2010; 6(1):49–52.

36. Poole R, Kennedy OJ, Roderick P, Fallowfield JA, Hayes PC, Parkes J. Coffee consumption and health: umbrella review of meta-analyses of multiple health outcomes. BMJ. 2017;359:j5024.

37. Reissig CJ, Strain EC, Griffiths RR. Caffeinated energy drinks-a growing problem. Drug Alcohol Depend. 2009;99:1–10.

38. Rodrigues IM, Klein LC. Boiled or filtered coffee? Effects of coffee and caffeine on cholesterol, fibrinogen and C-reactive protein. Toxicol Rev. 2006;25(1):55–69.

39. Smit HJ. Theobromine and the pharmacology of cocoa. Handb Exp Pharmacol. 2011;200:201–34.

40. Smit HJ, Gaffan EA, Rogers PJ. Methylxanthines are the psycho-pharmacologically active constituents of chocolate. Psychopharmacology (Berl). 2004;76(3–4):412–9.

41. Somerville LL. National Heart Lung and Blood Institute (NHLBI). Theophylline revisited. Allergy Asthma Proc. 2001;22(6):347–51.

42. Striley CW, Swain MJ. Interventions for excessive energy drink use. Curr Opin Psychiatry. 2019;32(4):288–92.

42. Vercammen KA, Koma WJ, Bleich SN. Trends in energy drink consumption among U.S. adolescents and adults, 2003–2016. Am J Prev Med. 2019;56(6):827–33. https://doi.org/10.1016/j.amepre.2018.12.007. PMID: 31005465

43. Wolk BJ, Ganetsky M, Babu KM. Toxicity of energy drinks. Curr Opin Pediatr. 2012;24(2):243–51.

Further Reading

Barranco Quintana JL, Allam MF, Serrano Del Castillo A, Fernández-Crehuet Navajas R. Alzheimer's disease and coffee: a quantitative review. Neurol Res. 2007;29(1):91–5.

Beaudoin MS, Graham TE. Methylxanthines and human health: epidemiological and experimental evidence. Handb Exp Pharmacol. 2011;200:509–48.

Berg JE, Høstmark AT. Cardiovascular risk factors in young drug addicts. Addict Biol. 1996;1(3):297–302.

Bronstein AC, Spyker DA, Cantilena LR Jr, Green JL, Rumack BH, Giffin SL. 2009 annual report of the American Association of Poison Control Centers' National Poison Data System (NPDS): 27th annual report. Clin Toxicol (Phila). 2010;48(10):979–1178.

Childs E, de Wit H. Subjective, behavioral, and physiological effects of acute caffeine in light, nondependent caffeine users. Psychopharmacology (Berl). 2006;185(4):514–23.

Cornish HH, Christman AA. A study of the metabolism of theobromine, theophylline, and caffeine in man. J Biol Chem. 1957;228(1):315–23.

Costa J, Lunet N, Santos C, Santos J, Vaz-Carneiro A. Caffeine exposure and the risk of Parkinson's disease: a systematic review and meta-analysis of observational studies. J Alzheimers Dis. 2010;20(Suppl 1):S221–38.

Dai B, Liu Y, Fu L, Li Y, Zhang J, Mei C. Effect of theophylline on prevention of contrast-induced acute kidney injury: a meta-analysis of randomized controlled trials. Am J Kidney Dis. 2012;60(3):360–70.

Freedman ND, Everhart JE, Lindsay KL, Ghany MG, Curto TM, Shiffman ML, Lee WM, Lok AS, Di Bisceglie AM, Bonkovsky HL, Hoefs JC, Dienstag JL, Morishima C, Abnet CC, Sinha R, HALT-C Trial Group. Coffee intake is associated with lower rates of liver disease progression in chronic HCV. Hepatology. 2009;50:1360–9.

Freedman ND, Curto TM, Lindsay KL, Wright EC, Sinha R, Everhart JE, HALT-C TRIAL GROUP. Coffee consumption is associated with response to peginterferon and ribavirin therapy in patients with chronic hepatitis C. Gastroenterology. 2011;140(7):1961–9.

Huxley R, Lee CM, Barzi F, Timmermeister L, Czernichow S, Perkovic V, Grobbee DE, Batty D, Woodward M. Coffee, decaffeinated coffee, and tea consumption in relation to incident type 2 diabetes mellitus: a systematic review with meta-analysis. Arch Intern Med. 2009;169(22):2053–63.

Larsson SC, Wolk A. Coffee consumption and risk of liver cancer a meta-analysis. Gastroenterology. 2007;132:1740–5.

Larsson SC, Männistö S, Virtanen MJ, Kontto J, Albanes D, Virtamo J. Coffee and tea consumption and risk of stroke subtypes in male smokers. Stroke. 2008;39:1681–7.

Larsson SC, Virtamo J, Wolk A. Coffee consumption and risk for stroke in women. Stroke. 2011;42:908–12.

Lucas M, Mirzaei F, Pan A, Okereke OI, Willett WC, O'Reilly ÉJ, Koenen K, Ascherio A. Coffee, caffeine, and risk of depression among women. Arch Intern Med. 2011;171(17):1571–8.

Malik VS, Popkin BM, Bray GA, Després JP, Willett WC, Hu FB. Sugar-sweetened beverages and risk of metabolic syndrome and type 2 diabetes: a meta-analysis. Diabetes Care. 2010;33(11):2477–83.

Sharwood LN, Elkington J, Meuleners L, Ivers R, Boufous S, Stevenson M. Use of caffeinated substances and risk of crashes in long distance drivers of commercial vehicles: case-control study. BMJ. 2013;346:f1140.

Wikoff D, Welsh BT, Henderson R, Brorby GP, Britt J, Myers E, Goldberger J, Lieberman HR, O'Brien C, Peck J, Tenebein M, Weaver C, Harvey S, Urban J, Doepker C. Systematic review of the potential adverse effects of caffeine consumption in healthy adults, pregnant women, adolescents, and children. Food Chem Toxicol. 2017;109(Pt 1):585–648.

Yew D. Caffeine toxicity. 2018. Medscape. https://emedicine.medscape.com/article/821863-overview. Accessed 7 July 2019.

Khat Addiction

17

Michael Odenwald, Axel Klein, and Nasir Warfa

Contents

Abstract

Khat leaves are traditionally consumed in African and Arab countries around the Horn of Africa. The central and peripheral stimulant alkaloid cathinone (S-(-)-a-aminopropiophenone) is considered to be the main psychoactive compound in the khat leaves. The leaves and tender stems are usually chewed and kept in a tight wad in the cheek pocket. Within about 15–30 minutes, the user experiences physiological excitability, euphoria, talkativeness, and flow of ideas. While khat production and consumption is popular in traditional user countries and use patterns swiftly change to excessive usage, particularly in East Africa, the substance is treated as illegal in the rest of the world. Today, cathinone is listed in Schedule I of the 1971 International Convention on Psychotropic Substances, although the leaves

M. Odenwald (✉)
Department of Psychology, Konstanz University, Konstanz, Germany
e-mail: michael.odenwald@uni-konstanz.de

A. Klein
Global Drug Policy Observatory, University of Swansea, Swansea, UK

N. Warfa
Maltepe University, Maltepe/İstanbul, Turkey

of khat are not internationally controlled. Khat use is associated with a number of mental health problems. A problem with diagnosis of khat use disorders is that established criteria are not easily applicable. Since the first edition of this textbook, some research has been done on khat; however, the current empirical knowledge base is still limited on prevalence and use patterns; most studies that associate khat use with mental and physical health problems have weak designs and treatment studies are rare. There is a need to build up research and treatment capacities in the main khat use countries. There is also a need to develop adequate legal regulations, monitoring systems, and public health responses that moderate between economic, cultural, and health viewpoints.

Keywords

Khat · Qat · Miraa · *Catha edulis* · Cathinone

17.1   Introduction

Khat refers to the young and tender leaves and shoots of the khat tree (*Catha edulis*). It is an evergreen tree of the Celastraceae family. It grows to 6 m in height, and 25 m under warm equatorial climate. *Catha edulis* can be found in the Abyssinian highlands, East Africa and in the southern Arab peninsula [64]. Khat has many names including *qat* (Yemen), *jad/chat* (Ethiopia, Somalia), *miraa* (Kenya), and *marungi* (Kenya, Uganda). The leaves and twigs of khat have been consumed for centuries for their mildly stimulating properties. Khat has several alkaloids and more than 40 known different chemical compounds. The alkaloid cathinone (S-(-)-a-aminopropiophenone) is considered to be the main psychoactive compound. It is unstable as it swiftly decomposes soon after harvesting. Cathinone resembles amphetamine in chemical structure and has a stimulating effect on the central and peripheral nervous system and behavior

similarly [33]. In the anthropological literature, the effect of khat as well as its cultural integration has often been compared to coffee and caffeine. Recently, synthetic cathinone derivates such as mephedrone constitute a large group among the "novel psychoactive substances" that are known as "legal highs" [24]. More stable compounds of the khat leaves are cathine (S,S-(+)-norpseudoephedrine) and other alkaloids which are at the same time metabolites of cathinone and less potent central and peripheral stimulants.

While consumers prefer chewing fresh leaves, dried leaves are used when no fresh khat is available or is too expensive. Soon after harvesting, the fresh twigs, leaves, and shoots of khat are artfully rolled into bundles and wrapped into banana leaves to retain their moisture. Such bundles form the standard unit of consumption, though leaves of lower quality are also sold in plastic bags. Traditionally, khat is used in group sessions in private homes and at specific khat establishments ("marfrish") that start from early afternoon and finish evening hours. During these chewing hours, some users accompany khat with cigarettes, water pipe, carbonated soft drinks, and sometimes chewing gums. Consumers pick off leaves and tender stems and form a tight wad in their cheek pocket where they are slowly chewed over hours. Within the first 15–30 minutes, the effects reach the "mirqaan" (high), a psychological state marked by euphoria, talkativeness, and a flow of ideas. This is followed by a quieter and introvert phase, often accompanied by irritability, anxiousness or depression, and then a gradual come-down. The experience may disturb sleeping patterns in the following night and is liable to produce hangover the next morning. In order to balance off these unwanted feelings, some khat chewers carry on chewing for prolonged longer sessions.

The khat research field is still in its infancy. Although scientific literature on khat is steeply increasing, the quantity of peer-reviewed papers, however, is small compared to the use prevalence [69]. The quality of the research, methods, and methodologies is not consistent, and key khat studies have not yet been replicated. One important challenge for the external validity of khat research is that main user populations are deprived, and studies need to control for potential confounding factors. There is a great need to build up research capacity in the traditional khat use countries.

17.2   The Khat Controversy

The legal, economic, social, and religious controversies around khat, and the question of whether it is a drug or a part of cultural heritage, are as old as the existence of khat itself [42]. Medieval writings and ancient legend anecdotes narrate the ambivalent attitudes toward its effects that are sometimes described as helpful and joyful, noxious, and damaging at other times [42]. It has been condemned by the Ethiopian Orthodox Church and Islamic Scholars who consider it to be harmful or "haram." On the other hand, some moderate Islamic scholars in Somalia and Ethiopia integrated khat use into religious rituals. For moderate Sufi Muslims, the justification made is to stay awake at night time in order to cite religious texts, particularly during the month of Ramadan in order to stay awake until late in the evening. The use of khat is controversial as it regularly stirs emotions across diverse secular, religious, cultural, and economic groups (e.g., [13, 64]). During the colonial era, arguments about moral degeneration, falling economic productivity, and the association of khat use with political unrest motivated officials to ban khat in countries like Somalia or Yemen, but these attempts led to political opposition and were largely unsuccessful (Klein, Beckerleg and Hailu 2009; [25, 39]). Likewise, strong pro-khat movements prevented the introduction of legal restrictions in the traditional khat-producing and khat-consuming countries.

Similarly, the scientific discourse on khat is dominated by disagreements along the lines of various competing academic disciplines [55]. Medical and pharmacological research approach khat from the underlying assumption that it is analogous to other harmful psychoactive drugs.

Consequently, these studies focus on the pharmacology of psychoactive compounds, as well as the mental and physical health problems linked with khat use. Since the current khat studies lack rigorous study designs, some social scientists warn against the medicalization of khat-related problems. Overall, the negative and positive roles khat play in social, cultural, and economic factors are much debated. One aspect of the literature highlights how khat is consumed for sustaining cultural functions and traditional values [10]. There is an ongoing international debate that these cultural and traditional functions of khat are often overlooked or not fully taken into account by medical research. Others argued that such concepts as addiction are Western and that these do not grasp the philosophy of the mostly non-Western khat users.

This ambiguity is also found in the way khat is seen from a legal perspective. Attempts have been made to include khat leaves and its psychoactive compounds in international and national drug legislation. Cathinone is listed in Schedule I and cathine in Schedule III of the 1971 International Convention on Psychotropic Substances. Fresh khat leaves and twigs, however, are not controlled under the Convention. On national levels, most producer countries allow khat production, use, and trade, e.g. Ethiopia, Kenya, and Yemen. While these countries have put in place some restrictions and taxation schemes, in recent time the official classification of khat has gradually moved from a psychoactive substance to a cash crop. Some of the neighboring countries (e.g., Tanzania) and most of the Western countries, however, have imposed legal restrictions and treat khat as illegal drug [27]. Recently, the UK and the Netherlands (two countries which had been used as transit ports for khat transportation to rest of EU countries and North America) prohibited khat. The objectives behind such prohibitions and the aims of public health protection were questioned from social scientific perspectives [40]. Several countries implemented ambiguous politics, e.g., Saudi Arabia, where khat is banned but its production and use are tolerated in Jazan region neighboring Yemen.

17.3 From a Niche Crop to a Cash Crop

Historically, khat use was confined to certain cultural or ethnic groups. It was used socially during cultural ceremonies and rituals. The elites were stated to chew khat for social purposes but also to get inspirations for artistic expressions in poetry and song composition. They would gather in dedicated rooms within private households and/or in communal places called Marfrish. Other groups who are known for khat use are khat farmers, distance travelers, and university students. These groups are reported to use khat for staying alert or to overcome tiredness. From these earlier times, khat misuse was rarely observed. Outside the few traditional producing areas, khat use was rare. Khat use for medical purposes was noticed by early European travelers, for example, the Swedish botanist Peter Forsskal (1732–1763). By 1900, new patterns of khat use and misuse begin to emerge, which was partly linked to increased availability. In countries like Somalia and Yemen, groups of men from all walks of life would meet to discuss politics, business, and social issues over khat sessions [65]. In the second part of the century, frequent and excessive use has become a regular part of social life for a large number of people in East Africa. With no or limited legal restrictions, the historical and cultural significance of usage gradually eroded, replaced by practices of khat misuse.

Transport innovations, the invention of fast railway networks, road haulages, and affordability of air cargo have facilitated greater commodification and branding. This has created a regional market with attractive conditions for the producers and the development of a whole new industry around khat. All these emerging developments have made khat a popular cash crop from its previous niche markets. To this date, khat is sold and consumed in several regions and countries beyond East Africa and Arabia. New varieties of khat have emerged in response to new khat markets, partly encouraged by immigrants living in the West and elsewhere. After decades of rapid production, the economic significance of the khat sector has dramatically increased. The khat economy provides significant employment and income to farmers, pickers, packers, sellers, and other associated traders in East Africa and the Arab Peninsula [10, 25]. It has been identified as an example of an economic success story for African agricultural producers without any support by development actors and involvement of multinational companies [39]. Consequently, the recent bans in the Netherlands and the UK had negative effects on incomes of khat farmers in Africa [41]. As production has risen in response to increasing demands, new social, health, and ecological challenges have emerged particularly over the use of finite resources. For example, water irrigation for khat production was identified as one of the major factors that contribute to the groundwater decline in Yemen, as well as a contributing factor to deforestation in Ethiopia.

17.4 Development from Traditional Use to Binge Patterns

Despite the growing scientific data on khat, only limited population surveys are available. It is estimated that more than ten million globally use khat for recreational purposes on any 1 day [56]. In Yemen, the pre-civil war estimates vary between 60% and 90% of adult males and 10% and 50% of adult women [25]. Different surveys indicated that Yemeni households spent 9–10% of their income on khat (on average), with low-income groups spending as much as 40% [25]. In Ethiopia, two representative national surveys [30, 62] revealed a current prevalence use of 15–16%, with regional variations of 50% (khat production regions) and 1–3% (in a region where khat is traditionally not consumed); furthermore, male gender, Muslim faith, living in rural areas, wealth, and lower education were positively related to khat use. A recent meta-analysis [26] estimated a national prevalence rate of 23.2% among high school and university students, with considerable regional variations (18.1–31.6%). In Kenya, no prevalence data for the general population is available. A survey conducted from a khat-growing region put a prevalence estimate of 36.8% (lifetime 44.6%; [58]). Other studies of treatment-seeking patients revealed a lifetime prevalence rate of 10.7–30% [48]. From the last population survey carried out in Somalia, regular (or current) khat use was estimated to be between 31% and 64% of adult males in the north of the country and 21% in the South, with excessive khat use patterns found among militia members [22]. In the West, khat use is almost exclusively limited to immigrant groups from khat-producing or khat-consuming countries.

The pattern of khat use has changed significantly over recent decades due in part to the combined consequences of urbanization, commodification, and rapid social changes [10]. The dissolution of traditional and cultural use of khat together with the lack of government regulations has led to the rise of more excessive and extensive use, including early morning use, prolonged binge sessions, as well as the emergency of new patterns of risky use, for example, khat chewing while taking other drugs and substances, e.g., alcohol or benzodiazepines [44, 58, 62]. This illustrates that like other stimulant users, the functional use of "downers," e.g., in order to be able to sleep, has become common among khat users which may be indicative of a shift in the patterns of use and integration into functional lifestyles. Furthermore, today khat chewers frequently smoke tobacco (cigarettes or shisha) during khat sessions [6]. The age in which people start chewing khat also changed. Traditionally, chewers were exposed to the habit from about the age of 20 years, whereas now children as young as 8 years old are reported to use it [56]. Furthermore, what has previously been considered an exclusively male habit is increasingly practiced by women, with a recent study showing significant evidence of khat use by pregnant women in Ethiopia [46].

17.5   What Is Known About Khat Addiction?

While there have been reports of excessive patterns of khat consumption and description of addictive behaviors since colonial times [28], experts consider the harm associated with khat use mild when compared to other psychoactive substances, i.e., similar to MDMA (3,4-methylenedioxy-metham-

phetamine; "Ecstasy") [51]. This is one of the reasons why the WHO Expert Committee on Drug Dependence has repeatedly decided that the misuse potential is too low to merit international controls [68], at least, on medical grounds.

Without firm database, it is believed that prolonged and excessive khat use can potentially produce psychological dependence comparable to amphetamine [68].

Mild and brief withdrawal symptoms upon discontinuation are reported, unless khat is used excessively for extended periods of time [68]. Withdrawal symptoms include profound lassitude, anergia, difficulty in initiating normal activity, mild trembling, and nightmares of paranoid nature, for example, vivid or unpleasant dreams of being attacked, strangled, or followed by strangers (e.g., [38]). Recent studies provided first data on the prevalence of withdrawal symptoms among chewers (any symptom 68.2%; [3]; 28% meeting core requirements for stimulant withdrawal, [21]) and about the course of withdrawal symptoms in the weeks after quit attempts [19].

In the same token, today it is generally believed that with regular consumption over extended periods of time khat chewers become habituated to the physical effect, a process described as "tolerance," often associated with increased levels of consumption [68]. It has been argued that the chewing mode of ingestion limits the possible amount to consume in a certain time, and, thus, tolerance development is usually prevented. This view can be criticized based on recent definitions of tolerance. Among stimulant users, tolerance development, the upward shift in the set point for reward, and the subsequent dysphoria ("opponent process") are closely related to the development of "binge" consumption patterns: Users need to increase the dose and the frequency of drug administration in order to experience the desired psychological effects. Thus, khat tolerance development might not only include increases in the amount of consumption per time unit but rather the extension of the time spent for consuming it which leads to an increase of the absolute amount ingested. Recent studies and personal observations indicate that a growing group of binge users consume khat for more than

24 h in a row in such large quantities a novice would never manage [45, 66, 67]. While the development of tolerance to physiological effects was reported [50], no study has ever directly targeted the topic of tolerance to desired psychological effects, e.g., euphoria. In contrast to the medical view of tolerance development, social scientists highlight that among khat-using populations who are frequently exposed to violence, deprivation, and injustice, increasing levels of khat use are mechanisms of coping with adverse living conditions and of strengthening social and cultural identity. Studies are needed to disentangle the social mechanisms from the pure somatic processes.

Other features of khat addiction that have been the focus of research are craving, the urge to consume khat, and the continuous need to use the substance despite harmful effects and unsuccessful attempts at reducing consumption (e.g., [62]). The dynamic around khat use is illustrated by typical scenes from khat markets where there are situations of heightened euphoria, nervousness, and aggressiveness during or before khat is delivered [29].

Furthermore, observational data confirm the existence of a specific nomenclature for psychological states experienced by Somali khat users, e.g., "jibane" ("eye opener," i.e., early morning use of khat in a group setting in order to reduce aversive symptoms) or "xaraaro" (feelings of urge to chew and nervousness), which point to use-specific reflection on shared experience and a cumulative learning.

A recent study reported that khat chewers enhance the experience of euphoria and other emotional benefits by stepping up consumption of tobacco [35], but studies on co-use of other psychoactives, particularly tea and sugar, are still missing.

17.6 Measurement and Diagnosis of Khat Addiction

A problem with diagnosis of khat use disorders is that established criteria are not easily applicable as is the case for other traditional sub-

stances. Besides the previously mentioned limited knowledge on withdrawal and tolerance, some of the other criteria outlined in DSM-5 (or ICD research criteria) might need further specification to adapt to societies where daily social khat use is rather the rule than the exception and where social khat use is the most widely practiced social and leisure activity, i.e., "… The individual may spend a great deal of time obtaining the substance, using the substance, or recovering from its effects… Important social, occupational, or recreational activities may be given up or reduced because of substance use" [11, p. 483]. In general, the adaption of criteria seems necessary in order to avoid overdiagnosis. Although research has started to address this problem [44], it needs more studies to understand khat-related cultural conventions that establish the range for socially acceptable consumption as well as sanctions for excess, including stigmatization and social exclusion. Recently, studies showed the applicability of the diagnostic criteria as defined by DSM and, at the same time, the skewed distribution highlighting the above-mentioned problem: in the UK, 31% of 204 khat users of Yemeni origin fulfilled the DSM-IV criteria for dependence [37]; in an Ethiopian university student convenience sample ($N = 400$), 10.5% were diagnosed with mild, 8.8% with moderate, and 54.5% with severe khat use disorder according to DSM-5 (using an adapted version of the AUDADIS-IV; [21]).

Limited evidence-based information is emerging from cross-sectional studies on the prevalence of khat use disorders as defined by ICD or DSM criteria. An Ethiopian study [12] used the WHO's Composite International Diagnostic Interview to measure the prevalence of khat dependence according to ICD-10 in a representative sample drawn in a traditional khat-producing area, reporting 5% among males and 1.3% females. Using a structured clinical interview, in a representative sample of 242 Somali refugees in Nairobi, the criteria for substance abuse according to DSM-IV were applied to khat and were fulfilled in 15.3% of khat users [49]. In selected patient or user samples, khat dependence reached much higher levels (e.g., [66]). These studies should be interpreted with caution, because studies developed their own conventions to adapt diagnostic criteria to the reality of khat use.

Validated self-report instruments to screen for and to assess aspects of khat addiction are rare, and few standardized questionnaires have ever been applied in khat users. A general problem is the missing cross-cultural validation of instruments that originally had been developed in Western countries. A khat version of the Severity of Dependence Scale (SDS), a five-item instrument thought to measure the psychological component of dependence, was developed [34] and validated for the study of khat addiction in various languages, including Arab and Amharic [47]. The SDS score correlated with DSM-5 SUD symptoms [18], with more khat-related behaviors and higher khat alkaloid levels in saliva [36]. Furthermore, the Alcohol, Smoking and Substance Involvement Screening Test (ASSIST) was adapted to khat use [67] as well as the Drug Abuse Screening Test-10 (DAST-10; [2]).

17.7 Neurocognitive Deficits and Comorbid Disorders

A common characteristic of chronic central stimulant use is a neurocognitive deficit syndrome. Several studies found poorer working memory among heavy khat users compared to controls [16, 31]. Other studies reported impaired memory functions [32], impaired executive functions, inhibitory control [15], cognitive inflexibility [16], lack of cognitive control [17], as well as problems with perception processing and motor speed [31, 32]. Cognitive deficits among khat chewers, however, were related to age and education [32], and in general, studies did not control for potential confounding factors, i.e., like chronicity of use, recent use, or withdrawal states.

17.8 Comorbid Disorders

Khat use has been associated with the presence of mental distress and psychiatric and physical disorders (for overview [57]) – with heterogeneous assumptions on the type of underlying association.

Comorbidities of khat use with depression, posttraumatic stress disorder, psychotic symptoms, and suicide ideas have been reported [64]. Recent cross-sectional studies found associations between khat use and occurrence of psychotic symptoms (e.g., [5, 21, 58]) as well as with measures of mental distress (e.g., [1]). Functional khat use to counteract symptoms of depression, posttraumatic stress disorder (e.g., [54]), and antipsychotic medication side effects has been described (e.g., [61]). While there is no evidence for a simple causal-effect relationship, khat use per se doesn't seem to be related to the development of psychiatric disorders in healthy individuals, in contrast to specific patters of use, e.g., excessive or prolonged use, but longitudinal studies are missing in order to quantify khat use patterns as specific risk factors. Several studies on brief khat-induced psychotic episodes (for overview, [53]) reported excessive khat use before the onset and violent behavior in the course of the acute psychiatric development; complete remission was observed after 2–4 weeks when abstinence is maintained, but such episodes tended to occur repeatedly. Also the exacerbation of psychotic symptoms and antipsychotic nonadherence in patients with preexisting psychotic disorders have been reported [14, 23, 61]. A few and weak studies found first support in favor of the hypothesis that early, chronic, and severe khat use might be a risk factor for the development of chronic psychotic disorders [52].

The problems of this literature are the cross-sectional design and the use of self-report measures and screening instruments instead of gold standard assessments and biological data.

Besides psychiatric sequelae, numerous physical health problems have been attributed to khat use (for review, see [7, 57]). Observed somatic consequences associated to khat use include mucosal problems, hypertension, cardiovascular complications, duodenal ulcers, sexual dysfunction, hepatoxicity, and problems related to pregnancy and birth (e.g., [9, 59, 60]). Efforts to establish khat consumption as risk factor for physical health problems remain inconclusive because it has not been possible to differentiate between the effects of khat itself, the pesticide contents in khat leaves, and comorbid tobacco smoking and because of other problems related to research design. As with mental health, moderate khat use seems not to be noxious in most users, and adverse effects are commonly linked with the currently growing excessive use. Additionally, some studies showed that khat users (like other substance users) have lower adherence to treatment of physical disorders and infectious diseases (e.g., HIV, [43]).

By the same token, the argument for possible medicinal uses has only been touched on, e.g., probiotic effects.

17.9   Treatment of Khat Addiction

According to the UNODC's annual World Drug Reports, khat users constitute the largest group of patients in substance treatment facilities in Ethiopia and the second largest group in Kenya [63]. However, the UNODC statistics have to be treated with caution, e.g., because the absolute numbers of provided treatments are very small in these countries. Treatment offered to individuals with khat use disorders in traditional khat use countries is usually nonspecific standard psychiatric treatment. Specialized khat addiction programs or treatment facilities are nonexistent. Additionally, some nongovernmental organizations offer counseling.

In Western countries, khat users almost exclusively belong to minority groups from the original khat use countries, and individuals with khat use disorder have been integrated into general treatment programs for illegal substances. Some local initiatives in Western countries (e.g., the UK, Sweden) gained experience in psychosocial support for khat users showing the multifaceted problems of khat-using individuals that seem to be similar to other groups of illegal substance users. Unique has been the building up of a specialized khat addiction treatment center in

Stockholm; however, the utilization and acceptance of this service by the target group was weak.

A recent review [57] revealed the scarcity of scientific studies on psychiatric and psychological treatment offered to individuals with khat use disorders. A problem is the high mental health comorbidity of khat users due to violence in traditional khat use countries. One recent case series reported on a combined treatment of khat dependence according to DSM-IV and comorbid PTSD in Somali refugees with encouraging outcomes [4]. Several studies report on the reduction of khat use in nonclinical groups: In a retrospective study, former khat users reported reasons why they stopped using it [8]. Using the quit date paradigm, 60 healthy Ethiopian university students chewing khat at least three times per week for 2 years with high motivation to stop their use were followed up for 28 days: While 93.2% lapsed, only 6.8% achieved continuous abstinence [20]. One controlled study used Screening and Brief Intervention with 330 Somali khat users from the community (adapted version of the ASSIST-linked Brief Intervention; [67]): The intervention group showed decreased khat use time compared to a control group who just received assessment; among participants without comorbid psychopathology (depression, PTSD), khat use reduction was more pronounced.

17.10   Conclusion

The economic significance of khat production and its use are growing in one of the poorest regions of the world, barely noticed by international health policies, losing sight of the potential public health consequences. The topic of khat use and its related social, mental, and physical health complications urgently need empirical studies. The current empirical knowledge base is weak, while the use of khat is becoming widespread, and patterns of use are changing. Khat research capacities need to be built up in the traditional use countries. Future studies will have to get the full picture of current khat use and to disentangle khat effects from confounding effects (e.g., psychosocial and socioeconomic, environmental effects) using strong methods and designs.

Current evidence supports the hypothesis that khat is used because of its euphorigenic effects and in order to alleviate symptoms of mental distress and that excessive and prolonged khat use can contribute to the development of a range of mental and physical health problems, including khat use disorder. The question of khat-related withdrawal and tolerance needs further studying as well as the neurocognitive consequences of chronic use. For the application of diagnostic criteria for khat use disorder, conventions are lacking plus the development of culturally validated psychodiagnostic measures. The current knowledge base about the treatment for khat use disorders is poor especially as its users rarely utilize or demand for addiction treatment services. The development of commonly accepted, effective, and culturally adequate treatment concepts to be applied in the traditional khat use countries and among khat-using immigrant communities is highly demanded.

It is time for a balanced approach to khat, overcoming the controversies of the past and the romanticized or sensationalist approaches to its use that too often had been deemed an exotic or peculiar habit. Instead, empirical evidence is needed to guide national and international policies and to support law and public health strategies in order to strike a balance between khat-related health and social issues and cultural and economic interests.

References

1. Abbay AG, Mulatu AT, Azadi H. Community knowledge, perceived beliefs and associated factors of mental distress: a case study in northern Ethiopia. Int. J. Environ. Res. Public Health 2018;15:2423. https://doi.org/10.3390/ijerph15112423.
2. Abdelwahab SI, Alsanosy RM, Rahim BEA, Mohan S, Taha S, Elhassan M, El-Setouhy M. Khat (Catha edulis Forsk.) dependence potential and pattern of use in Saudi Arabia. BioMed Res Int. 2015;2015:604526.
3. Abdeta T, Tolessa D, Adorjan K, Abera M. Prevalence, withdrawal symptoms and associated factors of khat chewing among students at Jimma University, Ethiopia. BMC Psychiatry. 2017;17:142.
4. Abednego M, Veltrup C, Warsame AH, Isse MM, Widmann M, Ndetei D, Mutisu V, Odenwald M. Developing an integrated treatment for PTSD and khat dependence: results from a case series among Somali refugees. Paper presented at the XIV conference of European Society for Traumatic Stress Studies, 10–13 June 2015, Vilnius, 2015.
5. Adorjan K, Odenwald M, Widmann M, Tesfaye M, Tessema F, Toennes S, Suleman S, Papiol S, Soboka M, Mekonnen Z, Rockstroh B, Rietschel M, Pogarell O, Susser E, Schulze TG. Khat use and occurrence of psychotic symptoms in the general male population in Southwestern Ethiopia: evidence for sensitization by traumatic experiences. World Psychiatry. 2017;16(3):323. https://doi.org/10.1002/wps.20470.
6. Al'Absi M, Grabowski J. Concurrent use of tobacco and khat: added burden on chronic disease epidemic. Addiction. 2012;107(2):451–2.
7. Al-Motarreb A, Al-Habori M, Broadley KJ. Khat chewing, cardiovascular diseases and other internal medical problems: the current situation and directions for future research. J Ethnopharmacol. 2010;132(3):540–8.
8. Alsanusy R, El-Sethouhy M. Why would khat chewers quit? An in-depth qualitative study on Saudi khat quitters. Subst Abus. 2013;34:389–95. https://doi.org/10.1080/08897077.2013.783526.
9. Al-Shahethi AH, Zaki RA, Al-Serouri AWA, Awang Bulgiba A. Maternal, prenatal and traditional practice factors associated with perinatal mortality in Yemen. Women Birth. 2019;32(2):e204–5. https://doi.org/10.1016/j.wombi.2018.06.016.
10. Anderson D, Beckerleg S, Hailu D, Klein A. The Khat controversy: stimulating the debate on drugs. Oxford: Berg; 2007.
11. American Psychiatric Association. Diagnostic and statistical manual of mental disorders, fifth edition (DSM-5). Washington, D.C.: American Psychiatric Association; 2013.
12. Awas M, Kebede D, Alem A. Major mental disorders in Butajira, southern Ethiopia. Acta Psychiatr Scand. 1999;397(Suppl):56–64.
13. Beckerleg S. What harm? Kenyan and Ugandan perspectives on khat. Afr Aff. 2006;105(419):219–41. https://doi.org/10.1093/afraf/adi105.
14. Bimerew MS, Sonn FCT, Korlenbout WP. Substance abuse and the risk of readmission of people with schizophrenia at Amanuel Psychiatric Hospital, Ethiopia. Curationis. 2007;30(2):74–81.
15. Colzato LS, Ruiz M, van den Wildenberg WP, Bajo M, Hommel B. Long-term effects of chronic khat use: impaired inhibitory control. Front Psychol. 2010;1:129.
16. Colzato LS, Ruiz MJ, van den Wildenberg WP, Hommel B. Khat use is associated with impaired working memory and cognitive flexibility. PLoS One. 2011;6(6):e20602.

17. Colzato LS, Ruiz MJ, van den Wildenberg WP, Hommel B. Khat use is associated with increased response conflict in humans. Hum Psychopharmacol Clin Exp. 2012;27(3):315–21.

18. Duresso SW, Matthews AJ, Ferguson SG, Bruno R. Using the severity of dependence scale to screen for DSM-5 khat use disorder. Hum Psychopharmacol Clin Exp. 2018;33:e2653. https://doi.org/10.1002/hup.2653.

19. Duresso SW, Bruno R, Matthews AJ, Ferguson SG. Khat withdrawal symptoms among chronic khat users following a quit attempt: an ecological momentary assessment study. Psychol Addict Behav. 2018;32(3):320–6.

20. Duresso SW, Bruno R, Matthews AJ, Ferguson SG. Stopping khat use: predictors of success in an unaided quit attempt. Drug Alcohol Rev. 2018;37(Suppl 1):235–9. https://doi.org/10.1111/dar.12622.

21. Duresso SW, Matthews AJ, Ferguson SG, Bruno R. Is khat use a valid diagnostic entity? Addiction. 2016;111:1666–76.

22. Elmi AS. The chewing of khat in Somalia. J Ethnopharmacol. 1983;8(2):163–76.

23. Eticha T, Teklu A, Ali D, Solomon G, Alemayehu A. Factors associated with medication adherence among patients with schizophrenia in Mekelle, northern Ethiopia. PLoS One. 2015;10(3):e0120560. https://doi.org/10.1371/journal.pone.0120560.

24. European Monitoring Centre for Drugs and Drug Addiction. European drug report: trends and developments. Luxembourg: Publication Office of the European Union; 2018.

25. Gatter P. Politics of Qat: the role of a drug in ruling Yemen. Wiesbaden: Reichert; 2012.

26. Gebrie A, Alebel A, Zegeye A, Tesfaye B. Prevalence and predictors of khat chewing among Ethiopian university students: a systematic review and meta-analysis. PLoS One. 2018;13(4):e0195718. https://doi.org/10.1371/journal.pone.0195718.

27. Griffiths P, Lopez D, Sedefov R, Gallegos A, Hughes B, Noor A, Royuela L. Khat use and monitoring drug use in Europe: the current situation and issues for the future. J Ethnopharmacol. 2010;132(3):578–83.

28. Halbach H. Medical aspects of the chewing of khat leaves. Bull World Health Organ. 1972;47(1):21–9.

29. Hansen P. The ambiguity of khat in Somaliland. J Ethnopharmacol. 2010;132(3):590–9.

30. Haile D, Lakew Y. Khat chewing practice and associated factors among adults in Ethiopia: further analysis using the 2011 demographic and health survey. PLoS One. 2015;10(6):e0130460.

31. Hoffman R, al'Absi M. Working memory and speed of information processing in chronic khat users: preliminary findings. Eur Addict Res. 2012;19(1):1–6.

32. Ismail AA, El Sanosy RM, Rohlman DS, El-Setouhy M. Neuropsychological functioning among chronic khat users in Jazan region, Saudi Arabia. Subst Abus. 2014;35:235–44.

33. Kalix P. Pharmacological properties of the stimulant khat. Pharmacol Ther. 1990;48(3):397–416.

34. Kassim S, Islam S, Croucher R. Validity and reliability of a severity of dependence Scale for khat (SDS-khat). J Ethnopharmacol. 2010;132(3):570–7.

35. Kassim S, Islam S, Croucher RE. Correlates of nicotine dependence in U.K. resident Yemeni khat chewers: a cross-sectional study. Nicotine Tob Res. 2011;13:1240.

36. Kassim S, Hawash A, Johnston A, Croucher R. Validation of self-reported khat chewing amongst khat chewers: an exploratory study. J Ethnopharmacol. 2012;140(1):193–6.

37. Kassim S, Croucher R, al'Absi M. Khat dependence syndrome: a cross sectional preliminary evaluation amongst UK-resident Yemeni khat chewers. J Ethnopharmacol. 2013;146(3):835–41.

38. Kennedy JG, Teague J, Fairbanks L. Qat use in North Yemen and the problem of addiction: a study in medical anthropology. Cult Med Psychiatry. 1980;4(4):311–44.

39. Klein A, Beckerleg S, Hailu D. Regulating Khat – dilemmas and opportunities for the international drug control system. Int J Drug Policy. 2009;20(6):509–13.

40. Klein A. The Khat ban in the UK. What about the 'scientific' evidence? Anthropol Today. 2013;29(5):6–8.

41. Klein A. Framing the chew: narratives of development, drugs and danger with regard to khat (catha edulis). In: Labate BC, Cavnar C, editors. Prohibition, religious freedom, and human rights: regulating traditional drug use. Berlin/Heidelberg: Springer; 2014.

42. Krikorian AD. Kat and its use: an historical perspective. J Ethnopharmacol. 1984;12:115–78.

43. Lifson AR, Workneh S, Shenie T, Ayana DA, Melaku Z, Bezabih L, Waktola HT, Dagne B, Hilk R, Winters KC, Slater L. Frequent use of khat, an amphetamine-like substance, as a risk factor for poor adherence and lost to follow-up among patients new to HIV care in Ethiopia. AIDS Res Hum Retrovir. 2017;33(10):995–8. https://doi.org/10.1089/aid.2016.0274.

44. Mihretu A, Nhunzvi C, Fekadu A, Norton S, Teferra S. Definition and validity of the construct "Problematic Khat Use": a systematic review. Eur Addict Res. 2019;25(4):161–71. https://doi.org/10.1159/000499970.

45. Nabuzoka D, Badhadhe FA. Use and perception of khat among young Somalis in a UK city. Addict Res. 2000;8(1):5–26.

46. Nakajima M, Jebena MG, Taha M, Tesfaye M, Gudina E, Lemieux A, Hoffman R, al'Absi M. Correlates of khat use during pregnancy: a cross-sectional study. Addict Behav. 2017;73:178–84.

47. Nakajima M, Dokam A, Alsameai A, AlSoofi M, Khalil N, al'Absi M. Severity of Khat dependence among adult Khat chewers: the moderating influence of gender and age. J Ethnopharmacol. 2014;155(3):1467–72.

48. Ndetei DM, Khasakhala LI, Ongecha-Owuor FA, Kuria MW, Mutiso V, Kokonya DA. Prevalence of

substance abuse among patients in general medical facilities in Kenya. Subst Abus. 2009;30(2):182–90.

49. Ndetei DM, Khasakhala L, Mathai M, Mutiso V, Mbwayo A, Warsame A, Isse M, Mohamud RO, Mursal BM, Abdi MH. Mental health needs assessment of Somali urban refugees. A monograph of Africa Mental Health Foundation. Nairobi: Africa Mental Health Foundation; 2014.

50. Nencini P, Ahmed AM, Amiconi G, Elmi AS. Tolerance develops to sympathetic effects of khat in humans. Pharmacology. 1984;28(3):150–4.

51. Nutt D, King LA, Phillips LD. Drug harms in the UK: a multicriteria decision analysis. Lancet. 2010;376:1558–65.

52. Odenwald M, Neuner F, Schauer M, Elbert TR, Catani C, Lingenfelder B, Hinkel H, Hafner H, Rockstroh B. Khat use as risk factor for psychotic disorders: a cross-sectional and case control study in Somalia. BMC Med. 2005;3(1):5.

53. Odenwald M. Chronic khat use and psychotic disorders: a review of the literature and future prospects. Sucht. 2007;53(1):9–22. https://doi.org/10.1463/2007.01.03.

54. Odenwald M, Hinkel H, Schauer E, Schauer M, Elbert T, Neuner F, Rockstroh B. Use of khat and posttraumatic stress disorder as risk factors for psychotic symptoms: a study of Somali combatants. Soc Sci Med. 2009;69(7):1040–8.

55. Odenwald M, Klein A, Warfa N. Introduction to the special issue: the changing use and misuse of khat (Catha edulis)–tradition, trade and tragedy. J Ethnopharmacol. 2010;132(3):537–9.

56. Odenwald M, Warfa N, Bhui K, Elbert T. The stimulant khat–another door in the wall? A call for overcoming the barriers. J Ethnopharmacol. 2010;132(3):615–9.

57. Odenwald M, al'Absi M. Khat use and related addiction, mental health and physical disorders: the need to address a growing risk. East Mediterr Health J. 2017;23(3):236–44.

58. Ongeri L, Kirui F, Muniu E, Manduku V, Kirumbi L, Atwoli L, Agure S, Wanzala P, Kaduka L, Karimi M, Mutisya R, Echoka E, Mutai J, Mathu D, Mbakaya C. Khat use and psychotic symptoms in a rural Khat growing population in Kenya: a household survey. BMC Psychiatry. 2019;19:137.

59. Orlien SMS, Sandven I, Berhe NB, Ismael NY, Ahmed TA, Stene-Johansen K, Gundersen SG, Morgan MY, Johannessen A. Khat chewing increases the risk for developing chronic liver disease: a hospital-based case-control study. Hepatology. 2018;68(1):248–57.

60. Suwaidi JA, Ali WM, Aleryani SL. Cardiovascular complications of Khat. Clin Chim Acta. 2013;419:11–4.

61. Teferra S, Hanlon C, Alem A, Jacobsson L, Shibre T. Khat chewing in persons with severe mental illness in Ethiopia: a qualitative study exploring perspectives of patients and caregivers. Transcult Psychiatry. 2011;48(4):455–72.

62. Teklie H, Gonfa G, Getachew T, Defar A, Bekele A, Bekele A, Gelibo T, Amenu K, Tadele T, Taye G, Getinet M, Chala F, Mudie K, Guta M, Feleke Y, Shiferaw F, Tadesse Y, Yadeta D, Gbebremichael M, Girma Y, Kebede T, Teferra S. Prevalence of Khat chewing and associated factors in Ethiopia: findings from the 2015 national non-communicable diseases STEPS survey. Ethiop J Health Dev. 2017;31(Special Issue):320–30.

63. United Nations Office on Drugs and Crime. World drug report 2012. New York: United Nations; 2012.

64. Warfa N, Klein A, Bhui K, Leavey G, Craig T, Stansfeld SA. Khat use and mental illness: a critical review. Soc Sci Med. 2007;65:309–18.

65. Weir S. Qat in Yemen: consumption and social change. London: British Museum Publications Limited; 1985.

66. Widmann M, Warsame AH, Mikulica J, von Beust J, Isse MM, Ndetei D, al'Absi M, Odenwald M. Khat use, PTSD and psychotic symptoms among Somali refugees in Nairobi – a pilot study. Front Public Health. 2014;2:71.

67. Widmann, M., Apondi, B., Musau, A., Warsame, A.H., Isse, M. M., Mutiso V,·Veltrup C, Ndetei D, Odenwald M. Comorbid psychopathology and everyday functioning in a brief intervention study to reduce khat use among Somalis living in Kenya: description of baseline multimorbidity, its effects of intervention and its moderation effects on substance use. Soc Psychiatry Psychiatr Epidemiol, 2017, 52, 1425–1434.

68. World Health Organization. WHO expert committee on drug dependence, thirty-fourth report, WHO technical report series no. 942. Washington, D.C.: World Health Organization; 2006.

69. Zyoud SH. Bibliometric analysis on global Catha edulis (khat) research production during the period of 1952–2014. Glob Health. 2015;11:39.

Further Reading

Klein A, Beckerleg S, Hailu D. Regulating Khat – dilemmas and opportunities for the international drug control system. Int J Drug Policy. 2009;20(6):509–13.

Mihretu A, Nhunzvi C, Fekadu A, Norton S, Teferra S. Definition and validity of the construct "Problematic Khat Use": a systematic review. Eur Addict Res. 2019;25(4):161–71. https://doi.org/10.1159/000499970.

Odenwald M, Warfa N, Bhui K, Elbert T. The stimulant khat–another door in the wall? A call for overcoming the barriers. J Ethnopharmacol. 2010;132(3):615–9.

Odenwald M, al'Absi M. Khat use and related addiction, mental health and physical disorders: the need to address a growing risk. East Mediterr Health J. 2017;23(3):236–44.

Opioid Addiction and Treatment

18

Marta Torrens, Francina Fonseca,
Fernando Dinamarca, Esther Papaseit,
and Magi Farré

Contents

M. Torrens (✉) · F. Fonseca
Institut de Neuropsiquiatria i Addiccions,
Hospital del Mar, Barcelona, Spain

IMIM (Institut Hospital del Mar d'Investigacions
Mèdiques), Barcelona, Spain

Universitat Autònoma de Barcelona,
Barcelona, Spain
e-mail: mtorrens@parcdesalutmar.cat

F. Dinamarca
Institut de Neuropsiquiatria i Addiccions,
Hospital del Mar, Barcelona, Spain

IMIM (Institut Hospital del Mar d'Investigacions
Mèdiques), Barcelona, Spain

E. Papaseit · M. Farré
Universitat Autònoma de Barcelona,
Barcelona, Spain

Hospital Universitari Germans Trias i Pujol (IGTP),
Badalona, Spain

© Springer Nature Switzerland AG 2021
N. el-Guebaly et al. (eds.), *Textbook of Addiction Treatment*,
https://doi.org/10.1007/978-3-030-36391-8_18

Abstract

Opioid use disorder continues to be an important public health concern, reaching epidemic ranges in some countries as well as the consequences associated with consumption. A review of the pharmacology of different opioid drugs available is presented. Also, a current state of the art in the treatment of opioid-related disorders is reviewed. Opioid overdose is a potentially fatal medical emergency that can be reversed with naloxone, an antagonist of opioid receptors, in different doses and routes depending on the opioid that caused the intoxication. For opioid use disorders, the main pharmacological approach is substitution treatment (methadone, buprenorphine, slow-release oral morphine) with the objective of neurochemical stabilization, avoiding the reinforcing effect, and decreasing withdrawal symptoms and craving; there is also a naltrexone depot formulation approved for relapse prevention, associated with psychosocial interventions that seek to restore functionality and prevent relapse. In this chapter, the authors review the current state of knowledge in the field focused on clinical practice.

Keywords

Opioid · Dependence · Overdose · Methadone Buprenorphine · Naloxone

18.1 Introduction

Opioid use disorder (OUD) is a chronic relapsing disease with high costs to individuals and society. In this chapter the term opioids will include all-natural plant alkaloids from opium, such as morphine and codeine, and many semisynthetic derivatives as heroin and methadone as well as totally synthetic substances as fentanyl and others. OUD may involve the use of illicitly manufactured opioids, such as heroin or street fentanyl or the nonmedical use of prescribed opioid medications.

There were an estimated 34.3 million past-year users of opioids globally in 2016, corresponding to 0.7 per cent of the global population aged 15–64 years. The prevalence of past-year use of opioids among the population aged 15–64 years is high in North America (4.2 per cent) and Oceania (2.2 per cent). Among users of opioids, 19.4 million were past-year users of heroin or opium, corresponding to 0.4 per cent of the population aged 15–64 years, with high prevalence rates of past-year use of these opioids in Central Asia and Transcaucasia (0.9 per cent), Eastern and Southeastern Europe (0.7 per cent), and North America (0.8 per cent). WHO estimates that there were 167,750 deaths associated with drug use, with 76 per cent of deaths from drug use disorders related to the use of opioids. Also, it is important to take into account the deaths indirectly attributable to opioid use, such as those related to HIV and HCV acquired through unsafe injecting or from suicides [1].

The high level of misuse of pharmaceutical opioids remains a major concern in North America, where there is also resurgence in heroin use in the past 4 years, particularly in the USA. Together with the use of fentanyl and its analogues, the interlinked epidemic of prescription opioids and heroin has generated a high number of fatal overdoses associated with their use. There are also increasing signs of misuse of pharmaceutical opioids in Western and Central Europe. While not at the same level as in North America, overdose deaths related to fentanyl and its analogues have also been reported in Western and Central Europe [1]. The misuse of pharmaceutical opioids such as tramadol is reported in many countries in Africa (particularly West and North Africa) and in some countries of the Near and Middle East.

This chapter is aimed at updating knowledge about OUD. After a review of the main pharmacological characteristics of opioids, mainly focused in the new synthetic opioids, a state-of-the-art treatment of opioid-related disorders, including opioid intoxication, opioid withdrawal, and opioid use disorder including pharmacological and psychosocial interventions, is presented.

18.2 Pharmacology of Opioids

Opioids exert their pharmacological effects through the endogenous opioid system. The endogenous opioid system is constituted by opioid receptors, mu, kappa, and delta, which are widely distributed in the brain, and the endogenous opioids that include different peptides as endorphins, enkephalins, and dinorphins, which are the ligands of these receptors and play a central role in establishing habits and responses for survival and pain relief.

The opioid endogenous system plays an important role in opioid addiction [2], and also it has been implicated in the pathophysiology of dependence of alcohol and cocaine [3].

The three opioid receptors belong to the G protein receptor family. Depending on the capacity to promote changes in the G protein, ligands are classified into full opioid agonists, partial agonists, antagonists, and agonists–antagonists:

- An agonist or full agonist is a substance that is capable of binding to a receptor, producing their activation and causing a biochemical or cellular response.
- An antagonist is the opposite of an agonist in the sense that it also binds to a receptor, but does not activate the receptor and blocks its activation by agonists.
- A partial agonist binds and activates the receptor, but does not cause complete effect as a full agonist, and has a ceiling of maxim effect inferior than the agonist. They can display antagonism when used in conjunction with a full agonist.

Opioids can be classified according to their affinity on opioid receptors (Table 18.1) as:

- *Pure agonist or full agonist:* opioid agonists at receptor mu fundamentally, with high efficacy (intrinsic activity). This is the group of morphine, heroin, pethidine, methadone, fentanyl, and its derivatives.
- *Mixed agonist–antagonists:* act as agonists in one receptor (kappa) and as partial agonists or antagonists in another (mu). When adminis-

Table 18.1 Classification of pharmacological opioid ligands based on their affinity for the opioid receptors (mu, delta, and kappa)

	Mu	Delta	Kappa	Others
Morphine	Ag+++	Ag+	Ag+	
Diacetyl-morphine	Ag+++	Ag+	Ag+	
Methadone	Ag+++	Ag+	Ag++	NMDA antagonist
Codeine	Ag++			
Buprenor-phine	PA	An+++	An+++	
Fentanyl	Ag+++			
Oxycodone	Ag+++			
Hydro-morphone	Ag+++		Ag+	
Hydro-codone	Ag+++			
Meperidine (pethidine)	Ag+++	Ag+	Ag+	Serotonergic activity
Pentazocine	An+	Ag+	Ag+	Norepinephric and serotonergic activity
Tramadol	Ag+			Norepinephric activity
Tapentadol	Ag+			
Naloxone	An+++	An+	An++	
Naltrexone	An+++	An+	An+++	
Nalmefene	An+++	An+	PA	

The number of symbols "+" is an indication of potency
Ag agonist, *PA* partial agonist, *An* antagonist

tered together with a pure mu agonist, it may antagonize the effects and may reduce or eliminate their analgesic effect. In opioid-dependent subjects, agonists (heroin) cause withdrawal symptoms. This is the group of pentazocine, butorphanol, or nalorphine.

- *Partial agonists:* act on mu receptors with lower efficacy than pure agonists. They are analgesic when administered alone but antagonize the effects of a pure agonist. The most characteristic of this group is buprenorphine.
- *Pure antagonists:* possess affinity for the receptors but not exhibit intrinsic effect. Inhibit or reverse the action of the agonists and do not have analgesic effects. In subjects with opioid dependence, withdrawal symp-

toms occur. They are used in cases of poisoning or overdose by its ability to reverse the effects of exogenous opioids. They are naloxone and naltrexone.

In the brain, mu receptors are highly concentrated in regions that are part of the pain and reward networks and in brainstem regions that regulate breathing. Then the agonist actions at mu receptors are responsible for the rewarding effects of opioids and analgesia, and respiratory depression, which is the main cause of death from opioid overdoses.

The main pharmacodynamic effects of opioid agonists at the mu-opioid receptor are:

- Sedation: can produce drowsiness and cognitive impairment, and at higher doses, they could produce stupor, sleep, and coma. They worsen the psychomotor performance. At very high doses, convulsions can appear.
- Euphoria: feeling of euphoria, pleasure, and a well-being feeling and reduces anxiety. The euphoria has been linked to reinforcing, abuse potential, and addiction of opioids.
- Analgesia: reduction of the sensorial and affective components of pain. They can relieve and suppress acute and chronic pain. This action is mediated by with the mu agonist action; mu receptors control the pain pathways in the medulla. Also, it has actions in the limbic and cortical systems that reduce the negative perception of pain.
- Respiratory depression: reduction of the sensitivity to CO_2 and hypoxemia at the pontine respiratory center. It reduces the number of breaths per minute and can cause an apnea. This effect is dose dependent.
- Antitussive: depression of the cough reflex at least in part by a direct effect on the cough center in the medulla. This mechanism is not well known and has no relation with analgesia or respiratory depression.
- Miosis: the pupillary constriction is related with the disinhibition of the Edinger–Westphal nucleus at the oculomotor nerve. This effect does not show tolerance and could be adequate to detect recent use of opioids.

- Nausea and vomiting: they are observed more frequently after the first administrations. It is caused by direct stimulation of the chemoreceptor trigger zone for emesis in the area postrema of the medulla.
- Neuroendocrine actions: morphine actions in the hypothalamus inhibit the release of gonadotropin-releasing hormone and corticotropin-releasing hormone, producing a decrease in the luteinizing hormone, follicle-stimulating hormone, adrenocorticotropic hormone (ACTH), and beta-endorphin. It also stimulated the secretion of the antidiuretic hormone (ADH). By its effects in the hypothalamus, also a central hypothermia is observed.
- Muscular tone: myoclonus is a rare side effect, ranging from mild twitching to generalized spasm. In anesthetic use muscular rigidity can be observed.

The main peripheral actions are a reduction in the gastrointestinal motility, which clinically is related with constipation; some hypotension by its action in the vasomotor center and by vasodilatation; histamine release in the face, neck, and upper thorax, with a feeling of heat, flushing, and pruritus; and an increase of the tone of the detrusor muscle of the bladder.

The pharmacokinetic properties of main opioids are summarized in Table 18.2; some of them present a low oral bioavailability. The pharmacokinetics varies, depending on the route of administration (oral, intravenous, intramuscular, cutaneous, etc.) and metabolization.

Opioids are biotransformed mainly by hepatic glucuronidation and through the CYP450. Genetic differences among CYP2D6 involved in the metabolization and also the activity of major metabolites must be taken into account for possible interactions of the different opioids with other drugs. Some opioids as tramadol or codeine are transformed to its active opioid metabolites (desmetramadol or O-desmethyltramadol and morphine, respectively) by the CYP2D6, and genetic polymorphisms in CYP2D6 produce inability to convert to the active metabolites, thus making these drugs ineffective as an analgesic for

Table 18.2 Pharmacokinetic properties of main opioids

Opioid	Oral bioavailability (%)	Elimination half-life (h)	Plasma protein binding (%)	Duration of action (h)	10 mg morphine equivalence (analgesia)	
					im	po
Morphine	35–75	2–3	35	4–6	10	30–60
Slow-release oral morphine	35–75	2–3	35	12–24 h		
Diacetylmorphine	20–50	0.1	35	3–6	5	20
Methadone	70–80	15–40	80	24	10	20
Codeine	50	2–4	7	4	130	75
Buprenorphine	50(sl)/90(td)	3–5	96	6–8	0.3	0.8 (sl)
Fentanyl	20–50(po)/90(td)	2–4	80–85	1–2(im)	0.002	
Oxycodone	60–87	3–4	45	12	–	6.7
Hydromorphone	30–40	5	8–19	3–5	1.5	7.5
Hydrocodone	25	4–6	20–50	4–8	–	30
Meperidine	50	3	60	1.5–3	100	300
Pentazocine	10	2–3	60	3–6	60	150
Tramadol	68	6	4	4–6	100	100
Tapentadol	32	4–5	20	4–6	–	100–200
Naloxone	5–10	1–2	NA	0.5–2	–	–
Naltrexone	5–20	4–13a	20	24–72	–	–
Nalmefene	41	13	30	24	–	–

Im intramuscular, *po* oral administration, *sl* sublingual, *td* transdermal
[a]Half-life for 6-β-naltrexol

about 7–10% of the Caucasian population. Table 18.3 summarizes the metabolism and interactions of main opioids.

Also, other medications that can be used in patients under opioid treatments are drugs for HIV and HCV infections. In relation to antiretroviral treatment (ART) for HIV, patients on nevirapine, efavirenz, and ritonavir (including lopinavir/ritonavir and darunavir/ritonavir combinations) may require higher methadone doses [4]. The combination regimen of paritaprevir/ombitasvir/ritonavir has many interactions with psychotropics drugs including opioids as buprenorphine, fentanyl, and hydrocodone that should be used with caution (probably because ritonavir is a strong inhibitor of CYP3A). The combination regimen voxilaprevir/velpatasvir/sofosbuvir also has a caution recommendation regarding the coadministration with buprenorphine, and finally there is a warning in relation to ledipasvir/sofosbuvir that could increase dose of buprenorphine because of mild/moderate

inhibition of P-gp [5]. Because of the continued update of reports of new antivirals and other medications, we suggest checking interactions of prescriptions in webs as https://www.drugs.com.

Short- and long-term opioid use is also characterized by the development of different neuroadaptative processes including tolerance, physical dependence, and addiction. Physiological dependence is manifested with the emergence of withdrawal symptoms when use of opioids is abruptly discontinued or an antagonist is administered. Symptoms include insomnia, cramps, diarrhea, nausea, vomiting, and body aches, as well as dysphoria, anxiety, and irritability. The severity of these symptoms varies, depending on chronicity, the opioid drug in question (symptoms are stronger for more potent and shorter-acting drugs), and individual variability [2].

All patients treated with opioids or misusing them will develop physical dependence, and withdrawal symptoms usually resolve promptly

Table 18.3 Metabolism of main opioids

Opioid	Phase I metabolism	Phase II metabolism	Major metabolites	Clinical effects and drug interactions
Morphine	CYP3A	UGT2B7	Morphine-3-glucuronide (M3G) Morphine-6-glucuronide (M6G)[a]	Cimetidine reduces metabolism Increase of metformin (lactic acidosis risk) Caution in renal failure (accumulation)
Diacetylmorphine			6-Monoacetylmorphine (6-MAM)[a] Morphine[a]	
Methadone	CYP3A4 CYP2B6 CYP2D6		EDDP EMDP	QT prolongation Interactions with rifampin, carbamazepine, phenytoin (>metabolism) and fluconazole, voriconazole, ciprofloxacin, fluoxetine (<metabolism)
Codeine	CYP2D6 CYP3A	UGT2B7	Morphine[a]	Risk of accumulation in renal failure 7–10% are poor metabolizers
Buprenorphine	CYP3A4 CYP2C8	UGT1A1 UGT1A3 UGT2B7	Norbuprenorphine[a] Buprenorphine-3-glucuronide Norbuprenorphine-3-glucuronide	Could precipitate withdrawal symptoms if other agonist is present Higher dose of naloxone are required in respiratory depression
Fentanyl	CYP3A4		Noralfentanil N-Phenylpropionamide	Bradycardia and hypotension with amiodarone
Oxycodone	CYP2D6 CYP3A		Oxymorphone[a] Noroxycodone[a]	7–10% are poor metabolizers Risk of accumulation in renal failure
Hydromorphone		UGT2B7 UGT1A3	Hydromorphone-3-glucuronide	Risk of accumulation in renal failure
Hydrocodone	CYP3A4 CYP2D6		Norhydrocodone Hydromorphone[a]	Risk of accumulation in renal failure
Meperidine	CYP2D6 CYP3A CYP2C19		Normeperidine[a]	Neurotoxic metabolite, not indicated for chronic treatment Risk of accumulation in renal failure
Tramadol	CYP2D6 CYP3A4		Nortramadol O-Desmethyltramadol[a]	Risk of serotoninergic syndrome (antidepressants) 7–10% are poor metabolizers
Tapentadol	CYP2D6 CYP2C9 CYP2C19	UGT1A9 UGT2B7	Hydroxy tapentadol N-Desmethyltapentadol	Risk of interactions with other drugs that affect noradrenergic system
Naltrexone		UGT2B7	6-β-Naltrexol	Could increase liver enzymes (dose related) Theoretical interactions with zidovudine (AZT)

[a]*Active metabolite*

within a few days but can sometimes last weeks after use is discontinued. Dependence can lead to opioid seeking as individuals attempt to avoid withdrawal symptoms, contributing to addiction by perpetuating repeated exposures.

Pharmacologic characteristics of more used opioids in opioid addiction and their treatment are described with more detail.

18.2.1 Morphine

Morphine is a natural product of the seeds of the poppy plant and the most important compound found in opium. Morphine is the prototype for opioid agonist actions.

Slow-Release Oral Morphine (SROM) has been used in some countries as an alternative maintenance pharmacotherapy for treatment of opioid dependence with retention rates similar to methadone, with a better safety profile and greater improvements in several patient-reported outcomes, including tolerability, treatment satisfaction, and mental symptoms, as well as alleviation of cravings and withdrawal symptoms [6].

18.2.2 Diacetylmorphine (Diamorphine, Heroin)

Heroin is synthesized from morphine and is twice more active than morphine at equivalent doses due to its higher lipophilic properties. Heroin is the world's most widely misused opioid, and frequently associated with intravenous administrations, with an increased risk of bloodborne disease transmission (such HIV and hepatitis B and C) and overdoses, because of the narrow margin between recreational and lethal doses and the variations in street drug purity [7].

There are several types of heroin in the market depending on its origin and characteristics:

(a) Base heroin or Tsao-ta: comes from Southeast Asia. Its color is white or dark and is used for injection or smoking.
(b) The brown sugar: is the heroin used to be smoked. It has been mixed with other substances as caffeine, strychnine, sugars, etc. Contents vary from 25% to 50%.
(c) White heroin or hydrochloride: is also known as the Thai heroin. Its use is predominantly intravenous. It has the higher active content, sometimes more than 90%.
(d) Black heroin or black tar heroin: as its name indicates, its aspect is similar to tar; it is a black and sticky substance. It comes from America and its purity is around 20%. It is used for injection.

Heroin itself has no intrinsic opioid activity; but it is a very effective prodrug and metabolized in humans to active opioid compounds first by deacetylation to the active 6-monoacetylmorphine (6-MAM) and then by further deacetylation to morphine, when administered by parenteral route

[8]. Heroin has an average half-life in blood of 3 min after intravenous administration; the half-life of 6-monoacetylmorphine in humans appears to be 3–10 min. The use of intranasal, intramuscular, and subcutaneous heroin all produces peak blood levels of heroin or 6-monoacetylmorphine within 5 min; however, intranasal use has about half the relative potency [9].

Diacetylmorphine is also used for treatment in opioid users previously not responding adequately to methadone or other opioid treatments in some countries as Switzerland, the Netherlands, Germany, Canada, and England [10]. The prescription is under special programs.

18.2.3 Methadone

Methadone is a semisynthetic opioid agonist that is used in the chronic treatment of pain and in the OUD. It has been used as a maintenance treatment for heroin addiction since the first years of the 1960s [11]. Methadone is rapidly absorbed after an oral dose, it can be detected in the blood at 15–45 min after oral administration, and peak plasma concentrations occur at 2–4 h after dosing [12]. The oral bioavailability of methadone was found to be around 70–80% in a range of doses of 10–60 mg with great interindividual variability. Methadone is highly bound to plasma proteins. Enantiomeric differences are also relevant in protein binding (the unbound fraction for (S)-methadone is 10% while for the (R)-enantiomer is 14%) and its metabolic disposition [12]. All these variables might contribute to interindividual response differences to methadone treatment. Methadone undergoes N-demethylation by multiple cytochrome P450 (CYP) enzymes including CYP3A4, CYP2B6, CYP2C19, CYP2D6, CYP2C9, and CYP2C8 [13]. Its main metabolite (2-ethylidene-1,5-dimethyl-3,3-diphenylpyrrolidine (EDDP)) is inactive. (R)-Methadone has a longer half-life than (S)-methadone (38 vs. 29 h, respectively). After chronic administration, a reduction in half-life (from 55 to 22 h) has been detected because it induces its own metabolism regulated by cytochrome P450 CYP3A4 [12, 14]. Also, many studies have demonstrated genetic variability in the coding genes involved in the pharmacokinetics of methadone metabolism and transport. These genetic variables must be considered to improve the clinical management of methadone [15]. Chronic administration of methadone leads to the gradual development of tolerance to the effects on hypothalamic-releasing factors, with resumption of normal menses and return of plasma levels of testosterone to normal within 1 year as well as return to normal levels and activity of anterior pituitary-derived ACTH and beta-endorphin and normal ACTH stimulation in approximately 3 months. Prolactin levels still rise after oral methadone dosing; however, both peak plasma levels of methadone and also prolactin are found at 2–4 h after dosing; prolactin levels usually do not exceed the upper limit of normal [16].

There are two important adverse events related to methadone: the risk of respiratory depression and the risk of cardiac rhythm disorders related to QT interval prolongation. Methadone at high doses can increase the QT interval. A QT interval longer than 500 ms increases the risk of polymorphic ventricular tachycardia, such as torsade de pointes (TdP) [17]. The mechanism of this increase has been related to the inhibitory action of methadone on the hERG voltage-gated potassium channel and also could be related to the blockade of calcium channels in the cardiac myocyte membrane and the induction of bradycardia. Risk factors that increase prolonged QTc interval in patients on methadone maintenance are female gender, cardiac disease, high doses of methadone, HIV infection chronic, and hepatitis C-induced cirrhosis [18].

In order to detect and minimize the risk for cardiac adverse events related to methadone, clinicians should follow some recommendations: (a) to obtain a complete clinical history about background related to personal and familiar heart disease; (b) to inform patients of arrhythmia risk with methadone; (c) to obtain a basal electrocardiogram with QTc measure, to detect patients with a possible congenital long QTc syndrome, and also an annual electrocardiogram and additional if doses are above 100 mg/day with every dose change; (d) in cases with QTc interval between 450 and 499 ms, patients should be monitored more frequently; (e) in cases with QTc interval equal or above 500 ms, consider to switch to another opioid substitution treatment with reduced risk of QTc enlargement (slow-release morphine, buprenorphine); and (f) potential interactions should be always taken into account, with drugs that could prolong the QTc interval and those that increase methadone plasma concentrations [19].

18.2.4 Codeine

Codeine is one of several naturally occurring alkaloids found in opium. It is more lipophilic than morphine and thus crosses the blood–brain barrier faster. Its oral bioavailability is greater than that of morphine. Codeine has very low affinity for opioid receptors; it is active only because a 10% of it is metabolized to morphine, while other metabolites are mostly inactive and excreted in the urine. Codeine is commonly used in combination to non-opioid analgesics in moderate pain (before using strong opioids) and to suppress cough via a central mechanism, at doses lower than used for analgesia [14, 20].

18.2.5 Buprenorphine

Buprenorphine is a semisynthetic opioid that it is primarily mu-opioid receptor partial agonist and a kappa antagonist. Buprenorphine has high affinity for, but low intrinsic activity at, mu receptors and displaces some full opioid agonists from receptors. For this reason, and because of buprenorphine's higher affinity for the mu receptor, full agonists cannot displace it and therefore will not exert a dose-related opioid effect on the receptors already occupied by buprenorphine, and also it can induce a withdrawal syndrome in subjects using full opioid agonists. Owing to its ceiling effect, increasing doses in humans beyond 32 mg sublingually has no greater opioid agonist effect. Two important properties of buprenorphine are relevant: (a) its apparent lower severity of withdrawal signs and symptoms on cessation, compared with heroin and methadone, and (b) its reduced potential to produce lethal overdose when used alone in opiate-naive or nontolerant persons because of its partial agonist properties. However, it is not clear whether there is a ceiling for this effect; the respiratory depression and other effects of buprenorphine can be prevented by prior administration of naloxone, but they are not readily reversed by high doses of naloxone once the effects have been produced [21]. This suggests that buprenorphine dissociates very slowly from opioid receptors. This very slow dissociation from mu-opioid receptor seems to be responsible for its long duration of action (24–48 h) when administered on a chronic basis. In relation to the antagonist properties at the kappa-opioid receptor of buprenorphine, and its important role in mood regulation, new clinical studies about the possible antidepressant effects of buprenorphine are in development [22].

Buprenorphine has poor oral bioavailability and fair sublingual bioavailability. FDA-approved formulations of the drug for the treatment of opioid addiction are in the form of sublingual tablets that are held under the tongue and absorbed through the sublingual mucosa. After the report in many countries of the buprenorphine diversion and the intravenous misuse, a formulation in combination with naloxone was developed. In this formulation, naloxone will not precipitate withdrawal when taken sublingually because of its limited oral bioavailability; however, it may block the initial euphoric effects of buprenorphine if abused by the intravenous route and may also then precipitate acute withdrawal [23]. In the last years, with the objective of diminishing the risk of misuse, sustained-release buprenorphine formulations (a 6-month subdermal implant and a monthly injectable sustained-release; already approved by the FDA) have been developed with apparently good efficacy and safety profile [24].

18.2.6 Fentanyl

Fentanyl is a synthetic opioid synthesized in 1974 by Paul Janssen. The actions of fentanyl and its congeners (sufentanil, remifentanil, and alfentanil) are similar to other mu-opioid receptor agonists, although its potency is 50–100 fold more potent than morphine and 24–40 than heroin. It produces analgesia, drowsiness, and euphoria, the last effect less than heroin and morphine. Its half-life is not affected significantly in the case of hepatic impairment, and in renal impairment, fentanyl excretion is less affected than other opioids [25]. There are several fentanyl formulations including sublingual tablets, nasal sprays, transmucosal lozenges, transdermal patches, and injectables, which are used as anesthetic agents but also as treatment for chronic pain and supplemental medications for breakthrough pain in oncologic patients [24]. In the last years there has been a growing concern in relation to the illicitly manufactured fentanyl in the USA being used as an adulterant to heroin (for the lower cost of production and transportation because it is so potent) with a rise in overdose deaths [26]. Fentanyl, fentanyl analogues, and other new synthetic opioids (NSO) have arrived onto the illegal drug market as new psychoactive substances (NPS). They are often sold as heroin. These derivatives are more potent than fentanyl and represent a third of the opioids causing acute intoxication in the USA (Opioid Overdose Crisis).

18.2.7 Oxycodone

Oxycodone is a semisynthetic opioid with agonist activity, primarily at mu receptors. It is combined with aspirin or acetaminophen for moderate pain and is available orally without co-analgesic for severe pain. It is a popular drug of abuse, especially in the controlled-release formulation, which can be crushed for a potentially toxic, rapid "high" comparable to the effects of the immediate-release formulation [27].

18.2.8 Tramadol

Tramadol is a synthetic codeine and morphine analogue that is a weak mu agonist. It also exerts some capacity to inhibit the uptake of norepi-nephrine and serotonin [28]. It is more effective in the treatment of mild and moderate pain than in the treatment of severe and chronic pain [18]. Misuse, diversion, physical dependence, abuse, addiction, and withdrawal have been reported in conjunction with the use of tramadol. The phar-macological effects are similar to those of mor-phine, and the main adverse effects include nausea, vomiting, dizziness, dry mouth, seda-tion, and headache. Respiratory depression and constipation are mild compared to morphine. Tramadol can cause seizures and possibly exac-erbate seizures in patients with predisposing factors; also there is a risk of serotoninergic syndrome, especially with the use of other sero-toninergic medications [28]. Recent reports indicate that it is one of the most abused opioids in Africa.

18.2.9 Naloxone

Naloxone is competitive antagonist at all opioid receptors, but with great affinity for mu recep-tors. Naloxone is usually administered in the streets and emergency department to revert her-oin overdoses and also as an aid to distinguish causes of coma (if patient does not respond to naloxone, a non-opioid cause should be consid-ered) [29, 30].

Naloxone is widely distributed and rapidly achieves effective concentrations in the CNS after parenteral administration. Plasma and brain concentrations fall precipitously because of rapid redistribution. The drug is rapidly cleared by hepatic biotransformation, mainly to the 3-glucuronide. The clearance is high which suggests that extrahepatic elimination may be occurring. The terminal half-life is 1–2 h. The onset of antagonist effect is extremely rapid, but the duration of action is quite brief. The dura-tion of naloxone is nearly always shorter than that of the opioids whose effects it is intended to antagonize. It has to be taken into account that opioid reversal can sometimes have important hemodynamic consequences. Increases in sys-temic pressure, heart rate, and plasma levels of catecholamines can occur. Oral or sublingual administration of naloxone has very low sys-temic bioavailability due to marked hepatic first-pass metabolism. Enteral naloxone can block opioid action at the intestinal receptor level but has no general effects [20]. Naloxone is available in different formulations: as a solu-tion for intravenous, intramuscular, and orotra-cheal injection and as a spray for nasal administration [25].

18.2.10 Naltrexone

Naltrexone is an opioid antagonist, chemically related to naloxone. Compared to naloxone, it has higher oral bioavailability and a longer dura-tion of action that allows its administration by oral route. Naltrexone has been used for relapse prevention in opioid dependence because of its ability to antagonize all the actions of opioids. Also, there is evidence that naltrexone blocks activation by alcohol of dopaminergic pathways in the brain that are thought to be critical to reward, so it is used also in the treatment of alco-hol dependence, as relapse prevention substance. The most common side effect of naltrexone is nausea. An increase of transaminases could be observed, so it is contraindicated in hepatitis or hepatic failure [30].

Naltrexone is rapidly absorbed and undergoes an extensive first-pass metabolism to 6-b-naltrexol. This is an active metabolite that probably accounts for most of the naltrexone activity. The metabolite accumulates during chronic treatment and has a terminal half-life of 13 h, so significant antagonist effects may persist for 1–3 days after naltrexone is stopped [30].

A depot formulation of naltrexone that pro-vides 30 days of medication after a single injec-tion has been approved for the treatment of alcoholism and heroin dependence in detoxified patients. This formulation eliminates the neces-sity of daily pill-taking and prevents relapse when the recently detoxified patient leaves a pro-tected environment [31].

18.2.11 Nalmefene

Nalmefene is another long-lasting, opioid antagonist. It is the 6-methylene derivative of naltrexone. It is an antagonist at the mu- and delta-opioid receptors and a partial agonist at the kappa receptors; there is no evidence of activity in any other receptor (Tables 18.1 and 18.2). There have been described some advantages over naltrexone, including greater oral bioavailability; rapidly absorbed, longer duration of action; and lack of dose-dependent liver toxicity [32]. In Europe, nalmefene has been approved as an anticraving treatment for alcohol use disorder [33].

18.3 Opioid-Related Disorders

According to the fifth edition of *Diagnostic and Statistical Manual of Mental Disorders* (DSM-5) [34], the main opioid-related disorders are opioid intoxication, opioid withdrawal, opioid use disorder, and opioid-induced disorders (psychosis, bipolar, depression, anxiety, sleep, sexual dysfunctions, delirium, and neurocognitive).

Opioid use disorder (OUD) includes physiological, behavioral, and cognitive symptoms, ending in a repeated use of opioid drugs, despite significant problems related to such use, and is characterized by compulsion to seek and take the drug; as in other drug dependence, there is a loss of control in limiting the intake and emergence of a negative emotional state (i.e., dysphoria, anxiety, irritability) reflecting a motivational withdrawal syndrome when access to the drug is prevented [2]. OUD can be mild, moderate, or severe depending on the number of criteria fulfilled.

In the next section we present the main disorders related to opioid use with main pharmacological and psychosocial strategies used.

18.4 Treatment of Opioid-Related Disorders

Pharmacological strategies used in the treatment of opiate overdose, withdrawal, and addiction are described in Table 18.4.

18.4.1 Opioid Acute Intoxication

Acute opioid intoxication could result from clinical overdosage, accidental overdosage, or attempts of suicide. Opioid intoxication is a life-threatening emergency. Typical triad signs are depressed consciousness or coma, depressed respiration, and miotic or pinpoint pupils. The treatment goal is to sustain or restore vital functions and to immediately reverse the overdose with an opioid antagonist (naloxone).

First, it is essential to maintain the air pathway, and then, to avoid aspiration, put the

Table 18.4 Main pharmacological strategies in opioid-related disorder treatment

	Type	Objective	Process	Pharmacological treatment
Opioid acute intoxication	Opioid intoxication	Decrease mortality	Revert opioid intoxication	Naloxone
Opioid withdrawal	Opioid detoxification	Avoid withdrawal syndrome	Detoxification	Methadone Buprenorphine Clonidine/lofexidine
Opioid use disorder	Total abstinence oriented	Remove the opioid	Detoxification + Continued total abstinence	Methadone Buprenorphine Clonidine/lofexidine +/− Naltrexone
	Opioid substitution treatment	Stabilization	To stabilize brain neurochemistry	Agonist maintenance treatment
		Harm reduction	Functional improvement	Needle exchange and other risk reduction strategies

patient in lateral decubitus position; if necessary, in case of cardiopulmonary arrest, mechanical ventilation should be applied [29]. The administration of naloxone 0.2–0.4 mg intravenously will begin to reverse the effects of an opiate overdose within 1 min. If there is no response to the initial dose, repeat doses may be administered every 2–3 min (0.5 mg, 2 mg, 4 mg, and 10 mg). If the patient has no response to 10 mg, then an opioid likely is not responsible for the respiratory depression [29]. Finally, once the consciousness level is reverted, it is important to investigate a possible suicide intention risk of the patient and to perform a psychiatric assessment.

Increasing access to naloxone is a major component to reverse the overdose epidemic, and with the increase in overdoses from fentanyl and other synthetic opioids, multiple naloxone doses are necessary for reversal. There have been developed various strategies like community educational overdose prevention programs, injectable and nasal self-administered kit formulations with higher dose, and also the use of new technologies with apps that monitor a person's respiratory rate and trigger an alert when diminished breathing is detected, and a device is being developed that automatically administers naloxone in response to a reduction in respiratory rate or oxygen saturation [35].

18.4.2 Opioid Withdrawal

The withdrawal syndrome for short-acting opioids (heroin or morphine) begins 6–12 h after last use. Early symptoms include opiate craving, anorexia, anxiety, and irritability. These are coupled with clinical signs of increased respirations and blood pressure, sweating and yawning, rhinorrhea, lacrimation, piloerection (gooseflesh), tremor, and dilated pupils. After 48–72 h, the symptoms progress to include nausea, vomiting, diarrhea, insomnia, tachycardia, abdominal cramps, and involuntary muscle spasms and limb movements. Signs subside over 5–7 days. Signs and symptoms associated with withdrawal from long-acting opioids such as methadone are simi-

lar to those described above, but they may not begin until 24–48 h after the last dose and may last for 2–3 weeks or more. Withdrawal syndrome of buprenorphine is usually less intense and of shorter duration. Withdrawal can also appear when an opioid antagonist, such as naloxone or naltrexone, is provided to a subject under any opioid agonist drug use; this is called precipitated withdrawal.

18.4.3 Opioid Use Disorder

Opioid use disorder includes physiological, behavioral, and cognitive symptoms, ending in a repeated use of opioid drugs, despite significant problems related to such use, and is characterized by compulsion to seek and take the drug; as in other drug dependence, there is a loss of control in limiting the intake and emergence of a negative emotional state (i.e., dysphoria, anxiety, irritability) reflecting a motivational withdrawal syndrome when access to the drug is prevented [2]. Opioid addiction can be mild, moderate, or severe depending on the number of criteria fulfilled. OUD presents high rates of comorbidity (psychiatric disorders, infections such as HIV and hepatitis C), mortality (overdose), and legal and social problems [1]. There are two main therapeutic strategies in opioid addiction: abstinence-oriented treatment and medication assisted treatment (MAT).

18.4.3.1 Abstinence-Oriented Treatments
In the abstinence-oriented, the goal is to remove the abused opioid in a controlled fashion, with a complete eradication of the opioid agonist treatment. Abstinence is usually achieved in two stages: detoxification and continued total abstinence.

18.4.3.2 Detoxification
Detoxification involves the substitution of the abused opioid by other long half-life opioid agonist or partial agonist (methadone or buprenorphine, usually) or an alpha2-adrenergic agonist (clonidine or lofexidine) and a progressive reduc-

tion in order to reduce the intensity of the withdrawal syndrome [36–38].

In general, the use of long-acting opioids (such as methadone) is recommended in opioid detoxification, with a long and slow tapering, medical supervision, ancillary medications, and psychosocial treatment to improve the outcomes and reduce the risk of relapse. Offering withdrawal management as a stand-alone option to patients is neither sufficient nor appropriate. Rapid and ultra-rapid protocols for detoxification are also not recommended. Methadone detoxification guidelines recommend starting with an initial dose of 10–45 mg/day, orally, depending on the severity of opioid withdrawal symptoms. Every 2 h it is necessary to assess the intensity of withdrawal and ensure that the dose will not exceed 60 mg/day. The same dose of the first day should be administered for 2–3 days and then reduced to 5–10 mg/day until total suppression. The detoxification usually lasts 10–20 days.

When buprenorphine (or buprenorphine–naloxone) is used in the detoxification treatment, initial doses of 4–6 mg of buprenorphine are recommended, and then increase the dose until 8–10 mg/day. After 2–3 days, the recommendation is to reduce the dose to 2 mg every 1–2 days until complete suppression. It is important to administer the first dose 24 h after the last heroin use, when the first withdrawal symptoms appear, in order to avoid a precipitated withdrawal.

Alpha2-adrenergic agonists (clonidine or lofexidine) are also effective for reducing the severity of opioid withdrawal symptoms and increasing the probability of completing withdrawal management, but compared to methadone, alpha2-adrenergic agonists are somewhat less effective in mitigating withdrawal symptoms and are more likely to present adverse effects such as hypotension, specially clonidine (not US FDA approved for withdrawal); they could be used as adjunctive therapy [39].

18.4.3.3 Continued Total Abstinence

After complete opioid detoxification, naltrexone is a pharmacologic alternative to maintain the abstinence. The main advantages of naltrexone include the following: decrease in opioid craving, can be administered in a standard outpatient office setting, and the absence of abuse potential. Also, it is well tolerated with few adverse effects, except for the risk of increase of liver enzymes. Despite all these advantages, naltrexone has shown low rates of efficacy, with poor retention and high relapse rates. To improve the described problems with retention and relapse with naltrexone, an injectable sustained-release formulation has been developed with a recent trial that shows a similar safety and efficacy compared to buprenorphine, but naltrexone had a substantial induction hurdle with a lower rate of participants that succeed in the induction [40]. Only one study has compared the efficacy of depot naltrexone versus methadone maintenance treatment [41] in 46 volunteers in a prison setting. The study was randomized, and the results showed similar reductions in the use of heroin and benzodiazepines and criminality 6 months after prison release. In conclusion, depot formulations of naltrexone seem to be promising in order to improve outcomes in opioid dependence disorder in less well-integrated subjects with a strong motivation to become totally abstinent. Oral naltrexone is a treatment option for patients also with a strong motivation to become totally abstinent of all opioid agonists and very well integrated.

18.4.3.4 Medication Assisted Treatment: Opioid Substitution Treatments (OST)

The objective is to stabilize brain neurochemistry by replacing a short-acting opioid with a long-term acting opioid that has relatively steady-state pharmacokinetics, such as methadone or buprenorphine. Opioid agonist maintenance treatment has a minimal euphoric effect, blocks the euphoria associated with the administration of exogenous opioids, and eliminates the phenomenon of opioid withdrawal [2]. The most frequently studied medications for maintenance treatment are methadone and buprenorphine and, to a lesser extent, sustained-release morphine, diacetylmorphine (heroin), and (R)-methadone.

Methadone Maintenance Treatment (MMT)

In general, methadone maintenance treatment (MMT) has been considered the first-line treatment for opioid dependence. MMT has demonstrated its efficacy in retaining patients in treatment and decreasing illicit opioid use, decreasing risk behaviors related to the HIV/sexually transmitted diseases, decreasing criminal behavior related with drug use, reducing the risk of fatal overdose, and improving health-related quality of life. Methadone dosing should be based on clinically guided dose titration. The main problem with methadone has been described in the first part of this chapter and is related with an increased risk of QTc prolongation, so the electrocardiogram monitoring previously to initiate is mandatory in these patients. Methadone dosing should be based on clinically guided dose titration. Usual maintenance dosage of methadone is 60–100 mg/day; some patients achieve abstinence or are free of withdrawal symptoms when treated with less than 40 mg/day of methadone. Some studies suggest that methadone doses of 60–100 mg/day or higher are more effective than lower doses for reducing or stopping illegal opioid self-administration in opioid-dependent patients. Regarding the duration of maintenance treatment, there are no clear recommendations; however, the literature shows better improvements with longer treatments, so the advice is to favor indefinite treatments and start the suppression when significant changes in lifestyle have been made [42].

(R)-Methadone Maintenance Treatment

(R)-Methadone (or L-methadone or Polamidon®) is the active component of the racemic methadone, and it is used in Germany as the maintenance treatment of opioid use disorder. As described previously, (R)-methadone shows more affinity of the mu receptors and has more analgesic potency than racemic (R,S)-methadone. Efficacy studies show no differences between the (R)-enantiomer and the racemate [43]. As the cardiac side effects of methadone reside in the (S)-enantiomer, the substitution of the racemate by the (R)-methadone has demonstrated a reduc-

tion in the QTc interval [44], reducing the risk of sudden death in methadone-maintained patients. Unfortunately, the direct costs of the treatment with (R)-methadone are much higher than the use of the racemate.

Buprenorphine Maintenance Treatment

Buprenorphine is, after methadone, the most widely used opioid for maintenance. Buprenorphine is a partial opioid agonist, with a ceiling effect for respiratory depression and with reduced abuse potential [42]. Buprenorphine is commercialized alone or in combination with naloxone, to decrease abuse risk. The commercialization of buprenorphine in combination with naloxone is as sublingual tablets (4:1 ratio, sublingual tablets containing buprenorphine 2 and 8 mg and naloxone 0.5 and 2 mg) or as soluble film (sublingual film containing buprenorphine 2, 4, 8, or 12 mg and naloxone 0.5, 1, 2, or 3 mg).

To initiate buprenorphine or buprenorphine–naloxone treatment successfully and to avoid a precipitated withdrawal, it is essential to determine that the patient is opioid-free for at least 24 h (in case of short-acting opiates) and observe the presence of opioid withdrawal symptoms. The recommended initial dose is 4 mg sublingually and should be administered at the clinic, and the patient should remain under observation for 2 h. Supplemental doses can be given if withdrawal symptoms persist, with a maximum recommended first-day dose of 8 mg. The dose can be raised in 2–4 mg increments over the next 2–3 days. Doses of 8–16 mg buprenorphine are superior to lower doses, and doses of 12–24 mg are preferable for maintenance treatment. Doses should not exceed a maximum single daily dose of 24 mg. Because of the ceiling effect, there is no pharmacological justification for daily doses over 32 mg.

The main advantages of buprenorphine compared to methadone maintenance treatment are the lower risk of fatal respiratory depression during intoxication, the quick induction to full doses, its cardiac safety because it has no effect on the QTc interval, the lower risk of interactions, and the destigmatization of patients compared to methadone [42].

Slow-Release Oral Morphine (SROM)

In the last years, maintenance treatment with SROM for opioid dependence disorder had captured more interest as an alternative to methadone, with a better safety profile (non-QTc prolongation and lower risk of drug–drug interactions), good tolerability, treatment satisfaction, and retention [6], being included in the Canadian treatment guidelines [36]. However, in terms of efficacy, there are contradictory results in the studies performed [45]. The major concerns with SROM treatment are the risk of misuse; the severe adverse event, such as overdose; and the risk of diversion. Another problem associated with SRMO treatment is the difficulty to monitor illicit opioid abstinence as SRMO and heroin will give a positive test in the screening tests.

Diacetylmorphine (Diamorphine, Heroin) Maintenance

Diacetylmorphine maintenance has also been studied in patients with a history of unsuccessful agonist treatment in specific programs in a few countries with good acceptance by patients and public opinion [10]. The treatment has been usually prescribed alongside methadone and has demonstrated an increase in treatment retention and reduced engagement in illegal activities in patients who previously failed in other maintenance programs. The main problem is related with the rate of serious adverse events, mainly the risk of overdose; for that reason, the treatment is only recommended in patients refractory to other substitution treatments and should be provided in settings with proper medical assistance [46].

18.4.3.5 Psychosocial Interventions in Opioid Use Disorder

Psychosocial treatments are those that use any psychological or social strategy to achieve an improvement or a behavioral change. Opioid treatment guidelines (as the WHO guidelines 2009) [47] recommend the use of psychosocial treatments.

Interventions at a psychological level range from unstructured supportive psychotherapy and motivational interviewing techniques to highly structured psychological techniques. The main psychological strategies in OUD are cognitive behavioral therapy (CBT) and contingency management. Cognitive approaches primarily aim to change addictive behaviors by changing faulty cognitions that serve to maintain behavior or by promoting positive cognitions or motivation to change behavior. Behavioral approaches aim primarily to modify behaviors underpinned by conditioned learning, that is, by classical and operant conditioning. Contingency management rewards or punishes specific types of behaviors using a structured, transparent approach that increases learning of desired behaviors. Also, there is scarce knowledge about the effectiveness of psychosocial interventions alone or in combination with pharmacological strategies and which intervention is the most effective. A Cochrane review performed by Amato and cols in 2011 [48] showed no evidence that any intervention improves outcomes with opioid agonist therapy. But in a recent study [49], John Marsden and colleagues report the results of randomized controlled study where 273 patients in methadone or buprenorphine were randomly assigned to a group with a weekly psychosocial interventions (as a flexible approach performed by assistant psychologists) and medical management or to a group of treatment as usual, setting as objective the absence of unprescribed drug use. Fewer than 20% of participants met that goal, but differences where significative (being better for psychosocial intervention group), and authors conclude that overall, the intervention was cost-effective.

In terms of social interventions, the main interventions used in substance use disorders are as follows: vocational training, which includes a range of programs designed to help patients find and retain employment; housing services that can vary from group accommodation for the homeless to more stable, affordable, long-term accommodation; the referral to participate in activities, such as enjoying leisure activities of their choice; and self-help groups, which, in the context of opioid use disorder, are voluntary, small-group structures formed by peers to assist each other in their struggle with opioid dependence. Usually abstinence oriented, they often provide both material assistance and emotional support and promulgate an ideology or values through which members may attain a greater sense of personal identity. Social skills training refers to methods that use the principles of learning theory to promote the acquisition, generalization, and durability of skills needed in social and interpersonal situations. Training should take place in the context of real everyday life experiences, not in closed, unrealistic settings.

In opioid use disorder, the efficacy of psychosocial interventions has little evidence due to the difficulty in the design of controlled trials.

18.4.3.6 Harm Reduction Strategies

Broadly defined, harm reduction refers to policies, programs, and practices that aim to reduce the adverse health, social, and economic consequences of licit and illicit substance use. It includes programs of needle/syringe exchange, overdose prevention with take-home naloxone, and supervised injection or consumption services. Harm reduction strategies could be perceived by patients or wider public with concern generating possible barriers, but there is no evidence that these actions could promote the consumption; rather to the contrary, the research has shown that this approach could even promote entry into addiction treatments besides the reduction of risky behaviors, HIV and HCV infection, and overdose deaths [36].

18.5 Conclusion

This chapter has reviewed the last evidence and clinical practice recommendations in relation to opioid-related disorders. In the context of the current opioid crisis, there is a growing concern about how to mitigate the impact and avoid further losses, and in that sense, naloxone remains a fundamental tool to prevent deaths from overdoses, with development of different programs and studies to improve the accessibility of this drug. Methadone, buprenorphine, and, to a lesser degree, naltrexone are effective drugs for the treatment of long-term maintenance, with new

formulations that probably will facilitate compliance by the patient avoiding relapses. It is necessary to study the inclusion of alternatives such as SROM and diacetylmorphine, already available in some countries, and also to elucidate with greater clarity the best recommendation of psychosocial interventions in patients with opioid use disorder.

Acknowledgments This work was supported by the following projects: Red de Trastornos Adictivos-RTA RD16/0017/0003 and RD16/0017/0010, integrated in the National RCDCI and funded by the ISCIII and the European Regional Development Fund (FEDER), European Commission action grants (Directorate-General for Migration and Home Affairs, Grant Agreement number: 806996-JUSTSO-JUST-2017-AGDRUG), and grants from Suport Grups de Recerca AGAUR Gencat (2017SGR 316 and 2017SGR 530) and Instrumental Action for the Intensification of Health Professionals-Specialist practitioners (PERIS: SLT006/17/00014).

References

1. United Nations Office on Drugs and Crime. World drug report 2018, Vienna; 2018.
2. Volkow ND, Jones EB, Einstein EB, Wargo EM. Prevention and treatment of opioid misuse and addiction: a review. JAMA Psychiat. 2019;76(2):208–16.
3. Kreek MJ, Zhou Y, Butelman ER, Levran O. Opiate and cocaine addiction: from bench to clinic and back to the bench. Curr Opin Pharmacol. 2009;9(1):74–80.
4. Fanucchi L, Springer SA, Korthuis PT. Medications for treatment of opioid use disorder among persons living with HIV. Curr HIV/AIDS Rep. 2019;16(1):1–6.
5. Roncero C, Villegas JL, Martínez-Rebollar M, Buti M. The pharmacological interactions between direct-acting antivirals for the treatment of chronic hepatitis c and psychotropic drugs. Expert Rev Clin Pharmacol. 2018;11(10):999–1030.
6. Socías ME, Wood E. Evaluating slow-release oral morphine to narrow the treatment gap for opioid use disorders. Ann Intern Med. 2017;168(2):141–2.
7. Dinis-Oliveira RJ. Metabolism and metabolomics of opiates: a long way of forensic implications to unravel. J Forensic Legal Med. 2019;61:128–40.
8. Inturrisi CE, Max MB, Foley KM, Schultz M, Shin SU, Houde RW. The pharmacokinetics of heroin in patients with chronic pain. N Engl J Med. 1984;310(19):1213–7.
9. Cone EJ, Holicky BA, Grant TM, Darwin WD, Goldberger BA. Pharmacokinetics and pharmacodynamics of intranasal "snorted" heroin. J Anal Toxicol. 1993;17(6):327–37.

10. Strang J, Groshkova T, Uchtenhagen A, van den Brink W, Haasen C, Schechter MT, Lintzeris N, Bell J, Pirona A, Eugenia Oviedo-Joekes E, Simon R, Metrebian N. Heroin on trial: systematic review and meta-analysis of randomised trials of diamorphine-prescribing as treatment for refractory heroin addiction. Br J Psychiatry. 2015;207(1):5–14.

11. Dole VP, Nyswander ME, Kreek MJ. Narcotic blockade. Arch Intern Med. 1966;118(4):304–9.

12. Eap CB, Buclin T, Baumann P. Interindividual variability of the clinical pharmacokinetics of methadone: implications for the treatment of opioid dependence. Clin Pharmacokinet. 2002;41(14):1153–93.

13. Volpe DA, Xu Y, Sahajwall CG, Younis IR, Patel V. Methadone metabolism and drug-drug interactions: in vitro and in vivo literature review. J Pharm Sci. 2018;107(12):2983–91.

14. Mercadante S. Opioid metabolism and clinical aspects. Eur J Pharmacol. 2015;769:71–8.

15. Fonseca F, Torrens M. Pharmacogenetics of methadone response. Mol Diagn Ther. 2018;22(1):57–78.

16. Kreek MJ. Medical safety and side effects of methadone in tolerant individuals. JAMA. 1973;223(6):665–8.

17. Toce MS, Chai PR, Burns MM, Boyer EW. Pharmacologic treatment of opioid use disorder: a review of pharmacotherapy, adjuncts, and toxicity. J Med Toxicol. 2018;14(4):306–22.

18. Fonseca F, Marti-Almor J, Pastor A, Cladellas M, Farre M, de la Torre R, Torrens M. Prevalence of long QTc interval in methadone maintenance patients. Drug Alcohol Depend. 2009;99(1–3):327–32.

19. Krantz MJ, Martin J, Stimmel B, Mehta D, Haigney MC. QTc interval screening in methadone treatment. Ann Intern Med. 2009;150(6):387–95.

20. Yaksh TL, Wallace MS. Opioids, analgesia and pain management. In: Brunton LL, Hilal-Dandan R, Knollmann BC, editors. Goodman and Gilman's the pharmacological basis of therapeutics. 13th ed. New York: McGraw Hill; 2018.

21. Wiegand TJ. The new kid on the block — incorporating buprenorphine into a medical toxicology practice. J Med Toxicol. 2016;12(1):64–70.

22. Saxena PP, Bodkin JA. Opioidergic agents as antidepressants: rationale and promise. CNS Drugs. 2019;33(1):9–16.

23. Mendelson J, Jones RT. Clinical and pharmacological evaluation of buprenorphine and naloxone combinations: why the 4:1 ratio for treatment? Drug Alcohol Depend. 2003;70(2 Suppl):S29–37.

24. Coe MA, Lofwall MR, Walsh SL. Buprenorphine pharmacology review: update on transmucosal and long-acting formulations. J Addict Med. 2019;13(2):93–103.

25. Pérez-Mañá C, Papaseit E, Fonseca F, Farré A, Torrens M, Farré M. Drug interactions with new synthetic opioids. Front Pharmacol. 2018;9:1145.

26. Comer SD, Cahill CM. Fentanyl: receptor pharmacology, abuse potential, and implications for treatment. Neurosci Biobehav Rev. 2018;pii:S0149-7634(18):30207–0.

27. Webster LR, Bath B, Medve RA, Marmon T, Stoddard GJ. Randomized, double-blind, placebo-controlled study of the abuse potential of different formulations of oral oxycodone. Pain Med. 2012;13(6):790–801.

28. Miotto K, Cho AK, Khalil MA, Blanco K, Sasaki JD, Rawson R. Trends in tramadol: pharmacology, metabolism, and misuse. Anesth Analg. 2017;124(1):44–51.

29. Boyer EW. Management of opioid analgesic overdose. N Engl J Med. 2012;367(2):146–55.

30. Barnett V, Twycross R, Mihalyo M, Wilcock A. Opioid antagonists. J Pain Symptom Manag. 2014;47(2):341–52.

31. Noble F, Marie N. Management of opioid addiction with opioid substitution treatments: beyond methadone and buprenorphine. Front Psych. 2019;9:742.

32. Soyka M, Rosner S. Nalmefene for treatment of alcohol dependence. Exp Opin Investig Drugs. 2010;19(11):1451–9.

33. Shen WW. Anticraving therapy for alcohol use disorder: a clinical review. Neuropsychopharmacol Rep. 2018;38:105–16.

34. American Psychiatric Association. Diagnostic and statistical manual of mental disorders. 5th ed. Arlington: American Psychiatric Association; 2013.

35. Fairbairn N, Coffin PO, Walley A. Naloxone for heroin, prescription opioid, and illicitly made fentanyl overdoses: challenges and innovations responding to a dynamic epidemic. Int J Drug Policy. 2017;46:172–9.

36. British Columbia Centre on Substance Use and B.C. Ministry of Health. A guideline for the clinical management of opioid use disorder. Published June 5, 2017. Available at: http://www.bccsu.ca/care-guidance-publications/.

37. World Health Organization. Guidelines for the psychosocially assisted pharmacological treatment of opioid dependence. 2009. http://www.who.int/substance_abuse/publications/opioid_dependence_guidelines.pdf.

38. Kampman K, Jarvis M. American Society of Addiction Medicine (ASAM) national practice guideline for the use of medications in the treatment of addiction involving opioid use. J Addict Med. 2015;9(5):358–67.

39. Gowing L, Farrell M, Ali R, White JM. Alpha2-adrenergic agonists for the management of opioid withdrawal. Cochrane Database Syst Rev. 2016;(5):CD002024.

40. Lee JD, Nunes EV Jr, Novo P, Bachrach K, Bailey GL, Bhatt S, et al. Comparative effectiveness of extended-release naltrexone versus buprenorphine-naloxone for opioid relapse prevention (X:BOT): a multicentre, open-label, randomised controlled trial. Lancet. 2018;391(10118):309–18.

41. Lobmaier PP, Kunøe N, Gossop M, Katevoll T, Waal H. Naltrexone implants compared to methadone: outcomes six months after prison release. Eur Addict Res. 2010;16(3):139–45.

42. Dematteis M, Auriacombe M, D'Agnone O, Somaini L, Szerman N, Littlewood R, Alam F, Alho H, Benyamina A, Bobes J, Daulouede JP, Leonardi C, Maremmani I, Torrens M, Walcher S, Soyka M. Recommendations for buprenorphine and methadone therapy in opioid use disorder: a European consensus. Expert Opin Pharmacother. 2017;18(18):1987–99.

43. de Vos JW, Ufkes JG, Kaplan CD, Tursch M, Krause JK, van Wilgenburg H, Woodcock BG, Staib AH. L-methadone and D, L-methadone in methadone maintenance treatment: a comparison of therapeutic effectiveness and plasma concentrations. Eur Addict Res. 1998;4(3):134–41.

44. Ansermot N, Albayrak O, Schläpfer J, Crettol S, Croquette-Krokar M, Bourquin M, De'glon JJ, Faouzi M, Scherbaum N, Eap CB. Substitution of (R, S)-methadone by (R)-methadone: impact on QTc interval. Arch Intern Med. 2010;170(6):529–36.

45. Ferri M, Minozzi S, Bo A, Amato L. Slow-release oral morphine as maintenance therapy for opi-oid dependence. Cochrane Database Syst Rev. 2013;6:CD009879.

46. Ferri M, Davoli M, Perucci CA. Heroin maintenance for chronic heroin-dependent individuals. Cochrane Database Syst Rev. 2011;(12):CD003410.

47. World Health Organization. Guidelines for the psychosocially assisted pharmacological treatment of opioid dependence. Geneva. 2009. Available: https://www.ncbi.nlm.nih.gov/books/NBK143185.

48. Amato L, Minozzi S, Davoli M, Vecchi S. Psychosocial combined with agonist maintenance treatments versus agonist maintenance treatments alone for treatment of opioid dependence. Cochrane Database Syst Rev. 2011;(10):CD004147.

49. Marsden J, Stillwell G, James K, Shearer J, Byford S, Hellier J, Kelleher M, Kelly J, Murphy C, Mitcheson L. Efficacy and cost-effectiveness of an adjunctive personalised psychosocial intervention in treatment-resistant maintenance opioid agonist therapy: a pragmatic, open-label, randomised controlled trial. Lancet Psychiatry. 2019;6(5):391–402.

Addiction of Hallucinogens, Dissociatives, Designer Drugs and "Legal Highs": Update on Potential Therapeutic Use

19

Magi Farré, Esther Papaseit, Francina Fonseca, and Marta Torrens

Contents

M. Farré (✉) · E. Papaseit
Universitat Autònoma de Barcelona,
Barcelona, Spain

Hospital Universitari Germans Trias i Pujol (IGTP),
Badalona, Spain
e-mail: mfarre.germanstrias@gencat.cat

F. Fonseca · M. Torrens
Universitat Autònoma de Barcelona,
Barcelona, Spain

Institut de Neuropsiquiatria i Addiccions, Hospital
del Mar, Barcelona, Spain

IMIM (Institut Hospital del Mar d'Investigacions
Mèdiques), Barcelona, Spain

Abstract

Hallucinogenic drugs have as their primary effect the production of disturbances of perception. Hallucinogens can be classified according to their chemical structure as indoleamines (similar to serotonin), phenethylamines (similar to catecholamines), dissociatives (phencyclidines) and others (including salvinorin, dextromethorphan, muscarinic antagonists and cannabinoids). The hallucinogenic effects appear to be related to the agonistic action on 5-HT2A receptors in the cortex. These actions seem to cause a functional imbalance at various levels (cortical areas, limbic system, which is a group of brain structures involved in emotional regulation), contributing to distort the integrative action. Hallucinogens produce substance use disorder, induce acute tolerance to its effects and do not present withdrawal syndrome. The novel psychoactive substances (NPS) can induce substance use disorder, intoxication and in some cases withdrawal syndrome (for those with psychostimulant properties). Depending on the substance and pharmacological effects, the DSM-5 diagnostic criteria for hallucinogens or stimulants can be applied. The therapeutic aim in these cases is to reduce consumption and achieve the abstinence. There are no specific drugs for treating the addiction caused by these substances. Some hallucinogens are under evaluation for its therapeutic use in different mental disorders.

Keywords

Hallucinogens · LSD · Psilocybin · Mescaline
MDMA · Esketamine · Therapeutic use
Substance use disorder · New psychoactive
substances

19.1   Introduction

This chapter is a review of the different families of hallucinogenic, dissociative and novel psychoactive substances. It provides a brief historical introduction, origin, chemistry and mechanism of action, its pharmacological and adverse effects and the relevant psychiatric clinical aspects. In addition, an update on its potential therapeutic use is included.

Hallucinogenic drugs have as their primary effect the production of disturbances of perception, thought or mood at low doses with minimal effects on memory and orientation. A hallucination is defined as a sensory perception without objective reality. An illusion is a perceptual distortion of an actual stimulus in the environment; it is a distortion of the perceived. Hallucinations can develop in any sensory modality but most commonly are visual or auditory in nature.

Subjects with hallucinations induced by acute consumption of a hallucinogenic are aware that the experience is caused by the substance and are able to maintain a sense of reality. There are a variety of widely accepted synonyms for hallucinogens, including the terms psychedelics and psychotomimetics.

Hallucinogens include a diverse group of substances with different chemical structures, including natural products and synthetic drugs. Hallucinogens can be classified (Table 19.1)

according to their chemical structure as indoleamines (similar to serotonin), phenethylamines (similar to catecholamines), dissociative (phencyclidines) and others (including salvinorin, dextromethorphan, muscarinic antagonists and cannabinoids). Hallucinogens can be found natu-

Table 19.1 Classification of hallucinogens

Indoleamides	LSD derivatives	Lysergic acid amides: ergine, isoergine Lysergic acid diethylamide (LSD-25 or Lysergide)
	Substituted tryptamines	Psilocybin Psilocin O-Acetylpsilocin (4-acetoxy-DMT) Dimethyltryptamine (DMT) Bufotenine (cebilcin, 5-OH-DMT) Diethyltryptamine (DET) 5-Bromo-N,N-dimethyltryptamine (5-Bromo-DMT) 5-Methoxy-N,N-dimethyltryptamine (5-methoxy-DMT) 5-Methoxy-dimethyltryptamine (5-MeO-DMT) Ibogaine Ayahuasca (contains DMT)
Phenethylamines	Methoxyamphetamines "hallucinogenic amphetamines"	Mescaline (3,4,5-trimethoxyphenethylamine) 4-Bromo-2,5-dimethoxyamphetamine (DOB) 4-Methyl-2,5-dimethoxyamphetamine (DOM, serenity, tranquility and peace or STP) 2,4,5-Trimethoxyamphetamine (TMA-2) paramethoxyamphetamine (PMA) 4-Bromo-2,5-dimethoxyphenylamphetamine (2CB-MFT) 2,5-Dimethoxy-4-bromo-phenethylamine (2-CB, nexus) 2,5-Dimethoxy-4-iodophenethylamine (2C-I) 2,5-Dimethoxy-4-ethylthiophenethylamine (2C-T-2) 2,5-Dimethoxy-4-(n)-propylthiophenethylamine (2C-T-7) 8-Bromo-2,3,6,7-benzo-dihydrodifuran-ethylamine (2CB-Fly) Bromo-benzodifuranyl-isopropylamine (bromo-dragonfly)
	Methylenedioxyamphetamines "entactogen amphetamines"	3,4-Methylenedioxymethamphetamine (MDMA, "ecstasy", "Adam") 3,4-Methylenedioxyamphetamine (MDA, "love pill") 3,4-Methylenedioxyethylamphetamine (MDEA or MDE, "Eve") N-Methyl-1-(3,4-methylenedioxyphenyl)-2 butanamine (MBDB) 3,4-Methylenedioxymethcathinone (methylone, "explosion") 4-Methyl methcathinone (mephedrone) β-keto-N-methylbenzodioxolylpropylamine (bk-MBDB, butylone)

(continued)

Table 19.1 (continued)

Dissociatives (phencyclidines)	Phencyclidine (PCP) Ketamine Methoxetamine 3-Methoxyphencyclidine (3-MeO-PCP)	
Others	Opioid derivatives Anticholinergics Salvinorin A Thujones Muscimol and ibotenic acid Cannabinoids	Dextromethorphan Atropine, scopolamine, trihexyphenidyl *Salvia divinorum* (contains salvinorin A)

rally in some plants and animals and can be synthesized in the laboratory. Some hallucinogen drugs are included in the category of designer drugs, legal highs and new psychoactive substances [1, 2].

19.2 Classical Hallucinogens

19.2.1 Origin and Synthesis

Hallucinogenic substances are among the oldest substances used by human kind. Many cultures recorded using certain plants specifically to induce visions or alter the perception of reality. Often these hallucinations were part of a religious or initiation experience. In this context they are referred to as entheogens. Shamans in Siberia were known to eat the hallucinogenic mushroom *Amanita muscaria*. Peyote, a cactus found in the southwestern United States and Mexico, was used by native peoples, including the Aztecs, to produce visions.

The modern synthetic drug era began in the late 1930s with the synthesis of lysergic acid diethylamide (LSD) by the Swiss chemist, Albert Hoffman. Some years later in 1943, after accidentally absorbing a small amount, he experienced its psychoactive effects. After World War II, there was an explosion of interest in hallucinogenic drugs in psychiatry, on either it's potential for psychotherapeutic applications or on its use to produce a "controlled psychosis", in order to understand psychotic disorders. LSD was marketed by Sandoz

laboratories under the trade name Delysid ® as a potential tool for psychotherapy in the 1950s. The growing popularity of LSD in the 1960s associated with the hippie movement resulted in its ban in the United States in 1967. In recent years, there is a new interest in the investigation of therapeutic use of hallucinogens [3, 4].

19.2.2 Epidemiology and Pattern of Consumption

For a number of years, the overall prevalence levels of LSD and hallucinogenic mushroom use in Europe have been generally low and stable. Among young adults (15–34 years), national surveys report last-year prevalence estimates of less than 1% for both substances in 2017 or most recent survey year, with the exception of Finland (1.9%) and the Netherlands (1.6%) for hallucinogenic mushrooms and Norway (1.1%) and Finland (1.3%) for LSD [5].

The lifetime prevalence of LSD use in the United States in students on the 12th grades is among 4.9–5.1 in the past 3 years and similar for hallucinogens other than LSD. The trend in annual prevalence in young adults (30 years) is lower, among 0.2–0.9% in the last 3 years [6].

In the United States, of all substance use disorders, other hallucinogen use disorder (exclude dissociative) is one of the rarest. The 12-month prevalence is estimated to be 0.2% among 12- to 17-year-olds and 0.4% among adults age 18 and older in the United States [7].

19.2.3 Mechanism of Action

LSD activity is predominantly on serotonin receptors (5-HT), but also on dopamine receptors. LSD as other classical hallucinogens are partial agonist on serotonin 5-HT2 receptors and also on the 5-HT1A/1C receptors, both presynaptic and postsynaptic. There is a good correlation between the relative affinity of these compounds for 5-HT2 receptors and their potency as hallucinogens in humans.

The hallucinogenic effects appear to be related to the agonistic action on 5-HT2A receptors in the cortex. Ketanserin, a 5-HT2 antagonist, blocks some of the specific effects of LSD and other hallucinogens. It also activates the dopaminergic receptors and causes glutamatergic activation. All these actions seem to cause a functional imbalance at various levels (cortical areas, limbic system, which is a group of brain structures involved in emotional regulation), contributing to distort the integrative action. At a peripheral level, it acts as a serotonergic antagonist and also has an action in dopaminergic system (D1 and D2 at least) and is alpha adrenergic. Most classical hallucinogens share actions of LSD, but dissociative anaesthetics and dextromethorphan are NMDA receptor antagonists (N-methyl-D-aspartate or NMDA), and salvinorin A is a potent kappa-opioid receptor agonist. Some anticholinergic derivatives (*Amanita muscaria* mushroom, plants containing atropine derivatives) at high doses can induce an intoxication with hallucinations due to its action as antagonists of the muscarinic receptor in the CNS [1, 8, 9].

19.2.4 LSD

LSD is an extremely potent substance; active doses are between 0.5 and 2 microgram/kg (50–150 micrograms per dose). LSD is well absorbed by the gastrointestinal tract. It is rapidly metabolized, and only 1% of the dose is excreted in urine without being biotransformed. It undergoes hydroxylation (addition of a group-OH) and conjugation with glucuronic acid in the liver. Its half-life is about 3 hours (2–5 hours), but its effects last longer [2, 10].

Psychoactive effects peak at 2–4 hours and can last for up to 12 hours depending on dose, tolerance, body weight and age. Users of LSD typically experience autonomic symptoms within several minutes and psychoactive effects approximately 10 minutes later. The autonomic symptoms are mainly sympathomimetic, such as elevated blood pressure and pulse, diaphoresis, piloerection, nausea, hyperreflexia and tremor. Anisocoria (unequal pupils) and hippus (rhythmically dilating pupils) are not uncommon [10].

Sensory effects generally appear 1 hour after administration. Initially there are fluctuations or changes in brightness or illumination, shapes are distorted and the colours are more intense and bright and constantly vary in pitch and intensity. Auditory distortions are less common. At higher doses, synesthesia may occur (perceiving a sensation in a different modality such as hearing colours). Distortions regarding the perception of time include time halting, stretching, repeating and ceasing to exist. The sense of self can change dramatically, even to depersonalization. It feels as if the mind left the body and there was a union of the self with the universe. There are frequent religious, philosophical or mystical experiences. Psychological symptoms include multiple mood alterations, ranging from happy to sad. When the overall experience is perceived as enlightening or emotionally stimulating, it is referred to as a "good trip". Other times the experience might be nightmarish, with fears of insanity or losing control and anxiety. Such negative experiences are referred to as "bad trips". The cause of good trips versus bad trips is not known. The psychic experience generally lasts 8–12 hours and is often followed by a pleasant "psychic numbness" [1, 2, 10].

19.2.5 Hallucinogen Use Disorder

Long-term hallucinogen use is not common. Tolerance to the psychological effects of LSD and other hallucinogens, but not the physiological effects, develops quickly. In contrast to highly addictive drugs such as cocaine and heroin, they do not produce physical dependence or withdrawal syndrome upon cessation of consumption.

Usually, there is a clear and accurate memory of what happened during the hallucinogenic experience [1, 2, 8].

19.2.6 Intoxication of Hallucinogens

Patients have symptoms of sympathetic activation, perceptual changes, and psychiatric symptoms (agitation, anxiety, panic, psychosis). There are also frequent "bad trips" that present with psychiatric symptoms (anxiety or important panic reaction). Intoxications are occasionally accompanied by delirium (is a separate diagnostic category). The elimination of the substance gradually improves symptoms. There are no documented fatalities from LSD use, but fatal accidents and suicides have occurred during intoxication.

19.2.7 Hallucinogen Persisting Perception Disorder

It is defined as "the transient recurrence of disturbances in perception that are reminiscent of those experienced during one or more earlier Hallucinogen Intoxications". Flashbacks are referred to as hallucinogen persisting perception disorder by the DSM-5 when they cause significant distress [11].

The most common phenomena are visual distortions such as colour confusion, geometric hallucinations and trailing, but the content of the flashback may involve any of the senses. It is not known what causes flashbacks. Theories include persisting damage to visual processing systems, dysfunction of inhibitory cortical interneurons, reverse tolerance and that they are an atypical dissociative state. Flashbacks may occur several days to several years after the antecedent use of LSD and have been reported with mescaline, phencyclidine and marijuana. Some users find these episodes pleasant and even refer to them as "free trips". For others they are terrified about it and they recur frequently. An antecedent good trip does not predict a good flashback. It is unclear what determines who will experience

flashbacks and whether or not the experience will be pleasant.

Flashbacks have reportedly been induced by many situations including stress, exercise, pregnancy, sexual intercourse, dark environments, flashing lights, monotony and use of other psychoactive drugs. It is estimated that anywhere from 15% to 60% of LSD users experience flashbacks. The flashback experience is often precipitated by psychiatric illness as well as another drug use. Regardless of treatment, the frequency of flashbacks tends to decrease with time. Suicidal behaviour, major depressive disorder and panic disorders are potential complications [2, 12].

19.2.8 Persistent Psychosis Related to Mental Illness

Occasionally, LSD appears to precipitate a "persistent psychosis" characterized by visual hallucinations, mania, grandiosity and religiosity. It is estimated to occur in 0.08–4.6% of people who have used lysergic acid diethylamide.

Chronic effects include descriptions of permanent schizoid disorders and subsequent or prior ingestion associated with LSD. Although the association between the occurrence of permanent psychosis and LSD is well established in various publications, it is not known precisely what the actual risk is. It seems that LSD would not be the direct cause of the development of permanent disorders, but LSD intake would act as a trigger of a preexisting disease state [2, 8].

19.2.9 Hallucinogen-Induced Affective Disorders

While feeling overwhelmed, scared and afraid of losing control occurs in panic attacks, LSD intoxication is further characterized by dramatic and persistent perceptual distortions. As with any altered mental state, the clinician should have a low threshold for suspecting delirium. Unlike delirium, there is no fluctuation level consciousness with LSD intoxication. There is no specific pharmacological treatment for this disorder. When the patients stop the consumption, anxious-depressive syndrome may appear requiring symptomatic treatment [2, 8].

19.2.10 Somatic Complications of Hallucinogens

Although LSD and other hallucinogens are considered relatively safe when compared with other drugs of abuse, there are case reports of respiratory failure, hyperthermia and coagulopathies associated with massive doses. Early on a relationship between lysergic acid diethylamide and chromosomal damage was suspected, but this has been consistently refuted and lysergic acid diethylamide does not appear to be teratogenic. LSD, however, does induce uterine contractions which could disrupt pregnancy.

19.2.11 Treatment of Hallucinogen Use Disorder

The aim is to reduce consumption and achieve the abstinence. It is easy to stop consuming initially, because there is no physical dependence, but abstinence is more difficult at long term. Often bad trips facilitate abstinence or not to repeat the experience. As in the other drug addiction programmes, psychiatric and psychological support components are used.

There are no specific drugs for treating disorders caused by these substances. Psychotropic drugs will be used according to the patient's symptoms (benzodiazepines, antipsychotics, antidepressants). The "bad trip" generally does not require inpatient hospitalization because of its limited time course and quick recovery. The patient should be placed in a quiet, non-stimulating environment and provided continuous reassurance that his or her state of mind is drug induced and will not result in permanent brain damage. When medications are needed, benzodiazepines are probably the best choice, as long as delirium has been ruled out. The use of neuroleptics should be reserved for instances

where none of the aforementioned efforts have succeeded. High-potency (less anticholinergic) neuroleptics should be used because anticholinergics have been associated with paradoxical reactions such as hypotension and anticholinergic crises. The use of haloperidol and chlorpromazine has a high potential risk of favouring the occurrence of seizures [1, 2, 8].

19.2.12 Mescaline

Mescaline is the 3,4,5-trimethoxyphenethylamine. It is a phenethylamine hallucinogen found in several species of North and South American cacti, including peyote (*Lophophora williamsii*) and San Pedro. Mescaline was first isolated from peyote cacti in 1896 and was synthesized approximately 20 years later.

Natural peyote has a bitter taste. It is dried and chewed, soaked in water and drank or injected. The hallucinogenic dose is approximately 5 mg/kg (0.3–0.5 g). Each button contains about 50–100 mg of mescaline, and users typically ingest 3–8 buttons. Within the first 30 minutes, before the onset of psychological symptoms, users can experience nausea, vomiting, restlessness and headaches. By 1–2 hours, however, these unpleasant physiologic symptoms dissipate, and the psychic phase characterized by euphoria, sensory distortions, and feelings of confidence begins. The entire experience lasts up to 12–14 hours. As in the case with LSD and the other serotonergic hallucinogens, tolerance develops rapidly, and physical dependence does not occur. Treatment of acute intoxication and adverse consequences as with LSD and psilocybin involves reassurance and use of benzodiazepines if necessary [1, 2, 4].

19.2.13 Tryptamines

There are a number of noncontrolled tryptamines that are used for their psychedelic properties. They have effects similar to the tryptamines already controlled such as psilocybin (found in *Psylocybe* mushrooms or "magic mushrooms") or dimethyltryptamine (DMT). Tryptamines can be synthesized, although they also exist in plants, fungi and animals [1].

Albert Hoffman isolated and then synthesized psilocybin. It was marketed by Sandoz laboratories under the trade name Indocybin ® as a potential tool for psychotherapy in the 1960s. The mushrooms can be eaten fresh, dried or brewed. They are usually ingested orally. Psilocybin is a prodrug that is converted in the body into the pharmacologically active compound psilocin by a dephosphorylation reaction. Typical doses of psilocybin range from 4 to 20 mg (40 µg/kg) corresponding to 1–2 g of dried mushrooms. Sympathomimetic symptoms occur at lower doses (3–5 mg), and psychological effects are elicited by doses above 8 mg. Psychological effects begin within 30 minutes of ingestion, peak at 2–3 hours and dissipate by 12 hours. Psilocybin occasioned mystical-type experiences. Only one third of "magic mushrooms" bought on the street actually contain psilocybin (many are simply store-bought mushrooms laced with phencyclidine), and there are many wild poisonous mushrooms. Adulteration and misidentification are the most common causes of serious adverse outcomes. As with the other serotonergic hallucinogens, tolerance develops quickly but physical dependence does not occur [1, 13, 14].

19.2.14 Dextromethorphan

Dextromethorphan is the dextro isomer of levorphanol, a codeine derivative, used as a cough suppressant at doses between 15 and 30 mg orally every 6–8 hours. It is marketed in single or in multicomponent medicines for the treatment of symptoms associated with the common cold or flu. It is a hallucinogen when administered at high doses of 240–480 mg.

Dextromethorphan hallucinogenic effects are due to its antagonistic action on NMDA glutamate receptors. It has no opioid activity.

Readily absorbed orally, it is metabolized to dextrorphan, which is the active ingredient in cough by cytochrome P450 CYP2D6. Up to 5–10% of Caucasians have a deficiency of this isoenzyme and therefore cannot metabolize dextromethorphan to dextrorphan (poor metabolizers). The elimination half-life is 1.5–4 hours for dextromethorphan in extensive metabolizers. It is a minority used substance, commonly used as ketamine to provoke feelings of mind-body separation and the so-called near-death experiences. Poisoning presents with light-headedness, fatigue, nausea and vomiting and ataxia. Also described are nystagmus, mydriasis or even coma and death, plus cases of psychosis, dystonia and serotonin syndrome. In case of poisoning, supportive measures and symptomatic treatment are recommended [1, 15].

19.2.15 Salvia divinorum

Salvinorin A is the psychoactive substance in the plant *Salvia divinorum*. It can induce dissociative effects and is a potent producer of visual and other hallucinatory experience. Salvinorin A appears to be the most potent naturally occurring hallucinogen. Salvinorin A is present in the dried plant at about 0.18%. It is a potent and selective κappa-opioid receptor agonist; in addition, it is a potent D2 receptor partial agonist, and it is likely this action plays a significant role in its effects as well. *Salvia divinorum* is usually smoked and produces rapid and intense effects with a short action (15–30 minutes). Its effects include various psychedelic experiences, including past memories (such as revisiting places from childhood memory), merging with objects and overlapping realities (such as the perception of being in several locations at the same time). In contrast to other drugs, its use often prompts dysphoria, i.e. feelings of sadness and depression, as well as fear. In addition, it may prompt a decreased heart rate, slurred speech, lack of coordination and possibly loss of consciousness.

Differing studies suggest no overall consensus so far with regard to the long-term effects of *Salvia* on mood [1, 2].

19.2.16 Ayahuasca

Ayahuasca, also commonly called *yagé*, is a hallucinogenic brew of various psychoactive infusions or decoctions prepared with the *Banisteriopsis caapi* vine (that contains the beta-carboline alkaloids harmaline and harmine). It is either mixed with the leaves from the genus *Psychotria* (*Psychotria viridis*), which contains dimethyltryptamine (DMT). DMT is not absorbed by oral route because it is metabolized by deamination enzymes in the gut, but when the two plants are ingested together, the beta-carboline alkaloids inhibit the deamination enzymes that ordinarily degrade DMT (monoamine oxidase, MAO). Ayahuasca is used largely in religious rituals. The psychedelic effects of ayahuasca include visual and auditory stimulation, the mixing of sensory modalities and psychological introspection that may lead to great elation, fear or illumination. It produces intense vomiting and occasional diarrhoea. In native or religious communities using ayahuasca, there is no evidence of psychological maladjustment, mental health deterioration or cognitive impairment [4, 16, 17].

19.2.17 Ibogaine

Ibogaine is an indole alkaloid found in plants as *Tabernanthe iboga*. The plant originates in Africa and traditionally is used in sacramental initiation ceremonies. Ibogaine is a hallucinogen at the 400-mg dose range. Ibogaine is a tryptamine that acts as an agonist for the 5-HT2A receptor. In addition it also acts as an antagonist of the NMDA receptor set and an agonist for the kappa-opioid receptor. Ibogaine is metabolized in the human body by cytochrome P450 CYP2D6, and the major metabolite is noribogaine (12-hydroxyibogamine). Noribogaine is most potent as a serotonin reuptake inhibitor and acts as a moderate kappa-opioid receptor antagonist and weak mu-opioid receptor full agonist. In recent years ibogaine has been studied and even patented as a pharmacotherapy for opiate and other addictions involving doses that range as high as 1500 mg orally. There are not well-controlled studies in humans assessing its efficacy in opiate detoxification. The ingested material is taken from the plant or pure powder. Ibogaine can produce a QT-interval prolongation and induce ventricular tachycardia after initial use. Fatalities following ibogaine ingestion are documented in the medical literature [18–20].

19.3 Dissociatives

Dissociatives include phencyclidine (PCP, angel dust), ketamine (Special K), esketamine and other recent derivatives that sometimes are classified in the novel psychoactive substances category (as methoxetamine, methoxydine or 4-MeO-PCP, among others). Chemically, dissociatives are arylcyclohexylamine derivatives. These substances were developed as anaesthetics. Phencyclidine quickly was discarded because of a high frequency of postoperative delirium with hallucinations. It was classified as a dissociative anaesthetic because, in the anaesthetized state, the patient remains conscious with analgesia, with staring gaze, flat facies and rigid muscles. The use of ketamine persists, especially in animals and humans, as analgesic and anaesthetic.

19.3.1 Phencyclidine

Phencyclidine is just consumed in Europe but is very common in the United States. In the United States, 2.5% of those ages 12 and older acknowledged ever using PCP. The highest lifetime prevalence was in those aged 26–34 years (4%), whereas the highest proportion using PCP in the last year was in those aged 12–17 years (0.7%) [6, 7].

PCP is injected intravenously, smoked, snorted or ingested orally. It is a substance that causes medical complications resulting in often more toxic than LSD. It is estimated that up to 3% of deaths in drug users in the United States are due to phencyclidine.

Phencyclidine is an antagonist of NMDA glutamate receptors. It also activates dopaminergic ventral tegmental area, the area starting in the reward pathway. There is tolerance to the effects, but not physical dependence. Only a small percentage of daily users tend to use it infrequently. The elimination half-life is 21 hours. At low doses (less than 5 mg), ataxia, dysarthria, blurred vision, nystagmus and weakness are produced. At higher doses (5–10 mg), hypertonia, hyperreflexia, hypertension, tachycardia, sweating, fever, vomiting, stereotyped movements and muscle stiffness appear. Often there is emergence of aggressive and transient confusional episodes (with psychomotor agitation, belligerence and impulsivity). Also it induces changes in perception, disorganized thinking and feeling of unreality. And at even higher doses, it produces analgesia, amnesia and coma.

The intoxication is a medical emergency because it can be severe and life-threatening. Hyperpyrexia, muscle stiffness, seizures, severe hypertension, intracerebral bleeding and respiratory depression can be observed. Patients go to the emergency room with high hostility, aggressiveness, agitation, anxiety and self-injurious behaviour. It is the substance that produces more pictures of psychosis. It is symptomatically with the administration of anxiolytics (diazepam) and antipsychotics (haloperidol) [2, 8].

19.3.2 Ketamine

Ketamine has two optical isomers: S and R; the S-(+) isomer is more potent than the R(−) isomer. Ketamine is used by intramuscular or intravenous route as analgesic and anaesthetic. Ketamine has been evaluated for the therapy of treatment-resistant depression. Recently, the S-isomer or esketamine has been recently marketed in some countries for the treatment of treatment-resistant depression in conjunction with an oral antidepressant [21].

The recreational use of ketamine has been reported among subgroups of drug users in Europe for the last two decades. National estimates, where they exist, of the prevalence of ketamine use in adult and school populations remain low. In 2017, last-year prevalence of ketamine use among young adults [16–34] was estimated at 0.6% in Denmark and 1.7% in the United Kingdom [5]. In the United States the past-year use of ketamine appears to decline among 12th graders (1.2–0.7% over the past 3 years) [6].

Although the pharmaceutical presentation is injectable solution, it is transformed and crystallized in powder to consume. The illegal use of ketamine (Special K, Super K, kit kat, K) has been increasing in recent years and is part of the so-called club drugs, drugs used in electronic music parties. Another type of consumption is related to the search for new sensations. Consumers also use ecstasy and gamma hydroxybutyrate (GHB). Like PCP, ketamine is an antagonist of the NMDA glutamate receptors. It is administered by injection (intramuscular or intravenous), orally, smoked and inhaled. The elimination half-life of ketamine is 2–3 hours. The effects are fast, short-lasting and dose-dependent and can cause perceptual changes (from dissociation body sensation to near-death experiences) and psychopathological reactions similar to those of phencyclidine [21].

Appealing effects described by users include visual hallucinations and out-of-body experiences; undesirable effects include memory loss and decreased sociability. General central nervous system depressant effects include poor concentration and poor recollection similar to alcohol intoxication, which is not unexpected for an anaesthetic drug. Ketamine effects include profound changes in consciousness and psychotomimetic effects such as changes in body image (feeling that the body is made of wood, plastic or rubber) and possible feelings of spiritual separation from the body, including out-of-body experiences. At low doses, users describe mild dissociative effects, distortion of time and space and hallucinations. At large doses, users experience severe dissociation with intense detachment such that their perceptions seem to be located deep within their consciousness and reality is far off in the distance; this is called the "K-hole". The analgesic and dissociative effects may result in injury or even death in users.

Tolerance develops rapidly to the desired effects, resulting in reduced length of the subjective experience and requiring an increase in dose to maintain the expected effects. Users escalate the amount used to achieve the full hallucinogenic experience, up to seven times the original amount. Use of higher recreational doses can result in more adverse effects, especially physiological side effects. Use of very high doses can result in onset of full anaesthetic effects, which may result in an overdose situation for a recreational user. Continued use of ketamine or phencyclidine despite experiencing these consequences constitutes addiction (using the phencyclidine use disorder criteria). Some people develop compulsive consumption, recalling more the type of use of cocaine or psychostimulants [2].

The clinical symptoms of intoxication from ketamine are tachycardia, altered consciousness, disorganized speech and nystagmus. Treatment consists of supportive measures. Some ketamine users suffer urinary symptoms such as urinary frequency, urgency, dysuria and haematuria, which improve or disappear after cessation of use [8, 22].

19.4 Designer Drugs and "Legal Highs": MDMA and New Psychoactive Substances

19.4.1 Definitions

The emergence of new psychoactive substances that are not controlled under existing drug laws is not a new phenomenon. Over the last 20 years, a variety of terms and definitions have been used for new psychoactive substances that emerge on the market and are not under international control. Actually, the preferred term is new/novel psychoactive substances (NPS).

The emergence started in the 1970s with the denominated "designer drugs". They were defined as a psychoactive substance produced from chemical precursors in a clandestine laboratory, which, by slight modification of the chemical structure, has been intentionally designed to

mimic the properties of known psychoactive substances and which is not under international control (Buchanan and Brown 1988). Over the past few years, the globalization and the massive use of the Internet allowed the unprecedented growth in both the number and availability of these substances. In the European Union (EU), 24 novel psychoactive substances were identified for the first time in 2009, 71 in 2013, 98 in 2015 and 51 in 2017 [23].

More recently, "legal highs" has been used as an umbrella term for unregulated novel psychoactive substances, or products claiming to contain them, which are intended to mimic the effects of controlled drugs. The term includes a wide range of synthetic and/or plant-derived substances and products. These may be marketed as "legal highs" (emphasizing "legality"), "herbal highs" (stressing the natural/plant origin), as well as "research chemicals" and "party pills". "Legal highs" are usually sold via the Internet or in bricks and "head shops" or "smart shops". In most cases they are intentionally mislabelled with regard to their intended use (e.g. labelled as "not for human consumption", "plant food", "bath salts", "room odourizers", "incenses") and the active substances that they contain. This "legal highs" market can be distinguished from other drug markets by the speed at which suppliers circumvent drug controls by offering new alternatives to restricted products.

The NPS is defined by the United Nations Office on Drugs and Crime as "substances of abuse, either in a pure form or a preparation, that are not controlled by the 1961 Convention on Narcotic Drugs or the 1971 Convention on Psychotropic Substances, but which may pose a public health threat". The term "new" does not necessarily refer to new inventions—several NPS were first synthesized 40 years ago—but to substances that have recently become available on the market [24].

19.4.2 Origin and Synthesis

As mentioned above, the term "designer drug" was coined in the 1980s. It originally referred to various synthetic opioids, mostly based on modifications of fentanyl (alfa-methyl-fentanyl) and pethidine [25]. The term entered widespread use when 3,4-methylenedioxymethamphetamine (MDMA, "ecstasy") experienced a boom in the mid-1980s, first in the United States, followed by Europe in the 1990s, and then in other parts of the world. Another term that emerged in the late 1990s and early 2000s is "research chemicals" (RC). The term was coined by some marketers of designer drugs, specifically, psychedelic drugs of the tryptamine and phenethylamine families. The idea was that by selling the chemicals for so-called scientific research rather than for human consumption (they included an advice of "not for human use or consumption"), drug laws could be circumvented. The same strategy was behind the marketing of some of the cathinone-related substances as "bath salts" not intended for human consumption.

Substances sold as "legal highs" are mainly manufactured in chemical laboratories in Asia, according to the International Narcotics Control Board and the Europol, although some manufacture also takes place in Europe, the Americas and other regions. They are legally imported, either as chemicals or as packaged products [5].

New psychoactive substances can be classified as shown in Table 19.2.

Phenethylamine, including MDMA, and tryptamine derivatives are shown in Table 19.1 (see Sect. 19.1. Introduction).

19.4.3 Epidemiology and Pattern of Consumption

The use of NPS has grown rapidly over the past decade, in contrast to the prevalence rates for the use of internationally controlled drugs, which seem generally to have stabilized in the same time period [26].

According to United Nations, the number of stimulant NPS identified over the period 2009–2017 increased more than fourfold, from 48 substances in 2009 to a peak of 206 in 2015, a number that has remained stable since then [24].

Table 19.2 Classification of substances categorized as NPS based on the systems used by UNODC and EMCDDA. Some substances of each class are included as examples

Group	Substances
Synthetic cannabinoids	JWH-018 JWH-073 JWH-200 JWH-250 AM-694 CP 47,497 Cannabicyclohexanol CP 55,940 HU-210 THC-O-acetate AB-PINACA AB-FUBINACA UR-144 XLR-11
New synthetic opioids	Fentanyl and derivatives, carfentanil, isotonitazene
Synthetic cathinones	Cathinone Methcathinone (ephedrone) 4-Methylmethcathinone (mephedrone) Methylenedioxypyrovalerone (MDPV) Pyrovalerone Naphyrone (naphthylpyrovalerone, NRG-1) Ethylone (see Table 19.1 entactogens) Methylone (see Table 19.1 entactogens) Butylone (see Table 19.1 entactogens)
Phenethylamines	See Table 19.1 Paramethoxymethamphetamine (PMMA) 2,5-Dimethoxy-4-iodophenethylamine (2C-I) 2,5-Dimethoxy-4-methyl-phenethylamine (2C-D) 2,5-Dimethoxy-4-iodoamphetamine (DOI) 2,5-Dimethoxy-4-bromophenethylamine (2C-B) 4-Methylthioamphetamine (4-MTA) 25B-NBOMe
Piperazines	1-Benzylpiperazine (BZP) 1-(3,4-Methylenedioxybenzyl) piperazine (MDBP) 1-(3-Chlorophenyl)piperazine (mCPP) 1-(3-Trifluoromethylphenyl) piperazine (TFMPP) 1-(4-Methoxyphenyl)piperazine (MeOPP)

Table 19.2 (continued)

Group	Substances
Ketamine and phencyclidine-type substances	See Table 19.1 Ketamine N-Ethylnorketamine 3-Methoxyphencyclidine (3-MeO-PCP) 4-Methoxyphencyclidine (4-MeO-PCP) Eticyclidine (PCE, CI-400, N-ethyl-1-phenylcyclohexylamine) 2-(3-methoxyphenyl)-2-(ethylamino)cyclohexanone (methoxetamine) Rolicyclidine (PCPy; 1-(1-phenylcyclohexyl) pyrrolidine) Tenocyclidine (TCP; 1-(1-(2-thienyl)cyclohexyl) piperidine) 2-(3-Methoxyphenyl)-2-(ethylamino)cyclohexane (3-MeO-PCE)
Tryptamines	See Table 19.1
Plant-based psychoactive substances	Kratom (*Mitragyna speciosa*) *Salvia divinorum* Khat (*Catha edulis*)
Other:	
Aminoindanes	2-Aminoindane (2-AI) 5,6-Methylenedioxy-N-methyl-2--aminoindane (MDMAI) 5,6-Methylenedioxy-2-aminoindane (MDAI) 5-Methoxy-6-methyl-2--aminoindane (MMAI)
Benzofuranes	5-(2-Aminopropyl)-2,3-dihydrobenzofuran (5-APDB, 3-Desoxy-MDA, EMA-4) 6-(2-Aminopropyl)-2,3-dihydrobenzofuran (6-APDB, 4-Desoxy-MDA, EMA-3)
Piperidines	Pipradrol Desoxypipradrol (2-diphenylmethylpiperidine, 2-DPMP)
Synthetic cocaines	Dimethocaine 4-Fluorotropacocaine
Medicines	Phenazepam Etizolam Ethylphenidate Phenibut 4-Methylphenmetrazine

Well-known examples of NPS include substances such as synthetic cannabinoids contained in various herbal mixtures, new synthetic opioids, piperazines, products sold as "bath salts" (i.e. cathinone-type substances such as mephedrone and methylenedioxypyrovalerone (MDPV)) and various phenethylamines. From 2004 onwards, synthetic cannabinoids such as Spice appeared in the market, followed by synthetic cathinones and other emerging groups of NPS.

Among young adults (aged 15–34), last-year prevalence of use of these substances ranged from 0.1% in Norway to 3.2% in the most recent findings from the Netherlands, in 2016, with 4-fluoroamphetamine (4-FA) being the most commonly used. Survey data on the use of mephedrone are available for the United Kingdom (England and Wales). In the most recent survey (2017), last-year use of this drug among 16- to 34-year-olds was estimated at 0.2%, down from 1.1% in 2014/2015. In their most recent surveys, last-year estimates of the use of synthetic cannabinoids among 15- to 34-year-olds ranged from 0.1% in the Netherlands to 1.5% in Latvia [5]. The annual prevalence of use of bath salts among 12th-grade students fell by half between 2012 and 2018 [6].

The consumption of ecstasy is associated with attending electronic-dance music events or raves. It is estimated that 13.7 million adults in the European Union (aged 15–64), or 4.1% of this age group, have tried MDMA/ecstasy during their lives. Recent data about use among young adults suggest that 2.1 million young adults [15–34] used MDMA in the last year (1.7% of this age group), with national estimates ranging from 0.2% in Portugal and Romania to 7.1% in the Netherlands [5].

In North America, it is estimated that 0.9% of the population aged 15–64 were past-year "ecstasy" users in 2017. The annual prevalence of "ecstasy" use was reportedly highest among young adults aged 18–25, who accounted for 400,000 past-year users [24].

19.4.4 Pharmacological Properties and Consequences of the Use of MDMA (Ecstasy)

3,4-Methylenedioxymethamphetamine (MDMA) is a ring-substituted amphetamine structurally similar to methamphetamine and mescaline. MDMA has become widely known as "ecstasy" (shortened to "E", "X" or "XTC").

MDMA acts as a potent releaser and/or reuptake inhibitor of presynaptic serotonin (5-HT), dopamine (DA) and norepinephrine. MDMA is more potent and active on serotonergic neurons. MDMA is also a mild inhibitor of monoamine oxidase (MAO) and also has some direct actions in several types of receptors including the 5-HT2 receptor, the M1 muscarinic receptor, the 2-adrenergic receptor and the histamine H1 receptor [27].

Ecstasy is presented for use as tablets-pills, capsules or powder (crystal). Some wrap the powder in a cigarette paper and swallow it (bomb, bombing). It is usually taken orally, but some user snorted the contents. The MDMA content of pills or tablets varies widely between regions and different brands of pills and fluctuates. Pills may contain other active substances meant to stimulate in a way similar to MDMA, such as amphetamine, mephedrone, methamphetamine, ephedrine or caffeine. In some cases, tablets sold as ecstasy do not even contain any MDMA [28].

In general, users begin reporting subjective effects within 30–60 minutes of consumption, a peak appear at about 75–120 minutes, reaching a plateau that lasts about 3.5 hour. This is followed by a comedown feeling of a few hours. The usual dose is 50–125 mg with additional doses along the recreative session. The most frequent effects after MDMA administration are euphoria, well-being, happiness, stimulation, increased energy, extroversion, feeling close to others, increased empathy, increased sociability, enhanced mood, mild perceptual disturbances, somatic symptoms related to its cardiovascular (increase in blood pressure and heart rate) and autonomic effects (dry mouth, sweating, tremor, mydriasis tremor, jaw clenching and restlessness) and moderate derealization but not hallucinations. Some of the effects differential from those elicited by classical amphetamines (e.g. feeling close to others, increased empathy, increased sociability) are collectively termed as empathetic or entactogenic, and MDMA is considered the prototypical drug producing such effects [29–31].

MDMA-induced acute toxic effects are in relation to its pharmacologic actions. Mild toxicity signs include nausea, vomiting, restlessness, tremor, hyperreflexia, irritability, pallor, bruxism, trismus and palpitations. Moderate intoxication signs include hyperactivity, aggressive behaviour, panic attack, psychosis, confusion, muscle tension, tachycardia, arterial hypertension and increase in body temperature. Severe intoxication can include delirium, coma, seizures hypotension, tachydysrhythmias, hyperthermia (>40 °C) and renal failure associated with rhabdomyolysis. A serotonin syndrome (increased muscle rigidity, hyperreflexia and hyperthermia). Intracranial haemorrhage has been described. Heat stroke is a severe complication that can cause death; it includes hyperthermia, rhabdomyolysis, myoglobinuria, disseminated intravascular coagulation and renal failure. Fulminant hepatitis and hepatic necrosis have been described. Hyponatremia is an uncommon complication associated with inappropriate antidiuretic hormone (SIADH) secretion and excessive water intake. Its chronic use is linked to a progressive neurodegeneration of the serotonergic neurotransmission system [3, 32].

Two main pathways are involved in MDMA metabolic clearance: (1) O-demethylation partially regulated by CYP2D6 followed by catechol-O-methyltransferase (COMT)-catalyzed methylation (HMMA) and/or glucuronide/sulfate conjugation and (2) N-dealkylation leading to 3,4-methylenedioxyamphetamine (MDA), further subject to similar metabolic reactions than MDMA (O-demethylation and O-methylation). MDMA metabolic clearance accounts for about 75% of plasma clearance, and 30% of its metabolism is regulated by CYP2D6. In addition MDMA is a competitive inhibitor of CYP2D6; after a single dose, most hepatic

CYP2D6 is inactivated within 2 hours and returning to a basal level of CYP2D6 activity after at least 10 days. Other isoenzymes of cytochrome P450 and a relevant contribution of renal excretion play part in their clearance. Globally, the clinical relevance of CYP2D6 polymorphism is lower than that predicted by in vitro studies [32–34].

In addition, there is some evidence that MDMA produces in the mid-long-term selective long-lasting serotonergic neurotoxicity in animal models when administered at highly relative doses and/or after repeated administrations. The direct extrapolation of these results from animal to human is difficult [27, 33, 35, 36].

MDMA therapeutic use is under investigation. Few recent randomized, controlled trials of MDMA-assisted psychotherapy for post-traumatic stress disorder have been published showing some therapeutic efficacy [37–39].

MDMA can induce use-abuse, but it is not clear and, in some cases, it produces drug dependence but not drug withdrawal. Users reported tolerance to its desired effects and tend to cease spontaneously the consumption. MDMA can cause intoxication, and in this case the DSM-5 diagnostic criteria for stimulants can be applied [11]. There are no specific drugs for treating disorders caused by MDMA. Psychotropic drugs will be used according to the patient's symptoms (benzodiazepines, hypnotics, antipsychotics, antidepressants). As in the other drug addiction programmes, psychiatric and psychological support are used.

19.4.5 Consequences of the Use of "Legal Highs" and New Psychoactive Substances

NPS can induce substance use disorder, intoxication and in some cases withdrawal syndrome (for those with psychostimulant properties). Depending on the substance and pharmacological effects, the DSM-5 diagnostic criteria for hallucinogens or stimulants can be applied [11].

The clinical picture of the intoxication by NPS depends on the class of substances; in the case of cathinones and phenethylamines, the symptoms and signs are similar to an intoxication by a stimulant (amphetamine, MDMA). Synthetic cannabinoids can induce severe toxic effects including psychosis, respiratory depression, cardiac events including cardiac arrest, nephrotoxicity, gastrointestinal problems including hyperemesis, severe rhabdomyolysis, hyperthermia, acute cerebral ischaemia and seizures. In the case of tryptamines, the intoxication is similar to other hallucinogens [3, 40].

The use of ephedrone (methylcathinone) has recently been associated with symptoms like those seen in patients with Parkinson's disease (manganism) due to the compound manganese dioxide which is a by-product of synthesis with permanganate [41].

The use of MDPV was, in a number of cases, associated with highly bizarre behaviour, including a number of suicides, deaths associated with MDPV delirium and highly violent homicides [42].

Mephedrone is consumed intravenously in some countries as a substitute of heroin. Mephedrone is a common substance used in "chem-sex" to facilitate sexual sessions lasting several hours or days with multiple sexual partners. Mephedrone is usually taken by oral route but in some cases intravenous ("slamming"). Other substances used in "chem-sex" sessions are γ-hydroxybutyrate (GHB), γ-butyrolactone (GBL) and crystallized methamphetamine or cocaine [43].

The therapeutic objective is to reduce consumption and reach the abstinence. In some cases of NPS stop consuming can be easy because there is no physical dependence, in other cases (more psychostimulant profile) some symptoms of withdrawal syndrome can be observed. There are no specific drugs for treating disorders caused by these substances. Required of psychotropic drugs will be used according to the patient's symptoms (benzodiazepines, hypnotics, antipsychotics, antidepressants). As in the other drug addiction programs are used psychiatric and psychological support components [2].

It is very important to perform a psychiatric evaluation by a specialist to detect, if present, the comorbidity with other psychiatric diseases and evaluate the need for an early pharmacological treatment. It is important to be aware that cases of poisoning can be by NPS, not yet known pharmacodynamics and their effect. Also, they cannot be detected by usual urinary tests. It is recommended storing samples for study.

19.5 Update on Therapeutic Use of Hallucinogens

In the 1950s and 1960s, there was a scientific interest in psychedelic compounds, and they were studied as tools to understand the neurobiology of mental functions and as therapeutic agents for mental disorders, including substance abuse, depression, personality disorders (e.g. antisocial) and palliative care, and as adjuncts to psychotherapy. The scientific investigation of these substances was overshadowed by their widespread recreational use, criminalization and its inclusion in the schedule I class by the United Nations Convention on Psychotropics Substances of 1971. Schedule I substances are considered to have high abuse potential, poor safety and no therapeutic indication. Over the past decade, there has been a resurgence of scientific interest in psychedelic drugs [1, 4].

19.5.1 LSD

Early studies from the 1950s to 1970s indicated that LSD may have antidepressant and anxiolytic properties [4, 17]. LSD-assisted psychotherapy was often performed in patients with anxiety and cancer and in patients with depression or related disorders [4]. Due to methodological issues, these studies need a replication in the future. One recent study assessed the effects of LSD-assisted psychotherapy on anxiety in 11 patients with life-threatening diseases (eight with cancer). The study found nonsignificant decreases in depression and increases in quality of life [44]. A follow-up study at 12 months in nine patients reported sustained decreases in anxiety, an increase in quality of life and no lasting adverse

reactions after LSD, but there was no report of long-lasting effects and no control group [4]. Single or few doses of LSD reduced cluster headache intensity and induced remission more effectively than conventional medications; however, no controlled studies have been conducted. LSD was also well studied as treatment for alcohol use disorder [45]. The study identified 6 controlled eligible trials, including 536 participants. There was evidence for a beneficial effect of LSD on alcohol misuse (OR, 1.96; 95% CI, 1.36–2.84), although the results should be read with precaution because of risk of different biases.

19.5.2 Psilocybin

Psilocybin has been recently evaluated for obsessive-compulsive disorder in a trial including nine subjects; a reduction of symptoms was reported. A double-blind, randomized, placebo-controlled study assessed the safety and potential therapeutic effects of psilocybin in the treatment of psychological distress associated with the existential crisis of terminal disease. The trial included 11 subjects, and significant decreases were observed in anxiety scores at the 1- and 3-month follow-up [4, 17]. Psilocybin obtained from the FDA the Breakthrough Therapy Designation in 2018. This is a process designed to expedite the development and review of drugs that are intended to treat a serious condition, and preliminary clinical evidence indicates that the drug may demonstrate substantial improvement over available therapy on a clinically significant endpoint(s).

Two recent studies recently reported the efficacy of psilocybin in the treatment of anxiety and depression associated with life-threatening cancer. In a double-blind, placebo-controlled, crossover trial, 29 patients with cancer-related anxiety and depression were randomly assigned and received treatment with single-dose psilocybin (0.3 mg/kg) or niacin, both in conjunction with psychotherapy. In conjunction with psychotherapy, single moderate-dose psilocybin produced rapid, robust and enduring anxiolytic and antidepressant effects in patients with cancer-related psychological distress [4]. The effects of psilocybin were studied in 51 cancer patients with life-threatening diagnoses and symptoms of depression and/or anxiety. This randomized, double-blind, crossover trial investigated the effects of a very low (placebo-like) dose (1 or 3 mg/70 kg) vs. a high dose (22 or 30 mg/70 kg) of psilocybin administered in counterbalanced sequence with 5 weeks between sessions and a 6-month follow-up. High-dose psilocybin produced large decreases in clinician- and self-rated measures of depressed mood and anxiety, along with increases in quality of life, life meaning and optimism and decreases in death anxiety. At 6-month follow-up, these changes were sustained, with about 80% of participants continuing to show clinically significant decreases in depressed mood and anxiety [46].

In an open-label feasibility trial, 12 patients (six men, six women) with moderate-to-severe, unipolar, treatment-resistant major depression received two oral doses of psilocybin (10 mg and 25 mg, 7 days apart) in a supportive setting. Psychological support was provided before, during and after each session. Relative to baseline, depressive symptoms were markedly reduced 1 week and 3 months after high-dose treatment. Marked and sustained improvements in anxiety and anhedonia were also noted. Symptom improvements remained significant 6 months posttreatment in a treatment-resistant cohort [47, 48].

19.5.3 MDMA

In the late 1970s and early 1980s, psychiatrists/psychologists who employed MDMA in combination with psychotherapy described that it exerted therapeutic effects, especially by promoting subjects to talk openly and honestly about themselves and their early relationships without defensive conditioning intervening, even in individuals who were chronically constricted and apprehensive. Psychiatric attention with respect to therapeutic MDMA has especially focused on post-traumatic stress disorder (PTSD) and, more recently, on social anxiety in autistic adults and anxiety associated with life-threatening illness [32, 37, 39].

Six double-blind, randomized, placebo-controlled phase II clinical trials have demonstrated initial safety and efficacy for MDMA-assisted psychotherapy in the treatment of resistant PTSD [38, 39] and were conducted from April 2004 to February 2017. Active doses of MDMA (75–125 mg, $n = 72$) or placebo/control doses (0–40 mg, $n = 31$) were administered to individuals with PTSD during manualized psychotherapy sessions in two or three 8-hours sessions spaced a month apart. Three non-drug 90-minutes therapy sessions preceded the first MDMA exposure, and three to four followed each experimental session.

Results showed that after two blinded experimental sessions, the active group had significantly greater reductions in symptoms in the Clinician-Administered PTSD Scale (CAPS-IV) in comparison to placebo. After two experimental sessions, more participants in the active group (54.2%) did not meet CAPS-IV PTSD diagnostic criteria than the control group (22.6%). All doses of MDMA were well tolerated. Although the results are promising, it is relevant to take into account the small sample size. These studies supported expansion into phase III trials and led to FDA granting Breakthrough Therapy Designation for this promising treatment in 2017 [38, 39].

19.5.4 Esketamine

Ketamine has been assessed for the therapy of depression [49]. Similar to ketamine, esketamine appears to be a rapid-acting antidepressant. It received a Breakthrough Therapy Designation from the FDA for treatment-resistant depression (TRD) in 2013 and major depressive disorder (MDD) with accompanying suicidal ideation in 2016. The drug was studied for its use in combination with an oral antidepressant in people with TRD who had been unresponsive to treatment. Six phase III clinical trials for this indication were conducted in 2017. It is available as a nasal spray [50, 51].

Esketamine's efficacy and safety in treatment-resistant depression were evaluated in three 4-week, placebo-controlled, parallel-group studies and one longer-term randomized withdrawal study. Long-term safety was also evaluated in a 12-month open-label safety study. For esketamine, the positive short-term trial and the positive randomized withdrawal trial provided substantial evidence of effectiveness, although two short-term studies failed to demonstrate a statistically significant treatment effect. A major safety concern is esketamine's abuse potential [50]. In February 2019, FDA approved the nasal spray version of esketamine provided that it be administered in a clinical setting, with patients remaining on-site for at least 2 hours after administration (because some patients temporarily experienced sedation, visual disturbances, trouble speaking, confusion, numbness and feelings of dizziness/faintness during the period immediately after administration) [50].

19.5.5 Ayahuasca

The number of adequate therapeutic studies with ayahuasca is very limited; scientists from Brazil, the United States and Spain have performed observational studies to evaluate its therapeutic potential. In a parallel, double-blind, randomized, placebo-controlled trial with 35 patients with treatment-resistant MDD [52], a single ayahuasca dose induced significant reduction in depressive symptoms from 1 to 7 days after its intake. Tolerability of ayahuasca was good; the common adverse reactions were nausea (71%), vomiting (57%), anxiety (50%), restlessness (50%) and headache (42%). Although results are promising, the sample size and only one controlled trial are important limitations. Future studies should explore the use of ayahuasca in anxiety and mood disorders using different multiple doses, to assess efficacy and safety [17].

19.6 Conclusion

Hallucinogens are a heterogeneous group of substances that have as their primary effect the production of disturbances of perception. The hallucinogenic effects appear to be related to the agonistic action on 5-HT2A receptors and antagonism at NMDA receptors and agonist at opioid-kappa receptors. Hallucinogens produce substance use disorder, with acute tolerance but not withdrawal syndrome. Novel psychoactive substances (NPS) can induce substance use disorder, intoxication and in some cases withdrawal syndrome (for those with psychostimulant properties). The therapeutic objective for hallucinogen use disorder is to reduce consumption and achieve the abstinence. There are no specific drugs for treating the addiction caused by these substances. Some hallucinogens are under evaluation for its therapeutic use in different mental disorders (LSD, psilocybin, ayahuasca and the designer drug MDMA).

Acknowledgements This work was supported by the following grants: Instituto de Salud Carlos III (PI17/01962, JR16/0020) and Red de Trastornos Adictivos-RTA RD16/0017/0003 and RD16/0017/0010, integrated in the National RCDCI and funded by the ISCIII and the European Regional Development Fund [FEDER], European Commission action grants (Directorate-General for Migration and Home Affairs, Grant Agreement number: 806996-JUSTSO-JUST-2017-AGDRUG), Suport Grups de Recerca AGAUR Gencat (2017SGR 316 and 2017SGR 530) and Instrumental Action for the Intensification of Health Professionals-Specialist practitioners (PERIS: SLT006/17/00014).

References

1. Nichols DE. Psychedelics. Pharmacol Rev. 2016;68(2):264–355. https://doi.org/10.1124/pr.115.011478.
2. Bogenschutz MP, Ross S. Hallucinogen-related disorders. In: Sadock BJ, Sadock VA, Ruiz P, Sadock BJ, editors. Kaplan & Sadocks concise textbook of clinical psychiatry. Philadelphia: Wolters Kluwer; 2017.
3. Hill S, Thomas S. Clinical toxicology of newer recreational drugs. Clin Toxicol. 2011;49(8):705–19. https://doi.org/10.3109/15563650.2011.615318.

4. Rucker JJ, Iliff J, Nutt DJ. Psychiatry & the psychedelic drugs. Past, present & future. Neuropharmacology. 2018;142:200–18. https://doi.org/10.1016/j.neuropharm.2017.12.040.

5. European Monitoring Centre for Drugs and Drug Addiction – EMCDDA (2019), European Drug Report 2019: Trends and Developments, Luxembourg. Retrieved from http://www.emcdda.europa.eu/system/files/publications/11364/20191724_TDAT19001ENN_PDF.pdf.

6. Miech RA, Johnston LD, O'Malley PM, Bachman JG, Schulenberg JE, Patrick ME. Monitoring the future national survey results on drug use, 1975–2018: Volume I, Secondary school students. Ann Arbor: Institute for Social Research, The University of Michigan; 2019. Retrieved from http://monitoringthefuture.org/pubs.html#monographs.

7. Substance Abuse and Mental Health Services Administration-SAMHSA. Key substance use and mental health indicators in the United States: results from the 2017 National Survey on Drug Use and Health (HHS Publication No. SMA 18-5068, NSDUH Series H-53). Rockville: Center for Behavioral Health Statistics and Quality, Substance Abuse and Mental Health Services Administration; 2018. Retrieved from https://www.samhsa.gov/data/.

8. O'Brien C. Drug use disorders and addiction. In: Brunton LL, Knollmann BC, Hilal-Dandan R, editors. Goodman & Gilmans: the pharmacological basis of therapeutics. New York: McGraw Hill Medical; 2018. p. 433–42.

9. Sibley DR, Hazelwood LA, Amara SG. 5-Hydroxytryptamine (Serotonin) and dopamine. In: Brunton LL, Knollmann BC, Hilal-Dandan R, editors. Goodman & Gilmans: the pharmacological basis of therapeutics. New York: McGraw Hill Medical; 2018. p. 225–42.

10. Liechti ME. Modern clinical research on LSD. Neuropsychopharmacology. 2017;42(11):2114–27. https://doi.org/10.1038/npp.2017.86.

11. American Psychiatric Association. Diagnostic and statistical manual of mental disorders. 5th ed. Arlington: Author; 2013.

12. Lerner AG, Gelkopf M, Skladman I, Oyffe I, Finkel B, et al. Flashback and hallucinogen persisting perception disorder: clinical aspects and pharmacological treatment approach. Isr J Psychiatry Relat Sci. 2002;39(2):92–9.

13. Griffiths RR, Johnson MW, Richards WA, Richards BD, Mccann U, Jesse R. Psilocybin occasioned mystical-type experiences: immediate and persisting dose-related effects. Psychopharmacology. 2011;218(4):649–65. https://doi.org/10.1007/s00213-011-2358-5.

14. Johnson MW, Hendricks PS, Barrett FS, Griffiths RR. Classic psychedelics: an integrative review of epidemiology, therapeutics, mystical experience, and brain network function. Pharmacol Ther. 2019;197:83–102. https://doi.org/10.1016/j.pharmthera.2018.11.010.

15. Carbonaro TM, Johnson MW, Hurwitz E, Griffiths RR. Double-blind comparison of the two hallucinogens psilocybin and dextromethorphan: similarities and differences in subjective experiences. Psychopharmacology. 2017;235(2):521–34. https://doi.org/10.1007/s00213-017-4769-4.

16. Bouso JC, González D, Fondevila S, Cutchet M, Fernández X, Barbosa PC, et al. Personality, psychopathology, life attitudes and neuropsychological performance among ritual users of Ayahuasca: a longitudinal study. PLoS One. 2012;7(8):e42421. https://doi.org/10.1371/journal.pone.0042421.

17. Dos Santos RG, Bouso JC, Alcázar-Córcoles MÁ, Hallak JE. Efficacy, tolerability, and safety of serotonergic psychedelics for the management of mood, anxiety, and substance-use disorders: a systematic review of systematic reviews. Expert Rev Clin Pharmacol. 2018;11(9):889–902. https://doi.org/10.1080/17512433.2018.1511424.

18. Alper KR, Stajić M, Gill JR. Fatalities temporally associated with the ingestion of ibogaine. J Forensic Sci. 2012;57(2):398–412. https://doi.org/10.1111/j.1556-4029.2011.02008.x.

19. Brown T. Ibogaine in the treatment of substance dependence. Curr Drug Abuse Rev. 2013;6(1):3–16. https://doi.org/10.2174/15672050113109990001.

20. Corkery JM. Ibogaine as a treatment for substance misuse: potential benefits and practical dangers. Prog Brain Res. 2018;242:217–57. https://doi.org/10.1016/bs.pbr.2018.08.005.

21. Morgan CJ, Curran HV. Ketamine use: a review. Addiction. 2011;107(1):27–38. https://doi.org/10.1111/j.1360-0443.2011.03576.x.

22. Abanades S, Peiró AM, Farré M. Club drugs: old medicines as new party drugs. Med Clin. 2004;123(8):305–11. https://doi.org/10.1016/s0025-7753(04)74499-1.

23. European Monitoring Centre for Drugs and Drug Addiction – EMCDDA (2018). EMCDDA–Europol 2017 Annual Report on the implementation of council decision 2005/387/JHA, implementation reports, Publications Office of the European Union, Luxembourg. Retrieved from http://www.emcdda.europa.eu/system/files/publications/9282/20183924_TDAN18001ENN_PDF.pdf.

24. United Nations Office on Drugs and Crime (2019). World Drug Report 2019. Retrieved from https://wdr.unodc.org/wdr2019/prelaunch/WDR-2019-Methodology-FINAL.pdf.

25. Buchanan JF, Brown CR. Designer drugs. Med Toxicol Adverse Drug Exp. 1988;3(1):1–17. https://doi.org/10.1007/bf03259928.

26. Papaseit E, Farré M, Schifano F, Torrens M. Emerging drugs in Europe. Curr Opin Psychiatry. 2014;27(4):243–50. https://doi.org/10.1097/yco.0000000000000071.

27. Green A, King M, Shortall S, Fone K. Lost in translation: preclinical studies on 3,4-methylenedioxymethamphetamine provide information on mechanisms of action, but do not allow accurate prediction of adverse events in humans. Br

J Pharmacol. 2012;166(5):1523–36. https://doi. org/10.1111/j.1476-5381.2011.01819.x.

28. Papaseit E, Farré M, Pérez-Mañá C, Torrens M, Ventura M, Pujadas M, et al. Acute pharmacological effects of 2C-B in humans: an observational study. Front Pharmacol. 2018;9 https://doi.org/10.3389/ fphar.2018.00206.

29. de la Torre R, Farré M, Roset PN, Pizarro N, Abanades S, Segura M, et al. Human pharmacology of MDMA: pharmacokinetics, metabolism, and disposition. Ther Drug Monit. 2004;26(2):137–44. https://doi. org/10.1097/00007691-200404000-00009.

30. Farré M, Torre RD, Mathúna BÓ, Roset PN, Peiró AM, Torrens M, et al. Repeated doses administration of MDMA in humans: pharmacological effects and pharmacokinetics. Psychopharmacology. 2004;173(3–4):364–75. https://doi.org/10.1007/ s00213-004-1789-7.

31. Farre M, Abanades S, Roset PN, Peiro AM, Torrens M, Omathuna B, et al. Pharmacological interaction between 3,4-Methylenedioxymethamphetamine (ecstasy) and paroxetine: pharmacological effects and pharmacokinetics. J Pharmacol Exp Ther. 2007;323(3):954–62. https://doi.org/10.1124/ jpet.107.129056.

32. Papaseit E, Torrens M, Pérez-Mañá C, Muga R, Farré M. Key interindividual determinants in MDMA pharmacodynamics. Expert Opin Drug Metab Toxicol. 2018;14(2):183–95. https://doi.org/10.1080/1742525 5.2018.1424832.

33. de la Torre R, Farré M. Neurotoxicity of MDMA (ecstasy): the limitations of scaling from animals to humans. Trends Pharmacol Sci. 2004;25(10):505–8. https://doi.org/10.1016/j.tips.2004.08.001.

34. Pardo-Lozano R, Farré M, Yubero-Lahoz S, O'Mathúna B, Torrens M, Mustata C, et al. Clinical pharmacology of 3,4-Methylenedioxymethamphetamine (MDMA, "ecstasy"): the influence of gender and genetics (CYP2D6, COMT, 5-HTT). PLoS One. 2012;7(10):e47599. https://doi.org/10.1371/journal. pone.0047599.

35. de Sola Llopis S, Miguelez-Pan M, Peña-Casanova J, Poudevida S, Farré M, Pacifici R, et al. Cognitive performance in recreational ecstasy polydrug users: A two-year follow-up study. J Psychopharmacol. 2008;22(5):498–510. https://doi. org/10.1177/0269881107081545.

36. Müller F, Brändle R, Liechti ME, Borgwardt S. Neuroimaging of chronic MDMA ("ecstasy") effects: a meta-analysis. Neurosci Biobehav Rev. 2019;96:10–20. https://doi.org/10.1016/j. neubiorev.2018.11.004.

37. Mithoefer MC, Grob CS, Brewerton TD. Novel psychopharmacological therapies for psychiatric disorders: psilocybin and MDMA. Lancet Psychiatry. 2016;3(5):481–8. https://doi.org/10.1016/ s2215-0366(15)00576-3.

38. Mithoefer MC, Feduccia AA, Jerome L, Mithoefer A, Wagner M, Walsh Z, et al. MDMA-assisted psychotherapy for treatment of PTSD: study design

and rationale for phase 3 trials based on pooled analysis of six phase 2 randomized controlled trials. Psychopharmacology. 2019;236:2735. https://doi. org/10.1007/s00213-019-05249-5.

39. Sessa B, Higbed L, Nutt D. A review of 3,4-methy lenedioxymethamphetamine (MDMA)-Assisted psychotherapy. Front Psychiatry. 2019;10 https://doi. org/10.3389/fpsyt.2019.00138.

40. Schifano F, Orsolini L, Papanti GD, Corkery JM. Novel psychoactive substances of interest for psychiatry. World Psychiatry. 2015;14(1):15–26. https://doi.org/10.1002/wps.20174.

41. De Bie RM, Gladstone RM, Strafella AP, Ko J, Lang AE. Manganese-induced parkinsonism associated with methcathinone (Ephedrone) abuse. Arch Neurol. 2007;64(6):886. https://doi.org/10.1001/ archneur.64.6.886.

42. Murray BL, Murphy CM, Beuhler MC. Death following recreational use of designer drug "bath salts" containing 3,4-Methylenedioxypyrovalerone (MDPV). J Med Toxicol. 2012;8(1):69–75. https:// doi.org/10.1007/s13181-011-0196-9.

43. Papaseit E, Moltó J, Muga R, Torrens M, Torre RD, Farré M. Clinical pharmacology of the synthetic cathinone mephedrone. Curr Top Behav Neurosci. 2016:313–31. https://doi.org/10.1007/7854_ 2016_61.

44. Gasser P, Holstein D, Michel Y, Doblin R, Yazar-Klosinski B, Passie T, Brenneisen R. Safety and efficacy of lysergic acid diethylamide-assisted psychotherapy for anxiety associated with life-threatening diseases. J Nerv Ment Dis. 2014;202(7):513–20. https://doi.org/10.1097/nmd.0000000000000113.

45. Krebs TS, Johansen P. Lysergic acid diethylamide (LSD) for alcoholism: meta-analysis of randomized controlled trials. J Psychopharmacol. 2012;26(7):994– 1002. https://doi.org/10.1177/0269881112439253.

46. Griffiths RR, Johnson MW, Carducci MA, Umbricht A, Richards WA, Richards BD, et al. Psilocybin produces substantial and sustained decreases in depression and anxiety in patients with life-threatening cancer: a randomized double-blind trial. J Psychopharmacol. 2016;30(12):1181–97. https://doi. org/10.1177/0269881116675513.

47. Carhart-Harris RL, Bolstridge M, Rucker J, Day CM, Erritzoe D, Kaelen M, et al. Psilocybin with psychological support for treatment-resistant depression: an open-label feasibility study. Lancet Psychiatry. 2016;3(7):619–27. https://doi.org/10.1016/ s2215-0366(16)30065-7.

48. Carhart-Harris RL, Bolstridge M, Day CM, Rucker J, Watts R, Erritzoe DE, et al. Psilocybin with psychological support for treatment-resistant depression: six-month follow-up. Psychopharmacology. 2017;235(2):399–408. https://doi.org/10.1007/ s00213-017-4771-x.

49. Rot MA, Zarate CA, Charney DS, Mathew SJ. Ketamine for depression: where do we go from here? Biol Psychiatry. 2012;72(7):537–47. https://doi. org/10.1016/j.biopsych.2012.05.003.

50. Kim J, Farchione T, Potter A, Chen Q, Temple R. Esketamine for treatment-resistant depression — first FDA-approved antidepressant in a new class. N Engl J Med. 2019;381(1):1–4. https://doi.org/10.1056/nejmp1903305.

51. Popova V, Daly EJ, Trivedi M, Cooper K, Lane R, Lim P, et al. Efficacy and safety of flexibly dosed esketamine nasal spray combined with a newly initiated oral antidepressant in treatment-resistant depression: a randomized double-blind active-controlled study. Am J Psychiatr. 2019;176(6):428–38. https://doi.org/10.1176/appi.ajp.2019.19020172.

52. Palhano-Fontes F, Barreto D, Onias H, Andrade KC, Novaes MM, Pessoa JA, et al. Rapid antidepressant effects of the psychedelic ayahuasca in treatment-resistant depression: a randomized placebo-controlled trial. Psychol Med. 2018;49(4):655–63. https://doi.org/10.1017/s0033291718001356.

Inhalant Addiction

20

Tania Real, Silvia L. Cruz,
María Elena Medina-Mora, Rebeca Robles,
and Hugo González

Contents

T. Real · R. Robles · H. González
National Institute of Psychiatry Ramón de la Fuente
Muiz, Mexico City, Mexico

S. L. Cruz
Department of Pharmacobiology, CINVESTAV,
Mexico City, Mexico

M. E. Medina-Mora (✉)
Mental Health Global Research Center, National
Institute of Psychiatry Ramón de la Fuente Muiz/
UNAM, Mexico City, Mexico

© Springer Nature Switzerland AG 2021
N. el-Guebaly et al. (eds.), *Textbook of Addiction Treatment*,
https://doi.org/10.1007/978-3-030-36391-8_20

Abstract

This chapter is divided into seven sections, beginning with a general overview of this group of substances, their definitions, and the current classification of the disorders associated with their use. This is followed by a description of prevalence, the groups of the population affected, and the patterns of use in different regions of the world. Particular attention is paid to use among vulnerable groups, to inhalant effects and consequences, the social determinants that underlie the problem, and opportunities for solution. These sections are followed by a brief overview of the evidence for prevention and treatment strategies currently in use. This chapter ends with a discussion on policies to address the problem.

Keywords

Inhalant · Effects · Special population
Recovery potential · Policy

Inhalants are a special class of drugs that require attention from health and social welfare experts and policy makers. Many products that are misused are easily available. Although there are legal restrictions to sell and distribute certain products to minors [35], inhalants are not included in Drug International Regulations. These substances also less frequently targets for health and social interventions, as well as for research and funding.

Inhalants are the only drugs of abuse defined by the route of administration rather than by its attributes, specifically similar mechanism of actions or common pharmacological effects. They include a wide group of substances with different uses, short- and long-term negative effects, and consequences. These products have legal uses in industry and households and are therefore easily available. Inhalants are used by the general population saliently among persons in vulnerable conditions, mainly children and adolescents from poor sectors of society, young students (specially but not exclusively, those under 17 years of age), some indigenous groups, workers that use solvents for their everyday work (e.g., varnishers, house painters, anesthesiologists, etc.), and heavy drug users, especially when they do not have access to other substances, among other groups.

20.1   Definition and Classification

A working definition proposed by Balster and colleagues states:

Abused inhalants contain volatile substances that are self-administered as gases or vapors to induce a psychoactive or mind-altering effect. These volatile substances are available in legal, relatively inexpensive and common household products which can be gases, liquids, aerosols or, in some cases, solids [7].

NIDA [73] includes in its definition the main issues that characterize this varied group of substances and their effects: the intentionality of their use, due to the chemicals' mind-altering effects; the nature of the short-term effects most of them producing a rapid high that resembles alcohol intoxication; the effects when sufficient amounts are inhaled, as nearly all solvents and gases produce a loss of sensation and even unconsciousness; the long-term irreversible effects that can include hearing loss, limb spasms, bone marrow, and brain damage; and, finally, the risk of mortality when sniffing high concentrations of inhalants that may result in death from heart failure or suffocation.

A wide variety of substances are grouped together into this class, which by its own nature challenges definitions and classifications. Inhalants include (1) solvents (liquids or semisolid substances that evaporate and include glue, shoe polish, toluene, and gasoline), (2) aerosol sprays (volatile substances or gases such as spray paints, hair sprays, cleaners for computers, etc.), (3) gases (anesthetics for medical use such as ether, chloroform, butane, and refrigeration products), and (4) nitrites that include products containing butyl nitrite and amyl nitrite, known as "poppers," locker room deodorizers, or "rush," and nitrous oxide known as "whippets."

From the physicochemical point of view, members of this group (a) are gases or can easily become vapors at room temperature (without heating), (b) are nonpolar molecules with high affinity for lipids and can therefore cross all biological membranes, (c) are flammable, and (d) mostly are lighter than water in their liquid form, but as vapors are heavier than air, which means that they are not easily dispersed from rooms where they have been inhaled [25].

Because many substances can meet these criteria, they can be classified on the basis of their chemical structure (hydrocarbons, ethers, ketones, etc.), commercial use (solvents, anesthetics, propellants, etc.), physical state (gases, liquids, aerosols), or effects (central nervous system) (depressants, vasodilators, etc.). Each classification has its own limitations and some substances may fit into several categories. For example, butane is a hydrocarbon gas used both as fuel and as propellant; nitrous oxide is a propellant and also an aesthetic gas used in dentistry.

Moreover, a single substance can have different names such as toluene, methylbenzene, phenylmethane, or toluol. This contributes to the difficulties associated with inhalant research. Table 20.1 shows some commonly misused compounds, their synonyms, and chemical structure, examples of commercial products, threshold limit values (TLV: maximum average concentration to which workers can be exposed 8 h/day, 5 days/week, without experiencing significant adverse health effects), and vapor concentrations in air that are dangerous to life and health (IDHL). This table also includes the CAS number, a unique chemical abstract service number that can be used to obtain the most important information on individual compounds. A detailed table of the physicochemical properties of main inhalants can be found elsewhere [20].

Although there is not enough evidence to establish a scientific-based pharmacological classification of inhalants, it is possible to distinguish at least three different categories with various mechanisms of actions: (a) solvents, fuels, and anesthetics; (b) nitrous oxide; and (c) volatile alkyl nitrites. The first one is the most extensive group and includes inhalants that are misused throughout the world in the form of gasoline, industrial solvents, adhesives, paints, sprays, inks, pen markers, and many other commercial products. Among solvents, toluene is the most frequently misused and the best-studied inhalant compound. It is the main component of paint thinners (mixed with xylene, ethylbenzene, and other solvents in different proportions), inks, adhesives, and degreasing agents. Commercial xylene (a mixture of the three isomers: ortho-, metha-, and para-xylene) is used in the leather

Table 20.1 Inhalants: synonyms, products, and safety limits

Class	Compound	Structure	Synonyms	CAS#	Products	TLV (ppm)	IDLH (ppm)
Hydrocarbon, acyclic	n-Hexane		Hexyl hydride, dipropyl	110-54-3	Gasoline, solvents, glues, varnishes	50	1100
Hydrocarbon, alicyclic	Cyclohexane		Hexamethylene, hexanaphtene	110-82-7	Lacquers, resins, varnish removers, solvents, cigarette smoke	300	1300
Hydrocarbons, aromatic	Benzene		Benzol, phenyl hydride, cyclohexatriene	71-43-2	Gasoline	0.5	500
	Toluene		Toluol, methyl-benzene, phenylmethane	108-88-3	Solvents, paints, thinners, glues, lacquers, gasoline, inks, cigarette smoke	50	500
	Xylene		Xylol, dimethyl-benzene, methyl toluene	1330-20-7	Cleaning agents, thinner. Used in printing, rubber, and leather industries	100	900
	Ethylbenzene		Phenyl ethane, ethyl benzol	100-41-4	Gasoline, paints, inks. Used as styrene precursor	100	800
	Propylbenzene		Phenyl propane, isocumeme	103-65-1	Gasoline. Used in textile dyeing and printing	N.E.	N.E.
Hydrocarbons, halogenated	1,1,1-TCE		Trichloroethane. TCE, perchloroethylene, tetrachloroethane, methyl chloroform	71-55-6	Cleaning products, paints, correction fluids, degreasers	350	700
	1,1,2-Trichloroethylene		TCE	79-01-6	Solvents, dry cleaning products, degreasers (car parts) Plastic spray fixative	50	1000
	Diethylether		Ethyl ether, octapentane, ethoxy ethane	60-29-7	Anesthetic, solvents, fuels	400	1900
	Chloroform		Trichloromethane, methyl trichloride	67-66-3	Anesthetic, spot removers, precursor for refrigerants	10	500
	Halothane		Fluothane	151-67-7	Anesthetic	50	N.E

Inorganic	Nitrous oxide		Dinitrogen monoxide	10024-97-2	Anesthetic, laughing gas, propellant (hair sprays, whipped cream, cooking spray), engine combustion enhancer	50	N.E
Hydrocarbon, acyclic	Propane		Dimethyl methane, LP gas	74-98-6	Industrial fuel, refrigerant, aerosol propellant	1000	2100
	Butane		Methylethyl ethane, Freon 600 LP gas	106-97-8	Lighter fuel, gas tanks for cooking, refrigerant, aerosol propellant (deodorant sprays)	800	N.E.
Hydrocarbons, halogenated	1.1-difluoroethane		Ethylene fluoride, Freon 152a, R152a, HCF152a, Dymel	75-37-6	Propellant (PC duster), refrigerant (air conditioning)	1000	N.E.
	1,1,1.2-Tetrafluoroethane		Freon 134 R134	811-97-2	Propellant (PC duster), refrigerant (car air-conditioning systems)	N.E.	N.E.

Sources: PubChem, NIOSH ICSC (International Chemical Safety Cards), ATSDR (Agency for Toxic Substances and Disease Registry), Household Products Database, and Haz Map

CAS# Chemical Abstract Service number, TLV threshold limit value, IDLH immediately dangerous to life and health and rubber industries and in histology laboratories. 1,1,1-TCE or trichloroethylene is another solvent present in correction fluids, but it is no longer produced in most developed countries because it is harmful to the ozone layer. Gasoline is a mixture of several solvents, which can or cannot contain lead. Several anesthetic gases such as halothane, ether, and chloroform are included in the same group with solvents because they share some of the effects and mechanism of actions of misused solvents.

Nitrous oxide constitutes a class of its own due to its unique pharmacological profile and affinity for specific receptors. It is used as a propellant in whipped cream products and as an anesthetic gas for dental procedures. As for nitrites, they are smooth muscle relaxant and vasodilator drugs rather than depressant substances and are inhaled from small bottles, some of which "pop" when opened (hence the name "poppers") [24].

20.2 Disorders Due to Use of Volatile Inhalants in ICD-11

In an important effort to aligning the World Health Organization's classification of disorders due to substance use with global service needs, the *International Classification of Diseases* 11th Revision (ICD-11) includes several changes based on a public health approach. This involved a greater specification of different harmful patterns of substance use, as well as a new category to denote single episodes of harmful use of all substances, including inhalants [80]. These changes allow for the early detection and intervention of people in risk to develop a problem related with the use of a substance.

Thus, according to the ICD-11 beta platform (https://icd.who.int/browse11/l-m/en), disorders due to use of volatile inhalants are classified, given the pattern and consequences of their use, in (i) volatile inhalant intoxication, (ii) volatile inhalant dependence, (iii) volatile inhalant withdrawal when inhalant use is reduced or discontinued, (iv) single episode of harmful use of volatile

inhalants or unintentional exposure (e.g., occupational exposure), and (v) harmful pattern of use of volatile inhalants, which is evident over a period of at least 12 months if substance use is episodic or at least 1 month if use is continuous (i.e., daily or almost daily).

Definitions of "harmful use" and "harmful pattern" clarify that, in both conditions, a damage to physical or mental health of the substance user and/or other person has been caused by the substance itself or by the consequent behavior of the substance user. Harm to health of the individual occurs due to one or more of the following: (1) behavior related to intoxication, (2) direct or secondary toxic effects on body organs and systems, or (3) a harmful route of administration; and that harm to health of others includes any form of physical harm, including trauma, or mental disorder that is directly attributable to behavior due to volatile inhalant intoxication on the part of the person to whom the diagnosis applies.

Additionally, several volatile inhalant-induced mental disorders are recognized, including (i) volatile inhalant-induced delirium; (ii) volatile inhalant-induced psychotic disorder; (iii) volatile inhalant-induced mood disorder, which could be with depressive symptoms, with maniac symptoms, or mixed; and (iv) volatile inhalant-induced anxiety disorder.

Moreover, in the block for neurocognitive disorders (characterized by primary clinical deficits in cognitive functioning that are acquired rather than developmental), categories for amnestic disorder and dementia due to use of volatile inhalants have been included. Amnestic disorder due to volatile inhalant misuse is defined as a syndrome of memory impairment with specific features of amnestic disorder that is judged to be the direct consequence of the use of this type of substance.

Dementia due to use of volatile inhalants is characterized by the development of persistent cognitive impairments (e.g., memory problems, language impairment, and an inability to perform complex motor tasks) that are judged to be a direct consequence of inhalant use or exposure and that persist beyond the usual duration of action or withdrawal syndrome associated with the substance.

It should be added that all ICD-11 definitions of mental and neurocognitive disorders due to use of volatile inhalants (and all substances) specified that produced symptoms persist beyond the usual duration of volatile inhalant intoxication or withdrawal; that the amount and duration of volatile inhalant use must be enough to be capable of producing them; and that they are not better accounted for by a disorder that is not due to use of volatile inhalants [81].

20.3 Epidemiology: How Widespread Is Its Use?

Inhalant misuse worldwide has mainly spread among young people. In some countries, the phenomenon appears among some adults and seniors, working in the formal and informal economies, as well as among some members of rural and indigenous groups [97].

In the Americas in general population, since 12–65 years, past-year prevalence rates vary around the world, around 0.1% or lower in half of the region countries. Some places stand out for higher use: as the United States (0.6%), Belize (1%), Bolivia (0.3%), and Barbados (0.8%); and use is higher in males than females, except for Guyana and Jamaica; also, there are variations in use according to age groups. In Guyana and Jamaica, inhalant misuse has been reported in young adults from 18 to 34 years, but in El Salvador, Bolivia, and Costa Rica, use is prevalent among those between 12 and 17 years of age [75].

According to a study on secondary students from 8th to 12th grade in the United States [53], inhalant misuse increased from the late 1970s to the mid-1990s, especially in the 8th, 10th, and 12th grades. Trends have changed since 2001, when use began to decrease. The last measurement in 2018 shows that annual prevalence is 8.7% in 8th grade, 6.5% in 10th grade, and 4.4% in 12th grade. Despite variations, the trend is for use to decline, and it is believed that this decrease may have been associated with information campaigns.

In Canada, the Ontario Student Drug Use and Mental Health Survey [14] indicates that among students in 7th and 12th grade, inhalants occupy the 11th place of use in the last year, with 3.4% prevalence (3.0% for females and 3.7% for males). Between 1999 and 2017, inhalant misuse in this population decreased from 8.9% to 3.4%. It is worth mentioning that inhalant treatment centers are spread among Canada, specifically addressing native indigenous groups among which volatile solvent use was prevalent [32].

According to OAS/CICAD Report [75], in most Latin American and Caribbean countries excluding tobacco and alcohol, inhalants are the most commonly used substance after cannabis, especially among high school students, although there are countries where it is the number one drug of choice. In general population, the lowest prevalence of the last year of use of inhalants among general population was reported in the Dominican Republic (0.03%), versus the highest in Belize (1%), Barbados (0.8%), the United States (0.6%), and Bolivia (0.3%). In other countries for which information is available, the prevalence rate is around 0.1%. Inhalant use is higher among males than females in every country except Guyana and Jamaica. Higher prevalence of inhalant use is among young people aged 12–17 in Chile, Mexico, Colombia, Ecuador, Panama, the United States, and Uruguay. In Guyana and Jamaica, inhalant use has been reported only among young adults (18–34).

Among secondary school students, the highest rates of past-year inhalant are found in Caribbean countries: Saint Lucia, Saint Vincent and the Grenadines, Barbados, Grenada, Saint Kitts and Nevis, Trinidad and Tobago, Jamaica, Antigua, and Barbuda, with rates between 7.5% and 11%. The lowest prevalence is in the Dominican Republic (0.5%) which is also in this subregion, followed by Costa Rica and Honduras (below 1%), Peru (1%), and Canada (1.4%). Largest differences by sex are in Panama and the Dominican Republic, where for every female who used inhalants in the past year, three males did so. Among eighth-grade students is greater than or equal to that of the tenth and twelfth graders.

Consumption in university students comes from eight countries: Andean Community and Brazil, El Salvador, Panama, and Uruguay. Brazil reports the highest rates, 6.5%, and the other countries' rates are below 0.5%. In Ecuador and Peru, inhalant use is higher among females.

In Mexico, inhalant misuse has shown fluctuations among students in various regions, for instance, annual prevalence increased from 4.4% in 2006 to 7.5% in 2009 and decreased to 5.8% in 2016 among high school students [99, 101]. According to the National Household Survey 2017 conducted among population 12–65 years of age, annual prevalence of use in the last year was still low, 0.2%, but higher than the 0.1% in 2008 [51]; this same trend is reported by the System of Epidemiological Surveillance that gathers information from cases attending treatment in nongovernmental organizations: Inhalants occupy the fourth place as a starting drug, followed by alcohol, tobacco, and marijuana. In 6.9% of the population, inhalants can be considered the impact drug that leads to treatment.

Data from university students show that Brazil's past-year prevalence was 6.5%. Panama, El Salvador, Peru, Colombia, Ecuador, Bolivia, and Uruguay throw data with prevalences below 0.5%.

In Russia, Koposov et al. [55] reported that the prevalence of inhalant use was 6.1% among boys and 3.5% among girls of sixth- to tenth-grade students in public schools in Arkhangelsk city. Of these, 3.6% ($n = 41$) of boys and 2.4% ($n = 39$) of girls used inhalants irregularly, while 2.5% ($n = 28$) of boys and 1.0% ($n = 16$) of girls reported using inhalants several times a week.

The European School Survey Project on Alcohol and Other Drugs [38] reported that the average prevalence of lifetime inhalant use was 7%, and the country with the highest rate was Croatia (25%), followed by Slovenia (14%). The lowest prevalence rates (1–2%) were found in the Faroes, the former Yugoslav Republic of Macedonia, and Moldova. The use of inhalants shows generally stable lifetime prevalence rates over the observed period. The gender-specific trends reveal a narrowing of the gender gap, with

rates among boys slightly decreasing but rather unchanged rates among girls.

For Arabian countries, Bassiony [8] reports in eight studies found that the prevalence of inhalant use among Saudi patients ranged from 0.9% to 17.9%. It has also been reported in Asia; in a survey in Thailand, Verma et al. [98] report that 20% of adolescents in middle and high schools have experimented with inhalants. In Japan in general population (15–64) survey, the lifetime prevalence of drug use was 1.5% for organic solvents [91]. Also in a systematic review of substance use among young people in China during their lifetime, ever having used solvents was 4.8% [103, 104]. A study in the Republic of Uzbekistan to assess drug use among young people (students in the 9th grade) found low levels of drug use, about 0.5% of the students indicated that they had consumed cannabis and inhalants, once or twice in their life [39].

20.4 Use Among Special Populations

Studies conducted in different parts of the world show that drug use among adolescents differs from place to place. The highest rates of inhalant misuse are associated with low-income, chaotic, fractured, or abusive households and living on the streets [108]. According to SAMSHSA [85], in the United States, past-year inhalant use among adolescents was 2.7% for Blacks, 2.6% for Whites and adolescents of two or more races, and 4.6% among American Indians or Alaska Natives.

Villatoro et al. [100] analyzing data from the National Household Survey in Mexico found that those drug users that reported having ever inhaled a substance, as compared to cannabis users that had not experimented with these substances, came more often from more disorganized and violent communities; users also report having been involved in fights, selling drugs, and other problem behaviors more often. Ortiz and colleagues [76], also in Mexico, reported the misuse of solvents in the context of a religious festivity among street children. The respondents reported consuming between 10 and 30 "monas" (a piece of cloth soaked with a thinner-type solvent) a day. Ortiz and colleagues studied groups of children, adolescents, and young people living on the street and described certain dynamics around consumption such as presence of a dealer a privileged role and is able to wield power over the group, sellers who worked for the dealer. Drug distribution is part of a complex system of theft and transportation. Sometimes migrants are received by streetchildren groups and become part of the groups, street children from newborn to 50 and older, and people with a variety of professions such as windshield washers, construction workers, PET collectors, and sex workers coexist, which implies a complex social interaction.

In India, Gigengack [44] reported that children from street families, children of the street, ragpickers, and part-time street children use a diluter and whitener. Interviews suggest that children are seeking intoxication in pursuit of pleasure despite the harm that comes with it.

This practice has also been reported across indigenous communities in Australia; a survey of school students showed that around 23% of indigenous students (12–15) had use illicit substances in their lifetime, compared with 11% of all students. Twenty-four percent of the indigenous students had use inhalants [47].

Swaim and Stanley [93] reported time prevalence of inhalant use between 8th-, 10th-, and 12-grade American Indian students was 13.2%, 10.7%, and 10.8% compared with 7.7%, 6.6%, and 5.0% from a national sample of US adolescents.

Other studies have focused on the association of inhalant misuse with risky behaviors and HIV infection, as in the case of nitrite use among males that have sex with males [103, 104].

20.5 Patterns of Use

As is the case with other drugs, inhalers can be classified as experimenters, regular users, heavy users, and persons with dependence. Among students, especially among those in early adolescence, the most common pattern is of experi-

mentation with a low proportion of regular users and even smaller proportion of students that have developed dependence. For instance, among American and Australian students, experimental inhalant use rates during early adolescence are high (26% of 12-year-old students), whereas the proportion that report inhaling on a regular basis is more than six times smaller (4%) [52, 105]. In Mexico City, and Jalisco, rates of experimentation (use one to five times) among young students (7–9 years of school) are also considerably higher (66% and 76%, respectively) than those that report having used on over five occasions (44% and 24%) of all persons that have ever used [21, 99]. This pattern differs from the one observed among adolescents living on the streets who are heavily involved in inhalation, with daily heavy use being the most common pattern combined with periods of complete abstinence [63].

Few studies report rates of dependence; Perron et al. [78], using data from the National Epidemiologic Survey on Alcohol and Related Conditions (NESARC) household sample of persons 18 years of age and older in the United States, documented that 19.5% of the lifetime inhalant users met the criteria for DSM-IV inhalant use disorder (abuse 17.2% or dependence, 2.3%).

Inhalants are usually "sniffed" directly from container to nose, but inhaling fumes through mouth ("huffing" or "chroming") is also common. The open tube of glue, nail polish, etc. is usually placed close to the nose and the fumes are inhaled. Sometimes users heat substances to accelerate the vaporization process which increases the risks of gas explosions; other forms of use include inhaling from damp rags or shirt sleeves or from plastic bags or paper bags ("bagging"). Fatal accidents may occur when the inhaler places the complete bag over his head; balloons filled with substances such as nitrous oxide have also been reported [71]. Some authors have reported that the route of administration is related to environmental factors such as the presence of police and the need to disguise use [64]. A case study in India reports petrol inhalation by a 10-year-old boy who started to inhale it accidentally by applying his face against the keyhole of the petrol tank of his father's motorbike [9].

Preference for specific substances varies according to the characteristics of the groups that use them and their effects. Takagi et al. [94], for example, when assessing preferences for type of paint among inhalers in Australia, found that the chrome-using group compared to non-chrome users was more likely to report deliberately inhaling to experience altered perceptions (such as visual and auditory hallucinations). A greater proportion of chrome users reported that the perceptual alterations they experienced after sniffing paint differed between paint colors, with more vivid hallucinations being produced with chrome colors. Similarly, Leal [57] reported that children living in the streets in downtown Mexico City preferred pure toluene for its psychotropic effects and lower level of toxicity. Cruz and Dominguez [26] have also reported hallucinations among heavy inhalers in Mexico that use toluene or a mixture of solvents.

Common choices for solvents among American Indian youth and Alaskan natives are gasoline (28%), glue (23%), paint removers and nail polish remover (18%), and paint sprays (17%). In this group as is often also the case of street children [64], most of the substances inhaled contain mixtures of chemicals, making it almost impossible to determine which compounds are responsible for the effects experienced by the abuser and observed by therapists [10].

Trotter [95] reported that inhalant abuse was sometimes combined with drinking the liquid residue left in aerosol cans after sniffing the propellant [95]. Hillabrant [49] reports interviews with Navajo adolescents who report the fad of drinking hair spray, users of which faint after five bottles in an hour.

Some groups in Mexico use "compressed air" at special gatherings known as "perreos" or "grinding, booty dancing, bumping, or housing" in the Caribbean. Inhalants and alcohol are the substances used; attendees might buy a piece of rag soaked with toluene that has been flavored. Risky sexual behavior and fights are common [45]. In Brazil, lança perfume (chloroform/ether)

is used [68], mainly by higher social class students [86]. Also in Mexico a study to determine factors that differentiate inhalant users from other drug users and those who do not consume any drugs reported that inhalant users are primarily secondary students, have a low perception of risk of illegal drug use and have easy access to them, compared with non-users or consumers of other substances. In addition, users of inhalants have greater impulsiveness, have more friends with antisocial problems, have a family member who is a consumer of drugs, and are in a social context in which peers tolerate the use of substances [67].

Medina-Mora et al. [66] reported inhalation is more prevalent among youth coming from low socioeconomic; it is almost four times higher among males of 12–17 years of age and 20 times higher among females that do not work or study (2.3% and 4%) as compared to those enrolled in school or working (1% and 0.2%). It is also more frequent among students that do not attend school.

20.6 Health Effects

Inhalants Short-term effects are similar to alcohol and other central nervous system inhibitors, initial stimulation, and persistence. They act as anxiolytics, antidepressants, and anticonvulsants and are associated with impaired motor coordination, emotional lability and difficulty speaking. Chronic effects include neurotoxicity, cognitive impairment, headaches, diminished sensorial abilities (loss of vision, audition, and coordination), and an increase in mental disorders and sleep disturbances.

There is evidence that the more widely used inhalants share cellular mechanisms and have similar effects to other drugs, particularly depressors of the central nervous system [25], but the use of these substances has also been associated with illusions and hallucinations [26]. When used by pregnant rats, they affect development and irregular heartbeat during intoxication has also been described [23]. Unfortunately, a significant shortage of information remains, despite the increase in research projects addressing the neurobiology of inhalants; the majority are still conducted on toluene. Little is known of abstinence, and researchers do not know the extent to which cognitive and other effects can be reversible, though some laboratory experiments with enriched environments have provided some evidence of reversibility [59].

20.6.1 Acute Effects

Inhalants vary in their chemical composition and consequently in how and where they act. In fact, it is rather surprising that such a dissimilar group of substances should have common effects, although this is partly due to their common administration route. Misusing inhalants implies introducing gases other than air into the body causing poor brain oxygenation (hypoxia) and the deleterious consequences associated with it. This happens with all inhalants regardless of their pharmacological profile and is a significant health hazard in itself.

Once in the body, inhaled vapors rapidly reach various specific molecular targets to induce a state of intoxication similar to that produced by other central nervous system depressant drugs such as alcohol and barbiturates. The pulmonary route is highly efficient as an administration route because the lungs are profusely irrigated and have extensive absorption surface. This results in a rapid intoxication, which is, however, short-lived due to inhalants' high volatility. In order to maintain the effects, users repeat the experience every few minutes to maintain the desired level of active substance in the brain.

Several solvents and fuels produce a transient state of excitation followed by a more persistent sedation, lack of motor coordination (ataxia), slurred speech, cognitive impairment, and slow reactivity toward stimuli [89]. At high concentrations illusions and hallucinations are common and are known to play an important role in the motivation to inhale and socialize [26, 61]. When anesthetic gases are intentionally used, sedative effects on top of psychoactive actions can be extreme.

Other effects depend on the type of compound inhaled. Let us consider the case of solvents. The respiratory system is the first to come into contact with the irritant vapors of these substances, producing coughing, frequent nose bleeding, rashes, and dry skin around the nose and mouth. Irritation is frequent in all the parts (usually hands and arms) that come into contact with rags or tissue papers soaked with solvents because—as degreasing agents—solvents damage the dermal lipid layer. Among this type of inhalants, apparently only toluene produces notorious detrimental effects in acoustic perception, initially described as a strong buzz and chronically associated with inner ear damage. On the other hand, if the gas inhaled is nitrous oxide (also known as laughing gas), hilarity, mood swings, altered perception, and anesthesia may occur. Inhalation of 1,1-difluoroethane, a gas used as propellant in computer dusters, can cause frostbite in the tongue, mouth, larynx, and other soft tissues in addition to its psychoactive actions.

Volatile alkyl nitrites differ from all other inhalants because they produce vasodilation and smooth muscle relaxation rather than cognitive effects. Amyl nitrite was introduced as medication for the treatment of angina pectoris until it was subsequently replaced by nitroglycerine. Amyl, butyl, and isobutyl nitrites are sought as sexual enhancers due to their ability to increase genital irrigation. These compounds decrease blood pressure, increase heart rate, and, under some circumstances, can cause syncope. These harmful cardiovascular effects may be enhanced if alkyl nitrites are combined with phosphodiesterase-5 inhibitors, the active ingredients of medications used to treat erectile dysfunction.

20.6.2 Chronic Effects

Repeated inhalant use produces chronic irritation of respiratory airways with breathing difficulties and increased frequency of respiratory illnesses, anosmia (decreased capacity to detect odors), and general cognitive impairment. Chronic inhalant users have higher incidence of neurobiological abnormalities including diffuse cerebral and cerebellar atrophy, enlarged brain ventricles, and general white matter damage. These abnormalities have been correlated with attention dysfunction, impaired motor control, and memory loss along with reduced speed of information processing, among other detrimental effects [110]. Inhalation of toluene-based products can cause hearing loss, visual impairment, and severe ataxia [40].

Benzene, a component of gasoline, produces anemia and leukemia because it impairs blood cell formation in the bone marrow. The toxicity associated with gasoline inhalation can be related not only to benzene but also to the presence of lead in countries that do not use unleaded gasoline. Hexane, another organic solvent used in inks and other products, causes peripheral neuropathy because it is metabolized to 2,5-hexanedione, a highly toxic compound.

Halogenated compounds, that is, those containing chloride, fluoride, or bromide in their structure such as 1,1,1-trichloroethane, trichloroethylene (a degreasing agent and spot remover), halothane (a liquid anesthetic), or 1,1-difluoroethane (PC duster) can produce liver and kidney failure as well as cardiac arrest.

Repeated exposure to nitrous oxide produces a vitamin B_{12} deficiency, which can lead to damage to the neuron's myelin sheath manifested as ascending lower extremity weakness and numbness [58]. As to nitrites, chronic users of this compound can experience bilateral vision loss due to retinal damage [4].

20.6.3　Prenatal Effects

The fact that the gender gap is getting smaller poses specific challenges for service providers and researchers owing to the harmful effects of inhalants in women of reproductive age. A fetal solvent syndrome, similar to that caused by alcohol, has been described in babies born from mothers that used inhalants during pregnancy, and this syndrome includes facial anomalies, delays in growth, and impaired neurobehavioral development [19]. Low weight at birth and craniofacial abnormalities have also been documented both in clinical and preclinical studies [46]. Follow-up studies of children exposed to inhalants during gestation have shown growth retardation, learning impairment, cerebellar dysfunction (affecting balance) language deficiencies and hyperactivity. It is worth mentioning that some of these studies cannot rule out the use of other drugs and, in fact, it is fairly common for inhalants to be used in combination with other psychoactive substances. However, animal studies in which environmental conditions are controlled and only solvents are used to support these findings.

20.6.4　Molecular Effects

The available evidence indicates that toluene, the best-studied misused solvent, has a complex mechanism of action, which includes effects on diverse molecular targets. A detailed description of toluene's mechanism of action is beyond the scope of this chapter and has been reviewed elsewhere [18], but a few relevant data might be worth noting. Toluene inhibits the function of certain channels activated by excitatory neurotransmitters such as the glutamatergic NMDA receptors [22] and nicotinic receptors [5]. At similar concentrations, toluene enhances the function of inhibitory neurotransmitter receptors such as GABA [6] and glycine [13]. Calcium channels, potassium channels, and sodium channels are also affected by toluene [23, 30, 88]. Like other drugs of abuse, toluene increases dopamine release in key areas of the dopaminergic mesolimbic system Less data are available on other solvents, but the evidence indicates that at least the effects on GABAergic and glutamatergic systems are common to many substances including the majority of inhaled gases.

20.6.5　Morbidity and Mortality

Mortality is associated with this practice. Sudden sniffing death is a rare but serious complication that can occur at any moment, even after single use, that is, it is not necessarily associated with repeated or prolonged exposure. Death can be due to a combination of factors including poor oxygen supply, a direct cardiac effect (arrhythmias) and sensitization to catecholamine stimulatory effects. Sudden death can occur when an intoxicated user is startled because catecholamines are released, the heart function is increased, and cardiac arrest becomes more probable [19]. It has also been reported as a result of an adrenaline surge. It can occur during abuse or in the subsequent few hours because solvents, dissolved in lipid-rich cell membranes, dissipate slowly.

Other causes are derived from the interaction between the substances abused, the user, the route of administration, and the environment. Suffocation and trauma may occur when the user puts a plastic bag sprayed with a solvent over the head to enhance the amount inhaled; the plastic bag may occlude the airway if the user loses consciousness. Death by aspiration usually of vomit is similar to that observed for alcohol and other depressants and results from a combination of a decreased level of consciousness and the loss of protective airway reflexes. Risk of accidents is high as users become less inhibited and less alert and oriented, which facilitates engagement in risky behaviors [106].

Lifestyles of some subgroups as street children raise the burden related to violence and increased risk of HIV from sexual abuse and prostitution [64]. In a survey conducted in 100 cities in Mexico among working children and adolescents from 6 to 17 years of age, Medina-Mora found that less than 1% declared prostitution as their source of income. Increased risk of seroconversion among street population has been reported [83].

The toxic exposure surveillance system database of the American Association of Poison Control Centers showed 63 deaths in 11,670 cases of intentional inhalant abuse reported from 1996 to 2001 to poison control centers in that country, linked to gasoline inhalation (45%), air fresheners (26%), and propane/butane (11%) [92]. In two particular states, Virginia and Texas, a higher rate was found, 39 and 144, respectively, the majority linked to fuel inhalation.

There is a wide range of diseases linked to this practice that includes ichthyosis-like dermatitis on the extremities, decreased visual acuity, toxic hepatitis, distal renal tubular acidosis, metabolic acidosis, leukemia, and aplastic anemia.

There is also evidence of tolerance, dependence, and withdrawal, among many others: despite this evidence, there is insufficient data to allow the assessment of the proportion of the global burden of disease related to this behavior [29].

20.7 Correlates

In a review published in 2008, Medina-Mora and Real found evidence of high rates of psychiatric comorbidity, mood, anxiety, and personality disorders being common among lifetime inhalant users; they also reported a higher prevalence of lifetime dysthymia and anxiety disorders among female inhalant users, but a lower prevalence of antisocial personality disorder. Among inhalant users with comorbid disorders, those who developed social or specific phobia had experienced the onset of these disorders prior to the initiation of inhalant use; all other mood and anxiety disorders usually developed following the onset of inhalant use. Odds of psychiatric disorders were higher for inhalant users who were women, poor, and less educated, with an early onset of inhalant use, family histories of psychopathology, and personal histories of substance abuse treatment.

These same authors also concluded from their review of literature that among incarcerated youth, inhalant users as compared to users of other substances showed significantly higher levels of criminal behavior, antisocial attitudes, current psychiatric symptoms, earlier onset of offending and substance use, and more extensive histories of head injury, kidney disease, hormonal problems, mental illness, suicidality, trauma, and substance-related problems [65]. Mustonen et al. [70] reported recurrent inhalant use (five times or more) in adolescence and subsequent onset of psychosis.

The complex nature of this problem requires (a) holistic, cultural sensitive interventions at the individual, family, and community level to public policies aimed at reducing the risk associated with the substances themselves; (b) control of inhalant availability, with special focus on children and adolescents; (c) changes of social determinants that underlie this disorder; and (d) reduction of health disparities.

20.8   Prevention

Prevention incorporates different strategies, including education, skill building, environmental changes, and policy development. In the school setting prevention, some programs suggest that everyone should be involved: students, teachers, administrators, school nurses, guidance counselors, school social workers, school psychologists, librarians, parent volunteers, school police or safety officers, coaches, clerical staff, cafeteria workers, custodians, and bus drivers [102].

Other authors suggest efforts to prevent volatile substance abuse focused on interventions with community. Specially disseminate information to health workers, educators, media representatives, and parents.

Many strategies focus on educating very young children informing about dangers of inhalants and disseminating messages that show inhalants like poison. In Texas, some of these programs have tried to redefine the problem as a public health rather than a substance abuse issue; these visions facilitate the involvement of community partners, nurses, emergency room personnel, medical associations, and poison centers.

Other prevention interventions developed and provided educational materials and resources to families, school, and media. Products include staff training and curricula for schools and resources to teach parents skills [72].

Some populations require special attention like Indian population in different countries. Alaska Natives have developed school programs aimed at making students aware of the dangers of inhalants [49].

A program for young migrants from Morocco aimed at covering basic needs and detecting early those persons recently involved with inhalants. A

change of demand is expected by means of workshops on health promotion and promotion of sport activities and art activities [42].

As in treatment, prevention includes teaching and helping children and teenagers to build strengths, increase cultural self-identity, and develop social and emotional skills and also helping families [31].

20.9   Treatment

Considering the wide variety of compounds included in the inhalants' category, several approaches are required to provide effective treatment to chronic users.

20.9.1   Recovery Potential and Treatment

Despite the impact of the negative effects of inhalant misuse reviewed in this chapter, there is some evidence on the recovery potential of cognitive and neurological deleterious effects that occur following abstinence from solvent misuse, pending on the extension and duration of inhalant misuse [33]. Bowen and Cruz [20] described evidence indicating that the myeloneuropathy associated with chronic use of nitrous oxide improves with inhalant discontinuation and vitamin B_{12} supplementation [2] and that retinal damage produced by chronic nitrite inhalation can recover after cessation [4]. Unfortunately, some negative sequelae, such as benzene-induced leukemia or liver toxicity produced by halogenated compounds, seem to be more devastating. Support with behavioral cognitive therapy, attention to organic damage (e.g., hearing or sight loss), and treatment of psychiatric comorbid disorders when needed are important components to successful treatment programs.

In this same review, Cruz concludes that to date, there is no available pharmacological therapy for treating this substance use disorder, but found some evidence of limited success, such as using risperidone to control the paranoid psychosis in a male who had been inhaling gasoline and carburetor cleaner daily for 5 years [69]. Other authors have reported that inhalant-induced psychotic disorder was reduced in the severity of symptoms when treated with either carbamazepine or haloperidol [48]. Also, daily administration of lamotrigine decreased craving in a 21-year-old male with a 4-year history of inhalant misuse [90]. More investment in research is needed to develop better pharmacological treatment for this population.

Psychosocial interventions have proven to be effective; these include housing, programs aimed at promoting school attendance and retention, activity-based programs (to engage drug users in therapeutic relationships, develop skills and provide alternatives to substance misuse, e.g., art activities), counseling, outreach of children in risk of becoming street children [37], family therapy (focused either on addressing family dynamics or dysfunctional family behaviors), and indigenous-led residential approaches [62].

As can be seen, effective psychological interventions are directed to increment personal, educational/vocational, and social functioning and to reduce risk behaviors, which are valid and desirable results of the treatment of disorders related to drug use. Treatment and rehabilitation services should not focus exclusively on the ultimate goal of abandonment of the use of drugs; instead, they should consider the intermediate objectives of reducing drug use and its harmful consequences as an integral part of the whole rehabilitation and social reinsertion process [96]. For such purpose, the support and participation of the community and patient orientation is a crucial principle for effective treatment of disorders due to the use of drugs [96], especially in the case of inhalant users, which are generally vulnerable individuals who are socioeconomically disadvantaged and marginalized.

Good treatment models are an important factor for improving quality of life of those affected and reducing the costs for society, and availability of services and service utilization complete the equation. We know from the World Mental Health Survey that the treatment gap for mental disorders including substance use disorders is important, between 35.5% and 50.3% in devel-

oped countries and 76.3% and 85.4% in developing countries [34], and that the treatment gap in some countries as in Mexico is similar for substance use disorders [16], but few studies report rates of service utilization by type of substance, among those with dependence to inhalants.

Perron and colleagues [78] within the National Epidemiologic Survey on Alcohol and Related Conditions (NESARC) documented that among those with dependence (2.3%), 66% used some sort of service, mainly 12 step programs (68.5%) followed by drug rehabilitation programs (61.2%) and private practitioners (55.6%); 15% reported at least one barrier to receiving services, with the low-income group reporting more barriers (22.8%). The most common treatment barriers reported were related to a lack of understanding of what dependence means; between 41% and 43% gave argument thoughts that *the individual should be strong enough to handle it alone* or *that the problem would get better by itself.* The same proportion (42%) reported that they didn't want to go; and in around one third (28.8%) barriers were related to stigma: *feeling too embarrassed to discuss it with anyone.* Lack of resources was reported by one-fifth of those with dependence (23.2%). This information highlights the need to introduce policies to increase both, coverage of treatment and service utilization.

20.10 Evaluation of Biomedical Conditions and Their Complications

20.10.1 Physical Exam

In the physical examination of a patient who was recently exposed to solvents, clinical signs and behavioral changes can be found that may suggest this diagnosis. The characteristic odor is an important fact because it can persist in the breath or in the clothes for several hours after its last use. In users who have been chronically exposed, it is common to find very dry skin and mucous membranes, which facilitates bacterial infection, resulting in perinasal or perioral pyoderma. Irritation of mucous membranes causes users to cough, sneeze, pant, or salivate frequently. Conjunctival epistaxis and irritation can also be observed. More severe cases may present with dyspnea and tachycardia, nausea, vomiting, diarrhea, and abdominal pain [56]. These symptoms usually resolve in about 2 or 3 h. The neurological symptoms of intoxication go from an initial stage of euphoria and disinhibition to a state of confusion, sputtering language, and weakness. In severe poisonings, the user could present ataxia, decreased reflexes, and nystagmus [36, 56].

Hypokalemia is the main risk among inhalant users exposed to toluene-based products. When potassium levels are low, numbness, fatigue, muscle weakness, and cramps occur. This condition can lead to cardiac infarction and kidney failure and is one of the main causes of death. Treatment consists of parenteral potassium replenishment [28].

20.10.2 Evaluation of the Presence of Cognitive Impairment: Mini-Mental State Examination

A relevant aspect when evaluating a patient with problems due to the use of solvents and other substances is to evaluate the cognitive state. In the case of chronic consumers, it is possible that there are various types of deficits, including dementia, so the use of a rapid test can help to suspect the presence of these states from the first evaluation. The "Mini-Mental State Examination" test is a fast application instrument developed by Folstein et al. [41] that has been validated in the Mexican population [11]. Its use is suggested for the assessment of dementia in several clinical guidelines [12] although it is widely used in other populations to assess mental status. This test qualifies several areas, with a maximum score of 30, and is easy to apply per clinician in a short period of time. A score higher than 27 indicates a normal cognition, while a lower score represents a mild cognitive impairment (19–26 points), moderate (10–18 points), or severe (<10 points). Based on the experience of the First Nations Youth Residential Treatment Centers in Canada,

the Mini-Mental or any other diagnostic test should be applied to inhalant users only after a short (1- or 2-week) recovery period, with appropriate sleep and nourishment (Debra Dell, Youth Solvent Addiction Committee; personal communication). Otherwise, neurocognitive impairment is usually overestimated.

20.10.3 History and Current Status of Substance Use

Information on the history and current use of substances should include information on the substance or substances of preferential use as well as the use of secondary substances. Explore about consumption of susbtance for medical use (tranquilizers, stimulants, etc.). For each of the substances used, describe the age of initiation, frequency and amount of use, patterns of low and high consumption, reasons for its use, context including the way in which it obtains or purchases the substance, periods of abstinence and how it achieved them, and history of previous relapses [79].

20.10.4 Evaluation Instruments

Addiction Severity Index (ASI). The Severity Index of Addiction (ASI) is a semi-structured instrument of 200 items, widely used in various scenarios, designed to evaluate 7 areas of potential problems in patients with substance use disorders: medical status, employment, drug use, alcohol use, legal status, family and social status, and psychiatric status. Each area receives a rating which is useful for clinical and research purposes. ASI investigates current status and various problems throughout life. It has been used in diverse populations and its application requires specific training [60]. There is a Spanish translation of the sixth version in English [15]. It is an instrument with adequate validity and reliability.

According to the Clinical Practice Guideline (GPC) prevention and detection of the use of inhalable substances in adolescents in the first level of care, the Inhalant Substance Use Evaluation Card can be applied.

Laboratory tests Laboratory tests that should be done to users with acute solvent poisoning include a blood count, oxygen saturation, serum electrolytes, liver function tests, creatinine, urea nitrogen, glucose, and urine [56]. The detection analysis of drug metabolites in urine is useful to rule out exposure to other drugs, since solvent tests are not routinely found in hospitals.

Cabinet auxiliary studies Chest X-ray plates and an electrocardiogram may be useful especially in patients with cardiological or pulmonary manifestations of solvent exposure [56]. Magnetic resonance imaging of the skull is a very suitable way to assess the damage caused by the abuse of toluene and other compounds. However, it is not as sensitive to detect incipient data, so when they are apparent in studies, the changes are usually very advanced and irreversible after 5–7 years or more of chronic abuse [17].

In brain images, the most characteristic feature is atrophy, which may include cerebellar atrophy, ventricular dilatation, widening of the sulcus and grooves and enlargement of the basal cistern, brain stem atrophy in particular in the pontine area, generalized cerebral atrophy, atrophy of the hippocampus, and atrophy of the optic nerve. Also in 20% of the patients a thinning of the corpus callosum can be observed [17]. Diffuse alterations in the white matter and loss of the boundaries between the white and gray matter are also frequently found. Twenty percent of chronic abusers can present T2 hyperintensities in the thalamus. Unlike other processes that cause atrophy, injuries due to the use of solvents are bilateral, as in alterations due to opioid abuse or metabolic processes [17].

The most prominent finding in chronic toluene abusers is diffuse hyperintensities in white substance in T2 being found in about 46% of patients. The most affected areas are the periventricular white matter, the centrum semiovale, and the cerebellar white matter. Other areas affected to a lesser extent are the internal capsule and the bridge. There is a concordance between the extension of T2 hyperintensities and neurological deficits [17].

20.11 Psychiatric Medical Evaluation

20.11.1 Subtypes of Consumers of Inhalable Solvents

In a study of incarcerated adolescents, it was sought to identify subgroups among users of solvents based on their reasons for using them. Through an analysis of latent classes, three subtypes of solvent consumers were identified: the experimenters, with occasional and limited use, active consumers, and consumers for "self-medication" who use solvents primarily to cope with feelings of sadness, loneliness, anger, etc. [43]. The subgroups did not differ in terms of demographic characteristics but did so in clinical measures such as the presence of anxiety, problems associated with the use of substances, overall severity of the symptoms, and number of different types of solvents used. The results showed heterogeneity for the reasons of use and distress associated with consumption [77].

20.11.2 Comorbid Mental Disorders

The active use of inhalants, in particular solvents, can induce acute secondary or induced psychiatric symptoms. According to the DSM-V psychiatric classification, solvent poisoning can be associated with acute psychotic disorders, mood disorders, and anxiety disorders [3]. On the other hand, in epidemiological studies, it has been found that there is a high comorbidity of the abuse and dependence of inhalants with various psychiatric disorders throughout life. A study in the United States with epidemiological data of 43, 093 adults from 18 to 98 years of age of which 664 (1.7% of the sample) reported use at some time in the life of inhalants (88% abuse criteria, 12% dependency criteria), 60% began consumption before 18 years. In this studied sample, there was a high comorbidity with other psychiatric disorders at some point in life: 48% mood disorders, 36% anxiety disorders, and 45% personality disorders. In addition, there was also a high frequency of major depression (41%), dysthymia (18%), manic episodes (15%), specific phobias (18%), obsessive-compulsive personality disorder (17%), and antisocial disorder (32%). A high percentage presented several psychiatric disorders throughout their lives [109]. These data reflect the importance of assessing the current or past presence of psychiatric disorders.

In adolescents who misuse solvents, a high presence of comorbid disorders has also been found. In a study of 847 adolescents admitted to treatment, it was found that those with abuse or dependence on solvents were more likely to present abuse or dependence on alcohol, hallucinogens, nicotine, cocaine, and amphetamines. In addition, 40% had suffered from major depression and one third had ever attempted suicide [84].

20.11.3 Anxiety Disorders

In this epidemiological study, a higher lifetime prevalence of some psychiatric disorders in women was found, for example, anxiety disorder in 53% (30% in men), panic disorder without agoraphobia in 25% (11% in men), and specific phobias in 28% (14% in men). When assessing the presence of disorders in the last year, the prevalence of anxiety disorders remained high with 25% of the sample [109].

Clinically, anxiety disorders are very frequent and are usually a reason for requesting attention. The individual experiences these states as unpleasant, and in many cases, they are accompanied by physical symptoms such as tachycardia and sweating. The Hamilton Anxiety Scale, which is an instrument applied by the clinician, can be used to determine the severity of anxious symptoms

20.11.4 Affective Disorders

In the case of affective disorders, women had a higher percentage of dysthymia throughout their lives (24% vs. 16% in men). Regarding the age of onset of consumption, those who started before the age of 18 had greater percentage of manic

episodes (10%) than those with late onset (4%), and subjects with early onset and 54% of early initiators had a major depressive episode at some point in their lives. Twenty-six percent of the sample reported having had an affective disorder in the last year, and subjects with previous treatments for substance abuse had a higher percentage of affective disorders (47% vs. 24% in those who did not attend previous treatments) [109].

Depressive disorders are very frequent in the general population and even more frequent in patients with substance use disorders, so it is necessary to evaluate the presence of them from the general diagnostic interview. Depressive disorders are characterized by a low mood, decay, irritability, subjective feeling of discomfort, and impotence. In addition, to a greater or lesser degree, symptoms of cognitive, volitional, and somatic type are present. Sometimes it can be associated with suicidal ideas, which must always be assessed and managed.

The Hamilton Depression Scale is useful to assess the severity of depressive symptoms and allows to determine in a very short time the current severity of depression.

20.11.5 Psychotic Disorders

The psychotic disorders in consumers of solvents are usually of acute type, with an important hallucinatory component. This has been reported since the 1960s, with a high proportion of visual hallucinations and, to a lesser extent, auditory hallucinations. In a qualitative study with adolescents using solvent based on toluene, Cruz and Dominguez [26] found that the use of solvents was clearly associated with hallucinatory experiences, these being visual, auditory, tactile, and olfactory. They also expressed a continuum between dreams, illusions, and complex hallucinations [25].

20.11.6 Personality Disorders

Among abusers of volatile substances, there is a higher prevalence of antisocial behaviors, interpersonal violence, mood disorders, anxiety, personality disorders, use of other substances, and treatment in mental health services in the last year compared to non-users of volatile substances [43].

20.12   Exploration of Medical Complications

20.12.1   Kidney

At the renal level, the use of solvents, especially toluene, is associated with renal tubular acidosis, urinary stones, glomerulonephritis, and renal failure [59].

20.12.2   Kidney Tubular Acidosis

Compounds with toluene are especially nephrotoxic since it is assumed that toluene inhibits the secretion of protons in the distal tubules. The subsequent renal tubular acidosis (TKA) is characterized by a hyperchloremic metabolic acidosis with a strong loss of potassium and phosphates, which can cause weakness, muscle spasticity, and cardiac arrhythmias. Renal tubular acidosis is also associated with recurrent urinary stone formation [56].

Liver. It has been documented that the use of solvents can produce toxic hepatitis and liver failure [59]. The vapors of chlorinated hydrocarbons and chloroform are known to be hepatotoxic that can cause toxic hepatitis. Sometimes some metabolites released by the kidney and liver are free radicals that cause damage to the membranes of the hepatocytes, and in some individuals complete liver and kidney failure have been observed after exposure to inhaled solvents [56].

20.12.3   Other Organs and Tissues

Benzene has been associated with suppression of the bone marrow and with the subsequent development of leukemia, lymphomas, and aplastic anemia [56, 59].

Lungs The most direct pulmonary effects are related to direct damage to the lung tissue or are related to asphyxia, since volatile solvents can displace oxygen and produce hypoxia and loss of consciousness. There are some solvents that can produce chemical pneumonitis [56, 59].

In an epidemiological study in the United States among adults between 35 and 45 years of age, it was found that the duration of inhalant abuse was positively and significantly associated with a higher probability of suffering from tuberculosis, bronchitis, asthma, and sinusitis. These diseases are necessary [50]. On the other hand, it has been reported that the inhalation of gases from hydrocarbons such as butane can cause laryngeal edema and laryngospasm [19].

20.12.4   Heart

Adverse cardiac effects have been reported in acute intoxication by toluene and other solvents, whose cardiotoxicity can cause severe arrhythmias and death [40]. The syndrome of sudden death by solvents was described by Bass in 1970 and is caused by cardiac arrhythmias, apparently due to a sensitization of the myocardium to catecholamines (adrenaline, noradrenaline), so that when feeling scared or agitated a user has a rapid increase of these substances and can cause ventricular fibrillation [56, 59].

At low doses, hydrocarbons can produce hypotension due to peripheral vasodilatation and reflex tachycardia, while increasing the dose produces an increase in cardiac output and bradycardia. In the case of nitrates, they cause vasodilatation with stagnation of blood in the lower extremities, which can cause orthostatic hypotension and syncope [56].

20.12.5   Pregnancy

In animal models, prenatal exposure to toluene is associated with malformations, growth retardation, slow reflexes, and decreased attention. There is evidence that these negative effects are increased if the experimental animals are exposed to stress [27].

In humans, the use of inhalants in pregnancy has been associated with multiple risks such as miscarriage and premature birth, reaching frequencies of up to 9% of the products of mothers who had exposure to toluene during pregnancy [19]. There have also been reports of withdrawal symptoms in the neonate characterized by very acute crying, insomnia, overactive Moro reflex, tremor and hypotonia, and difficulty feeding [19].

20.12.6 Fetal Solvent Syndrome

Since the use of inhalants is prevalent in young women of childbearing age, it is important to highlight the possibility of pregnancy, which is accompanied by a series of characteristic complications. The use of toluene during pregnancy in humans has been linked to congenital malformations including craniofacial deformations similar to those found in fetal alcohol syndrome such as cleft palate, micrognathia, microcephaly) as well as developmental delay [56, 59]. In addition, on many occasions, the effects of the consumption of other substances are added [19].

The monitoring of these infants up to 3 years has documented alterations in development such as growth retardation, hyperactivity, language disorders, and cerebellar dysfunction characterized by lack of coordination [19].

20.13 Psychiatric Medical Intervention

20.13.1 Pharmacological Management of Disorders Due to the Use of Solvents

The psychiatric medical treatment of the addiction to solvents follows the general lines of the treatment of other addictions. In a Cochrane systematic review, no adequate studies were identified, observational or experimental controlled and prospective studies, limited to reports of isolated cases, so they conclude that there is insufficient evidence to recommend any pharmacological treatment for this type of abuse [54].

20.13.2 Management of Damage to Organs and Systems

Acute poisoning Solvent users are usually brought to medical attention only when they are in a life-threatening situation or when there have been injuries. The intervention can save the user's life and must include assessment of the airway, breathing, and circulation. Cardiorespiratory monitoring is recommended because of the risk of sudden death or profound depression of the central nervous system. Life support includes oximetry and hydration with saline and close observation [56].

20.13.3 Policy Options

As reviewed in this chapter, inhalant misuse is a phenomenon characterized by significant inequalities, regarding the social context of the most affected users who tend to come from more poor, disorganized, or isolated communities, who are differentially exposed to low-quality substances, violence, and other adverse experiences; who have lower opportunities of education and work; who are differential; and who have worst health outcomes and socioeconomic consequences such as school dropout, unemployment, informal labor, stigma, and barriers to accessing health care. This scenario calls for the inclusion of intervention efforts to reduce these social determinants within a framework of community interventions.

Some recommended measures include attending needs of education and employment; ensuring access to health systems for different needs such as vaccination, nutrition, and acute and chronic disorders including mental health disorders; and providing alternatives to inhalation such as sports and other recreational, artistic activities along with active search of persons in risk or using substances and counseling [66, 82]. Community interventions aimed at reducing disorganization and violence include environmental design, urbanization, participation of organizations that provide support to families, prevention programs that promote group cohesion and conflict resolution without violence, and in general empowering communities to make accurate diagnosis, develop action plans, formalize process, and monitor progress [107, 111].

Good example of policies aimed at reducing the risk associated with the toxicity of substances was the development, in Australia, of Opal fuel which contains very low levels of the aromatic compound that causes intoxication, benzene, toluene, and xylene, making it less attractive for inhalation. Other examples of this type of interventions are the modifications to the formula aerosol spray paints replacing aromatic chemicals toluene and xylene to less intoxicating ones [1] and the development of glues based on water for use at schools.

Control of availability with special focus on children and adolescents in supermarkets, hardware stores, or service stations and integrating commerce organizations in avoiding selling inhalants to these groups of the population are other examples.

Harm reduction interventions aimed at educating about the special dangers associated with certain substances and ways of administration, reducing risk of accidents and mortality, are controversial but can be considered when approaching heavy using populations as a first step.

Legislation can provide governments, retailers, and community and health workers means to address misuse such as to remove products from users or stores, move users to safe places, mandate treatment, restrict packaging and sale of inhalants, etc. The existing laws generally do not make illegal the possession of inhalants [1].

Training of frontline health workers, teachers, police, and community counselors requires appropriate training in identifying those at risk, interventions based on evidence, and referral to services.

Provide information to parentes, teachers, police, and community organizations on the substances with an abuse liability, identification of persons that are abusing, adequate handling, and referral of cases.

More invesment on basic and applied reseach on susbtance misuse is required, ensuring translational research from the molecular to the clinical level and to the community.

1. The term inhalants refers to:
   (a) Industrial products of easy access, which are inhaled to produce a psychoactive effect
   (b) Solvent products
   (c) Gases, nitrites, aerosols, and solvents
2. People seeking treatment due to inhalant use:
   (a) They have no chance of recovery; it is preferable to focus on prevention.
   (b) They could go to treatment centers that include CBT, care for organic damage, and comorbidity.
   (c) Treatment in organic damage reduction is the only one that has proven to be effective.
3. The modifications made to the ICD-11, which include the consumption of inhalants, are due to:
   (a) Need to describe more precisely consumption and damage patterns, for a better intervention
   (b) The increasing number of substances of abuse
   (c) Increasing global prevalence of inhalant use
4. Sudden Sniffing Death can be a consequence when:
   (a) The person consumes inhalants daily
   (b) It can occur in a first attempt
   (c) It is a consequence of the consumption of other substances but not of inhalants
5. Examples of successful public policies are those that include:
   (a) Those policies that guarantee that the industry withdraws the most toxic products from market
   (b) Policies aimed at harm reduction, teaching children resistance substance use skills
   (c) Those policies that include combined strategies of industry support, modification of legislation, harm reduction, availability control, and psychoeducation

References

1. Alcohol and other Drug Council of Australia, Policy Position, Inhalants. 2010. http://www.healthinfonet. ecu.edu.au/key-resources/organisations?oid=403.
2. Alt RS, Morrissey RP, Gang MA, Hoffman RS, Schaumburg HH. Severe myeloneuropathy from acute high-dose nitrous oxide (N2O) abuse. J Emerg Med. 2011;41(4):378–80. https://doi.org/10.1016/j. jemermed.2010.04.020.
3. American Psychiatric Association. Guía de consulta de los criterios diagnósticos del dsm-5: American Psychiatric Publishing; 2014.
4. Audo I, El Sanharawi M, Vignal-Clermont C, Villa A, Morin A, Conrath J, Fompeydie D, Sahel JA, Gocho-Nakashima K, Goureau O, Paques M. Foveal damage in habitual poppers users. Arch Ophthalmol. 2011;129(6):703–8. https://doi.org/10.1001/ archophthalmol.2011.6.
5. Bale AS, Meacham CA, Benignus VA, Bushnell PJ, Shafer TJ. Volatile organic compounds inhibit human and rat neuronal nicotinic acetylcholine receptors expressed in Xenopus oocytes. Toxicol Appl Pharmacol. 2005a;205(1): 77–88.
6. Bale AS, Tu Y, Carpenter-Hyland EP, Chandler LJ, Woodward JJ. Alterations in glutamatergic and gabaergic ion channel activity in hippocampal neurons following exposure to the abused inhalant toluene. Neuroscience. 2005b;130(1):197–206.
7. Balster RL, Cruz SL, Howard MO, Dell CA, Cottler LB. Classification of abused inhalants. Addiction. 2009;104(6):878–82. https://doi. org/10.1111/j.1360-0443.2008.02494.x.
8. Bassiony M. Substance use disorders in Saudi Arabia: review article. J Subst Use. 2013;18(6):450–66. https://doi.org/10.3109/14659891.2011.606349.
9. Basu D, Jhirwal OP, Singh J, Kumar S, Mattoo SK. Inhalant abuse by adolescents: a new challenge for Indian physicians. Indian J Med Sci. 2004;58:245–9.
10. Beauvais F, Oetting ER. Indian youth and inhalants: an update. NIDA Res Monogr. 1988;85:34–48. Epidemiology of inhalants abuse: an update.
11. Becerra B, Ortega-Soto H, Torner C. Validez y reproductibilidad del examen cognoscitivo brebe (Mini-mental State Examination) en una unidad de cuidados especiales de un hospital psiquiátrico. Salud Mental. 1992;15(4):41–5.
12. Becerra Pino M, Calleja Olvera J, Lozano Dávila M, Sosa Ortiz A, Trujillo de los Santos Z. Guía de Consulta para el Médico de Primer Nivel de Atención Alteraciones de la Memoria en la Persona Adulta Mayor. Centro Nacional de Programas Preventivos y Control de Enfermedades. Secretaría de Salud; 2010
13. Beckstead MJ, Weiner JL, Eger EI 2nd, Gong DH, Mihic SJ. Glycine and gamma-aminobutyric acid(A) receptor function is enhanced by inhaled drugs of abuse. Mol Pharmacol. 2000;57(6):1199–205.
14. Boak A, Hamilton HA, Adalf EM, Mann RE. Drug use among Ontario students. 1977-2017. Highlights from the Ontario student drug use and Health Survey (OSDUHS) (CAMH Research Document Series No. 46) Toronto: Center for Addiction and Mental Health; 2017. Available at: https://www.camh.ca/-/ media/files/pdf%2D%2D-osduhs/drug-use-among- ontario-students-1977-2017%2D%2D-detailed- findings-from-the-osduhs.pdf?la=en&hash=2B434 CDAAD485834497E3B43F2264BDEB255F29F.
15. Bobes J, Bascarán MT, Bobes-Bascarán MT, Carballo JL, Díaz Mesa EM, Flórez G, García Portilla MP, Sáiz PA. Valoración de la gravedad de la adicción: aplicación a la gestión clínica y monitorización de los tratamientos. Madrid: Delegación del Gobierno para el Plan Nacional sobre Drogas; 2007. Available at: http://www.fundacioncsz.org/ ArchivosPublicaciones/214.pdf.
16. Borges G, Wang P, Medina-Mora ME, Lara C, Chiu W. Delay of first treatment of mental and substance use disorders in Mexico. Am J Public Health. 2007;97(9):1638–43.
17. Borne J, Riascos R, Cuellar H, Vargas D, Rojas R. Neuroimaging in drug and substance abuse part II: opioids and solvents. Top Magn Reson Imaging. 2005;16(3):239–45.
18. Bowen SE, Batis JC, Paez-Martinez N, Cruz SL. The last decade of solvent research in animal models of abuse: mechanistic and behavioral studies. Neurotoxicol Teratol. 2006;28(6):636–47.
19. Bowen SE. Two serious and challenging medical complications associated with volatile substance misuse: sudden sniffing death and fetal solvent syndrome. Subst Use Misuse. 2011;46(1):68–72. https://doi.org/10.3109/10826084.2011.580220.
20. Bowen SE, Cruz SL. Inhalants: addiction and toxic effects in the human. In: Madras B, Kuhar M, editors. The effects of drug abuse on the human nervous system, Book 2 in the Neuroscience-net master reference book series (ebook); 2012. Available at: http://neuroscience.com/books/ book-2-effects-drug-abuse-human-nervous-system.
21. Chávez J, Villatoro J, Robles L, Bustos M, Moreno M, Olivia N, Fregoso D, Gómez G, Medina-Mora ME, Paredes A. Encuesta escolar sobre adicciones en el Estado de Jalisco 2012. Consejo Estatal contra las Adicciones de Jalisco. México: Instituto Nacional de Psiquiatría Ramón de la Fuente Muñiz; 2013.
22. Cruz SL, Mirshahi T, Thomas B, Balster RL, Woodward JJ. Effects of the abused solvent toluene on recombinant N-methyl-D-aspartate and non-N-methyl-D-aspartate receptors expressed in Xenopus oocytes. J Pharma Exp Therap. 1998;286(1):334–40.
23. Cruz SL, Orta-Salazar G, Gauthereau MY, Millan-Perez Pena L, Salinas-Stefanon EM. Inhibition of cardiac sodium currents by toluene exposure. Br J Pharmacol. 2003;140(4):653–60.
24. Cruz SL, Bowen, SE Inhalant abuse. In: Ubach MM, Mondragon-Ceballos R, editors. Neural mechanisms of action of drugs of abuse and natural reinforcers.

(ISBN 978-81-308-0245-9) Pandalai, Managing editor, Research Signpost, Kerala, India; 2008. p. 181.

25. Cruz SL. The latest evidence in the neuroscience of solvent misuse: an article written for service providers. Subst Use Misuse. 2011;46(Suppl 1):62–7.

26. Cruz SL, Dominguez M. Misusing volatile substances for their hallucinatory effects: a qualitative pilot study with Mexican teenagers and a pharmacological discussion of their hallucinations. Subst Use Misuse. 2011;46(Suppl 1):84–94. https://doi.org/10.3109/10826084.2011.580222.

27. Cruz SL, Rivera-García MT, Woodward JJ. Review of toluene actions: clinical evidence, animal studies, and molecular targets. J Drug Alcohol Res. 2014;3:1–8. Available at: https://www.ncbi.nlm.nih.gov/pmc/articles/PMC4211428/.

28. Cruz SL. Inhalant misuse management. The experience in Mexico and a literature review. J Subst Use. 2018;23(5):485–91. https://doi.org/10.1080/14659891.2017.1405090.

29. Degenhardt L, Hall W. Extent of illicit drug use and dependence, and their contribution to the global burden of disease. Lancet. 2012;379(9810):55–70. https://doi.org/10.1016/S0140-6736(11)61138-0.

30. Del Re AM, Dopico AM, Woodward JJ. Effects of the abused inhalant toluene on ethanol-sensitive potassium channels expressed in oocytes. Brain Res. 2006;1087(1):75–82.

31. Dell C, Ogborne A, Begin P. Youth residential solvent treatment program design: an examination of the role of program length and length of client stay. Ottawa: Canadian Center on Substance Abuse; 2003.

32. Dell D, Hopkins C. Residential volatile substance misuse treatment for indigenous youth in Canada. Subst Use Misuse. 2011;46(S1):107–13. https://doi.org/10.3109/10826084.2011.580225.

33. Dingwall KM, Cairney S. Recovery from central nervous system changes following volatile substance misuse. Subst Use Misuse. 2011;46(1):73–83. https://doi.org/10.3109/10826084.2011.580221.

34. Demyttenaere K, Bruffaerts R, Posada-Villa J, Gasquet I, Kovess V, Lepine J, Angermeyer MC, Bernert S, de Girolamo G, Morosini P, Polidori G, Kikkawa T, Kawakami N, Ono Y, Takeshima T, Uda H, Karam EG, Fayyad JA, Karam AN, Mneimneh ZN, Medina-Mora ME, Borges G, Lara C, de Graaf R, Ormel J, Gureje O, Shen Y, Huang Y, Zhang M, Alonso J, Haro JM, Vilagut G, Bromet EJ, Gluzman S, Webb C, Kessler RC, Merikangas KR, Anthony JC, Von Korff MR, Wang PS, Brugha TS, Aguilar-Gaxiola S, Lee S, Heeringa S, Pennell BE, Zaslavsky AM, Ustun TB, Chatterji S, World Mental Health Survey Consortium WHO. Prevalence, severity and unmet need for treatment of mental disorders in the World Health Organization World Mental Health (WMH) surveys. JAMA. 2004;291(21):2581–90.

35. Drug Enforcement Administration. Drugs of abuse. Inhalants. 2015 EDITION: a DEA resource guide. 2015. Available at: https://portal.ct.gov/-/media/DCF/Substance_Abuse/pdf/Inhalentspdf.pdf?la=en.

36. Duncan JR, Lawrence AJ. Conventional concepts and new perspectives for understanding the addictive properties of inhalants. J Pharmacol Sci. 2013;122(4):237–43.

37. Echeverría C, Tavera S. Matlapa. Redes de atención para la infancia en situación de calle. México: Instituto Nacional de Desarrollo Social; 2007.

38. ESPAD. Report 2015. Results from the European School Survey Project on Alcohol and Other Drugs. European Monitoring Center for Drugs and Drug Addiction; 2016.

39. European Monitoring Center for Drugs and Drug Addiction. Country overview: Uzbekistan [Internet]. 2015. Available at: http://www.emcdda.europa.eu/publications/country-overviews/uz#gps.

40. Filley CM, Halliday K, Kleinschmidt-DeMasters BK. The effects of toluene on the central nervous system. J Neuropathol Exp Neurol. 2004;63(1):1–12.

41. Folstein M, Folstein S, McHugh P. "Mini-mental state". A practical method for grading the cognitive state of patients for the clinician. J Psychiatr Res. 1975;12(3):189–98.

42. Fundación SEARCH. Guía para profesionales sobre abuso de sustancias volátiles. Fundación Search Comunidad Europeas. 2002. Available at: http://www.lwl.org/ks-download/downloads/searchII/Solvents-Guide_span.pdf.

43. Garland EL, Howard MO. Volatile substance misuse: clinical considerations, neuropsychopharmacology and potential role of pharmacotherapy in management. CNS Drugs. 2012;26(11):927–35. https://doi.org/10.1007/s40263-012-0001-6.

44. Gigengack R. "My body breaks. I take solution." Inhalant use in Dheli as pleasure seeking at a cost. Int J Drug Policy. 2014;25(4):810–8. https://doi.org/10.1016/j.drugpo.2014.06.003.

45. Gutiérrez R, Vega L, Medina-Mora ME. La infancia "callejera" en México. In: Echeverría C, Tavera S, editors. Matlapa. Redes de atención para la infancia en situación de calle. 1st ed. México: nstituto Nacional de Desarrollo Social; 2007. pp.17–34.

46. Hannigan JH, Bowen SE. Reproductive toxicology and teratology of abused toluene. Syst Biol Reprod Med. 2010;56(2):184–200. https://doi.org/10.3109/19396360903377195.

47. Health Performance Framework. Health performance framework report. Determinants of Health. Drug and other substance use including inhalants. Australian Government. Department of the Prime Minister and Cabinet Aboriginal and Torres Strait Islander; 2014.

48. Hernandez-Avila CA, Ortega-Soto HA, Jasso A, Hasfura-Buenaga CA, Kranzler HR. Treatment of inhalant-induced psychotic disorder with carbamazepine versus haloperidol. Psychiatr Serv. 1998;49(6):812–5.

49. Hillabrant W, Woodis P, Navratil C, McKenzie J, Rhoades M. Inhalant abuse in Indian country. Indian

Health Service. Support Services International, Inc.; 2001

50. Howard MO, Bowen SE, Garland EL, Perron BE, Vaughn MG. Inhalant use and inhalant use disorders in the United States. Addict Sci Clin Pract. 2011;6(1):18–31.

51. Instituto Nacional de Psiquiatría Ramón de la Fuente Muñiz, Instituto Nacional de Salud Pública, Comisión Nacional Contra las Adiciones, Secretaría de Salud. Encuesta Nacional de Drogas, Alcohol y Tabaco 2016–2017: Reporte de drogas. Ciudad de México: INRF; 2017.

52. Johnston LD, O'Malley PM, Bachman JG. Monitoring the future national survey results on drug use, 1975–2002. Volume I: secondary school students (NIH Publication no. 03-5375) Bethesda: National Institute on Drug Abuse; 2003.

53. Johnston LD, Miech RA, O'Malley PM, Bachman JG, Schulenberg JE, Patrick ME. Monitoring the future national survey results on drug use 1975–2018: overview, key findings on adolescent drug use. Ann Arbor: Institute for Social Research, University of Michigan; 2019.

54. Konghom S, Verachai V, Srisurapanont M, Suwanmajo S, Ranuwattananon A, Kimsongneun N, Uttawichai K. Treatment for inhalant dependence and abuse. Cochrane Database Syst Rev. 2010;8(12) https://doi.org/10.1002/14651858.CD007537.pub2.

55. Koposov R, Stickley A, Ruchkin V. Inhalant use in adolescents in northern Russia. Soc Psychiatry Psychiatr Epidemiol. 2018;53(7):709–16. https://doi.org/10.1007/s00127-018-1524-z.

56. Kurtzman T, Otsuka K, Wahl R. Inhalant abuse by adolescents. J Adolesc Health. 2001;28(3):170–80.

57. Leal H, Mejía L, Gómez I, Salinas de Valle O. Estudio naturalístico sobre el fenómeno del consumo de inhalantes en niños de la Ciudad de México. Contreras C (comp) En Inhalación Voluntaria de Disolventes Industriales, Trillas, México; 1977. p. 442–459.

58. Lin RJ, Chen HF, Chang YC, Su JJ. Subacute combined degeneration caused by nitrous oxide intoxication: case reports. Acta Neurol Taiwanica. 2011;20(2):129–37.

59. Lubman DI, Yücel M, Lawrence AJ. Inhalant abuse among adolescents: neurobiological considerations. Br J Pharmacol. 2008;154(2):316–26. https://doi.org/10.1038/bjp.2008.76.

60. McLellan AT, Luborsky L, O'Brien CP, Woody GE. An improved evaluation instrument for substance abuse patients: the addiction severity index. J Nerv Ment Dis. 1980;168(1):26–33.

61. MacLean S. Global selves: marginalised young people and aesthetic reflexivity in inhalant drug use. J Youth Stud. 2007;10(4):399–418. https://doi.org/10.1080/13676260701360691.

62. MacLean S, Cameron J, Harney A, Lee NK. Psychosocial therapeutic interventions for volatile substance use: a systematic review. Addiction. 2012;107(2):278–88. https://doi.org/10.1111/j.1360-0443.2011.03650.x.

63. Medina-Mora ME, Berenzon S. Epidemiology of inhalant abuse in Mexico. NIDA Res Monogr. 1995;148:136–74.

64. Medina-Mora ME, Gutiérrez R, Vega L. What happened to street kids? An analysis of the Mexican experience. Subst Use Misuse. 1997;32(3):293–316.

65. Medina-Mora ME, Real T. Epidemiology of inhalant use. Curr Opin Psychiatry. 2008;21(3):247–51. https://doi.org/10.1097/YCO.0b013e3282fc9875.

66. Medina-Mora ME, Vilatoro J, Fleiz C, Domínguez M, Cruz S. Challenges to neuroscience and public policy derived from new trends and patterns of inhalant misuse. J Int Drug Abuse Res Soc. 2014;3:1–8. https://doi.org/10.4303/jdar/235842.

67. Medina-Mora ME, Rafful C, Villatoro J, Robles NO, Bustos M, Moreno M. Diferencias sociodemográficas entre usuarios de inhalables, usuarios de otras drogas y adolescents no consumidores en una muestra Mexicana de estudiantes. Rev Int Inv Adicciones. 2015;1(1):6–15. https://doi.org/10.28931/riiad.2015.1.02.

68. Mesquita AM, de Andrade AG, Anthony JC. Use of the inhalant lança by Brazilian medical students. Subst Use Misuse. 1988;33(8):1667–80.

69. Misra LK, Kofoed L, Fuller W. Treatment of inhalant abuse with risperidone. J Clin Psych. 1999;60(9):620.

70. Mustonen A, Niemelä S, McGrath JJ, Murray GK, Nordström T, Mäki P, Miettunen J, Scott JG. Adolescent inhalant use and psychosis risk - a prospective longitudinal study. Schizophr Res. 2018;201:360–6. https://doi.org/10.1016/j.schres.2018.05.013.

71. National Inhalant Prevention Coalition. News briefs: CADCA announces National Leadership Forum; Press Conference Marks New Inhalant PSA & Survey. 1997.

72. National Institute of Drug Abuse. Inhalant abuse among children and adolescents: consultation on building an international research. 2005.

73. National Institute of Drug Abuse. The science of drug abuse. 2012. Available at: http://www.drugabuse.gov/drugs-abuse/inhalants.

75. Organization of American States, Inter American Drug Abuse Control Commission. (OEA/CICAD). Report on drug use in the Americas 2019. Washington, DC: Inter American Drug Abuse Control Commission; 2019. Available at: http://www.cicad.oas.org/oid/Report%20on%20Drug%20Use%20in%20the%20Americas%202019.pdf.

76. Ortiz A, Domínguez M, Palomares G. Solvent inhalants use in the San Judas Tadeo feast. Salud Mental. 2015;38(6):423–8. https://doi.org/10.17711/SM.0185-3325.2015.057.

77. Perron BE, Howard MO. Perceived risk of harm and intentions of future inhalant use among ado-

lescent inhalant users. Drug Alcohol Depend. 2008;97(1–2):185–9. https://doi.org/10.1016/j.drugalcdep.2008.04.005.

78. Perron B, Mowbray O, Bier S, Vaughn M, Krentzman A, Howard M. Service use and treatment barriers among inhalant users. J Psychoactive Drugs. 2011;43(1):69–75. https://doi.org/10.1080/0279107 2.2011.566504.

79. Peters RH, Peyton E. Guideline for drug courts on screening and assessment. Prepared for the American University, Justice Programs Office, in association with the U.S. Department of Justice, Office of Justice Programs, Drug Courts Program Office. 1998. Available at: https://www.ncjrs.gov/pdffiles1/bja/171143.pdf.

80. Poznyak V, Reed GM, Medina-Mora ME. Aligning the ICD-11 classification of disorders due to substance use with global service needs. Epidemiol Psychiatr Sci. 2018;27(3):212–8. https://doi.org/10.1017/S2045796017000622.

81. Ridenour TA, Halliburton AE, Bray BC. Does DSM-5 nomenclature for inhalant use disorder improve upon DSM-IV? Psychol Addict Behav. 2015;29(1):211–7. https://doi.org/10.1037/adb0000007.

82. Rodgers D. Youth gangs and violence in Latin America and the Caribbean, A literature survey. LCR Sustainable development working paper No.4. Washington DC: World Bank; 1999

83. Roy E, Leclerc P, Cédras L, Weber A, Claessens C, Boivin J. HIV incidence among street youth in Montreal, Canada. AIDS. 2003;17:1071–5.

84. Sakai JT, Hall SK, Mikulich-Gilbertson SK, Crowley TJ. Inhalant use, abuse, and dependence among adolescent patients: commonly comorbid problems. J Am Acad Child Adolesc Psychiatry. 2004;43(9):1080–8.

85. SAMHSA. The CBHSQ Report. Understanding adolescent inhalant use. National Survey on Drug Use and Health. 2017. Available at: https://www.samhsa.gov/data/sites/default/files/report_3095/ShortReport-3095.html.

86. Sanchez Z, Noto A, Anthony J. Social rank and inhalant drug use: the case of lança perfume use in São Paulo, Brazil. Drug Alcohol Depend. 2012;131(1–2):92–9. https://doi.org/10.1016/j.drugalcdep.2012.12.001.

87. Secretaría de Salud Sistema de Vigilancia Epidemiológica de las Adicciones (SISVEA). Informe 2011. Secretaría de Salud. Subsecretaría de Prevención y Promoción de la Salud. México: Dirección General de Epidemiología; 2016

88. Shafer TJ, Bushnell PJ, Benignus VA, Woodward JJ. Perturbation of voltage-sensitive Ca2+ channel function by volatile organic solvents. J Pharma Expe Therapeutics. 2005;315(3):1109–18.

89. Sharp CW, Rosenber N, Beauvais F. Inhalant- related disorders. In: Tasman A, Kay J, Lieberman JA, First MB, Maj M, editors. Psychiatry. 3rd ed. New Jersey: John Wiley & Sons: 2008. p. 1127–48.

90. Shen YC. Treatment of inhalant dependence with lamotrigine. Prog Neuropsychopharmacol Biol Psychiatry. 2007;31(3):769–71.

91. Shimane T. Annual Report 2015 Nationwide General Population Survey on Drug Use in Japan. Health and Labour Sciences Research Grants 2015. Research on Regulatory Science of Pharmaceuticals and Medical Devices. H27-Iyaku A-Ippan-001 (2017).

92. Spiller HA. Epidemiology of volatile substance abuse (VSA) cases reported to US poison centers. Am J Drug Alcohol Abuse. 2004;30(1):155–65.

93. Swaim RC, Stanley LR. Substance use among American Indian youths on reservations compared with a National Sample of US adolescents. JAMA Netw Open. 2018; https://doi.org/10.1001/jamanetworkopen.2018.0382.

94. Takagi M, Yücel M, Lubman D. The dark side of sniffing: paint colour affects intoxication experiences among adolescent inhalant users. Drug Alcohol Rev. 2010;29:452–5. https://doi.org/10.1111/j.1465-3362.2009.00162.x.

95. Trotter R, Rolf J, Baldwin L. Cultural models for inhalant abuse among Navajo youth. Drugs Society. 1997;10(1–2):39–59.

96. United Nations. Informe de la Junta Internacional de Fiscalización de Estupefacientes correspondiente a 2017. Viena: United Nations; 2018.

97. Vega L, Rendón A, Gutiérrez R, Villatoro J, Vargas A, Juárez A, Severiano E, Sánchez V, Trejo S. Estudio sobre patrones de consumo de sustancias psicoactivas en población indígena residente y originaria de la ciudad de México. México: INP-IAPA; 2015.

98. Verma R, Balhara YPS, Dhawan A. Inhalant abuse: an exploratory study. Psychiatry J. 2011;20(2):103–6. https://doi.org/10.4103/0972-6748.102493.

99. Villatoro J, Gaytán F, Moreno M, Gutiérrez ML, Olivia N, Bretón M, López MS, Bustos M, Medina-Mora ME. Consumo de Alcohol, Tabaco y otras Drogas en la Ciudad de México. Medición 2009. México: Instituto Nacional de Psiquiatria Ramón de la Fuente; 2010.

100. Villatoro J, Medina-Mora ME, Fleiz C, Moreno M, Oliva R, Bustos A, Fregoso D, Gutiérrez ML, Amador N. El consumo de drogas en México: Resultados de la Encuesta Nacional de Adicciones, 2011. Salud Mental. 2012;34:447–57.

101. Villatoro J, Medina-Mora ME, Martín del Campo R, Fregoso D, Bustos M, Reséndiz E, Mujica R, Bretón M, Soto I, Cañas V. El consumo de drogas en estudiantes de México: tendencias y magnitud del problema. Salud Mental. 2016;39(4):193–203.

102. Virginia Department of Education. Inhalant abuse prevention: staff education and student curriculum. Richmond: Division of Special Education and Student Services; 2007.

103. Wang RJ, Wang YT, Ma J, Liu MX, Su MF, Lian Z, Shi J, Lu L, Bao YP. Substance use among young people in China: a systematic review and meta-

analysis. Lancet. 2017a;390(14):01. https://doi.org/10.1016/S0140-6736(17)33152-5.

104. Wang X, Li Y, Wu Z, Tang Z, Reilly KH, Nong Q. Nitrite inhalant use and HIV infection among Chinese men who have sex with men in 2 large cities in China. J Addict Med. 2017b;11(6):468–74. https://doi.org/10.1097/ADM.0000000000000347.

105. White V, Hayman J. Australian Secondary Students' Use of Over-the-Counter and Illicit Substances in 2002. Canberra: Australian Government Department of Health and Ageing; 2004. National Drug Strategy Monograph series no.56.

106. Williams J, Storck M, and the Committee on Substance Abuse and Committee on Native American Child Health Pediatrics 2007; 119–10009. https://doi.org/10.1542/peds.2007-0470. http://pediatrics.aappublications.org/content/119/5/1009.full.html.

107. World Bank. Crimen y Violencia en Centroamérica Un Desafío para el Desarrollo. Washington DC: Banco Mundial; 2011. www.bancomundial.org.lac.

108. World Drug Report. Global overview of drug demand and supply. Latest trends, cross-cutting issues. United Nations publication, Sales No. E.18.XI.9. 2018. Available at: https://www.unodc.org/wdr2018/prelaunch/WDR18_Booklet_2_GLOBAL.pdf.

109. Wu LT, Howard MO. Psychiatric disorders in inhalant users: results from The national epidemiologic survey on alcohol and related conditions. Drug Alcohol Depend. 2007;88(2–3):146–55. Available at: http://www.pubmedcentral.nih.gov/articlerender.fcgi?artid=1934509&tool=pmcentrez&rendertype=abstract.

110. Yucel M, Takagi M, Walterfang M, Lubman DI. Toluene misuse and long-term harms: a systematic review of the neuropsychological and neuroimaging literature. Neurosci Biobehav Rev. 2008;32(5):910–26. https://doi.org/10.1016/j.neubiorev.2008.01.006.

111. Zakocs RC, Edwards EM. What explains community coalition effectiveness?: a review of the literature. Am J Prev Med. 2006;30(4):351–61.

Anabolic Steroid Use Disorders: Diagnosis and Treatment

21

Gen Kanayama and Harrison G. Pope Jr

Contents

Abstract

The anabolic-androgenic steroids (AAS) are a family of hormones that comprise the natural male hormone testosterone and its many synthetic relatives. Once used almost exclusively by elite athletes, AAS have now spread to the general population, with some tens of millions of users worldwide. Contrary to popular belief, most AAS users are not competitive athletes, but take these drugs simply to gain muscle. Because widespread AAS use did not arise until the 1980s in the United States and about a decade or more later in

other countries, even the oldest AAS users – individuals who started AAS as youths in the 1980s or 1990s – are only now reaching middle age. Thus, the long-term adverse effects of AAS are only beginning to be recognized, as more individuals enter the age of risk for these effects.

AAS users rarely disclose their drug use to clinicians and often come to clinical attention only because of adverse effects such as cardiovascular complications, AAS-withdrawal hypogonadism, and various effects on other organ systems. Because AAS users rarely seek treatment, little is known about optimal treatment strategies for this form of substance use disorder. The limited available data suggest that treatment should focus on underlying body image disorders, correction of AAS-withdrawal hypogonadism, and possible

G. Kanayama · H. G. Pope Jr (✉)
Biological Psychiatry Laboratory, McLean Hospital, Belmont, MA, USA

Harvard Medical School, Boston, MA, USA
e-mail: hpope@mclean.harvard.edu

© Springer Nature Switzerland AG 2021
N. el-Guebaly et al. (eds.), *Textbook of Addiction Treatment*,
https://doi.org/10.1007/978-3-030-36391-8_21

therapeutic attempts to address the hedonic properties of AAS. Data on treatment of AAS-induced mood syndromes are also limited, although general principles for treatment of both hypomanic and depressive episodes are probably appropriate when these syndromes arise from AAS use.

Keywords

Anabolic-androgenic steroids · Testosterone · Body image · Hypogonadism · Men

21.1 Introduction

The anabolic-androgenic steroids (AAS) are the family of drugs that include the natural male hormone testosterone, together with numerous synthetic derivatives of testosterone that have been created over the last 80 years (Table 21.1). AAS could also correctly be called simply "androgens" [37], but the term "anabolic-androgenic steroids" has become the more common term and will be used here. When taken in supraphysiologic doses, AAS can allow individuals to gain large amounts of muscle mass and lose body fat, often well beyond the limits of what can be attained naturally [58, 61]. Because of these properties, the use of AAS has grown into a major worldwide substance use disorder. Since AAS use is arguably the newest of the world's major substance use disorders, many aspects of AAS still remain poorly understood, both by clinicians and by investigators. However, the last two decades have seen substantial advances in our understanding of this form of substance use, as summarized in this chapter.

The history of AAS, illustrated in Fig. 21.1, begins at about the time of the Second World War [37]. Testosterone was first identified in Germany in the 1930s, and hundreds of synthetic AAS were quickly created thereafter. By the early 1950s, elite athletes began to discover that these drugs could greatly improve performance, especially in sports requiring muscle strength. As early as 1954, the Russian team was found to be using AAS at the weightlifting championships in Vienna, and over the course of the next decade, AAS spread rapidly through the elite athletic world. By the late 1960s, drug testing for AAS had been instituted at the Olympics and similar elite events. Also in the 1960s and 1970s, in the so-called golden age of bodybuilding, AAS were widely used by competition bodybuilders, who performed for a general public largely unaware that the muscular prowess that they were seeing was attributable to use of drugs. Even most clinicians also remained unaware of the powerful muscle-building effects of AAS. For example, in 1977, the American College of Sports Medicine issued a position paper stating that there was no conclusive evidence that AAS were actually

Table 21.1 Examples of frequently used anabolic-androgenic steroids (AAS)

Compounds administered orally	Compounds injected intramuscularly
Stanozolol (Winstrol)	Stanozolol (Winstrol-V[a])
Mesterolone (Mesteranum, Proviron)	Testosterone esters blends (Sustanon, Sten)
Oxymetholone (Anadrol, Hemogenin)	Testosterone cypionate (Depo-testosterone)
Oxandrolone (Anavar)	Testosterone enanthate (Delatestryl)
Fluoxymesterone (Halotestin, android-F, Ultandren)	Testosterone propionate (Testoviron, Androlan)
Methyldrostanolone (Superdrol)	Drostanolone propionate (Masteron)
Mibolerone (Cheque drops[a])	Trenbolone acetate (Finajet, Finaplix[a])
Methandienone (formerly called methandrostenolone) (Dianabol)	Trenbolone hexahydrobenzylcarbonate (Parabolan)
Methyltestosterone (android, Testred, Virilon)	Nandrolone decanoate (Deca-Durabolin)
Compounds administered transdermally	Methenolone enanthate (Primobolan depot)
Testosterone gel (AndroGel, Testim, Axiron)	Boldenone undecylenate (Equipoise[a])

[a]Veterinary preparation

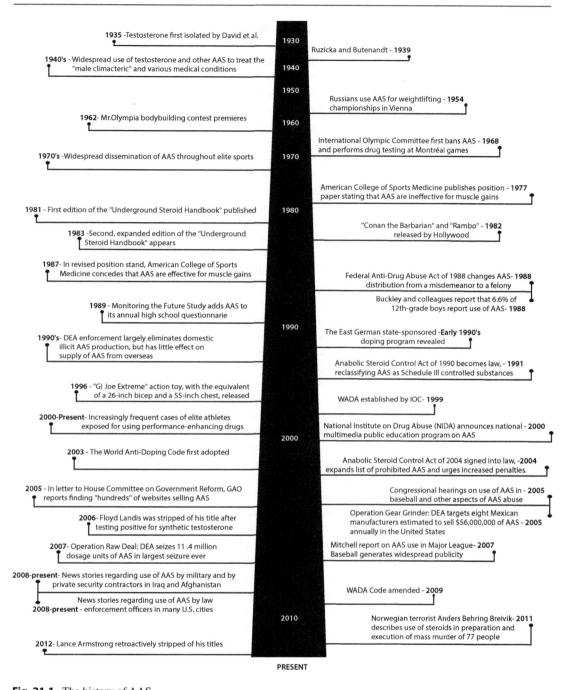

1935 -Testosterone first isolated by David et al.

Ruzicka and Butenandt - **1939**

1930

1940's - Widespread use of testosterone and other AAS to treat the "male climacteric" and various medical conditions

1940

1950

Russians use AAS for weightlifting - **1954** championships in Vienna

1962- Mr.Olympia bodybuilding contest premieres

1960

International Olympic Committee first bans AAS - **1968** and performs drug testing at Montréal games

1970's -Widespread dissemination of AAS throughout elite sports

1970

American College of Sports Medicine publishes position - **1977** paper stating that AAS are ineffective for muscle gains

1981 - First edition of the "Underground Steroid Handbook" published

1980

1983 -Second, expanded edition of the "Underground Steroid Handbook" appears

"Conan the Barbarian" and "Rambo" - **1982** released by Hollywood

1987- In revised position stand, American College of Sports Medicine concedes that AAS are effective for muscle gains

Federal Anti-Drug Abuse Act of 1988 changes AAS- **1988** distribution from a misdemeanor to a felony

Buckley and colleagues report that 6.6% of 12th-grade boys report use of AAS- **1988**

1989 - Monitoring the Future Study adds AAS to its annual high school questionnarie

1990's- DEA enforcement largely eliminates domestic illicit AAS production, but has little effect on supply of AAS from overseas

1990

The East German state-sponsored -**Early 1990's** doping program revealed

Anabolic Steroid Control Act of 1990 becomes law, - **1991** reclassifying AAS as Schedule III controlled substances

1996 - "GI Joe Extreme" action toy, with the equivalent of a 26-inch bicep and a 55-inch chest, released

WADA established by IOC- **1999**

2000-Present- Increasingly frequent cases of elite athletes exposed for using performance-enhancing drugs

National Institute on Drug Abuse (NIDA) announces national - **2000** multimedia public education program on AAS

2000

2003 - The World Anti-Doping Code first adopted

Anabolic Steroid Control Act of 2004 signed into law, -**2004** expands list of prohibited AAS and urges increased penalties.

2005 - In letter to House Committee on Government Reform, GAO reports finding "hundreds" of websites selling AAS

Congressional hearings on use of AAS in - **2005** baseball and other aspects of AAS abuse

2006- Floyd Landis was stripped of his title after testing positive for synthetic testosterone

Operation Gear Grinder: DEA targets eight Mexican manufacturers estimated to sell $56,000,000 of AAS - **2005** annually in the United States

2007- Operation Raw Deal: DEA seizes 11 .4 million dosage units of AAS in largest seizure ever

Mitchell report on AAS use in Major League- **2007** Baseball generates widespread publicity

2008-present- News stories regarding use of AAS by military and by private security contractors in Iraq and Afghanistan

WADA Code amended - **2009**

News stories regarding use of AAS by law **2008-present** - enforcement officers in many U.S. cities

2010

Norwegian terrorist Anders Behring Breivik- **2011** describes use of steroids in preparation and execution of mass murder of 77 people

2012- Lance Armstrong retroactively stripped of his titles

PRESENT

Fig. 21.1 The history of AAS

effective for gaining muscle mass – a statement that was to prove seriously erroneous [37].

Starting in about the 1980s in the United States, and about a decade thereafter in many other Western countries, AAS began to percolate out of the elite athletic world and onto the street. One catalyst for this transition was the appearance of various "underground guides" in the

United States, starting in the early 1980s, explaining how to obtain and use AAS, how to perform self-injections, and how to deal with side effects [37]. Also fueling enthusiasm for AAS use in the 1980s was a growing Western focus on male body image [56, 65]. Soon, growing numbers of ordinary rank-and-file weightlifters in local gymnasiums around the United States began to use AAS. Most of these individuals were not competitive athletes at all, but simply were using AAS to enhance personal appearance. Despite the widening use of these drugs, AAS still remained little understood by the general public, and most clinicians still had little or no experience with diagnosing or treating AAS users.

By the late 1980s and early 1990s, the US government began to recognize the problem of illicit AAS use, and in 1991, the US Congress passed the Steroid Trafficking Act, reclassifying AAS as controlled substances. However, possession and use of AAS without a doctor's prescription has remained legal in many countries around the world. Even in countries where AAS are illegal, users can readily purchase these drugs through Internet websites and receive shipments of AAS with little risk of interception [9]. Consequently, AAS use has become a relatively common substance use disorder in many countries, especially in Scandinavia, the United Kingdom, other British Commonwealth countries, and Brazil. Other countries on the European continent are now also showing growing rates of AAS use, whereas AAS use in Eastern Asian countries, such as China, Korea, and Japan, remains extremely rare. The uneven distribution of AAS use around the world appears likely attributable to cultural factors, as we have detailed in previous reports [33, 77].

21.2 Epidemiology of AAS Use

It has been difficult to estimate accurately the number of persons who have used AAS in various countries. Although there are numerous published surveys of AAS use among various student populations, especially high school students in the United States, these surveys have been vul-

nerable to the problem of false-positive responses to questions about "steroid" use. Specifically, if respondents on a questionnaire are asked whether they have used, say, heroin or cocaine, they will know almost certainly that they either have or have not used these drugs (although they may of course elect not to disclose this use). But when asked on an anonymous survey whether they have used "steroids," many respondents, especially those of high school age, may misinterpret the question and answer that they have used "steroids" when in fact they have been administered corticosteroids by a physician or have purchased an over-the-counter preparation in a supplement store that they erroneously believed was a "steroid." In a detailed analysis of this issue [25], we have shown that most American surveys of high school students have almost certainly produced grossly inflated estimates of the prevalence of AAS use as a result of false-positive questionnaire responses.

These false-positive survey responses have led to several widespread misconceptions about the epidemiology of AAS use. First, many surveys have created the impression that AAS use was not uncommon in teenage girls, and this belief has become a subject for popular reports in the news media and even for hearings conducted by the US Congress in which one of the authors of this chapter (HGP) was called to testify [57]. In fact, however, AAS use is virtually nonexistent in teenage girls, and the survey findings to this effect represent almost entirely false-positive responses [25]. Indeed, we are unaware of any published study in the last 25 years that has reported even a single female teenage AAS user who was actually evaluated in person by the investigators. Moreover, we are aware of only one study in the last 25 years dedicated specifically to female AAS users [21]. In this study, which was conducted by our laboratory, we spent 2 years advertising in three American cities and located only 25 female AAS users. In a recent analysis of five studies published since the year 2000 that surveyed AAS users without regard to gender [58, 61], it was found that of 1157 AAS users in the studies collectively, only 25 (1.8%) were female (95% confidence interval: 0.8%, 2.7%). In summary, therefore, AAS use is overwhelmingly concentrated in men. Upon reflection, this is hardly surprising, since women rarely aspire to look extremely muscular and women are also vulnerable to the various masculinizing side effects of AAS, such as beard growth, deepening of the voice (which may be permanent), and masculinization of secondary sexual characteristics.

A second misconception arising from high school surveys is that AAS use is a common phenomenon in teenagers. Again, however, this misconception arises largely from false-positive responses generated by anonymous surveys. In an analysis of nine studies around the world published since the year 2000 that assessed the age of onset of AAS use in 3218 individuals collectively, less than 1% began AAS use prior to their 16th birthday, and the median age of onset was approximately 23 [58, 61]. Therefore, although the problem of teenage AAS abuse should not be dismissed, the evidence suggests that the vast majority of AAS users are young adults in their 20s and 30s.

A third misconception, widely shared by both clinicians and members of the general public, is that AAS use occurs primarily among athletes. This misconception is likely fueled by the numerous reports in the popular media about various elite athletes believed to have used these drugs for performance purposes. In fact, however, the great majority of AAS users are not competitive athletes at all, and they have used these drugs purely for the purposes of increasing strength and enhancing personal appearance. For example, in a recent study at our center, in which we recruited men from gymnasiums in Massachusetts, Florida, and California, USA, only 6 (6%) of 94 AAS users who were questioned responded that they had used AAS primarily for athletic purposes. Another 13 (14%) reported that they had used AAS partially for athletic purposes, and the remaining 75 reported that they had never used AAS for any athletic purpose [55]. Similarly, in a recent Internet study of 500 AAS users, 392 (78%) were classified as non-athletes [49]. In summary, therefore, the great majority of AAS users are *male, over the age of 18, and not involved in any competitive athletics*.

How many AAS users exist in various countries? National household surveys in the United Kingdom [5, 10], Australia [6], and Brazil [19] have suggested a lifetime prevalence of 0.5% to 2.0% among men in these countries. In the United States, no household surveys of the general population have been conducted since 1994, at which time the American National Household Survey estimated that about 1,000,000 Americans had used AAS [72]. A recent review, combining American household survey data with more recent American studies involving college students and young adults, has estimated that between 2.9 and 4.0 million American men have used AAS at some time in their lives [58, 61].

Given that AAS use affects many millions of people worldwide, one might ask why there is not a larger literature of clinical and research studies on AAS use. Several factors may account for this paucity of research. First, as mentioned earlier, AAS use is a relatively new phenomenon, in contrast to use of other types of drugs such as cannabis and opiates that have existed for millennia. Furthermore, the great majority of AAS users are still relatively young; even most older users – those individuals who first started using AAS as youths in the 1980s and 1990s, when AAS first entered the general population – are only now approaching middle age. Thus, most AAS users are still too young to have exhibited long-term adverse effects from AAS exposure and hence have not come to the attention of the clinical community. AAS use has also escaped clinical attention because it rarely precipitates acute toxic reactions that bring patients to the emergency room, in the manner of opiate overdoses or severe alcohol intoxication. Thus, drug detection systems based on emergency room visits, such as the American DAWN network [73], rarely detect AAS abuse. For all these reasons, a large population of AAS users exists outside the view of most clinicians and researchers.

Further compounding this situation, AAS users rarely seek treatment and rarely disclose their AAS use to physicians in any event. In one study, 56% of AAS users reported that they had never disclosed their AAS use to any physician that they had seen [62]. This statistic is particularly striking when it is considered that it was obtained from a group of men who had already volunteered to participate in a psychiatric interview study. Thus, these men were likely more candid than AAS users as a whole, and therefore the 56% figure probably underestimates the actual degree of nondisclosure by AAS users.

Finally, clinicians should be aware that many so-called dietary supplements, sold over the counter in supplement stores or available through the Internet, may contain surreptitious AAS, other potentially performance-enhancing drugs, and other untested substances of unknown toxicity [20, 47, 66, 75]. Not only are these surreptitious ingredients often of unknown efficacy and toxicity, but the identity and dose of these ingredients may not correspond to that specified on the label. Thus, the population of known AAS users has been augmented with substantial numbers of unwitting AAS users who have ingested these drugs through dietary supplements.

21.3   Adverse Effects of Long-Term AAS Use

Cardiovascular effects Given that AAS use is relatively recent, often undetected, and inadequately studied, our understanding of the adverse effects of these drugs remains limited. However, several important adverse effects have begun to emerge as areas of primary concern. Perhaps the most worrisome consequence of long-term AAS exposure is its effect on the cardiovascular system [1, 58, 61]. This problem has been suggested by numerous case reports, emerging over the last 20 years, describing premature death from myocardial infarction in young men who were apparently using AAS. One study followed up 62 leading Finnish powerlifters for 10–15 years after the time that they had competed; these men had all likely used AAS [50]. The investigators found that 8 (13%) of the powerlifters had died on follow-up – a rate significantly higher than in matched individuals from the general population. Three of the eight deaths in the powerlifter group

were attributed to myocardial infarction. It appears likely that most of the cases of myocardial or cerebral infarction in young AAS users are attributable to premature atherosclerotic disease, likely caused by the fact that AAS – especially orally active 17-alkylated AAS – produce markedly adverse effects on lipid profiles [35]. The potential consequences of this atherogenic profile are illustrated by one pilot study of 14 competition bodybuilders that found markedly elevated levels of coronary artery calcium relative to that expected for men of comparable age [68]. More recently, in the largest study to date of the cardiovascular adverse effects of AAS exposure, our group compared 86 long-term AAS users and 54 otherwise similar weightlifters reporting no history of AAS [7]. Using computed tomography coronary angiography, we found that the AAS users exhibited significantly elevated atherosclerotic plaque in the coronary arteries as compared to the nonusers, and the degree of plaque, as well as other measures of atherosclerotic disease, was signally associated with lifetime duration of AAS exposure. Three of the 86 AAS users recruited for the study had experienced a myocardial infarction prior to the age of 45.

A growing literature has also demonstrated that AAS may commonly cause cardiomyopathy. In our recent study just cited, AAS users displayed impaired systolic function, as reflected by significantly decreased mean left ventricular ejection fraction, as well as impaired diastolic function, as shown by significantly decreased early left ventricular relaxation velocity [7]. Interestingly these impairments of systolic and diastolic function were much more prominent in individuals currently taking AAS at the time of evaluation and less serious among AAS users who were currently off-drug at the time of evaluation. Many other smaller studies have also demonstrated similar evidence of cardiomyopathy among AAS users (e.g., [4, 14, 42]).

AAS may also produce other toxic effects on the cardiovascular system, including hypertension, cardiac arrhythmias, and coagulation abnormalities [1]. These effects likely combine with the effects described above to increase rates of cardiac morbidity and mortality in AAS users [46]. At present, the overall prevalence of cardiac disease in AAS users is unknown but is likely rising as increasing numbers of long-term AAS users are now moving into the age of increased risk for these phenomena.

Neuroendocrine effects Exogenous AAS suppress the function of the hypothalamic-pituitary-testicular (HPT) axis in men, leading to decreased gonadotropin production from the hypothalamus, decreased luteinizing hormone and follicle-stimulating hormone from the pituitary, and consequent decreases in testicular production of testosterone and spermatozoa [15]. Therefore, when a man discontinues AAS use, especially after a prolonged course of AAS, he will likely exhibit AAS-withdrawal hypogonadism [74]. Normally, this interval of hypogonadism will be self-limited, because the HPT axis will gradually return to normal function and restore natural testosterone production. However, a growing literature has suggested that some men may exhibit very prolonged hypogonadism after discontinuing AAS, sometimes lasting more than a year, and in some cases perhaps becoming irreversible [13, 30, 31, 67]. The mechanism in these cases remains poorly understood, but may reflect a direct toxic effect of AAS on the testis itself. As with most other forms of AAS-induced adverse effects, the prevalence of prolonged or irreversible hypogonadism remains unknown. This is a matter of serious concern, since hypogonadism may lead to loss of libido, impaired sexual function, infertility, and in some cases severe depression. These effects may induce AAS users to quickly resume AAS to "self-treat" these dysphoric symptoms, thus leading to repeated cycles of AAS use and ultimately to AAS dependence syndromes. We discuss this issue in greater detail below.

Psychiatric effects AAS use and withdrawal may precipitate major mood disorders in some susceptible individuals. During periods of AAS use, especially use at very high doses, some individuals will develop hypomanic or manic syndromes characterized by increased self-confidence, irritability, aggressiveness, hyperactivity, and impaired judgment [22, 58, 61]. In rare cases, these syndromes may be associated with psychotic symptoms, such as grandiose or paranoid delusions [64]. In some individuals, hypomanic syndromes may also be associated with violent behavior, often entirely uncharacteristic of the individual's premorbid personality, and sometimes leading to acts of attempted or actual murder. Over the last 25 years, a number of reports have described individuals with no prior history of a major psychiatric disorder, no history of violence, and no criminal record, who committed murder or attempted murder during an episode of AAS use [22, 52, 58, 61]. At first, it was widely speculated that aggressive or violent behavior by AAS users might simply reflect the premorbid personalities of individuals prone to use AAS or might be due to expectational factors. However, several placebo-controlled double-blind studies have now been conducted in which supraphysiologic doses of AAS were given to normal volunteers [64]. In four of these studies, doses of testosterone or testosterone-equivalent equal to 500 mg per week or greater were administered to normal volunteers under blinded conditions. In these four studies collectively, 5 (4.8%) of 105 men administered AAS exhibited manic or hypomanic syndromes, but none exhibited such syndromes on placebo. These findings indicate that psychological factors alone cannot account for these mood effects and suggest that some individuals apparently harbor a biological predisposition to AAS-induced mood symptoms – although the nature of this biological predisposition remains unknown [64]. Very likely the 4.8% prevalence of hypomanic or manic syndromes observed in these blinded studies represents an underestimate of the true rate of such symptoms in the field for several reasons. First, many AAS users ingest doses far higher than the equivalent of 500 mg of testosterone week, sometimes rising to the range of several thousand milligrams per week, and thus are likely at increased risk for mood-altering effects (see below). Second, the above-cited studies recruited participants who had been screened to be free of major psychiatric or medical problems; illicit AAS users in the field do not screen themselves with such care. Third, AAS users may ingest additional drugs of abuse in conjunction with AAS that potentiate AAS-induced psychiatric effects. Alcohol, in particular, may act in conjunction with AAS to precipitate more severe behavioral effects that would be observed with comparable doses of either drug alone [58, 61].

AAS-induced mood symptoms appear to be idiosyncratic, with a majority of AAS users exhibiting little or no mood change and only a small minority exhibiting pronounced pathology. These effects may be more common in individuals ingesting higher doses of AAS. One study found that major mood disorders were uncommon in men ingesting less than the equivalent of 1000 mg of testosterone per week (a dose equivalent to about 15–20 times the normal male endogenous production of testosterone) but became more frequent at levels above 1000 mg of testosterone-equivalent per week [63]. Aside from this observation, however, it remains unclear why certain individuals are unusually susceptible to AAS-induced psychiatric effects; for example, these effects have not been convincingly demonstrated to be associated with prior history of psychiatric disorders or with any identified predisposing biological factor.

In the same manner that AAS exposure appears to precipitate hypomanic symptoms in some individuals, it has also been found that AAS withdrawal may precipitate depressive symptoms. AAS-withdrawal depression may occasionally be severe and has even been an apparent cause of suicide attempts or completed suicide [58, 61, 64]. Again, however, these mood effects appear highly idiosyncratic, with most men experiencing little or no depression on AAS withdrawal, while an occasional man develops profound depression. This idiosyncratic pattern has been observed even under laboratory conditions in a study where normal male volunteers were rendered deliberately hypogonadal by administration of the gonadotropin-releasing hormone agonist leuprolide [69]. Under these conditions, all men experienced loss of libido and other mild nonspecific symptoms, but only a small subgroup of about 10% of the men experienced prominent depressive symptoms. As with

hypomanic symptoms, the mechanism of these idiosyncratic depressive responses remains poorly understood.

Other adverse effects AAS have also been associated with a variety of other less serious or less common adverse effects on other organ systems [53, 58, 61]. For example, some users occasionally develop severe truncal acne, and many develop gynecomastia caused by estrogenic metabolites of AAS. These are both largely cosmetic issues that rarely deter young AAS users from continued use. AAS have also been implicated in occasional cases of hepatotoxicity, including peliosis hepatis (the formation of blood-filled cysts in the liver), and rare cases of hepatic adenomas, adenocarcinomas, and other tumors. However, these hepatic effects are rare. In our experience, there appears to be a widespread misconception among clinicians that serious hepatotoxicity with AAS is relatively common. This misconception is likely attributable to the fact that AAS users frequently exhibit marked elevations of so-called liver enzymes, such as aspartate aminotransferase (AST) and alanine aminotransferase (ALT). However, these same enzymes are also present in muscle tissue and hence will be elevated in muscular individuals undergoing intense resistance training. Thus, elevations of these enzymes in AAS users are generally a consequence of muscle trauma, rather than evidence of liver disease [16, 53]. Genuine liver disease should generally be suspected only in cases where aminotransferases are elevated in the *absence* of an elevation in creatine kinase (CK; an enzyme which is rapidly elevated in the presence of muscle trauma) or in the *presence* of an elevation of gamma-glutamyl transferase (GGT; an enzyme that is present exclusively in the liver and not in the muscle). In these latter cases, the possibility of a concomitant alcohol use disorder should be considered.

Musculoskeletal complications of AAS use include tendon rupture, which may occur as a result of disproportionately strengthened muscles and possibly weakened tendons [30, 31, 40]. Recent evidence has also implicated AAS in cases of focal segmental glomerulosclerosis [23] and possibly other cases of renal failure [40, 51]. By contrast, there is little evidence that AAS tend to precipitate or exacerbate prostate cancer, with only two cases of prostate cancer in possible AAS users reported in the entire literature, both of which were published more than 20 years ago [27, 32]. The absence of such reports in more recent years, despite much larger numbers of aging AAS users, suggests that there may be little or no association between AAS use and prostate cancer – an observation consistent with recent work questioning the belief that increased testosterone can cause prostate cancer or contribute to prostate cancer flares [45].

Finally, a new and worrisome possibility is that prolonged exposure to high levels of AAS may lead to apoptosis of brain cells. Testosterone-induced apoptosis of human neuronal cells was first demonstrated in vitro in 2006 [18], with some of these effects occurring at testosterone concentrations within the range that might be attained by humans using very large doses of AAS. This observation caused the investigators to speculate that long-term high-dose AAS users might eventually experience cerebral apoptotic effects similar to those demonstrated in the laboratory. In the first study, to our knowledge, to pursue this hypothesis in humans, our group administered a battery of neuropsychological tests to 31 AAS users and 14 non-AAS-using weightlifters in the United Kingdom [34]. Although the two groups exhibited comparable performance on reaction time, a continuous performance task, and on verbal memory, the long-term AAS users showed significant deficits compared to nonusers on two tests of visuospatial memory. Furthermore, performance on one of these visuospatial tests showed a highly significant association with total lifetime dose of AAS exposure. A subsequent study in the United States, using magnetic resonance spectroscopy, demonstrated deficits in levels of scyllo-inositol in a group of eight AAS users compared to ten non-AAS-using weightlifters [39]. Scyllo-inositol prevents clumping and deposition of β amyloid, and therefore this deficit, if demonstrated in a larger sample, might represent a risk factor for early-onset dementia. A recent study in Norway found widespread cortical thinning and smaller neuroanatomical volumes, including total gray matter, cerebral cortex, and putamen, in AAS users as compared to nonusing weightlifters [8]. These differences related significantly after adjustment for several potentially confounding variables, and the magnitude of these differences appeared to be associated with cumulative lifetime AAS exposure.

21.4 AAS Dependence Syndromes

It is now well established that AAS can cause a dependence syndrome, characterized by chronic AAS use that may persist despite adverse effects [26, 28]. In an analysis of 10 studies that used criteria adapted from the American Psychiatric Association *Diagnostic and Statistical Manual of Mental Disorders* [3, 26, 28] to diagnose AAS dependence in 1248 AAS users collectively, the mean prevalence of AAS dependence across all studies was approximately 33% [58, 61]. Thus, it would follow that some millions of men around the world have experienced or are currently experiencing AAS dependence, with a consequently increased risk for the adverse effects enumerated above. As mentioned earlier, AAS use in women is rare, and AAS dependence in women is consequently extremely rare, with only two female cases documented to our knowledge in the world literature [12, 44].

AAS dependence may arise as part of a larger picture of dependence upon performance- and image-enhancing drugs in general [24]. This issue has been discussed in detail by Hildebrandt and colleagues, who have noted that many individuals may exhibit not only pathological use of AAS but also use of other potentially anabolic substances (e.g., human growth hormone and insulin), thermogenic ("fat-burning") substances (e.g., clenbuterol, thyroid hormones, and sympathomimetic drugs), and drugs used to counteract the side effects of AAS (e.g., aromatase inhibitors). Individuals using these various performance- and image-enhancing drugs may also display a characteristic cluster of symptoms of body image disturbance, together with symptoms of potentially pathological dieting and exercising behavior. Hildebrandt and colleagues have proposed a more detailed set of diagnostic criteria to capture these various aspects of a broader dependence syndrome [24].

AAS dependence is associated not only with use of other performance- and image-enhancing drugs but also frequently with use of classical drugs of abuse as well. Recent studies have increasingly documented that AAS use may arise as but one of many forms of drug use in the midst of a pattern of polydrug abuse and dependence [17, 35, 70]. These observations further contradict the popular notion that AAS use is primarily a phenomenon among athletes pursuing a lifestyle of health and fitness. To the contrary, AAS is often simply another form of drug use seen in polysubstance abusers.

Despite the increasing overlap between AAS use and abuse of classical drugs, it must be recognized that AAS possess certain unique features. Classical drugs are typically ingested because they produce an immediate "reward" in the form of acute intoxication (a "high") shortly after ingestion. Addiction to classical drugs often occurs because individuals come to use the drugs more frequently and in higher doses to obtain the intoxicating effect. AAS, on the other hand, deliver very little sense of acute intoxication and instead deliver a delayed reward of increased muscularity and decreased body fat. Thus, it may initially seem puzzling that AAS would be prone to producing a dependence syndrome in such a large proportion of users. However, several mechanisms may contribute to the high prevalence of AAS dependence. Specifically, we have hypothesized that there are three pathways that collectively contribute to AAS dependence: an "anabolic" pathway, an "androgenic" pathway, and a "hedonic" pathway (Fig. 21.2). These three pathways may contribute to AAS dependence in different degrees in different individuals, and each

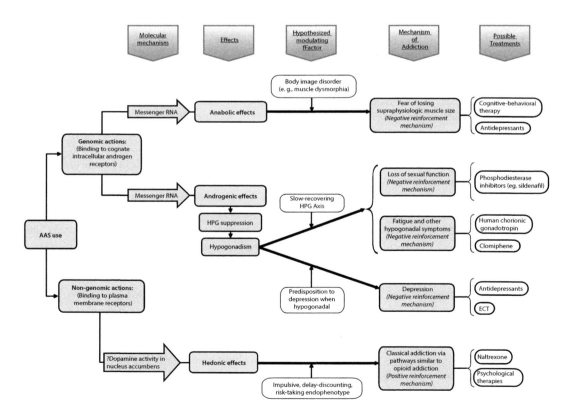

Fig. 21.2 AAS dependence: an "anabolic" pathway, an "androgenic" pathway, and a "hedonic" pathway

of these pathways may dictate particular treatment strategies as detailed in the next section.

The "anabolic" pathway refers to the ability of AAS to build muscle and decrease fat, thereby enhancing body image. Individuals with prominent body image concerns, especially those with a form of body dysmorphic disorder called "muscle dysmorphia," may be drawn to AAS use because of a pathological concern that they are not sufficiently muscular [36, 71]. Indeed, we have shown in one recent study that adolescent concerns about muscularity represented perhaps the strongest predictor of eventual AAS use among men who lift weights [55]. AAS users with body image concerns may gain large amounts of muscle mass by weightlifting and use of AAS, but paradoxically they may often grow even more concerned about their muscularity as time passes. As a result, they become anxious about discontinuing AAS, fearing that they may lose some muscle mass, and may quickly resume taking AAS after stopping a prior course because of these fears.

The "androgenic" pathway refers to the fact, discussed earlier, that exogenous AAS suppress the HPT axis. Upon stopping AAS, especially after a prolonged course of use, many men will experience profound AAS-withdrawal hypogonadism, with associated loss of libido, fatigue, and occasional pronounced depression [74]. Men experiencing these dysphoric symptoms may be prompted to rapidly resume AAS to restore themselves to normal mood and sexual functioning. This potential cause of AAS dependence was proposed some 30 years ago by Kashkin and Kleber [38] as a potential "anabolic steroid addiction hypothesis."

Finally, it has become increasingly clear that there is also a "hedonic" pathway to AAS dependence, apparently mediated by subtle hedonic effects of AAS. Unlike the anabolic and androgenic effects of AAS, which are mediated by binding to cognate intracellular androgen receptors, the hedonic effects appear to be mediated by binding to plasma membrane receptors. Thus, the hedonic effects of AAS likely arise via a mechanism similar to that induced by classical drugs, perhaps as a result of increased dopaminergic activity in the nucleus accumbens. Strong evidence for a hedonic pathway to AAS dependence arises from animal studies, which have shown that rats and mice will exhibit conditioned place preference for testosterone administration and that male hamsters will self-administer testosterone to the point of death [76]. Interestingly, self-administration of testosterone is blocked in hamsters by administration of the opioid antagonist naltrexone [76]. This is one of several lines of evidence suggesting that opioidergic mechanisms may be involved in the hedonic pathway to AAS dependence. Although a full discussion of these issues is beyond the scope of this chapter, a recent review by Nyberg and Hallberg provides an excellent summary of current knowledge in this area [48].

21.5 Treatment of AAS Abuse and Dependence

AAS users rarely seek treatment from clinicians, as mentioned above, and hence the available literature regarding treatment remains minimal. There are several reasons for this, many of which have been discussed above. First, AAS users are typically concerned with their body image, often to a pathological degree, and are reluctant to discontinue a drug that has allowed them to achieve a muscular physique. Thus, for an AAS user to approach a clinician for help in discontinuing AAS would be somewhat analogous to a patient with anorexia nervosa approaching a clinician with a request that she wants to gain body weight. In both cases, seeking treatment effectively contradicts the underlying disease. Furthermore, unlike the analogy of anorexia nervosa, where patients may develop life-threatening symptoms that bring them to clinical attention, AAS users rarely develop severe adverse effects in the early stages of AAS use and hence have little motivation to seek clinical care. As noted earlier, widespread illicit AAS use did not develop until the 1980s and 1990s, and thus most of the world's AAS users are still below the age of 50 and have not entered the age of risk for long-term medical complications of the types described above.

Finally, it should be reiterated that AAS users often have little faith in clinicians and feel that clinicians are poorly informed about AAS effects – an attitude confirmed in surveys of AAS users [62] and abundantly illustrated in AAS- and bodybuilding-related sites on the Internet [9].

For all of these reasons, clinicians should remain alert for possible AAS use when seeing younger male patients, even if these patients do not disclose AAS use on interview. Young men who seem unusually muscular, while still having low levels of body fat, may be particularly likely to represent surreptitious AAS users. As we have noted in prior publications, there is a relatively clear upper limit of muscularity that can be obtained by men while still retaining low body fat, and men above this limit are very likely lying if they claim that they have not used drugs [41, 59]. Other possible clues to surreptitious AAS use in muscular young males are prominent acne, gynecomastia, and findings of abnormal cholesterol profiles or unusually high hematocrit. We [59, 60] and others [11] have detailed these and other possible clues to AAS use in previous publications. Note that testosterone levels in surreptitious AAS users may be either grossly elevated (in cases where the individual is self-administering high doses of testosterone) or grossly depressed (in cases where an individual is self-administering other AAS, but not testosterone, thereby suppressing his own endogenous testosterone production). Thus, any testosterone level markedly below or markedly above the normal range should raise suspicion of surreptitious AAS use.

It should also be reiterated that the great majority of AAS users are not athletes. Thus, individuals reporting no competitive athletic activity may nevertheless be AAS users. Similarly, it should be remembered that AAS use is increasingly documented as a component of polysubstance abuse, and thus the possibility of AAS use should always be considered in young male patients reporting abuse of other substances. For example, in 1 study of 223 consecutive men admitted to a substance abuse treatment unit [29], it was found that 29 (13%) reported a past history of AAS use but that AAS had been documented by the admitting clinician in only 4 of these 29 cases.

Despite the above barriers to recognition and treatment of AAS users, our impression is that growing numbers of AAS users will be seen for treatment over the next decade. The prime reason for this trend, we believe, is that large numbers of AAS users are only now beginning to move into middle age and developing cardiac, neuroendocrine, and other complications that bring them to the attention of clinicians. In particular, our research group has recently seen various AAS users, generally over the age of 35, who have exhibited problems including myocardial infarction occurring prior to the age of 45, cardiomyopathy sufficient to produce symptoms of congestive heart failure, chronic hypogonadism with loss of libido and erectile function, evidence of renal failure discovered on laboratory testing, and "brittle" mood disorders with abrupt swings between episodes of hypomanic irritability and aggressiveness and episodes of depression with suicidal ideation. Often, these AAS users had never disclosed their AAS use to a physician prior to developing an adverse effect that brought them to clinical attention.

Once a clinician has identified an AAS user, and once that individual has decided that he wants help in discontinuing AAS use, what treatment options can be offered? As we have discussed in our previously referenced paper on treatment of AAS dependence [27, 32], the possible treatments will be dictated to some extent by the three different pathways that we have postulated as causes of AAS dependence. First, in men with muscle dysmorphia, who are pathologically afraid of loss of muscularity upon stopping AAS, it would seem appropriate to use treatments that have been successfully applied for other forms of body dysmorphic disorder. These include antidepressants such as selective serotonin reuptake inhibitors and clomipramine, which have been shown effective in controlled trials in patients with body dysmorphic disorder, even though these agents have not been specifically studied in muscle dysmorphia per se [54]. Body dysmorphic disorder has also been shown to respond to cognitive behavioral therapies [54], and therefore it seems likely that cognitive behavioral approaches would be helpful for AAS users who have to develop pathological concerns with body image.

Second, it is imperative to address the neuroendocrine effects of AAS, since the dysphoric effects of AAS-withdrawal hypogonadism may often prompt AAS users to resume their drug use. Treatment of AAS-withdrawal hypogonadism should ideally be handled by an endocrinologist familiar with this population. Typically, treatment would consist of administration of human chorionic gonadotropin (HCG), which mimics the effects of pituitary-luteinizing and follicle-stimulating hormones, thus stimulating the testis to resume production of testosterone and spermatozoa. HCG may be started weeks before actually discontinuing AAS in order to "jumpstart" testicular function. In addition, clomiphene is usually added because this drug mimics the effects of hypothalamic gonadotropin-releasing hormone and thus stimulates the pituitary to begin its own natural production of luteinizing and follicle-stimulating hormones. Clomiphene exists in two isomers, the *trans* isomer (enclomiphene) and the *cis* isomer (zuclomiphene). Enclomiphene is an estradiol antagonist and is responsible for stimulating pituitary gonadotropin release; zuclomiphene is an estradiol agonist and hence does not contribute to this effect or even antagonizes this effect. Therefore, an estrogen antagonist such as tamoxifen or letrozole may be administered in conjunction with clomiphene to neutralize its estrogenic effects. More detailed discussions of these treatment strategies are available in endocrinological publications [74].

Finally, clinicians may need to address the hedonic aspects of AAS dependence. Here it seems likely that the possible treatment modalities should resemble those found effective for classical drugs of abuse, whose dependence-inducing properties are often largely based on hedonic mechanisms. There are virtually no available studies of treatment of AAS dependence using classical substance abuse treatment modalities, but we have offered speculations on possible treatment options in a recent paper [27, 32]. It is conceivable, for example, that long-acting preparations of intramuscular naltrexone might be of some value for treatment of AAS dependence, given that this modality has been shown effective for other forms of substance dependence and has also been shown to be effective at preventing testosterone dependence in animal models as mentioned above. Also, psychological therapies shown effective in treating other forms of substance dependence might well prove helpful in AAS dependence, especially in cases where AAS dependence occurs in the context of polysubstance use or dependence. Thus, motivational therapies designed to encourage commitment to treatment may be of value, and once treatment is initiated, modalities such as contingency management, supportive-expressive therapy, and behavioral couples therapy might be effective. The last approach might be particularly indicated in AAS users, since women may be abused by AAS-using men and be eager to encourage these male partners to abstain from subsequent use.

In conclusion, it should be noted that much of the above discussion remains speculative, since so few AAS users have actually sought and received a clinical treatment to date. However, our knowledge of treating AAS use will likely expand over the next decade as increasing numbers of users come to clinical attention and thus enter treatment.

21.6 Treatment of AAS-Associated Psychiatric Syndromes

As detailed above, most of the adverse effects of long-term AAS use are medical and fall outside the domain of clinicians who treat substance abuse disorders. Individuals displaying such effects will therefore likely require referral to appropriate specialists, most often cardiologists or endocrinologists. However, the psychiatric effects of AAS use and withdrawal can typically be managed by clinicians with mental health expertise. Although there is very little published literature on the treatment of AAS-induced hypomania or mania, the first priority of treatment is clearly the removal of the offending agent. Thereafter, in our experience, standard treatment for manic symptoms (e.g., antipsychotics, valproate, and lithium) appears appropriate – although this has not been formally assessed in clinical trials. Major depressive episodes associated with AAS withdrawal will typically require endocrinological intervention to restore HPT function, as discussed above. In addition, based on our experience, standard psychiatric treatments for depression, including antidepressant medications and electroconvulsive therapy, may well be indicated. Again, we are aware of no clinical trials of psychiatric treatments for AAS-withdrawal depression, although one case series has reported success with fluoxetine [43] and one case report has described success with electroconvulsive therapy in an AAS user who failed to respond to tricyclic antidepressants and fluoxetine [2]. In AAS-withdrawal depression requiring treatment, it seems likely that treatment can be discontinued once neuroendocrine parameters have returned to normal – but we are not aware of longitudinal studies addressing this issue.

21.7 Conclusion

Most drugs of abuse have been ingested by humans for centuries or millennia, but AAS misuse represents perhaps the newest of the world's major forms of substance abuse and dependence. Although elite athletes began using AAS as far back as the 1950s, widespread AAS use by rank-and-file AAS users did not begin until the 1980s in the United States and even later in most other Western countries. Thus, even most of the world's older AAS users – those who first tried AAS as youths in the 1980s and 1990s – are only now reaching middle age and entering the age of risk for adverse cardiac, neuroendocrine, and other effects of AAS exposure. Consequently, scientific knowledge about the effects of AAS use and appropriate treatment strategies for AAS dependence remain limited. However, this situation seems poised to change over the next decade or two, as larger numbers of aging AAS users develop adverse effects that bring them to clinical

attention and treatment. It is to be hoped that clinicians will become increasingly conscious of the possibility of AAS use when evaluating male patients and will be sensitized to the physical and laboratory signs of AAS use mentioned above. Similarly, it is to be hoped that increasing research will better delineate the frequency, severity, and duration of AAS-induced adverse effects.

References

1. Achar S, Rostamian A, Narayan SM. Cardiac and metabolic effects of anabolic-androgenic steroid abuse on lipids, blood pressure, left ventricular dimensions, and rhythm. Am J Cardiol. 2010;106(6):893–901.
2. Allnutt S, Chaimowitz G. Anabolic steroid withdrawal depression: a case report. Can J Psychiatr. 1994;39(5):317–8.
3. American Psychiatric Association. Diagnostic and statistical manual of mental disorders, fourth edition, text revision (DSM-IV-TR). Washington, DC: American Psychiatric Association; 2000.
4. Angell PJ, Ismail TF, Jabbour A, Smith G, Dahl A, Wage R, et al. Ventricular structure, function, and focal fibrosis in anabolic steroid users: a CMR study. Eur J Appl Physiol. 2015;114(5):921–8.
5. APS Group Scotland. 2010/11 Scottish Crime and Justice Survey: Drug Use: Scottish Government Social Research. 2012. Available online at: http://www.scotland.gov.uk/Topics/Statistics/Browse/Crime-Justice/crime-and-justice-survey. Accessed 30 Jan 2019.
6. Australian Institute of Health and Welfare. National Drug Strategy Household Survey Report 2016. 2017. Available online at: https://www.aihw.gov.au/reports/illicit-use-of-drugs/2016-ndshs-detailed/data. Accessed 30 Jan 2019.
7. Baggish AL, Weiner RB, Kanayama G, Hudson JI, Lu MT, Hoffmann U, Pope HG. Cardiovascular toxicity of illicit anabolic-androgenic steroid use. Circulation. 2017;135(21):1991–2002.
8. Bjornebekk A, Walhovd KB, Jorstad ML, Due-Tonnessen P, Hullstein IR, Fjell AM. Structural brain imaging of long-term anabolic-androgenic steroid users and nonusing weightlifters. Biol Psychiatry. 2017;82(4):294–302.
9. Brennan BP, Kanayama G, Pope HG. Performance-enhancing drugs on the web: a growing public-health issue. Am J Addict. 2013;22:158–61.
10. British Home Office. Drug misuse: findings from the 2017/2018 crime survey for England and Wales. 2018. Available online at: https://assets.publishing.service.gov.uk/government/uploads/system/uploads/attach-

ment_data/file/729249/drug-misuse-2018-hosb1418. pdf. Accessed 30 Jan 2019.

11. Brower KJ. Anabolic steroid abuse and dependence in clinical practice. Phys Sportsmed. 2009;37:1–11.

12. Copeland J, Peters R, Dillon P. Anabolic-androgenic steroid dependence in a woman. Aust N Z J Psychiatry. 1998;32(4):589.

13. Coward RM, Rajanahally S, Kovac JR, Smith RP, Pastuszak AW, Lipshultz LI. Anabolic steroid induced hypogonadism in young men. J Urol. 2013;190(6):2200–5.

14. D'Andrea A, Caso P, Salerno G, Scarafile R, De Corato G, Mita C, et al. Left ventricular early myocardial dysfunction after chronic misuse of anabolic androgenic steroids: a Doppler myocardial and strain imaging analysis * commentary. Br J Sports Med. 2007;41(3):149–55. https://doi.org/10.1136/bjsm.2006.030171.

15. de Souza GL, Hallak J. Anabolic steroids and male infertility: a comprehensive review. BJU Int. 2011;108:1860–5.

16. Dickerman RD, Pertusi RM, Zachariah NY, Dufour DR, McConathy WJ. Anabolic steroid-induced hepatotoxicity: is it overstated? Clin J Sport Med. 1999;9(1):34–9.

17. Dodge T, Hoagland MF. The use of anabolic androgenic steroids and polypharmacy: a review of the literature. Drug Alcohol Depend. 2011;114(2–3):100–9.

18. Estrada M, Varshney A, Ehrlich BE. Elevated testosterone induces apoptosis in neuronal cells. J Biol Chem. 2006;281(35):25492–501.

19. Galduróz JCF, Noto AR, Fonseca AM, Carlini EA. Levantamento Nacional Sobre o Consumo de Drogas Psicotrópicas entre Estudantes do Ensino Fundamental e Médio da Rede Pública de Ensino nas 27 Capitais Brasileiras- 2004. São Paulo: Centro Brasileiro de Informações sobre Drogas Psicotrópicas; 2004. Available online at: http://www.cebrid.epm.br/levantamento_brasil2/index.htm; Accessed 30 Jan 2019.

20. Garcia-Cortes M, Robles-Diaz M, Ortega-Alonso A, Medina-Caliz I, Andrade RJ. Hepatotoxicity by dietary supplements: a tabular listing and clinical characteristics. Int J Mol Sci. 2016;17(4):537.

21. Gruber AJ, Pope HG. Psychiatric and medical effects of anabolic-androgenic steroid use in women. Psychother Psychosom. 2000;69(1):19–26.

22. Hall RC, Hall RC, Chapman MJ. Psychiatric complications of anabolic steroid abuse. Psychosomatics. 2005;46(4):285–90.

23. Herlitz LC, Markowitz GS, Farris AB, Schwimmer JA, Stokes MB, Kunis C, et al. Development of focal segmental glomerulosclerosis after anabolic steroid abuse. J Am Soc Nephrol. 2010;21:163–72.

24. Hildebrandt T, Lai JK, Langenbucher JW, Schneider M, Yehuda R, Pfaff DW. The diagnostic dilemma of pathological appearance and performance enhancing drug use. Drug Alcohol Depend. 2011;114(1):1–11.

25. Kanayama G, Boynes M, Hudson JI, Field AE, Pope HG. Anabolic steroid abuse among teenage girls: an illusory problem? Drug Alcohol Depend. 2007;88(2–3):156–62; PMCID 1978191.

26. Kanayama G, Brower KJ, Wood RI, Hudson JI, Pope HG. Anabolic-androgenic steroid dependence: an emerging disorder. Addiction. 2009;104:1966–78. PMCID 2780436.

27. Kanayama G, Brower KJ, Wood RI, Hudson JI, Pope HG. Treatment of anabolic-androgenic steroid dependence: emerging evidence and its implications. Drug Alcohol Depend. 2010;109:6–13; PMCID 2875348.

28. Kanayama G, Brower KJ, Wood RI, Hudson JI, Pope HG Jr. Issues for DSM-V: clarifying the diagnostic criteria for anabolic-androgenic steroid dependence. Am J Psychiatry. 2009;166(6):642–5; PMCID 2696068.

29. Kanayama G, Cohane GH, Weiss RD, Pope HG. Past anabolic-androgenic steroid use among men admitted for substance abuse treatment: an underrecognized problem? J Clin Psychiatry. 2003;64(2):156–60.

30. Kanayama G, DeLuca J, Meehan WP 3rd, Hudson JI, Isaacs S, Baggish A, et al. Ruptured tendons in anabolic-androgenic steroid users: a cross-sectional cohort study. Am J Sports Med. 2015;43(11):2638–44.

31. Kanayama G, Hudson J, DeLuca J, Isaacs S, Baggish A, Weiner R, et al. Prolonged hypogonadism in males following withdrawal from anabolic-androgenic steroids: an underrecognized problem. Addiction. 2015;110(5):823–31.

32. Kanayama G, Hudson JI, Pope HG. Illicit anabolic-androgenic steroid use. Horm Behav. 2010;58(1):111–21; PMCID 2883629.

33. Kanayama G, Hudson JI, Pope HG Jr. Culture, psychosomatics and substance abuse: the example of body image drugs. Psychother Psychosom. 2012;81(2):73–8. https://doi.org/10.1159/000330415.

34. Kanayama G, Kean J, Hudson JI, Pope HG. Cognitive deficits in long-term anabolic-androgenic steroid users. Drug Alcohol Depend. 2013;130:208–14.

35. Kanayama G, Pope HG. Illicit use of androgens and other hormones: recent advances. Curr Opin Endocrinol Diabetes Obes. 2012;19:211–9.

36. Kanayama G, Pope HG Jr. Gods, men, and muscle dysmorphia. Harv Rev Psychiatry. 2011;19:95–8.

37. Kanayama G, Pope HG. History and epidemiology of anabolic androgens in athletes and non-athletes. Mol Cell Endocrinol. 2018;464:4–13.

38. Kashkin KB, Kleber HD. Hooked on hormones? An anabolic steroid addiction hypothesis. JAMA. 1989;262(22):3166–70.

39. Kaufman MJ, Janes AC, Hudson JI, Brennan BP, Kanayama G, Kerrigan AR, et al. Brain and cognition abnormalities in long-term anabolic-androgenic steroid users. Drug Alcohol Depend. 2015;152:47–56.

40. Kersey RD, Elliot DL, Goldberg L, Kanayama G, Leone JE, Pavlovich M, Pope HG. National athletic trainers' association position statement: anabolic-androgenic steroids. J Athl Train. 2012;47(5):567–88.

41. Kouri EM, Pope HG Jr, Katz DL, Oliva P. Fat-free mass index in users and nonusers of anabolic-androgenic steroids. Clin J Sport Med. 1995;5(4):223–8.

42. Luijkx T, Velthuis BK, Backx FJ, Buckens CF, Prakken NH, Rienks R, et al. Anabolic androgenic steroid use is associated with ventricular dysfunction on cardiac MRI in strength trained athletes. Int J Cardiol. 2013;167:664–8.

43. Malone DA Jr, Dimeff RJ. The use of fluoxetine in depression associated with anabolic steroid withdrawal: a case series. J Clin Psychiatry. 1992;53(4):130–2.

44. Malone DA Jr, Dimeff RJ, Lombardo JA, Sample RH. Psychiatric effects and psychoactive substance use in anabolic-androgenic steroid users. Clin J Sport Med. 1995;5(1):25–31.

45. Morgentaler A. Testosterone and prostate cancer: an historical perspective on a modern myth. Eur Urol. 2006;50(5):935–9.

46. Nascimento JH, Medei E. Cardiac effects of anabolic steroids: hypertrophy, ischemia and electrical remodelling as potential triggers of sudden death. Mini Rev Med Chem. 2011;11(5):425–9.

47. Navarro VJ, Khan I, Bjornsson E, Seeff LB, Serrano J, Hoofnagle JH. Liver injury from herbal and dietary supplements. Hepatology. 2017;65(1):363–73.

48. Nyberg F, Hallberg M. Interactions between opioids and anabolic androgenic steroids: implications for the development of addictive behavior. Int Rev Neurobiol. 2012;102:189–206.

49. Parkinson AB, Evans NA. Anabolic androgenic steroids: a survey of 500 users. Med Sci Sports Exerc. 2006;38(4):644–51.

50. Parssinen M, Kujala U, Vartiainen E, Sarna S, Seppala T. Increased premature mortality of competitive powerlifters suspected to have used anabolic agents. Int J Sports Med. 2000;21(3):225–7.

51. Pendergraft WF, Herlitz LC, Thornley-Brown D, Rosner M, Niles JL. Nephrotoxic effects of common and emerging drugs of abuse. Clin J Am Soc Nephrol. 2014;9(11):1996–2005. https://doi.org/10.2215/CJN.00360114.

52. Perry PJ, Kutscher EC, Lund BC, Yates WR, Holman TL, Demers L. Measures of aggression and mood changes in male weightlifters with and without androgenic anabolic steroid use. J Forensic Sci. 2003;48(3):646–51.

53. Pertusi R, Dickerman RD, McConathy WJ. Evaluation of aminotransferase elevations in a bodybuilder using anabolic steroids: hepatitis or rhabdomyolysis? J Am Osteopath Assoc. 2001;101(7):391–4.

54. Phillips KA, Didie ER, Feusner J, Wilhelm S. Body dysmorphic disorder: treating an underrecognized disorder. Am J Psychiatry. 2008;165(9):1111–8.

55. Pope H, Kanayama G, Hudson J. Risk factors for illicit anabolic-androgenic steroid use in male weightlifters: a cross-sectional cohort study. Biol Psychiatry. 2012;71:254–61.

56. Pope H, Phillips K, Olivardia R. The Adonis complex: the secret crisis of male body obsession. New York: Simon & Schuster; 2000.

57. Pope HG. Widespread anabolic steroid use in American girls and women: an illusion? Paper presented at the Testimony before the United States House of Representatives Committee on Government Reform, Washington, D.C.; 15 June 2005.

58. Pope HG, Wood RI, Rogol A, Nyberg F, Bowers L, Bhasin S. Adsverse health consequences of performance-enhancing drugs: an Endocrine Society scientific statement. Endocr Rev. 2014;35(3):341–75.

59. Pope HG, Kanayama G. Can you tell if your patient is using anabolic steroids? Curr Psychiatry Prim Care. 2005;1:28–34.

60. Pope HG, Kanayama G. Treatment of anabolic-androgenic steroid related disorders. In: Galanter M, Kleber H, Brady K, editors. The American Psychiatric Publishing textbook of substance abuse treatment. 5th ed. Washington, D.C.: American Psychiatric Association; 2015, pp. 263–76.

61. Pope HG, Kanayama G, Athey A, Ryan E, Hudson JI, Baggish A. The lifetime prevalence of anabolic-androgenic steroid use and dependence in Americans: current best estimates. Am J Addict. 2014;23:371–7.

62. Pope HG, Kanayama G, Ionescu-Pioggia M, Hudson JI. Anabolic steroid users' attitudes towards physicians. Addiction. 2004;99(9):1189–94.

63. Pope HG, Katz DL. Psychiatric and medical effects of anabolic-androgenic steroid use. A controlled study of 160 athletes. Arch Gen Psychiatry. 1994;51(5):375–82.

64. Pope HG, Katz DL. Psychiatric effects of exogenous anabolic-androgenic steroids. In: Wolkowitz OM, Rothschild AJ, editors. Psychoneuroendocrinology: the scientific basis of clinical practice. Washington, D.C.: American Psychiatric Press; 2003. p. 331–58.

65. Pope HG, Olivardia R, Gruber A, Borowiecki J. Evolving ideals of male body image as seen through action toys. Int J Eat Disord. 1999;26(1):65–72.

66. Rahnema CD, Crosnoe LE, Kim ED. Designer steroids – over-the-counter supplements and their androgenic component: review of an increasing problem. Andrology. 2015;3(2):150–5. https://doi.org/10.1111/andr.307.

67. Rasmussen JJ, Selmer C, Ostergren PB, Pedersen KB, Schou M, Gustafsson F, et al. Former abusers of anabolic androgenic steroids exhibit decreased testosterone levels and Hypogonadal symptoms years after cessation: a case-control study. PLoS One. 2016;11(8):e0161208.

68. Santora LJ, Marin J, Vangrow J, Minegar C, Robinson M, Mora J, Friede G. Coronary calcification in body builders using anabolic steroids. Prev Cardiol. 2006;9(4):198–201.

69. Schmidt PJ, Berlin KL, Danaceau MA, Neeren A, Haq NA, Roca CA, Rubinow DR. The effects of pharmacologically induced hypogonadism on mood in healthy men. Arch Gen Psychiatry. 2004;61(10):997–1004.

70. Skarberg K, Nyberg F, Engstrom I. Multisubstance use as a feature of addiction to anabolic-androgenic steroids. Eur Addict Res. 2009;15(2):99–106.

71. Sreshta N, Pope H, Hudson J, Kanayama G. Muscle dysmorphia. In: Phillips K, editor. Body dysmorphic disorder. New York: Oxford University Press; 2016.

72. Substance Abuse and Mental Health Services Administration. (SAMHSA). National Survey on Drug Use and Health (formerly called the National Household Survey). United States Department of Health and Human Services. Available online at: http://www.oas.samhsa.gov/nhsda.htm; data for 1994-B survey available online at: http://www.icpsr.umich.edu/cgi-bin/SDA/SAMHDA/hsda?samhda+nhsda94b. Accessed 30 Jan 2019.

73. Substance Abuse and Mental Health Services Administration. The DAWN report: highlights of the 2011 drug Abuse warning network (DAWN) findings on drug-related emergency department visits. 2012. Available online at: http://www.samhsa.gov/data/emergency-department-data-dawn; Accessed 30 Jan 2019.

74. Tan RS, Scally MC. Anabolic steroid-induced hypogonadism--towards a unified hypothesis of anabolic steroid action. Med Hypotheses. 2009;72(6):723–8.

75. Van Wagoner RM, Eichner A, Bhasin S, Deuster PA, Eichner D. Chemical composition and labeling of substances marketed as selective androgen receptor modulators and sold via the Internet. JAMA. 2017;318(20):2004–10. https://doi.org/10.1001/jama.2017.17069.

76. Wood RI. Anabolic-androgenic steroid dependence? Insights from animals and humans. Front Neuroendocrinol. 2008;29(4):490–506; PMC 2585375.

77. Yang CF, Gray P, Pope HG Jr. Male body image in Taiwan versus the west: Yanggang Zhiqi meets the Adonis complex. Am J Psychiatry. 2005;162(2):263–9.

Prescription Drug Abuse: Risks, Diversion, and Prevention

22

Jørgen G. Bramness

Contents

Abstract

Abuse of and dependence on prescription drugs is an increasing problem and is closely related to the increasing use of prescription drugs worldwide. The problem of prescription drug abuse includes both weak and strong opioids for pain management; sedating drugs like benzodiazepines, barbiturates, and newer hypnotics; and stimulant drugs used for the treatment of narcolepsy and attention-deficit/hyperactivity disorder (ADHD). Several other prescription drugs also have the potential for abuse. This chapter focuses on the epidemiology, the diagnostics, the treatment, and the prevention of prescription drug abuse.

J. G. Bramness (✉)
Norwegian Competence Centre for Dual Diagnosis
Innland Hospital Trust, Hamar, Norway

Norwegian Institute of Public Health, Oslo, Norway

Institute of Clinical Medicine, UiT, The Arctic
University of Norway, Tromsø, Norway
e-mail: j.g.bramness@medisin.uio.no

Keywords

Prescription drugs · Abuse · Opioids · Benzodiazepines · Central simulants · Doctor shopping

22.1   Introduction

As long as we have had medicinal drugs, there has been abuse. The problem is probably increasing [67]. All health-care workers need to be aware of this, but prescribing doctors need to pay particular attention.

All prescription drugs that seek market authorization need to have their abuse potential investigated. Guidelines for such testing exist [31]. But many of today's drugs were marketed long before these modern prerequisites. Furthermore, even with careful premarket testing, the real abuse potential of many drugs may not be fully recognized. Before marketing, drugs are usually tested on smaller, selected (non-abuser) populations under strictly controlled conditions, which do not allow for inappropriate use. Thus, postmarketing surveillance is needed to reveal abuse of drugs; many drugs are not fully recognized for their abuse potential until they have been on the market for many years [4].

Even though many drugs have abuse potential, the same drugs obviously also have therapeutic benefit. If abuse potential is discovered, the drug can be scheduled with restrictions on its use. We must weigh the risks against the benefits. If the risks are perceived to be greater than the benefits, action should be taken. Ultimately, this could mean withdrawing the market authorization of a drug, but often more modest action will serve the purpose.

This backdrop is useful to keep in mind when encountering prescription drug abuse, be it as a doctor worried about prescribing drugs that could be used for reasons other than therapeutic, a therapist encountering a patient with abuse or dependence problems because of these drugs, or when contemplating using known drugs of abuse for the benefit of seriously ill patients.

22.2   Epidemiology of Prescription Drug Abuse

It is not easy to get an overview of the epidemiology of prescription drug abuse. In surveys, responders tend not to answer questions truthfully. Some are reluctant to admit breaking the law. Often, the people of most interest are not available for answers; they may be imprisoned or in treatment. Some seldom open their mailbox or do not even have an address. If you choose to do your research in a prison or a treatment institution, you will face the problem of selection bias. Not all abusers or dependants will be under treatment or imprisoned. The study of the epidemiology of abuse thus needs to draw on a variety of sources to aggregate comprehensive data. This is no less true for prescription drug abuse.

There are two main types of data that we can get from epidemiological studies. The first is signals of abuse in drugs not previously recognized as drugs of abuse. Case reports and case series often give the first signals of such abuse potential [4, 43]. These signals must be followed up by a second kind of studies with more systematic and broader data collection. This is done to substantiate the signal and to investigate the *extent* of the abuse. The different sources of data below may serve as providers of both types of information.

22.2.1 Monitoring Populations or Patients

Population Surveys Despite the mentioned drawbacks of population surveys, they can provide information on the extent of the prescription drug abuse problem. Surveys have shown us that nonprescribed use of prescription drugs is quite common. The National Comorbidity Survey showed that more than 7% of adults reported having used non-prescribed sedatives [39]. A survey, also from the United States, showed that during the previous month, around 2% of the total population (≈ 6 million people) had abused pain medication, 0.7% tranquilizers (mostly benzodiazepines), 0.4% stimulants (attention-deficit/hyperactivity disorder (ADHD) medication), and 0.1% sedatives in 2008 [85]. Several studies show that figures vary a lot [80]. Being male, being older, having a parent who has done the same, and reporting more psychiatric symptoms increased the risk [17, 22]. From other studies, we know that people with alcohol or drug-use problems have a higher risk of abusing prescription drugs [59].

Patient Surveys Such monitoring programs will provide information both on the size of a problem and will give signals of drugs to be monitored. The Drug Abuse Warning Network (DAWN) gathered information on drugs mentioned at emergency room visits across the United States from 1974 to 2011 and served as a source of information about the extent of prescription drug abuse and gave signals on new drugs of abuse [19]. The 2010 figures showed that 30% of the mentions for prescription drugs were benzodiazepines and 40% were opioids. The drugs were mentioned in 20% and 18% of all emergency room visits respectively, and prescription drugs were mentioned almost as often as narcotics. It is also valuable to get information from patients entering treatment for drug abuse [49].

Adverse Effects Databases Signals of prescription drug abuse often come from national or international adverse effects databases, such as the WHO in Uppsala Monitoring Centre Adverse Effects Database. Such databases have given us information on the abuse liability of drugs like pregabalin [35] or quetiapine [20].

Forensic Data Data from driving under the influence (DUI) cases, from autopsies, or from prisons may be useful in determining whether drugs are abused or even which drugs are popular in the catchment area [9].

22.2.2 Monitoring Sources of Drugs

Sales Statistics As described above, US doctors started treating non-malignant pain with opioids in the mid-1990s, and a sharp increase in abuse of the drug has followed. As seen in the total consumption model, the sales of the drugs can tell us something about the amount of problematic use (and other adverse events; see Fig. 22.1). The large sales of opioids in the United States are closely related to high levels of abuse. For example, among 12th graders in the United States, non-medical use of prescription drugs (opioids) is the second most common form of abuse [60]. Sales data should include area and/or country because this gives useful hints on specific abuse trends.

Prescription Data Prescription data is another source of information. Such data could stem from claims databases in insurance institutions, national prescription databases, such as those found in many countries in northern Europe, or through pharmacy records. Basically, two types of information, both important, can stem from these sources. First, we can gain information about the abuse liability of a drug by looking at phenomena like "doctor shopping": the more doctors a drug seeker is willing to go to in order to get hold of the drug, the higher the abuse liability [74]; forged prescriptions: if many prescriptions for a drug are forged, the higher the abuse potential [33]; high use of a drug indicating some people are using it for recreational purposes [34, 72]; or skewness in use, i.e., if a large proportion of the drug is consumed by a few individuals, this is indicative of abuse liability [36, 44]. Second, these sources of information might tell us directly how many individuals show overuse of the drugs in an area [12]. These data point to the fact that drugs like carisoprodol, clonazepam, flunitrazepam, alprazolam, and all opioids are attractive abuse drugs.

Other Legal/Gray Sources Surveys in the normal population have shown that the most prevalent sources of prescription drugs for abuse are friends and family [64]. This US study showed how pain medication was most often obtained; it may be different in other countries. Having a drug problem, using a lot of alcohol, or having peers with use increased the risk. Still, we know that many individuals start to abuse through drugs prescribed to a family member [8].

Illegal Sources Prescription drugs, be it opioids, benzodiazepines, or others, are found on the black market. They are diverted illegally from people who have them prescribed, do not use them, but sell them. They are also sold after thefts from patients, pharmacies, or factories. Thus, drug abuse situations can be monitored by looking at seizures of drugs by the police or customs.

Novel Channels of Drugs The Internet is a novel source of drugs and very difficult to control. Only a small share of the drugs bought are

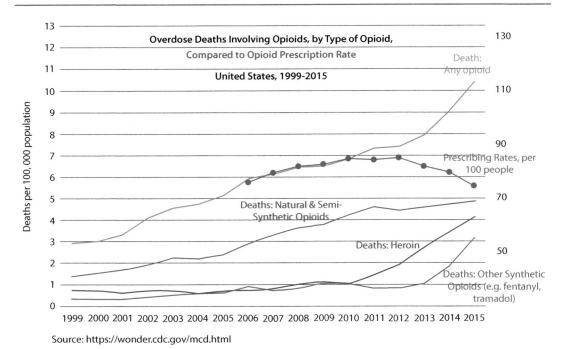

Fig. 22.1 The North American opioid epidemic. Data from Centers for Disease Control and Prevention (https://wonder.cdc.goc/med.html) showing prescription rates for opioids and deaths by medical opioids, heroin, and fentanyls

ever discovered by customs. But turning it the other way around, monitoring the Internet can be a way of picking up new trends. One such project is the European Union–funded Psychonaut Web Mapping Project that has been successful in identifying ever-increasing numbers of novel substances [27]. But data can also be collected by looking at websites for information or online reports of abuse [87].

Wastewater Analysis A novel approach that might give results in the future is to look at the presence of prescription drugs in wastewater (sewage analysis) [79]. By comparing sales statistics with findings in wastewater, one could get an idea of the black market for a drug, but also looking at weekly temporal variations in drugs, one might get a feeling how much is used for recreational use (most at weekends and less during weekdays) and how much is used on a regular basis (more evenly distributed).

In summary, we cannot today seriously say we know the extent of the problem of prescription drug abuse. No single source of data can substantiate all drugs that are abused or the extent of this abuse. Some data (surveys) will be flawed by information and selection bias; some data (databases) will not be able to identify the clinical features of abuse or dependence. We are therefore stuck with several estimates. And what do these tell us?

- These drugs are often used, but most use is clinically correct and well founded.
- Prescription drugs are, however, often abused, and the problem of abuse is increasing.
- The size of the problem is related to total sales of the drug; increased use always comes at the price of increased abuse. Countries with a high prescribing rate (such as the United States) have a substantial problem. In such countries, the problems following prescription drug abuse may equal those following the use of narcotic drugs.
- Some drugs have a higher abuse potential than others. As with other drugs of abuse, prescription drugs with high potency and a rapid effect will be more attractive to abusers.

- Patients who have legitimate use of these drugs are also at risk of abuse, but use according to the doctor's recommendations can also be problematic. Doctors should review their patient lists and act when necessary.
- Specific populations will have more risk of abuse of prescription drugs than others. These include drug abusers, psychiatric patients, but also patients with somatic problems such as pain.
- It often takes a long time from when a drug is first marketed until its true abuse potential is revealed, even with modern requirements for pre-marketing investigations. Always be open to signals of a drug's abuse potential.

22.3 Prescription Drugs of Abuse

22.3.1 Sedative Drugs

This group of drugs covers many different compounds (Table 22.1). They mainly belong to four groups: benzodiazepines, z-hypnotics, barbiturates, and barbiturate-like drugs. They are all agonist to receptor sites on the gamma-aminobutyric acid (GABA) receptor, subtype A. GABA is our main inhibitory neurotransmitter and is widespread throughout the CNS. The GABA$_A$ receptor complex is a ligand-gated ion channel. This transmembrane chloride channel is a pentamer with several different combinations of α (six subtypes), β (three subtypes), or γ (three subtypes) subunits and some other possible variants. To a large extent, the α subunit configuration determines a drug's abuse potential [5, 92]. While the barbiturates and barbiturate-like drugs can influence the receptor even in the absence of GABA, benzodiazepines and the z-hypnotics are dependent on the presence of GABA to perform their action. The consequence is that while barbiturates and barbiturate-like drugs are more dangerous and may more easily be overdosed, benzodiazepines and benzodiazepine-like drugs have a ceiling effect and thus a broad therapeutic window of use. The literature gives few, if any, examples of lethal overdoses of benzodiazepines taken alone in otherwise healthy individuals.

It is thus safe to say that when benzodiazepines were introduced at the end of the 1950s and in increasing numbers in the 1960s and 1970s, they were seen as a better and safer alternative to the barbiturates that had caused so many deaths and so much dependence [56]. The true abuse potential of these drugs was not revealed until the late 1960s and early 1970s.

Different benzodiazepines are basically the same regardless of their main indication. It is often arbitrary which indication the market authorization was filed for. It is most often a question of dosage whether a benzodiazepine is used as an anxiolytic (lower dose), a hypnotic (medium dose), or an antiepileptic drug (high dose). What differs between the compounds is their potency (mainly dependent on lipid solubility) and their pharmacokinetics. Table 22.1 shows this through the dosing and the terminal elimination half-life ($T_{1/2}$). It must be remembered that dosing in this table (and in much of the literature) is for the main use the drug is registered for. Taking the example of diazepam, doses would be 5–10 mg for anxiety, 10–20 mg for sleep, and up to 40 mg per day as an antiepileptic. Equipotency for benzodiazepines is thus a complex term. However, some are more potent than others (alprazolam, lorazepam, flunitrazepam, and clonazepam) and thus more attractive among abusers [6, 40, 45], partly because clinicians have a tendency to underestimate the differences in potency and subsequently dose high potency benzodiazepines relatively more highly. The $T_{1/2}$ is another parameter which varies between the benzodiazepines. It must however be remembered that owing to the phenomenon of acute tolerance (tolerance occurring within the same dosing), $T_{1/2}$ is not a good parameter for judging the time of effect for benzodiazepines. But the *relative* duration of action between the different benzodiazepines is roughly judged by this parameter. A short duration of action often also implies a short time between intake and effect, a parameter important for the reinforcing effects of a drug. Again, we see alprazolam, lorazepam, flunitrazepam, and clonazepam scoring highly on this parameter.

Z-hypnotics (zaleplon, zopiclone, eszopiclone, and zolpidem) are not benzodiazepines in

Table 22.1 Some commonly used sedatives marketed in many countries

	Compound (generic name)	Main use	Mean usual dose main use (mg)	Mean terminal half-life (hours)	Abuse potential
Benzodiazepines	Alprazolam	Anxiolytic	1	12	***
	Bromazepam	Anxiolytic	9	16	**
	Lorazepam	Anxiolytic	4	12	***
	Oxazepam	Anxiolytic	30	10	*
	Chlordiazepoxide	Anxiolytic	30	27	**
	Clobazam	Anxiolytic	30	18	**
	Diazepam	Anxiolytic	5	40	**
	Lorazepam	Hypnotic	1	12	***
	Temazepam	Hypnotic	15	14	**
	Flunitrazepam	Hypnotic	1	25	***
	Nitrazepam	Hypnotic	5	28	**
	Flurazepam	Hypnotic	15	60	***
	Clonazepam	Antiepileptic	4	36	***
Benzodiazepine-like hypnotics	Zaleplon	Hypnotic	10	1.5	*
	Zopiclone	Hypnotic	7,5	4.5	**
	Eszopiclone	Hypnotic	6	6	**
	Zolpidem	Hypnotic	5	2.5	**
Barbiturates	Barbital	Antiepileptic	750	30	***
	Phenobarbital	Antiepileptic	200	80	***
Barbiturate like drugs	Chlormethiazole	Muscle relaxant	600	6	**
	Meprobamate	Muscle relaxant	200	10	***
	Methaqualone	Muscle relaxant	150	74	***
	Chlormezanone	Muscle relaxant	200	40	**
	Orphenadrine	Muscle relaxant	100	16	**
	Chlorzoxazone	Muscle relaxant	750	1	**
	Carisoprodol	Muscle relaxant	700	2	***

Not all drugs will be marketed in all countries

their chemical structure. When introduced, their manufacturers wanted to have them introduced as "benzodiazepine-free hypnotics." However, their similarity to benzodiazepines in pharmacological effects are striking, and there is no longer doubt they can be abused. These drugs probably have a lesser capacity to relieve anxiety, and the role of anxiety in a drug's abuse potential should not be underestimated. It is thus true to state that the abuse potential of these drugs *may* be lower than for benzodiazepines, but the difference is likely to be marginal. We still see that zolpidem is a very popular drug of abuse in many countries. A distinct metal taste following the intake of zopiclone (also after i.v. intake) is probably preventive for abuse. Despite many claims to the contrary, eszopiclone has no advantages over zopiclone and probably none over benzodiazepines in terms of abuse potential. These drugs can be and are abused [43, 49].

Benzodiazepines are hugely popular among injecting drug addicts. Heroin users use them to prolong their intoxication and prevent withdrawal [82]. This may also contribute significantly to overdose deaths [24]. Users of central stimulants will use benzodiazepines at the end of a binge or a run to "land" [52].

Barbiturates and barbiturate-like drugs are much less abused today than they were before. That does not mean that they cannot be abused. These drugs really taught us what prescription drug abuse is, with methaqualone (Quaalude®) as a prominent example. Their high lipid solubility and resulting potential to cross the blood-brain barrier quickly, and their ever-increasing effects with higher doses and no ceiling effect, even if marked tolerance triggered massive dose escalations made them very popular as drugs of abuse. When this was acknowledged, heavy restrictions were put on their prescribing, and these drugs were withdrawn in many countries, but they are still on the market in many others.

Carisoprodol is a barbiturate-like drug that has been around since the late 1950s. It is a prodrug of meprobamate, a highly abused barbiturate-like drug [70]. Carisoprodol, however, has effects itself, including being highly toxic [13]. A negative utility to risk ratio led to the market withdrawal of carisoprodol in the EU in 2008, leading to a drop in intoxications with the drug [47]. The drug is still marketed in the United States [78].

It is a point of discussion whether buspirone should be listed here. We have opted not to do so because of the low abuse potential shown for this drug in several studies. This is not to say that it cannot be abused in some situations or by some patients.

22.3.1.1 Analgesics

The mechanism of action and other pharmacological points concerning opioid analgesics, including those which are prescribed, are as described elsewhere in this book. There are at least two different groups of prescription opioid abusers. First, we have the pain patient who has aberrant use of his or her medication [93]. It is difficult to predict who the patients at risk seem to be. Second, we have the abusers without a prescription. This group includes anyone from the teenager who accesses a relative's pain medication to the marginalized heroin abuser adding prescription opioids to his or her abuse. The

delineation between these two groups has become increasingly unclear in the light of the modern-day epidemic of opioids in the United States. The nonmedical use of prescription opioids in the United States is around 4% of the population [94].

Pain is a very common condition with potentially very severe consequences, such as reduced quality of life but also depression and suicide. The last three decades have seen an unprecedented emergence and culmination of a prescription opioid epidemic in the United States, and there is worry that other countries could follow. Until the mid-1980s, opioids were correctly viewed as a useful, but still problematic, tool of pain control that should be used with caution, most often only for cancer pain and acute pain conditions. From 1987 until the mid-1990s, a series of unfortunate events and statements paved the way for uncontrolled overprescribing of opioids in the United States. This included the misunderstanding that if opioids were used for pain, the patients could not become addicted [73, 76]. This huge misunderstanding paved the way for "ethics" campaigns stating that it was morally questionable to allow a patient to experience unbearable pain and that opioids needed to be used aggressively [63, 98]. Until around the year 2000, many advocated increased use of opioids in the management of nonmalignant pain [26]. Typically, the nomenclature of addiction was questioned and phrases like "pseudo-addiction" appeared [63, 76], and the American Pain Society was able to introduce pain as a "fifth vital sign" [26]. The US "direct to consumer" advertising, not found anywhere else in the world, increased the pressure on prescribing even more. It has been shown that the pharmaceutical company Purdue Pharma holding the patent for OxyContin played a major role in promoting these "alternative professional views" and the prescribing of OxyContin [96]. The company made a lot of money as the prescribing of opioids for non-cancer pain increased by a factor of 10 over a period of a few years. The increase in prescribing of opioids increased until around 2010 [25]. It must be added that foreign researchers visiting US colleagues during these years were a bit stunned by the fact that US epidemiologists were asking themselves *why* they had so many problems with prescription opioid abuse. The obvious overprescribing was followed by increasing number of overdoses and overdose deaths [99]. There was drug diversion [21] and non-prescribed use of the same opioids. Around 2010, many people addicted to prescription opioids turned to heroin.

Prescription opioids were becoming harder to obtain, and they were expensive. In this wave, we saw a very high increase in overdose deaths due to heroin, with at least two-thirds those addicted to heroin in this wave having started with prescription opioids [53]. A third wave of opioid use with worrisome effects was the increasing use of the extremely potent fentanyl opioids [32, 50]. All this is shown in Fig. 22.1.

The North American opioid epidemic has, to a large degree, been contained to this continent, but some of the misconceptions underlying the epidemic are finding their way to other parts of the world [46]. There have been smaller increases in the use of opioids in several European countries [10], but the situation is not comparable to the United States and Canada. However, the authors urge for vigilance [95, 100]. There have been reports of fentanyl deaths in some European countries, but these reports are some years old, and it is uncertain whether or not they are related to the current opioid problem [54].

Opioid substitution treatment (OST) has been used effectively for opioid-dependent patients for more than 60 years [66] and has considerable advantages in increasing adherence to treatment programs [18], promoting rehabilitation [58], and preventing illnesses and death [23]. Worldwide methadone and buprenorphine (with or without addition of naloxone) are mostly used for the substitution treatment, but in principle, any opioid could be used. There is increasing use of long-acting morphine variants and even heroin [91]. There is always a risk that opioids given to patients will be diverted. Many different strategies have been put in place to try to avoid this with actions such as observed intake and no take-home medicines [102]. No strategy that is achievable can prevent all diversion, but reasonable measures should be taken. Some patients should be observed taking the drug. It is possible

to measure serum methadone levels to make sure the drug is taken, but for other drugs, this is more difficult. Some countries have seen considerable diversion of opioids from their OST programs and overdose deaths in the wake of this [57]. For a comprehensive review of the subject, see Alho [3] (Table 22.2).

22.3.1.2 Central Stimulants

During recent years, there has been an enormous increase in the prescribing of central stimulating drugs for treating attention-deficit/hyperactivity disorder (ADHD). Using central stimulants to treat ADHD is an effective treatment in children [11] and probably also in adults [101], but not all these drugs are used as prescribed; some are also abused. This is partly true because patients with ADHD have an extra vulnerability to becoming involved in drug use [42]. The drugs can be abused by saving a whole week's worth of pills for a simultaneous intake to get a stimulant high or by selling the drugs to friends or on the black market. Epidemiological studies using wastewater indicate that methylphenidate is used as a party drug [84]. A typical therapeutic use of methylphenidate would involve using 10–30 mg, but 50–150 mg would be common in abuse. It is debatable whether bupropion should be listed here. We have opted not to do so because of the low abuse potential of this drug shown by several studies. This is not to say that it cannot be abused in some situations or by some patients.

Abuse of central stimulants includes using them as cognitive enhancers. This means otherwise healthy people take them in order to optimize cognitive abilities, using them to increase school performance or to stay awake and work for prolonged periods, be it as a student, soldiers in the field, or a truck driver with long shifts. Surveys show varying degrees of use, but quite a few students report having tried them to increase performance. Studies have found that central stimulants reduce errors and improve working memory even in those not disadvantaged [7, 77]. Some have found more mixed results and possible indications of genetic variability [90] Long-term memory may be positively influenced [62] with an increase in total recall [7]. There is more

Table 22.2 Some commonly used opioids marketed in many countries

Compound	Main use	Mean terminal half-life (hours)	Abuse potential	Comment
Morphine	Pain relief	2–3	***	
Ethyl morphine	Cough suppression	?	**	
Codeine	Pain relief	3–4	*	10% metabolized to morphine by CYP2D6
Fentanyl	Anesthesia	1–6	***	Mostly used as a transdermal patch
Hydrocodone	Pain relief	4–6	**	
Oxycodone	Pain relief	3–5	**	
Oxymorphone	Pain relief	1–2	**	
Dextropropoxyphene	Pain relief	8–24	***	
Hydromorphone	Pain relief	2–3	**	
Meperidine/pethidine	Pain relief	3–5	**	
Diphenoxylate	Constipating drug	12–14	*	
Methadone	Substitution in opioid dependence	6–8	**	High doses make once daily intake possible
Buprenorphine	Substitution in opioid dependence	20–73 hours	**	Strong binding (covalent) to receptor makes once daily intake possible

Not all drugs will be marketed in all countries

solid evidence of improved cognitive performance in periods of prolonged wakefulness, a fact that the world's many coffee drinkers can verify. Research in the combat field has, however, shown that the use of stronger central stimulants may not be optimal. In this area of research, there is interest in a wide variety of drugs stimulating the noradrenergic, serotonergic, and glutaminergic receptor systems. Such drugs could potentially be effective treatments for the cognitively impaired, such as patients with Alzheimer's disease (Table 22.3).

22.3.1.3 Other Drugs

Many prescription drugs can be abused. No complete list could ever be compiled. As prescribers, we always need to work with others to produce early warnings and to remain up to date on the possible dangers of prescribing different drugs. We must remember that abuse potential is often not revealed until a drug has been on the market for a very long time.

Several studies have shown the abuse potential of the antiepileptic GABA-ergic analogs pregabalin [88] and possibly also gabapentin [29]. This may be one reason why use of pregabalin may

reduce the use of benzodiazepines [15]. Even so, a signal of abuse should not deter prescribing totally but should be included as one of many arguments to be included in the weighing of benefits and risks of prescribing.

There have been increasing reports on the abuse of the antipsychotic drug quetiapine. This is (contrary to what been believed) not only a product of marginal use on groups who have difficulties in getting hold of drugs but reflects a true abuse potential of the drug [55, 68, 75]. The extent of the abuse and the dangers associated with it are not clear, but abuse does happen.

A last group that has therapeutic potential but also an abuse potential are the $GABA_B$-receptor agonists. These include the highly abusable gamma hydroxybutyrate (GHB) [51] used for the treatment of AUD (both withdrawal and abstinence maintenance) mostly in Italy [61]. Phenibut was developed in the 1960s in the Soviet Union to enhance wakefulness in the armed forces but has a clear abuse potential [2]. The abuse potential of the most used AUC drug in France, Lioresal [1], is yet undetermined, but probably low [81] (Table 22.4).

Table 22.3 Some commonly used central stimulating drugs marketed in many countries

Compound	Main use	Mean usual dose main use (mg)	Mean terminal half-life (hours)	Abuse potential
Methylphenidate	ADHD and narcolepsy	20–30	2–3; 7–12 for extended release	**
Amphetamine	ADHD and narcolepsy	20	13	***
Dextroamphetamine	ADHD and narcolepsy	20	10	***
Ephedrine	Cough medicine	20–50	3–6	*
Diet pills	Weight loss	Varying	Varying	Varying
Caffeine	Narcolepsy and in combination for migraine	50–300 mg	Varying	Low
Melanotan	Illegal tanning product	10–30	1–2	?
Modafinil	Narcolepsy and to prolong wakefulness	200–400	15	*

Not all drugs will be marketed in all countries

Table 22.4 Miscellaneous drugs that have been reported abused

Compound	Main use	Abuse potential	Comment
Marinol and other synthetic cannabinoids	Pain and muscle spasms in MS patients	***	Being a synthetic cannabinoid with very high potency, it has a high abuse potential
Sativex (cannabis extract)	Pain and muscle spasms in MS patients	*	Abuse potential as with other cannabis products
Pregabalin	Antiepileptic	**	Case reports and reviews confirm the abuse potential of the drug [88]
Gabapentin	Antiepileptic	*	An increasing number of case reports point to the abuse potential of this GABA analog [29]
Ketamine	Anesthetic	**	This anesthetic is an antagonist to the glutamatergic NMDA receptor giving vivid hallucinations as one of its main effects [86]
Quetiapine	Antipsychotic	*	An increasing number of case reports point to the abuse potential of this antipsychotic drug [68, 75, 55]
Xyrem	GHB treatment of alcohol dependence and withdrawal	***	As for GHB [51]
Phenibut	GABAB agonist	**	Developed by the Russians in the 1960s and appears increasingly in the European market [2]
Lioresal	GABAB agonist also used for AUD treatment in France	?	This centrally acting muscle relaxant can possibly be abused in higher doses, but the euphoric and psychomotor effects are weak [1, 81]

Not all drugs will be marketed in all countries

22.4 Terminology and Diagnosis

In the face of prescription drug abuse, it is important to remember that most use of prescription drugs is legitimate and therapeutically wise. The overwhelming majority of those who receive a prescription for analgesics or for hypnotics or sedatives use these drugs for a limited period to get through a time of pain, insomnia, or life stress. However, problems can and do arise.

Some use too much. Some increase their dose. Others use the drugs for too long, after their original problem is over, in order to avoid the discomforts of discontinuation and withdrawal. The drugs can be taken for the wrong reasons. They are not meant to be used recreationally or as part of an addiction. And some people mix different drugs. This can be done for several reasons but increases the addictive potential of the drugs and increases the chances of intoxication, even lethal.

Use that is not in line with the doctor's recommendation is worrisome, but even drugs used as prescribed may become problematic. A prescription is no guarantee against harm. All prescription drug use even if used for good reasons or as prescribed may become problematic. Abuse, dependence, or addiction should be diagnosed according to the usual tools using ICD-10 or DSM-5 diagnostic criteria. A diagnosis of harmful use (abuse), dependence, or addiction is not different for prescription drugs than for other substance use disorders. However, some problematic use of prescription drugs does not fit into these categories, and other typical patterns may be visible that challenge our understanding of problematic use and the diagnostic systems. Some of these more archetypical prescription drug use patterns are listed here:

Pseudo-therapeutic Long-Term Use Sedating drugs are meant for short-term use only. The manufacturer, authority, and society guidelines say that the drugs should be used only for 3–4 weeks. Still, many patients continue to use the drugs for longer periods of time [16]. This group of patients may cause concern at the doctor's office because of discussions about the re-prescribing of the drugs. Many patients feel that their honesty is being questioned, and many doctors feel that they are being "forced" into prescribing for longer than necessary. These patients, however, are not true abusers. They certainly use the drugs for longer than intended, but seldom at high doses, most often at lower doses than prescribed, and they seldom increase their doses. These users are often termed quasi-therapeutic long-term users [41]. They are mentioned here because they are quite prevalent and clearly violate recommendations but may not represent a true problem.

Self-Medicating Pain/Anxiety/Insomnia Patients Patients with anxiety disorders and also patients with other psychiatric disorders may use different prescription drugs to self-medicate or treat their symptoms [65]. It is important to acknowledge that anxiety disorders, major depression, post-traumatic stress disorder, personality disorders, and pain conditions may lead to overuse of prescription drugs. The possibility of abuse should not stop the doctor from introducing effective and necessary treatment, but the dangers of overuse should be kept in mind. Even when drugs are used as prescribed, the patient may encounter problems such as tolerance, abstinence, abuse, and dependence (see below).

True Prescription-Drug Abuser Some patients can be labeled true prescription-drug abusers. These are patients with no or marginal reasons to use these drugs, who keep using the drugs, often in increasing dosages. They are involved in drug-seeking behaviors such as doctor shopping, prescription forging, and diversion of drugs prescribed to others. The doctor should be aware of these individuals, even though it is not a large group. These patients resemble the next group.

Polydrug Abuse Many users of heroin or central stimulants use prescription opioids as part of their addiction [37]. Benzodiazepines are used to increase the high but also to postpone withdrawal in heroin users or to end a binge in users of central stimulants. When such combination use occurs, it is often labeled as polydrug abuse, but it can be argued that it in fact represents a kind of self-medication in drug abusers who have a main drug problem, be it heroin or central stimulants. This distinction may be important for treatment choices.

22.5 Strategies for Prevention

Making drugs available only on prescription is a preventive measure. The process of prescribing came into place to increase the doctor's ability to monitor effects and adverse events, including abuse. Other measures have been introduced to send out signals about the abuse liability of medicinal drugs. How this is done will vary between countries, but basically there are two ways. First, there can be rules and regulations on specific drugs within the prescribing system, under the laws of medicinal drugs. This could imply different rules and regulations for prescribing these drugs compared to other drugs.

- The use of special prescribing.
- Only one doctor can prescribe to one patient.
- Only one pharmacy can deliver the drug.
- Only a specialist in a certain field can prescribe the drug.
- Special forms should be used for prescribing certain drugs.
- Special authorities should be informed and can perform controls/audits.
- Only certain package sizes can be prescribed.
- No telephone or Internet prescribing allowed for certain drugs.

Second, some medicinal drugs could be placed on narcotics lists and lists of controlled or prohibited substances. This puts the drug under jurisdiction outside the health-care system and makes it police business. In many country's legislative systems, these boundaries are not so clear, and (often for historical reasons) illegal drugs and

medicinal drugs are regulated by the same laws. The scheduling system in the United States is such a system (Table 22.5). The different degrees of scheduling can be followed by different rules or regulations for prescribing as mentioned in the examples above.

Prescriptions are no guarantee against aberrant use. Abuse, dependence, or overconsumption is seen despite these precautions. Research has shown us that the occurrence of overuse follows the sales of the drug in the community or group and the prevalence of abuse can be predicted by sales, following the total consumption model. This model states that there is a close relationship between the population mean of a health variable, in this case prescribing of drugs with abuse potential, and the prevalence of individuals at high risk concerning this variable [89]. The model applies for alcohol consumption and heavy drinkers and for the availability of narcotic drugs and has now been shown to apply for prescriptions drugs [14]. This understanding is important for two reasons. First, a lot about aberrant drug use in a group or a country can be learned from sales statistics. We do not always need clinical investigations to look for aberrant drug use: the sales figures can give a good indication of the problem. And second, preventive measures can

Table 22.5 Prescription drugs are, according to US health authorities, classified after their potential for harm, including abuse

Schedule	Definition	Most central drugs included
I	Drugs with no currently accepted medical use in treatment in the United States and high potential for abuse and dependence	Cathinone, GHB, heroin, LSD, marijuana, MDMA, most hallucinogens, methaqualone (Quaalude)
II	Drugs with currently accepted medical use in treatment with severe restrictions in the United States and high potential for abuse and dependence	Cocaine, amphetamines, other opiates than heroin, some opioids, some synthetic cannabinoids, barbiturates
III	Drugs with currently accepted medical use in treatment in the United States and with a lower risk for abuse than drugs in schedules I and II and low to moderate dependence risk	Anabolic steroids, some barbiturates, buprenorphine, codeine, ketamine, GHB as Xyrem, some synthetic cannabinoids
IV	Drugs with an accepted medical use in treatment in the United States and with a low risk for abuse and dependence (lower than III)	Benzodiazepines, benzodiazepine-like z-hypnotics, some barbiturates, carisoprodol
V	Drugs with a currently accepted medical use in treatment in the United States and with a low risk for abuse and dependence (lower than IV)	Codeine, pregabalin, lacosamide, atropine

Some but not all drugs in this list are prescription drugs

be any procedure that will limit the prescribing and sales of a drug. Such measures must always be weighed against what is good treatment. But this also teaches us that guidelines which allow for liberal practices may have this downside.

We know that some doctors, independently of the profile of their patients, prescribe more drugs with abuse potential than others. This can be due to local traditions and to countrywide regulations but also has to do with the doctor's own beliefs and ideas. Doctors with a liberal view on these drugs tend to prescribe more. This is also reflected in the doctors' own use of these drugs; doctors more willing to use these drugs themselves are also more willing to prescribe them to their patients [83].

Prescription drugs should only be prescribed after a consultation and a review of the patient's problems. There is, however, an increasing sale of prescription drugs via the Internet. The police and customs face an almost impossible task trying to stop this import. Patients who buy drugs from Internet pharmacies and the Internet pharmacies themselves are operating in a gray zone. We do not know the extent of this Internet market, but different estimates usually suggest large figures. There is a thin line between these sources and a true black market. The only way to deal with this is to appeal to people's reasoning and warn against the dangers of receiving a suboptimal product. Some of the products are of good quality, but others contain little or no active ingredient or even toxic material.

22.6 Treatment

The boundary between prevention and treatment is often obvious but can sometimes become unclear. Some preventive measures will be embedded in treatment, and some experiences and views from treatment will be reflected in prevention.

Tackling the Drug-Seeking Patient What kind of drug-seeking behavior physicians will encounter may vary according to their field, but also according to their place, region, or country of work. Some common features can, however, be mentioned. Beware of lost prescriptions, lost medicines, or other reasons patients give for needing a prescription earlier [38, 48]. Also be cautious prescribing drugs with abuse potential to patients you do not know. Optimally, only one doctor should prescribe drugs with abuse potential to the patient. If other doctors need to write prescriptions for patients that they do not know, they need to do a proper workup and confirm diagnosis. If prescriptions are given, prescribe drugs with the lowest abuse potential in the smallest possible quanta. Remember that you do not have to prescribe a whole package, even of the smallest package. The crux is to give your patients appropriate care. Withholding effective medication to needy patients is not an optimal alternative. Some institutions have policies for not prescribing drugs with an abuse potential to patients at certain times or under certain conditions. These institutions can report that they avoid a lot of drug-seeking patients because word often spreads quickly if you cannot get what you want, but the institutions also risk not providing adequate treatment in some cases.

Minimal Interventions If you are worried about a patient's use of prescription drugs, the first step is to discuss this with your patient. Open communication is of the essence. Even if the patient does not admit to problematic drug use, just verbalizing the issue may give them food for thought. Some doctors regularly review their patient lists and try to get a grip on who they should be concerned about. One strategy would be to send a letter or e-mail of concern to the patients in question, just informing them of the potentially problematic sides to their drug use. Such interventions have proven efficient in stopping or reducing aberrant drug use [69]. Further support may be needed ("stepped care"), and follow-up could include information meetings (pharmacology education), psycho-educative programs (information about the underlying disease and alternatives to pharmacological treatments), support groups, or even group therapy [97].

Tapering in the More Difficult Cases (Inpatient vs. Outpatient) Gradual tapering of the medication is preferable to abrupt discontinuation [28, 71]. The use of anticonvulsants like carbamazepine or valproate can be of use for benzodiazepine withdrawal and clonidine for opioid withdrawal. Also some authors suggest the use of benzodiazepines for withdrawal from opioids, even if this can mean substituting one addiction with another [30]. The main principle is to substitute short-acting drugs with longer-acting drugs in order to have more control over the withdrawal symptoms.

Tapering the Patients with Benzodiazepine Dependency A thorough evaluation of the dose should be done. All the different benzodiazepines and benzodiazepine-like drugs should be reduced to two different drugs at the most. Switch to a longer-acting drugs like diazepam (in most people) or a drug with fewer reinforcing effects like oxazepam (in drug abusers or the elderly). Remember that some benzodiazepines (e.g., alprazolam, clonazepam, and flunitrazepam) are 10–20 times more potent and need to be converted to equivalent diazepam doses. For good cooperation between you and your patient, you need to assure the patient that he/she will be adequately covered. For outpatient treatment, you may want to taper by reducing 20% of the total daily dose during the first months and then 10% of the dose later, reducing to 5% or less for the last weeks. Allow the patient to reach a steady state between dose reductions and allow for time to tackle the withdrawal symptoms. For adults with a $T_{1/2}$ of 1–1.5 days of diazepam, one step can be performed every second week, but for older people, the $T_{1/2}$ of diazepam increases, and more time should be allowed for each step. A lot of support and encouragement may be needed, sometimes in support groups, sometimes individually. For inpatient treatment, a more aggressive approach is recommended. Often, the patient will not be given enough time for a slow taper. The amount of withdrawal the patient needs to manage is constant either with short- or long-term tapering. Thus, in the inpatient situation, a tapering of the whole dose within 2–3 weeks is

recommended. You must then be aware of benzodiazepine delirium.

Tapering/Detoxifying the Patients with Opioid Dependency The tapering of prescription opioids should always be done after a thorough workup on pain and consideration of adequate pain management. For this, we refer to textbooks on pain management. Even if inadequate pain management is the cause of the patient's problem, reduction or removal of the drugs will be needed. This would involve tapering. Such tapering can be more manageable using a long-acting opioid such as methadone or buprenorphine as a tool, even supported by clonidine to tackle the worst withdrawal symptoms. For further information on opioid detoxification, we refer to other chapters in this book.

Intoxications Acute treatment of intoxications with prescription drugs should be handled as other emergencies. Life support including airways, breath, and circulation should be observed. Gastric lavage can be performed if necessary and when done within a limited amount of time. For opioids and benzodiazepines, there are antidotes such as naloxone and flumazenil. Otherwise, drugs should be given on indication.

Benzodiazepine Delirium This should be treated like an alcoholic delirium tremens. Reinstating benzodiazepines and tapering them at a slower pace would be the preferred mode.

22.7 Brief Summary

Many drugs can be abused, but sedatives, painkillers, and central stimulants are the most prevalent prescription drugs to be abused. We have seen an opioid epidemic, especially in the States during the latter years, mostly due to overprescribing and underestimation of the problematic sides of this. All prescription drugs with an abuse potential need to be used with care to ensure the right treatment for the maladies, avoiding use that could lead to addiction. Treatment is as for many other drugs, but special emphasis should be put on tapering from high doses.

References

1. Agabio R, Sinclair JM, Addolorato G, Aubin HJ, Beraha EM, Caputo F, Chick JD, De La Selle P, Franchitto N, Garbutt JC, Haber PS, Heydtmann M, Jaury P, Lingford-Hughes AR, Morley KC, Muller CA, Owens L, Pastor A, Paterson LM, Pelissier F, Rolland B, Stafford A, Thompson A, Van Den Brink W, De Beaurepaire R, Leggio L. Baclofen for the treatment of alcohol use disorder: the Cagliari statement. Lancet Psychiatry. 2018;5:957–60.

2. Ahuja T, Mgbako O, Katzman C, Grossman A. Phenibut (beta-phenyl-gamma-aminobutyric acid) dependence and management of withdrawal: emerging nootropics of abuse. Case Rep Psychiatry. 2018;2018:9864285.

3. Alho H. Opioid agonist diversion in opioid dependence treatment. In: El-Guebaly N, Carrà G, Galanter M, editors. Textbook of addiction treatment: international perspectives. New York: Springer; 2015.

4. Arfken CL, Cicero TJ. Postmarketing surveillance for drug abuse. Drug Alcohol Depend. 2003;70:S97–105.

5. Ator NA. Contributions of GABAA receptor subtype selectivity to abuse liability and dependence potential of pharmacological treatments for anxiety and sleep disorders. CNS Spectr. 2005;10:31–9.

6. Ator NA, Griffiths RR, Weerts EM. Self-injection of flunitrazepam alone and in the context of methadone maintenance in baboons. Drug Alcohol Depend. 2005;78:113–23.

7. Bagot KS, Kaminer Y. Efficacy of stimulants for cognitive enhancement in non-attention deficit hyperactivity disorder youth: a systematic review. Addiction. 2014;109:547–57.

8. Ballantyne JC. Opioid misuse in oncology pain patients. Curr Pain Headache Rep. 2007;11:276–82.

9. Benotsch EG, Martin AM, Koester S, Mason MJ, Jeffers AJ, Snipes DJ. Driving under the influence of prescription drugs used nonmedically: associations in a young adult sample. Subst Abus. 2015;36:99–105.

10. Birke H, Kurita GP, Sjogren P, Hojsted J, Simonsen MK, Juel K, Ekholm O. Chronic non-cancer pain and the epidemic prescription of opioids in the Danish population: trends from 2000 to 2013. Acta Anaesthesiol Scand. 2016;60:623–33.

11. Bloch MH, Panza KE, Landeros-Weisenberger A, Leckman JF. Meta-analysis: treatment of attention-deficit/hyperactivity disorder in children with comorbid tic disorders. J Am Acad Child Adolesc Psychiatry. 2009;48:884–93.

12. Bramness JG, Furu K, Engeland A, Skurtveit S. Carisoprodol use and abuse in Norway. A pharmacoepidemiological study. Br J Clin Pharmacol. 2007;64:210–8.

13. Bramness JG, Morland J, Sorlid HK, Rudberg N, Jacobsen D. Carisoprodol intoxications and serotonergic features. Clin Toxicol (Phila). 2005;43:39–45.

14. Bramness JG, Rossow I. Can the total consumption of a medicinal drug be used as an indicator of excessive use? The case of carisoprodol. Drugs Ed Prev Policy. 2010;17:168–80.

15. Bramness JG, Sandvik P, Engeland A, Skurtveit S. Does Pregabalin (Lyrica((R))) help patients reduce their use of benzodiazepines? A comparison with gabapentin using the Norwegian prescription database. Basic Clin Pharmacol Toxicol. 2010;107:883–6.

16. Bramness JG, Sexton JA. The basic pharmacoepidemiology of benzodiazepine use in Norway 2004-9. Nor Epidem. 2011;21:35–41.

17. Brunette MF, Noordsy DL, Xie HG, Drake RE. Benzodiazepine use and abuse among patients with severe mental illness an co-occuraing substance use disorder. Psychiatr Serv. 2003;54:1395–401.

18. Bukten A, Skurtveit S, Waal H, Clausen T. Factors associated with dropout among patients in opioid maintenance treatment (OMT) and predictors of re-entry. A national registry-based study. Addict Behav. 2014;39:1504–9.

19. Cai R, Crane E, Poneleit K, Paulozzi L. Emergency department visits involving nonmedical use of selected prescription drugs in the United States, 2004-2008. J Pain Palliat Care Pharmacother. 2010;24:293–7.

20. Chiappini S, Schifano F. Is there a potential of misuse for Quetiapine?: Literature review and analysis of the European Medicines Agency/European Medicines Agency Adverse Drug Reactions' Database. J Clin Psychopharmacol. 2018;38:72–9.

21. Clark DJ, Schumacher MA. America's opioid epidemic: supply and demand considerations. Anesth Analg. 2017;125:1667–74.

22. Clark RE, Xie HG, Brunette MF. Benzodiazepine prescription practices and substance abuse in persons with severe mental illness. J Clin Psychiatry. 2004;65:151–5.

23. Clausen T, Anchersen K, Waal H. Mortality prior to, during and after opioid maintenance treatment (OMT): a national prospective cross-registry study. Drug Alcohol Depend. 2008;94:151–7.

24. Clausen T, Waal H, Thoresen M, Gossop M. Mortality among opiate users: opioid maintenance therapy, age and causes of death. Addiction. 2009;104:1356–62.

25. Dart RC, Surratt HL, Cicero TJ, Parrino MW, Severtson SG, Bucher-Bartelson B, Green JL. Trends in opioid analgesic abuse and mortality in the United States. N Engl J Med. 2015;372:241–8.

26. Dayer LE, Painter JT, Mccain K, King J, Cullen J, Foster HR. A recent history of opioid use in the US: three decades of change. Subst Use Misuse. 2019;54:331–9.

27. Deluca P, Davey Z, Corazza O, Di Furia L, Farre M, Flesland LH, Mannonen M, Majava A, Peltoniemi T, Pasinetti M, Pezzolesi C, Scherbaum N, Siemann H, Skutle A, Torrens M, Van Der Kreeft P, Iversen E, Schifano F. Identifying emerging trends in recreational drug use; outcomes from the Psychonaut Web Mapping Project. Prog Neuro-Psychopharmacol Biol Psychiatry. 2012;39:221–6.

28. Denis C, Fatseas M, Lavie E, Auriacombe M. Pharmacological interventions for benzodiazepine

mono-dependence management in outpatient settings. Cochrane Database Syst Rev. 2006;(3):CD005194.

29. Evoy KE, Morrison MD, Saklad SR. Abuse and misuse of Pregabalin and gabapentin. Drugs. 2017;77:403–26.

30. Fatseas M, Auriacombe M. Why buprenorphine is so successful in treating opiate addiction in France. Curr Psychiatry Rep. 2007;9:358–64.

31. FDA. Guidance for industry assessment of abuse potential of drugs. Rockville: U.S. Department of Health and Human Services; 2010.

32. Fischer B, Vojtila L, Rehm J. The 'fentanyl epidemic' in Canada – some cautionary observations focusing on opioid-related mortality. Prev Med. 2018;107:109–13.

33. Frauger E, Nordmann S, Orleans V, Pradel V, Pauly V, Thirion X, Micallef J. Which psychoactive prescription drugs are illegally obtained and through which ways of acquisition? About OPPIDUM survey. Fundam Clin Pharmacol. 2012;26:549–56.

34. Frauger E, Pauly V, Thirion X, Natali F, Pradel V, Reggio P, Rouby F, Coudert H, Micallef J. Estimation of clonazepam abuse liability: a new method using a reimbursed drug database. Int Clin Psychopharmacol. 2009;24:318–24.

35. Gahr M, Freudenmann RW, Hiemke C, Kolle MA, Schonfeldt-Lecuona C. Pregabalin abuse and dependence in Germany: results from a database query. Eur J Clin Pharmacol. 2013;69:1335–42.

36. Gaist D, Andersen M, Aarup AL, Hallas J, Gram LF. Use of sumatriptan in Denmark in 1994-5: an epidemiological analysis of nationwide prescription data. Br J Clin Pharmacol. 1997;43:429–33.

37. Gambi F, Conti CM, Grimaldi MR, Giampietro L, De Bernardis B, Ferro FM. Flunitrazepam a benzodiazepine most used among drug abusers. Int J Immunopathol Pharmacol. 1999;12:157–9.

38. Gerhardt AM. Identifying the drug seeker: the advanced practice nurse's role in managing prescription drug abuse. J Am Acad Nurse Pract. 2004;16:239–43.

39. Goodwin RD, Hasin DS. Sedative use and misuse in the United States. Addiction. 2002;97:555–62.

40. Griffiths RR, Johnson MW. Relative abuse liability of hypnotic drugs: a conceptual framework and algorithm for differentiating among compounds. J Clin Psychiatry. 2005;66(Suppl 9):31–41.

41. Griffiths RR, Weerts EM. Benzodiazepine self-administration in humans and laboratory animals – implications for problems of long-term use and abuse. Psychopharmacology. 1997;134:1–37.

42. Groenman AP, Oosterlaan J, Rommelse N, Franke B, Roeyers H, Oades RD, Sergeant JA, Buitelaar JK, Faraone SV. Substance use disorders in adolescents with attention deficit hyperactivity disorder: a 4-year follow-up study. Addiction. 2013;108:1503.

43. Hajak G, Müller WE, Wittchen HU, Pittrow D, Kirch W. Abuse and dependence potential for the non-benzodiazepine hypnotics zolpidem and zopiclone: a review of case-reports and epidemiological data. Addiction. 2003;98:1371.

44. Hallas J, Støvring H. Templates for analysis of individual-level prescription data. Basic Clin Pharmacol Toxicol. 2006;98:260–5.

45. Hallfors DD, Saxe L. The dependence potential of short half-life benzodiazepines: a meta-analysis. Am J Public Health. 1993;83:1300–4.

46. Helmerhorst GT, Teunis T, Janssen SJ, Ring D. An epidemic of the use, misuse and overdose of opioids and deaths due to overdose, in the United States and Canada: is Europe next? Bone Joint J. 2017;99-B:856–64.

47. Hoiseth G, Karinen R, Sorlid HK, Bramness JG. The effect of scheduling and withdrawal of carisoprodol on prevalence of intoxications with the drug. Basic Clin Pharmacol Toxicol. 2009;105:345–9.

48. Isaacson JH. Preventing prescription drug abuse. Cleve Clin J Med. 2000;67:473–5.

49. Jaffe JH, Bloor R, Crome I, Carr M, Alam F, Simmons A, Meyer RE. A postmarketing study of relative abuse liability of hypnotic sedative drugs. Addiction. 2004;99:165–73.

50. Jannetto PJ, Helander A, Garg U, Janis GC, Goldberger B, Ketha H. The fentanyl epidemic and evolution of fentanyl analogs in the United States and the European Union. Clin Chem. 2019;65:242–53.

51. Johnson MW, Griffiths RR. Comparative abuse liability of GHB and ethanol in humans. Exp Clin Psychopharmacol. 2013;21:112–23.

52. Jones AW, Holmgren A. Amphetamine abuse in Sweden: subject demographics, changes in blood concentrations over time, and the types of coingested substances. J Clin Psychopharmacol. 2013;33:248–52.

53. Jones CM. Heroin use and heroin use risk behaviors among nonmedical users of prescription opioid pain relievers – United States, 2002-2004 and 2008-2010. Drug Alcohol Depend. 2013;132:95–100.

54. Jonsson AK, Holmgren P, Druid H, Ahlner J. Cause of death and drug use pattern in deceased drug addicts in Sweden, 2002-2003. Forensic Sci Int. 2007;169:101–7.

55. Klein-Schwartz W, Schwartz EK, Anderson BD. Evaluation of quetiapine abuse and misuse reported to poison centers. J Addict Med. 2014;8:195–8.

56. Lader M. History of benzodiazepine dependence. J Subst Abuse Tr. 1991;8:53–9.

57. Launonen E, Alho H, Kotovirta E, Wallace I, Simojoki K. Diversion of opioid maintenance treatment medications and predictors for diversion among Finnish maintenance treatment patients. Int J Drug Policy. 2015;26:875–82.

58. Lobmaier P, Gossop M, Waal H, Bramness J. The pharmacological treatment of opioid addiction--a clinical perspective. Eur J Clin Pharmacol. 2010;66:537–45.

59. Longo LP, Johnson B. Addiction: part I. benzodiazepines – side effects, abuse risk and alternatives. Am Fam Physician. 2000;61:2121–8.

60. Manchikanti L, Helm S, Fellows B, Janata JW, Pampati V, Grider JS, Boswell MV. Opioid epidemic in the United States. Pain Physician. 2012;15:ES9–38.

61. Mannucci C, Pichini S, Spagnolo EV, Calapai F, Gangemi S, Navarra M, Calapai G. Sodium oxybate therapy for alcohol withdrawal syndrome and keeping of alcohol abstinence. Curr Drug Metab. 2018;19:1056–64.

62. Marraccini ME. A meta-analysis of prescription stimulant efficacy: are stimulants neurocognitive enhancers? Sci Eng. 2016;76, No Pagination Specified.

63. Martino AM. In search of a new ethic for treating patients with chronic pain: what can medical boards do? J Law Med Ethics. 1998;26:332–49, 263

64. Mccabe SE. Misperceptions of non-medical prescription drug use: a web survey of college students. Addict Behav. 2008;33:713–24.

65. Mccabe SE, Boyd CJ, Teter CJ. Subtypes of nonmedical prescription drug misuse. Drug Alcohol Depend. 2009;102:63–70.

66. Mcelrath K, Joseph H. Medication-assisted treatment (MAT) for opioid addiction: introduction to the special issue. Subst Use Misuse. 2018;53:177–80.

67. Mchugh RK, Nielsen S, Weiss RD. Prescription drug abuse: from epidemiology to public policy. J Subst Abus Treat. 2015;48:1–7.

68. Montebello ME, Brett J. Misuse and associated harms of Quetiapine and other atypical antipsychotics. Curr Top Behav Neurosci. 2017;34:125–39.

69. Mugunthan K, Mcguire T, Glasziou P. Minimal interventions to decrease long-term use of benzodiazepines in primary care: a systematic review and meta-analysis. Br J Gen Pract. 2011;61:e573–8.

70. Olsen H, Koppang E, Alvan G, Morland J. Carisoprodol elimination in humans. Ther Drug Monit. 1994;16:337–40.

71. Parr JM, Kavanagh DJ, Cahill L, Mitchell G, Mc DYR. Effectiveness of current treatment approaches for benzodiazepine discontinuation: a meta-analysis. Addiction. 2009;104:13–24.

72. Pauly V, Frauger E, Pradel V, Nordmann S, Pourcel L, Natali F, Sciortino V, Lapeyre-Mestre M, Micallef J, Thirion X. Monitoring of benzodiazepine diversion using a multi-indicator approach. Int Clin Psychopharmacol. 2011;26:268–77.

73. Pawl R. Prescription narcotic drug abuse: "we have met the enemy and they are ourselves". Surg Neurol. 2008;69:538–41.

74. Peirce GL, Smith MJ, Abate MA, Halverson J. Doctor and pharmacy shopping for controlled substances. Med Care. 2012;50:494–500.

75. Pirog-Balcerzak A, Habrat B, Mierzejewski P. Misuse and abuse of quetiapine. Psychiatr Pol. 2015;49:81–93.

76. Portenoy RK. Opioid therapy for chronic nonmalignant pain: a review of the critical issues. J Pain Symptom Manag. 1996;11:203–17.

77. Ragan CI, Bard I, Singh I. What should we do about student use of cognitive enhancers? An analysis of current evidence. Neuropharmacology. 2013;64:588–95.

78. Reeves RR, Burke RS, Kose S. Carisoprodol: update on abuse potential and legal status. South Med J. 2012;105:619–23.

79. Reid MJ, Langford KH, Morland J, Thomas KV. Quantitative assessment of time dependent drug-use trends by the analysis of drugs and related metabolites in raw sewage. Drug Alcohol Depend. 2011;119:179–86.

80. Roland CL, Lake J, Oderda GM. Prevalence of prescription opioid misuse/abuse as determined by international classification of diseases codes: a systematic review. J Pain Palliat Care Pharmacother. 2016;30:258–68.

81. Rolland B, Labreuche J, Duhamel A, Deheul S, Gautier S, Auffret M, Pignon B, Valin T, Bordet R, Cottencin O. Baclofen for alcohol dependence: relationships between baclofen and alcohol dosing and the occurrence of major sedation. Eur Neuropsychopharmacol. 2015;25:1631–6.

82. Ross J, Darke S. The nature of benzodiazepine dependence among heroin users in Sydney, Australia. Addiction. 2000;95:1785–93.

83. Rosvold EO, Vaglum P, Moum T. Use of minor tranquilizers among Norwegian physicians. A nation-wide comparative study. Soc Sci Med. 1998;46:581–90.

84. Salvatore S, Roislien J, Baz-Lomba JA, Bramness JG. Assessing prescription drug abuse using functional principal component analysis (FPCA) of wastewater data. Pharmacoepidemiol Drug Saf. 2017;26:320–6.

85. SAMHSA. Results from the 2008 national survey on drug use and health: national findings. Rockville: U.S. Department of Health and Human Services; 2009.

86. Sassano-Higgins S, Baron D, Juarez G, Esmaili N, Gold M. A review of ketamine abuse and diversion. Depress Anxiety. 2016;33:718–27.

87. Schifano F, D'offizi S, Piccione M, Corazza O, Deluca P, Davey Z, Di Melchiorre G, Di Furia L, Farre M, Flesland L, Mannonen M, Majava A, Pagani S, Peltoniemi T, Siemann H, Skutle A, Torrens M, Pezzolesi C, Van Der Kreeft P, Scherbaum N. Is there a recreational misuse potential for pregabalin? Analysis of anecdotal online reports in comparison with related gabapentin and clonazepam data. Psychother Psychosom. 2011;80:118–22.

88. Schjerning O, Rosenzweig M, Pottegard A, Damkier P, Nielsen J. Abuse potential of Pregabalin: a systematic review. CNS Drugs. 2016;30:9–25.

89. Skog OJ. Total alcohol consumption and rates of excessive use: a rejoinder to Duffy and Cohen. Br J Addict. 1980;75:133–45.

90. Smith ME, Farah MJ. Are prescription stimulants "smart pills"? The epidemiology and cognitive neuroscience of prescription stimulant use by normal healthy individuals. Psychol Bull. 2011;137:717–41.

91. Strang J, Groshkova T, Uchtenhagen A, Van Den Brink W, Haasen C, Schechter MT, Lintzeris N, Bell J, Pirona A, Oviedo-Joekes E, Simon R, Metrebian N. Heroin on trial: systematic review and meta-analysis of randomised trials of diamorphine-prescribing as treatment for refractory heroin addictiondagger. Br J Psychiatry. 2015;207:5–14.

92. Tan KR, Rudolph U, Luscher C. Hooked on benzo-diazepines: GABAA receptor subtypes and addiction. Trends Neurosci. 2011;34:188–97.

93. Turk DC, Swanson KS, Gatchel RJ. Predicting opioid misuse by chronic pain patients: a systematic review and literature synthesis. Clin J Pain. 2008;24:497–508.

94. UNODC. World drug report 2011. Vienna: United Nations Office on Drugs and Crime; 2012.

95. Van Amsterdam J, Van Den Brink W. The misuse of prescription opioids: a threat for Europe? Curr Drug Abuse Rev. 2015;8:3–14.

96. Van Zee A. The promotion and marketing of oxycontin: commercial triumph, public health tragedy. Am J Public Health. 2009;99:221–7.

97. Voshaar RC, Couvee JE, Van Balkom AJ, Mulder PG, Zitman FG. Strategies for discontinuing long-term benzodiazepine use: meta-analysis. Br J Psychiatry. 2006;189:213–20.

98. Wanzer SH, Federman DD, Adelstein SJ, Cassel CK, Cassem EH, Cranford RE, Hook EW, Lo B, Moertel CG, Safar P, et al. The physician's responsibility toward hopelessly ill patients. A second look. N Engl J Med. 1989;320:844–9.

99. Webster LR. Risk factors for opioid-use disorder and overdose. Anesth Analg. 2017;125:1741–8.

100. Weisberg DF, Becker WC, Fiellin DA, Stannard C. Prescription opioid misuse in the United States and the United Kingdom: cautionary lessons. Int J Drug Policy. 2014;25:1124–30.

101. Wilens TE, Spencer TJ, Biederman J. A review of the pharmacotherapy of adults with attention-deficit/hyperactivity disorder. J Atten Disord. 2002;5:189–202.

102. Wright N, D'agnone O, Krajci P, Littlewood R, Alho H, Reimer J, Roncero C, Somaini L, Maremmani I. Addressing misuse and diversion of opioid substitution medication: guidance based on systematic evidence review and real-world experience. J Public Health (Oxf). 2016;38:e368–74.

Part III

Behavioural Approaches

Richard Rawson and Marc Galanter

Behavioral Approaches: An Introduction

Richard A. Rawson and Marc Galanter

Contents

Abstract

Behavioral approaches are the most widely used clinical strategies for treating individuals with substance use disorders (SUDs). This introduction provides an overview of the chapters in this section on behavioral approaches to SUDs, including motivational interviewing, cognitive behavioral therapy, contingency management, couples and family therapy, trauma-informed therapy, network therapy, community reinforcement approach, mindfulness, psychodynamic psychotherapy, group therapy, and physical exercise. In addition, this section includes chapters that describe strategies for managing the acute and chronic pain of individuals with SUD, address the application of technology in delivering behavioral treatments, and discuss the importance of adapting approaches in culturally sensitive ways while maintaining fidelity to the original model.

Keywords

Behavioral approaches · Therapies · Psychological approaches

R. A. Rawson (✉)
Vermont Center for Behavior and Health, University of Vermont, Burlington, VT, USA

Department of Psychiatry and Biobehavioral Sciences, University of California Los Angeles (UCLA), Los Angeles, CA, USA
e-mail: rrawson@mednet.ucla.edu

M. Galanter
Division of Alcoholism and Drug Abuse, Department of Psychiatry, NYU School of Medicine, New York, NY, USA
e-mail: marcgalanter@nyu.edu

23.1 Introduction

Behavioral approaches, including "talk therapies," are essential components in the development of treatment systems for treating individuals with substance use disorders (SUDs). In their most rudimentary form, behavioral treatments consist of advice-giving or commonsense generic counseling. While these nonspecific methods can serve as humane, compassionate activities, there is little, if any, evidence of their effectiveness in helping people reduce or eliminate their drug use. As the addiction treatment field has developed, there has been an increasing emphasis on promoting the use of behavioral strategies with empirical support for their effectiveness (aka "evidence-based practices").

In recent years, a collection of behavioral interventions and approaches, developed and evaluated in research trials, have gradually been adopted into a wide variety of treatment settings. As outpatient settings have increasingly become the primary setting for SUD services, two key guiding principles in assessing the impact of these approaches are: do they retain people in treatment and do they help people reduce/eliminate their unhealthy use of drugs and alcohol? Unlike the harsh, confrontational approaches previously used in the early years of addiction treatment, many of the approaches described in this section make extensive use of positive reinforcement to enable behavioral change, including retention in treatment.

The behavioral approaches and strategies described in the section now represent the foundational treatment paradigm for much of the SUD treatment delivered in the world. For the treatment of SUDs that have effective pharmacotherapies, including the treatment of opioid and alcohol dependence, these behavioral approaches are frequently employed in combination with these medications. For other SUDs, such as stimulant dependence, these approaches are the only empirically supported techniques currently available. A limiting factor to increasing access to these therapies is the need for a well-trained workforce, requiring a significant training effort necessary for the successful transfer of the knowledge and skills needed to deliver these treatments.

Section IV includes a comprehensive set of chapters on the behavioral approaches that have been developed and evaluated for the treatment of SUDs. During the past 25 years, three behavioral approaches, motivational interviewing, cognitive behavioral therapy, and contingency management, have been the most extensively researched, evaluated, and widely disseminated behavioral approaches. Motivational interviewing (MI), conceived and first presented in a 1991 text authored by Miller and Rollnick, is reviewed

in Chap. 24 by Kouimtsidis and colleagues. MI is arguably the most important behavioral strategy ever developed for the treatment of SUDs, as it has been applied in a very extensive array of settings and with a wide variety of patient populations. Chapter 24 reviews the rationale for MI and the skills needed by therapists to effectively employ the MI approach. In Chap. 25, Lee and colleagues review the learning-theory underpinnings of cognitive behavioral therapy (CBT), some of the practical considerations for the use of CBT, and the skills needed by therapists to effectively deliver CBT. They also provide a comprehensive array of CBT models and variations as developed by various authors/researchers, and Lee et al. review the evidence that supports the efficacy of CBT. In Chap. 29, Roll and colleagues describe the operant-conditioning foundational principles for contingency management (CM) and theoretical rationale for methods used to apply CM principles in the treatment of addiction. They review some prototypic examples of how CM has been practically applied in clinical settings. Of all the behavioral approaches, CM has the strongest empirical evidence of efficacy. Roll and colleagues organize their review of the research evidence to reflect the key factors that impact the effectiveness of CM interventions. They finish their review by addressing the implementation barriers and limitations of CM and new work on the implementation of CM using technology to deliver CM remotely.

Two of the chapters in Section IV describe behavioral approaches where there are multiple individuals involved in participating in the treatment process. In many parts of the world, group therapy plays a major role in addiction treatment. In Chap. 30, McHugh and colleagues review the variety of group therapies used in SUD treatment and the data that supports the value of group therapy. They provide practical information on which models of group therapy are appropriate for which patient groups, including for patients with co-occurring psychiatric disorders. In Chap. 31, Klosterman and O'Farrell present a review of couples and family therapy. They discuss the impact of substance abuse on the family, and they describe the models, techniques, and principles of couples and family therapy that have been used with substance-abusing patients, their partners, and extended family members. They also discuss the potential barriers to implementing partner- and family-involved approaches for substance use and explore future directions with respect to partner- and family-involved therapies for SUD.

Section IV also includes three chapters that describe multi-element outpatient approaches. In Chap. 32, Galanter describes the rationale and elements of network therapy and the importance of employing the support of family and close friends for the treatment of addictive disorders. The chapter provides clinical examples of how network therapy is applied and research to support the approach, as well as a role for the use of twelve-step facilitation in conjunction with this approach. In Chap. 33, Roozen and Smith describe the Community Reinforcement Approach (CRA) and Community Reinforcement and Family Training (CRAFT) therapy models. These models are predicated on the behavioral principle that a non-drinking/non-drug using lifestyle must be experienced by individuals as rewarding in order for them to choose it consistently over substance use. The chapter describes elements of the approaches and how they can be applied with unmotivated individuals and with adolescents. Research evidence on the efficacy and effectiveness of the approaches is also presented. In Chap. 28, Brown provides a comprehensive review of the role of trauma as a contributing factor to SUD and mental health disorders. Brown describes the rationale and techniques used in trauma-based therapy and trauma-informed care. She also describes how traditional treatment methods can re-traumatize patients (and staff) and how this can be avoided. Data are presented on the benefits of trauma-based care.

Two innovative behavioral techniques that are generating considerable interest are mindfulness meditation and physical exercise. In Chap. 27, McClintock and Marcus describe the foundations and types of activities that make up mindfulness. They describe numerous therapy models in which mindfulness is a component and a variety of applications for mindfulness approaches. They review the research evidence for mindfulness as it is applied to specific SUDs. In Chap. 34, Mooney and Rawson review the extensive set of research that documents the robust positive health benefits of exercise. The chapter documents the rapid expansion of exercise research on exercise for SUD and provides a summary of the research findings. They describe in detail the study methodology and results of a randomized clinical trial of exercise for individuals in early recovery from methamphetamine.

In Chap. 26, Khantzian describes how drugs and alcohol are used to cope with suffering and emotional pain. Psychodynamic psychotherapy has long been used to understand how people use drugs and alcohol to modify hedonic states and self-regulate moods. The chapter describes the concept of "disordered self-care" and the implications of this concept to the psychotherapeutic process. In addition, the chapter emphasizes the importance of the therapeutic alliance as an important element in promoting change and describes the key elements of this alliance as kindness, support, empathy, respect, patience, and instruction. In Chap. 37, Krashin and colleagues describe the complex and challenging interface between pain and its treatment and SUDs and their treatment. They recommend a multimodal approach that is personalized for each individual. They review current treatment recommendations for the treatment of acute and chronic pain within SUD settings and for different patient populations. They provide a discussion of palliative care and strategies for risk management in the use of opioid medications.

In Chap. 35, Lemle and Marsch provide an excellent overview of the new world of technology applications to the treatment of SUDs. Because there are a variety of factors that limit access to in-person clinical service delivery (e.g., distance, cost, lack of trained personnel), digital strategies to bring treatment information and programming via digital technology are being rapidly developed and implemented. The chapter presents a review of the types of interventions developed and an overview of the research evidence concerning their effectiveness. In Chap. 36,

Castro and colleagues have contributed a chapter on the importance of culturally adapting behavioral approaches in a systematic manner for their application in other languages and cultures. They describe a systematic methodology for balancing the fidelity to the original evidence-based model while allowing for adaptation of the model to address specific cultural issues of importance. They describe the challenges of effective language translation as well and cautions about misadaptation. This chapter is of tremendous value in assisting in the adaptation of evidence-based practices developed in Western cultures to other parts of the world.

23.2 Summary

Section IV includes a collection of chapters, written by experts in the topic areas that provide a comprehensive overview of the major evidence-based behavioral approaches to the treatment of SUD. This is an area of tremendous change as extensive work continues to develop, scientifically examine the efficacy and effectiveness of new approaches, and implement these strategies in applied treatment settings around the world.

Motivational Interviewing, Behaviour Change in Addiction Treatment

24

Christos Kouimtsidis, Claudia Salazar, and Ben Houghton

Contents

C. Kouimtsidis (✉)
Imperial College, London, UK

C. Salazar
Central North West London NHS Foundation Trust, London, UK

B. Houghton
St George's University of London, London, UK

Abstract

In this chapter, we discuss the concept of addiction and the most influential theories of behaviour change under a common theory framework, including theories on motivation such as the PRIME theory.

© Springer Nature Switzerland AG 2021
N. el-Guebaly et al. (eds.), *Textbook of Addiction Treatment*,
https://doi.org/10.1007/978-3-030-36391-8_24

Motivational interviewing (MI) has been an influential therapeutic approach proposed by Miller in 1983. MI is a way of interviewing people with an addiction problem, which goal is directed and aims to empower the person to explore their ambivalence, mixed feelings, and thoughts about their addictive behaviour and develop their own plan of action to address it. We discuss the main components of MI and how to use it in everyday clinical practice.

MI is the major ingredient of brief interventions for alcohol use disorder and other substance use disorders. MI can also be a component of other structured psychological interventions (such as cognitive behavioural therapy) for people with dependence on alcohol or other substances. Finally, we discuss the evidence supporting the effectiveness of MI from the early individual trials to the most recent systematic reviews.

Keywords

Addiction · Addiction theories · Motivation
Motivational interviewing

24.1 Introduction

What is the best way that we can help people change behaviour has been and still is one of the major challenges for health and social care professionals. In substance use disorder treatment, the role of motivation and the professionals' skills in influencing change are central across all approaches. Motivational interviewing (MI) was described by the psychologist William Miller [1] and later expanded on though collaboration with Stephen Rollnick. Through consultation with other researchers and clinicians working in the 1980s, there were concerns about confrontational and cohesive approaches that were commonplace in addiction treatment, that were based on little evidence and that were observed to have poor outcomes. Miller and Rollnick collaborated in combining the emerging evidence about motivation and behaviour change research as well as their

experience in psychology and counselling those with substance use disorders. They put forward their approach in their first edition of their book that focused mainly on illicit substance and alcohol treatment, describing the approach and techniques involved in having a different kind of conversation about change that avoided conflict and judgement of the person. As MI became more widely applied and processes better understood across a range of health and social care settings, in their second edition, they include applications across a wide range of problem areas and begin to propose possible mechanisms on how MI works. In their third edition [2], they bring together the key evidence from randomised controlled trials in the intervening decade, and they clarify and redefine some of the skills and processes involved, in particular emerging evidence on the importance of paying selective attention to particular types speech MI that strengthens commitment to change.

24.2 Addiction and Choice Theories of Behaviour Change

Addiction is a social phenomenon. Across diagnostic classification systems and across the years, the definition has three main components/aspects. It is described as (i) a reward-seeking behaviour, (ii) that has become out of control and (iii) which impaired control is leading to harm [3]. To that effect, addiction includes any behaviour that satisfies the above three criteria, such as substance use, drinking alcohol, smoking, gambling, gaming and others. The above behaviours per se do not equal addiction unless there is loss of control and associated harm. It could be argued that addiction sits at the core of human species, defined as a 'social animal' by Aristotle. Addiction is an inherent biological phenomenon, related with the existence of the brain pathways of reward, aiming to maximise the chances of the individual to survive and multiply within a challenging physical and social environment.

Over the years, several theories were developed with the aim to understand and explain the aforementioned components of the definition of addiction. The multitude of existing theories is an example of pluralism of approaches. This pluralism is necessary for further development of our understanding of addiction. Furthermore, it is considered important that phenomena are understood under the framework of a single theory because fewer axioms have to be accepted as true, concepts can be shared, and testable hypotheses can be generated. To that effect for human behaviour, the theory of evolution is considered the master theory that provides the framework to acknowledge the reciprocal and dynamic interaction between living organisms/humans and the environment. All theories trying to understand a specific phenomenon (such as addiction) should be conceived under and be compliant with the theory of evolution.

All the theories of addiction that aim to explain the process of how the reward-seeking behaviour is initiated, then becomes out of control and is maintained irrespective of the harm experienced could be seen under a common theory framework that focuses on the principle of choice. The therapeutic interventions (pharmacological, psychological or social) based on these theories conceive addiction as a decision-making process which is conscious to start with, later on becomes unconscious and in order to be modified needs to become conscious again. For this theory framework to be consistent with the evolution theory, there is a need to identify and understand the potential advantage of having reward pathways that become out of control and the cognitive process of choice becoming unconscious.

Under the common framework of choice theories, we could include early basic theories and their more recent adaptations such as operational conditioning [4], as well as the very influential social learning theory [5], and the expectancy theory.

Social learning theory is a generic theory of human behaviour and focuses on the individual and his/her choices within a social environment. Behaviour is regarded as the result of a continuous interaction between personal and environmental variables. Social learning theory introduces two main concepts: (i) outcome expectations, which are 'the person's estimate that a given behaviour will lead to certain outcomes', and (ii) efficacy expectations (or self-efficacy), which refer to a person's belief 'that one can successfully execute the behaviour required to produce outcomes' ([5], p.193). Self-efficacy is relevant to all stages and aspects of human development (family environment, school, career development and pursuits, health-promoting behaviour). The theory was expanded later to the social cognitive theory in order to conceive the person as an agent of change that affects the person and the social environment [6].

Originally, expectancy theory placed emphasis on initial conscious cognitive processes, which are related to the experience of craving. Evidence though suggested that subjective report of craving is only moderately linked with substance use and relapse. As addiction progresses, substance use is regulated by automatic cognitive processes, while craving represents the activation of non-automatic processes. These non-automatic processes are activated to either aid in completing interrupted substance use or block automatic substance use sequences [7]. As addiction develops, the expectancy-based control system of behaviour becomes unconscious, and therefore, behaviour is influenced less by conscious expectancies involving controlled processes and more by unconscious expectancies involving automatic processes. Furthermore, cognitive bias theory introduces the concept of biases that affect conscious functions such as beliefs, attention and memories as well as unconscious processes in information recall from memory [8]. Over time, activation of one part of the 'network' (e.g. alcohol representations) automatically triggers propositional links in other parts (e.g. relaxation concepts) and vice versa; however, it is hypothesised that this information is less accessible and relies more on effortful and non-automatic cognitive processes; therefore, its moderating impact on behaviour is compromised [9].

Hybrid models which provide a synthesis between biological and psychological models could be placed under the choice framework. Such models include the hedonic homeostatic dysregulation model [10] and more recent ones such as the incentive-sensitisation model [11] and the inhibition dysregulation model [12], which attempt to explain the progress from choice to compulsive use.

In summary and in order to address the question of the evolutionary advantage of addiction, it could be argued that the phenomenon of addiction is related with the ability of humans to test new behaviours, those considered important for surviving to become automatised and therefore replicated fast without ongoing review of their appropriateness. Therefore, it could be argued that addictive behaviours are the price paid by humans for having the ability to learn and to adapt to environmental changes.

24.3 Theories of Motivation

24.3.1 Trans-theoretical Model of Change

The development of motivational interviewing coincided with the appearance of the extremely influential trans-theoretical model of behaviour change or stages of change model, developed by Prochaska and DiClemente in 1986. The focus of this model is the motivation to change and the process of change itself. Although it is described as a model, it proposes new theory concept; therefore, it could be seen as a theory.

'Stages of change' (as it is often referred to) has been used in everyday clinical practice alongside MI although MI was never based on this model as argued by Miller and Rollnick in the second edition of their book in 2009. People are rarely in a state where they do not view some aspect of their substance use or other behaviour to be problematic, or in need of change, even more so when they are encouraged to reflect on the impact of the addictive behaviour on their life. To that effect, stages of change helps the person to define or acknowledge the state of their commitment to change.

The model proposes that the process of recovery from an addictive behaviour involves transi-

tion through five stages: (i) pre-contemplation stage in which no change is contemplated; (ii) contemplation in which change is contemplated for the near future; (iii) preparation, in which plans are made on how to change behaviour in a definite way; (iv) action stage in which the plans are put into action and change takes place; and (v) maintenance in which the new pattern of behaviour emerges, establishes and is maintained. There is a sixth stage, that of termination, which was added more recently and in some way overlaps with the maintenance stage. In this stage, the individual has adopted and consolidated the new behaviour. The model proposes that individuals can move forwards or backwards through the stages.

The model has enjoyed great popularity although it has received major criticism. The popularity might be explained by the seemingly scientific approach of diagnosing the stage of change and the perceived relation to a specific treatment plan, as well as the provision of categories to place people rather than use everyday language. The criticism relates to several aspects of the model, such as the definition and validity of the proposed stages, the proposed linear progress through the stages as well as the inability of the model to account for the unconscious decision-making processes [3].

24.3.2 Identity Shift Theory

Identity shift theory [13] takes into account the principle of unstable preferences, which is considered a fundamental feature of human motivation, and proposes that increasing distress caused by behaviours results to value conflict. This prompts to a small step towards behaviour change, which if successful begins to lead to an identity shift. Increased self-awareness and self-confidence then fuel continued change. At the core of the model is the ongoing evaluation of benefits, costs and the build-up of dissatisfaction with the current situation. Then a trigger, small or major, results in an immediate and unplanned step of change that initiates the process of behaviour change.

24.3.3 PRIME Theory of Motivation

West [3] proposed a new theory of motivation called PRIME, an acronym standing for the proposed five levels of motivation: plans, responses, impulses/inhibitory forces, motives and evaluations. Although it is described as a theory of motivation, it could be regarded as a theory of addiction in general. According to this theory, addiction is conceived as a chronic condition of the motivational system in which the reward-seeking behaviour has become out of control. This is a synthetic theory that aims to encompass all the elements of the previously discussed theories. The levels of motivation are hierarchical from low levels of responses that involve reflexes and automatic behaviours to higher responses that include evaluations, plans involving expectancies and the concept of identity.

The theory proposes that there are three types of abnormalities of motivation: (i) abnormalities of the motivational system that exist independently of the addictive behaviour such as a predisposition to anxiety or depression; (ii) abnormalities of the motivational system resulting from the development of the addictive behaviour itself, meaning the process of developing a habit; and (iii) abnormalities in the individual's social or physical environment such as the presence of strong social or other pressures to engage in an activity such as drinking or drug taking. This means that an activity becomes addictive if it affects an already unbalanced system (comorbid anxiety, traits of impulsivity) which operates within an unbalanced environment (belonging to a social group that activity is considered normal), in such a way of undermining the normal checks and balances that operate to prevent undesirable behaviour (activity becoming continuously rewarding).

The theory is based on the principles of chaos theory. This means that the motivational system is inheritably unstable in the sense that it is susceptible to continuous influence of smaller or bigger internal and external stimuli. This notion can explain both the development of an addictive behaviour and the need for change. Therefore, any event that could be seen as significant or insignificant can potentially send an individual down to a specific path (use of a substance) or could set up an environment which is liable to facilitate for the addictive behaviour to develop. The theory also accounts for the co-occurrence of several addictive behaviours as long as they are mutually reinforcing in terms of their effect on the balance of the motivational system or the individual's environment. According to the theory, triggers for urges (impulses) or desires are not simply the consequence of associative learning but are responsive to higher level expectations and interpretations.

24.4 About Ambivalence

Ambivalence is a natural part of change process for humans, and the way people have to talk to themselves and others about the benefits and costs of change influences those decisions to make that change or not to. Having a dilemma about change is common in people facing psychological difficulties. Statements about *wanting* to change (change talk) and *not wanting* to change (sustain talk) coexist, and for some people, this ambivalence can go on for a long time [2]. It is natural for those working in alcohol and other substance use treatment to want to persuade or convince the person on the arguments for change, but instead this has the opposite effect and provokes people to voice arguments against change. Humans do not like to see other people suffering, especially when they are visibly so unwell, and there can be a want to 'fix it'. This is referred to as the 'righting reflex', a person's desire to help urging the giving of immediate advice without permission, voicing of the counter-arguments with the effect of increasing the sustain talk. The behaviour of the practitioner predicts the outcome, and the more directive and confrontational the practitioner becomes, the more resistance this raises from the person being helped [2]. What influences change is complicated and fluid. Change is not easy, people change when they think change is of value and achievable, and often, change requires several attempts to do so, with lapses and relapses being necessary for success to be achieved [14]. People are more persuaded by their own arguments, and the skill of the practitioner is to develop a style of communication, characterised by active listening and avoiding being directive, that helps the person make decisions for themselves. This is referred to as a guiding style of communication [15]. The practitioner's task is to support a person led shift in favour of behavioural change and to recognise the discrepancy between their view of self and their behaviour.

24.5　What Is Motivational Interviewing?

MI has evolved from the person-centred approach of Carl Rogers [16], but it is distinct from the 'non-directive' role of counselling as it has direction in that it is goal orientated with an intentional focus towards change. Using this guiding style of communication (somewhere between a directive and non-directive style), the practitioner pays selective attention to certain forms of speech (change talk). The more the practitioner is able to recognise, draw out, reflect and amplify change talk, the more likely this is to strengthen commitment to change that in turn predicts positive outcomes [17]. This needs to be done in a particular atmosphere that requires specific attitudes as well as skills.

The technical definition:

> Motivational interviewing is a collaborative, goal orientated style of communication with particular attention to the language of change. It is designed to strengthen personal motivation for and commitment to a specific goal by eliciting and exploring the person's own reasons for change within an atmosphere of acceptance and compassion [2].

24.6　How to Create Atmosphere for Change?

The values and attitude of the practitioner, referred to as the 'spirit', are the central component of this way of interacting. In the early applications of MI, researchers and practitioners focused on improving fidelity to the approach by structuring the techniques into structured feedback or manualised treatment such as motivational enhancement therapy. However, manualised and structured approaches have been found to be less effective [18], so over the last decade, the practice has refocused on the relational components in the interaction as having the most impact [19]. There are four vital aspects of the 'spirit' [2]:

Partnership The practitioner always involves the person in every aspect of the process, from deciding on what to change and then how to go about this; information and advice are offered but not imposed, with the understanding that the solutions and ideas lie as much with the person as with the practitioner. The practitioner is honest about what could be focused on and what has been noticed but involves the person in deciding the next step.

A question such as 'I would like to know what your thoughts are about your drinking' would help to open a dialogue and an assessment process.

> Should we look into this in more detail?
>
> What do you think you should do about this? What do you think might be possible for you to achieve?

Acceptance The practitioner's focus should be on the person's strengths, affirming their efforts and intentions, staying neutral and avoiding either positive or negative judgements. The practitioner should have empathy towards the person and believe the person to be trustworthy, emphasising their freedom to choose and the ability to make the best decisions for themselves.

> I don't have a ready-made recipe of how to resolve your challenge. We can understand this together. You know yourself better, what you can do and what might be extremely difficult to do at this point.

Compassion Actively promoting the other person's welfare, acting in their best interest, and maintaining hope that change is possible. This is fundamental for ethical practice.

I could help you though using my science and my experience of what might be easier or advisable. Two people working together is better than one.

Evocation The practitioner role is to draw out ideas and thoughts from the person, believing in their wisdom and the importance for the person to voice their thoughts and to listen to their own change talk, as being crucial. The practitioner avoids taking the expert role, as the belief is that people are the best experts in their experience and they have the best ideas and solutions that will work for them. The practitioner role is one that facilitates the exploration of answers that lay within the individual.

So let us start with what do you think has worked for you in the past. What are your observations?

These four elements describe the way of being, the values that an MI practitioner working with substance use disorders should seek to establish to maintain collaborative and empathic relationships with the people they are trying to help. Continuing working throughout the lapses and relapses, believing in their ability to change and succeed in maintaining change, affirming their strength to persevere, normalising how hard change is and helping them maintain the hope that they will succeed.

24.7   The Processes and Skills in MI

In the practice of MI, there is now an understanding that there are four processes in the journey of helping people change and that the practitioner guides the person through them [2]. Each process is a stepping stone to the next that helps the practitioner concentrate on the skills and techniques to guide the person through each step beginning with engaging them to ultimately making a robust plan for change. The core skills are known by the acronym of *OARS, open-ended questions, affirming, reflecting and summarising*, and are derived from person-centred counselling. These skills are used throughout the

four processes in developing and maintaining momentum, forming a central part of becoming a skilled practitioner [20].

Planning
'How to change?'

Evoking
'Why change?'

Focusing
'What to change?'

Engaging
'Shall we work together?'

24.7.1 Engaging

The first task is establishing a good therapeutic relationship to develop trust and collaboration as quickly as possible. The first few minutes of any interaction can be crucial in this process [21], and it requires the practitioner to concentrate on active listening skills and focus on the OARS.

Open-ended questions This type of questions cannot be answered by 'yes', 'no' or a 'fact' but is explorative. These questions are encouraging the respondent to think and elaborate and to voice their wisdom, their *change talk*. In engagement, we want to understand their perspective without pursuing particular answers or assuming that the person has made a decision to change.

'How long have you had an alcohol problem?' is a closed question that is already labelling a problem as opposed to 'Tell me about your drinking?' which is an open question that is encouraging the person to tell you their story.

Affirming MI is strength focused and requires the practitioner to concentrate on valuing the person's perspective, with the practitioner making a conscious bias to notice and voice the person's strengths, insights and abilities to promote engagement, reduce defensiveness and raise confidence. There is active effort not to focus on what is wrong, the pathology, errors or deficits [22]. Making people feel better about themselves enables them to have the strength to address their problems and retains people in treatment. Acknowledging the potential embarrassment associated with the realisation that the behaviour is self-inflicted is important. Be clear about having no right to make judgements as we are all made from an evolutionary point of view to develop habits and addictions. Emphasise that what matters is the willingness to consider change.

Reflecting Listening Reflective statements are a key skill in MI, allowing the practitioner to voice their guess at what the person means, to check understanding, to convey empathy as well as to allow the person to hear their thoughts and ideas. Hearing reflections makes people feel encouraged to continue talking. The skill of forming reflections is key, from simply reflecting what the person said to more complex reflections that attempt to convey an understanding of meaning and feeling. There is a selective use of reflections, and so the ability to recognise and reflect *change talk* is key to encourage the person to decide to commit to change.

Simple Reflection: One strategy is simply to reflect what the client is saying. This sometimes has the effect of eliciting the opposite and balancing the picture.

Client:	*I'm fed up of talking about my drinking!*
Practitioner:	*You're fed up of talking about your drinking. Ok what else would you like to talk about?*

(The aim is to return to a discussion about the drinking through a different indirect route.)

Reflection with Amplification: A modification is to reflect but exaggerate or amplify what the client is saying to the point where the client is likely to disavow it. There is a subtle balance here because overdoing an exaggeration can elicit hostility.

Client:	*But I'm not an alcoholic or anything like that.*
Practitioner:	*I understand. You don't want to be labelled. There is no need for labels, but what do you mean about being an alcoholic? What alcoholics do?*
Client:	*I don't think I have a drinking problem.*
Therapist:	*So you think there haven't really been any problems or harm caused by your drinking.*
Client:	*Well. I wouldn't say that.*
Practitioner:	*I see; you don't like the idea that you have a drinking problem (pause); but you think your drinking has caused you problems. Could we investigate this?*

Double-Sided Reflections:

Client:	*But I can't stop drinking. All my friends do it!*
Practitioner:	*It's difficult for you to imagine not drinking with your friends (pause); but you also worry what it's doing to you. I think that I understand.*

Then you might want to break down the two components (friends and stopping) of the above statement and see what would be easier and more productive to challenge. For example, *Are there situations that you don't drink with your friends? May I ask if your drinking is similar or different to this of your friends? Maybe we don't need to stop drinking. Maybe reducing the amount would be easier. What do you think?*

Summarising Bringing together key statements voiced by the person is particularly important; a summary can help collect various statements together to help clarify ideas. Often, if there is ambivalence when you are trying to engage with the person, it is very helpful to summarise the arguments that they have voiced for and against change. Summarising not only helps clarify their thoughts but can make them more real and conveys the desire to understand their dilemma.

> Let me see if I got this right. So far you have told me that you don't think you are an alcoholic but you think that your drinking has caused you some problems.

A part of the engagement process, Miller and Rollnick [2] describe how important it is to avoid various traps that may interfere and lead to disengagement from treatment, such as *assessment trap* (focusing gathering of facts), *expert trap* (having all the answers), *premature focus trap* (working on solutions before you have engagement), *labelling trap* (*diagnostic labelling*), *blame trap* (focusing on who might be to blame) and *chat trap* (not having a focus to the session).

24.7.2 Focusing

Once good rapport has been established and there is engagement, it is important to clarify the change direction towards defining a specific goal. Often, a person may be facing several areas in their lives they are considering changing and feel overwhelmed, for example, it may be illicit substance or alcohol use, smoking or domestic violence, or conversely, they may be unclear about what needs to be changed. The 'agenda mapping' tool may be used to explore possible options for change to help prioritise what may be most important. The key is to maintain a guiding style to decide collaboratively on a change direction and help the person maintain this.

'So what would you like to talk about? Should we make a list together?'

24.7.3 Evoking

Drawing out the person's motivations for change is a process that is most unique to MI. There is a need to explore how *important* the change is and how *confident* the person feels about making a change, and this may need to be strengthened if it is low. For change to happen, the change has to matter to the person, and they need to have the confidence to do so. The focus is to ensure, through selective use of OARS, that there is an increase in the amount of change talk and any self-expressed language that is an argument for change [2] whilst paying attention to the different types of change talk that indicates a person is ready to make changes [23]. Amrhein differentiates *preparatory change talk*, statements that express *desire*, *ability*, *reason* or *need* to change from *mobilising change talk*, statements that indicate that the person has made a *commitment* 'I will stop' or activation 'I am ready to set a quit date' or *taking steps* 'I've started cutting down'. By listening and affirming change talk, the practitioner strengthens commitment to change. Miller and Rollnick [2] suggest that those people who present to treatment ready to make changes may need to go straight to planning and skip evoking.

24.7.4 Planning

The final step in the process is guiding the person to develop a specific plan, and this is seen as the beginning of change. For some, the plan may be about how to take the first step that will begin a process. Some people may have a clear plan, others may need to consider choices as part of the process, and some may need to start from scratch as it may be all new. The important practice point is to stay within the collaborative spirit and actively listen. It is important to allow the person to lead and choose from options and for practitioners to avoid becoming directive and prescriptive, remaining open to new ideas. The practitioner may offer suggestions, information or ideas, but most importantly, they should help the person explore theirs first. Miller and Rollnick [2] suggested a template for change plan that has the component to have a guided discussion to help someone arrive at a robust plan.

Miller and Rollnick [2] initially described five basic motivational interviewing practices underlying such an approach:

1. Express empathy
2. Develop discrepancy
3. Avoid argument
4. Roll with resistance
5. Support self-efficacy

24.7.4.1 Express Empathy

Empathy refers to the ability of the practitioner to make sense of the person's experience. Contrasted with approval or identification, empathy is the process of communicating to the person that the behaviour in question has its own rationale. This is different from sympathy, which implies a sense of inevitability and feeling sorry for the person. Empathy is communicated by the practitioner through reflective listening and selective reinforcement, through affirmation and the way that the practitioner summarises a person's position.

24.7.4.2 Develop Discrepancy

Motivation for change occurs when people perceive a discrepancy between where they are and where they want to be. The approach seeks to enhance and focus the person's attention on such discrepancies with regard to drinking. In certain cases, it may be necessary first to develop such discrepancy by raising the person's awareness of the personal consequences of the behaviour. Such information, properly presented, can precipitate a crisis of motivation for change. As a result, the individual may be more willing to enter into a frank discussion of change options in order to reduce the perceived discrepancy and retain emotional equilibrium.

24.7.4.3 Avoid Argument

If handled poorly, ambivalence about the current behaviour and discrepancy between the consequences of the behaviour and person goals or aspirations result in defensive coping strategies that reduce discomfort but do not alter the behav-

iour and related risks. An attack on the person's drinking or substance using behaviour tends to evoke defensiveness and opposition and suggests to the person that the practitioner 'does not really understand'. MI explicitly avoids direct argument. No attempt is made to have the person accept or admit a diagnostic label. The practitioner does not seek to prove or convince by force of argument. Instead, the practitioner employs other strategies to assist the person to see accurately the negative consequences of the behaviour and to begin devaluing the perceived positive aspects of it. In essence when MI is conducted properly, *the person and not the practitioner* voices arguments for change [2].

> You are worried about having to decide right now. Let's just carry on understanding together where you are at the moment (pause). Later on, we can worry about what, if anything, you want to do about it.

24.7.4.4 Roll with Resistance

How the practitioner handles person resistance is a crucial and defining characteristic of MI. Motivational strategies do not meet resistance head on but rather roll with the momentum, with a goal of shifting person perceptions in the process. New ways of thinking about problems are invited but not imposed. Ambivalence is viewed as normal, not pathological, and is explored openly. Solutions are usually evoked from the person unless specifically requested of the practitioner.

> Okay, that's where you're at now (pause). That it's too difficult to make a change. Maybe you'll decide that you want to keep on drinking. That's up to you.

24.7.4.5 Support Self-Efficacy

People who are persuaded that they have a serious problem will still not move towards change unless there is hope for success. Self-efficacy is a critical determinant of behaviour change (see social learning theory above). In this case, people must be convinced that it is possible for them to change their own drinking and thereby reduce related problems. Unless this element is present, a discrepancy crisis is likely to resolve into defensive coping (e.g. denial, rationalisation) to reduce discomfort without changing behaviour. This is a natural and understandable protective process. If one has little hope that things could change, there is little reason to face the problem.

Learning practising motivational interviewing requires practitioners to acquire skills identified in 12 learning tasks that are illustrated and explained in detail in the third edition of the textbook [2]:

1. Understanding the underlying spirit
2. Developing skill of reflective listening and person-centred OARS skills
3. Identifying change goals towards which to move
4. Exchanging information and providing advice in MI style
5. Being able to recognise sustain talk and change talk
6. Evoking change talk
7. Responding to change talk to strengthen it
8. Responding to sustain talk and discord so it does not increase
9. Developing hope and confidence
10. Timing and negotiating change plan
11. Strengthening commitment
12. Flexibility in integrating MI with other clinical skills and practices

24.8 About Information and Advice

Interactions in healthcare often require practitioners to give information and advice that often makes the practitioner assume the expert role and employ a directive style. In MI, there is an acknowledgement that clinical interactions involve information exchange but that this needs to be done skilfully. Principles of good practice outlined by Miller and Rollnick [2] start with suggestions that we need to make this process personalised and strength driven, starting with finding out what the person already knows and offering information on what they would like or need to know whilst encouraging autonomy on

decision-making. One strategy for information exchange is termed 'elicit-provide-elicit':

- *Elicit* – Ask the person to offer information, finding out what the person already knows and what they would like to know.
- *Provide* – Prioritise the information that the person is asking for. Be clear, use everyday language and avoid jargon, presenting information in a neutral manner avoiding the need for the person to interpret.
- *Elicit* – Ask the person what they think about the information, allowing time to process and ask further questions.

Offering **advice** is a special kind of information, as it usually involves recommendations that suggest action to be taken, for example, reducing alcohol consumption to low risk levels. For advice to be heard and followed, this needs to be offered following the elicit-provide-elicit strategy and can only be given if you have engagement with the emphasis of personal choice and control.

24.9 How Effective Is Motivational Interviewing for Substance Use Disorders?

An early body of evidence exists about the effectiveness on motivational interviewing, how it works and how it compares with other approaches. The original research mainly focused on those with alcohol problems and the positive effect of one session of MI on follow-up [24]. Brief intervention studies in alcohol across the world were showing positive outcomes, and a review of controlled trials found brief interventions in alcohol to be better than no treatment and as effective as more intensive interventions [25]. This review highlighted common components that were further developed MI practice. A feedback component was added to subsequent MI research that was defined as an adaptation of MI (AMI). Significant benefits have been also found in outcomes in drug treatment, and single-session interventions also continue to demonstrate effectiveness [26].

Two major randomised controlled trials (RCT) in the alcohol use disorder have taken place in the 1990s and merit special mention. Project MATCH [27] was the first multisite RCT in the USA. It has used a feedback-based approach referred to as *motivational enhancement therapy*, which combined the clinical style of MI with structured assessment feedback in four sessions over 12 weeks. This was compared to 12 sessions of 12-step facilitation and 12 sessions of CBT, with all three showing similar outcome measures. Another multisite RCT in the UK, trial in the late 1990s [28], compared outcomes of MI with other two approaches, and although no differences in efficacy were found, MI was just as good as more intensive, evidence-based interventions.

More recently, though, Cochrane systematic reviews did not support the efficacy of MI for substance use disorders. A consistent finding across these Cochrane reviews was the low quality of evidence available. This limitation is common across research for all psychological interventions in the field of substance use disorders. There are two points of note: (a) MI is a tool to be used to resolve ambivalence, and studies do not identify whether participants are ambivalent; therefore, it may not be the right tool to be used which would skew efficacy data; (b) MI was developed for alcohol use disorders which is where the evidence for efficacy appears strongest from individual studies.

For example, in smoking cessation, a systematic analysis including 15,000 participants found insufficient and low-quality evidence to recommend MI as a tool to aid smoking cessation despite a slight increase in likelihood to quit smoking if MI was provided [29]. In benzodiazepine, no efficacy was found for MI [30], whereas in gambling behaviour, there is preliminary evidence for the use of MI although CBT would appear to be more effective [31]. Very low-quality evidence was also found for the efficacy of MI versus other treatments in Cochrane review of people who inject drugs with concurrent alcohol use. Within this review, one study of 187 participants found that a brief motivational intervention

reduced alcohol use versus assessment only [32]. Furthermore, MI for people with severe mental illness and substance use disorders may increase attendance at aftercare appointments but does not seem to have an advantage against other treatments in reducing dropout rates or abstaining from substances other than alcohol [33]. There were no observable changes in mental state following MI in this population though it should be noted the quality of evidence included in analysis was thought to be very low. These results were replicated in a review of drug-using offenders with co-occurring mental disorders [34]. Similarly, Cochrane review of 84 trials in young adults aged between 15 and 24 years with alcohol-related problems concludes that MI does not appear to have substantive and meaningful benefit, despite limited efficacy for reducing alcohol-related problems, but no effect for binge drinking or drink driving was found [35].

In contrast to Cochrane reviews that consistently found methodological quality a concern with MI studies, a review by DiClemente and colleagues [36], which included six Cochrane reviews, concluded that there was strong evidence of effectiveness for motivational enhancement interventions with alcohol and tobacco users, brief interventions showing the strongest efficacy. There was some efficacy in gambling and strong support with cannabis use but insufficient evidence for methamphetamine and opiate use disorders. Critically, this review was not recommending MI above other therapies but simply concluded it was more effective than no therapy at all.

Another systematic review regarding the efficacy of MI for adult behaviour change in health and social care settings comprising 104 reviews and 39 meta-analyses also found low-quality evidence. Evidence was graded moderate for the short term (<6 months) statistically significant beneficial effects for reduced binge drinking, frequency and quantity of alcohol consumption and substance abuse in people with dependency or addiction [37].

Beyond conventional face-to-face delivery of MI, there is promising efficacy in alternate methods such as telephone, Internet based and text messaging [38]. Whilst the latter two findings remain controversial and inconclusive given the small number of studies, telephone-based delivery of MI may be considered a viable alternative for substance use disorders.

24.10 Clinical Relevance

- MI is a general way of approaching the interaction with our client and less so a detailed therapy model. It is more about how we do something rather than what we do. It is about how we approach an assessment appointment, how we develop an understanding of the given problem, how we develop and how we implement a change plan. This 'WE' involves the practitioner, the individual and when appropriate their immediate social environment.
- MI is not just a technique but instead an integrated set of interviewing skills, centred on particular values and attitudes to be conducted with the person in guiding them towards change and choice.
- MI is the main component of any brief or extended brief intervention, which could be the sole intervention for smoking, non-dependent alcohol use or a light to moderate drug misuse and can be implemented by any professional not necessarily a specialist. For more severe substance use disorders or other behavioural disorders, MI could be an important component at all stages of treatment.
- Use of MI can be challenging for professionals, as they might have to distant themselves from approaches and attitudes well impeded into their basic professional training, especially doctors, when they are called to resolve a problem using an authoritarian approach. It could be though equally challenging for a counsellor who s/he might over-rely on his/her model or a peer mentor in recovery who can only share his/her way of changing his life. For the professional to develop an MI-based approach, he or she needs to accept the relative effectiveness of his/her treatment approach and to appreciate the fundamental role of the individual who needs and decides to change.

24.11 Conclusion

In motivational interviewing (MI), the aim is to walk alongside the person to the point where they propose goals to change their addictive behaviour, through a process of helping them to explore the positive and negative aspects of the behaviour, recognising the discrepancy between their view of self and their behaviour with the aim to enhance the need for action to change the addictive behaviour and hence resolving this discrepancy. This process is similar to the cognitive restructuring process of cognitive behavioural therapy models which put major emphasis on evaluation of positive expectancies and negative effects and expectations of the addictive behaviour.

Despite the mixed evidence for its efficacy and the link with the process of change model, which has received major criticism, MI has been proven extremely popular and influential. It has helped the field of addictions to move away from the concept of 'denial', to reduce barriers for accessing treatment and open the door to professionals, specialists in addictions or not, to work with persons not ready yet to commit to major change of their lifestyle. It has somehow shifted the responsibility from the person with the addictive behaviour to find a way to commit to a change towards the professional who now has the tools to facilitate this change. MI has provided an easy way to intervene earlier and with populations not considered appropriate for more structured and expensive treatment options.

References

1. Miller WR. Motivational interviewing with problem drinkers. Behav Psychother. 1983;11:147–72.
2. Miller WR, Rollnick S. Motivational interviewing – helping people change. 3rd ed. New York: Guildford Press; 2013.
3. West R. Theory of addiction. London: Blackwell Publishing; 2006.
4. Sue D, Sue DW, Sue S. Understanding abnormal behaviour. 7th ed: Houghton Mifflin; 2003.
5. Bandura A. Self-efficacy: toward a unifying theory of behavioral change. Psychol Rev. 1977;84: 191–215.

6. Bandura A. Social cognitive theory: an agentic perspective. Annu Rev Psychol. 2001;52:1–26.

7. Tiffany ST, Conklin CA. A cognitive processing model of alcohol craving and compulsive alcohol use. Addiction. 2000;95(8 Supplement 2):145–53.

8. Ryan F. Detected, selected, and sometimes neglected: cognitive processing of cues in addiction. Exp Clin Psychopharmacol. 2002;10(2):67–76.

9. McCusker CG. Cognitive biases and addiction: an evolution in theory and method. Addiction. 2001;96:47–56.

10. Koob GF, leMoal M. Drug abuse: hedonic homeostatic dysregulation. Science. 1997;278:52–8.

11. Robinson TE, Berridge KC. The psychology and neurobiology of addiction: an incentive-sensitization view. Addiction. 2000;(Supplement 2):S91–S117.

12. Lubman DI, Yucel M. Addiction, a condition of compulsive behaviour? Neuroimaging and neuropsychological evidence of inhibitory dysregulation. Addiction. 2004;99(12):1491–502.

13. Kearney MH, O'Sullivan J. Identity shifts as turning points in health behaviour change. West J Nursing Res. 2003;25:134–52.

14. Kok G, Van den Borne B, Dolan-Mullen P. Effectiveness of health education and health promotion: meta-analyses of effect studies and determinants of effectiveness. Patient Educ Couns. 1997;30:19–27.

15. Rollnick S, Miller W, Butler C. Motivational interviewing in health care – helping patients change behaviour. New York: Guilford Press; 2008.

16. Rogers CR. A theory of therapy, personality, and interpersonal relationships as developed in the client-centered framework. In: Koch S, editor. Psychology: the study of a science, Formulations of the person and the social contexts, vol. 3. New York: McGraw-Hill; 1959. p. 184–256.

17. Moyers TB, Martin T. Therapist influence on client language during motivational interviewing sessions: support for a potential causal mechanism. J Subst Abus Treat. 2006;30:245–51.

18. Hettema J, Steele J, Miller WR. Motivational interviewing. Annu Rev Clin Psychol. 2005;1:91–112. https://doi.org/10.1146/annurev.clinpsy.1.102803.143833.

19. Moyers TB. The relationship in motivational interviewing. Psychotherapy (Chic). 2014;51(3):358–63. https://doi.org/10.1037/a0036910. Review.

20. Rosengren DB. Building motivational interviewing skills – a practitioner workbook. New York: Guildford Press; 2009.

21. Ashton M. The motivational hallo. Drug Alcohol Findings J. 2005;(13):23–30.

22. Arkowitz H, Westra H, Miller W, Rollnick S, editors. Motivational interviewing in the treatment of psychological problems. New York: Guilford Press; 2008.

23. Amrhein PC. The comprehension of quasi-performance verbs in verbal commitments: new evidence for componential theories of lexical meaning. J Mem Lang. 1992;31:756–84.

24. Miller WR, Zweben A, DiClemente CC, Rychtarik RC. Motivational enhancement therapy manual: a clinical research guide for therapists treating individuals with alcohol abuse and dependence, Project MATCH monograph series, vol. 2. National Institute on Alcohol Abuse and Alcoholism: Rockville; 1992.

25. Bien TH, Miller WR, Boroughs JM. Motivational interviewing with alcohol outpatients. Behav Cogn Psychother. 1993;21:347–56.

26. Strang J, McCambridge J. The efficacy of single session motivational interviewing in reducing drug consumption and perceptions of drug- related risk and harm among young people: results from a multi-site cluster randomised trial. Addiction. 2004;99:39–52.

27. Project MATCH Research Group. Matching alcohol treatment to client heterogeneity: project MATCH post-treatment drinking outcomes. J Stud Alcohol. 1997;58:7–29.

28. UKATT Research Team. Effectiveness of treatment for alcohol problems: findings of the randomised UK alcohol treatment trial (UKATT). Br Med J. 2005;11:1–5.

29. Lindson N, Thompson TP, Ferrey A, Lambert JD, Aveyard P. Motivational interviewing for smoking cessation. Cochrane Database Syst Rev. 2019;(7):CD006936. https://doi.org/10.1002/14651858.CD006936.pub4.

30. Darker CD, Sweeney BP, Barry JM, Farrell MF, Donnelly-Swift E. Psychosocial interventions for benzodiazepine harmful use, abuse or dependence. Cochrane Database Syst Rev. 2015, 2015;(5):CD009652. https://doi.org/10.1002/14651858.CD009652.pub2.

31. Cowlishaw S, Merkouris S, Dowling N, Anderson C, Jackson A, Thomas S. Psychological therapies for pathological and problem gambling. Cochrane Database Syst Rev. 2012, 2012;(11):CD008937. https://doi.org/10.1002/14651858.CD008937.pub2.

32. Klimas J, Fairgrieve C, Tobin H, Field CA, O'Gorman CSM, Glynn LG, Keenan E, Saunders J, Bury G, Dunne C, Cullen W. Psychosocial interventions to reduce alcohol consumption in concurrent problem alcohol and illicit drug users. Cochrane Database Syst Rev. 2018;(12):CD009269. https://doi.org/10.1002/14651858.CD009269.pub4.

33. Hunt GE, Siegfried N, Morley K, Sitharthan T, Cleary M. Psychosocial interventions for people with both severe mental illness and substance misuse. Cochrane Database Syst Rev. 2013;(10):CD001088. https://doi.org/10.1002/14651858.CD001088.pub3.

34. Perry AE, Neilson M, Martyn-St James M, Glanville JM, Woodhouse R, Godfrey C, Hewitt C. Interventions for drug-using offenders with co-occurring mental illness. Cochrane Database Syst Rev. 2015;(6):CD010901. https://doi.org/10.1002/14651858.CD010901.pub2.

35. Foxcroft DR, Coombes L, Wood S, Allen D, Almeida Santimano NML, Moreira MT. Motivational interviewing for the prevention of alcohol misuse in young adults.

Cochrane Database Syst Rev. 2016;(7):CD007025. https://doi.org/10.1002/14651858.CD007025.pub4.

36. DiClemente CC, Corno CM, Graydon MM, Wiprovnick AE, Knoblach DJ. Motivational interviewing, enhancement, and brief interventions over the last decade: a review of reviews of efficacy and effectiveness. Psychol Addict Behav. 2017;31(8):862–87.

37. Frost H, Campbell P, Maxwell M, O'Carroll RE, Dombrowski SU, Williams B, et al. Effectiveness of motivational interviewing on adult behaviour change in health and social care settings: a systematic review of reviews. PLoS One. 2018;13(10):e0204890.

38. Jiang S, Wu L, Gao X. Beyond face-to-face individual counseling: a systematic review on alternative modes of motivational interviewing in substance abuse treatment and prevention. Addict Behav. 2017;73:216–35.

Cognitive Behavioural Therapies for Alcohol and Other Drug Use Problems

25

Nicole K. Lee, Paula Ross, and Richard Cash

Contents

N. K. Lee (✉)
National Drug Research Institute (NDRI), Curtin
University, Bentley, WA, Australia

360Edge, Melbourne, VIC, Australia
e-mail: nicole@360edge.com.au

P. Ross · R. Cash
360Edge, Melbourne, VIC, Australia
e-mail: paula@360edge.com.au;
richard@360edge.com.au

© Springer Nature Switzerland AG 2021
N. el-Guebaly et al. (eds.), *Textbook of Addiction Treatment*,
https://doi.org/10.1007/978-3-030-36391-8_25

Abstract

Cognitive behavioural therapy is an umbrella term that describes an expansive group of therapies. Although many in number and broad in their approach, they have in common a focus on 'cognitions' (including thoughts, beliefs, schemas and metacognitions) as the central driver of, and the solution to, effective emotion regulation. The early cognitive behavioural therapy models grew from behaviour therapy and introduced the concept of cognition into the behavioural models. The most well-known of these models were developed by Aaron Beck (Cognitive Therapy) and Albert Ellis (Rational Emotive Behaviour Therapy). More recently, mindfulness-based therapies, such as Mindfulness-Based Relapse Prevention, Acceptance and Commitment Therapy and Dialectical Behaviour Therapy, have contributed to the evolution of cognitive behavioural therapies. This chapter describes how these models work and how they have been adapted to alcohol and other drug use treatment, ranging from intensive to brief and low-intensity interventions. The evidence shows that cognitive behavioural therapy is one of the most effective interventions for alcohol and other drug use issues, as well as for co-occurring alcohol and other drug use and mental health problems. It has been adapted and applied across a range of cultures and countries.

Keywords

Cognitive behavioural therapy · CBT · Alcohol and other drug treatment · Alcohol and other drug use disorder

We are what we think. All that we are arises with our thoughts. With our thoughts we make the world. Shakyamuni Buddha

25.1 Introduction

25.1.1 What Is Cognitive Behavioural Therapy and Where Did It Come from

Cognitive behavioural therapy (CBT) has evolved significantly since its beginnings in the 1950s. At that time, psychology more broadly had begun to shift from its psychoanalytic roots into a science-based discipline with an emphasis on the scientific method, and therefore the measurable. A branch of psychology called behaviour therapy began to form driven by scientific enquiry [76].

By the 1960s, two psychoanalytically trained therapists, psychiatrist Aaron Beck ('Cognitive Therapy') and psychologist Albert Ellis ('Rational Emotive Behaviour Therapy', usually referred to as simply REBT), had almost simultaneously began to look beyond behavioural principles to the role of interpretation of events, drawing on ideas from cognitive psychology [53] and social learning theory [4]. What most people refer to as traditional 'CBT' is usually some version of one of these two styles.

The next major development began in the 1990s with the mindfulness-based therapies such as Dialectical Behaviour Therapy (DBT) [41], Mindfulness-Based Relapse Prevention (MBRP) [13] and later Acceptance and Commitment Therapy (ACT) [27].

Thus, cognitive behavioural therapy is not a single therapy. It is an umbrella that encompasses a large group of therapies that have in common a focus on cognitions and behaviour as both the cause of, and the means to resolve, emotional and behavioural dysregulation. Perhaps more accurately referred to as cognitive behavioural therapies, this group of therapies is based on well-researched theoretical models; they share the underlying assumption that our thoughts, behaviours and emotional reactions are learned and that the path to well-being is through managing thoughts and beliefs and to some extent behaviour.

Cognitive behavioural therapies are the most researched group of therapies in the world, and due to the extensive evidence base, they have become a core competency for people in the alcohol and other drug workforce.

25.2 Assumptions Behind Cognitive Behavioural Therapies

25.2.1 Thoughts, Behaviours and Emotions Are Learned

From a cognitive behavioural perspective, alcohol and other drug use, and dependence is complicated by genetic, biological and temperamental factors, but these are risk factors rather than determinants. In much the same way as certain people may have a biological or genetic history of heart disease that puts them at higher risk of heart problems, environmental and learned factors such as eating habits, ability to control stressors, and exercise can prevent or lead to the development of a heart condition.

Both alcohol and other drug use and dependence are considered to be learned behaviours that emerge over time and can therefore be 'unlearned' [50]. They are assumed to operate within a context of a range of environmental influences, including family and friends, availability of alcohol and other drugs and sociodemographic circumstances. Cognitions and emotional responses are also considered to be learned.

25.2.2 Therapeutic Alliance Is a Necessary but Not Sufficient for Change

Cognitive behavioural therapies are often accused of ignoring the therapeutic alliance, but this is not the case. It is true that, unlike the analytic style therapies, cognitive behavioural therapies do not rely on the therapeutic alliance to create change. It is viewed as a necessary (but not sufficient) condition for change [8]. Leahy [39] describes it like an anaesthetic in surgery. Without it, surgery would be difficult and painful, but if you *only* had the anaesthetic, the problem would not be rectified.

Cognitive behavioural therapies build alliance in multiple subtle ways. Collaboration and active participation by individuals in their own treatment is viewed as essential and an important vehicle to developing a positive therapeutic alliance.

Clients' negative attitudes to treatment predict poor alliance in cognitive behavioural therapy [6], so a good effective treatment experience can improve therapeutic alliance. Cognitive behavioural therapies are goal oriented and problem-resolution focused. Whilst treating the whole person is important, addressing the client's immediate goals through developing problem-solving skills is the initial focus of treatment. In the process of resolving the client's problems, therapeutic alliance is naturally developed.

In addition, alleviating the clients' problems, good counselling skills, a flexible adapting style, a collaborative approach and seeking feedback from the client all contribute to the development of therapeutic alliance [8].

25.2.3 Focus on the Here and Now

Cognitive behavioural therapies emphasise the present, at least initially. This is especially important because for many people who have problems with alcohol and other drugs, focusing on resolving past difficulties, especially those associated with the development of alcohol and other drug problems, is often of little benefit unless the day-to-day issues of drug use are addressed [50]. For example, there is little benefit in addressing childhood trauma, which may have contributed to the development of a drug problem, if the client is attending sessions intoxicated.

25.2.4 The Client as Their Own Therapist and the Importance of Homework

Cognitive behavioural therapies focus on developing skills in the client to enable them to be, in a sense, their own therapist. The session is designed to help clients to develop skills in reflection and self-management, and the emphasis of therapy is what happens outside the session, rather than in it. Hence, skill practice (sometimes referred to as 'homework') in between sessions is critical.

In one meta-analysis, the overall effect size between homework compliance and treatment outcome was 0.26; completing homework is associated with improved treatment outcome [47]. This effect size is similar to the effect of therapeutic alliance on outcomes [33], further emphasising the importance of homework.

25.2.5 Guided Discovery as a Self-Reflection Tool

Guided discovery, based on Socratic questioning, is the primary tool of cognitive behavioural therapists to support self-reflection. Socratic

questioning is drawn from Socrates' teaching method of asking questions to promote thinking and reflection. The key difference between Socratic questioning and guided discovery is that Socrates usually had an end in mind, whilst this is not necessary for guided discovery. In fact, guided discovery requires genuine collaboration and curiosity [56] which preclude having an outcome in mind. The assumption behind the use of guided discovery is that the client has the answer to their problems, or at least the means to find answer. The therapist's role is as a guide or coach rather than the expert.

25.2.6 The Scientist-Practitioner Approach and Collaborative Empiricism

Cognitive behavioural therapies are driven by the scientist-practitioner approach. That is, the practitioner applies the scientific method to understanding and addressing client issues. Therefore, there is a constantly evolving cognitive behavioural case formulation that poses hypotheses that are then collaboratively tested. This is referred to as 'collaborative empiricism'.

The scientist-practitioner approach also necessitates undertaking and utilising research about outcomes, which is why cognitive behavioural therapies are the most researched group of therapies. In the scientist-practitioner approach, cognitive behavioural therapists use science in their practice, continually review science to maintain best practice and contribute to science through research [66].

25.3 Cognitive Behavioural Therapy in Practice

25.3.1 Length

In general, cognitive behavioural therapies are relatively brief (usually not more than 12–16 sessions), and even briefer versions have been developed that are designed for delivery between one and six sessions [3].

25.3.2 Structure

Typically, cognitive behavioural therapies use a structured session plan broken into three or four interconnected sections. Within those sections, the work is tailored to the client's needs, so the session format is both structured and flexible.

Carroll [14] uses the '20-20-20 rule': 20 minutes on review of the week, homework tasks and issues arising during the week; 20 minutes on discussion and practice of a particular skill or topic linked to an issue from initial assessment or something that has arisen during the week (e.g. 'since you've had a couple of close shaves this week, I thought we'd talk about high-risk situations today'); and then 20 minutes on recapping the session, agreeing on homework tasks and planning for the next week. In reality, sometimes the middle 20 minutes takes up slightly more time than the first and third 20 minutes, and it may become a 15-30-15 rule.

Mitcheson et al. [50] use a four-part structure: (1) setting the agenda and recap of previous session, (2) dealing with the specific agenda items (the focus of the session), (3) planning for the next session and (4) session review.

Structure of some sort is needed because often clients do not have well-developed skills in structuring their own lives, and this serves as a model to assist them to learn these skills. The structure is outlined to, and agreed with, the client at the beginning of each session. This practice is referred to as 'setting an agenda'.

'Structured' does not mean 'inflexible'. If issues arise, they are incorporated into the agenda as appropriate. Practitioners still need to use their clinical judgement and skills to determine what happens within the structure and when the structure may need to adapt to the immediate circumstances.

The purpose of the structure is both to help the client learn how to apply structure to their own world and to focus the session to ensure critical therapeutic work is being done, so the session is not just general counselling, or a chat.

25.4 Key Cognitive Behavioural Therapies for Alcohol and Other Drug Problems

There is extensive evidence for the effectiveness of cognitive behavioural therapies for a range of mental health problems, including alcohol and other drug disorders. McHugh et al. [48] showed moderate effect sizes (on average $d = 0.45$) with the largest treatment effects found for cannabis use disorders, followed by cocaine, opioids and then polysubstance dependence. Magill and Ray [43] showed similar results.

Overall, cognitive behavioural therapies appear to be both effective and long lasting when compared with general drug counselling, treatment as usual and no treatment controls and are effective in both individual and group formats [48].

25.4.1 Relapse Prevention

Relapse Prevention [45] is one of the earliest cognitive behavioural approaches developed specifically for alcohol and other drug problems. Its main goal is to develop skills to identifying and preparing for high-risk situations that lead to relapse to problematic alcohol or other drug use. Relapse is influenced by numerous factors including self-efficacy, outcome expectancies, craving, motivation, coping, emotional states and interpersonal factors, as well as lifestyle factors, and specific interventions also deal with each of these risk factors.

A number of studies have examined Relapse Prevention, including a systematic review of psychosocial interventions for alcohol and other drug use disorders [48], which included five studies that showed positive outcomes on retention in treatment and use. Compared to other types of behavioural therapies, Relapse Prevention was most effective in maintaining abstinence post-treatment (39% abstinent post-treatment), suggesting if abstinence is the treatment goal, relapse prevention may be the treatment of choice.

In a review of cognitive behavioural therapy, relapse prevention and contingency management, Dutra et al. [21] found that the group referred to as 'CBT therapies' (which included Cognitive Therapy and similar therapies such as Dialectical Behaviour Therapy) had lower dropout rates (35%) than relapse prevention (57%), equivalent effect sizes, but lower abstinence rates post-treatment.

Other treatments that draw heavily from the relapse prevention model have also been found to be effective. The Matrix Model [60], for example, is a 16-week manualised group focused outpatient intervention that includes many components of relapse prevention, plus a range of other behavioural interventions such as contingency management. It has been found to be effective for a range of people who use alcohol and other drugs, including amphetamine and cocaine users [64].

25.4.2 Cognitive Therapy

Cognitive Therapy of Substance Abuse, was first developed by Aaron Beck et al. [7], based on the general Cognitive Therapy model. Cognitive Therapy is often used interchangeably with the term cognitive behavioural therapy. Cognitive Therapy is a type of cognitive behavioural therapy but is not synonymous with it. Typically, in the literature, an intervention described as 'cognitive behavioural therapy' is a pure or modified form of Cognitive Therapy, or sometimes a pure or modified form of Relapse Prevention.

Not dissimilar to Relapse Prevention, the theory of Cognitive Therapy focuses on 'proximal situational factors', such as cognitive, behavioural, emotional and physiological variables that are immediate triggers for alcohol and other drug use, and 'distal background factors', such as personal history, long-standing cognitive and behavioural variables and personality traits that provide a context or set of vulnerabilities for alcohol and other drug use and may act as maintaining factors [71].

25.4.3 Coping Skills Therapy

The four main components of Coping Skills Therapy are relapse prevention training, social and communication skills training, training in coping with urges and cravings and mood management. Monti and Rohsenow [51] also used Cue Exposure Therapy to extinguish alcohol-related cues and to enable an environment to test out coping skills.

Although there are several positive studies linking cues to relapse, cue exposure has not shown the same effectiveness in alcohol and other drug use treatment as it has in other mental health areas, such as post-traumatic stress, obsessive-compulsive and panic disorders (e.g. Kavanagh et al. [36]).

Project MATCH, the largest alcohol treatment outcome study, used a modified version of Coping Skills Therapy as the cognitive behavioural arm of the study [51] and found it equally as effective as Motivational Enhancement and 12-Step Facilitation.

25.4.4 Mindfulness-Based Cognitive Behavioural Approaches

Mindfulness interventions are derived from the Buddhist practice of 'mindfulness' which involves purposeful attention to the present and an openness to accept things as they are [65]. There are a number of mindfulness-based therapies that are part of the cognitive behavioural therapy family.

Mindfulness-Based Relapse Prevention (MBRP) was developed specifically for substance use and integrates traditional relapse prevention with mindfulness-based meditation practices [74]. In a review of Mindfulness-Based Relapse Prevention [23], found significant improvements on withdrawal and craving symptoms, and negative consequences of substance use with Mindfulness-Based Relapse Prevention compared to Relapse Prevention, health education, Cognitive Therapy and treatment as usual. Studies have shown reductions in alcohol and other drug use and craving and increases in acting with awareness and acceptance using mindfulness strategies [19].

Although Acceptance and Commitment Therapy has shown some good outcomes [40], there have been few well-conducted empirical studies from which to draw conclusions. Dialectical Behaviour Therapy, which blends traditional cognitive behavioural approaches with Zen buddhism was oroginally developed for people with borderline personality didorder but has also been found to be effective for people with alcohol and other drug problems [25].

There is a limited, but growing, research base for mindfulness-based therapies more generally. Hofmann et al. [31] argue that the proposed differences between mindfulness-based and traditional cognitive behavioural therapies do not require a separate classification of these treatments and have shown that the outcomes from both are about equivalent.

25.5 Variations in Cognitive Behavioural Therapies for Alcohol and Other Drug Problems

25.5.1 Brief Cognitive Behavioural Therapies

A number of brief cognitive behavioural interventions have been developed, primarily based on relapse prevention or coping skills therapy. In general, brief cognitive behavioural interventions are best utilised for moderate- to high-risk use and with people who are dependent but are not ready to engage in intensive treatment. They have been found to be effective for a range of people who use alcohol and other drugs, including those who are severely dependent.

Brief cognitive behavioural interventions have also been shown to assist with cocaine, alcohol and polydrug dependences and with drug-related problems such as insomnia (see [43] for a review) and drug-related harms [18].

A brief six-session intervention for cannabis dependence [34] has also been developed in Australia, using a combination of Motivational Interviewing and Relapse Prevention. Sessions include goal setting, planning to quit, dealing with lapses and relapses, refusal skills, managing withdrawal and cognitive and coping skills.

In addition, a range of brief therapies (one to two sessions) and brief interventions (5–20 minutes) for moderate- to high-risk drinking have been developed, based on social learning and cognitive behavioural therapy principles, including coping skills and relapse prevention strategies [67].

In Australia, Baker et al. [3] developed an intervention for people who use amphetamines that combined Motivational Interviewing with two or four sessions of brief Relapse Prevention, including coping with cravings and lapses, controlling thoughts about using (triggers, seemingly irrelevant decisions and pleasant activity scheduling) and relapse prevention (refusal skills and relapse planning). People with methamphetamine related problems can be difficult to engage and retain in treatment, and a briefer intervention may be more desirable for this group.

25.5.2 Low-Intensity Cognitive Behavioural Therapies

'Low-intensity' interventions are those that are low intensity for the practitioner or service and sometimes, but not always, less intensive for the client. They can be delivered face to face, usually by non-specialists in the field, for example, by medical practitioners delivering screening, brief intervention and referral to treatment (SBIRT), and through psychoeducational groups and 'advice clinics'. However, they are often delivered using a range of remote and self-directed technologies, such as books and paper-based materials, CD-ROMs and computers, and online media such as the Internet [54].

Low-intensity interventions have an advantage of increasing 'reach', access, flexibility and responsiveness, patient choice and cost-effectiveness of evidence-based intervention [61] and can be used to address a range of alcohol and other drug use problems from prevention to tertiary treatment. Cognitive behavioural therapies are ideally suited to the low-intensity environment because they are typically brief, structured and easily manualised.

A number of different types of low-intensity interventions have been developed in recent years. Advice clinics, for example, operate in mental health services in the UK [72] as a one-off 30-minute appointment with a clinician.

Guided self-help cognitive behavioural therapies [38] involve either paper-based or Internet-based self-directed learning materials that are supplemented by lower-intensity guidance from a practitioner as required. The practitioner is available to answer questions about the material, but otherwise, the client works through a brief programme essentially on their own.

25.5.3 Digital Cognitive Behavioural Therapies

Despite the established efficacy of interventions for alcohol and other drug use disorders, a range of factors continue to limit their impact. Leaving aside considerations of quality and fidelity of treatment delivery, a range of barriers restrict the extent to which clients can access and engage with treatment. For many clients, barriers to accessing treatment stem from the availability or practical accessibility of services [17] and from considerations of anonymity and autonomy, from difficulties with recognising problematic alcohol and other drug use behaviours and from experiences of shame [57].

Digital treatments (also known as computer-delivered interventions and computer-assisted interventions) offer a means for mitigating the impact of some or all of these barriers to care. Digital treatments offer several potential advantages over traditional delivery modalities, not least being their ability to help a greater number of people access treatment [5].

Digital treatments promise much lower barriers to accessing services, facilitated via the increasingly ubiquitous availability of the Internet, and the proliferation of Internet-capable digital devices able to deliver digital treatments (computers, tablets, and smartphones). These accessibility and resourcing advantages have driven much of the enthusiasm for digital treatment approaches and are seen as methods for reaching a larger proportion of people who would benefit from alcohol and other drug use treatment but do not access it (a 2011 US survey put this number at 90%) [68].

Barriers relating to stigma and concerns around privacy and confidentiality can likewise be moderated by decoupling treatment from interactions with clinicians and services and the anonymity of accessing information online. Finally, digital treatments may assist with delivering treatments of greater consistency and fidelity, ensuring that any individual accessing treatment receives the same quality of service.

Several early reviews of computer-delivered interventions for a range of high-prevalence mental health disorders (e.g. depression and anxiety) were promising, suggesting that this modality offered similar efficacy to traditional face-to-face delivery [5]. This early enthusiasm has been tempered by methodological issues with much of the available literature, not least the large variation in how digital treatment interventions are operationalised, delivered and evaluated.

The overwhelming majority of substance disorder-focused digital treatments have been based on cognitive behavioural therapy foundations [2], albeit with considerable variation in how cognitive behavioural therapy has been implemented and how faithfully the treatment has been represented. This variation includes the format for delivery – structured as 'sessions' that are accessed at discrete times, or more frequent, less intensive interactions. Similarly, treatments can be offered in sequential, linear formats or offer a variety of modules that users can access flexibly [22]. Some digital treatments offer only targeted components (e.g. psychoeducation, goal setting, intake monitoring and motivational enhancement [28, 55, 70]), whilst others offer more complete translations of traditional cognitive behavioural therapy [15].

Digital treatment approaches also vary in the degree of involvement of a clinician. Programs can be provided as completely self-guided activities (similar to traditional self-help approaches) or as combined self-guided/clinician-supported modalities. Clinician support is provided as structured or ad hoc contact via face to face, telephone- or video-based sessions, or text-based interactions. Digital treatment resources can also play a role as adjunctive elements supporting traditional face-to-face interventions (e.g. assisting with treatment adherence and homework compliance).

There have been a number of systematic reviews of the effectiveness of digital treatment approaches for alcohol and other drug use disorders, indicating broad preliminary support for these interventions as effective means for reducing rates of alcohol and other drug use compared to treatment-as-usual approaches [10, 46, 52].

It is difficult to estimate the overall effectiveness of cognitive behavioural therapy-based digital treatments for alcohol and other drug use disorders. The applicability of the available evidence is hampered by several factors. Firstly, there is a wide variety of digital intervention types, structures, populations and alcohol and other drug use types targeted. Secondly, there are variations in the terminology used to describe these interventions in the literature. Thirdly, whilst cognitive behavioural therapy or elements of cognitive behavioural therapy form the basis for most interventions, the degree to which any given intervention is faithfully translating cognitive behavioural therapy to a digital application varies, according to the treatment's intent and the inherent limitations of the digital technology being used. Finally, assessments of the actual effectiveness of digital modalities are complicated by whether or not clinician guidance or input is involved (although one recent meta-analytical review of guided and unguided low-intensity interventions for alcohol use found

overall small effect sizes for these interventions overall, with no significant differences between clinician guided or unguided approaches [62]).

There may be differential effectiveness for these programmes based on substance type. A 2017 meta-analysis of the effectiveness of digital treatments for illicit substances found that when viewed across all substance types, Internet-based interventions demonstrated small but significant effect sizes in terms of decreasing use compared to control conditions, and these effects appeared to be retained at follow-up, but there was too few high-quality studies to be confident that their effectiveness was uniform across specific drug types [11]. Where meta-analyses exist for specific drug types are available, they tend to echo these findings (few high-quality studies and small but significant effect sizes). For example, a 2013 review identified only ten studies of sufficient quality assessing effectiveness of digital interventions for cannabis use and reported small effect sizes post-treatment [69]. A similar systematic review in 2016 included four studies using cognitive behavioural therapy and motivational interviewing for cannabis use and also reported a small mean effect size [29].

The evidence base for digital interventions for alcohol and other drug use disorders exhibits some methodological weaknesses, including comparatively weak or inconsistent (wait list/information/treatment as usual) control conditions and comparatively infrequent reporting of follow-up outcomes. Despite enthusiasm for the potential of digital modalities to reach larger numbers of individuals requiring treatment, and indications that these modalities are somewhat effective in modifying alcohol and other drug use behaviour, the current state of the evidence supports a prudent approach be taken to their widespread adoption as stand-alone methods of treatment.

In addition, interventions have been developed for mobile phone text messaging [63], mail [35] and online-facilitated peer support [24] (see www.theshedonline.org.au for an example).

25.6   The General Application of Cognitive Behavioural Therapies to Alcohol and Other Drug Treatment

Clients rarely present to alcohol and other drug treatment with *only* alcohol and other drug disorders. Up to 80% of clients seen in alcohol and other drug treatment have co-occurring mental health issues [32], up to 80% have been exposed to at least one traumatic event in their life with nearly half screening positive for some post-trauma symptoms [49], and an estimated 50–80% have some level of functional cognitive impairment [20].

Cognitive behavioural therapies are ideally suited to alcohol and other drug treatment populations with comorbid disorders because they are highly structured, enabling those with cognitive deficits to gain benefit from the treatment, and have been well researched both in populations where these disorders are primary and in populations where these disorders co-occur with alcohol and other drug problems.

25.6.1 A General Cognitive Behavioural Model for Alcohol and Other Drug Disorders

We use a generic cognitive behavioural model that is heavily drawn from traditional models but flexible enough to accommodate newer cognitive behavioural therapies. Our cognitive behavioural model is outlined in Fig. 25.1. This model allows clinicians to develop a clear formulation of a problem and flexibly implement a variety of strategies and techniques.

The model assumes that all six elements – early experience, beliefs and schemas, triggers, and a cycle of thoughts, feelings and behaviours – are important and influence each other. Understanding each element and the relationships between them is crucial in enabling change.

Despite being mostly present-focused, cognitive behavioural therapies do recognise that *early experience* is important in the develop-

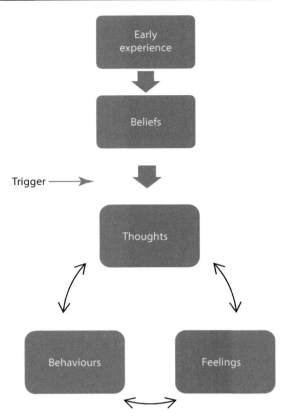

Fig. 25.1   General cognitive behavioural therapy model

ment of our fundamental beliefs. Family, social, community, environmental and personal experiences early in life all contribute to people developing core beliefs about themselves, others and the world.

Everybody's early experiences are different, even those from the same family, and the development of beliefs will therefore be highly individual. These beliefs may be 'beliefs' or 'core beliefs' or 'schemas' and can be positive or negative and often feel like facts or truths to the person.

At various times, our core beliefs may be triggered by people, places or events (external) or emotions (internal) that lead to the day-to-day thoughts that are connected to our feelings and behaviours. In this model, feelings may be feelings, emotions or sensations. There is a strong influential relationship between thoughts, feelings and actions.

25.6.2 Triggers

Careful identification of triggers and the patterns of thoughts, feelings and behaviour following the triggers maximises the selection of appropriate interventions. Assisting clients to manage triggers can be a useful first step for clients to make changes and develop some sense of control over their reactions and behaviour.

Relapse prevention, one of the most well-known forms of cognitive behavioural therapy for alcohol or other drugs problems, has an emphasis on triggers. The original focus of relapse prevention [45] was to address the important issue of relapse after cessation of alcohol and other drug use [44], although it is now used in cases of controlled use and among people who use alcohol and other drugs who are not yet abstinent.

The primary focus of relapse prevention is to identify and understand 'triggers' or 'high-risk situations' (which may be locations, people and emotions) and for the client to develop behavioural coping strategies for those situations. This may involve avoiding or changing certain triggers, for example, changing activities or routines or access to substance using paraphernalia or money.

25.6.3 Thoughts and Beliefs

Substance-related thoughts and beliefs are an important focus of investigation and intervention. Broadly, the three categories of thought and belief-based interventions are *analysing*, *challenging*, and *accepting*. Clinicians need to identify problematic thoughts and beliefs with clients and then choose in collaboration with the client the approach that best suits the situation.

Analysing approaches involve identifying thoughts and beliefs and their relationship to feelings and behaviour and considering the helpfulness or unhelpfulness of these thoughts and beliefs. Traditional cognitive therapy (Beck) and rational emotive behaviour therapy (Ellis) are examples of this approach where problematic thoughts and beliefs that maintain alcohol and other drug use, 'cognitive biases', would be identified. There are a number of categories of substance-related thoughts and beliefs that may be worthy of the clinician's attention including coping and self-efficacy (e.g. ability to cope without a substance generally or in specific situations), positive outcome expectancy (e.g. enhancement of functioning as a result of alcohol and other drug use or relief from negative internal experiences such as pain or distress) and craving and withdrawal (e.g. ability to tolerate these states).

Relapse prevention approaches consider salient beliefs about the effects of using alcohol and other drugs. Thoughts such as 'I can only relax if I have a drink' can increase the risk of lapse and relapse in specific situations, for example, during periods of high stress [50]. Therefore, self-efficacy (one's belief in one's ability to achieve a goal – in this case abstinence or controlled use) and expectancies (beliefs about the effects of alcohol and other drug use) become very important and one of the main targets of treatment.

Challenging approaches involve analysing the thoughts and beliefs as described above and utilising challenging strategies such as asking for evidence for the beliefs and looking for exceptions and contradictions and then developing modified or alternative thoughts and beliefs.

An example of this approach from relapse prevention involves identifying the thoughts and beliefs that might occur should a client lapse (one instance of alcohol and other drug use following a period of abstinence) and find themselves moving towards a relapse (return to fully using alcohol and other drugs), a phenomenon known as the 'abstinence violation effect'. Thoughts underlying an abstinence violation effect are usually associated with perceived loss of control and self-blame, for example, 'I've blown it so I might as well use whatever I want...'. A challenging approach would in advance identify these thoughts and beliefs, challenge their accuracy and develop alternative less risky beliefs.

Accepting approaches involve noticing and accepting thoughts and beliefs without judgement or necessary further action. This approach is consistent with Acceptance and Commitment Therapy that grew from the same radical behaviourist perspective as applied behaviour analysis [26]. The central components are cognitive diffusion (i.e. learning not to place a high importance on thoughts), acceptance of thoughts without judgement and commitment to action based on one's core values. It is also used in other more traditional cognitive behavioural therapies.

25.6.4 Feelings

A criticism levelled at cognitive behavioural therapies has been that the role of emotions has been undervalued. However, as stated earlier, in our model, 'feelings' are considered an essential element that influences and is influenced by the other elements. Likewise, in the relapse prevention model, negative emotional states are a focus as they both trigger and maintain alcohol and other drug use and are considered one of the main predictors of relapse [75]. Therefore, clinicians need to explore feeling states with clients and have strategies to intervene with feelings as required.

If feelings have been identified as an area requiring intervention, a number of strategies can be utilised. These include understanding emotions, identifying the relationship between emotions and alcohol and other drug use (including emotions as a trigger for and a consequence of alcohol and other drug use), emotion regulation, distress tolerance (including mood and urge surfing) and mindfulness.

Our model can be utilised to assist clients with alcohol and other drug issues to understand and identify emotions by selecting an example of the presenting issue, exploring the elements of the model and asking clients about the feeling element. We find clients may need coaching and psychoeducation about feeling states and mood monitoring homework is often of use.

With regard to emotion regulation and distress tolerance, clinicians can draw on strategies from Dialectical Behaviour Therapy, a combination of standard cognitive behavioural therapy strategies for emotion regulation and four mindfulness-oriented modules of mindfulness, distress tolerance, emotion regulation and interpersonal effectiveness. Although Dialectical Behaviour Therapy was originally developed for borderline personality disorder (BPD), it has been recommended by its developers as most suitable for very complex alcohol and other drug use disorder presentations. This includes people with co-occurring alcohol and other drug use and BPD, alcohol and other drug use disorder and chronic suicidality, and alcohol and other drug use disorder that has not responded to traditional cognitive behavioural therapy over time, especially if emotional regulation is a key factor in relapse. It is not considered a first-line treatment for uncomplicated alcohol and other drug use disorder.

Mindfulness approaches focusing on the cultivation of acceptance of negative feelings and relaxation strategies to regulate affect may also be useful where the clinician has identified that intervention is required with a client's 'feeling' states.

25.6.5 Behaviour

It is essential that clinicians consider a client's behaviour when attempting to assist them to change a pattern of ongoing alcohol and other drug use. Intervening at the behavioural level can focus on the substance using behaviour itself or on behaviours strongly associated with the alcohol and other drug use. Behavioural change can not only reduce health risks for a client but can also increase their sense of efficacy.

There are a number of alcohol and other drug specific approaches that focus on behaviour. As described above, relapse prevention identifies triggers with the purpose of changing or modifying behaviour to reduce or eliminate the impact of the trigger, for example, planning a different route home not past the bottle shop, or not listening to music associated with alcohol and other drug use. Relapse prevention approaches emphasise behavioural strategies to manage cravings, for example, relaxation, distraction or attention switching.

Coping skills therapy was developed by Monti and Rohsenow [51], initially in conjunction with cue exposure therapy, and has many similarities to relapse prevention. Like relapse prevention, it is based on social learning theory [51] but focuses more heavily on learning behavioural coping skills, and less on cognitive skills, in high-risk situations. It also teaches specific social skills to both improve relationships that have been damaged through alcohol or other drug use and to help develop healthy, non-using social networks [4].

Other cognitive behavioural approaches, not specific to alcohol and other drugs, are often useful for clients with alcohol and other drug use issues, including activity scheduling, and anger, depression and anxiety management (particularly when mood has been identified as a trigger for alcohol and other drug use).

25.7 International Considerations

Cognitive behavioural therapies have their origins in the developed world and are heavily based on western concepts and models of illness [59]. However, it is a broad and flexible model of care based on a well-grounded treatment formulation that can accommodate cultural and other influences and as a result has been adapted and successfully used across a number of cultures.

For example, in some cultures, such as many Indigenous groups, collective history is an important component of their world view [59], or in cognitive behavioural terms, 'core beliefs'. Although cognitive behavioural therapies do not delve deeply into the past to routinely reappraise it, past issues are not precluded when they are driving or maintaining current problems, and cognitive behavioural therapies can easily accommodate these types of cultural differences.

Hodges and Oei [30] have examined the compatibility of cognitive behavioural therapies with Chinese values and have identified a number of potential issues, including the value Chinese and other Asian cultures place on conformity, certainty and discipline, persistence and a strong work ethic, and respect for authoritarian systems. In Asia more broadly, there is also a high level of stigma around mental health issues and a tendency for somatisation (expressing mental health issues as physical symptoms).

Hodges and Oei [30] argue that because cognitive behavioural therapies are structured and can be adapted to a more instructive rather than collaborative style, it may suit cultural contexts needing a more directive style. This adaptation may suit the need for certainty and authority in these cultures and can also reduce the stigma of mental health treatment by using a 'coaching' style of therapy. Finally, they note that with the expansion of cognitive behavioural therapy using Eastern and Buddhist mindfulness strategies, cognitive behavioural therapies are well suited to Asian cultures.

Cognitive behavioural therapy for mental health problems has been applied successfully in a range of diverse cultures and countries including, but not limited to, Pakistan [37], Japan [12, 42], China [58], among Latina women in the USA [16], Muslims [73] and Indigenous Australians [1] using a more narrative style of delivery, sometimes referred to as 'bush Cognitive Behaviour Therapy' [9]. Although many of these studies are not specifically related to alcohol and other drug use disorders, the cross-cultural applications still apply.

25.8 Summary

Cognitive behavioural therapies encompass a wide range of therapies that have in common a focus on thoughts and beliefs as the central driver of, and the solution to, effective emotion regulation.

They tend to be relatively brief and highly collaborative, the latter the focus of the development of the therapeutic alliance, an essential component of the application of cognitive behavioural therapy. They come in a wide range of formats, including group and individual therapy, longer-term and brief therapy and low-intensity interventions such as computerised cognitive behavioural therapy.

They are among the most researched treatments in the world; both traditional and newer models have shown effectiveness for treating alcohol and other drug use disorders. The structured and theoretical base makes it ideally suited to issues that co-occur with alcohol and other drug use problems, including common mental health problems, cognitive impairment and trauma.

It has been adapted and applied across a range of cultures and countries. Cognitive behavioural therapy is ideal for adaptation to non-Western cultures because of its flexible collaborative style and its reliance on effective case formulation.

References

1. Amaro H, Magno-Gatmaytan C, Meléndez M, Cortés DE, Arevalo S, Margolin A. Addiction treatment intervention: An uncontrolled prospective pilot study of spiritual self-schema therapy with Latina women. Subst Abus. 2010;31(2):117–25.
2. Andersson G. The internet and CBT: a clinical guide. Boca Raton: CRC Press; 2014.
3. Baker A, Kay-Lambkin F, Lee NK, Claire M Jenner L. A brief cognitive behavioural intervention for regular amphetamine users – a treatment guide. Australian Government Department of Health and Ageing: Canberra; 2003.
4. Bandura A. Social learning theory. Englewood Cliffs: Canberra: Prentice Hall; 1977.
5. Barak A, Hen L, Boniel-Nissim M, Shapira NA. A comprehensive review and a meta-analysis of the effectiveness of internet-based psychotherapeutic interventions. J Technol Hum Serv. 2008;26(2–4):109–60. https://doi.org/10.1080/15228830802094429.
6. Barrowclough C, Haddock G, Wykes T, Beardmore R, Conrod P, Craig T, et al. Integrated motivational interviewing and cognitive behavioural therapy for people with psychosis and comorbid substance misuse: randomised controlled trial. BMJ. 2010;341:c6325. https://doi.org/10.1136/bmj.c6325.
7. Beck AT, Wright FD, Newman CF, Liese BS. Cognitive therapy of substance Abuse. New York: The Guilford Press; 1993.
8. Beck JS. Cognitive therapy: basics and beyond. New York: The Guilford Press; 2011.
9. Beshai S, Clark CM, Dobson KS. Conceptual and Pragmatic Considerations in the Use of Cognitive-Behavioral Therapy with Muslim Clients. Cogn Ther Res 2013;37:197–206.
10. Bickel WK, Christensen DR, Marsch LA. A review of computer-based interventions used in the assessment, treatment, and research of drug addiction. Subst Use Misuse. 2011;46(1):4–9. https://doi.org/10.3109/10826084.2011.521066.
11. Boumparis N, Karyotaki E, Schaub MP, Cuijpers P, Riper H. Internet interventions for adult illicit substance users: a meta-analysis. Addiction. 2017;112(9):1521–32. https://doi.org/10.1111/add.13819.
12. Bowen S, Chawla N, Collins SE, Witkiewitz K, Hsu S, Grow J, et al. Mindfulness-based relapse prevention for substance use disorders: a pilot efficacy trial. Subst Abus. 2009;30(4):295–305.
13. Bowen S, Chawla N, Marlatt GA. Mindfulness-based relapse prevention for addictive behaviors: a Clinician's guide. New York: The Guilford Press; 2010.
14. Carroll KM, Manual 1. 'A cognitive-behavioral approach: treating cocaine addiction' N. I. o. D. Abuse therapy manuals for drug addiction. Rockville: National Institue on Drug Abuse; 1998.
15. Carroll KM, Ball SA, Martino S, Nich C, Babuscio TA, Nuro KF, et al. Computer-assisted delivery of cognitive-behavioral therapy for addiction: a randomized trial of CBT4CBT. Am J Psychiatry. 2008;165(7):881–8. https://doi.org/10.1176/appi.ajp.2008.07111835.
16. Chen J, Nakano Y, Ietzugu T, Ogawa S, Funayama T, Watanabe N, et al. Group cognitive behavior therapy for Japanese patients with social anxiety disorder: preliminary outcomes and their predictors. BMC Psychiatry. 2007;7(1):69.
17. Clarke D. Intrinsic and extrinsic barriers to health care: implications for problem gambling. Int J Ment Heal Addict. 2007;5(4):279–91. https://doi.org/10.1007/s11469-007-9089-1.
18. Copeland J, Swift W, Roffman R, Stephens R. A randomized controlled trial of brief cognitive–behavioral interventions for cannabis use disorder. J Subst Abus Treat. 2001;21(2):55–64.
19. Currie SR, Clark S, Hodgins DC, El-Guebaly N. Randomized controlled trial of brief cognitive–behavioural interventions for insomnia in recovering alcoholics. Addiction. 2004;99(9):1121–32.
20. Dore G, Mills K, Murray R, Teeson M, Farrugia P. Post-traumatic stress disorder, depression and suicidality in inpatients with substance use disorders. Drug Alcohol Rev. 2011;31(3):294–302.
21. Dutra L, Stathopoulou G, Basden S, Leyro T, Powers M, Otto M. A meta-analytic review of psychosocial interventions for substance use disorders. Am J Psychiatr. 2008;165(2):179–87.
22. Fairburn CG, Patel V. The impact of digital technology on psychological treatments and their dissemination. Behav Res Ther. 2017;88:19–25. https://doi.org/10.1016/j.brat.2016.08.012.
23. Grant S, Colaiaco B, Motala A, Shanman R, Booth M, Sorbero M, Hempel S. Mindfulness-based Relapse Prevention for Substance Use Disorders: A Systematic Review and Meta-analysis. J Addict Med. 2017 Sep/Oct;11(5):386–396.

24. Griffiths KM, Reynolds J. Online mutual support bulletin boards. In: Bennett-Levy J, Richards D, Farrand P, Christensen H, Griffiths KM, Kavanagh DJ, et al., editors. Oxford guide to Low intensity CBT Interventions. New York: Oxford university press; 2010.

25. Haktanır A, Callender KA. (2020). Meta-analysis of dialectical behavior therapy (DBT) for treating substance use. Research on Education and Psychology (REP), 4(Special Issue), 74–87.

26. Hayes SC. Acceptance and commitment therapy and the new behavior therapies: mindfulness, acceptance and relationship. In: Hayes SC, Follette VM, Linehan M, editors. Mindfulness and acceptance: expanding the cognitive behavioral tradition. New York: The Guilford Press; 2004. p. 1–29.

27. Hayes SC, Strosahl KD. Acceptance and commitment therapy, second edition: the process and practice of mindful change. New York: The Guilford Press; 2011.

28. Hester RK, Delaney HD, Campbell W. The college drinker's check-up: outcomes of two randomized clinical trials of a computer-delivered intervention. Psychol Addict Behav. 2012;26(1):1–12. https://doi.org/10.1037/a0024753.

29. Hoch E, Preuss UW, Ferri M, Simon R. Digital interventions for problematic Cannabis users in non-clinical settings: findings from a systematic review and meta-analysis. Eur Addict Res. 2016;22(5):233–42. https://doi.org/10.1159/000445716.

30. Hodges J, Oei TP. Would Confucius benefit from psychotherapy? The compatibility of cognitive behaviour therapy and Chinese values. Behav Res Ther. 2007;45(5):901–14.

31. Hofmann SG, Sawyer AT, Fang A. The empirical status of the "new wave" of CBT. Psychiatr Clin North Am. 2010;33(3):701.

32. Hoppes K. The application of mindfulness-based cognitive interventions in the treatment of co-occurring addictive and mood disorders. CNS Spectr. 2006;11(11):829.

33. Horvath AO, Del Re AC, Fluckiger C, Symonds D. Alliance in individual psychotherapy. Psychother. 2011;48(1):9–16. https://doi.org/10.1037/a0022186.

34. Kadden R, Carroll K, Donovan D, Cooney N, Monti P, Abrams D, et al. Cognitive Behavioral Coping Skills Therapy Manual – A Clinical Research Guide for Therapists Treating Individuals With Alcohol Abuse and Dependence M. E. Mattson *Project Match Monograph Series*. Rockville: U.S.Department of Health and Human Services Public Health Service National Institutes of Health; 2003.

35. Kavanagh DJ, Connolly J, White A, Kelly A, Parr J. Low intensity CBT by mail. In: Bennett-Levy J, Richards D, Farrand P, Christensen H, Griffiths KM, Kavanagh DJ, et al., editors. Oxford guide to Low intensity CBT Interventions. New York: Oxford University Press; 2010.

36. Kavanagh DJ, Sitharthan G, Young RM, Sitharthan T, Saunders JB, Shockley N, et al. Addition of cue exposure to cognitive-behaviour therapy for alcohol misuse: a randomized trial with dysphoric drink-ers. Addiction. 2006;101(8):1106–16. https://doi.org/10.1111/j.1360-0443.2006.01488.x.

37. Kay-Lambkin FJ, Baker AL, Lewin TJ, Carr VJ. Computer-based psychological treatment for comorbid depression and problematic alcohol and/or cannabis use: a randomized controlled trial of clinical efficacy. Addiction. 2009;104(3):378–88.

38. Kenwright M. Introducing and supporting written and internet-based guided CBT. In: Bennett-Levy J, Richards D, Farrand P, Christensen H, Griffiths KM, Kavanagh DJ, et al., editors. Oxford guide to Low intensity CBT Interventions. New York: Oxford university press; 2010.

39. Leahy R. Roadblocks in cognitive-behavioral therapy: transforming challenges into opportunities for change. New York: Guilford Press; 2003.

40. Lee EB, An W, Levin ME, Twohig MP. An initial meta-analysis of acceptance and commitment therapy for treating substance use disorders. Drug Alcohol Depend. 2015;155:1–7. https://doi.org/10.1016/j.drugalcdep.2015.08.004.

41. Linehan M. Borderline personality disorder: concepts, controversies, and definitions. *Cognitive-Behavioral Treatment of Borderline Personality Disorder*. New York: The Guildord Press; 1993.

42. Luoma JB, Kohlenberg BS, Hayes SC, Bunting K, Rye AK. Reducing self-stigma in substance abuse through acceptance and commitment therapy: model, manual development, and pilot outcomes. Addict Res Theory. 2008;16(2):149–65.

43. Magill M, Ray LA. Cognitive-behavioral treatment with adult alcohol and illicit drug users: a meta-analysis of randomized controlled trials. J Stud Alcohol Drugs. 2009;70(4):516–27.

44. Marlatt AG, Donovan DM. Relapse prevention: maintenance strategies in the treatment of addictive behaviors. New York: The Guilford Press; 2005.

45. Marlatt AG, Gordon JR. Relapse prevention: maintenance strategies in the treatment of addictive behaviors. New York: The Guilford Press; 1985.

46. Marsch LA, Dallery J. Advances in the psychosocial treatment of addiction: the role of technology in the delivery of evidence-based psychosocial treatment. Psychiatr Clin North Am. 2012;35(2):481–93. https://doi.org/10.1016/j.psc.2012.03.009.

47. Mausbach BT, Moore R, Roesch S, Cardenas V, Patterson TL. The relationship between homework compliance and therapy outcomes: an updated meta-analysis. Cogn Ther Res. 2010;34(5):429–38. https://doi.org/10.1007/s10608-010-9297-z.

48. McHugh RK, Hearon BA, Otto MW. Cognitive-behavioral therapy for substance use disorders. Psychiatr Clin North Am. 2010;33(3):511.

49. Mills K, Deady M, Proudfoot H, Sannibale C, Teesson M, Mattick R, et al. Guidelines on the management of co-occuring mental health conditions in alcohol and other drug treatment settings. Sydney: National Drug and Alcohol Research Centre, University of New South Wales; 2009.

50. Mitcheson L, Maslin J, Meynen T, Morrison T, Hill R, Wanigaratne S, et al. Applied cognitive and behavioural approaches to the treatment of addiction: a practical treatment guide. Chichester: Wiley; 2010.

51. Monti PM, Rohsenow DJ. Coping-skills training and cue-exposure therapy in the treatment of alcoholism. Alcohol Res Health. 1999;23(2):107–15.

52. Moore BA, Fazzino T, Garnet B, Cutter CJ, Barry DT. Computer-based interventions for drug use disorders: a systematic review. J Subst Abus Treat. 2011;40(3):215–23. https://doi.org/10.1016/j.jsat.2010.11.002.

53. Neisser U. Cognitive psychology. New York: Appleton-Century-Crofts; 1967.

54. NICE. 'Generalised anxiety disorder in adults: management in primary, secondary and community care' N. C. C. f. M. Health. Leicester: Tthe British Psychological Society & The Royal College of Psychiatrists National Clinical Guideline Number 113; 2011.

55. Ondersma SJ, Chase SK, Svikis DS, Schuster CR. Computer-based brief motivational intervention for perinatal drug use. J Subst Abus Treat. 2005;28(4):305–12. https://doi.org/10.1016/j.jsat.2005.02.004.

56. Padesky CA. Socratic questioning: changing minds or guiding discovery? Invited keynote address presented at the 1993 European Congress of Behavioural and Cognitive Therapies. London; 1993. Available at: http://padesky.com/newpad/wp-content/uploads/2012/11/socquest.pdf.

57. Priester MA, Browne T, Iachini A, Clone S, DeHart D, Seay KD. Treatment access barriers and disparities among individuals with co-occurring mental health and substance use disorders: An integrative literature review. J Subst Abus Treat. 2016;61:47–59. https://doi.org/10.1016/j.jsat.2015.09.006.

58. Rahman A, Malik A, Sikander S, Roberts C, Creed F. Cognitive behaviour therapy-based intervention by community health workers for mothers with depression and their infants in rural Pakistan: a cluster-randomised controlled trial. Lancet. 2008;372(9642):902.

59. Rathod S, Kingdon D. Cognitive behaviour therapy across cultures. Psychiatry. 2009;8(9):370–1.

60. Rawson RA, Shoptaw SJ, Obert JL, McCann MJ, Hasson AL, Marinelli-Casey PJ, et al. An intensive outpatient approach for cocaine abuse treatment: the matrix model. J Subst Abus Treat. 1995;12(2):117–27.

61. Rees V, Copeland J, Swift W, Technical Report No. 64. A brief cognitive-behavioural intervention for cannabis dependence: Therapists' treatment manual. Sydney: National Drug and Alcohol Research Centre University of New South Wales; 1998.

62. Riper H, Blankers M, Hadiwijaya H, Cunningham J, Clarke S, Wiers R, et al. Effectiveness of guided and unguided low-intensity internet interventions for adult alcohol misuse: a meta-analysis. PLoS One. 2014;9(6):e99912. https://doi.org/10.1371/journal.pone.0099912.

63. Shapiro JR, Bauer S. Use of the short message services (SMS)-based interventions to enhance low intensity CBT. In: Bennett-Levy J, Richards D, Farrand P, Christensen H, Griffiths KM, Kavanagh DJ, et al., editors. Oxford guide to Low intensity CBT Interventions. New York: Oxford University Press; 2010.

64. Shoptaw S, Rawson RA, Worley M, Lefkowith S, Roll JM. Psychosocial and behavioral treatment of methamphetamine dependence. In: Roll JM, Rawson RA, Ling W, Shoptaw S, editors. Methamphetamine addiction: from basic science to treatment. New York: The Guilford Press; 2009. p. 185.

65. Siegel RD, Germer CK, Olendzki A. Mindfulness: What Is It? Where Did It Come From?. In: Didonna F. (eds) Clinical Handbook of Mindfulness. Springer, New York, NY; 2009.

66. Stoltenberg CD, Pace TM. The scientist-practitioner model: now more than ever. J Contemp Psychother. 2007;37(4):195–203. https://doi.org/10.1007/s10879-007-9054-0.

67. Substance Abuse and Mental Health Services Administration 34. 'Quick guide for clinicians based on TIP 34 – brief interventions and brief therapies for substance abuse'. Center for substance abuse treatment quick guide for clinicians based on TIP 34. Substance Abuse and Mental Health Services Administration Center for Substance Abuse Treatment; 2012.

68. Substance Abuse and Mental Health Services Administration. Results from the 2011 national survey on drug use and health: summary of national findings. NSDUH series H-44. Rockville: Substance Abuse and Mental Health Services Administration HHS Publication No. (SMA) 12-4713; 2012.

69. Tait RJ, Spijkerman R, Riper H. Internet and computer based interventions for cannabis use: a meta-analysis. Drug Alcohol Depend. 2013;133(2):295–304. https://doi.org/10.1016/j.drugalcdep.2013.05.012.

70. Walters ST, Ondersma SJ, Ingersoll KS, Rodriguez M, Lerch J, Rossheim ME, et al. MAPIT: development of a web-based intervention targeting substance abuse treatment in the criminal justice system. J Subst Abus Treat. 2014;46(1):60–5. https://doi.org/10.1016/j.jsat.2013.07.003.

71. Wenzel A, Liese BS, Beck AT, Friedman-Wheeler DG. Group cognitive therapy for addictions. New York: The Guilford Press; 2012.

72. White J. The STEPS model: a high volume, multi-level, mulit-purpose approach to address common mental health problems. In: Bennett-Levy J, Richards D, Farrand P, Christensen H, Griffiths KM, Kavanagh DJ, et al., editors. Oxford guide to low intensity CBT interventions. New York: Oxford University Press; 2010.

73. Williams M, Foo K, Haarhoff B. Cultural considerations in using cognitive behaviour therapy with Chinese people: a case study of an elderly Chinese woman with generalised anxiety disorder. N Z J Psychol. 2006;35(3):153.

74. Witkiewitz K, Bowen S, Douglas H, Hsu SH. Mindfulness-based relapse prevention for substance craving. Addict Behav. 2013;38(2):1563–1571.

75. Witkiewitz K, Marlatt GA. Relapse prevention for alcohol and drug problems: that was Zen, this is Tao. Am Psychol. 2004;59(4):224–35. https://doi.org/10.1037/0003-066x.59.4.224.

76. Wolpe J. The practice of behavior therapy. New York: Pergamon Press; 1973.

Key Reading

Beck JS. Cognitive therapy: basics and beyond. New York: The Guilford Press; 2011.

Bowen S, Chawla N, Marlatt GA. Mindfulness-based relapse prevention for addictive behaviors: a clinician's guide. New York: The Guilford Press; 2010.

Bennett-Levy J, Richards D, Farrand P, Christensen H, Griffiths KM, Kavanagh DJ, Klein B, Lau MA, Proudfoot J, Ritterband L, White J, Williams C. Oxford guide to low intensity CBT interventions. New York: Oxford University Press; 2010.

Mitcheson L, Maslin J, Meynen T, Morrison T, Hill R, Wanigaratne S. Applied cognitive and behavioural approaches to the treatment of addiction: a practical treatment guide: Wiley; 2010.

Witkiewitz K, Marlatt GA. Relapse prevention for alcohol and drug problems: that was Zen, this is Tao. Am Psychol. 2004;59(4):224–35.

Psychodynamic Psychotherapy for the Treatment of Substance Use Disorders

26

E. J. Khantzian

Contents

Abstract

An understanding of addiction to drugs and alcohol and their treatment is reviewed from a modern-day psychodynamic perspective drawing on ego/self-psychology and object relations and attachment theory. The author places emphasis on addictions as a self-regulation disorder. Deficits in regulating emotions, self-esteem, relationship, and self-care interact variably and cause individuals so affected to relieve their pain and suffering associated with these deficits with addictive substances and to become addicted to them. The author considers addictive drugs to be appealing not so much as pleasure producing but rather as agents that create and foster comfort and contact for individuals who are discomforted and disconnected. Alcohol and drugs, short term, relieve and/or change states of anhedonia, dysphoria, and unbearable painful emotional states. Individuals so affected discover that depending on the particular emotional pain with which they suffer, they discover a preference for a particular class of drugs. The action of each class of drugs is linked to how individuals discover these specific effects in relation to the suffering associated with their self-regulation problems. Appreciating these vulnerabilities and in contrast to outmoded psychoanalytic modes of detachment, passivity, and more strictly interpretive approaches, the author considers, from a contemporary perspective, important therapeutic elements and attitudes necessary to address the vulnerabilities such as being more

E. J. Khantzian (✉)
Department of Psychiatry, Harvard Medical School, Boston, MA, USA
e-mail: drejk26@comcast.net

© Springer Nature Switzerland AG 2021
N. el-Guebaly et al. (eds.), *Textbook of Addiction Treatment*,
https://doi.org/10.1007/978-3-030-36391-8_26

interactive and to incorporate attitudes of kindness, support, empathy, respect, patience, and instruction in order to build and maintain a strong therapeutic alliance.

Keywords

Psychodynamics · Affects · Self-medication · Self-regulation

26.1 Introduction

Psychodynamic psychotherapy rests on the principle that important psychological factors are at the root of addictive behaviors and that these factors can be identified, targeted, and modified in the treatment relationship and thus eliminate or make less likely a reliance on addictive substances. We have reviewed elsewhere [5] early psychoanalytic formulations, that with a few exceptions, emphasized the use of addictive drugs as a regressive, pleasurable adaption, whereas more contemporary formulations have placed emphasis on a progressive adaptation where addictive substances serve to cope with painful internal states and conditions and overwhelming external realities. Contemporary psychodynamic psychiatrists dating back to the 1960s and 1970s have reported on the nature of addictive vulnerability based on an appreciation of factors from structural, ego/self, and object relations perspectives. These perspectives underscore how disturbances and vulnerabilities in experiencing and processing emotions, sense of self/self-esteem, interpersonal relations, and behaviors are important if not essential factors for the development and maintenance of addiction to substance of abuse. Although there is empirical data supporting the efficacy of psychodynamic psychotherapy for a range of psychiatric disorders, including treatment of addictive disorders [4, 13, 21], there is a rich clinical literature describing how an appreciation of the underlying dynamics of addictive behavior can be fathomed and targeted in individual and group therapy to help addicted individuals understand and modify

these dynamics and overcome their addictive attachments and behaviors [4]. Although individual psychotherapy is the primary focus here, this treatment modality should not or need not compete with complimentary or alternative treatments when psychodynamic findings indicate the need for additional or alternative treatment as will be discussed subsequently.

What is reviewed in this chapter derives mainly from clinical work with drug-dependent individuals. This chapter rests on the assumption that the case method and the treatment relationship (practice-based evidence) yields rich data that illuminates the nature of addictive disorders and provides keys to understand and treat patients who suffer with addictive illness. We will emphasize the more contemporary formulations that provide a basis to appreciate the vulnerabilities that underlie reliance on addictive substance and behaviors, and how individual and group psychotherapy can ameliorate addictive suffering and modify addictive behavior.

26.2 Addiction as a Self-Regulation Disorder

Addictive disorders are rooted in suffering – not pleasure seeking or self-destructive motives as early psychodynamic formulations suggested. The suffering is mainly a consequence of addicted individual's inability to regulate their emotions, self-esteem, relationships, and behavior, especially their self-care [13]. From the earliest phases of infancy through early adult development, environmental influences around parenting, safety, comfort, traumatic abuse/neglect, and peer relationships are crucial in influencing self-regulation capacities; and significantly, experiences from earliest phases of development, for which there are no memories or symbolic representations, have some of the most profound influences [8, 17, 20]. In this respect, these developmental factors weave their way through addictively prone individuals' ways of experiencing their emotions, sense of self, relationships, and behaviors to make addictions more likely. In what follows, I will elaborate on these self-regulation problems and how appreciation of the dynamics involved can guide effective individual and group therapeutic responses.

26.2.1 Disordered Emotions

Contemporary psychodynamic views have placed heavy emphasis on how addictively prone individuals suffer in the extreme with their emotions. Affect life at one extreme is perplexing, elusive, cut-off, or absent, and at the other extreme, feelings are overwhelming and unbearable. Terms such as alexithymia, disaffected, anhedonia, and non-feeling states have been adopted to capture how feelings are not available, elusive, and disconnected, thus causing individuals so effected to feel empty, cut-off, and unable to use their emotions to guide their reactions and behavior [17–19]. Krystal and Raskin [18] appreciated some of the bases of these deficits when they described how feeling life has a normal developmental line (and potential for arrest or regression secondary to trauma or neglect) and how at the outset of life feelings are undifferentiated (i.e., anxiety cannot be distinguished from depression), that feelings are somatized, and without words (alexithymic). Addictively prone individuals at the other extreme suffer because feelings are intense, overwhelming, and unbearable. In this respect, more recent psychoanalytic investigators stressed defects in affect and drive defense and deficits in psychological structure to explain how substance-dependent individuals adopt addictive drugs to make intolerable feelings more bearable, especially those involving rage and aggression [10, 23, 24].

These same investigators have elaborated on how addictive drugs can stimulate and enliven individuals who are cut-off or feel vacuous or help to contain disorganizing and intense emotions when such affect is threatening or overwhelming. In these reports, the activating properties of stimulants and the releasing effects of low to moderate doses of depressants are described as correctives for individual experiencing their feelings as cut-off or vacuous [9, 11,

12]. Weider and Kaplan [23] coined the term "drug-of-choice," elaborating on how individuals self-select addictive drugs as a "prosthetic" to cope with overwhelming adolescent anxiety. The works of Wurmser [24] and Khantzian [11] emphasized the calming or muting action of opiates or obliterating doses of alcohol, especially for feelings of rage and aggression. What should be emphasized here is that these reports better focused on and appreciated how addictive drugs were used not for pleasure or self-destructive motives as early psychoanalytic studies stressed, but more precisely to selectively alleviate or make more tolerable affects that were confusing, unbearable, or intolerable.

More recently, Khantzian (2002, 2012) has considered some of the more subtle psychodynamics of addictive behavior that are insufficiently considered, namely, why so much of addictive behavior unfortunately continues to be linked to pleasure seeking (especially by neuroscientists) and how and why seeking relief from addictive drugs most usually produces more suffering than it relieves yet addicted individuals persist in their use of their drugs. In the former instance, especially those who are alexithymic and confused about their feelings, addicted individuals wittingly and unwittingly substitute the suffering which they perpetuate and control with use for the suffering they do not understand or control. The operative changes from simply relieving suffering, for one of control where they better understand and control it. In the second case, Khantzian [13] has speculated, based on clinical observations, that addicted individuals often suffer with pervasive anhedonia and that the often magical relief they first experience with their drug of choice is experienced as euphoric, which is interpreted as pleasure, when in fact it is the result of relief of the anhedonia.

26.2.2 Disordered Relations with Self and Others

Dating back to the seminal contributions of self-psychologist Heinz Kohut [15, 16], recent formulations have underscored the faulty and troubled ways addictively inclined individuals suffer with troubled inner states of discomfort about self. Inner states of cohesion and well-being are lacking and lead to periodic and/or chronic feelings of helplessness, fragmentation, impoverishment, shame, and a low sense of self-worth; as a consequence, feelings of rage and defensive postures of omnipotence and bravado often result to mask underlying feelings of emptiness and inadequacy [13]. Dodes [2, 3] has emphasized how feelings of helplessness and compensatory narcissistic rage are major factors leading to drug use and relapse. On this basis, he formulated that addictions are a compulsive disorder and thus subject to traditional psychodynamic psychotherapy. Along similar lines, Director [6] focused on feelings of powerlessness, unimportance, and compensatory reactions of omnipotence to explain recurrent relapse to addictive drugs in her work with two addicted women.

The importance of these perspectives is that clinicians must be sensitive and fine tune to the troubled sense of self and painful lack of self-regard drug dependent struggle with and to be appreciative of how the off-putting defensive characteristics can be understood as necessary postures to avoid narcissistic collapse. Furthermore, these findings indicate the significance of appreciating how such dynamics basically interweave with the compulsion to self-medicate the emotional pain such dynamics engender.

Troubled sense of self and self-esteem issues powerfully interact with relational difficulties for substance-dependent individuals. The early psychoanalytic literature linked addictions to pathological or problematic dependency. In contrast, contemporary psychodynamic views underscore problems of interpersonal isolation and counterdependence. Although drug-dependent individuals suffer from enduring troubled, disrupted, and often traumatizing histories, experiencing or expressing their needs for connection and comfort with others that they so desperately need cannot be dared or accepted. As a consequence, feeling lonely, cut off, and alienated becomes a tragic way of life. Psychodynamic explorations of these attachment problems, more often infan-

tile in origin, reveal how such adaptation is powerfully connected to addictive use of substance to deal with the associated distress and the pain perpetuating defenses of self-sufficiency, disavowal of need, and counterdependence ([7, 13, 22], Weegmann 2004).

Considering how these problems with sense of self, self-worth, and relational difficulties cause drug-dependent individuals so much pain and difficulty in tolerating distress and interactions with others, it should not be surprising the action of addictive drugs provides temporary relief and "solutions" to their intrapsychic and interpersonal pain and difficulties. Stimulants can counter states of helplessness, enfeeblement, and deflation in narcissistically injured individuals as well as provide a psychic boost for deflated self-esteem; or opiates can contain or offset the dysphoria that comes with disorganizing rage and make connections to others less threatening [2, 12, 13]. Low to moderate doses of alcohol can help shamefully restricted individuals, briefly, and therefore tolerably, to breakthrough and connect with others [18].

These examples offer support for the recurrent clinical observation of why and how addictive substances become so compelling in individuals who suffer with an injured sense of self, poor self-esteem, and problematic interpersonal relations.

26.2.3 Disordered Self-Care[1]

Khantzian [13] and Khantzian and Mack [14] have described a fundamental ego function involved in life and in addictive vulnerability, namely, a capacity for self-care. Self-care functions insure safety, well-being, and survivability. They are underdeveloped or deficient in substance-dependent individuals. Early in his career, Khantzian [13] cites his experience working with intravenous heroin users in a methadone program wherein he describes his powerful subjective reaction to the idea of injecting oneself with illicit drugs; he realized that his reaction of

---

[1]The following sections on self-care and treatment are based in part on a recent report by Khantzian [14].

repugnance to that idea was one of counter-transference (modern theorists would call it an "intersubjective" response, namely, patients getting the therapist to feel something that the patient is unaware or incapable of). Tactfully sharing his recoil and discomfort with the many patients he was evaluating, Khantzian consistently and monotonously elicited reactions of little or no emotions or concerns of alarm about crossing the so-called needle barrier. Subsequently, working with abstinent drug or alcohol-dependent patients in psychotherapy, Khantzian was struck by how such lack of worry or thought persisted when no longer substance dependent. He observed these deficiencies to be involved in interpersonal and physical mishaps, slip-ups around management of important matters of unpaid premiums, lapsed licenses, and preventable medical and dental problems. It is in this context that he began to conclude that a major contributing factor to the development of addictions involved deficits in a capacity for self-care. Namely, addictively prone individuals think and feel differently about potential and real situations of harm and danger. Anxiety, fear, worry, and apprehension are deficient or absent and fail to guide such individuals in risky or self-harmful situations. There is a failure to draw cause/consequence relationship in the face of risk. Where anticipatory shame and guilt might guide when self-care capacities are better developed, in addictively prone people, shame and guilt come after the fact (e.g., "I felt stupid and bad when I did that" [rather than] "I will feel stupid and bad if I do that"). It is the combination of self-care deficits interacting with the pain and suffering involved in self-regulation difficulties that make vulnerable individuals more likely to develop addictive disorders.

26.3 Implications for Psychodynamic Psychotherapy

Treating clinicians need to constantly appreciate the underlying dynamics and vulnerabilities that govern addictive behavior. Considering the diffi-

culties addicted individuals have with regulating their emotions, sense of self/self-esteem, relationships, and self-care, therapists need to think about therapeutic elements and attitudes that would best attune and respond to the suffering and dysfunction with which patients struggle. Old psychoanalytic approaches of passivity, therapeutic detachment, and strictly interpretive methods, therefore, would not be the order of the day. In fact, such approaches could perpetuate the confusion, shame, alienation, and disconnect with which addicted patients suffer. Thus, a contemporary psychotherapist needs to be more interactive (balance talking and listening) and incorporate attitudes of kindness, support, empathy, respect, patience, and instruction in the service of building and maintaining a strong treatment alliance. These elements are essential in order to deal with and overcome the problems with inaccessible or intense emotions, shame, broken self-esteem/relationships, and poor self-care [13]. Confrontation should be avoided and used only rarely such as concerns about safety but done in a way that preserves self-esteem.

Given recent developments in use of medications in managing substance use disorders, I should emphasize here that it is clearly evident that medication-assisted treatments (MATs) are crucially important and life-saving. They should be employed to curtail and prevent the dangers of overdose, loss of control, and the emotional and behavioral instability associated with drug-alcohol problems. They also provide beneficial prosthetic support and control to safely allow the psychodynamic explorations and therapeutic interventions reviewed in this chapter.

The psychodynamic findings that have been outlined previously are considered in what follows, not only in reference to individual psychotherapy but also as they apply to considering other treatments, especially psychodynamic group therapy, as they can enhance individual therapy or be considered as alternatives when there are psychodynamic indications to do so.

Remembering how cut-off addicted patients can be with their thoughts and feelings, therapists can help significantly with these dysfunctions by actively drawing out, identifying, and labeling feelings that begin to surface or seem evident to the therapist. When patients protest they do not know what they are feeling, treating clinicians should avoid concluding it is resistance or denial but rather use such interactions to invite and support the patient to consider the challenge of exploring, discovering, and understanding their feelings and emotions. Allen, Fonagy and associates [1] (2008) have coined the term *mentalization* to emphasize one of the most basic aspects of psychotherapeutic work in general, but the concept preeminently applies to work with addicted patients, namely, to persistently focus on helping patients to access feelings, put them into words, and sustain them. Beyond individual therapy, the narrative and storytelling traditions that occur in group therapy and 12-step meetings are often very beneficial in helping patients to develop a capacity to recognize, express, and practice their own thoughts and feelings.

For those patients who struggle with and self-medicate intense and threatening emotions, particularly anger and rage, considerations and efforts should be made to help them contain and moderate the feelings that can feel so dangerous to self and others. It is worth noting how the positive treatment relationship and the therapist's concern for the safety of the patient is in and of itself a containing influence. For those whose rage and violent feeling derive from trauma and neglect, it is crucial to acknowledge and validate the legitimacy of such reactions and help them to understand how and why they have resorted to addictive drugs to contend with such intense emotions. Carefully timed and gentle explorations of the experiences that engender such emotions can gradually diminish or resolve such intense affect. In this context, judicious use of legitimate psychotropic medications targeting these affects can significantly attenuate the intensity to make the working through of these affects in psychotherapy more doable.

The support and empathy exhibited by the therapist in response to drug patients' pervasive sense of shame and broken self-esteem (predisposing and consequential) is a vital element in engaging and retaining such patients in psychotherapy. Such an approach helps in gaining inroads on the confusing and elusive ways in which the sense of self and others is experienced by substance users. Openings are created to focus on and help identify and resolve feeling of powerlessness, defensive rage, and reactions of omnipotence that are experienced and often surface in treatment. Patience, support, and kindness remain of paramount importance and allow for opportunities to therapeutically address and help the patient and the therapist, understand, and better work out problems with off-putting characteristics. These characteristics are more often reactive and defensive secondary to feelings of helplessness as well as feelings of unimportance [2, 6]. And for those who are seemingly void of emotions and disengaged, the therapist may draw on their own energy and liveliness to help activate and enliven patients who are so affected. Again, group therapy experiences often can be invaluable in this respect in instilling and validating a better sense of self/self-esteem.

The issue of low self-esteem of substance abusers is related to their tendency to be avoidant of relationships and interpersonally isolated. They feel undeserving of the care and connection to others. Remaining interactive, engaging, and empathic is an important element in responding to patients' fear of and ambivalence about relationship. Impassivity and detached interpretations can be counter-therapeutic and devastating. Tactful focus on the ambivalence can materially stimulate possibilities of beneficial connections to others. It is in this respect that the connections stimulated by individual and group therapy are extraordinarily helpful in addressing and ameliorating the attachment difficulties and sense of alienation with which substance-dependent individuals struggle.

The thoughtless and unfeeling behaviors of substance-dependent patients that are characteristic of self-care deficits become manifest in the treatment relationship by the alarm stirred in the therapist by patients' risky or dangerous behaviors. Such reactions and interactions can alert the therapist and patient to how such deficits are major factors for patients to use and relapse to additive behaviors. The therapist should be unhesitant in using their reactions of alarm and concern that patients stir to identify the lack of such reaction in the patient. Constant attention to patients' poor self-care can help instill a growing awareness of how their self-care deficits continuously leave those so affected continuously in harm's way, especially those involved with the harm and dangers associated with addictive substances. Long-term therapy often helps in getting at and understanding the developmental and environmental roots of these deficits, but a here-and-now, active, instructive approach is essential in order to stimulate and better develop a better capacity to recognize, anticipate, and avoid self-harm, particularly related to addictive substances. Finally, "We need to help patients use self-respect, feelings of apprehension/worry, relationships with others, and thoughtfulness as a guide for safe behavior and self-preservation" ([13], p.278).

26.4 Summary and Conclusion

Contemporary psychoanalytic understanding of addictive disorders has generated and documented observable, developmental, structural, ego/self, and object relations disturbances that predispose to and maintain addictive behaviors and attachments. These findings provide a basis to identify the ways in which these disturbances affect feelings, self-esteem, relationships, and self-care. They provide a basis to guide therapists in targeting these problems psychotherapeutically. Impassive and strictly interpretive approaches are contraindicated if not damaging. Modern psychotherapeutic treatments employ more interactive, supportive, and empathic attitudes and techniques to help patients and therapist to focus on vulnerabilities and dysfunction that perpetuate addictive suffering and pain. This contemporary perspective provides understanding, hope, and more effective means to overcome the compelling, self-defeating, and tragic causes and consequences of addictive disorders.

References

1. Allen JG, Fonagy P, Bateman AW. Mentalizing in clinical practice. Washington, DC: American Psychiatric Publishing, Inc; 2008.
2. Dodes LM. Compulsion and addiction. J Am Psychoanal Assoc. 1996;44:815–35.
3. Dodes LM. The heart of addiction. New York: Harper Collins; 2002.
4. Dodes LM, Khantzian EJ. Individual psychodynamic psychotherapy. In: Mack AH, Brady KT, Miller SI, Frances RJ, editors. Clinical textbook of addictive disorders. 4th ed. New York: Guilford Press; 2016. p. 548–62.
5. Dodes LM, Khantzian EJ. Individual psychodynamic psychotherapy. In: Frances RJ, Miller SI, Mack AH, editors. Clinical textbook of addictive disorders. 3rd ed. New York: Guilford Press; 2005. p. 457–73.
6. Director L. Encounters with omnipotence in the psychoanalysis of substance users. Psychoanal Dialog. 2005;15:567–86.
7. Flores PJ. Addiction as an attachment disorder. New York: Jason Aronson; 2004.
8. Gedo J. Conceptual issues in psychoanalysis: essays in history and method. Hillsdale: The Analytic Press; 1986.
9. Khantzian EJ. Self-selection and progression in drug dependence. Psychiatry Dig. 1975;10(1):9–22.
10. Khantzian EJ. The ego, the self and opiate addiction: theoretical and treatment considerations. Int Rev Psychoanal. 1978;5:189–98.
11. Khantzian EJ. The self-medication hypothesis of addictive disorders. Am J Psychiatr. 1985;142:1259–64.
12. Khantzian EJ. The self-medication hypothesis of substance use disorders: a reconsideration and recent applications. Harv Rev Psychiatry. 1997;4:231–44.
13. Khantzian EJ. Reflections on treating addictive disorders: a psychodynamic perspective. Am J Addict. 2012;21:274–9.
14. Khantzian EJ, Mack JE. Self-preservation and the care of the self: ego instincts reconsidered. Psychoanal Study Child. 1983;38:209–32.
15. Kohut H. The analysis of the self. New York: International Universities Press; 1971.
16. Kohut H. The restoration of the self. New York: International Universities Pres; 1977.
17. Krystal H. Integration and self-healing: affect, trauma alexithymia. Hillsdale/New Jersey: The Analytic Press; 1988.
18. Krystal H, Raskin HA. Drug dependence: aspects of ego functions. Detroit: Wayne State University Press; 1970.
19. McDougall J. The 'disaffected' patient: reflections on affect pathology. Psychoanal Q. 1984;53:386–409.
20. Lichtenberg JD. Psychoanalysis and infant research. Hillsdale/New Jersey: The Analytic Press; 1983.
21. Shedler J. The efficacy of psychodynamic psychotherapy. Am Psychol. 2010;65(2):98–109.
22. Walant KB. Creating the capacity for attachment: treating addictions and the alienated self. New York: Jason Aronson; 2002.
23. Weider H, Kaplan E. Drug use in adolescents. Psychoanal Study Child. 1969;24:399–431.
24. Wurmser L. Psychoanalytic considerations of the etiology of compulsive drug use. J Am Psychoanal Assoc. 1974;22:820–43.

Mindfulness-Based Approaches in Addiction Treatment

27

Andrew S. McClintock and Marianne Marcus

Contents

Abstract

Substance use disorders (SUDs) are prevalent and persistent psychiatric conditions that have damaging consequences on physical and psychological health. Recently, mindfulness-based interventions (MBIs) have been developed and tested in the treatment of SUDs. In this chapter, we discuss mindfulness concepts and practices and review the empirical literature on the efficacy of MBIs for SUDs. Our review suggests that there is substantial meta-analytic evidence that SUD populations generally benefit from MBIs. Nevertheless, when examining effects on a specific SUD (e.g., tobacco, alcohol, or opioid use disorder), the evidence base is more limited and inconsistent. Literature

A. S. McClintock (✉)
University of Wisconsin-Madison,
Madison, WI, USA
e-mail: asmcclintock@wisc.edu

M. Marcus
The University of Texas Health Science Center
at Houston, Houston, TX, USA
e-mail: marianne.t.marcus@uth.tmc.edu

© Springer Nature Switzerland AG 2021
N. el-Guebaly et al. (eds.), *Textbook of Addiction Treatment*,
https://doi.org/10.1007/978-3-030-36391-8_27

shortcomings and suggestions for future research are provided.

Keywords

Addiction · Substance use disorder · Mindfulness · Mindfulness-based intervention · Review · Efficacy

27.1 Introduction

Addiction is a chronic disease characterized by craving and impairments in behavioral control [1]. Addiction is thought to hijack reward, motivation, and memory neural circuitry [1] and, like other chronic diseases, often involves cycles of remission and relapse. Although addictions can be formed to a range of objects (e.g., gambling, sex), addictions to psychoactive substances are particularly prevalent and deleterious to physical and psychological health. The 12-month prevalence of substance use disorders (SUDs) is approximately 7.6% among US adults, with about 5.7% meeting criteria for an alcohol use disorder, 2.8% an illicit drug use disorder, and 0.8% an opioid use disorder [41]. Substance abuse is a leading cause of disability and lost work productivity and costs the United States more than $740 billion annually [36]. Moreover, each year, about 88,000 Americans die from alcohol-related causes [37], and 70,000 die from drug overdose [8]. Of particular concern is the recent mortality spike attributable to heroin, commonly prescribed opioids (e.g., oxycodone), and other synthetic opioids (e.g., fentanyl). In the United States, opioid overdose claims about 130 lives every day [8].

Given the prevalence of SUDs and the impact of SUDs on the user, those close to him or her, and society as a whole, it is imperative that SUDs be treated with demonstrably effective interventions. Over the past 25 years, there has been increasing clinical and empirical interest in the application of mindfulness-based interventions (MBIs) for SUDs. In this chapter, we will discuss the concept and practice of mindfulness, high-light the most commonly used MBIs in the treatment of SUDs, and review the evidence on the effectiveness of MBIs for reducing substance misuse and preventing substance relapse.

27.2 Mindfulness

Mindfulness refers to a mode of awareness characterized by curiosity, nonjudgment, and a present-moment focus [24]. Mindfulness involves enhanced awareness and acceptance of immediate, moment-to-moment experiences (e.g., sounds, smells, thoughts, bodily sensations). Mindfulness skills and abilities are typically developed through repeated engagement in mindfulness meditation practices [24]. During mindfulness meditation, the practitioner typically sustains attention on a meditative object (e.g., breath), notes distractions when they occur (e.g., worries about a future event), and then returns attention to the meditative object. As indicated by Segal et al. [39], if the mind wanders a hundred times during meditation practice, then the task is to simply bring it back a hundred times; the issue "is not learning to switch thoughts off, but how best we can change the way we relate to them: seeing them as they are, simply, streams of thinking, events in the mind, rather than getting lost in them" (p. 134).

There are many reasons why mindfulness may help in addiction treatment. For instance, mindfulness might facilitate increased attentional disengagement from substance-related stimuli [13], reduced cognitive preoccupation with future use [48, 49], and decreased stress, guilt, and other emotional states associated with use and relapse [4]. Importantly, mindfulness may foster *decentering* from cravings, such that cravings can be observed in a wider field of awareness, with more objectivity and less reactivity [26].

27.3 Mindfulness-Based Interventions

Over the past 40 years, mindfulness-based interventions (MBIs) have been introduced to treat various psychological and behavioral problems.

The introduction of MBIs has radically altered the trajectory of clinical theory, research, and practice. Hayes and Wilson [22] assert that mindfulness-based approaches "are not just a different way of treating traditionally conceptualized problems [...] They imply a redefinition of the problem, the solution, and how both should be measured" (p. 165). As an alternative to traditional cognitive-behavioral therapies, which focus on modifying the *content* of thoughts, MBIs aim to help patients to change how they *relate* to their thoughts [11].

Among the most popular MBIs are mindfulness-based stress reduction (MBSR; [24]), mindfulness-based cognitive therapy (MBCT; [39]), dialectical behavior therapy (DBT; Linehan,1993), and acceptance and commitment therapy (ACT; [21]). While MBSR, MBCT, DBT, and ACT have been employed in the treatment of SUDs, they were originally developed for non-SUD conditions. In contrast, mindfulness-based relapse prevention (MBRP; [4]) and mindfulness-oriented recovery enhancement [12] were specifically designed for SUD populations and explicitly target the symptoms and problems associated with SUDs. Descriptions of these approaches are provided below.

27.3.1 Mindfulness-Based Stress Reduction (MBSR)

MBSR is a psychoeducational program that provides rigorous training in mindfulness meditation to improve health and well-being. Originally designed to relieve stress in medical patients, MBSR has since been applied in a variety of settings and for a variety of conditions. The traditional MBSR program is structured as an 8-week course for groups of up to 30 participants who meet weekly for 2.5 hours and a full-day session during the sixth week. Mindfulness meditation is considered to be the main therapeutic technique in MBSR [24]. Patients receive extensive training in four formal mindfulness practices: (1) sitting meditation, which involves awareness of the breath and various contents of consciousness, (2) body scan, which involves sequential focus on

sensations in different parts of the body, (3) mindful hatha yoga, which involves mindful awareness of the body in movement, and (4) mindful walking, which involves mindfulness of sensations associated with walking. To foster mindfulness skills, patients are asked to engage in formal mindfulness practices at least 45 minutes per day, 6 days per week. Minimum qualifications for MBSR instructors include a master's degree in a mental health field, attendance at 2-week-long silent meditation retreats, an ongoing daily meditation practice, 3 years of hatha yoga experience, 2 years of experience teaching stress reduction, and attendance at a 5- or 7-day residential MBSR professional training [24].

27.3.2 Mindfulness-Based Cognitive Therapy (MBCT)

MBCT unites elements of MBSR and cognitive-behavioral therapy and is designed to prevent depressive relapse in patients in remission from recurrent major depressive disorder. Like MBSR, MBCT is delivered in a group format over eight weekly sessions and provides training in sitting meditation, body scan, mindful hatha yoga, and mindful walking. A primary goal of MBCT is to teach patients to recognize thoughts associated with depressed mood and to relate to them as passing, transient events in the mind, rather than to identify with them or regard them as accurate reflections of reality [39]. In this way, depression-related cognitions may continue to arise, though they may not exacerbate depressed mood or lead to a depressive relapse [39].

27.3.3 Dialectical Behavioral Therapy (DBT)

DBT was originally designed for suicidal patients and was later developed and refined for patients with borderline personality disorder. The traditional DBT format entails weekly individual therapy and group-based skills training and typically requires a 6- or 12-month commitment from the patient. While mindfulness meditation is thought to be the main ingredient in MBSR and MBCT, it plays a considerably smaller role in DBT. That is, DBT teaches numerous skills in addition to mindfulness, including emotion regulation, distress tolerance, and interpersonal effectiveness skills, rendering the contribution of mindfulness to be somewhat diluted. Nevertheless, mindfulness is the first set of skills taught and is integrated in the other facets of the treatment [27, 28]. The central dialectic in DBT pertains to the tension between acceptance and change, whereby the patient reaches synthesis by accepting the self while working toward change and personal development. Several modifications can be made to DBT when working with SUD populations [10]. Specifically, DBT clinicians can help patients: (a) identify the antecedents and consequences of drug use; (b) avoid drug cues; (c) improve regulation of urges, cravings, and emotions associated with drug use; and (d) increase engagement in healthy behaviors. Manuals are available to guide the individual therapy [27] and group-based skills training [28] components of the treatment.

27.3.4 Acceptance and Commitment Therapy (ACT)

ACT is a manualized behavioral treatment that has been delivered in both individual and group formats [21]. Derived from a contextual theory of language and cognition known as relational frame theory, ACT employs mindfulness techniques to promote psychological flexibility and value-oriented behavior. ACT stresses the notion that attempts to control or avoid unwanted experiences (e.g., anxiety) are ineffective and counterproductive, in that they actually serve to exacerbate the distress. Thus, clients are encouraged to embrace life fully by increasing awareness and acceptance of the full range of subjective experiences, including unpleasant cognitions, emotions, and sensations [21]. Like DBT, ACT teaches a myriad of skills and emphasizes mindfulness training to a somewhat lesser extent than MBSR and MBCT.

27.3.5 Mindfulness-Based Relapse Prevention (MBRP)

Patterned after MBSR and MBCT, MBRP was developed to specifically reduce risk and severity of SUD relapse. MBRP is typically administered in a group format in eight weekly 2-hour treatment sessions. Participants are introduced to several formal mindfulness practices (e.g., sitting mindfulness of breath) and are encouraged to apply mindfulness when encountering addiction-related triggers in day-to-day life (e.g., practicing "urge surfing" and "SOBER" [stop, observe, breath, expand awareness, and respond mindfully]). The mindfulness practices embedded in MBRP aim to raise awareness of internal (e.g., cognitions, emotions, sensations) and external (e.g., friends, physical environments) cues associated with substance use and to help patients engage in more skillful, healthy behaviors. Clinicians who provide MBRP in clinical trials typically hold at least a master's degree in psychology or related discipline and have experience with cognitive-behavioral therapy and mindfulness meditation [4].

27.3.6 Mindfulness-Oriented Recovery Enhancement (MORE)

Mindfulness-oriented recovery enhancement (MORE) is a manualized, integrative treatment that is delivered in eight to ten 2-hour group sessions. MORE draws on mindfulness training, positive psychology concepts, cognitive-behavioral therapy strategies, and insights from cognitive neuroscience to address an array of factors that underpin addictive behaviors and chronic pain. Psychoeducation, experiential exercises, and at-home mindfulness practice are emphasized. Mindfulness training is thought to serve numerous functions in MORE, including (a) greater awareness of attentional fixation on pain or addiction-related cues, (b) improved ability to shift from affective to sensory processing of pain or craving sensations, (c) increased psychological flexibility, (d) enhanced ability to reappraise maladaptive cognitions associated with negative emotions and addictive behaviors, and (e) greater savoring of naturally rewarding experiences (e.g., watching a sunset). Relative to other MBIs, MORE is unique in its focus on reward processing and eudaimonic growth. A step-by-step MORE intervention manual is available [12].

27.4 Effectiveness of Mindfulness-Based Interventions for SUD-Related Issues

A growing body of research has investigated the effectiveness of MBIs in alleviating SUD-related problems. While many studies test MBI's effects on a specific SUD (e.g., opioid use disorder), others enroll a heterogenous sample involving multiple SUDs (e.g., opioid, alcohol, and amphetamine use disorders) and test effects collapsing across SUDs. Below, we review evidence of MBI's effectiveness with heterogenous SUDs and then with the specific SUDs most commonly studied in this area of work: tobacco, alcohol, and opioid use disorders.

27.4.1 Heterogenous Substance Use Disorders

Several recent meta-analyses have documented the effectiveness of MBIs when collapsing across various SUDs. In a meta-analysis of data from 900 participants, Goldberg et al. [18] found that MBIs were superior to active control conditions in addiction-related outcomes (d = 0.27). Similarly, Li et al.'s [26] meta-analysis showed that MBIs have small-to-medium effects in reducing craving (d = 0.63) and substance misuse (d = 0.33) relative to comparison conditions.

Regarding specific interventions, Grant et al. [20] conducted a meta-analysis of nine randomized controlled trials (RCTs) that evaluated MBRP for adult participants diagnosed with SUDs (total of 901 participants). Results suggested that MBRP outperforms comparison con-

ditions on withdrawal/craving symptoms and negative consequences of substance use but not on relapse rates, frequency of use, or treatment dropout. One recent study may help to explain some of these null effects; Roos et al. [38] found that MBRP outperformed comparators among participants with highly severe affective and SUD symptoms but did not outperform comparators among participants with less severe affective and SUD symptoms. It is possible that for patients high in affective and SUD symptom severity, MBRP may help to decouple the link between emotional distress and craving [46], resulting in fewer distress-induced cravings and relapses over time.

Lee et al. [25] performed a meta-analysis of ten RCTs that assessed the impact of ACT on SUDs. Relative to active treatment comparisons (e.g., cognitive-behavioral therapy, pharmacotherapy), ACT produced small-to-medium effects on substance use outcomes at post-treatment (g = 0.29) and follow-up (g = 0.43). Importantly, ACT has demonstrated higher abstinence rates than cognitive-behavioral therapy at 18-month follow-up [19]. Luomam et al. [31] found that an ACT intervention designed to reduce shame associated with substance-related problems was effective in reducing shame and increasing long-term treatment engagement and days of abstinence among adults in a residential SUD treatment center. Results further suggested that the effects of the ACT intervention on long-term treatment engagement were mediated by levels of shame, in that those who became less ashamed about their substance-related problems later exhibited greater treatment engagement.

Regarding other MBIs, DBT has yielded better treatment retention and substance use outcomes than treatment-as-usual (TAU) in a small sample of women with SUDs and borderline personality disorder (N = 27; [30]). There is also evidence that DBT remains effective for SUDs when it is delivered with cultural adaptations; a DBT intervention that incorporated American Indian/Alaska Native cultural and spiritual practices produced a large pre-post effect (d = 1.3) on psychosocial distress among 229 adolescents in a residential SUD treatment center [2]. Garland et al. [16] recently evaluated the efficacy of MORE with homeless men with SUDs. Participants were randomized to 10 weeks of group treatment with MORE ($n = 64$), cognitive-behavioral therapy ($n = 64$), or TAU ($n = 52$). MORE was found to outperform cognitive-behavioral therapy on substance craving, post-traumatic stress, and negative affect and outperform TAU on posttraumatic stress and positive affect. Additionally, MORE was shown to have indirect effects on craving and posttraumatic stress via mindfulness skills, implying that an improvement in mindfulness skills may be at least partly responsible for some of MORE's beneficial effects [16].

Mindfulness techniques have also been incorporated into substance recovery therapeutic communities, which are highly structured groups that use social learning to promote changes in self-image, worldview, and addiction-related behaviors [9]. Mindfulness-based therapeutic communities have demonstrated significant reductions in salivary cortisol in a pre-post study with 21 participants receiving inpatient treatment for SUDs [33] and significantly greater reductions in self-reported muscle tension and emotional irritability relative to TAU at 3-month follow-up in a large quasi-experimental study ($N = 459$; [34]).

27.4.2 Tobacco Use Disorder

A recent meta-analysis [32] synthesized data from ten RCTs evaluating MBIs for smoking cessation. Results indicated that MBIs did not significantly differ from comparators in their effects on abstinence or cigarettes smoked per day. Notably, of the ten studies included in Maglione et al.'s [32] meta-analysis, only one [43] was deemed to be of good methodological quality. Vidrinee et al. [43] compared the efficacy of an MBCT intervention adapted for smoking cessation, group cognitive-behavioral therapy, and brief individual counseling in an RCT with 412 adults who smoked an average of at least five cigarettes per day over the prior year. Biochemically verified abstinence rates did not significantly differ across intervention conditions

at 4- and 26-week follow-ups. However, among participants who were smoking at the end of the treatment, MBCT participants were more likely to be abstinent at the follow-ups relative to participants in the other conditions. This finding implies that MBCT adapted for smoking cessation may be more effective than cognitive-behavioral therapy and brief individual counseling in promoting recovery from smoking lapses.

In the aforementioned Lee et al. [25] meta-analysis, subgroup analysis revealed that ACT was superior to active treatment comparisons in facilitating smoking cessation ($g = 0.42$; total of five studies). Importantly, there is evidence that the smoking cessation effects associated with bupropion can be augmented with the addition of an ACT-style behavioral intervention [17]. Also of note, ACT has produced promising smoking cessation rates when delivered by telephone [5], website [7], and smartphone application [6].

27.4.3 Alcohol Use Disorder

A burgeoning scientific literature has focused on the application of MBIs for alcohol misuse. Some studies have tested MBIs with individuals in remission from alcohol misuse, while others have been conducted with individuals with active, ongoing alcohol misuse. With regard to the latter, a recent pilot RCT [45] evaluated an 8-week Internet-delivered DBT skills training intervention for suicidal individuals who engage in heavy episodic drinking to regulate emotions. Participants who received the DBT intervention showed faster reductions in alcohol use relative to participants in the waitlist control [45]. Another pilot RCT [35] evaluated a brief MBI with 76 undergraduates who regularly binge drink. The mindfulness group reported significantly fewer binge episodes and alcohol-related consequences and higher dispositional mindfulness and self-efficacy than did a no-intervention control group [35].

There is also some evidence that MBIs can help persons in remission to avoid alcohol relapse. Preliminary evidence has been obtained from pre-post designs pilot testing MBRP adapted for the prevention of alcohol relapse (MBRP-A; [50]) and an MBI incorporating elements of MBSR, MBCT, MBRP, and ACT [44]. Building on the pilot pre-post study, Zgierska et al. [48] recently assessed the efficacy of MBRP-A in an RCT with 123 adults in early recovery from AUD. Participants received either the 8-week, group-based MBRP-A intervention plus TAU or TAU alone. Both groups exhibited improvements in drinking and related consequences over the 26-week study period, though no significant between-group differences were detected. Notably, within the MBRP-A plus TAU group, session attendance and at-home mindfulness practice time were correlated with drinking outcomes, suggesting that greater adherence to mindfulness training may be associated with less alcohol misuse [48, 49]. In another trial using RCT methodology, Garland et al. [13] compared ten sessions of MORE to ten sessions of support group with 53 low-income adults with AUD who had resided in a therapeutic community for at least 18 months. MORE was found to reduce stress and alcohol thought suppression to a significantly greater degree than did the support group. Additionally, MORE appeared to decrease alcohol-related attentional bias and increase physiological recovery from alcohol cues [13]. Thekiso et al. [42] examined whether ACT plus TAU improved outcomes relative to TAU with inpatients with AUD and a comorbid mood disorder, who at baseline were abstinent from alcohol for an average of about 50 days. Although not randomized, the two groups were matched according to diagnosis, age, and gender. The ACT intervention was an intensive (i.e., five sessions/week over 4 weeks) manualized group-based treatment tailored to problems associated with AUD and mood disorders (e.g., targeting the experiential avoidance that underpins these conditions). Compared to TAU, ACT plus TAU yielded significantly better drinking, craving, anxiety, and depression outcomes at 3-month follow-up and significantly better drinking, anxiety, and depression outcomes at 6-month follow-up [42].

27.4.4 Opioid Use Disorder

Although the effects of MBIs on opioid misuse and opioid use disorder have not been meta-analyzed to date, a few studies have investigated this topic. One RCT [29] randomized 23 opioid-dependent women with borderline personality disorder to 12 months of either DBT or nondirective therapy plus a 12-step support group. Results of urinalyses showed that opiate reductions were better maintained in the DBT group than the support group [29]. Stotts et al. [40] conducted a Stage I pilot study examining ACT as an aid in opioid detoxification. In this trial, 56 methadone-treated opioid-dependent adults were randomly assigned to 24 individual therapy sessions of either ACT or education-based drug counseling. Fear of withdrawal during detoxication was found to decrease significantly in the ACT group only. About 37% of ACT participants met criteria for successful detoxification (i.e., opioid negative urine drug screen and discontinuation of methadone treatment) compared to 19% of drug counseling participants, although this difference did not reach statistical significance ($p = 0.17$), which could be attributable to the study's small sample size [40]. Hayes et al. [23] randomized 138 opiate-addicted adults to 16 weeks of either (1) methadone maintenance alone, (2) ACT plus methadone maintenance, or (3) 12-step support program plus methadone maintenance. The ACT plus methadone maintenance group had significantly higher percentages of opiate (61%) and total drug (50%) abstinence at a 6-month follow-up urinalysis assessment relative to the methadone-maintenance-only group (28% for opiate and 12% for total drug abstinence). The ACT plus methadone maintenance group did not significantly differ from the 12-step support program plus methadone maintenance group on any of the drug outcomes [23].

Two studies [14, 47] have investigated the effects of MBIs on opioid use with non-cancer chronic pain patients, who have been shown to be at elevated risk for developing opioid use disorder [3]. Zgierska et al. [47] conducted a 26-week pilot RCT with adults with chronic low back pain who had been treated with daily opioid therapy (at least 30 mg/day of morphine-equivalent dose) for at least 3 months. Participants were randomized to either continued opioid therapy ($n = 14$) or continued opioid therapy with a group-based MBI ($n = 21$). The MBI entailed eight weekly 2-hour treatment sessions and included MBRP techniques adapted for pain management (e.g., a "pain wave surfing" exercise, adapted from MBRP's "urge surfing"). On average, opiate use declined by about 7 mg/day (morphine equivalent dose) from baseline to post-MBI and about 10 mg/day from baseline to 18 weeks post-MBI (compared to average decreases of 1.4 and 0.2 mg/day in the control condition). However, given relatively low power due to small sample size, the conditions did not differ significantly in opiate use reduction [47]. A larger study [14, 15] randomized 115 opioid-treated chronic pain patients (72% met criteria for opioid use disorder) to 8 weeks of either MORE or a support group. Compared with support group participants, MORE participants reported significantly greater reductions in desire for opioids ($d = 0.50$) and were significantly less likely to meet criteria for opioid use disorder at post-treatment, although these between-group effects were not sustained at 3-month follow-up [14, 15]. Subsequent analyses with laboratory data [14] revealed that, relative to the support group, MORE led to significantly greater pre-post treatment reductions in heart rate response and self-reported craving to opioid cues, implicating reduced opioid cue reactivity as a potential mechanism underlying MORE's effects.

27.5 Conclusion

SUDs are prevalent and have serious personal and societal consequences. Accordingly, it is imperative that we identify effective treatments for SUDs through rigorous controlled research. At present, there is substantial meta-analytic evidence that heterogenous SUD populations benefit from MBIs generally [18, 26] and MBRP [20] and ACT [25] specifically. Between-group effects in heterogenous SUD populations typically fall in the small-to-medium range, suggesting modest

yet reliable addiction-related improvements in MBIs relative to comparison conditions.

MBIs have been less frequently studied in the context of specific SUDs. Extant research does not convincingly show that MBIs are superior to comparators in the treatment of tobacco use disorder/smoking cessation [32]. MBIs have demonstrated some promising results in the treatment of alcohol use disorder [13, 42] and opioid use disorder [14, 15, 23], yet these bodies of evidence are still limited and inconsistent, and as such, inconclusive.

More rigorous scrutiny, using powerful, well-designed clinical trials, is needed to answer questions about the effectiveness and "active ingredients" of MBIs in SUD populations. In particular, the effects of MBIs on cannabis, benzodiazepine, and amphetamine use disorders are virtually unknown and deserving of future empirical attention. Additionally, because few studies have found maintenance of addiction-related effects over time, long-term follow-ups are needed and recommended for future research. Other study limitations include small sample size, reliance on self-reported drug use, and utilization of pre-post designs and inactive/waitlist controls, which do not adequately control for extraneous factors. Neuroimaging of the correlates of mindfulness-induced changes in addictive behaviors offers an important avenue for future research. We would also recommend the following: (1) additional standardization of treatment manuals to facilitate data pooling and replication, (2) measurement of the time participants spend in mindfulness practice to assess dose-response relationships, and (3) analysis of biomarkers of substance use, which may reveal different patterns of use than are suggested by self-report.

This review focused on a treatment for SUDs that is relatively safe and inexpensive. Past research has produced some positive results suggesting that MBIs may hold some promise in the treatment of SUDs. While more rigorous, large-scale studies are needed before unequivocally recommending MBI as a first-line treatment for specific SUDs, the clinical implications of employing a form of mental training to attenuate substance misuse is of unique practicality to clinicians and attractiveness to patients seeking safe substance abuse treatment.

References

1. American Society of Addiction Medicine. Definition of addiction. Accessed in 2019 at: http://www.asam.org/for-the-public/definition-of-addiction.
2. Beckstead DJ, Lambert MJ, DuBose AP, Linehan M. Dialectical behavior therapy with American Indian/Alaska native adolescents diagnosed with substance use disorders: combining an evidence based treatment with cultural, traditional, and spiritual beliefs. Addict Behav. 2015;51:84–7.
3. Boscarino JA, Rukstalis MR, Hoffman SN, Han JJ, Erlich PM, Ross S, Gerhard GS, Stewart WF. Prevalence of prescription opioid-use disorder among chronic pain patients: comparison of the DSM-5 vs. DSM-4 diagnostic criteria. J Addict Dis. 2011;30:185–94.
4. Bowen S, Chawla N, Marlatt GA. Mindfulness-based relapse prevention for addictive behaviors: a Clinician's guide. New York: Guilford Press; 2011.
5. Bricker JB, Bush T, Zbikowski SM, Mercer LD, Heffner JL. Randomized trial of telephone-delivered acceptance and commitment therapy versus cognitive behavioral therapy for smoking cessation: a pilot study. Nicotine Tob Res. 2014;16:1446–54.
6. Bricker JB, Mull KE, Kientz JA, Vilardaga R, Mercer LD, Akioka KJ, Heffner JL. Randomized, controlled pilot trial of a smartphone app for smoking cessation using acceptance and commitment therapy. Drug Alcohol Depend. 2014;143:87–94.
7. Bricker J, Wyszynski C, Comstock B, Heffner JL. Pilot randomized controlled trial of web-based acceptance and commitment therapy for smoking cessation. Nicotine Tob Res. 2013;15:1756–64.
8. Centers for Disease Control and Prevention. Understanding the epidemic. Accessed in 2019 at: http://www.cdc.gov/drugoverdose/epidemic/index.html.
9. De Leon G. The therapeutic community: theory, model, and method. New York: Springer Publishing; 2000.
10. Dimeff LA, Linehan MM. Dialectical behavior therapy for substance abusers. Addict Sci Clin Pract. 2008;4:39–47.
11. Fruzzetti AE, Erikson KM. Acceptance based interventions in cognitive-behavioral therapies. In: Dobson L, editor. Handbook of cognitive-behavioral therapies. 3rd ed. New York: Guilford; 2009. p. 347–72.
12. Garland EL. Mindfulness-oriented recovery enhancement for addiction, stress, and pain. Washington, DC: NASW Press; 2013.
13. Garland EL, Gaylord SA, Boettiger CA, Howard MO. Mindfulness training modifies cognitive, affec-

tive, and physiological mechanisms implicated in alcohol dependence: results of a randomized controlled pilot trial. J Psychoactive Drugs. 2010;42:177–92.
14. Garland EL, Manusov EG, Froeliger B, Kelly A, Williams JM, Howard MO. Mindfulness-oriented recovery enhancement for chronic pain and prescription opioid misuse: results from an early-stage randomized controlled trial. J Consult Clin Psychol. 2014;82:448.
15. Garland EL, Froeliger B, Howard MO. Effects of mindfulness-oriented recovery enhancement on reward responsiveness and opioid cue-reactivity. Psychopharmacology. 2014;231:3229–38.
16. Garland EL, Roberts-Lewis A, Tronnier CD, Graves R, Kelley K. Mindfulness-oriented recovery enhancement versus CBT for co-occurring substance dependence, traumatic stress, and psychiatric disorders: proximal outcomes from a pragmatic randomized trial. Behav Res Ther. 2016;77:7–16.
17. Gifford EV, Kohlenberg BS, Hayes SC, Pierson HM, Piasecki MP, Antonuccio DO, Palm KM. Does acceptance and relationship focused behavior therapy contribute to bupropion outcomes? A randomized controlled trial of functional analytic psychotherapy and acceptance and commitment therapy for smoking cessation. Behav Ther. 2011;42:700–15.
18. Goldberg SB, Tucker RP, Greene PA, Davidson RJ, Wampold BE, Kearney DJ, Simpson TL. Mindfulness-based interventions for psychiatric disorders: a systematic review and meta-analysis. Clin Psychol Rev. 2018;59:52–60.
19. González-Menéndez A, Fernández P, Rodríguez F, Villagrá P. Long-term outcomes of acceptance and commitment therapy in drug-dependent female inmates: a randomized controlled trial. Int J Clin Health Psychol. 2014;14:18–27.
20. Grant S, Colaiaco B, Motala A, Shanman R, Booth M, Sorbero M, Hempel S. Mindfulness-based relapse prevention for substance use disorders: a systematic review and meta-analysis. J Addict Med. 2017;11:386–96.
21. Hayes SC, Strohsal K, Wilson KG. Acceptance and commitment therapy. New York: Guilford Press; 1999.
22. Hayes SC, Wilson KG. Mindfulness: method and process. Clin Psychol Sci Pract. 2003;10:161–5.
23. Hayes SC, Wilson KG, Gifford EV, Bissett R, Piasecki M, Batten SV, Byrd M, Gregg J. A preliminary trial of twelve-step facilitation and acceptance and commitment therapy with polysubstance-abusing methadone-maintained opiate addicts. Behav Ther. 2004;35:667–88.
24. Kabat-Zinn J. Full catastrophe living: using the wisdom of your body and mind to face stress, pain and illness. New York: Random House; 2013.
25. Lee EB, An W, Levin ME, Twohig MP. An initial meta-analysis of acceptance and commitment therapy for treating substance use disorders. Drug Alcohol Depend. 2015;155:1–7.
26. Li W, Howard MO, Garland EL, McGovern P, Lazar M. Mindfulness treatment for substance misuse: a

systematic review and meta-analysis. J Subst Abus Treat. 2017;75:62–96.

27. Linehan MM. Cognitive-behavioral treatment of borderline personality disorder. New York: Guilford Press; 1993.

28. Linehan MM. DBT skills training manual. New York: Guilford Press; 2014.

29. Linehan MM, Dimeff LA, Reynolds SK, Comtois KA, Welch SS, Heagerty P, Kivlahan DR. Dialectical behavior therapy versus comprehensive validation therapy plus 12-step for the treatment of opioid dependent women meeting criteria for borderline personality disorder. Drug Alcohol Depend. 2002;67:13–26.

30. Linehan MM, Schmidt H, Dimeff LA, Craft JC, Kanter J, Comtois KA. Dialectical behavior therapy for patients with borderline personality disorder and drug-dependence. Am J Addict. 1999;8:279–92.

31. Luoma JB, Kohlenberg BS, Hayes SC, Fletcher L. Slow and steady wins the race: a randomized clinical trial of acceptance and commitment therapy targeting shame in substance use disorders. J Consult Clin Psychol. 2012;80:43–53.

32. Maglione MA, Maher AR, Ewing B, Colaiaco B, Newberry S, Kandrack R, Shanman RM, Sorbero ME, Hempel S. Efficacy of mindfulness meditation for smoking cessation: a systematic review and meta-analysis. Addict Behav. 2017;69:27–34.

33. Marcus MT, Fine PM, Moeller FG, Khan MM, Pitts K, Swank PR, Liehr P. Change in stress levels following mindfulness-based stress reduction in a therapeutic community. Addict Disord Treat. 2003;2:63–8.

34. Marcus MT, Schmitz J, Moeller G, Liehr P, Cron SG, Swank P, Bankston S, Carroll DD, Granmayeh LK. Mindfulness-based stress reduction in therapeutic community treatment: a stage 1 trial. Am J Drug Alcohol Abuse. 2009;35:103–8.

35. Mermelstein LC, Garske JP. A brief mindfulness intervention for college student binge drinkers: a pilot study. Psychol Addict Behav. 2015;29:259.

36. National Institute on Drug Abuse. Trend & statistics. Accessed in 2019 at: https://www.drugabuse.gov/related-topics/trends-statistics#supplemental-references-for-economic-costs.

37. National Institute on Alcohol Abuse and Alcoholism. Alcohol facts and statistics. Accessed in 2019 at: https://www.niaaa.nih.gov/alcohol-health/overview-alcohol-consumption/alcohol-facts-and-statistics.

38. Roos CR, Bowen S, Witkiewitz K. Baseline patterns of substance use disorder severity and depression and anxiety symptoms moderate the efficacy of mindfulness-based relapse prevention. J Consult Clin Psychol. 2017;85:1041–51.

39. Segal ZV, Williams JMG, Teasdale JD. Mindfulness-based cognitive therapy for depression: a new approach to preventing relapse. New York: Guilford Press; 2002.

40. Stotts AL, Green C, Masuda A, Grabowski J, Wilson K, Northrup TF, Moeller FG, Schmitz JM. A stage I pilot study of acceptance and commitment therapy for methadone detoxification. Drug Alcohol Depend. 2012;125:215–22.

41. Substance Abuse and Mental Health Services Administration. 2017 National survey on drug use and health (NSDUH). Accessed in 2019 at: https://www.samhsa.gov/data/sites/default/files/cbhsq-reports/NSDUHDetailedTabs2017/NSDUHDetailedTabs2017.htm#tab5-6B.

42. Thekiso TB, Murphy P, Milnes J, Lambe K, Curtin A, Farren CK. Acceptance and commitment therapy in the treatment of alcohol use disorder and comorbid affective disorder: a pilot matched control trial. Behav Ther. 2015;46:717–28.

43. Vidrine JI, Spears CA, Heppner WL, Reitzel LR, Marcus MT, Cinciripini PM, Waters AJ, Li Y, Nguyen NT, Cao Y, Tindle HA. Efficacy of mindfulness-based addiction treatment (MBAT) for smoking cessation and lapse recovery: a randomized clinical trial. J Consult Clin Psychol. 2016;84:824.

44. Vieten C, Astin JA, Buscemi R, Galloway GP. Development of an acceptance-based coping intervention for alcohol dependence relapse prevention. Subst Abus. 2010;31:108–16.

45. Wilks CR, Lungu A, Ang SY, Matsumiya B, Yin Q, Linehan MM. A randomized controlled trial of an internet delivered dialectical behavior therapy skills training for suicidal and heavy episodic drinkers. J Affect Disord. 2018;232:219–28.

46. Witkiewitz K, Bowen S. Depression, craving, and substance use following a randomized trial of mindfulness-based relapse prevention. J Consult Clin Psychol. 2010;78:362–74.

47. Zgierska AE, Burzinski CA, Cox J, Kloke J, Stegner A, Cook DB, Singles J, Mirgain S, Coe CL, Bačkonja M. Mindfulness meditation and cognitive behavioral therapy intervention reduces pain severity and sensitivity in opioid-treated chronic low back pain: pilot findings from a randomized controlled trial. Pain Med. 2016;17:1865–81.

48. Zgierska A, Burzinski CA, Mundt MP, McClintock AS, Cox J, Coe C, Miller M, Fleming M. Mindfulness-based relapse prevention for alcohol dependence: findings from a randomized controlled trial. J Subst Abus Treat. 2019;100:8–17.

49. Zgierska A, Rabago D, Chawla N, Kushner K, Koehler R, Marlatt A. Mindfulness meditation for substance use disorders: a systematic review. Subst Abus. 2019;30:266–94.

50. Zgierska A, Rabago D, Zuelsdorff M, Coe C, Miller M, Fleming M. Mindfulness meditation for alcohol relapse prevention: a feasibility pilot study. J Addict Med. 2008;2:165.

A Trauma-Informed Approach to Enhancing Addiction Treatment

28

Vivian B. Brown

Contents

Abstract

Research during the past two decades has shown that a large percentage of clients in addiction treatment have experienced multiple traumas from childhood into adulthood. Trauma is the expectation, not the exception. This chapter describes two major studies and their impact on the movement toward trauma-informed care: the Adverse Childhood Experiences (ACE) study and the Women with Co-occurring Disorders and Violence

Study. In addition to the high prevalence of trauma experienced by our client population, some of the procedures/practices in addiction treatment can be triggering or re-traumatizing. Also, staff may experience secondary traumatization or re-traumatization, particularly if they have previously experienced trauma themselves. By addressing the issue of trauma, which can lead clients to leave treatment and/or relapse, a trauma-informed program can improve engagement and retention and lead to successful outcomes. This chapter also explains the difference between trauma-specific interventions and trauma-informed care; describes the core values of a trauma-informed program; and details the components

V. B. Brown (✉)
Prototypes: Centers for Innovation in Health, Mental Health, and Substance Use Disorders, Pittsboro, NC, USA

© Springer Nature Switzerland AG 2021
N. el-Guebaly et al. (eds.), *Textbook of Addiction Treatment*,
https://doi.org/10.1007/978-3-030-36391-8_28

of trauma-informed care, including screening for trauma, multileveled training for all staff, stage-oriented treatment, trauma-sensitive supervision, and implementation of staff care/self-care. In a trauma-informed practice, staff members understand the prevalence of trauma in their clients and its impact, incorporate this knowledge into service delivery, and avoid re-traumatizing those who are seeking our help.

Keywords

Trauma · Trauma-informed care · Integrated treatment · Safety · Addiction treatment

This chapter is intended to support the work of addiction treatment providers in becoming trauma informed. Trauma-informed practice is not an additional program; rather, it is a shift in program culture and approach to service delivery. By addressing the trauma(s) that can lead clients to leave treatment and/or relapse, trauma-informed care can improve engagement and retention and lead to more successful outcomes.

Research during the past two decades has demonstrated that a large percentage of clients in drug treatment have experienced trauma at some point(s) in their lives. As defined by the Substance Abuse and Mental Health Services Administration, trauma is "an event, series of events, or set of circumstances that is experienced by an individual as physically or emotionally harmful or life threatening and that has lasting adverse effects on the individual's functioning and mental, physical, social, emotional, or spiritual well-being" [37, p. 9]. Estimates of lifetime exposure to traumatic events in the general population in the USA range from 60% to 70% [20]. In substance abuse populations, estimates range from 60% to 90% [15, 22, 33]. Overall, 20–30% of those exposed to trauma will develop post-traumatic stress disorder (PTSD). The more one is exposed to trauma, in terms of severity and duration, the higher the likelihood of a PTSD diagnosis (e.g., veterans' exposure to heavy levels of combat and trauma). However, millions of individuals who are experiencing PTSD and other sequelae of trauma go unrecognized and untreated.

This chapter begins with a focus upon two major studies from the USA and their impact on the movement toward implementation of trauma-informed care. While trauma-informed practices were developed in the USA, they are now receiving global attention, particularly in the following countries: Canada, the United Kingdom, Australia, New Zealand, and Scotland [1, 19, 21, 28, 38].

28.1 ACE Study

The most widely disseminated study of the relationship between stressful and traumatic events in childhood and long-term health effects is the Adverse Childhood Experiences (ACE) study [13], a collaborative effort between Kaiser Permanente (Felitti) in San Diego and the Centers for Disease Control and Prevention (CDC) (Anda). The study was conducted from 1995 to 1997 among 17,337 Kaiser Health Plan members. The purpose of the study was to determine the prevalence among this group of ten traumatic childhood (before the age of 18) events and the long-term effects of these experiences. The average age of the study participants was 52. The sample was almost evenly divided among men and women. Approximately 80% were White (Hispanic and non-Hispanic), 10% were Black, and 10% were Asian.

The prevalence among the group for the ten ACEs was as follows:

Psychological abuse (by parent)	11%
Physical abuse (by parent)	28%
Sexual abuse (by anyone)	22% (28% for women; 16% for men)
Emotional neglect	15%
Physical neglect	10%
Alcoholism or drug use in home	27%
Divorce or loss of a biological parent	23%
Depression or mental illness in family	17%
Mother treated violently	13%
Household member in prison	6%

An ACE score for each individual study participant was calculated by adding the number of categories of adverse events reported. Women were 50% more likely than men to have a score of 5 or higher. It should be noted that multiple incidents within a category are not scored beyond 1. This has the effect of definitely understating the findings. In addition, experiences such as encountering explicit racism and community violence were not included.

Felitti and Anda then looked at the correlation between these scores and a variety of health and behavioral health issues and risk behaviors in adulthood. In the area of addiction, the strongest relationship seen was between ACE scores and the injection of street drugs. At an ACE score of 6, there was a 46-fold increased likelihood of later becoming an injection drug user, as compared to an ACE Score of 0. The relationships between ACE scores and depression, suicidality, and chronic anxiety were also studied and showed similar results. The findings of the ACE study made it clear that traumatic events experienced in childhood have a cumulative effect on emotional state and health status, including liver disease, chronic obstructive pulmonary disease (COPD), coronary artery disease, and autoimmune disease. Later, the original ACE questions were extended to add items relevant for children living in Philadelphia, a racially diverse population. The added items were on racial discrimination and exposure to community violence. These ACE scores were higher than in the Kaiser Permanente population [40].

28.2 Women with Co-occurring Disorders and Violence Study (WCDVS)

The Women with Co-occurring Disorders and Violence Study (WCDVS), a five-year study funded by the Substance Abuse and Mental Health Services Administration (SAMHSA), was designed to look at the best practices for women who were diagnosed with substance abuse and mental illness who had also experienced violence or trauma histories. The sample, drawn from nine sites around the USA, was 2729 women, all of whom had had two or more previous treatment episodes. The women were provided either integrated services (integrating mental health, substance use, and trauma) or, in the comparison sites, treatment-as-usual (TAU).

WCDVS was one of the first studies to implement and evaluate the effectiveness of trauma-specific interventions and trauma-informed care in addressing the needs of consumer/survivors. A cross-site methodology evaluated the effectiveness of the trauma integrated interventions. Trauma integrated interventions were defined as the simultaneous provision of substance abuse, mental health, and trauma services to women in the intervention condition. Outcome measures were levels of PTSD/trauma, substance use, and mental health symptoms. Service utilization and consumer satisfaction were also measured.

The lessons learned included: (1) integrated care showed significant results in reducing substance use by 6 months and reduction in mental health and post-traumatic symptoms by 12 months; (2) consumer/peer staff played important roles in providing care and in participating in research design; (3) trauma-specific interventions showed significant results in outcomes; and (4) trauma-informed practice led to increased engagement and increased retention [3].

Morrissey and colleagues [26] also studied the characteristics of all participants to identify person-level characteristics that moderated outcomes and found that women with more severe baseline measures on behavioral health tended to report better outcomes at 6 months. At 12 months, mental health symptoms and PTSD severity showed statistically significant reductions in the intervention group. Further analyses [11] confirmed that at 12 months, treatment effects were largest for women with the most severe substance abuse and PTSD presentation.

Some specific WCDVS site data also adds to the accumulating knowledge about trauma integration into service programs. In the PROTOTYPES site [14], the rate of retention in treatment was significantly higher in the trauma-informed integrated treatment group than in the comparison group. Dropout was higher in the comparison condition than in the intervention condition throughout the first 12 weeks of treatment. In addition, the PROTOTYPES site added a measure of coping skills. In the intervention group, women's use of coping skills increased from baseline to 12 months, but in the comparison group, women's use of these skills decreased slightly from baseline to 12 months. Three-way repeated measures ANOVA results suggested that improvement on coping skills mediated improvements in emotional distress and substance use outcomes.

28.3 Why Attend to Trauma in Substance Abuse Treatment System

The substance abuse treatment system deals with high prevalence of clients with trauma. Many individuals entering the substance use disorders treatment system have been survivors of trauma from childhood through adulthood; that is, many have experienced childhood traumatic events but also have experienced additional trauma as they participated in the drug culture. These include women forced into sex work, who experienced trauma as a result of that; those who have been in jail and/or prison and experienced significant traumatic events in those settings; those who have witnessed the death of "running buddies" from overdoses, bad drug deals, hepatitis C, or HIV; and those who themselves have been diagnosed with HIV. Many have also experienced community violence. Trauma is the expectation, not the exception, for our clients.

Kessler et al. [20] showed, using the National Comorbidity Survey (NCS) data, that PTSD was significantly associated with a diagnosis of drug abuse or dependence. In addition, they found that PTSD was more often the primary or first diagnosis. The NCS generated a lifetime PTSD prevalence estimate of 5% among men and 10.4% among women and yielded far higher estimates of lifetime prevalence of trauma exposure and of the risk of developing PTSD. Lifetime prevalence of trauma exposure was estimated to be 60.7% among men and 51.2% among women.

The majority of those who reported any trauma experience reported multiple traumas. Combat was most frequently associated with PTSD in men; sexual assault was most frequently associated with PTSD in women.

More recent data show that 90% of drug users report having experienced at least one traumatic event and, often, many more than one [32]. In addition, post-trauma exposure further increases the risk for re-exposure. Peirce and colleagues [34] found that 27% of participants (registrants of Baltimore Needle Exchange Program) were re-exposed to a traumatic event each month. Women injecting drug users were more than twice as likely to report traumatic event re-exposure as were men, placing them at higher risk of developing PTSD. In a subsequence study [33] that looked at clients enrolled in methadone maintenance treatment, results showed that 97% had at least one lifetime traumatic event, with a total average of 18 traumatic events. Women were more likely than men to report histories of sexual assault at any age and interpersonal violence, as well as other threats (e.g., sexual harassment and stalking). Men were more likely than women to endorse histories of physical assault and witnessing physical assault. Traumatic re-exposure was common, with an average of 18% of participants reporting a new event each month during the study. Women were more likely than men to meet criteria for PTSD at study entry (31% vs 13%). An increase of 10% in PTSD symptom severity was associated with a 36% increased risk of treatment interruption. Interventions to reduce re-exposure or at least to ameliorate the negative effects of re-exposure on treatment would be beneficial.

With regard to opioids and trauma, the lifetime history of PTSD was 41% among individuals with opioid use disorder (OUD) seeking treatment [25]. In 2017, 70,237 Americans died from an opioid-related overdose [7]. Medication-assisted treatment (MAT), including methadone, buprenorphine, and naltrexone, shows improved retention and decreased relapse rates for the treatment of opioid use disorder. A total of 20–50% of OUD clients also meet the criteria for a PTSD diagnosis [12]. Despite successful outcomes documented in research studies, MAT is underutilized by many addiction treatment programs and drug courts.

Some substance abuse treatment procedures are triggering. Intense, aggressive confrontation in old-style therapeutic communities can trigger negative responses (e.g., depression, a sense of hopelessness, and re-traumatization) in clients with trauma histories, and clients will leave treatment early and relapse. Many other routine treatment procedures can be triggers as well, such as urine testing, night check-ins by counselors in residential treatment, co-ed programming, and reporting to courts and/or child welfare. With regard to urine testing, the need to have someone observing the testing can be quite "triggering" for survivors. It is important to explain that we are mandated to do observed testing and that it may feel uncomfortable for the client. We need to ask, "What can I do to make you feel more comfortable (e.g., step back, but still be able to observe)?" Also, there may be messages implicit in the manner of communication between staff member and client that can be triggering for a trauma survivor if s/he experienced boundary violation, betrayal, and/or powerlessness. Such a client may experience "power over" behavior by staff as disrespectful, coercive, and threatening.

Coping deficits associated with substance use disorder-PTSD lead to poorer treatment outcomes. Coping deficits have been associated with substance use disorder (SUD-PTSD in a number of studies. Ouimette et al. [30] found that problems from substance use at a 1-year follow-up were partially explained by SUD-PTSD patients' greater use of emotional discharge coping (e.g., risk-taking, yelling) and decreased expectations of benefits from abstinence. In a subsequent study [31], emotional discharge and cognitive avoidance coping (e.g., trying to forget about the trauma) both partially explained poorer 2-year substance use outcomes. In a third study, Brown et al. [5] found that individuals with unremitted PTSD had poorer substance use outcomes and poorer coping than those whose PTSD symptoms had remitted or those who had never been diagnosed with PTSD. The study also provided support for the critical role of coping in PTSD-SUD. The authors recommend that clinicians focus on helping these patients decrease their maladaptive coping strategies and learn more adaptive coping approaches.

Higher treatment burden leads to poor retention. I have discussed [3] a multileveled picture of the level of burden in clients and staff (see diagram), including the burden on the client of a number of problems (e.g., substance use, mental illness, trauma, cognitive impairments, physical problems, domestic violence, and poverty); the burdens of treatment (e.g., waiting times for appointments, triggering by procedures such as urine testing, medications, language/literacy issues, and turnover of staff); and the burdens on staff (e.g., time pressures, electronic health records, limits on amounts of service, new priorities, staff turnover, funding cutbacks, client emergencies, and angry/hostile clients). Therefore, it is important for providers to decrease all three types of burdens; increase the use of trauma-informed practices; give additional supports to clients to help them follow through on treatment plans; understand clients' angry, fearful, disassociated responses and respond to them in a caring, supportive way; and take care of ourselves as providers.

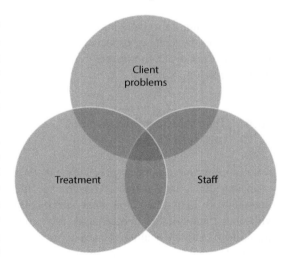

Levels of burden

Higher levels of burden, including those resulting from experiences of trauma, are related to lower levels of retention in treatment programs. For clients who have experienced trauma, it takes time to see reductions in the anxiety, fear, and mistrust that the clients bring with them into treatment. It also takes time for these clients to feel a positive connection to providers and to other clients in the program. Although the treatment program offers a safe and supportive environment, clients with trauma histories may feel overwhelmed by the need to participate with others, to behave in a structured way, and to comply with program rules and procedures. If clients have been cognitively impaired by domestic violence (mostly women), they may not be able to understand program rules or follow them. A mother who has experienced domestic violence and who has to come into residential treatment without her children will be fearful of what is happening to the children when she is not there protecting them; this can interfere with the woman's participation in treatment and recovery. This is why residential treatment programs for mothers and children are important for both.

Substance abuse treatment providers are at risk of secondary traumatization or re-traumatization and consequent burnout. Staff may themselves be trauma survivors and, therefore, acutely sensitive to trauma issues of clients. This can lead to a sensitivity and empathic response to trauma survivors but also can lead to secondary traumatization, especially if the staff member has not dealt with his/her trauma experiences (see below).

28.4 Trauma-Specific Interventions

Trauma-informed practices are different than trauma-specific interventions. Trauma-specific interventions help the client deal specifically with their traumatic experiences and teach coping skills to facilitate healing. As part of a trauma-informed organization/system, trauma-specific interventions need to be available, either on-site or by referral. These interventions directly address the effects of trauma on the client's life and facilitate trauma recovery by helping the client understand the connections between the

trauma and subsequent feelings and behaviors and teaching coping skills to help the client gain a sense of control, build more positive and safe relationships, and adopt safer behaviors. Trauma-specific interventions include both trauma-specific individual therapy and group interventions. For most treatment programs, groups are part of what they already do, so adding a new group should not be difficult.

Trauma-specific group interventions include two of the key components/principles of trauma recovery: empowerment and reconnection with others. The groups provide participants with opportunities to break down the isolating barrier of shame and to rebuild trust in others. The most frequently used trauma-specific interventions for adults are Stage 1 groups: *Seeking Safety* [27], *Trauma Recovery and Empowerment (TREM)* [16], *Beyond Trauma* [8, 10], and *Helping Men Recover* [9]. It is recommended that these groups have two co-facilitators, one of whom can be a trauma survivor or peer. This ensures that if a participant needs to leave the group because of becoming triggered, one facilitator can go with him/her. The groups also provide the learning of coping skills such as "grounding," which helps survivors calm themselves down when they are triggered by trauma memories. The secrecy and shame associated with a history of abuse may be more alleviated in a group setting than in individual treatment.

28.5 Trauma-Informed Practice

Trauma-informed practices are approaches that incorporate a thorough understanding of the prevalence and impact of trauma and are designed to avoid re-traumatizing those who seek care/help. SAMHSA has defined a trauma-informed approach as: "A program, organization, or system that is trauma-informed realizes the widespread impact of trauma and understands potential paths for recovery; recognizes the signs and symptoms of trauma in clients, families, staff, and others involved with the system; and responds by fully integrating knowledge about trauma into policies, procedures, practices, and seeks to actively resist re-traumatization" ([37], p. 9).

Trauma-informed practice expands the range of trauma sequelae; it goes beyond a focus only upon PTSD because we want to be able to prevent PTSD in patients who have already experienced trauma. It recognizes the strengths that survivors have used in dealing with interpersonal violence, i.e., that the specific symptoms such as substance abuse and/or hostility have helped the victim survive and manage the emotional and physical distress. The goal of this change in perspective is to move the fundamental question that we pose from "What's wrong with you?" to "What's happened to you?" and "How can we help?"

Harris and Fallot [17] defined the five core values or principles of a trauma-informed approach, viz., safety, trustworthiness, collaboration, empowerment, and choice.

- *Safety*. Patients/clients and staff feel physically, psychologically, and culturally safe. This means that the physical environment is safe and nurturing, that interactions between staff and client promote a sense of safety and respect, and that all procedures feel culturally safe to the patient. It is also important to be aware of the importance of language. We need to use terms that are not stigmatizing ("addicts," "borderlines"). Safe relationships are consistent, predictable, respectful, nonviolent, non-shaming, and non-blaming.
- *Trustworthiness*. Procedures are conducted with transparency; each step of the organization's processes from intake through treatment is explained in appropriate language, and patients are given enough time and respect to ask questions and receive appropriate answers; and confidentiality is explained and honored.
- *Collaboration*. There is sharing of power in decision-making between staff and clients, as well as collaboration between all providers in the system and the broader community network.
- *Empowerment*. The patient's strengths are recognized and validated, and the learning of new coping skills is provided in a respectful way. In addition, we normalize responses typically defined as "symptoms"; instead, they are seen as "adaptations." Survivors are not seen as manipulative, attention-seeking, or destructive, but as trying, instead, to cope using any means available to them. Recovery from trauma and addiction involves developing skills not only for managing intense feelings and situations but also for living a life that minimizes exposure to trauma triggers.
- *Choice*. Find ways to give clients choices. This is not "enabling" the client, as many staff in substance abuse treatment fear. Examples of choices are which groups s/he would like to start with (after all the groups available have been described) and how the client would prefer to be contacted (phone, email, or through a regular phone-in time set up for the client). Allowing the client to decide how contact with him/her will be made can be quite important for ensuring the safety of a client experiencing domestic violence. Another example is to have the client write down her/his treatment goals, while a staff member writes a separate set of goals s/he might suggest; then client and staff member work on developing the treatment plan together.

In addition to these core values, there are additional principles that are important for a trauma-informed practice. These include sensitivity to cultural issues and the inclusion of peer support.

Cultural Issues. As we have become more aware of the importance of taking culture into account as we provide care to the diverse populations in our systems, our ideas about how best to do so have moved through a continuum from cultural awareness to cultural competence to cultural humility to cultural safety. Cultural competency involves more than gaining factual knowledge about the different populations we serve; it also includes examining and changing our attitudes toward our clients. Cultural humility requires the provider to engage in continual self-reflection and to acknowledge "privilege" if that is relevant [39]. The provider must be able to overcome the natural tendency to view one's own beliefs and values as superior and, instead, be open to the beliefs and values of the client.

Cultural safety offers us one more step to enhance our understanding of the way culture affects our practices. The concept of cultural safety was first articulated in 1988 and emerged from the experiences of the indigenous people of New Zealand. The Nursing Council of New Zealand [29] furthered developed the concept: "Unsafe cultural practice comprises any action which diminishes, demeans or disempowers the cultural identity and well being of an individual." One of the key principles set forth by the Nursing Council is the need to recognize that both contemporary and historical inequities, including those resulting from colonization, affect healthcare interactions and can act as barriers to effective care. This principle, while developed for nursing, is applicable to addiction services.

This concept really helps us to understand safety through both a trauma lens and a cultural lens. There is no "post" or "past" traumatic stress when you feel your body is in danger because of your race, ethnicity, religion, gender, sexual orientation, etc. American Indian/First Nations peoples and African Americans may not feel safe when their lives can be taken by those who have been held up as their protectors. I believe that cultural safety is a key concept in understanding that although we are trying to help our patients through our addiction services, the patients may not experience our help or their safety. An essential feature of cultural safety is that the patient/client defines whether or not the practice, the provider, and the environment are culturally safe. What cultural safety asks us to do is to ask the client, "Do you feel safe here with me and in this place?"

A type of trauma that is often overlooked is historical trauma. It has been described as multigenerational trauma experienced by a specific cultural group over multiple generations. Among the many groups that have been identified as experiencing historical trauma are American Indians/First Nations people, African Americans, Jewish people, and Japanese-Americans. These populations have been traumatized by expulsion from their homelands, loss of economic status and self-sufficiency, removal of children and separations of families, loss of social ties, and torture

and murder. They have similarly experienced trauma; forced relocation(s) and migrations; stolen property (including land and homes); dehumanization; forced separations from family; mass incarceration, mass murder, and lynching; torture; medical experimentation; slavery; and internment. And while there can be the sense of a "community of suffering" among these groups, there is also a distrust of others outside the groups—particularly those from historically oppressive groups. This fear and mistrust can make it difficult to trust addiction treatment providers who are of a different group.

Peer Support Services. The concept of peers helping peers is not new for addiction treatment. In 1935, Alcoholics Anonymous, the oldest of the peer programs, came into being. It was viewed as a response to the limited effectiveness of traditional services and was intended to draw on the power on individuals to offer mutual support, solace, and learning. The achievements of self-help groups such as Alcoholics Anonymous were based on the principle that people who share a disease or disability have "something to offer each other that professionals can't provide."

Reiff and Reissman [35] described the use of "indigenous nonprofessionals" as "bridgemen," who bridged the social distance between those who need services (patients) and those providing services. They described the worker as a "peer of the client (who) shares a common background, language, ethnic origin, style, and group of interests" [35]. From the 1960s through the 1980s, persons with lived experience of drugs/alcohol began many of the addiction treatment programs. In the late 1980s and 1990s, during the early years of the AIDS epidemic, peers were hired to reach injecting drug users and their sexual partners to reduce risk-taking associated with needle-using and sexual behaviors [4]. Peers serve as role models, counselors, outreach workers, recovery coaches, advocates, case managers, trainers, co-facilitators, research assistants, and directors of addiction treatment programs. They have also come to play an important role in the delivery of services within Family Drug Treatment Courts. If a client is about to embark on a potentially stressful event (e.g., going to court or going to a medical appointment), sending a peer recovery specialist with her/him will help reduce stress.

28.6 What Does a Trauma-Informed Program Look like?

One of the consistent questions that agencies ask when they participate in trauma trainings is: "What does a trauma-informed program look like?" Because of the high prevalence of trauma within the populations entering their systems, organizations that work with children, youth, adults, and families should expect that the clients they serve have experienced some form of traumatic event.

In order to move toward trauma-informed practice in addiction treatment, there are a number of recommended organizational culture shifts and practice principles:

1. Trauma/PTSD and addiction are co-occurring disorders, and each condition is considered primary. Recovery involves moving through stages of change and phases of recovery for each condition (stabilization, motivational enhancement, active treatment, relapse prevention, recovery, continuing care) through an integrated program.
2. Implement a walk-through of your program. A trauma assessment and walk-through protocol [6] was developed and refined in the WCDVS study and a nationwide learning collaborative called the Network for the Improvement of Addiction Treatment (NIATx). The three authors of the protocol all participated in the WCDVS, and the first author was one of the first waves of NIATx grantees. Walk-throughs: enable organizations to better understand the experience of care from the clients' point of view, assist staff members to understand how they may be inadvertently re-enacting trauma dynamics, can uncover inconsistencies and limitations in systems, and generate ideas for improving organizational processes. The walk-through is a mutual data-gathering strategy that does not

resemble an "audit." Trainings and technical assistance grow out of the assessment and the action plan generated by the walk-through. The assessment allows the team (managers, staff, and senior clients) to walk through the agency procedures from the first call to the agency, to the intake process, and all the way through treatment.

3. Institute universal screening for trauma (see below).
4. The risk of re-traumatization should be minimized through:
   (a) Creating a safe treatment environment (physically and psychologically). This involves ensuring that the community surrounding the treatment program is safe (e.g., there is good lighting and adequate security). It also involves the treatment program: having policies about responding to acts of violence from clients; reducing "power over" behaviors by staff; restricting visitors who might be domestic violence perpetrators or otherwise "unsafe." In addition, the program environment needs to be calming, welcoming, and culturally sensitive.
   (b) Teaching grounding strategies and promoting resilience. A group session that teaches grounding skills is relevant to both substance use and trauma. Learning to regulate intense emotions can be empowering and promotes stability.
   (c) Implementing multileveled staff training. Workforce development, including training on trauma and trauma-informed practice, trauma-informed supervision, and strategies to address secondary trauma in staff and to promote self-care, is needed to begin transformation. Training should include all staff, including support staff (e.g., receptionists, cooks, maintenance, security guards, etc.). Training should be multileveled, so that everyone receives basic trauma training, clinical staff receive additional training including trauma-specific interventions, and supervisors receive training in responsive supervision.

(d) Considering stage-oriented treatment. Residential drug treatment programs are defined as stage-oriented and most use definitions of phases. In 1992, Herman proposed a three-stage model for trauma treatments [18]. The first stage is "safety", the second is "remembrance and mourning", and the third is "reconnection". A number of the trauma-specific group curricula that have been developed focus on Stage 1; these include *Seeking Safety*, *TREM*, and *Beyond Trauma*. In this first stage, the client is supported and helped to learn the connection between trauma and addiction, as well as to learn new coping strategies and methods of symptom containment. It is recommended that one of the Stage 1 trauma-specific group curricula be started within Phase 1. If a client begins to talk about trauma memories in detail, the group facilitator should state that clients may want to talk about their memories, but that "It isn't safe for you right now." It is important that clients have a period of stabilization (including medications) and that the interventions early in treatment focus upon psychoeducation and learning to regulate emotions and impulses. In the later stages, treatment is individualized, based on the patient's strengths, vulnerabilities, and cultural factors, and focuses more on the narrative of the survivor's trauma story.

5. Provide trauma-specific interventions. These include group interventions, such as *Seeking Safety*, *TREM*, *Beyond Trauma*, and *Helping Men Recover*, as well as individual interventions, such as *CBT* and *EMDR*) [23, 36].

6. Provide trauma-informed supervision for all direct treatment staff. Supervision can provide a physically and emotionally safe place for staff to examine their work with an experienced, supportive mentor. Ongoing supervision in trauma-informed care is recognized as a major protective factor in buffering against vicarious trauma.

7. Implement self-care strategies for staff to reduce potential for secondary trauma or burnout. An important part of being a trauma-informed provider organization is an awareness that providers may also have experienced trauma. Even if they have not, working with people who have survived traumatic experiences and listening to their stories can take an emotional toll and lead to secondary trauma. Secondary symptoms may include an increase in arousal and/or avoidance reactions, re-experiencing personal trauma, sleeplessness, fearfulness, and anger. Issues of self-care need to be included in the training of staff members. (See below.)

28.7 Screening

The patient/client pathway to services is extremely important in trauma-informed practice. By improving access to services and reducing waiting times and cumbersome procedures, we enhance the patient/client experience; by providing trauma-informed care, we improve the chances that s/he will follow through with treatment, feel safe and heard, and show improved outcomes.

Identification of a trauma history is critical if a provider/program is to be able to effectively respond to an individual. All clients should be screened for traumatic experiences. Those programs that routinely use the *Addiction Severity Index (ASI)* can begin by using the trauma items embedded within that instrument. Then, the program can decide on additional screening items. Some suggested screeners are *ACE Questionnaire* (which focuses on exposure before age 18), *PTSD Checklist (PCL-C)* (which focuses on recent symptoms), *Impacts of Events Scale-Revised (IES-R)*, *Trauma History Questionnaire (THQ)*, and *Life Stressor Checklist-Revised (LSC-R)*.

The screening needs to (1) determine imminent danger (as in the case of domestic or interpersonal violence); (2) communicate that the provider/program believes trauma and violence are significant events; (3) communicate openness to a discussion of painful events; (4) determine the most appropriate follow-up; and (5) open the possibility of later disclosure if the client is not ready at this time. Screenings are only beneficial if there are follow-up procedures in place and resources available for handling positive screens.

Survivors of childhood maltreatment and/or adult abuse and other traumatic experiences are often reluctant to talk about those experiences. If you have experienced trauma at the hands of another person, particularly someone who has been important to you and who you believed to be protective of you (e.g., parents, older siblings, teachers, coaches, clergymen), then you do not trust people—especially when they try to assure you that they want to help you and that you should trust them. For male clients, who have often learned not to show vulnerability or "weakness," ask about "exposure to violence," rather than abuse or trauma.

Facilitators for screening on trauma include the following:

1. Training providers on when and how to ask about trauma and how to respond to the answers given by patients/clients.
2. Identifying the person(s) on the treatment team who is best equipped to do the screening (e.g., intake person, admission clerk, nurse, medical assistant).
3. Keeping the screening questions short.

The reason for asking about trauma at the initial assessment is that if the questions are not asked then, they tend not to be asked at all. If the patient is too distressed at that point, then delaying the questions is appropriate. In those cases, it should be clearly recorded that the questions were not asked and the patient's file flagged for trauma screening at a later point. A trauma-informed introduction to screening might be, "I'm going to ask you some sensitive questions. If you don't want to answer, please tell me that. It's fine if you prefer not to answer" [2, 3].

There are two important points about that introduction. First, it prepares the client that there are some sensitive questions coming and that they have some importance to the provider. Second, if the client states s/he does not want to answer a question about interpersonal violence,

for example, this signals to the provider that the client probably has some problem with abuse and may have important reasons for not answering the questions at this time. Reasons for not answering may be that the abuser is sitting in the waiting room, and the client is afraid to speak about the abuse; s/he is afraid you will alert the authorities, that the abuser may then be punished, and that this will make him/her even more abusive; s/he is afraid you will alert the authorities and have the children taken away; and the client simply does not trust any providers yet. It is also important to ask about present abuse and to ensure a safety plan is in place if there is any danger to the patient and/or children.

With regard to responding, validation of the client's experience(s) and of their reaction to disclosure will communicate that you understand the importance of what has happened to them, that you care about what happened, and that you are nonjudgmental. Some recommendations include affirming that it was a good thing for the client to tell you, offering support, checking the client's emotional state at the end of the session, and offering follow-up.

28.8 Intake/Reception Procedures

Reception staff should be included in the trauma training, so that they understand how to assist anxious, fearful, or hostile patients/clients. Having pamphlets in the waiting room on sexual and physical abuse can convey to patients/clients that the practice/agency is aware of and ready to help with these issues. It is also critical to ensure that our intake processes are not burdensome, repetitive, or intrusive.

During intake, clients should be informed about policies, rules, and procedures. Knowing what to expect decreases anxiety and may prevent the patient from being triggered by unanticipated events. Rules and procedures need to be repeated. Each client has her/his own pattern of situations that can trigger her/him and her/his own pattern of things that can comfort her/him. As part of the intake, staff can ask clients what upsets them and what comforts them. This important data can be utilized by staff when the client becomes distressed. For the client, learning to recognize emotional triggers and soothing behaviors restores a sense of safety. For staff, this information can help prevent some of the disturbing events and/or help them comfort and stabilize the client when s/he is upset.

A trauma history may also impact medication adherence because the patient may fear that taking medications will result in a loss of control. Given that trauma has removed choice and control from them, whenever possible, clients should have choice and control in their treatment. For example, the provider can say: "For many people, this can all be overwhelming. We don't have to solve every problem right away. Is there one thing you would like to work on first?" Or, "We have a number of groups you could attend. Which one would you like to attend first?" And ask, "What can I do to make this easier for you?"

28.9 Reducing Re-Traumatization in Substance Abuse Treatment

When clients experience anything as a threat, the fight-flight-freeze response is triggered and results in a state of constant alertness or hyperarousal. The client is then reactive to any number of triggers. In a hyperarousal state, the individual can respond to benign stimuli as if they were life-threatening. For example, a veteran may hear a car backfire and drop to the ground, afraid he is about to be attacked as he was in combat. This prepares the individual to respond with "fight, flight, or freeze" responses; you may observe outbursts of anger (fight), clients leaving treatment early (flight), or a client with an appearance like "a deer in the headlights" (freeze). The last response is often seen in children who cannot, as easily as adults, fight or flee.

It should also be noted that, following traumatic events, survivors may also avoid "people, places, and things" associated with the event. This coping strategy is typically not available for victims of repeated child and intimate partner abuse, who are forced to continue to be engaged with the perpetra-

tors of the abuse. Many survivors use drugs and/or alcohol to modulate their arousal. For substance abuse treatment providers, this raises the issue of "triggers" that can increase the substance use. Triggers are quite relevant to trauma work, as well as to substance abuse treatment.

There are certain procedures that can be re-traumatizing for many clients, such as urine testing, aggressive confrontation, and sudden discharge from treatment. Supervised visits with children who may be in foster care and the presence of child welfare, combined with a trauma history and a fear of losing children, place parents, particularly mothers, at high risk for acute trauma responses. Some recommendations to drug abuse treatment staff to reduce re-traumatization and to become trauma-informed are as follows:

- *Motivational interviewing (MI)* [24] states that motivation for change is cultivated within the collaborative relationship between provider and client. The focus is understanding what each client values while evoking his/her reasons for change. *MI* is completely compatible with trauma-informed care.
- During urine testing, try not to stand too close to the client, assure the client you know this procedure can be uncomfortable, and ask, "What would make this more comfortable for you?"
- Have separate groups by gender.
- If a client is triggered in a group session, stop the action and introduce grounding strategies (see [8, 27]).
- Help decide on which trauma-specific intervention (e.g., *Seeking Safety*, *Beyond Trauma*, *TREM*) fits best in your program. Participate in the training for the intervention selected.
- Link "triggers" for using drugs and alcohol to "triggers" for re-experiencing traumatic events.
- Acknowledge client's strengths ("still standing").
- Ask, "Since the last time we spoke, has anything happened that was upsetting to you?"
- In residential treatment, prepare clients for staff entering the rooms at night (for monitoring).

Then, when monitoring, knock on the door; identify yourself; say, "I'm coming in," and ask if clients are okay.

- In addition to clients with co-occurring disorders, including trauma, clients with cognitive impairment may have diminished capacity to adhere to treatment rules and procedures. In our work at PROTOTYPES, we found that a number of our clients showed cognitive impairment when tested. This is not a topic typically discussed in addiction treatment. However, some treatment practices that can help these clients are providing clear explanations; using concrete language, short sentences, and visual aids (drawings, photos); and frequent repetition. In addition, assign an advanced residential client to read any written information to the client.
- Residential treatment offers a community experience with clear structure and a set of norms and boundaries. This can promote a sense of safety for some clients. For others, this environment may feel overwhelming and threatening. Behaviors such as hostility or aggression on the part of other clients can affect the group's feeling of safety.
- In outpatient treatment, it is extremely important to assess each client's safety at home/in the community. Also, safety plans for the children of clients need to be addressed.

colleagues and asking one another, "What was the hardest thing you had to handle today?"; becoming part of a team activity (e.g., sport); and being able to "leave work at work" and enjoy pleasant time with family and friends.

In conclusion, in order for addiction treatment to meet the needs of our clients, our approach needs to address the impact of trauma on clients' lives/substance use and on staff. The suggested practice changes discussed in this chapter are the beginning of a cultural change in our addiction treatment. Trauma-informed practices can address a variety of adversities that affect our clients. Addiction treatment can provide (1) a safe and supporting environment for clients and staff; (2) understanding of the link between trauma and substance use; (3) training in new coping skills; (4) parenting skills training to reduce the likelihood that clients' children will be impacted by child neglect or maltreatment; (5) assistance to the children in developing resilience; (6) training in developing positive relationships and connection; and (7) access to other supportive services, including employment, housing, education, and family treatment. As is discussed throughout this chapter, trauma-informed care incorporates gender-informed care, person-centered care, and cultural safety. It values continuous improvement and encourages staff and clients to propose ideas for improvement without fear.

28.10 Staff Care/Self-Care

There are a number of practices that can help in preventing and/or lessening secondary traumatization and burnout in staff members. First, the treatment agency needs to ensure that caseloads are balanced and *not overwhelming*; supervision is available to all staff and is trauma-sensitive; staff members have a place and time to debrief with colleagues and take breaks; and procedures are in place to assure safety for staff. In addition, staff members need training on self-care, including increasing self-awareness and the ability to process negative emotions; using supervision to share how it feels to work with certain clients; setting limits with clients; staying connected with

References

1. Atwool N. Challenges of operationalizing trauma-informed practice in child protection services in New Zealand. Child Fam Soc Work. 2019;24(1):1–8.
2. Brown VB. Integrated screening, assessment and training as critical components of trauma-informed care. In: Poole N, Greaves L, editors. Becoming trauma-informed. Toronto: Centre for Addiction and Mental Health; 2012. p. 319–27.
3. Brown VB. Through a trauma Lens: transforming health and behavioral health systems. New York: Routledge; 2018.
4. Brown BS, Beschner GM. At risk for AIDS—injection drug users and their sexual partners. Westport: Greenwood Press; 1993.
5. Brown PJ, Read JP, Kahler CW. Comorbid posttraumatic stress disorder and substance use disorders: treatment outcomes and the role of coping.

In: Ouimette P, Brown PJ, editors. Trauma and substance abuse: causes, consequences, and treatment of comorbid disorders. Washington, DC: American Psychological Association; 2003. p. 171–88.

6. Brown VB, Harris M, Fallot R. Moving toward trauma-informed practice in addiction treatment. J Psychoactive Drugs. 2013;45(5):386–93.

7. Centers for Disease Control and Prevention. Opioid overdoses. 2018. https://www.cdc.gov/drugoverdose/data/statedeaths.html.

8. Covington S. Beyond trauma: a healing journey for women. Center City: Hazelden; 2003.

9. Covington S, Griffin R, Dauer R. Helping men recover: a program for treating addiction. Hoboken: Wiley; 2011.

10. Covington SS. Beyond Trauma: A Healing Journey for Women (2nd Edition). Center City, MN: Hazelden. 2016.

11. Cusack KJ, Morrissey JP, Ellis AR. Targeting trauma-related interventions and improving outcomes for women with co-occurring disorders. Admin Pol Ment Health. 2008;35(3):147–58.

12. Ecker AH, Hundt N. Posttraumatic stress disorder in opioid agonist therapy: a review. Psychol Trauma. 2017;10(6):636–42.

13. Felitti VJ, Anda RF, Nordenberg D, Williamson DF, Spitz AM, Edwards V, Koss MP, Marks JS. Relationship of childhood abuse and household dysfunction to many of the leading causes of death in adults: the Adverse Childhood Experiences (ACE) Study. Am J Prev Med. 1998;14(4):245–58.

14. Gatz M, Brown V, Hennigan K, Rechberger E, O'Keefe M, Rose T, Bjelajac P. Effectiveness of an integrated trauma-informed approach to treating women with co-occurring disorders and histories of trauma: the Los Angeles site experience. J Community Psychol. 2007;35(7):863–77.

15. Gilbert LK, Breiding JJ, Merrick MT, Thompson WW, Ford DC, Dhingra SS, Parks SE. Childhood adversity and adult chronic disease: an update from ten states and the District of Columbia. Am J Prev Med. 2015;48:345–9.

16. Harris M, and the Community Connections Trauma Work Group. Trauma recovery and empowerment: a Clinician's guide for working with women in groups. New York: The Free Press; 1998.

17. Harris M, Fallot R, editors. Using trauma theory to design service systems. San Francisco: Jossey-Bass; 2001.

18. Herman JL. Trauma and recovery. New York: Basic Books; 1992.

19. IIMHL. Make it so: key national activities in trauma-informed care across IIMHL countries. Pakuranga/Aukland: Initial Initiative for Mental Health Leadership; 2012.

20. Kessler RC, Sonnega A, Bromet E, Hughes M, Nelson CB. Post-traumatic stress disorder in the National Comorbidity Survey. Arch Gen Psychiatry. 1995;52(12):1048–60.

21. Kezleman C, Stavropoulous P. Practice guidelines for treatment of complex trauma and trauma informed care and service delivery. Kirribilli: Adults Surviving Child Abuse; 2012.

22. Khoury L, Tang YL, Bradley B, Cubells JF, Ressler KJ. Substance use, childhood traumatic experience, and posttraumatic stress disorder in an urban civilian population. Depress Anxiety. 2010;27(12):1077–86.

23. McGovern MP, Lamber-Harris C, Alterman AI, Xie H, Meier A. A randomized controlled trial comparing integrated cognitive behavioral therapy versus individual addiction counseling for co-occurring substance use and post traumatic stress disorders. J Dual Diagn. 2011;7:207–27.

24. Miller WR, Rollnick S. Motivational interviewing: preparing people to change addictive behaviors. New York: Guilford Press; 1991.

25. Mills KL, Teeson M, Ross J, Darke S. The impact of post-traumatic stress disorder on treatment outcomes for heroin dependence. Addiction. 2007;102:447–54.

26. Morrissey JP, Jackson EW, Ellis AR, Amaro H, Brown VB, Najavits LM. Twelve-month outcomes of trauma-informed interventions for women with co-occurring disorders. Psychiatr Serv. 2005;56(10):1213–22.

27. Najavits LM. Seeking safety: a treatment manual for PTSD and substance abuse. New York: Guilford Press; 2002.

28. NHS Education for Scotland. Transforming psychological trauma: a knowledge and skills framework for the Scottish workforce. Edinburgh: NHS Education for Scotland; 2017.

29. Nursing Council of New Zealand. Guidelines for cultural safety, the treaty of Waitangi and Maori health in nursing education and practice. Wellington: Nursing Council of New Zealand; 2011.

30. Ouimette PC, Ahrens C, Moos RH, Finney JW. Posttraumatic stress disorder in substance abuse patients: relationship to 1-year posttreatment outcomes. Psychol Addict Behav. 1997;11(1):34–47.

31. Ouimette PC, Finney JW, Moos RH. Two-year posttreatment functioning and coping of substance abuse patients with posttraumatic stress disorder. Psychol Addict Behav. 1999;13(2):105–14.

32. Peirce JM, Burke CK, Stoller KB, Neufeld KJ, Brooner RK. Assessing traumatic event exposures: comparing the traumatic life events questionnaire to the structured clinical interview for DSM-IV. Psychol Assess. 2009;21(2):210–8.

33. Peirce JM, Brooner RK, King VL, Kidorf MS. Effect of traumatic event reexposure and PTSD on substance use disorder treatment response. Drug Alcohol Depend. 2016;158:126–31.

34. Pierce JM, Kolodner K, Brooner RK, Kidorf MS. Traumatic event re-exposure in injecting drug users. J Urban Health. 2011;89(1):117–28.

35. Reiff P, Reissman F. The indigenous non-professional: a strategy for change in community action and mental health programs, Community mental health journal monograph series, no. 1. New York: Behavioral Publications; 1965. p. 81.

36. Shapiro F. Eye movement desensitization and reprocessing (EMDR: principles, protocols, and procedures). 2nd ed. New York: Guilford Press; 2001.
37. Substance Abuse and Mental Health Services Administration (SAMHSA). SAMHSA's concept of trauma and guidance for a trauma-informed approach, HHS publication no (SMA) 14–4884. Rockville: Substance Abuse and Mental Health Services Administration; 2014.
38. Sweeney A, Clement S, Filson B, Kennedy A. Trauma-informed mental healthcare in the U.K.: what is it and how can we further its development? Ment Health Rev J. 2016;21:174–92.
39. Tervalen M, Murray-Garcia J. Cultural humility versus cultural competence: a critical distinction in defining physician training outcomes in multicultural education. J Health Care Poor Underserved. 1998;9(2):117–25.
40. Wade R, Shea JA, Rubin D, Wood J. Adverse childhood experiences of low-income urban youth. Pediatrics. 2014;134(1):e13–20. https://doi.org/10.1542/peds.2013-2475.

Contingency Management as a Behavioral Approach in Addiction Treatment

29

John M. Roll, Sterling M. McPherson, and Michael G. McDonell

Contents

Abstract

Contingency management is a well-documented intervention for initiating abstinence from abused drugs. The technique is rooted in a long tradition of operant psychology and has copious amounts of foundational and applied research supporting its use. This revised chapter describes the background research, reviews the history of using contingency management, and provides basic information on implementation. This revised chapter includes a new section on technology support for contingency management. The reader will hopefully find this chapter to be a useful basic introduction of the topic.

J. M. Roll (✉) · S. M. McPherson · M. G. McDonell
Washington State University, Spokane, WA, USA
e-mail: johnroll@wsu.edu; sterling.mcpherson@wsu.edu; mmcdonell@wsu.edu

Keywords

Behavioral treatment · Operant psychology · Supportive technology

29.1   Introduction

At its heart, drug abuse—addiction—is an easy concept to understand. People misuse drugs because the drugs make them feel good. This occurs either by inducing euphoria or by eliminating an unpleasant state, for example, pain or withdrawal. The effects of drugs are usually short-lived. That is to say that the euphoria or relief usually lasts for hours, not days. In order to regain the sought-after effect (feeling good), the drug must be taken repeatedly and over time. This repeated consumption quickly turns into addiction. Addiction is a vicious cycle in which the original efficacy of the drug is diminished, and the drug must be taken more frequently and at a higher dose to obtain similar efficacy (i.e., tolerance and habituation occurs).

Addiction is often further characterized by damage to the physiology of the person consuming the drug as a result of the drug's pharmacologic action. The lifestyle associated with compulsive drug seeking also damages the person—they do not take care of their personal health, and their relationships with others deteriorate and often are terminated. Compulsive users occasionally engage in dangerous behaviors to acquire drugs such as engaging in sex trade work or engaging in criminal activity, and they become less interested in maintaining their physical, psychologic, and spiritual health as they become more addicted to drugs. Unchecked, the person in the grasp of this vicious cycle of addiction will most often die or at best adopt what is essentially a palliative existence. This is true for virtually all drugs of abuse, even though the cycle may be faster for some drugs of addiction (e.g., acute methamphetamine use leading to a heart attack or an overdose resulting in death) compared to others (e.g., smoking cigarettes eventually leading to chronic obstructive pulmonary disease or eventually to lung cancer and death). These tragic outcomes result from a person simply wanting to feel euphoria or seeking relief from a negative state, something every human can relate to.

Characterizing this downward spiral that starts with the universal quest to feel good in terms of a scientific framework is important if we are to fully understand, effectively treat, and eventually prevent addiction. One of the best frameworks for characterizing addiction comes from the field of the Experimental Analysis of Behavior. While this field has its genesis in the distinguished work of scholars such as the British philosophers, Lloyd Morgan, Edward Thorndike, and others (e.g., [12]), it was essentially popularized and is most closely associated with the operant psychology of B. F. Skinner (e.g., [79]; see [68] for discussion of the history and evolution of operant psychology's influence on behavioral pharmacology).

One of the seminal events in the growth of operant pharmacology was the development of laboratory preparations (operant chamber, eponymously known as a Skinner box) for the convenient study of operant behavior. Briefly (see [41] for a detailed discussion of operant psychology), organisms could be put into the operant chamber, and under tightly controlled conditions, their behavior could be studied. A common example would be to place a hungry rat in the operant chamber and allow it to press a lever for food. Rate of responding for food will increase as the rat acquires the lever-pressing repertoire and then plateau as the rat masters the behavior. This change in rate across experimental sessions demonstrates learning. The food, which maintains the responding in the foregoing example, would be considered a reinforcer. A reinforcer can be defined as a stimulus that increases the behavior it follows. In this case, food reinforces lever pressing, and the lever pressing increases until the behavior has been mastered. Most would consider the food to be an example of positive reinforcement. That is to say, the behavior produces a stimulus (food) which increases the homeostatic "good" of the rat. Another type of reinforcement that can be demonstrated in a laboratory preparation is negative reinforcement. An example of this would be a rat placed in an operant chamber that receives a shock every 2 minutes regardless of what the rat did; in other words, the shock is inescapable. However, if a lever is placed in the box and the rat presses the lever, the next scheduled shock can be avoided. As in the positive reinforcement example, the rat will acquire the lever-pressing behavior over time until it has mastered the behavior and maintains it at a level that avoids shocks. Negative reinforcement, which is reinforcement that removes an aversive state, like this occurs when a behavior eliminates a noxious stimulus.

The forgoing is not merely a historical footnote. The use of the operant chamber opened many avenues for the study of how drugs influence behavior. Early examples of this work were conducted by Skinner and Heron [80] who examined how caffeine and amphetamine (Benzedrine) impacted food-reinforced behavior and the extinction of that behavior.

However, the aspect of operant psychology that is of most relevance to this chapter was the demonstration that naive animals would self-administer most of the same drugs abused by humans. In an early study, Thomson and Schuster demonstrated that drug-naive monkeys would self-administer morphine [86]. This was a seminal demonstration that drugs of abuse could serve as positive reinforcers analogous to other positive reinforcers like food and water. Since this demonstration, thousands of studies in which drugs are provided to organisms (human and nonhuman) contingent on an operant response have demonstrated the robustness of this phenomenon (e.g., [68]). It is one of the more unambiguous and well-accepted *facts* that drugs of abuse act as sources of positive reinforcement. Similarly, it has been demonstrated in laboratory paradigms that drugs of abuse can also serve as powerful sources of negative reinforcement (e.g., [31, 34, 46, 47, 87]). More specifically, drug-dependent organisms will increase their responding for a drug when they are in a state of withdrawal (see especially the body of work of Negus for discussion of this). That is, the animal, or person, will increase their consumption of a drug to escape from a negative state. In situations such as this, the drug functions as a negative reinforcer.

This observation, that drugs of abuse serve as sources of reinforcement, both positive and negative, has been an important observation in our quest to understand, treat, and prevent addiction. Many would argue that the goal of treatment (and prevention) efforts should be the diminution of the reinforcing efficacy of the drug of abuse.

To relate this operant framework back to the opening discussion about a drug user's quest to feel good, we can refine that description so that instead of describing a quest to feel good, we can describe a quest for reinforcement. This could be positive reinforcement, which some might equate with euphoria, or negative reinforcement, for example, the diminution of withdrawal symptoms. This conceptualization now allows us to place drug addiction and its associated sequela into the operant psychology framework.

To appreciate the utility of this operant framework for addressing addiction, one more point needs consideration. That is that primary, or naturalistic, reinforcers are biologically important for the survival of the organism and hence the species. Food, water, and sex are crucial to survival, and these are powerful sources of natural reinforcement. Human biology has evolved to be maximally sensitive to sources of reinforcement such as these. A detailed discussion of the neurobiology underpinning reinforcement is well beyond the scope of this chapter. Suffice it to say that an impressive array of neurobiological systems are at play. When a thirsty person takes a drink of water, it is a powerful source of reinforcement, and our neurobiology guarantees that in a similar state of thirst, we will again seek a drink of water. Unfortunately, most drugs of abuse interact with the same neurobiological system that governs our reinforcing relationship to primary sources of reinforcement. As popularized by a past director of the National Institute on Drug Abuse, Dr. Alan Leshner, drugs of abuse hijack this neurobiological system and insidiously shift a user's motivation toward a compulsive focus on drug-derived reinforcement. The result is that an addicted person develops a compulsive motivation to seek drug-based reinforcement and that that reinforcement is of exceptional strength.

While daunting, this conceptualization does point toward an effective treatment mechanism. In order to help an individual enter into recovery from drug addiction, it is necessary to reduce the reinforcing efficacy of the drug. We would argue that this is the goal of all drug abuse treatment efforts at some level. The cognitive behavior treatments seek to restructure thoughts about drugs or to reorganize a user's cognitions and skill set so that they conceptualize the negative aspects of drug use as being more salient than the positive aspects. Motivational therapies seek to alter the user's motivation to seek the drug reinforcement; pharmacologic and immunotherapeutic approaches seek to block the drug from ever interacting with the user's reward-related neurobiology. While some will surely disagree, we postulate that all successful treatment approaches can be couched in terms of lowering the abused drug's reinforcing efficacy. One approach that takes this as its stated goal is contingency management (CM). The remainder of this chapter will focus on this approach. We will briefly describe the basic science supporting the approach and discuss prototypic examples of how to use the approach, key factors to consider when using the approach, populations for which the approach has been used, barriers to implementation, technology supports for this approach, and finally potential limitations to the use of the approach. A series of meta-analyses supports the use of CM [1, 19, 39, 58]. The interested reader is encouraged to consult these publications as they are much more detailed than this chapter. There also exist a number of books on the topic of CM. This brief chapter can provide only a glimpse of the wealth of growing research on CM. Consulting these other texts is crucial prior to actual implementation of the procedure.

29.2   Underlying Logic of CM Approaches

One of the clearest demonstrations of the underlying principle of CM-based interventions is found in a study by Nader and Woolverton [45]. In this study, they allowed rhesus monkeys to make choices between intravenously delivered cocaine and food [45]. When the choice was between cocaine and one pellet of food, the monkeys showed a strong preference for self-administering the cocaine. However, when the dose of cocaine was held constant and the magnitude of the alternative source of reinforcement

(food) was increased to four pellets per choice, the monkeys chose to self-administer cocaine on only about half of the choice opportunities. Finally, when the magnitude of the alternative reinforcer was increased to 16 food pellets per choice, the monkeys selected the alternative reinforcer, food, almost exclusively. As discussed in Roll [68], this well-designed experiment demonstrates the powerful impact of arranging an environment so that the organism needs to make choices between a drug and a salient, high-magnitude, alternative source of reinforcement. This finding has been demonstrated by many investigators working with different drugs, different alternative reinforcers, and different animal species (e.g., [14]). When the magnitude of the alternative source of reinforcement is low, the drug has a powerful reinforcing efficacy. However, simply by elevating the magnitude of the available alternative sources of reinforcement, the reinforcing efficacy of the drug can be reduced to such a low level that it is not self-administered. That is to say, it is no longer an effective reinforcer.

It is reasonable to question how applicable these findings are to humans. In order to address this question, Higgins and colleagues conducted a similar study with human volunteers in which they investigated the impact of manipulating the magnitude of alternative reinforcers on cocaine self-administration [24, 25]. In this study, recreational cocaine users were recruited to participate in an outpatient study. Participants came to the laboratory where they made ten repeated choices between cocaine and money on a given day. Cocaine dose was 10 mg per choice and was held constant throughout the study. Money was used as an alternative source of reinforcement and was provided at three different levels: $0.50, $1.00, and $2.00. During a given session, monetary value was always held constant. In each experimental session, a participant made ten exclusive choices between cocaine and money. When the money value was low, participants elected to self-administer cocaine exclusively. As the value of the alternative source of reinforcement increased to $1.00, participants elected to receive about half of the available cocaine doses, and when the magnitude of the alternative was increased to $2.00, participants switched their preference—relative to that demonstrated with the low magnitudes of alternative reinforcement—and elected to decline cocaine and receive only money. This procedure has been replicated with other types of drugs besides cocaine (e.g., [74, 75]). Exactly as in the Nader and Woolverton study with monkeys, the penchant for humans to self-administer drugs typically decreases in an orderly and predictable fashion as the amount of the alternative source of reinforcement increases. These data demonstrate that providing a salient alternative source of reinforcement of sufficient magnitude reduces a drug's reinforcing efficacy. As noted, this is the hallmark of the successful treatment of drug addiction. Contingency-management approaches take advantage of this observation and seek to arrange a drug user's environment so that they can garner salient alternative sources of reinforcement when abstaining from drugs and forfeit that reinforcement when consuming drugs (Note: this section was adapted from [68]; also see [7]).

29.3 Prototypic Examples

Contingency management can take many forms, but in all cases, it is a technique that clinicians use to *engineer* a drug user's environment so that the drug user must choose between drug use (maintained by the drug's reinforcing efficacy) and other non-drug reinforcers. The salient non-drug reinforcers that have often been employed included access to housing [43]; access to employment [76]; provision of vouchers which can be exchanged for monetarily-based goods and services [24, 25]; access to prizes which are valued by the user (e.g., [55]); escape from judicial sanctions [57]; and access to one's monetary resources [66]. Several research groups have developed potential lists of other types of reinforcers that can be employed, and these include such things as reduced clinic fees, access to clinic-sponsored social events, reduced time in psychosocial counseling, fee rebates, and donated goods and services (e.g., [6, 70]).

While the CM class of interventions have been used for most types of drug abuse treatment [28], they have, in our opinion, been most successful for those types of addictions for which no viable pharmacotherapy exists. This largely excludes opioid addiction and nicotine addiction as both of these disorders are well-controlled with pharmacotherapy (e.g., opioids: [10]; nicotine: [8]). That is not to say that CM cannot be a useful adjunct for the management of opiate addiction or smoking cessation. For example, take-home doses of methadone delivered contingent on compliance with clinic regulations and the continued provision of drug-free urine tests is a relatively common practice (e.g., [84]). Contingency management may also have utility in treating nicotine addiction (e.g., [37]), but in our experience, CM is usually a secondary focus to the pharmacotherapy, which is the first-line treatment of these disorders. Please note that even when good pharmacotherapy is available, some populations such as pregnant women may not be able to use the pharmacotherapy. In cases such as this, CM may become a very important treatment modality (e.g., [29]). However, we still do not have accepted pharmacotherapies for psychostimulant addiction (excluding nicotine addiction), especially cocaine and methamphetamine. It is for these disorders that we believe CM is a useful first-line approach. There are two types of CM that are most commonly employed in the treatment of psychostimulant addiction. The first, popularized by Higgins (e.g., [24, 25]), is perhaps best described as voucher-based reinforcement therapy (VBRT), and the second, popularized by Petry (e.g., [55]), is variously referred to as the Fishbowl technique and prize-based CM but is more accurately known as Variable Magnitude of Reinforcement CM (e.g., [78]). Examples of each are provided below, and in the following section, the key factors related to the efficacy of the procedures are discussed.

Steve Higgins at the University of Vermont first demonstrated the efficacy of VBRT in a relatively large randomized clinical trial designed to assess the intervention's impact on cocaine using individuals [26]. The basic procedures for this type of intervention are as follows: Patients receive vouchers for the provision of biological samples (urine or breath) that indicate no recent drug use. Participants receive a voucher each time they test negative for the target drug. These vouchers can then be exchanged for goods or services. The initial voucher value is set at a low value (e.g., $2.50 USD). Each consecutive instance of abstinence increases the magnitude of the voucher by a small amount (e.g., $1.50 USD). Three consecutive abstinences result in the delivery of an additional bonus (e.g., $10.00 USD). A drug-positive urine sample, or failure to test, results in a reset of the voucher magnitude back to its original level (i.e., $2.50), from which the escalation can begin again.

The late Nancy Petry at the University of Connecticut popularized the variable magnitude of reinforcement procedure [48, 56]. This procedure involves making "draws" from a bowl of chips representing different prize/reinforcer magnitudes. These chips can be exchanged for goods that are available on-site. Typically, about half of the chips say "good job" and do not result in the delivery of any tangible reinforcement. 41.8% of the chips result in a small reinforcer (worth about $1.00 USD), 8% result in a large reinforcer (worth about $20.00 USD), and 0.2% result in a jumbo reinforcer (worth about $80.00 USD). Participants earn at least one draw for each urine sample submitted that is drug negative. The number of draws awarded at each urine collection escalates by one chip with consecutive instances of drug-negative urine tests. Missing or drug-positive urine samples result in a reset to one draw available when the next negative sample is submitted.

Both of these (VBRT and Variable Magnitude of Reinforcement) procedures are quite effective at treating psychostimulant addiction. In fact, the United States of America Veteran's Administration has recently adopted CM as a treatment modality for psychostimulant addiction [64]. Often, people wonder about the relative efficacy of the two procedures. It is important to note that there is substantial evidence suggesting that they both work. We are aware of no evidence demonstrating the superiority of one over the other. Both procedures have the advantage that they allow clinicians and

consumers of their services to celebrate success (e.g., drug abstinence) in a clinical session as opposed to focusing on failure (drug use). The Variable Magnitude of Reinforcement procedure has a potential advantage in that the prize drawing phase has an inherent excitement built into and an element of chance which many may find exciting. This may confer additional reinforcing efficacy to the prizes above and beyond that which can be accounted for via their monetary value via a process of conditioning (e.g., [4]). However, this suggestion is in need of empirical assessment. Some have suggested that on the face of it, this may resemble gambling and be a risk for pushing individuals who are seeking treatment for addiction to develop or exacerbate a pathological gambling problem. It is important to note that the Variable Magnitude of Reinforcement procedure is not gambling. The participant does not put up any of their own resources and does not have an opportunity for personal financial loss as is the case in gambling. In addition, we have studied those going through this type of CM procedure and found no evidence that they transition to or develop a gambling disorder [54].

A potential advantage of the VBRT procedure relative to the Variable Magnitude of Reinforcement procedure is that it allows a skillful clinician to engineer the voucher exchanges so that the consumer/patient comes into contact with powerful sources of non-drug reinforcement that exist in the consumer's natural environment. The goal is that these sources of reinforcement will come to exert control over the consumer's behavior as they initiate and maintain their recovery from their addiction. For example, exchanging vouchers for goods or services that allow the consumer to increase the reinforcement they get: from family interactions (e.g., exchanging a voucher so a mother can go roller skating with her daughter); from employment (e.g., exchanging a voucher for a set of clothes to wear at a job interview); or from engaging in a hobby (e.g., exchanging a voucher for a fishing license so that the consumer can engage in a hobby), all serve to increase the consumers contact with potentially powerful sources of non-drug reinforcement. In other words, the vouchers can act as behavioral vectors to draw the consumer's behavior into contact with non-drug reinforcers. It should be noted that in the Variable Magnitude of Reinforcement procedure, this can also be accomplished by tailoring the prizes that are available to consumers.

In summary, both of these procedures work well and have improved the lives of many individuals who have benefited from treatment that utilized these approaches. There is no immediate reason to prefer one approach over the other. Both are effective if delivered with high degrees of fidelity [48]. There is good evidence that the procedures work for most types of addiction [19, 23, 27, 39, 48, 58] and for many populations including adolescents [13], polysubstance abusers [18], pregnant women [29], and those afflicted with both substance use disorders and serious and persistent mental health issues [40]. There is also evidence that the procedures work best for those who rapidly initiate abstinence during treatment [90] and for those who begin treatment in a drug-free state [85]. The utility of the CM procedures for treatment in the criminal justice system is less compelling (e.g., [22]; although see [17]). This is perhaps not surprising as most criminal justice systems are punishment based. While punishment is usually to be avoided in therapeutic contexts because of the proclivity of the person being punished to escape the punisher (e.g., terminate the treatment interaction), that is not an option in a criminal justice setting in which the person is compelled to engage in treatment. Given these circumstances, contingent punishment should be quite effective in controlling behavior. For example, if a cocaine user is clearly informed that if they use cocaine they will be incarcerated, it is a powerful contingency management protocol based on punishment. This is the norm in many criminal justice systems (punishments range from mild sanction in some countries to death in others!). In such a milieu, it is unlikely that a reinforcement-based CM procedure will garner much additional control over a user's behavior unless very high-magnitude reinforcers are employed. In criminal justice systems where behavior is less controlled, however, CM interventions should be effective.

29.4 Key Factors

In this section, we briefly describe what we believe are four key factors for the successful implementation of any variety of CM. For a detailed discussion of these factors and others, please consult [48, 52, 88].

The first factor to consider is the procedure by which vouchers or prizes (henceforth both referred to as reinforcers) are disbursed. This is known in parlance of operant psychology as the schedule of reinforcement. Schedules of reinforcement have been extensively studied, and it has been repeatedly demonstrated that schedule changes can have profound impacts on behavior [20, 72]. Higgins developed the basic schedule that is routinely employed in CM procedures. This has two key components. First, as outlined in the examples in the previous section, there is an escalation in reinforcement magnitude for consecutive instances of abstinence. Second, as described above, there is a reset in reinforcer magnitude (voucher value or number of prize draws) following a failure to abstain. The combination of these components seems to provide the greatest likelihood for achieving a successful treatment outcome [71, 72]. While we do not precisely know why these components are operative, it is likely that they function to integrate individual instances of abstinence into a consecutive period of abstinence. If each abstinence were reinforced independently of those that preceded or followed it, the behavioral target would be individual instances of abstinence. By linking consecutive instances of abstinence via the escalation and reset procedure, the target becomes consecutive instances of abstinence, which should be the goal of all treatment efforts. Whenever it is possible, CM procedures should try to incorporate both of these schedule components to have the greatest likelihood of success.

The second factor to consider is the magnitude, or value, of the reinforcers used. There exists an extensive body of literature from both laboratory and clinical trials and with different species including humans that unambiguously demonstrates that higher magnitudes of reinforcement are better at controlling behavior [45,

50, 89]. Clinically, this means that the higher the value of the reinforcer employed, the more effective it is likely to be. Use of reinforcer magnitudes that are too low to control behavior (e.g., [50]) will result in failure of the intervention. Unfortunately, this could be interpreted as a failure of the CM protocol, when in fact it is a lack of fidelity to the protocol that is responsible for the failure. One should not expect a low-magnitude reinforcer procedure to be very effective. This often poses a significant challenge to the implementation of CM [73]. Treatment centers are often under-resourced and do not have the means to employ high-magnitude monetary reinforcers such as vouchers and prizes. In this case, other non-cash-based reinforcers can be used (as described above), or community donations can be sought (e.g., [5]). It is our belief that funders are beginning to embrace CM interventions as many insurance companies employ CM-based efforts to control health behaviors and as the United States Veterans Administration has adopted CM as a primary treatment strategy [63]. Hopefully, this will reduce the difficulty surrounding the provision of reinforcement of sufficient magnitude.

It should be noted that what is reinforcing for one person may not be reinforcing for another. Thus, when using non-cash-based reinforcers, it is incumbent on the clinician to find reinforcers that are salient to individual consumers. This can be done by identifying a functional relationship between behavior and reinforcers as described in Johnston and Pennypacker [33]. Also of note is that reinforcement magnitude can be changed during treatment, if necessary, to garner more control over a user's behavior. In a study by Robles and colleagues [67], it was demonstrated that even treatment-resistant cocaine users would abstain if high-magnitude vouchers (e.g., $100.00 US) were used.

The third factor to consider when developing, or delivering, a CM protocol is delay [50, 53, 75]. There are two types of delay that are common in CM protocols. The first is the delay between earning a reinforcer (e.g., providing biological evidence of drug abstinence) and receiving the reinforcer. That is, how long after someone provides a drug-negative urine sample until they receive their prize or voucher. In order to be maximally effective, this delay should be minimized. Another type of delay encountered when using vouchers is an exchange delay [32]. That is the delay between telling the counselor what you want to exchange your voucher for and the actual receipt of the item. Again, in order to maximize protocol efficacy, this delay should be minimized.

The fourth and final factor we wish to mention is intervention duration. While it is quite understandable that clinicians, consumers, their families, and funders want short, effective, treatment, it is important to remember that drug users spend a lifetime developing an addiction; it may not be reasonable to think that the behavioral patterns established in order to support compulsive drug-taking behavior can be terminated quickly. For this reason, we recommend that the longest possible duration of treatment be employed. There is evidence to suggest that longer treatments are more effective than shorter ones [69] and that long-term treatment is acceptable to consumers [77]. Notably, dozens of studies have shown that CM continues to decrease substance use as long as it is in place and ceases to work once it is removed, e.g., A-B-A, or return to baseline studies have shown this multiple times across various substances of abuse. Many have questioned the utility of CM because once the contingency is taken away, drug use often returns soon after. However, we view this as a strength of the CM approach. This is not unlike an ideal medication that works when it is taken with almost no side effects and does not work relatively soon after not being taken. Still, some have documented that the effects of CM can remain for up to 18 months after treatment.

29.5 Barriers

Given the widely accepted efficacy and relative ease of implementation, one could reasonably ask why CM is not more widely employed. To begin with, it is often employed although perhaps not as frequently as one would expect. In our experience, three common barriers are raised that hinder effective implementation of the procedure. These barriers have been discussed in detail, and interested readers should consult the literature for a thorough vetting (e.g., [64, 73]).

Primary among the barriers is the perceived cost of the CM interventions. We have touched on this in several of the above sections. Cost is an issue, but non-monetary reinforcers can be employed. Also, some of the most cited studies have shown that average cost can be between $100 and $200 in efficacious CM interventions [51, 56]. Some work has demonstrated unanticipated benefits such as decreased hospitalizations and improved comorbid psychiatric functioning [40] suggesting that potential cost offsets could be used to fund interventions. CM is cost-effective [44]; it is sometimes a matter of convincing payers of that efficacy.

An important issue to consider in this context as well is the cost of CM compared to other available treatments. Relative to most forms of psychosocial counseling that are available for psychostimulant use, for example, the cost should be evaluated carefully (e.g., societal costs, legal costs, emergency department costs) given the high costs associated with poorly performing treatments or a lack of available treatments as is the case for psychostimulants.

Another common concern is provider perceptions [11]. Providers sometimes argue that in order to be effective, treatment needs to engage a consumer's *intrinsic motivation* and not be based on a procedure that engineers the user's environment. The very existence of this construct (intrinsic motivation) is controversial. Moreover, when confronted with the efficacy of the CM interventions, most clinicians adopt a more conciliatory approach. Clinicians also have, on occasion, had personal experiences with substance use disorders and are themselves in recovery. In this case, they may believe that others need to follow the same strategies they used to obtain and maintain abstinence. Thankfully, this is an increasingly rare occurrence. It would be akin to a physician who suffered from bronchitis which was cured by antibiotic Z insisting that antibiotic Z is the only way to treat bronchitis based on her personal experience.

It has also been argued that CM protocols are too complex. Proponents of this argument claim that busy, poorly resourced clinicians do not have the time needed to calculate reinforcer value and carry out prize draws or voucher exchanges. While we certainly agree that clinicians are overworked and underpaid, we find this class of argument to be repugnant. It is akin to a surgeon declining to operate on someone because the surgical procedure was too complex, and they were too busy with other procedures. Again, it is important to consider the question of "too complex, compared to what?" Many psychosocial techniques are not easily deployed due to the intense training and fidelity needed. Even after being deployed after the therapist in question has achieved high enough fidelity, most clinicians agree that without consistent and ongoing trainings, there is a natural, therapeutic "drift" that occurs over time among many psychosocial treatments. Thus, the necessary training and monitoring is both costly and labor intensive and can also be magnitudes more complex than CM. Moreover, the advent of technology to aid clinicians with the delivery of CM (and the ability to conduct online voucher exchanges) [42] obviates most of these concerns. We discuss this in some detail below.

The final perception we wish to discuss is one of consumer resources. It has been suggested that CM-based interventions will only work for those who have limited financial resources. While it is undeniable that drug addiction eats away at a person's resources until they are depleted and that most abusers are financially deprived, we are aware of no data to suggest that CM efficacy is influenced by income level. In fact, research has shown the income level (both legal and illegal) does not impact CM efficacy [64]. That said, most treatment efforts and especially those involving clinical research protocols for substance abuse are populated by individuals of limited financial means. Further work is needed to assess the efficacy of the monetarily-based procedures in those with relative wealth.

29.6 Combining Experimental Technologies with Incentives for Behavior Change Remotely Monitoring Outcomes

As mentioned, one of the barriers to more widespread implementation and dissemination of CM has been the necessity of participants attending frequent clinic visits, driven mostly by the short half-life of point of care tests for drugs and alcohol. This is also driven by the need to deliver an immediate consequence consistent with evidence, or lack thereof, of a desired behavior. Notably, a strength of CM is that it can be administered by individuals with minimal training and no clinical credentials [38, 83]. This has led to new lines of research that seek to take advantage of novel, automated technologies that can streamline the delivery of incentives electronically and are paired with inexpensive biochemical monitoring [49]. As mobile phones are increasingly becoming a part of everyday life [81], this has generated much research activity focused on the virtual delivery of reinforcers to individuals that can be almost anywhere, including those dwelling in rural or otherwise remote locations that are essentially a "drug and alcohol use disorder treatment desert." Ironically, while CM has been criticized for years as being difficult to disseminate, as technology evolves, it appears that CM is becoming more portable than many other treatment modalities. Many of these technology-based CM strategies are in the feasibility stage, but significant progress has been made in remote monitoring of participants, intervention delivery, and delivery of reinforcers through technology.

In 2013, Alessi and colleagues published a randomized study that assessed the efficacy and feasibility of a CM intervention to reinforce alcohol abstinence using mobile technology [3]. This trial included 30 heavy drinking adults that were given a portable breathalyzer and a cell phone and were trained how to record a video of themselves provisioning breath samples prior to submitting the video in exchange for different incentives. Participants were randomized to two different groups: (1) a control group that received incentives for submitting breath samples, and payment was not contingent on the status of the sample, and (2) an active CM treatment group that received the same amount of incentives as the control group, but they also received escalating vouchers for the submission of alcohol-negative breath samples. Study staff communicated with participants through text messaging to send daily reminders for when the samples were due. This study demonstrated medium to large CM effects, showing that CM was significantly associated with (1) increased daily alcohol abstinence, (2) duration of abstinence from alcohol, and (3) decreases in self-reported drinking days and severity of drinking-associated problems during the intervention [3].

Another example from the smoking cessation literature is a trial that compared the effect of an online CM intervention to a non-CM, online monitoring, and goal-setting intervention [15]. The CM intervention significantly improved short-term smoking abstinence rates compared to the non-CM, online monitoring, and goal-setting intervention [15]. Similar to what Alessi and colleagues did in the above noted alcohol intervention, the distribution of incentives occurred virtually immediately after the submission of smoking-negative sample using carbon monoxide (CO; biochemical measure of recent smoking) as the biomarker [15]. A similar, "video-observed CO submission" online program was developed for adolescents dwelling in Appalachia. Adolescents in this area have smoking rates that are significantly elevated in comparison to the national average. Given that this population is harder to reach and is at higher risk, adapted CM interventions have the capacity to make a significant difference. In this study, 62 adolescents agreed to submit three videos each day showing the participants submitting the required breath samples using a portable CO breathalyzer. For adolescents in the CM group, provision of a smoking-negative sample would earn them virtual vouchers that could be exchanged for a variety of prizes. Those randomized to the monitoring and goal-setting condition received prizes for simply submitting the requisite video recordings. This trial was conducted almost entirely online, but it did require study staff to review the video to ensure that the appropriate person and sample had been collected before the vouchers were delivered [65].

Notably, a recent systematic review that examined 39 CM-based remote monitoring studies (18 targeted substance use; 11 targeted diet, exercise, or weight loss; 10 targeted medication adherence or in-home monitoring) found that 71% of the studies resulted in clinically and statistically significant treatment effects in favor of CM. These data support the benefits of adopting remote, technology-based CM interventions for both drug and alcohol use disorder but also for other health-impairing behaviors such as medication non-adherence [36]. In fact, the FDA has approved a mobile-based CM app for substance use disorders (SUDs) (Pear therapeutics, Inc. developed reSET) [59]. Other, related software applications are currently in development, some of which are supported through the National Institutes of Health's Small Business Innovation Research and Small Business Technology Transfer programs.

Beyond experimental software technologies that are under development, there are novel hardware technologies that could rapidly leverage the inherent strengths of CM, especially if paired with the optimal software applications that are simultaneously emerging. One example is BACTrack, a battery-operated breath alcohol capture analysis device that connects to a participants' cellphone through Bluetooth (KHN Solutions, San Francisco, CA, USA) [61]. This hardware has not been used in conjunction with CM yet in large demonstration project, but early pilot data indicate that it could be a valuable tool to monitor alcohol use similar to the portable CO breath analyzer noted in the studies above and utilized elsewhere for similar, remote monitoring studies of smoking cessation treatments. Another, more commonly researched tool for remotely monitoring alcohol use is a transdermal alcohol monitoring tool. This hardware eliminates any need for a clinician or staff member because it will passively collect patient samples. The Secure Continuous Remote Alcohol Monitoring

(SCRAM) continuously collects and monitors participants' alcohol consumption through an ankle monitor that collects and analyzes perspiration [2, 9]. This device has been used with CM, but in a recent investigation, there were no statistically significant differences in the primary outcomes of treatment attendance and alcohol abstinence between the CM and control groups [2]. However, there is some additional, more promising data published supporting the utility and feasibility of transdermal monitoring of alcohol use [2, 3].

29.7 Attendance and Medication Adherence Technologies

In the area of utilizing CM for promoting increased attendance and increased treatment adherence, there are also new technologies being designed including biosensors and pill bottle electronic reminder systems and monitors [21, 60]. The progress being made in this area is encouraging because treatment attendance, adherence, and medication adherence all have remained major barriers to the large-scale and consistent delivery of evidence-based treatments across drug and alcohol use therapeutic areas, but also in several other therapeutic areas [35]. For example, a recently published study by Raiff and colleagues assessed the feasibility of combining CM with a remote medication adherence monitoring system ("Wisepill") to target medication adherence among three adults with type 2 diabetes. Adherence to each patient's diabetes medication was remotely recorded in real time using the Wisepill device [60], a portable and electronically monitored pill dispenser. Patients received monetary incentives in exchange for time-window compliant evidence of daily tallied medication adherence. The results indicated that adherence was increased for all participants who were exposed to the CM intervention [15]. While the evidence is more dated, CM has also shown promise for improving medication adherence among HIV-positive methadone patients [82]. A 2007 published trial randomized participants to one of two groups: (1) a group that received medication-adherence coaching sessions on a biweekly basis or (2) a voucher group that received CM combined with the coaching sessions. The study found that the CM group experienced significantly higher medication adherence compared to the coaching session-only group [82].

A 2012 systematic review that focused on incentive-based interventions for targeting medication adherence concluded that while CM shows significant promise in the field and evidence is being accumulated that continues to support its use, it remains understudied [16]. A comparison between several studies demonstrated that CM adherence-based interventions increased medication adherence by 20% on average. However, the effect sizes varied greatly. This may have been the result of CM being applied non-uniformly and in some cases not as originally designed or intended in order to cause sustained behavior change [16]. While adherence to medications often diminished after the CM intervention was removed [16], this is not unlike most efficacious adherence interventions or treatments in the form of pharmacotherapies or other behavioral interventions. Further, it is important to note that a long-standing scientific principle for treatment development across therapeutic area is that a treatment works when it is in place and does not work when taken away. This is often associated with predictable and safe treatment effects that can be readily applied in the real world. However, long-term behavior change with CM and virtually all other SUD therapies with a comparable evidence base is an area that remains in need of investigation.

29.8 Limitations

While we are strong proponents for the use of CM-based interventions, we are also realistic. As of yet, there is no silver bullet for the treatment of psychostimulant addiction, including CM. In our experience however, CM is a great treatment modality for initiating abstinence. While some have demonstrated encouraging long-term maintenance of abstinence post-CM-based treatment (e.g., [30]), a perception lingers that long-term effects are difficult to demonstrate. As discussed

above, we believe that VBRT provides a mechanism for bringing consumers in contact with non-drug sources of reinforcement than can serve to maintain abstinence, but in our experience, this is not an automatic occurrence. Once individuals are treated for their addiction, they often find themselves right back in the same environment that occasioned their drug use in the first place. In this environment, the same pressures began to re-exert their influence and a risk of relapse is high. This brings us to our second limitation. We do not believe that CM should be a standalone intervention in most instances. Instead, we recommend pairing it with other evidence-based treatment. Drug abusers have complicated chaotic lives. They need help navigating affective, legal, and cognitive aspects of their addiction. While CM initiates abstinence and provides a sober client for the clinician to work with, it does nothing to inherently address these other concerns. These need to be addressed in the therapeutic relationship in order to maximize the likelihood of maintaining the abstinence which CM is so effective at initiating.

29.9 Conclusion

An impressive array of basic science research supports the notion that drugs of abuse serve as potent reinforcers. Further, the hallmark of successful drug abuse treatment is the diminution of the drug's reinforcing efficacy. CM is a very effective means for accomplishing this, especially in the treatment of psychostimulant addictions. Different types of CM appear to be generally effective and when delivered with high fidelity offer the clinician and the consumer perhaps their best chance for breaking the pernicious cycle of addiction.

References

1. Ainscough TS, McNeill A, Stang J, Clader R, Brose LS. Contingency management interventions for non-prescribed drug use during treatment for opiate addiction: a systematic review and meta-analysis. Drug Alcohol Depend. 2017;178:318–39.

2. Alessi SM, Barnett NP, Petry NM. Experiences with SCRAMx alcohol monitoring technology in 100 alcohol treatment outpatients. Drug Alcohol Depend. 2017;178:417–24.

3. Alessi SM, Petry NM. A randomized study of cell-phone technology to reinforce alcohol abstinence in the natural environment. Addiction. 2013;108(5):900–9.

4. Alessi SM, Roll JM, Reilly MP, Johanson CE. Establishment of a diazepam preference in human volunteers following a differential-conditioning history of placebo versus diazepam choice. Exp Clin Psychopharmacol. 2002;10(2):77–83. https://doi.org/10.1037//1064-1297.10.2.77.

5. Amass L, Kamien J. A tale of two cities: financing two voucher programs for substance abusers through community donations. Exp Clin Psychopharmacol. 2004;12(2):147–55.

6. Amass L, Kamien JB. Funding contingency management in community treatment clinics: use of community donations and clinic rebates. In: Contingency management in substance abuse treatment. New York: Guilford Press; 2008. p. 280–97.

7. Andrade LF, Petry NM. Contingency management. In: McSweeney FK, Murphy ES, editors. (in press). Wiley-Blackwell handbook of operant and classical conditioning. Oxford: Wiley-Blackwell; 2014.

8. Aubin H, Luquiens A, Berlin I. Pharmacotherapy for smoking cessation: pharmacological principles and clinical practice. Br J Clin Pharmacol. 2013. https://doi.org/10.1111/bcp.12116.

9. Barnett NP, Tidey J, Murphy JG, Swift R, Colby SM. Contingency management for alcohol use reduction: a pilot study using a transdermal alcohol sensor. Drug Alcohol Depend. 2011;118(2):391–9.

10. Bart G. Maintenance medication for opiate addiction: the foundation of recovery. J Addict Dis. 2012;31(3):207–25.

11. Benishek LA, Kirby KC, Dugosh KL, Padovano A. Beliefs about the empirical support of drug abuse treatment interventions: a survey of outpatient treatment providers. Drug Alcohol Depend. 2010;107(2):202–8.

12. Boakes RA. From Darwin to behaviourism: psychology and the minds of animals Cambridge [Cambridgeshire]. New York: Cambridge University Press; 1984.

13. Branson CE, Barbuti AM, Clemmey P, Herman L, Bhutia P. A pilot study of low cost contingency management to increase attendance in an adolescent substance abuse program. Am J Addict. 2012;21(2):126–9.

14. Carroll ME, Lac ST, Nygaard SL. A concurrently available nondrug reinforcer prevents the acquisition or decreases the maintenance of cocaine-reinforced behavior. Psychopharmacology. 1989;97(1):23–9.

15. Dallery J, Raiff BR, Kim SJ, Marsch LA, Stitzer M, Grabinski MJ. Nationwide access to an internet-based contingency management intervention to promote smoking cessation: a randomized controlled trial. Addiction. 2017;112(5):875–83.

16. DeFulio A, Silverman K. The use of incentives to reinforce medication adherence. Prev Med. 2012;55:S86–94.

17. DeFulio A, Stitzer M, Roll J, Petry N, Nuzzo P, Schwartz RP, Stabile P. Criminal justice referral and incentives in outpatient substance abuse treatment. J Subst Abus Treat. 2013;45(1):70–75.

18. Downey KK, Helmus TC, Schuster CR. Treatment of heroin-dependent poly-drug abusers with contingency management and buprenorphine maintenance. Exp Clin Psychopharmacol. 2000;8(2):176–84.

19. Dutra L, Stathopoulou G, Basden SL, Leyro TM, Powers MB, Otto MW. A meta-analytic review of psychosocial interventions for substance use disorders. Am J Psychiatry. 2008;165(2):179–87. https://doi.org/10.1176/appi.ajp.2007.06111851.

20. Ferster BF, Skinner CB, Ferster C. Schedules of reinforcement. New York: Appleton-Century-Crofts; 1957.

21. Flores GP, Peace B, Carnes TC, et al. Performance, reliability, usability, and safety of the id-cap system for ingestion event monitoring in healthy volunteers: a pilot study. Innov Clin Neurosci. 2016;13(9–10):12–9.

22. Hall EA, Prendergast ML, Roll JM, Warda U. Reinforcing abstinence and treatment participation among offenders in a drug diversion program: are vouchers effective? Crim Justice Behav. 2009;36(9):935–53.

23. Hartzler B, Lash SJ, Roll JM. Contingency management in substance abuse treatment: a structured review of the evidence for its transportability. Drug Alcohol Depend. 2012;122(1):1–10.

24. Higgins ST, Bickel WK, Hughes JR. Influence of an alternative Reinforcer on human cocaine self-administration. Life Sci. 1994;55(3):179–87. https://doi.org/10.1016/0024-3205(94)00878-7.

25. Higgins ST, Budney AJ, Bickel WK, Foerg FE, Donham R, Badger GJ. Incentives improve outcome in outpatient behavioral treatment of cocaine dependence. Arch Gen Psychiatry. 1994;51(7):568–76.

26. Higgins ST, Delaney DD, Budney AJ, Bickel WK, Hughes JR, Foerg F, Fenwick JW. A behavioral approach to achieving initial cocaine abstinence. Am J Psychiatry. 1991;148(9):1218–24.

27. Higgins ST, Silverman K. Motivating behavior change among illicit-drug abusers: research on contingency management interventions. Washington, DC: American Psychological Association; 1999.

28. Higgins ST, Silverman K, Heil SH. Contingency management in the treatment of substance use disorders: a science-based treatment innovation. New York: Guilford Press; 2008.

29. Higgins ST, Washio Y, Heil SH, Solomon LJ, Gaalema DE, Higgins TM, Bernstein IM. Financial incentives for smoking cessation among pregnant and newly postpartum women. Prev Med. 2012;55:S33–40.

30. Higgins ST, Wong CJ, Badger GJ, Ogden DEH, Dantona DL. Contingent reinforcement increases cocaine abstinence during outpatient

treatment and 1 year of follow-up. J Consult Clin Psychol. 2000;68(1):64–72. https://doi.org/10.1037//0022-006x.68.1.64.

31. Holz WC, Gill CA. Drug injections as negative reinforcers. Pharmacol Rev. 1975;27(3):437–46.

32. Hyten C, Madden GJ, Field PD. Exchange delays and impulsive choice in adult humans. J Exp Anal Behav. 1994;62(2):225–33.

33. Johnston JM, Pennypacker HS. Strategies and tactics of behavioral research. 2nd ed. Hillsdale: Lawrence Erlbaum Associates, Publishers; 1993.

34. Kandel DA, Schuster CR. An investigation of nalorphine and perphenazine as negative reinforcers in an escape paradigm. Pharmacol Biochem Behav. 1977;6(1):61–71.

35. Kimmel SE, Troxel AB. Novel incentive-based approaches to adherence. Clin Trials. 2012;9(6):689–95.

36. Kurti AN, Davis D, Redner R, et al. A review of the literature on remote monitoring technology in incentive-based interventions for health-related behavior change. Transl Issues Psychol Sci. 2016;2(2):128.

37. Ledgerwood DM. Contingency management for smoking cessation: where do we go from here? Curr Drug Abuse Rev. 2008;1(3):340–9.

38. Ledgerwood DM, Alessi SM, Hanson T, Godley MD, Petry NM. Contingency management for attendance to group substance abuse treatment administered by clinicians in community clinics. J Appl Behav Anal. 2008;41(4):517–26.

39. Lussier JP, Heil SH, Mongeon JA, Badger GJ, Higgins ST. A meta-analysis of voucher-based reinforcement therapy for substance use disorders. Addiction. 2006;101(2):192–203. https://doi.org/10.1111/j.1360-0443.2006.01311.x.

40. McDonell MG, Srebnik D, Angelo F, McPherson S, Lowe JM, Sugar A, Short RA, Roll JM, Ries RK. Randomized controlled trial of contingency management for stimulant use in community mental health patients with serious mental illness. Am J Psychiatr. 2013;170(1):94–101.

41. McSweeney FK, Murphy ESE. Wiley-Blackwell handbook of operant and classical conditioning. Oxford: Wiley-Blackwell; 2014.

42. Meredith SE, Dallery J. Investigating group contingencies to promote brief abstinence from cigarette smoking. Exp Clin Pschopharmacol. 2013;21(2):144–54. https://doi.org/10.1037/a0031707.

43. Milby JB, Schumacher JE, McNamara C, Wallace D, McGill T, Stange D, Michael M. Abstinence contingent housing enhances day treatment for homeless cocaine abusers. National Institute on Drug Abuse Research Monograph Series, 174. 1996.

44. Murphy SM, McDonell MG, McPherson S, Srebnik D, Angelo F, Roll JM, Ries RK. An economic evaluation of a contigency-management intervention for stimulant use among community mental health patients with serious mental illness. Drug Alcohol Depend. 2015;153:293–9.

45. Nader MA, Woolverton WL. Effects of increasing the magnitude of an alternative reinforcer on drug choice in a discrete-trials choice procedure. Psychopharmacology. 1991;105(2):169–74. https://doi.org/10.1007/Bf02244304.

46. Negus SS. Choice between heroin and food in non-dependent and heroin-dependent rhesus monkeys: effects of naloxone, buprenorphine, and methadone. J Pharmacol Exp Ther. 2006;317(2):711–23.

47. Negus SS, Banks ML. Medications development for opioid abuse. Cold Spring Harb Perspect Med. 2013;3(1).

48. Oluwoye O, Kriegel L, Alcover K, McPherson S, McDonell M, Roll J. Advances in the dissemination and implementation of contigency management of substance use disorders. Psychol Addict Behav. In Press.

49. Oluwoye O, Skalisky J, Burduli E, et al. Using a randomized controlled trial to test whether modifications to contingency management improve outcomes for heavy drinkers with serious mental illness. Contemp Clin Trials. 2018;69:92–8.

50. Packer RR, Howell DN, McPherson S, Roll JM. Investigating reinforcer magnitude and reinforcer delay: a contingency management analog study. Exp Clin Psychopharmacol. 2012;20(4):287–92.

51. Peirce JM, Petry NM, Stitzer ML, Blaine J, Kellogg S, Kellogg S, Satterfield F, Schwartz M, Krasnansky J, Pencer E, Silva-Vazquez L, Kirby KC, Royer-Malvestuto C, Roll JM, Cohen A, Copersino ML, Kolodner K, Li R. Effects of lower-cost incentives on stimulant abstinence in methadone maintenance treatment: a National Drug Abuse Teatment Clinical Trials Network Study. Arch Gen Psychiatry. 2006;63(2):201–8.

52. Petry N. Contingency management for substance abuse treatment: a guide to implementing this evidence based-practice. New York: Taylor and Francis Group; 2012.

53. Petry NM. A comprehensive guide to the application of contingency management procedures in clinical settings. Drug Alcohol Depend. 2000;58(1–2):9–25.

54. Petry NM, Kolodner KB, Li R, Peirce JM, Roll JM, Stitzer ML, Hamilton JA. Prize-based contingency management does not increase gambling. Drug Alcohol Depend. 2006;83(3):269–73.

55. Petry NM, Martin B. Low-cost contingency management for treating cocaine- and opioid-abusing methadone patients. J Consult Clin Psychol. 2002;70(2):398–405.

56. Petry NM, Peirce JM, Stitzer ML, Blaine J, Roll JM, Cohen A, Obert JL, Killeen T, Saladin ME, Cowell M. Effect of prize-based incentives on outcomes in stimulant abusers in outpatient psychosocial treatment programs: a national drug abuse treatment clinical trials network study. Arch Gen Psychiatry. 2005;62(10):1148.

57. Prendergast M, Hall E, Roll J, Warda U. Use of vouchers to reinforce abstinence and positive behaviors among clients in a drug court treatment program. J Subst Abus Treat. 2008;35(2):125–36.

58. Prendergast M, Podus D, Finney J, Greenwell L, Roll J. Contingency management for treatment of substance use disorders: a meta-analysis. Addiction. 2006;101(11):1546–60. https://doi.org/10.1111/j.1360-0443.2006.01581.x.

59. Press Announcements – FDA permits marketing of mobile medical application for substance use disorder. [Website]. 2017. https://www.fda.gov/NewsEvents/Newsroom/PressAnnouncements/ucm576087.htm. Accessed 3 Nov 2017.

60. Raiff BR, Jarvis BP, Dallery J. Text-message reminders plus incentives increase adherence to antidiabetic medication in adults with type 2 diabetes. J Appl Behav Anal. 2016;49(4):947–53.

61. Ran R, Mullins ME. Can handling E85 motor fuel cause positive breath alcohol test results? J Anal Toxicol. 2013;37(7):430–2.

62. Rash CJ, Andrade LF, Petr NM. Income received during treatment does not affect response to contingency management treatments in cocaine-dependent outpatients. Drug Alcohol Depend. 2013;132(3):528–34.

63. Rash CJ, DePhilippis D, McKay JR, Drapkin M, Petry NM. Training workshops positively impact beliefs about contingency management in a nationwide dissemination effort. J Subst Abus Treat. 2013;45(3):306–12.

64. Rash CJ, Petry NM, Kirby KC, Martino S, Roll J, Stitzer ML. Identifying provider beliefs related to contingency management adoption using the contingency management beliefs questionnaire. Drug Alcohol Depend. 2012;121(3):205–12.

65. Reynolds B, Harris M, Slone SA, et al. A feasibility study of home-based contingency management with adolescent smokers of rural Appalachia. Exp Clin Psychopharmacol. 2015;23(6):486.

66. Ries RK, Dyck DG, Short R, Srebnik D, Fisher A, Comtois KA. Outcomes of managing disability benefits among patients with substance dependence and severe mental illness. Psychiatr Serv. 2004;55(4):445–7.

67. Robles E, Silverman K, Preston KL, Cone EJ, Katz E, Bigelow GE, Stitzer ML. The brief abstinence test: voucher-based reinforcement of cocaine abstinence. Drug Alcohol Depend. 2000;58(1–2):205–12.

68. Roll JM. Behavioral pharmacology. In: McSweeney FK, Murphy ES, editors. Wiley-Blackwell handbook of operant and classical conditioning. Oxford: Wiley-Blackwell; 2014. p. 612–6.

69. Roll JM, Chudzynski J, Cameron J, Howell D, McPherson S. Duration effects in contingency management treatment of methamphetamine disorders. Addict Behav. 2013;38(9):2455–62.

70. Roll JM, Chudzynski JE, Richardson G. Potential sources of reinforcement and punishment in a drug-free treatment clinic: client and staff perceptions. Am J Drug Alcohol Abuse. 2005;31(1):21–33.

71. Roll JM, Higgins ST. A within-subject comparison of three different schedules of reinforcement of drug abstinence using cigarette smoking as an exemplar. Drug Alcohol Depend. 2000;58(1–2):103–9.

72. Roll JM, Higgins ST, Badger GJ. An experimental comparison of three different schedules of reinforcement of drug abstinence using cigarette smoking as an exemplar. J Appl Behav Anal. 1996;29(4):495–504. https://doi.org/10.1901/jaba.1996.29-495.

73. Roll JM, Medden GJ, Rawson R, Petry NM. Facilitating the adoption of contingency management for the treatment of substance use disorders. Behav Anal Pract. 2009;2(1):4–13.

74. Roll JM, Newton T. Contingency management for the treatment of methamphetamine use disorders. In: Higgins ST, Silverman K, Hiel SH, editors. Contingency management in substance abuse treatment. New York: The Guilford Press; 2008. p. 80–99.

75. Roll JM, Reilly MP, Johanson CE. The influence of exchange delays on cigarette versus money choice: a laboratory analog of voucher-based reinforcement therapy. Exp Clin Psychopharmacol. 2000;8(3):366–70. https://doi.org/10.1037//1064-1297.8.3.366.

76. Silverman K, DeFulio A, Sigurdsson SO. Maintenance of reinforcement to address the chronic nature of drug addiction. Prev Med. 2012;55:S46–53.

77. Silverman K, Robles E, Mudric T, Bigelow GE, Stitzer ML. A randomized trial of long-term reinforcement of cocaine abstinence in methadone-maintained patients who inject drugs. J Consult Clin Psychol. 2004;72(5):839–54.

78. Silverman K, Roll JM, Higgins ST. Introduction to the special issue on the behavior analysis and treatment of drug addiction. J Appl Behav Anal. 2008;41(4):471–80. https://doi.org/10.1901/jaba.2008.41-471.

79. Skinner BF. The behavior of organisms: an experimental analysis. Acton: Copley Publishing Group; 1938.

80. Skinner BF, Heron WT. Effects of caffeine and benzedrine upon conditioning and extinction. Psych Record. 1937;1:339–46.

81. Smith-Jackson T, Nussbaum M, Mooney A. Accessible cell phone design: development and application of a needs analysis framework. Disabil Rehabil. 2003;25(10):549–60.

82. Sorensen JL, Haug NA, Delucchi KL, et al. Voucher reinforcement improves medication adherence in HIV-positive methadone patients: a randomized trial. Drug Alcohol Depend. 2007;88(1):54–63.

83. Squires DD, Gumbley SJ, Storti SA. Training substance abuse treatment organizations to adopt evidence-based practices: the addiction technology transfer center of new England science to service laboratory. J Subst Abus Treat. 2008;34(3):293–301.

84. Stitzer ML, Iguchi MY, Felch LJ. Contingent take-home incentive: effects on drug use of methadone maintenance patients. J Consult Clin Psychol. 1992;60(6):927–34.

85. Stitzer ML, Petry N, Peirce J, Kirby K, Killeen T, Roll J, Hamilton J, Stabile PQ, Sterling R, Brown C, Kolodner K, Li R. Effectiveness of abstinence-based

incentives: interaction with intake stimulant test results. J Consult Clin Psychol. 2007;75(5):805–11.

86. Thompson T, Schuster CR. Morphine self-administration, food-reinforced, and avoidance behaviors in rhesus monkeys. Psychopharmacology. 1964;5(2):87–94.

87. Thompson T, Schuster CR. Behavioral pharmacology. Englewood Cliffs: Prentice Hall, Inc.; 1968.

88. Tuten M, Jones HE, Schaffer CM, Stitzer ML. Reinforcement-based treatment for substance use disorders: a comprehensive behavioral approach. Am J Addict. 2012;21(5):499–500.

89. Wong CJ, Sheppard J-M, Dallery J, Bedient G, Robles E, Svikis D, Silverman K. Effects of reinforcer magnitude on data-entry productivity in chronically unemployed drug abusers participating in a therapeutic workplace. Exp Clin Psychopharmacol. 2003;11(1):46–55.

90. Yoon JH, Higgins ST, Bradstreet MP, Badger GJ, Thomas CS. Changes in the relative reinforcing effects of cigarette smoking as a function of initial abstinence. Psychopharmacology. 2009;205(2):305–18.

Group Therapy for Substance Use Disorders

30

R. Kathryn McHugh, Jungjin Kim,
Sara Park Perrins, and Roger D. Weiss

Contents

Abstract

Group therapy is the predominant type of behavioral therapy offered in substance use disorder treatment settings. This chapter pro-

R. K. McHugh (✉) · J. Kim · R. D. Weiss
Division of Alcohol and Drug Abuse, McLean
Hospital, Belmont, MA, USA

Department of Psychiatry, Harvard Medical School,
Boston, MA, USA
e-mail: kmchugh@mclean.harvard.edu

S. P. Perrins
School of Environmental and Forest Sciences,
University of Washington, Seattle, WA, USA

vides an overview of the research literature on the efficacy of group therapy for substance use disorders and discusses research challenges and important future directions in the study of this topic. Research on the efficacy of group therapy for substance use disorders has generally found that group therapy is associated with superior outcomes compared to no treatment or treatment-as-usual. Studies examining the combination of group therapy with other forms of treatment, such as pharmacotherapy, have been mixed, with some studies finding additive benefits and others finding no benefit. However, group therapy appears to be

© Springer Nature Switzerland AG 2021
N. el-Guebaly et al. (eds.), *Textbook of Addiction Treatment*,
https://doi.org/10.1007/978-3-030-36391-8_30

equally as effective as individual therapy and may offer cost benefits relative to individual treatment. Group therapy for co-occurring substance use disorders and other psychiatric disorders, such as bipolar disorder and post-traumatic stress disorder, is associated with benefits for both disorders. Due to method-ological and logistical challenges of conduct-ing research on group therapy, this treatment modality remains understudied compared to individual therapy. Additional research is needed to identify the most effective types of group therapy and its optimal delivery method, either alone or in combination with other therapies.

Keywords

Group therapy · Substance use disorders · Co-occurring disorders · Cognitive-behavioral therapy

30.1 Introduction

Group therapy for substance use disorders (SUDs) is a treatment modality that entails the presence of at least two independent (i.e., not related) patients and a therapist who conducts meetings with the goal of eliminating or reducing substance use or SUD symptoms [1]. Group therapy formats can emphasize the interactions among members and the therapist (process or supportive therapy groups), the acquisition of information and skills (psychoeducational or behavioral therapy groups), or both. The content of group therapy also varies and might include components such as psycho-education, cognitive-behavioral or motivational interventions, "check-ins" about substance use and other symptoms, encouragement to attend 12-step or other mutual-help groups, relational interventions, skills training, and contingency management, among others.

The majority of SUD treatment programs offer group therapy (more than 94%) [2] and for many programs group therapy is their predomi-nant focus. The predominance of group therapy

in these settings may be attributable—at least in part—to the potential cost savings of a group rather than an individual approach. Cost analyses have found that group therapy is associated with substantially less therapist time per patient com-pared to individual therapy [3] and that it has both the lowest cost and best cost-effectiveness ratio of psychosocial treatment approaches [4, 5]. In addition, patients are generally satisfied with group therapy as indicated by similar (if not superior) retention rates compared to individual therapy and strong self-ratings of treatment satis-faction [3]. Studies of patient preference for group versus individual therapy are few; how-ever, group therapy has been shown to be pre-ferred over individual therapy by patients [6] and clinicians alike [7]. Thus, group therapy appears to be a highly acceptable and cost-effective approach to treating SUDs.

Despite its widespread use in the treatment of SUDs, group therapy has been studied far less extensively than individual therapy. In this review, we characterize the research on group therapy for patients with SUDs, with a focus on randomized controlled trials. We will limit our definition of group therapy to treatments that focus on sub-stance use or associated symptoms, and not on treatments targeted specifically to other symp-toms or co-occurring disorders (e.g., group cogni-tive-behavioral therapy (CBT) for depression in patients with SUDs). Where possible, we attempt to characterize the nature of the group therapy approach from content (e.g., cognitive-behavioral, psychoeducational), composition (e.g., targeted substance, single or mixed gender, dual diagno-sis), and timing (e.g., acute care, aftercare) per-spectives. We conclude with a commentary on limitations and challenges of conducting research on group therapy and provide an integration of findings from the extant literature.

30.2 Is Group Therapy Effective for the Treatment of SUDs?

Several studies have attempted to answer the basic question of whether group therapy is effec-tive for the treatment of SUDs. These studies either compare treatment-as-usual (usual care at a facility) to treatment-as-usual plus group therapy, or group therapy to no group therapy.

30.2.1 Comparing Group Therapy to Treatment-As-Usual or No Group Therapy

Studies of the effect of group therapy on SUD outcomes, in general, have suggested that group therapy is effective in reducing substance use and associated impairment. Stephens and colleagues [8] randomly assigned 291 individuals seeking treatment for marijuana to 14 sessions of group cognitive-behavioral therapy (CBT), 2 sessions of individual motivational treatment, or a waitlist control. Participants in both active treatment groups reported significantly greater reductions in marijuana use and consequences of use throughout treatment and at the 16-month follow-up than the waitlist control group. Group therapy and brief individual therapy were not significantly different on any outcomes. In a similar study, two sessions of group therapy were significantly more effective for reducing nicotine use in undergraduate smokers compared to a waitlist control group [9].

However, not all studies have yielded positive results. In a study of interventions to prevent relapse among abstinent smokers following 3 months of treatment with group therapy and/or nicotine replacement therapy, participants were randomly assigned to receive one of two counseling groups or no group treatment [10]. Abstinence rates were not significantly different across conditions after 12 months (range from 50% to 58%), suggesting that adding group counseling as a relapse prevention strategy after acute treatment may not be beneficial for increasing abstinence rates. Shorey and colleagues [11] randomized 117 post-detoxification patients at a residential treatment facility to receive adjunctive 8-session mindfulness and acceptance group therapy or treatment-as-usual. Groups were compared on the primary outcomes of drug craving and mindfulness, and no significant benefits of the group therapy relative to treatment-as-usual were observed.

30.2.2 Adding Group Therapy to Pharmacotherapy

Because pharmacotherapy is the first-line treatment for certain SUDs (e.g., opioid and nicotine use disorders), several trials have tested whether adding group therapy to medication can enhance outcomes.

A trial of adding 12 sessions of group CBT to the opioid antagonist naltrexone for opioid-dependent individuals found no difference between those who received group therapy and those who received naltrexone alone [12]. However, it is important to note in this study that fewer than 10% of the group therapy condition participants attended all group sessions. Moreover, participants in both conditions were permitted to engage in additional psychotherapy (including individual), with more than 85% of participants electing to do so. Thus, it is unclear whether the results reflect a failure of group therapy, an under-dosing of group therapy, or an effect of adjunctive treatment that was received by both groups (e.g., individual therapy).

Luthar and colleagues [13, 14] conducted two studies examining a relational psychotherapy group for mothers dependent on heroin. This relational intervention used a supportive approach focused on enhancing women's functioning and parenting. A study comparing this approach to methadone maintenance treatment as usual (including group counseling and case management) in 61 women found modest benefits of relational therapy for some parenting measures (e.g., risk of child maltreatment, affective interactions), but not others (e.g., limit setting, instrumental behaviors) [13]. Modest benefits were seen for depressive symptoms at post-treatment; however, this was no longer significant at follow-up. The relational group was associated with greater opioid abstinence, but not cocaine abstinence. This treatment was then examined in a larger study of 127 women receiving methadone maintenance compared to methadone maintenance plus a recovery training group therapy focused on psychoeducation and skills training [14]. Although the relational therapy was associated with some benefits at post-treatment, many of these benefits were reversed over a 6-month follow-up, with the comparison condition associated with better functional and child maltreatment outcomes.

Nyamathi et al. [15, 16] randomized 256 methadone-maintained adults who also used alcohol into (1) motivational interviewing (MI), delivered in group sessions, (2) motivational interviewing delivered individually, or (3) a nurse-led hepatitis health promotion group counseling. The nurse-led hepatitis health promotion counseling consisted of three 60-minute interactive psychoeducational groups focused on ways to promote liver health-promoting behaviors, including limiting alcohol and drug use. The motivational interviewing (MI) sessions were also three 60-minute sessions, delivered either individually or in a group format by MI-trained specialists. Self-reported alcohol use did not differ among the treatment groups, but the MI interventions—both group and individual—significantly reduced drug use, as measured by a 30-day recall, when compared to the nurse-led group counseling.

A qualitative literature review of studies of group therapy added to buprenorphine maintenance for opioid use disorder found that most studies in this area were not randomized trials (e.g., naturalistic studies), limiting the ability to draw conclusions about the efficacy of group therapy in this population [17]. Likewise, studies have often utilized very modest sample sizes (e.g., $N = 30$) [18], further complicating the ability to clearly interpret the effectiveness of group therapy for opioid use disorder.

Studies of the addition of group therapy to medication for nicotine dependence have also yielded mixed results. In a study of 154 nicotine-dependent women randomized to receive combinations of bupropion or placebo along with either cognitive-behavioral or supportive group therapy, a complex and mixed set of results emerged [19]. Specifically, CBT resulted in significantly higher abstinence rates than supportive therapy among those taking bupropion. However, supportive therapy was associated with superior outcomes among participants receiving placebo. Moreover, the combination of bupropion and CBT did not

result in better abstinence rates compared to either placebo condition [19].

A study by Smith and colleagues [20] randomized 677 smokers following a brief initial treatment (nicotine replacement therapy and 1 session of individual counseling) to 6 sessions of cognitive-behavioral group therapy, a motivational enhancement/supportive group therapy, or no group therapy; all participants also continued to receive nicotine replacement therapy. There were no significant differences among the three treatment conditions in terms of self-reported cigarette use; however, smokers who had not achieved abstinence during the initial treatment period had better outcomes in the motivational/supportive treatment relative to the cognitive-behavioral or no group conditions.

Overall, group therapy for SUDs appears to be superior to either waitlist or no treatment. Studies examining group therapy as an aftercare strategy or as added to pharmacotherapy are more mixed. In these studies, results imply that the effects of treatment may vary based on the subgroups (e.g., adding group therapy as aftercare may be effective for initial treatment non-responders) [20]. Additionally, mixed patterns of results regarding combination group therapy with pharmacotherapy imply that certain therapies may better complement certain medications; however, more studies are needed to understand whether such interactions exist and can be used to maximize outcomes.

30.3 Is Group Therapy as Good as Individual Therapy?

Several studies have tested whether therapy is more effective when delivered in a group or individual format. The largest well-controlled study of this association was conducted by Sobell and colleagues [3] in a sample of 264 individuals with "non-severe" alcohol and drug use problems (those with a history of severe dependence were excluded). Participants were randomly assigned to four sessions of a cognitive-behavioral motivational intervention in a group or individual format. Participants experienced significant reductions in self-reported alcohol and drug use and consequences of substance use. Results also indicated no differences in substance use outcomes for individual versus group administration for either alcohol or drug use and no differences in treatment retention.

In another study of group versus individual delivery of motivational therapy, John and colleagues [21] randomized 343 alcohol-dependent inpatients in German psychiatric hospitals to receive either 3 sessions of individual therapy or 9 sessions of group therapy for enhancing motivation for alcohol abstinence following detoxification. Those in the group therapy condition reported more self-help group attendance; however, there were no differences in other forms of treatment-seeking and overall service utilization between groups. There were also no differences in alcohol outcomes between these groups, with fewer than 30% in each group reporting abstinence at 6 months after detoxification.

Studies comparing individual and group cognitive-behavioral therapy have yielded similar results. A study of the use of 9 weeks (12 sessions) of cognitive-behavioral relapse prevention in group or individual format for 47 cocaine-dependent patients following inpatient treatment found similar outcomes for both groups over time on rates of abstinence as well as drug-related problems and measures of functioning [22]. By the end of treatment, fewer than 50% of both groups had remained abstinent, although gains in functioning and impairment were sustained over 24 weeks of follow-up; at the final assessment point, the average days of cocaine use in the previous month was low (2 days in the individual therapy condition; less than 1 day in the group therapy condition).

A similar study also compared individual to group relapse prevention as part of an aftercare program for 132 patients with alcohol and drug dependence [23]. Patients received 12 weekly sessions of either 45–60 minutes individual or 60–90 minutes group therapy. Group and individual therapies had similar outcomes for treatment adherence and retention and self-reported alcohol and drug use. However, group therapy was associated with better social support at 12-month follow-up. A study conducted in Brazil randomized 155 patients with alcohol and/or drug dependence to receive 17 sessions of cognitive-behavioral therapy in either group or individual format [24]. This study also found no significant differences in session attendance or in self-reported alcohol or drug use outcomes between groups when controlling for baseline levels of use.

A Norwegian study tested 12 weeks of 90-minute women-only group therapy or 7 hours of individual delivery of a short-term therapy focusing on skill acquisition toward individualized treatment goals (i.e., abstinence or harm reduction) [25]. Study participants who responded to advertisements and reported "alcohol problems" were randomized to one of these conditions and followed for 21 months. Although there was a higher rate of abstinence among women in individual therapy at the 3-month follow-up, there were no differences between groups at any subsequent time throughout the follow-up period. At the end of 21 months, almost 70% had reduced their alcohol consumption from pretreatment levels and half of the total sample reduced alcohol use by at least 50%.

In a more recent study [26], 155 women with alcohol use disorder were randomly assigned to 12 sessions of a manual-based women-only cognitive-behavioral-based group therapy or individual therapy. Both groups had a significant reduction in the percentage of drinking days and heavy drinking days, which was maintained at the 12-month follow-up. There were no significant differences in outcomes between the group and individual conditions. A subsequent cost-effectiveness analysis of this study showed greater cost-effectiveness for the group format [5].

Although relatively few studies have specifically tested individual versus group therapies using the same group content, the available research very clearly suggests that individual and group therapies are relatively equivalent in terms of both retention and clinical outcomes. Thus, it seems that high-quality treatment can be administered as effectively in group as in individually delivered formats.

30.4   What Types of Group Therapy Are Most Effective?

The majority of studies examining group therapy for SUDs have focused on comparing two or more types of group therapy that vary in terms of content or approach. For example, several studies have compared skills training to other group therapies and have yielded mixed results. Eriksen et al. [27] randomized 24 alcohol-dependent participants to 8 sessions of social skills training or counseling. The social skills training group reported fewer drinking days, drank less alcohol overall, and had better employment outcomes. A comparison of coping skills and interactional (interpersonal) groups for alcohol use disorder found no overall differences between the conditions in terms of alcohol use; however, individuals rating high on psychopathy had better outcomes with the coping skills group and those low on psychopathy had better outcomes in the interactional group, both following treatment [28] and a 2-year follow-up [29]. A later study by this group randomized 250 alcohol-dependent patients to either a random treatment assignment or matched treatment assignment based on the level of psychopathy [28]. Results of this study were mixed, with higher rates of abstinence in the randomized condition, but fewer alcohol-related consequences in the matched condition.

Several studies have compared cognitive-behavioral therapies to other therapies or control conditions. Kaminer et al. [30] randomized 88 adolescents presenting for outpatient substance abuse treatment to receive either cognitive-behavioral or psychoeducational group therapy. Results suggested an early benefit for cognitive-behavioral therapy; however, this was moderated by gender and age (with younger males responding better to cognitive-behavioral therapy) and the benefits were not maintained at 6-month follow-up. Both groups exhibited similar changes in substance use and functioning over time [30].

Similarly, mixed results were found by Pomerleau et al. [31] in a study of 32 alcohol-dependent men comparing behavioral therapy to psychodynamic group therapy. Results indicated better retention and less alcohol use in the behavioral therapy condition (consisting of several behavioral interventions, such as stimulus control and shaping), but higher rates of abstinence among completers of the psychodynamic therapy. A later study of male patients diagnosed with alcohol dependence in a Veterans Administration hospital found no differences between cognitive-behavioral and interpersonal therapies in alcohol use outcomes [32]. A study comparing 6 weeks of 12-step counseling (usual care) to behavioral skills training therapy, transactional analysis therapy, or their combination found that all conditions were associated with superior outcomes compared to transactional analysis alone [33].

A comparison of 6 sessions of cognitive-behavioral group therapy for smoking cessation compared to a health education control group plus nicotine replacement therapy in a sample of 154 African American smokers found greater rates of abstinence (past week) among those in the cognitive-behavioral therapy condition through 6 months of follow-up, with 31% versus 14% of participants abstinent at the end of follow-up [34].

Telch et al. [35] compared supportive therapy, behavioral therapy (covert sensitization), and a control therapy in 28 alcohol-dependent patients in an outpatient setting. Although those in the supportive therapy reported lower daily drinking, there were no differences among groups on alcohol craving or randomly collected blood-alcohol levels across the three conditions.

Mindfulness-based interventions are increasingly utilized in SUD treatment settings, and group therapy is no exception. Bowen and colleagues [36] randomized 286 patients who recently completed residential or intensive outpatient treatment for SUD into 8 weeks of a mindfulness-based relapse prevention group, a cognitive-behavioral relapse prevention group, or treatment-as-usual (involving psychoeducation and 12-step facilitation). Those assigned to mindfulness-based relapse prevention and cognitive-behavioral relapse prevention had significantly reduced risk of relapse to substance use or heavy drinking when compared to treatment-as-usual. The cognitive-behavioral group therapy outperformed mindfulness-based group therapy with regard to time to first drug use, but the mindfulness-based group had significantly fewer days of substance use and heavy drinking compared to both cognitive-behavioral group and treatment-as-usual at the 12-month follow-up.

Little research has compared group therapy to family therapy; however, a comparison of a process group therapy, family therapy, and family education for adolescents with SUDs suggested that family therapy was most effective in achieving drug abstinence [37].

Couples therapy may be the only setting wherein a group format has been shown yield worse substance-related outcomes than individual (i.e., single-couple). O'Farrell et al. [38] randomized 101 patients with alcohol dependence and their partners (without SUD) to either group behavioral couples therapy or the standard conjoint behavioral couples therapy. Substance use and relational outcomes were significantly worse for the group therapy cohort, suggesting that the standard one-couple therapy is superior to a multi-couple group format.

Overall, results comparing types of group therapy have been mostly inconclusive. Moreover, given dramatic variability across studies, it is difficult to make any generalizations based on the existing literature. Several studies have suggested that more skills-based therapies (e.g., cognitive-behavioral therapy) outperform less structured therapies, although this has not been consistently replicated, with other studies suggesting similar outcomes for other group therapy types. Several studies have suggested that there may be key moderators of treatment response (e.g., psychopathy, age); however, more research is needed to better understand what works best for whom. Accordingly, at this time, more well-controlled studies are needed to determine what types of group therapy are most effective.

30.5 Comparing Group Therapies for Co-Occurring Disorders

Other psychiatric disorders commonly co-occur with SUDs [39, 40]. Accordingly, numerous studies of group therapy for SUDs have examined therapies targeted to both the SUD and co-occurring psychiatric disorders.

Weiss et al. [41] compared usual care to usual care plus 12–20 sessions of an integrated group therapy for SUDs and bipolar disorder in a sample of 45 participants. Results indicated that group therapy was associated with significantly lower SUD severity, more months abstinent, and longer duration of abstinence relative to usual care alone. In a subsequent study, 62 outpatients with co-occurring bipolar disorder and substance dependence were randomly assigned to 20 sessions of either the integrated treatment or group drug counseling [42]. Patients in the integrated group therapy had fewer days of substance use following treatment and throughout 3 months of follow-up; however, mood outcomes were similar between groups. Weiss and colleagues [42] then tested the implementation of a 12-session version of the treatment with drug counselors without previous training in cognitive-behavioral therapy. Sixty-one participants were randomized to the integrated treatment or group counseling and results indicated better outcomes for both substance (e.g., likelihood of abstinence) and mood symptoms (e.g., greater reduction in risk for a mood episode) in the integrated treatment group.

In a study comparing dialectical behavioral therapy (DBT), which included a group therapy component, to treatment-as-usual for 28 women with co-occurring borderline personality disorder and substance dependence, there was significantly greater treatment adherence, more days abstinent, and more negative urine screens in the DBT group [43]. These findings suggesting the benefits of DBT were replicated in women with heroin dependence when compared to individual therapy [44].

In a study conducted in Australia, James et al. [45] randomized 63 participants with co-occurring alcohol or drug use and a psychotic disorder to receive either usual care and 1 session of substance use education or 6 sessions of an integrated treatment for both disorders. The integrated dual disorder treatment group was associated with significantly greater improvement in psychiatric symptoms, substance use, and SUD severity. In a similar study, Bellack et al. [46] randomized 129 outpatients with a diagnosis of drug dependence and serious mental illness (psychotic or major affective disorder) to receive an integrated behavioral treatment (Behavioral Treatment for Substance Abuse in Severe and Persistent Mental Illness) or supportive group discussion twice weekly for 6 months. Results indicated that the integrated treatment was associated with more negative urine screens as well as better treatment retention and functional outcomes (e.g., quality of life).

Results for co-occurring depression and anxiety disorders have been more mixed. Lydecker and colleagues [47] compared an integrated cognitive-behavioral therapy for co-occurring depression and SUDs to 12-step facilitation in a sample of 206 veterans with a current substance dependence diagnosis and a lifetime diagnosis of major depressive disorder. Both treatments were associated with significant improvements in both depression and substance use outcomes; however, there was evidence for better maintenance of substance use outcome gains in the integrated treatment group.

Studies comparing Seeking Safety, an integrated treatment for co-occurring SUDs and posttraumatic stress disorder, to usual care or alternative group treatments have found both positive results [48] and mixed results [49]. In a large trial of Seeking Safety, Hien et al. [50] randomized 353 women with posttraumatic stress disorder symptoms and a diagnosis of a drug or alcohol use disorder to receive either 12 sessions of Seeking Safety or a comparison health education treatment. Results indicated significant improvement in posttraumatic stress disorder symptoms in both groups with no differences between groups and no significant effects of treatment on either alcohol or drug use outcomes. A subsequent secondary analysis of this study showed that posttraumatic stress disorder symptoms in those in the Seeking Safety group displayed more rapid improvement than the comparison group, which was, in turn, associated with reduction in alcohol and cocaine use [51].

Intimate partner violence frequently co-occurs with SUDs. Easton et al. [52] examined whether group therapy could improve outcome in this population. They randomized 85 men with alcohol dependence and a history of domestic violence offense into either a 12-week CBT-based substance use and domestic violence group or a 12-step facilitation group. The substance use and domestic violence group outperformed the 12-step facilitation group on alcohol use outcomes, and this group trended toward less frequent physical violence over time in comparison to the 12-step group.

Group therapy targeting co-occurring SUDs and other disorders have been successful in some cases (e.g., bipolar disorder and psychotic disorders), with more mixed results for anxiety and depressive disorders. Nonetheless, integrated group therapies are promising for the reduction in symptoms of both SUDs and co-occurring disorders and are an important area for further study.

30.6 How Can We Maximize Outcomes in Group Therapy?

Because the evidence generally supports the effectiveness of group therapy for SUDs, recent research has begun to examine ways to maximize its effectiveness. Several studies have tested ways to enhance group therapy by adding adjunctive interventions or manipulating group factors.

30.6.1 Adjunctive Treatments

Contingency management involves providing patients with reinforcers (incentives such as money or vouchers) for engaging in beneficial behaviors, such as providing negative urine drug screens or attending treatment sessions. Several studies have examined the addition of contingency management to group therapy to enhance attendance. Petry et al. [53] examined the addition of a contingency management group to standard outpatient care (including group counseling and monitoring with urine toxicology screens) in community-based outpatient substance abuse treatment clinics. The addition of contingency management was associated with better program attendance (including more days of attendance and longer duration in treatment) and longer duration of drug abstinence. Other studies have similarly found benefits of adding incentives for attending group sessions [54, 55], although one study found only modest effects for attendance incentives [56].

Santa Ana et al. [57] randomized 101 dually diagnosed individuals from a detoxification unit of psychiatric hospital to receive 2 sessions of either a motivational enhancement group therapy or a group therapy control condition in addition to standard care, to enhance adherence to aftercare. Results indicated that group motivational enhancement resulted in more aftercare sessions attended and fewer drinking days and heavy drinking days.

Studies examining the addition of adjunctive individual therapy to group therapy suggest that the benefits of this approach are modest, at best. In a large study of behavioral therapies for cocaine dependence, 487 individuals were randomized to 1 of 4 treatments, including 24 sessions of group counseling alone, or in combination with 36 sessions of 1 of 3 individual therapies: cognitive therapy, supportive-expressive psychodynamic therapy, or 12-step oriented drug counseling [58]. The best outcomes on substance use were seen for the group drug counseling plus individual drug counseling intervention, followed by group drug counseling alone [59]. However, there were no differences among conditions on other functional outcomes (e.g., interpersonal functioning). Thus, the addition of individual drug counseling, and not other individual therapies, was associated with the enhancement of some group therapy outcomes. Another study examined group counseling compared to group counseling plus individual relapse prevention therapy for cocaine dependence [60]. Results at a 6-month follow-up indicated greater likelihood of cocaine abstinence in group therapy alone, but fewer days of cocaine use among those who were not abstinent in the group plus individual therapy condition.

Technology-based interventions for substance use disorders is a topic of emerging interest [61]. In a large, multisite trial, 507 substance-dependent patients entering treatment were randomized into either 12 weeks of treatment-as-usual (composed of individual and group therapies) or treatment-as-usual with adjunctive internet-based contingency management and community reinforcement approach modules [62]. The group receiving adjunctive treatment had a lower dropout rate and a higher abstinence rate than the treatment-as-usual group.

30.6.2 Intensity and Group Composition

Coviello et al. [63] randomized 94 patients with cocaine use disorder to group therapy programs of varying intensities over a 4-week treatment program, including either 6 hours of treatment (4 of which were group) or 12 hours of treatment (7 of which were group) per week [63]. There were no significant differences between study cohorts in terms of severity of substance use problems or other functional outcomes; on average, patients in both conditions improved on these measures.

Several studies have examined gender-specific group therapy for SUDs [64–66]. Greenfield et al. [66] compared a women-only relapse prevention group therapy, the Women's Recovery Group (WRG), to mixed-gender Group Drug Counseling. Results demonstrated higher satisfaction among women in the Women's Recovery Group and similar drug use outcomes between groups. The WRG also appeared to have better alcohol use outcomes and better maintenance of gains 6 months following treatment. Women in the WRG provided more frequent affiliative statements [67] and women in groups with high levels of affiliative statements had better substance use outcomes, particularly in the WRG condition [68]. Moreover, the WRG seemed to have particularly beneficial effects on substance use outcomes for women with high psychiatric severity [69].

Several considerations may be valuable in attempting to enhance group therapy outcomes. First, adding incentives for attendance appears to enhance retention, thereby ensuring a higher "dose" of therapy. Technology-based interventions have the potential to improve access to incentive-based treatments. Second, treatment targeted to a population of interest (e.g., women) may yield added benefits relative to more general group therapy. However, studies of the addition of individual to group therapy remain somewhat inconclusive and require more research. Results to date suggest that the type of individual therapy added to group therapy may be important to determining outcomes, and that those who are not able to achieve abstinence in group therapy alone may benefit from individual therapy. Nonetheless, additional research is needed to better understand the potential benefits of combining group and individual therapies.

30.7 Summary and Integration of the Literature

Although research on group therapy for SUDs varies widely in the types of group therapy, the substance of abuse, the population of interest, and timing and delivery of treatment, several trends emerge from the existing literature. In general, studies adding group treatment to minimal or no treatment suggest that group therapy is associated with improved substance use and often also functional outcomes [8, 41]. Although not all studies have found evidence for this effect [10], studies predominantly support group therapy as an effective intervention for SUDs. Results are mixed for adding group therapy to more powerful treatments (e.g., certain pharmacotherapies), with some evidence for no benefit of adding group therapy [12] and others finding benefits for some outcomes or in certain subgroups [13, 19]. However, many of these studies have been limited by either small sample sizes or uncontrolled designs (e.g., no limitations on additional adjunctive treatments); it thus remains unclear whether group therapy can achieve additive benefits when combined with pharmacotherapy.

Likewise, comparisons of different types of group therapy have generally yielded variable results. The relative effectiveness of different types of group treatment may depend on the fit of the intervention to the target population. For example, several integrated group therapies (such as those for SUD patients with co-occurring psychosis or bipolar disorder) have been associated with better outcomes than general alcohol and drug counseling therapies [42, 46]. Thus, the degree to which the treatment "fits" the population may be critical to understanding which treatment works best for whom.

Studies comparing individual to group-based delivery of substance abuse treatment (predominantly motivational enhancement or cognitive-behavioral therapy) have not found significant differences between individual and group therapies on substance use or other functional outcomes or differences in treatment retention. Although there is limited evidence for greater social functioning following group therapy [23] and greater patient preference for individual therapy [3], the evidence overall seems to support similar efficacy for group and individual therapies. Studies examining the mechanisms of these approaches may be of benefit to personalizing treatments for individuals. For example, group affiliation is a group-specific process that appears to confer outcome benefits [68].

Given the mixed findings on effectiveness, strategies to maximize outcomes are of particular importance. The addition of incentives for attending treatment appears to improve retention, maximizing the dose of therapy that patients receive. Because the findings examining the addition of individual therapy to group therapy have been mixed, contingency management (possibly using technology-based platforms) may be the best available strategy to enhance group therapy outcomes.

The mixed outcomes reported above are likely due in part to the heterogeneity of studies and populations, including the dosing (i.e., number of sessions) administered and the timing of when treatment occurs. In addition, many studies have used small sample sizes, which substantially limits the ability to identify differences in outcomes, particularly when comparing two active treatments, such as pharmacotherapy versus pharmacotherapy plus group therapy, or two types of group therapy. Thus, it is clear that more research is needed to understand what types of group therapy are most effective and under what conditions.

30.7.1 Why Is There So Little Research on Group Therapy for SUDs?

There are numerous study design considerations that are unique to conducting research on group therapy. Features such as open versus closed enrollment (i.e., whether all participants start treatment at the same time vs. "rolling" enrollment), group content/approach, and group composition (size and member characteristics) are all specific to group therapy research and are not relevant to studies of individual therapies. Additive designs may be of less concern than comparative designs for which conclusions about differential effects become more complicated. For example, comparing a single-gender group to a mixed-gender group might involve differences in both content (e.g., gender-specific group material) and composition (e.g., all women vs. men and women). Comparing individual to group therapy is even more challenging given the lack of clear guidance on equating the dosing of treatments. For example, if both group and individual sessions were 60 minutes, patients in individual therapy may gain a higher dose of therapy through more attention. However, if group sessions were longer, patients in group would be receiving more time in treatment. How to equivalently dose these types of therapy remains an open question (e.g., Is a 60-minute individual session equivalent to a 90-minute group session?).

The study of group therapy is also complicated by the number of potential variables that might contribute to the treatment's effectiveness. For example, active ingredients may include both the content of the group (e.g., the intervention components) and the format (i.e., group composition). Thus, studies can test one or both of these components, such as testing a group versus individual treatment or testing two types of group content or composition (e.g., single- vs. mixed-gender groups). Given the variability of studies conducted to date and—not surprisingly—variability in results, future well-designed research on group therapies will be important to improve treatments and to ultimately enhance outcomes for patients with SUDs.

30.7.2 Conclusion

Group therapy is the predominant method of delivery of psychosocial treatments for SUDs. This approach is associated with a lower cost than many other options as well as high satisfaction among patients. Evidence for the effectiveness of group therapy is mixed, and interpretation of the literature is limited by the heterogeneity of studies and the absence of many large, well-controlled studies. Nonetheless, as a whole, group therapy appears to be an effective treatment for a range of SUDs, particularly when the treatment is specific and well defined. Group treatment may be a particularly effective option for those with co-occurring psychiatric and substance use disorders. Studies suggest that group therapy is generally as effective as individual therapy, although the specific types of group therapy associated with the best outcomes remain unclear.

Acknowledgments Effort on this chapter was supported in part by awards K23 DA035297 (McHugh) and K24 DA022288 (Weiss) from the National Institute on Drug Abuse.

References

1. Weiss RD, Jaffee WB, de Menil VP, Cogley CB. Group therapy for substance use disorders: what do we know? Harv Rev Psychiatry. 2004;12(6):339–50. https://doi.org/10.1080/10673220490905723.
2. U.S. Department of Health and Human Services Center for Behavioral Health Statistics and Quality. National survey of substance abuse treatment services (N-SSATS): 2010. Data on substance abuse treatment facilities. 2010. Retrieved from http://www.samhsa.gov/data/DASIS/2k10nssats/NSSATS2010Index.htm.
3. Sobell LC, Sobell MB, Agrawal S. Randomized controlled trial of a cognitive-behavioral motivational intervention in a group versus individual format for substance us disorders. Psychol Addict Behav. 2009;23:672–83.
4. French MT, Zavala SK, McCollister KE, Waldron HB, Turner CW, Ozechowski TJ. Cost-effectiveness analysis of four interventions for adolescents with a substance use disorder. J Subst Abuse Treat. 2008;34(3):272–81. https://doi.org/10.1016/j.jsat.2007.04.008.
5. Olmstead TA, Graff FS, Ames-Sikora A, McCrady BS, Gaba A, Epstein EE. Cost-effectiveness of

individual versus group female-specific cognitive behavioral therapy for alcohol use disorder. J Subst Abuse Treat. 2019;100:1–7. https://doi.org/10.1016/j.jsat.2019.02.001.

6. Schmitz JM, Oswald LM, Baldwin L, Grabowski J. A survey of posthospitalization treatment needs and preferences in cocaine abusers. Am J Addict. 1994;3:227–35.

7. Daley DC, Stuart Baker MA, Donovan DM, Hodgkins CG, Perl H. A combined group and individual 12-step facilitative intervention targeting stimulant abuse in the NIDA clinical trials network: STAGE-12. J Groups Addict Recover. 2011;6(3):228–44. https://doi.org/10.1080/1556035X.2011.597196.

8. Stephens RS, Roffman RA, Curtin L. Comparison of extended versus brief treatments for marijuana use. J Consult Clin Psychol. 2000;68(5):898–908.

9. Omer H, Winch G, Dar R. Therapeutic impact in treatments for smoking and test-anxiety. Psychother Res. 1998;8:439–54.

10. Razavi D, Vandecasteele H, Primo C, Bodo M, Debrier F, Verbist H, et al. Maintaining abstinence from cigarette smoking: effectiveness of group counselling and factors predicting outcome. Eur J Cancer. 1999;35(8):1238–47.

11. Shorey RC, Elmquist J, Gawrysiak MJ, Strauss C, Haynes E, Anderson S, et al. A randomized controlled trial of a mindfulness and acceptance group therapy for residential substance use patients. Subst Use Misuse. 2017;52(11):1400–10. https://doi.org/10.1080/10826084.2017.1284232.

12. Tucker T, Ritter A, Maher C, Jackson H. A randomized control trial of group counseling in a naltrexone treatment program. J Subst Abuse Treat. 2004;27(4):277–88. https://doi.org/10.1016/j.jsat.2004.08.003.

13. Luthar SS, Suchman NE. Relational psychotherapy mothers' group: a developmentally informed intervention for at-risk mothers. Dev Psychopathol. 2000;12(2):235–53.

14. Luthar SS, Suchman NE, Altomare M. Relational psychotherapy mothers' group: a randomized clinical trial for substance abusing mothers. Dev Psychopathol. 2007;19(1):243–61. https://doi.org/10.1017/S0954579407070137.

15. Nyamathi A, Shoptaw S, Cohen A, Greengold B, Nyamathi K, Marfisee M, et al. Effect of motivational interviewing on reduction of alcohol use. Drug Alcohol Depend. 2010;107(1):23–30. https://doi.org/10.1016/j.drugalcdep.2009.08.021.

16. Nyamathi AM, Nandy K, Greengold B, Marfisee M, Khalilifard F, Cohen A, et al. Effectiveness of intervention on improvement of drug use among methadone maintained adults. J Addict Dis. 2011;30(1):6–16. https://doi.org/10.1080/10550887.2010.531669.

17. Sokol R, LaVertu AE, Morrill D, Albanese C, Schuman-Olivier Z. Group-based treatment of opioid use disorder with buprenorphine: a systematic review. J Subst Abuse Treat. 2018;84:78–87. https://doi.org/10.1016/j.jsat.2017.11.003.

18. Imani S, Atef Vahid MK, Gharraee B, Noroozi A, Habibi M, Bowen S. Effectiveness of mindfulness-based group therapy compared to the usual opioid dependence treatment. Iran J Psychiatry. 2015;10(3):175–84.

19. Schmitz JM, Stotts AL, Mooney ME, Delaune KA, Moeller GF. Bupropion and cognitive-behavioral therapy for smoking cessation in women. Nicotine Tob Res. 2007;9(6):699–709. https://doi.org/10.1080/14622200701365335.

20. Smith SS, Jorenby DE, Fiore MC, Anderson JE, Mielke MM, Beach KE, et al. Strike while the iron is hot: can stepped-care treatments resurrect relapsing smokers? J Consult Clin Psychol. 2001;69(3):429–39.

21. John U, Veltrup C, Driessen M, Wetterling T, Dilling H. Motivational intervention: an individual counseling vs a group treatment approach for alcohol-dependent in-patients. Alcohol Alcohol. 2003;38:263–9.

22. Schmitz JM, Oswald LM, Jacks SD, Rustin T, Rhoades HM, Grabowski J. Relapse prevention treatment for cocaine dependence: group vs. individual format. Addict Behav. 1997;22(3):405–18.

23. Graham K, Annis HM, Brett PJ, Venesoen P. A controlled field trial of group vs. individual cognitive-behavioural training for relapse prevention. Addiction. 1996;81:1127–39.

24. Marques AC, Formigoni ML. Comparison of individual and group cognitive-behavioral therapy for alcohol and/or drug dependent patients. Addiction. 2001;96:835–46.

25. Duckert F, Amundsen A, Johnsen J. What happens to drinking after therapeutic intervention? Br J Addict. 1992;87(10):1457–67.

26. Epstein EE, McCrady BS, Hallgren KA, Gaba A, Cook S, Jensen N, et al. Individual versus group female-specific cognitive behavior therapy for alcohol use disorder. J Subst Abuse Treat. 2018;88:27–43. https://doi.org/10.1016/j.jsat.2018.02.003.

27. Eriksen L, Bjornstad S, Gotestam KG. Social skills training in groups for alcoholics: one-year treatment outcome for groups and individuals. Addict Behav. 1986;11(3):309–29.

28. Kadden RM, Litt MD, Cooney NL, Kabela E, Getter H. Prospective matching of alcoholic clients to cognitive-behavioral or interactional group therapy. J Stud Alcohol. 2001;62(3):359–69.

29. Cooney NL, Kadden RM, Litt MD, Getter H. Matching alcoholics to coping skills or interactional therapies: two-year follow-up results. J Consult Clin Psychol. 1991;59(4):598–601.

30. Kaminer Y, Burleson JA, Goldberger R. Cognitive-behavioral coping skills and psychoeducation therapies for adolescent substance abuse. J Nerv Ment Dis. 2002;190(11):737–45. https://doi.org/10.1097/01.NMD.0000038168.51591.B6.

31. Pomerleau O, Pertschuk M, Adkins D, Brady JP. A comparison of behavioral and traditional treatment for middle-income problem drinkers. J Behav Med. 1978;1(2):187–200.

32. Ito JR, Donovan DM, Hall JJ. Relapse prevention in alcohol aftercare: effects on drinking outcome, change process, and aftercare attendance. Br J Addict. 1988;83(2):171–81.

33. Olson RP, Ganley R, Devine VT, Dorsey GC Jr. Long-term effects of behavioral versus insight-oriented therapy with inpatient alcoholics. J Consult Clin Psychol. 1981;49(6):866–77.

34. Webb MS, de Ybarra DR, Baker EA, Reis IM, Carey MP. Cognitive-behavioral therapy to promote smoking cessation among African American smokers: a randomized clinical trial. J Consult Clin Psychol. 2010;78(1):24–33. https://doi.org/10.1037/a0017669.

35. Telch MJ, Hannon R, Telch CF. A comparison of cessation strategies for the outpatient alcoholic. Addict Behav. 1984;9(1):103–9.

36. Bowen S, Witkiewitz K, Clifasefi SL, Grow J, Chawla N, Hsu SH, et al. Relative efficacy of mindfulness-based relapse prevention, standard relapse prevention, and treatment as usual for substance use disorders: a randomized clinical trial. JAMA Psychiatry. 2014;71(5):547–56. https://doi.org/10.1001/jamapsychiatry.2013.4546.

37. Joanning H, Thomas F, Quinn W, Mullen R. Treating adolescent drug abuse: a comparison of family systems therapy, group therapy, and family education. J Marital Fam Ther. 1992;18:345.

38. O'Farrell TJ, Schumm JA, Dunlap LJ, Murphy MM, Muchowski P. A randomized clinical trial of group versus standard behavioral couples therapy plus individually based treatment for patients with alcohol dependence. J Consult Clin Psychol. 2016;84(6):497–510. https://doi.org/10.1037/ccp0000089.

39. Conway KP, Compton W, Stinson FS, Grant BF. Lifetime comorbidity of DSM-IV mood and anxiety disorders and specific drug use disorders: results from the National Epidemiologic Survey on Alcohol and Related Conditions. J Clin Psychiatry. 2006;67(2):247–57.

40. Grant BF, Stinson FS, Dawson DA, Chou SP, Dufour MC, Compton W, et al. Prevalence and co-occurrence of substance use disorders and independent mood and anxiety disorders: results from the National Epidemiologic Survey on Alcohol and Related Conditions. Arch Gen Psychiatry. 2004;61(8):807–16. https://doi.org/10.1001/archpsyc.61.8.807.

41. Weiss RD, Griffin ML, Greenfield SF, Najavits LM, Wyner D, Soto JA, et al. Group therapy for patients with bipolar disorder and substance dependence: results of a pilot study. J Clin Psychiatry. 2000;61(5):361–7.

42. Weiss RD, Griffin ML, Jaffee WB, Bender RE, Graff FS, Gallop RJ, et al. A "community-friendly" version of integrated group therapy for patients with bipolar disorder and substance dependence: a randomized controlled trial. Drug Alcohol Depend. 2009;104(3):212–9. https://doi.org/10.1016/j.drugalcdep.2009.04.018.

43. Linehan MM, Schmidt H 3rd, Dimeff LA, Craft JC, Kanter J, Comtois KA. Dialectical behavior therapy for patients with borderline personality disorder and drug-dependence. Am J Addict. 1999;8(4):279–92.

44. Linehan MM, Dimeff LA, Reynolds SK, Comtois KA, Welch SS, Heagerty P, et al. Dialectical behavior therapy versus comprehensive validation therapy plus 12-step for the treatment of opioid dependent women meeting criteria for borderline personality disorder. Drug Alcohol Depend. 2002;67(1):13–26.

45. James W, Preston NJ, Koh G, Spencer C, Kisely SR, Castle DJ. A group intervention which assists patients with dual diagnosis reduce their drug use: a randomized controlled trial. Psychol Med. 2004;34(6):983–90.

46. Bellack AS, Bennett ME, Gearon JS, Brown CH, Yang Y. A randomized clinical trial of a new behavioral treatment for drug abuse in people with severe and persistent mental illness. Arch Gen Psychiatry. 2006;63(4):426–32. https://doi.org/10.1001/archpsyc.63.4.426.

47. Lydecker KP, Tate SR, Cummins KM, McQuaid J, Granholm E, Brown SA. Clinical outcomes of an integrated treatment for depression and substance use disorders. Psychol Addict Behav. 2010;24(3):453–65. https://doi.org/10.1037/a0019943.

48. Najavits LM, Gallop RJ, Weiss RD. Seeking safety therapy for adolescent girls with PTSD and substance use disorder: a randomized controlled trial. J Behav Health Serv Res. 2006;33(4):453–63. https://doi.org/10.1007/s11414-006-9034-2.

49. Zlotnick C, Johnson J, Najavits LM. Randomized controlled pilot study of cognitive-behavioral therapy in a sample of incarcerated women with substance use disorder and PTSD. Behav Ther. 2009;40(4):325–36. https://doi.org/10.1016/j.beth.2008.09.004.

50. Hien DA, Wells EA, Jiang H, Suarez-Morales L, Campbell AN, Cohen LR, et al. Multisite randomized trial of behavioral interventions for women with co-occurring PTSD and substance use disorders. J Consult Clin Psychol. 2009;77(4):607–19. https://doi.org/10.1037/a0016227.

51. Morgan-Lopez AA, Saavedra LM, Hien DA, Campbell AN, Wu E, Ruglass L, et al. Indirect effects of 12-session seeking safety on substance use outcomes: overall and attendance class-specific effects. Am J Addict. 2014;23(3):218–25. https://doi.org/10.1111/j.1521-0391.2014.12100.x.

52. Easton CJ, Mandel DL, Hunkele KA, Nich C, Rounsaville BJ, Carroll KM. A cognitive behavioral therapy for alcohol-dependent domestic violence offenders: an integrated substance abuse-domestic violence treatment approach (SADV). Am J Addict. 2007;16(1):24–31. https://doi.org/10.1080/10550490601077809.

53. Petry NM, Weinstock J, Alessi SM. A randomized trial of contingency management delivered in the context of group counseling. J Consult Clin Psychol. 2011;79(5):686–96. https://doi.org/10.1037/a0024813.

54. Ledgerwood DM, Alessi SM, Hanson T, Godley MD, Petry NM. Contingency management for attendance

to group substance abuse treatment administered by clinicians in community clinics. J Appl Behav Anal. 2008;41(4):517–26.

55. Petry NM, Weinstock J, Alessi SM, Lewis MW, Dieckhaus K. Group-based randomized trial of contingencies for health and abstinence in HIV patients. J Consult Clin Psychol. 2010;78(1):89–97. https://doi.org/10.1037/a0016778.

56. Alessi SM, Hanson T, Wieners M, Petry NM. Low-cost contingency management in community clinics: delivering incentives partially in group therapy. Exp Clin Psychopharmacol. 2007;15(3):293–300. https://doi.org/10.1037/1064-1297.15.3.293.

57. Santa Ana EJ, Wulfert E, Nietert PJ. Efficacy of group motivational interviewing (GMI) for psychiatric inpatients with chemical dependence. J Consult Clin Psychol. 2007;75(5):816–22. https://doi.org/10.1037/0022-006X.75.5.816.

58. Crits-Christoph P, Siqueland L, Blaine J, Frank A, Luborsky L, Onken LS, et al. Psychosocial treatments for cocaine dependence: National Institute on Drug Abuse Collaborative Cocaine Treatment Study. Arch Gen Psychiatry. 1999;56(6):493–502.

59. Crits-Christoph P, Siqueland L, McCalmont E, Weiss RD, Gastfriend DR, Frank A, et al. Impact of psychosocial treatments on associated problems of cocaine-dependent patients. J Consult Clin Psychol. 2001;69(5):825–30.

60. McKay JR, Alterman AI, Cacciola JS, Rutherford MJ, O'Brien CP, Koppenhaver J. Group counseling versus individualized relapse prevention aftercare following intensive outpatient treatment for cocaine dependence: initial results. J Consult Clin Psychol. 1997;65(5):778–88.

61. Sugarman DE, Campbell ANC, Iles BR, Greenfield SF. Technology-based interventions for substance use and comorbid disorders: an examination of the emerging literature. Harv Rev Psychiatry. 2017;25(3):123–34. https://doi.org/10.1097/HRP.0000000000000148.

62. Campbell AN, Nunes EV, Matthews AG, Stitzer M, Miele GM, Polsky D, et al. Internet-delivered treatment for substance abuse: a multisite randomized controlled trial. Am J Psychiatry. 2014;171(6):683–90. https://doi.org/10.1176/appi.ajp.2014.13081055.

63. Coviello DM, Alterman AI, Rutherford MJ, Cacciola JS, McKay JR, Zanis DA. The effectiveness of two intensities of psychosocial treatment for cocaine dependence. Drug Alcohol Depend. 2001;61(2):145–54.

64. Carroll KM, Chang G, Behr H, Clinton B, Kosten TR. Improving treatment outcome in pregnant, methadone-maintained women: results from a randomized clinical trial. Am J Addict. 1994;4:56–9.

65. Copeland J, Hall W, Didcott P, Biggs V. A comparison of a specialist women's alcohol and other drug treatment service with two traditional mixed-sex services: client characteristics and treatment outcome. Drug Alcohol Depend. 1993;32(1):81–92.

66. Greenfield SF, Trucco EM, McHugh RK, Lincoln M, Gallop RJ. The women's recovery group study: a stage I trial of women-focused group therapy for substance use disorders versus mixed-gender group drug counseling. Drug Alcohol Depend. 2007;90(1):39–47. https://doi.org/10.1016/j.drugalcdep.2007.02.009.

67. Sugarman DE, Wigderson SB, Iles BR, Kaufman JS, Fitzmaurice GM, Hilario EY, et al. Measuring affiliation in group therapy for substance use disorders in the women's recovery group study: does it matter whether the group is all-women or mixed-gender? Am J Addict. 2016;25(7):573–80. https://doi.org/10.1111/ajad.12443.

68. Valeri L, Sugarman DE, Reilly ME, McHugh RK, Fitzmaurice GM, Greenfield SF. Group therapy for women with substance use disorders: in-session affiliation predicts women's substance use treatment outcomes. J Subst Abuse Treat. 2018;94:60–8. https://doi.org/10.1016/j.jsat.2018.08.008.

69. Greenfield SF, Potter JS, Lincoln MF, Popuch RE, Kuper L, Gallop RJ. High psychiatric symptom severity is a moderator of substance abuse treatment outcomes among women in single vs. mixed gender group treatment. Am J Drug Alcohol Abuse. 2008;34(5):594–602. https://doi.org/10.1080/00952990802304980.

Couple and Family Therapy in Treatment of Alcoholism and Drug Abuse

31

Keith Klostermann and Timothy J. O'Farrell

Contents

Abstract

Historically, the prevailing wisdom in treating substance abuse was that it was a personal problem, best treated on an individual basis. However, the near myopic focus on individual-based treatment has slowly given way to a greater acknowledgment of the family's role in the development and maintenance of drug and alcohol misuse problems. Over the past four decades, the results of numerous studies have concluded that partner- and family-involved treatments produce better outcomes across several domains of functioning (e.g., reduced substance use, improved marital and family functioning) compared to individual-based interventions. The purpose of this chapter is to (a) discuss the impact of substance

K. Klostermann
Medaille College, Buffalo, NY, USA

T. J. O'Farrell (✉)
Harvard Medical School, Brockton, NY, USA
e-mail: timothy_ofarrell@hms.harvard.edu

© Springer Nature Switzerland AG 2021
N. el-Guebaly et al. (eds.), *Textbook of Addiction Treatment*,
https://doi.org/10.1007/978-3-030-36391-8_31

abuse on the family; (b) present the models, techniques, and principles of couples and family therapy that have been used with substance-abusing clients, their partners, and extended family members; (c) discuss the potential barriers to implementing partner- and family-involved approaches for substance use; and (d) explore future directions with respect to partner- and family-involved therapies for substance-abusing clients.

Keywords

Family · Treatment · Alcoholism · Drug abuse · Substance abuse

Historically, the prevailing wisdom in treating substance abuse was that it was a personal problem, best treated on an individual basis. This viewpoint characterized the thinking about treatment for much of the twentieth century [44]. However, the near myopic focus on individual-based treatment has slowly given way to a greater acknowledgment of the family's role in the development and maintenance of drug and alcohol misuse problems. Having an intimate partner with a substance use disorder creates stress and tension in the relationship and chaos in the family [29, 45] that may contribute to separation or divorce [1]. In response to the systemic implications of substance abuse, an increasing number of treatment providers are focusing on the individual and family as a way to reduce or eliminate substance abuse by one or more of its members.

Over the past four decades, the results of numerous studies have concluded that partner- and family-involved treatments produce better outcomes across several domains of functioning (e.g., reduced substance use, improved marital and family functioning) compared to individual-based interventions [60, 61]. Consequently, the Joint Commission on Accreditation of Health Care Organizations (JCAHO) standards for accrediting substance abuse treatment programs in the United States requires that an adult family member be included, at minimum, in the initial assessment phase of the treatment process [3].

The purpose of this chapter is to (a) discuss the impact of substance abuse on the family and describe the systemic principles that may aid in improving interactions among family members; (b) present the models, techniques, and principles of couples and family therapy that have been used with substance-abusing clients, their partners, and extended family members; (c) discuss the potential barriers to implementing partner- and family-involved approaches for substance use; and (d) explore possible future directions with respect to partner- and family-involved therapies with substance-abusing clients.

31.1 The Concept of Family

Given that societal norms and attitudes influence definitions of cultural constructs such as "family," coupled with the fact that cultures and beliefs are very dynamic, the definition of marriage and family continues to evolve. Consequently, family units may include the following configurations: (a) a traditional nuclear family in which members are cohabiting in the household; (b) a single-parent household; (c) a "blended" family resulting from divorce, separation, or remarriage; (d) lesbian or gay couples with or without custodial children; (e) a multigenerational household including grandparents, parents, and children; or (e) long-term cohabiting partners who are not romantically linked, but define themselves as a family [48]. Depending on the individual's conceptualization of family, coupled with his or her treatment needs, any of these configurations may be involved in the treatment process.

31.2 Co-dependence and Enabling

Originally developed by Alcoholics Anonymous (AA; [2]), the term co-dependency refers to help from family members, which either directly or indirectly supports the substance-abusing family member's addictive behaviors. Despite the often overwhelming stress and numerous relational complications resulting from the addicted family member's behavior, the co-dependent individual becomes intertwined with the individual's addiction and behaves in ways that contribute to sustaining the problematic behavioral patterns [59].

Enabling, a hallmark of co-dependency, is defined as behaviors that perpetuate the substance use [38] and may include activities and behaviors that make it easier for the individual to continue drinking or using or to protect him or her from the resulting negative consequences (e.g., personal, social, financial).

31.3 The Relationship Between Substance Use and Family Maladjustment

The relationship between substance use and relationship problems is not unidirectional with one causing the other. Rather, the link between problematic drinking or drug use and relationship distress appears to be bidirectional in nature, with each influencing the other. On one hand, families in which a member abuses substances may experience high levels of relationship dissatisfaction and be characterized by instability, conflict, sexual dissatisfaction, or psychological distress. On the other hand, several studies have also found relationship dysfunction to be strongly linked with substance use (e.g., [17, 20, 40]). Thus, the relationship between substance use and relationship problems is reciprocal with each serving as a precursor to the other; in other words, these couples end up stuck in a vicious cycle that can be difficult to break [62].

Although the misuse of alcohol and other psychoactive substances by adults has serious consequences (personal, financial, social), the secondary negative effects on children living in these homes are equally destructive [31]. Stress and the associated negative impacts on children and adolescents in these families have been associated with a greater likelihood of adolescent substance use [5].

The strong interrelationship between substance use and family interaction suggests that the role of family in developing and maintaining the issue should, at minimum, be considered as part of any intervention. Simply stated, couple- and family-therapy approaches share two primary objectives: (a) harness the power of the family and/or dyadic system to positively support the patient's recovery efforts, and (b) alter unhealthy interaction patterns to create a family environment more conducive to the individual's long-term recovery efforts, thus replacing the vicious cycle with a more virtuous one.

31.4 Foundational Frameworks

In general, three major approaches to family treatment of substance misuse have evolved: (1) family disease model, (2) family systems theory, and (3) behavioral family theory [49]. The family disease model proposes that both the individual and his or her family members have a disease. More specifically, substance misuse is considered a disease, and family members are believed to suffer from co-dependency. Family systems theory views substance misuse as a symptom of overall family dysfunction [70]. The presence or absence of alcohol or drugs becomes the organizing principle in family interactions. From the family systems perspective, substance use represents an unhealthy attempt to manage difficulties, which over time become homeostatic and regulates family transactions. Behavioral family therapy models are heavily influenced by operant and social learning theories in their conceptualization of the substance user within the family context. Simply stated, behavioral approaches assume that family interactions serve to reinforce alcohol- and drug-using behavior. From this vantage, substance-using behavior is learned in the context of social interactions (e.g., observing peers, parents, role models in the media) and reinforced by contingencies in the individual's environment.

31.5 Couples Therapy

A conjoint approach that has received extensive empirical support for the treatment of alcoholism and substance abuse is Behavioral Couples Therapy (BCT; [16]), which has also been referred to as Behavioral Marital Therapy and Learning Sobriety Together. During the last four decades, couples therapy for substance abuse has received extensive empirical scrutiny, with most research focusing on BCT. In general, these studies have compared BCT to some form of traditional individual-based treatment for substance abuse (e.g., coping skills therapy, 12-step facilitation). Findings from these studies have consistently found that participants who received BCT (a) experienced higher rates of abstinence and fewer drug- or alcohol-related problems (e.g., [18, 77, 78]), (b) have happier relationships [16], and (c) experienced a lower risk of relationship dissolution (e.g., separation, divorce; see [64]) compared to those in the individual treatment condition.

BCT is based on the assumption that substance use occurs in an interactional context, is maintained in part by interactions between the client and partner, and is changed most effectively by teaching partners individual coping skills and also by helping the couple change unhealthy interactions that serve to maintain or reinforce the problematic substance use patterns. Clients learn skills to help support abstinence and develop plans to support and maintain abstinence (i.e., continuing recovery plans); partners learn skills to enhance relationship functioning around the following domains: (1) caring behaviors, (2) communication, and (3) conflict resolution. Sessions are focused on reinforcing positive changes in client's behavior and decreasing behaviors that may trigger or reinforce drinking or drug use, and teaching (and rehearsing) new skills. The focus in BCT is twofold: (1) eliminate or decrease substance use, and (2) enhance relationship functioning.

Since the 1970s, the results of numerous studies have consistently revealed that involving the partner in treatment resulted in better outcomes for substance-misusing individuals and their families. Although BCT is a manualized treatment and the therapist is active and directive during treatment, it is also important to note that the therapist respects the clients' autonomy and need for self-determination [48]. Given the existing knowledge about the importance of client factors

in relation to outcome [79], the optimal stance is one of collaboration in exploring each partner goals and their thoughts about the means to achieve them.

Traditionally, the substance-abusing patient and his or her partner are seen together in BCT, typically for 12–20 sessions over 4–6 months. In those cases in which the identified patient is unwilling to engage in treatment, unilateral family therapy (UFT) may be an effective alternative. In UFT, the therapist works exclusively with the non-substance using partner in helping to engage the identified client into treatment [15]. This approach is described in detail later in this chapter.

31.6   Family Therapy Approaches

Some of the more common family therapy approaches utilized with substance-abusing patients are now described including family prevention models, community reinforcement and family training (CRAFT), Johnson intervention, unilateral family therapy, behavioral contracting, multisystemic family therapy (MFT), network therapy, solution-focused therapy (SFT), Stanton's therapeutic techniques, and Wegscheider-Cruse's approach. Although many of these approaches share similarities, they differ in terms of emphasis on the specific level of recovery (i.e., attainment of abstinence, adjustment to abstinence, and long-term maintenance; [22]) and areas of emphasis.

In general, the goal of most family-focused prevention-interventions is to strengthen the family's role in the positive development of children in the hope of decreasing future substance misuse problems within these children as they grow into adulthood [9]. The emphasis on family prevention programs may include parent-child interactions, communication skill training, child management principles, and parent training. Effective parenting skills are essential in preventing the development of child substance abuse and may be enhanced with additional training on topics such as setting limits, praising appropriate behavior, using clear expectations, and administering consistent (and appropriate) discipline [37]. Previous studies (e.g., [10, 11]) reveal parent training approaches are viable methods of preventing premature drug use among children.

Examples of successful family prevention/intervention models include the Focus on Families Project [4], Preparing for the Drug Free Years [21], Family Effectiveness Training [73], the Strengthening Families Program [39], and a universal prevention-intervention combining family and school programs [69]. The targeted children for these models range in age from 3 to 14 years.

In Community Reinforcement Training (CRT), changes in social reinforcement and contingencies are used to shape clients' behavior (e.g., [66]) in more positive ways with the goal of shifting the client's thinking to recognize abstinence as more rewarding than further substance misuse [54]. An offshoot of CRT, *Community Reinforcement and Family Training* (CRAFT; [67]) is an approach in which family members (e.g., spouses of substance abusers) are engaged in the individual's treatment process with the hope of increasing treatment compliance. As part of this process, family members are taught skills to use with the client including increasing motivation for change, improving communication, and safety skills. A more direct approach, the *Johnson Institute Intervention*, commonly referred to as the "intervention," involves training family members and significant others to confront the substance abuser, request that he or she seek treatment, and impose consequences for not seeking help [28]. The goal of this program is treatment engagement by the substance abuser. However, this approach has been widely debated and is controversial (on practical and ethical bases); moreover, there is limited evidence of effectiveness in engaging substance abusers into treatment [6]. Given the confrontational nature of this approach, coupled with the heterogeneity of substance abusers, this approach may not be a good fit for everyone.

In *Unilateral Family Therapy* (UFT; [74]), the therapist helps family members strengthen coping skills, improve family functioning, and create a family environment conducive to abstinence.

Family members engage in a series of formal steps before considering the possibility of confronting the substance abuser about his or her drinking or drug use and seeking formal treatment. Thomas et al. [75] found that participation in UFT was associated with increased likelihood that substance-misusing individuals would enter treatment or reduce their drinking. Rather than trying to motivate the substance-abusing partner to seek help, Dittrich [12] developed a group treatment program for wives of treatment-resistant substance abusers aimed at helping partners deal with the emotional distress resulting from client's problematic substance misuse. Similar to the principles of Al-Anon, this approach suggests family members should detach from the substance abuser in a gentle and caring way, accept they are powerless to control the substance abuser, and seek support from the Al-Anon community.

Similar to other behavioral approaches, *Behavioral Contracting* [71] involves the use of a collaboratively developed contract between the therapist and the client in which the client agrees to engage in recovery-related activities and behaviors as part of the treatment process. The contract may be helpful in developing clear, behaviorally specific, positive, and achievable goals and include rewards for goal attainment and consequences for non-compliance with agreed-upon activities. The key to successful behavioral contracts is to make sure the goals are small and achievable; given the instability among substance-abusing clients and challenges to remaining abstinent, goals must be small enough to be felt "do-able" otherwise, clients can become easily overwhelmed with the recovery process [57].

Based on social–ecological theory, *Multisystemic Family Therapy* (MFT; [27]) aims to alter the client's environment in ways that are more conducive to prosocial behaviors by focusing on multiple systems including family and peer domains. Families learn skills to increase cohesion and improve structure within the system. The role of the therapist is to identify family strengths and highlight competence while collaboratively developing feasible and achievable interventions. MFT is among the most heavily investigated family interventions [27].

Recognizing that the majority of change occurs in-between sessions and not within, *Network Therapy* [19] enlists the support of important family members and friends in the treatment process—not as clients, but as a support network capable of assisting the client during difficult times. The primary foci of treatment are twofold: attaining abstinence and relapse prevention. The client's network can serve as an important adjunct to office-based services and become an important resource and support during the recovery process.

Solution-Focused Therapy (SFT; [8]) is a strength-based approach in which clients are considered experts on their lives and are believed to possess the resources necessary for change. The role of the therapist is to identify and highlight client's strengths and resources and consider how they may be used in developing solutions to the presenting problem. Techniques such as identifying exceptions and the strategic use of compliments can be helpful in highlighting client's competence in similar areas. The therapist helps clients develop positive, small, concrete, and behaviorally descriptive goals and may use scaling questions as a way to identify next steps, assess progress, or measure a family member's level of commitment to the treatment process. The use of the miracle question is a creative way of identifying goals by asking clients to think about a future in which the presenting issue is less severe or non-existent. There is much debate about the usefulness of this approach with some believing the nearly exclusive focus on solutions rather than problems is too simplistic, while others believe the simplicity of the approach is what makes it so appealing to therapists and clients. Unfortunately, the empirical literature supporting the efficacy of this approach is less developed than some of the other models [65].

According to *Stanton's Therapeutic Techniques* [70], substance misuse is believed to result from a failed attempt at resolving a developmental milestone. The family tries to maintain homeostasis by indirectly reinforcing the substance-abusing behavior. According to Stanton, the primary goals for clients are (1) abstinence, (2) employment or attending school or a training program, and (3) independence. The therapist actively directs the course of treatment with the primary objective of altering problematic behavioral sequences and helping family members develop healthier boundaries. Thus, the therapist seeks to identify and disrupt the family's dysfunctional patterns in an effort to promote growth and behavioral change.

Wegscheider-Cruse's Theory [80] of family alcoholism proposes that family members take on various roles to maintain family balance and cope with the substance abuser's behavior. The *enabler* is the person emotionally closest to the client and may make excuses, protect the client from negative consequences, or take over the client's responsibilities. The enabler's behavior reinforces the client's problematic use. The *hero* is usually the oldest child in the family and outwardly appears to be well adjusted and successful, usually an overachiever. The *scapegoat* becomes the focal point for the family's problems and deflects attention away from the substance abuser. The lost child typically seeks to avoid trouble and blend into the background. This child's needs are often not met and his or her accomplishments typically go unnoticed. The *mascot* recognizes that something is wrong; however, it is convinced by other members within the system that things are fine. Thus, the role of the therapist is to create awareness of family roles and their impact on the substance-misusing patterns within the system. Similar to other approaches, treatment involves educating the family about substance misuses, challenging denial, and providing suggestions for help, which often includes self-help activities.

31.7 Family Treatments for Adolescent Substance Use Disorders

The bulk of clinical trials examining family treatments for substance abuse primarily examined adult clients and the impact of children growing up in these homes. However, it is also important to discuss available family treatments for adolescents who struggle with alcohol or drug problems. Two specific family therapy approaches have been developed for use with substance-abusing adolescents: (a) Brief Strategic Family Therapy (BSFT), and (b) Multidimensional Family Therapy (MDFT).

Brief Strategic Family Therapy (BSFT; [72]) integrates elements of structural and strategic family therapy to treat adolescent substance abuse in a systemic context [26]. More specifically, BSFT focuses on the here-and-now, and is problem focused with the goal of creating awareness of unhealthy relational patterns that contribute to adolescent substance use. The BSFT therapist is active and directive and strives to replace unhealthy interaction patterns with healthier ways of relating as a family unit. There are three underlying assumptions of BSFT: (1) family members are interrelated with one's behavior impacting the entire system; (2) families engage in unhealthy interactional patterns that become part of the family routine, despite not working or being unhealthy; and (3) the therapy process is problem focused, structured, and goal driven [25].

Similar to BSFT, *Multidimensional Family Therapy* (MDFT; [42]) combines elements of strategic and structural family therapy to treat adolescent problem behavior and emotional concerns. MDFT focuses on enhancing adolescent and family motivation for treatment, strengthening relationships and improving communication within the family, and developing conflict-resolution skills for managing interparental conflict or parent-child conflicts [24]. Adolescents are taught to recognize unhealthy people/situations, which may contribute to lapse or relapse and how to avoid slipping into other unhealthy behaviors. The goal of MDFT is to strengthen important social systems within the adolescent's life that may serve as protective factors against substance abuse and other problematic behaviors [41].

31.8 Barriers to Couple and Family Therapy

There are several clinically significant barriers unique to family interventions with substance-abusing patients and their families. One common and important impediment to couples and family treatment with a substance-abusing member is partner violence. O'Farrell and Murphy [63] report approximately 40% of men admitted into substance abuse treatment have perpetrated some form of violence toward their partner in the year preceding treatment. In cases where there is a risk of severe violence (i.e., aggression that has the potential to result in serious injury or is life threatening), the immediate intervention goal is safety; in these situations, partner and family therapy is contra-indicated (e.g., [35]). For some families, there may be also legal restrictions (i.e., restraining orders, no contact orders) that preclude conjoint family sessions.

Another barrier involves the presence of more than one active substance-misusing family member within the family, particularly if these individuals have formed a drinking or drug use partnership of some type [33]. These dual-using family systems may support continued use versus abstinence since shared recreational activities typically involve substance use. Research on family-based approaches for these family configurations is lacking and it is often recommended that individual therapy be used prior to engaging family members in treatment, especially when there are discrepant levels of commitment between partners toward recovery. Another demonstrated barrier to family interventions to treat substance abuse is the existence of high levels of blame and rumination from family members (usually the partner) toward the client [36]. Interestingly, there are also important practical and logistical barriers to partner or family intervention; these include (a) geographical distances among family members or among family members and the treatment provider; (b) family members who are divorced, incarcerated, or otherwise separated; (c) coordination of family members' and treatment providers' schedules; and (d) securing reimbursement for services delivered to multiple individuals in the context of formal treatment [32].

The simple fact is that couple and family approaches add a level of complexity to therapy—for clients, clinicians, and agencies [48]. Not only does the client have to agree to treatment, but also their partner must agree to attend and support their partner's recovery attempts, which for some may be difficult—especially when the partner does not see the systemic nature of the problem ("It's his problem—why do I have to go to therapy?"). Engaging and retaining clients in outpatient substance abuse treatment is challenging [14, 56, 68]. Although partner-involved substance abuse treatments are often shown to be more efficacious than individual treatments (e.g., [36]), they rely on the willingness of both partners to participate in treatment [30].

McCrady [46, 47] contends that a therapist's clinical experiences influence his or her beliefs about treatment and best practices. Couple and family treatment is more difficult than individual psychotherapy, which may explain why so many clinicians avoid involving significant others and family members in the treatment process. While the majority of clinicians (98%) conduct individual psychotherapy, only 49% work with couples and only 34% see families [58].

31.9 Future Directions

Despite recent advances in partner- and family-involved approaches for the treatment of alcoholism and drug abuse, there are several important gaps in both the research literature and clinical practice that reflect the next generation of research in this area. More specifically, the following four areas seem most pressing: (a) dissemination of evidence-based marital and family treatments to community-based treatment programs; (b) application of these approaches on specific populations; (c) examination of the mechanisms of action underlying the positive effects observed; and (d) exploring the use of partner- and family-involved models as part of a stepped care approach.

31.9.1 Dissemination

Despite often volumes of data supporting the effectiveness and efficacy of certain treatments or modalities, there is a discrepancy between the most commonly provided treatments in clinical practice and those with the strongest evidence for effectiveness [23, 53]. Although a number of couple and family approaches have demonstrated research support for their efficacy, very few have been widely adopted in community-based treatment. McGovern et al. [51] examined community addiction providers' (i.e., directors [n = 21] and clinicians [n = 89]) experiences, beliefs, and readiness to implement a variety of evidence-based practices. Results were mixed; providers reported more readiness to adopt 12-step facilitation, cognitive behavioral therapy, motivational interviewing, and relapse prevention, while less ready to implement contingency management, BCT, and pharmacotherapies. The investigators concluded that successful dissemination requires a clear rationale for the new service and leadership must demonstrate the relevance of the treatment to clinicians and staff, even if empirical support is already established. Other factors to consider include degree of difficulty in implementation, how closely (or not) the treatment is aligned with the therapist's preferred theoretical orientation or agency counseling approach, cost of providing treatment, and whether or not the treatment fills a perceived area of need for the clinic [34]. Each of these areas may serve as a potential barrier to successful dissemination of the treatment.

31.9.2 Specific Populations

Although the body of empirical literature supporting the use of couple and family therapy for substance abuse is substantial, it is critical to also recognize its limitations. Among these are the types of families that are typically the subject of such studies, which usually include largely White, male substance-abusing patients. Studies on the efficacy of marital and family therapy approaches for women with substance use disorders are far less common, although available evidence does suggest that they are efficacious [50]. Even fewer studies have examined partner- and family-involved interventions with same-sex couples [35]. Future studies are needed to examine gender orientation–specific factors as well as non-gender orientation–specific factors that may increase substance misuse among gay and lesbian individuals.

Furthermore, a great deal of research has been conducted related to both family therapy and culture and ethnicity, but very little of this has appeared in the family therapy literature on substance abuse. This represents what is likely the most important gap in the extant empirical literature to date. Among major life experiences that must be accounted for when treating families in which a member has a problem with drinking or drug use is how factors such as acculturation and ethnic identity influence the treatment process.

31.9.3 Mechanisms of Action

We now have confidence that many treatments are effective [55], but despite the successful efforts of substance abuse treatment researchers to conduct rigorous clinical trials and spell out in treatment manuals what the treatments consist of, little research has actually investigated what the active ingredients of these treatments are [43]. In other words, what are the mechanisms of action that make certain partner- and family-involved approaches curative? If these factors are identified, then these approaches can be modified to optimize their efficiency to create enhanced interventions.

31.9.4 Partner- and Family-Involved Treatment in the Context of Stepped Care

Despite the demonstrated efficacy of manualized marital and family approaches, there are large individual differences in patient response to treatment. As noted by McKay [52], even for the most efficacious treatments, there are a certain number of people who do not respond to treatment; yet in an effort to tightly control the intervention, non-responding

patients receive the same amount of manualized treatment as those who respond well. Research on standardized interventions to treat substance abuse disorders is beginning to shift away from a "one-size-fits-all" perspective and move toward adaptive interventions. Adaptive interventions, although standardized, call for different dosages of treatment to be employed strategically with patients and families across time. Given the heterogeneity in familial characteristics and response to treatment, future studies are needed to develop tailored interventions based on treatment algorithms that dictate treatment modifications triggered by the patient's initial response and changes in symptom severity. Thus, more flexible versions of marital and family treatments may be more easily disseminated to community providers and more palatable to patients receiving the intervention.

31.10 Conclusion

As has been well documented in scholarly journals and popular media, the emotional, economic, and societal toll of alcoholism and drug abuse is incalculable. The effects of substance use disorders affect not only the clients, but also those around them; in fact, those emotionally closest to the substance-abusing client often suffer the most. Over the past 40 years, the results of numerous studies have consistently supported the positive impact of involving supportive others and family in the client's treatment [7, 13, 76]. Therapists that do not include partners or family in the treatment process run the risk of not being helpful.

References

1. Amato PR, Previti D. People's reasons for divorcing: gender, social class, the life course, and adjustment. J Fam Issues. 2003;24(5):602–26.
2. Asher R, Brissett D. Codependency: a view from women married to alcoholics. Int J Addict. 1988;23(4):331–50.
3. Brown ED, O'Farrell TJ, Maisto SA, Boies K, Suchinsky R. Accreditation guide for substance abuse treatment programs. Newbury Park: Sage; 1997.
4. Catalano RF, Morrison DM, Wells EA, Gillmore MR, Iritani B, Hawkins JD. Ethnic differences in family

factors related to early drug initiation. J Stud Alcohol. 1992;53:208–17.

5. Chassin L, Curran PJ, Hussong AM, Colder CR. The relation of parent alcoholism to adolescent substance use: a longitudinal follow-up study. J Abnorm Psychol. 1996;105:70–80.

6. Connors GJ, Donovan DM, DiClemente CC. Substance abuse treatment and the stages of change: selecting and planning interventions. New York: Guilford; 2004.

7. Copello A, Williamson E, Orford J, Day E. Implementing and evaluating social behaviour and network therapy in drug treatment practice in the UK: a feasibility study. Addict Behav. 2006;31:802–10.

8. De Jong P, Berg IK. Interviewing for solutions. Belmont: Thomson Brooks/Cole Publishing Co.; 1998. Retrieved from http://search. ebscohost.com.ezproxy.medaille.edu/login. aspx?direct=true&db=psyh&AN=1998-06070- 000&site=ehost-live&scope=site.

9. DeMarsh JK, Kumpfer KL. Family, environmental, and genetic influences on children's future chemical dependency. J Child Contemp Soc. 1985;18:117–52.

10. Dishion TJ, Reid JB, Patterson GR. Empirical guidelines for a family intervention for adolescent drug use. In: Coombs RE, editor. The family context of adolescent drug use. New York: Haworth; 1988. p. 189–224.

11. Dishion TJ, Kavanaugh K. Intervening in adolescent problem behavior: a family-centered approach. New York: Guilford; 2005.

12. Dittrich JE. A group program for wives of treatment resistant alcoholics. In: O'Farrell TJ, editor. Treating alcohol problems: marital and family interventions. New York: Guilford; 1993. p. 78–114.

13. Dobkin PL, De Civita M, Paraherakis A, Gill K. The role of functional social support in treatment retention and outcomes among outpatient adult substance abusers. Addiction. 2002;97:347–56.

14. Dutra L, Stathopoulou G, Basden SL, Leyro TM, Powers MB, Otto MW. A meta-analytic review of psychosocial interventions for substance use disorders. Am J Psychiatry. 2008;165:179–87.

15. Edwards ME, Steinglass P. Family therapy treatment outcomes for alcoholism. J Marital Fam Ther. 1996;21:475–509.

16. Emmelkamp PM, Vedel E. Evidence-based treatment for drug and alcohol abuse. New York: Taylor and Francis Group; 2006.

17. Epstein EE, McCrady BS. Behavioral couples treatment of alcohol and drug use disorders: current status and innovations. Clin Psychol Rev. 1998;18:689–711.

18. Epstein EE, McCrady BS, Morgan TJ. Couples treatment for drug-dependent males: preliminary efficacy of a stand alone outpatient model. Addict Disord Treat. 2007;6:21–37.

19. Galanter M. Network therapy for addiction: a model for office practice. Am J Psychiatr. 1993;150:28–36.

20. Halford WK, Osgarby SM. Alcohol abuse in clients presenting with marital problems. J Fam Psychol. 1993;6(3):245–54.

21. Hawkins JD, Catalano RF, Brown EO, Vadasy PF, Roberts C, Fitzmahan D, Starkman N, Randsell M. Preparing for the drug (free) years: a family activity book. Seattle: Comprehensive Health Education Foundation; 1988.

22. Heath AW, Stanton MD. Family-based treatment: stages and outcomes. In: Frances RJ, Miller SI, editors. Clinical textbook of addictive disorders. 2nd ed. New York: Guilford; 1998. p. 496–520.

23. Holder H, Longabaugh R, Miller WR, Rubonis AV. The cost effectiveness of treatment for alcoholism: a first approximation. J Stud Alcohol. 1991;52(6):517–40.

24. Hoogeveen CE, Vogelvang B, Rigter H. Feasibility of inpatient and outpatient multidimensional family therapy for improving behavioral outcomes in adolescents referred to residential youth care. Resid Treat Child Youth. 2017;34(1):61–81.

25. Horigian V, Feaster D, Brincks A, Robbins M, Perez M, Szapocznik J. The effects of Brief Strategic Family Therapy (BSFT) on parent substance use and the association between parent and adolescent substance use. Addict Behav. 2015;42:44–50. https://doi. org/10.1016/j.addbeh.2014.10.024.

26. Horigian VE, Anderson AR, Szapocznik J. Taking brief strategic family therapy from bench to trench: evidence generation across translational phases. Fam Process. 2016;55(3):529–42.

27. Huey SJ Jr, Henggeler SW, Brondino MJ, Pickrel SG. Mechanisms of change in multisystemic therapy: reducing delinquent behavior through therapist adherence and improved family and peer functioning. J Consult Clin Psychol. 2000;68(3):451–67.

28. Johnson VE. Intervention: how to help someone who doesn't want help. Center City: Hazelden; 1986.

29. Joutsenniemi K, Moustgaard H, Koskinen S, Ripatti S, Martikainen P. Psychiatric comorbidity in couples: a longitudinal study of 202,959 married and cohabiting individuals. Soc Psychiatry Psychiatr Epidemiol. 2011;46(7):623–33.

30. Kelly S, Epstein EE, McCrady BS. Pretreatment attrition from couple therapy for male drug abusers. Am J Drug Alcohol Abuse. 2004;30(1):1–19. https://doi. org/10.1081/ADA-120029861.

31. Kelley M, Klostermann K, Doane AN, Mignone T, Lam KK, Fals-Stewart W, Padilla MA. The case for examining and treating the combined effects of parental drug use and intimate parental violence on children in their homes. Aggress Violent Behav. 2010;15:76–82.

32. Kennedy C, Klostermann K, Gorman C, Fals-Stewart W. Treating substance abuse and intimate partner violence: implications for addiction professionals. Couns Mag. 2005;6(1):28–34.

33. Klostermann K, Fals-Stewart W. Behavioral couples therapy for substance abuse. J Behav Anal Offender Vict. 2008;1(4):81–93.

34. Klostermann K, Kelley ML, Mignone T, Pusateri L, Wills K. Behavioral couples therapy for substance

abuse: where do we go from here? Subst Use Misuse. 2011;46:1502–9.

35. Klostermann K, Kelley ML, Milletich RJ, Mignone T. Alcoholism and partner aggression among gay, lesbian, and bisexual couples. Aggress Violent Behav. 2011;16:115.

36. Klostermann K, O'Farrell T. Couples' therapy in treatment of substance use disorders. In: Fitzgerald J, editor. Foundations for couples' therapy: research for the real world. New York: Routledge/Taylor & Francis Group; 2017. p. 404–14.

37. Kosterman R, Hawkins JD, Haggerty KP, Spoth R, Redmond C. Preparing for the drug free years: session-specific effects of a universal parent-training intervention with rural families. J Drug Educ. 2001;31(1):47–68.

38. Koffinke C. Family recovery issues and treatment resources. In: Daley DC, Raskin MS, editors. Treating the chemically and their families. Newbury Park: Sage; 1991.

39. Kumpfer K, Alvarado R. Family-strengthening approaches for the prevention of youth problem behaviors. The American Psychologist. 2003;58:457–65. https://doi.org/10.1037/0003-066X.58.6-7.457.

40. Lemke S, Brennan PL, Schutte KK. Upward pressures on drinking: exposure and reactivity in adulthood. J Stud Alcohol Drugs. 2007;68:437–45.

41. Liddle HA. Multidimensional family therapy: evidence base for transdiagnostic treatment outcomes, change mechanisms, and implementation in community settings. Fam Process. 2016;55(3):558–76.

42. Liddle HA, Hogue A. Multidimensional family therapy for adolescent substance abuse. In: Wagner EF, Waldron HB, editors. Innovations in adolescent substance abuse interventions. New York: Pergamon; 2001. p. 229–61.

43. Longabaugh R. The search for mechanisms of change in behavioral treatments for alcohol use disorders: a commentary. Alcohol Clin Exp Res. 2007;31:S1.

44. Mann K. One hundred years of alcoholism: the twentieth century. Alcohol Alcohol. 2000;35:10–5.

45. Marshal MP. For better or worse? The effect of alcohol use on marital functioning. Clin Psychol Rev. 2003;23(7):959–97.

46. McCrady BS. Behavioral marital therapy with alcoholics. In: Keller PA, Heyman SR, editors. Innovations in clinical practice: a source book, vol. 10. Sarasota: Professional Resource Press/Professional Resource Exchange; 1991. p. 117–39.

47. McCrady BS. Family and other close relationships. In: Miller WR, Carroll KM, editors. Rethinking substance abuse: what the science shows and what we should do about it. New York: Guilford; 2006.

48. McCrady BS. Alcohol use disorders: treatment and mechanisms of change. In: McKay D, Abramowitz JS, Storch EA, editors. Treatments for psychological problems and syndromes: Wiley-Blackwell; 2017. p. 235–47. https://doi.org/10.1002/9781118877142.ch16.

49. McCrady BS, Epstein EE. Theoretical bases of family approaches to substance abuse treatment. In: Rotgers F, Keller DS, Morgenstern J, editors. Treating substance abuse: theory and technique. New York: Guilford; 1996. p. 117–42.

50. McCrady BS, Epstein EE, Cook SM, Jensen N, Hildebrandt T. A randomized trial of individual and couple behavioral alcohol treatment for women. J Consult Clin Psychol. 2009;77:243–56.

51. McGovern MP, Fox TS, Xie H, Drake RE. A survey of clinical practices and readiness to adopt evidence-based practices: dissemination research in an addiction treatment system. J Subst Abuse Treat. 2004;26:305–12.

52. McKay JR. Treating substance use disorders with adaptive continuing care. Washington, D.C.: American Psychological Association; 2009.

53. Miller WR, Hester RK. Matching problem drinkers with optimal treatments. In: Miller WR, Heather N, editors. Treating addictive behaviors: processes of change. New York: Plenum Press; 1986. p. 175–203.

54. Miller WR, Meyers RJ, Tonigan JS. Engaging the unmotivated in treatment for alcohol problems: a comparison of three strategies for intervention through family members. J Consult Clin Psychol. 1999;67:688–97.

55. Miller WR, Wilbourne PL. Mesa grande: a methodological analysis of clinical trials of treatments for alcohol use disorders. Addiction. 2002;97:265–77.

56. Mitchell AJ, Selmes T. Why don't patients attend their appointments? Maintaining engagement with psychiatric services. Adv Psychiatr Treat. 2007;13:423–34.

57. National Institute on Drug Abuse. Principles of drug abuse treatment for criminal justice populations: a research-based guide. NIH pub. no. 06-5316. 2006. Retrieved from http://www.atforum.com/addiction-resources/documents/PODAT_CJ.pdf.

58. Norcross JC, Karpiak CP. Clinical psychologists in the 2010s: 50 years of the APA division of clinical psychology. Clinical Psychology: Science and Practice. 2012;19(1):1–12. https://doi.org/10.1111/j.1468-2850.2012.01269.x

59. Noriega G, Ramos L, Medina-Mora ME, Villa AR. Prevalence of codependence in young women seeking primary health care and associated risk factors. Am J Orthopsychiatry. 2008;78(2):199–210.

60. O'Farrell TJ, Clements K. Review of outcome research on marital and family therapy in treatment for alcoholism. J Marital Fam Ther. 2012;38:122–44.

61. O'Farrell TJ, Fals-Stewart W. Family-involved alcoholism treatment: an update. In: Galanter M, editor. Recent developments in alcoholism, volume 15: services research in the era of managed care. New York: Plenum Press; 2001. p. 329–56.

62. O'Farrell TJ, Fals-Stewart W. Behavioral couples therapy for alcoholism and drug abuse. New York: Guilford; 2006.

63. O'Farrell TJ, Murphy CM. Marital violence before and after alcoholism treatment. J Consult Clin Psychol. 1995;63:256–62.

64. Powers MB, Vedel E, Emmelkamp PM. Behavioral couples therapy (BCT) for alcohol and drug use disorders: a meta-analysis. Clin Psychol Rev. 2008;28:952–62.

65. Smock SA, Trepper TS, Wetchler JL, McCollum EE, Ray R, Pierce K. Solution-focused group therapy for level 1 substance abusers. J Marital Fam Ther. 2008;34:107–20.

66. Sisson RW, Azrin NH. Family member involvement to initiate and promote treatment of problem drinking. J Behav Ther Exp Psychiatry. 1993;17:15–21.

67. Smith JE, Meyers RJ. Community reinforcement and family training. In: Fisher GL, Roget's NA, editors. Encyclopedia of substance abuse prevention, treatment, and recovery. Thousand Oaks: Sage; 2009.

68. Snyder DK, Whisman MA. Treating difficult couples: helping clients with coexisting mental and relationship disorders. New York: Guildford; 2003.

69. Spoth RL, Redmond C, Trudeau L, Shin C. Longitudinal substance initiation outcomes for a universal preventive intervention combining family and school programs. Psychol Addict Behav. 2002;16(2):129–34.

70. Stanton MD, Todd TC, & Associates. The family therapy of drug abuse and addiction. New York: Guilford; 1982.

71. Steinglass P, Bennett LA, Wolin SJ, Reiss D. The alcoholic family. New York: BasicBooks; 1987.

72. Szapocznik J, Hervis O, Schwartz S. Therapy manuals for drug addiction: brief strategic family therapy for adolescent drug abuse. Bethesda: National Institute on Drug Abuse; 2003.

73. Szapocznik J, Santisteban D, Rio A, Perez-Vidal A, Santisteban D, Kurtines WM. Family effectiveness training: an intervention to prevent drug abuse and problem behaviors in hispanic adolescents. Hisp J Behav Sci. 1989;11:4–27.

74. Thomas EJ, Ager RD. Unilateral family therapy with spouses of uncooperative alcohol abusers. In: O'Farrell TJ, editor. Treating alcohol problems: marital and family interventions. New York: Guilford Press; 1993. p. 3–33.

75. Thomas EJ, Santa C, Bronson D, Oyserman D. Unilateral family therapy with spouses of alcoholics. J Soc Serv Res. 1987;10:145–62.

76. Tracy SW, Kelly JF, Moos RH. The influence of partner status, relationship quality and relationship stability on outcomes following intensive substance-use disorder treatment. J cStud Alcohol. 2005;66:497–50.

77. Walitzer KS. Family therapy. In: Ott PJ, Tarter RE, Ammerman RT, editors. Sourcebook on substance abuse: etiology, epidemiology, assessment, and treatment. Needham Heights: Allyn and Bacon; 1999. p. 337–49.

78. Walitzer KS, Dermen KH. Alcohol-focused spouse involvement and behavioral couples therapy: evaluation of enhancements to drinking reduction treatment for male problem drinkers. J Consult Clin Psychol. 2004;72(6):944–55. https://doi.org/10.1037/0022-006X.72.6.944

79. Wampold BE. The great psychotherapy debate: models, methods, and findings. London: Routledge Academic; 2010.

80. Wegscheider S. Another chance: hope and health for the alcoholic family. Palo Alto: Science and Behavior Books; 1981.

Network Therapy

32

Marc Galanter

Contents

M. Galanter (✉)
Division of Alcoholism and Drug Abuse, Department
of Psychiatry, NYU School of Medicine,
New York, NY, USA
e-mail: marcgalanter@nyu.edu

Abstract

Office-based practice for the treatment of
patients with substance use disorders is limited in important information obscured by a

© Springer Nature Switzerland AG 2021
N. el-Guebaly et al. (eds.), *Textbook of Addiction Treatment*,
https://doi.org/10.1007/978-3-030-36391-8_32

patient's denial of illness and lack of support for the patient in the face of potential relapse. This chapter provides a description of the rationale and technique for employing the support of family and close friends for the treatment of addictive disorders. This chapter provides clinical examples of how network therapy is applied, and research for validation of this approach, as well as a role for the use of Twelve-Step facilitation in conjunction with this approach.

Keywords

Addiction · Family therapy · Medication · Social support

32.1 Introduction

Psychotherapy for people dependent on alcohol and other drugs presents unique problems for the office-based practitioner. Among these are the ever-present vulnerability to relapse to substance use and high dropout rates. In order to address this problem, we can consider how engaging the input of people close to an addicted person can help in achieving a stable abstinence and deal with the vulnerability to dropout from treatment. To understand this option, it is first important to understand that certain conditioned drug-seeking behaviors may be extinguished if appropriate aversive stimuli are interposed after triggers to drug use are presented.

A drug user can become entangled in an interlocking web of self-perpetuating reinforcers that contribute to the persistence of drug abuse, despite compromising consequences, and the user's imperviousness to a traditional, psychodynamic psychotherapeutic approach does not necessarily take such conditioning factors into account. This is because neither the user nor the therapist is typically aware of their existence due to the unconscious nature of the conditioned response of drug-seeking. The therapist's attempt to alter the course of the stimulus–response sequence is therefore often not viable, even with the aid of a willing patient, as neither party is necessarily aware that a conditioned sequence is taking place.

Sufficient exploration, however, can reveal the relevant stimuli and their effect through conditioned sequences of drug-seeking behavior. An earlier publication described a technique for guided recall of relevant conditioned stimuli in a psychotherapeutic context, whereby the person with alcohol or substance use disorder may become aware of the sequence of circumstances that can precipitate relapse [16]. Once this is done, the patient's own distress at the course of the addictive process, generated by the patient's own motivation for escaping the addictive pattern, may be mobilized. This motivational distress then serves as an aversive stimulus. The implicit assumption behind this therapeutic approach is that the patient in question wants to alter his or her pattern of drug use and that the recognition of a particular stimulus as a conditioned component of addiction will then allow the patient, in effect, to initiate the extinction process. If a patient is committed to achieving abstinence from an addictive drug such as alcohol or cocaine but is in jeopardy of occasional slips, this cognitive labeling can facilitate consolidation of an abstinent adaptation.

As we shall see, the input of people close to the patient can help to reveal triggers to drugs use that may not be apparent to the patient. Such an approach is less valuable in the context of (a) a lack of motivation for abstinence, (b) fragile social supports, or (c) compulsive substance abuse unmanageable by the patient in the patient's usual social settings. Hospitalization or replacement therapy (e.g., methadone or buprenorphine) may be necessary in such cases, because ambulatory stabilization through psychotherapeutic support is often not feasible, even with the support of family and close peers. On the other hand, for willing patients, or ones whom family and friends have convinced to cooperate, the Network approach can be most valuable.

32.2 The Network Therapy Technique

This approach can be useful in addressing a broad range of addicted patients characterized by the following clinical hallmarks of addictive illness. When they initiate consumption of their addictive agent, be it alcohol, cocaine, opioids, or depressant drugs, they frequently cannot limit that consumption to a reasonable and predictable level; this phenomenon has been termed *loss of control* by clinicians who treat persons dependent on alcohol or drugs [26]. Second, they have consistently demonstrated relapse to the agent of abuse; that is, they have attempted to stop using the drug for varying periods of time but have returned to it, despite a specific intent to avoid it.

This treatment approach is not necessary for those with substance use disorder who can learn to set limits on their use of alcohol or drugs; their substance use may be treated as a behavioral symptom in a more traditional psychotherapeutic fashion. Nor is it directed at those patients for whom the addictive pattern is most unmanageable, such as addicted people with unusual destabilizing circumstances such as homelessness, severe character pathology, or psychosis. These patients may need special supportive care such as inpatient detoxification or long-term residential treatment.

32.2.1 Key Elements

Three key elements are integrated in the network therapy (NT) technique. The first is a cognitive–behavioral approach to relapse prevention, which has been considered valuable in addiction treatment [37]. Emphasis in this approach is placed on triggers to relapse and behavioral techniques for avoiding them, in preference to exploring underlying psychodynamic issues.

Second, support of the patient's natural social network is engaged in treatment. Peer support in AA has long been shown to be an effective vehicle for promoting abstinence, and the idea of the therapist's intervening with family and friends in

starting treatment was employed in one of the early ambulatory techniques specific to addiction [27]. The involvement of spouses [33] has since been shown to be effective in enhancing the outcome of professional therapy.

Third, the orchestration of resources to provide community reinforcement suggests a more robust treatment intervention by providing a support for drug-free rehabilitation [4]. In this relation, Khantzian pointed to the "primary care therapist" as one who functions in direct coordinating and monitoring roles in order to combine psychotherapeutic and self-help elements [30]. It is this overall management role over circumstances outside as well as inside the office session that is presented to trainees, in order to maximize the effectiveness of the intervention.

32.3 CBT and Social Support

Cognitive–Behavioral Therapy This format for treatment has been shown to be effective for a wide variety of substance use disorders, including alcohol [38], marijuana [44], and cocaine dependence [7]. It is premised on the original findings by Wikler [48] on conditioning models of drug-seeking in heroin-addicted subjects.

The *cognitive–behavioral therapy* (CBT) approach is goal oriented and focuses on current circumstances in the patient's life. In network therapy, reference in both individual and conjoint sessions can be made to salient past experiences. CBT sessions are typically structured, so, for example, patients begin each Network session with a recounting of recent events directly relevant to their addiction and recovery. This is followed by active participation and interaction of therapist, patient, and Network members in response to the patient's report. CBT emphasizes psychoeducation in the context of relapse prevention, so that circumstances, thoughts, and interpersonal situations that have historically precipitated substance use are identified, and the patient (and Network members as well) are taught to anticipate where such triggers can precipitate substance use.

The process of guided recall, noted previously, is particularly important because it allows the therapist both individual sessions with the patient alone—and network sessions—in conjunction with Network members along with the patient—to guide the patient to recognize a sequence of conditioned stimuli (triggers) that play a role in drug-seeking. Such triggers may not initially be apparent to the patient or Network members, but with encouragement and prompting, can emerge over the course of an exploration of the circumstances that have led, either in the past, or in a recent "slip," to substance use.

Social Support This issue has been studied in a variety of data sets in relation to the recovery from substance use disorders. For example, in the federal Project MATCH, three modalities, Twelve-Step facilitation (TSF), motivational enhancement, and cognitive–behavioral approaches, were compared. In a secondary analysis of findings from this multisite study, it was found [50] that certain aspects of social support were most predictive of abstinence outcomes. Two social network characteristics that had a positive effect on outcome were the size of the supportive social network in the person's life, and the number of members who were abstainers (or recovering from alcohol use disorder). I have found that nonproblem drinking participants are important to a long-term clinical outcome. In a matter of fact, a large number of Network members, when their participation is effectively maintained over time, can counter a variety of circumstances that may undermine a patient's abstinence. In addition, they can provide varied aspects of support relative to the patient's experience in recovery. And indeed, they should be free of substance-related problems. Of interest in this context, it has been reported that men are more typically encouraged by their wives to seek help, whereas women are more often encouraged by mothers, siblings, and children [6].

Community Reinforcement Family involvement in substance abuse treatment has long been shown to be effective in improving outcome, and

there are numerous approaches that make use of social network involvement in treatment, including Behavioral Couples Therapy [14], Marital Therapy [39], and the Community Reinforcement Approach [5, 36].

More specifically, the Community Reinforcement and Family Training (CRAFT) Program includes many aspects of treatment that are also employed in Network Therapy. The CRAFT approach was developed to encourage drinkers to enter therapy and reduce drinking, in part by eliciting support of concerned others as well as to enhance satisfaction with life among members of the patient's social network who were concerned about his or her drinking. As in Network Therapy, the CRAFT program includes a functional analysis of the patient's substance use, that is to say, understanding the substance use with respect to its antecedents and consequences. Like Network Therapy, it also serves to minimize reciprocal blaming and defensiveness among the concerned significant others, and to promote a patient's sobriety-oriented activities.

In one large trial in which concerned significant others were randomized to one of three conditions, a comparison was made between Al-Anon-facilitated therapy, an approach similar to the Johnson Institute interventions, and the CRAFT model [15]. The CRAFT intervention was more effective in engaging treatment-refusing people with alcohol use disorder as compared to the other two approaches. Similar positive findings were obtained in studies on CRAFT with illicit drug users [31, 35]. In another study, concerned significant others were successfully trained to apply a modified Johnson Intervention technique in the absence of a therapist, and this approach was found to be successful [32].

32.3.1 Initial Encounter: Starting a Social Network

The following approach is applicable, as appropriate, to patients with moderate to severe substance alcohol use disorder (F10.20) or similar severity of other substance use disorders [2]. It can be applied in ASAM levels of care 1–4, as appropriate [34].

How does one go about developing NT? The patient should be asked to bring his or her spouse or a close friend to the first session. Patients with alcohol use disorder often dislike certain things they hear when they first come for treatment and may deny or rationalize, even if they have voluntarily sought help. Because of their denial of the problem, a significant other is essential to both history taking and implementing a viable treatment plan. A close relative or spouse can often cut through the denial in a way that an unfamiliar therapist cannot and can therefore be invaluable in setting a standard of realism in dealing with the addiction.

Some patients make clear that they wish to come to the initial session on their own. This is often associated with their desire to preserve the option of continued substance abuse and is born out of the fear that an alliance will be established independent of them to prevent this. Although a delay may be tolerated for a session or two, it should be stated unambiguously at the outset that effective treatment can be undertaken only on the basis of a therapeutic alliance built around the addiction issue that includes the support of significant others and that it is expected that a network of close friends and/or relatives will be brought in within a session or two at the most.

The weight of clinical experience supports the view that abstinence is the most practical goal to propose to the addicted person for his or her rehabilitation [23, 24]. For abstinence to be expected, however, the therapist should ensure the provision of necessary social supports for the patient. Let us consider how a long-term support network is initiated for this purpose, beginning with availability of the therapist, significant others, and a self-help group.

In the first place, the therapist should be available for consultation on the phone and should indicate to the patient that he or she wants to be called if problems arise. This makes the therapist's commitment clear and sets the tone for a "team effort." It begins to undercut one reason for relapse, the patient's sense of being on the patient's own if unable to manage the situation. The astute therapist, however, will assure that he

or she does not spend excessive time on the telephone or in emergency sessions. The patient will therefore develop a support network that can handle the majority of problems involved in day-to-day assistance. This generally will leave the therapist to respond only to occasional questions of interpreting the terms of the understanding among himself or herself, the patient, and support network members. If there is a question about the ability of the patient and network to manage the period between the initial sessions, the first few scheduled sessions may be arranged at intervals of only 1–3 days. In any case, frequent appointments should be scheduled at the outset if a pharmacologic detoxification with benzodiazepines is indicated, so that the patient need never manage more than a few days' medication at a time.

What is most essential, however, is that the network be forged into a working group to provide necessary support for the patient between the initial sessions. Membership ranges from one to several persons close to the patient. Larger networks have been used by Speck [43] in treating schizophrenic patients. Contacts between network members at this stage typically include telephone calls (at the therapist's or patient's initiative), dinner arrangements, and social encounters and should be preplanned to a fair extent during the joint session. These encounters are most often undertaken at the time when alcohol or drug use is likely to occur. In planning together, however, it should be made clear to network members that relatively little unusual effort will be required for the long term, and that after the patient is stabilized, their participation will amount to little more than attendance at infrequent meetings with the patient and the therapist. This is reassuring to those network members who are unable to make a major time commitment to the patient as well as to those patients who do not want to be placed in a dependent position.

32.3.2 Defining the Network's Membership

Once the patient has come for an appointment, establishing a network is a task undertaken with active collaboration of the patient and the therapist. The two, aided by those parties who join the network initially, must search for the right balance of members. The therapist must carefully promote the choice of appropriate network members, however, just as the platoon leader selects those who will go into combat. The network will be crucial in determining the balance of the therapy. This process is not without problems, and the therapist must think in a strategic fashion of the interactions that may take place among network members.

32.3.3 Defining the Network's Task

As conceived here, the therapist's relationship to the network is like that of a task-oriented team leader, rather than that of a family therapist oriented toward insight. The network is established to implement a straightforward task, that of aiding the therapist in sustaining the patient's abstinence. It must be directed with the same clarity of purpose that a task force is directed in any effective organization. Competing and alternative goals must be suppressed, or at least prevented from interfering with the primary task.

Unlike family members involved in traditional family therapy, network members are not led to expect symptom relief for themselves or self-realization. This prevents the development of competing goals for the network's meetings. It also assures the members protection from having their own motives scrutinized and thereby supports their continuing involvement without the threat of an assault on their psychological defenses. Because network members have—kindly—volunteered to participate, their motives must not be impugned. Their constructive behavior should be commended. It is useful to acknowledge appreciation for the contribution they are making to the therapy. There is always a counterproductive tendency on their part to minimize the value of their contribution. The network must, therefore, be structured as an effective working group with high morale.

32.3.4 Use of Pharmacotherapy in the Network Format

For the person with alcohol use disorder, disulfiram may be of marginal use in assuring abstinence when used in a traditional counseling context [15], but becomes much more valuable when carefully integrated into work with the patient and network, particularly when the drug is taken under observation. A similar circumstance applies to the use of oral naltrexone for stabilizing abstinence in an opioid-dependent person. In the case of alcohol, it is a good idea to use the initial telephone contact to engage the patient's agreement to abstain from alcohol for the day immediately prior to the first session. The therapist then has the option of prescribing or administering disulfiram at that time. For a patient who is earnest about seeking assistance for alcoholism, this is often not difficult, if some time is spent on the phone-making plans to avoid a drinking context during that period. If it is not feasible to undertake this on the phone, it may be addressed in the first session. Such planning with the patient almost always involves organizing time with significant others and therefore serves as a basis for developing the patient's support network.

The administration of disulfiram under observation is a treatment option that is easily adapted to work with social networks. A patient who takes disulfiram cannot drink; a patient who agrees to be observed by a responsible party while taking disulfiram will not miss his or her dose without the observer's knowing. This may take a measure of persuasion and, above all, the therapist's commitment that such an approach can be reasonable and helpful.

As noted previously, individual therapists traditionally have seen the addicted person as a patient with poor prognosis. This is largely because in the context of traditional psychotherapy, there are no behavioral controls to prevent the recurrence of drug use, and resources are not available for behavioral intervention if a recurrence takes place—which it usually does. A system of impediments to the emergence of relapse, resting heavily on the actual or symbolic role of the network, must therefore be established. The therapist must have assistance in addressing any minor episode of drinking so that this ever-present problem does not lead to an unmanageable relapse or an unsuccessful termination of therapy.

32.3.5 Format for Medication Observation by the Network

1. Take the medication every morning in front of a network member.
2. Take the pill so that person can observe you swallowing them.
3. Have the observer write down the time of day the pills were taken on a list prepared by the therapist.
4. The observer brings the list in to the therapist's office at each network session.
5. The observer leaves a message on the therapist's answering machine on any day in which the patient had not taken the pills in a way that ingestion was not clearly observed.

32.3.6 Meeting Arrangements

At the outset of therapy, it is important to see the patient with the group on a weekly basis for at least the first month. Unstable circumstances demand more frequent contacts with the network. Sessions can be tapered off to biweekly and then to monthly intervals after a time.

To sustain the continuing commitment of the group, particularly that between the therapist and the network members, network sessions should be held every 3 months or so for the duration of the individual therapy. Once the patient has stabilized, the meetings tend less to address day-to-day issues. They may begin with the patient's recounting of the drug situation. Reflections on the patient's progress and goals, or sometimes on relations among the network members, then may be discussed. In any case, it is essential that network members contact the therapist if they are concerned about the patient's possible use of alcohol or drugs, and that the therapist contacts the network members if the therapist becomes concerned about a potential relapse.

32.3.7 Adapting Individual Therapy to the Network Treatment

As noted previously, network sessions are scheduled on a weekly basis at the outset of treatment. This is likely to compromise the number of individual contacts. Indeed, if sessions are held once a week, the patient may not be seen individually for a period of time. The patient may perceive this as a deprivation unless the individual therapy is presented as an opportunity for further growth predicated on achieving stable abstinence assured through work with the network.

When the individual therapy does begin, the traditional objectives of therapy must be arranged so as to accommodate the goals of the substance abuse treatment. For insight-oriented therapy, clarification of unconscious motivations is a primary objective; for supportive therapy, the bolstering of established constructive defenses is primary. In the therapeutic context that is described here, however, the following objectives are given precedence.

Of first importance is the need to address exposure to substances of abuse or exposure to cues that might precipitate alcohol or drug use [17]. Both patient and therapist should be sensitive to this matter and explore these situations as they arise. Second, a stable social context in an appropriate social environment—one conducive to abstinence with minimal disruption of life circumstances—should be supported. Considerations of minor disruptions in place of residence, friends, or job need not be a primary issue for the patient with character disorder or neurosis, but they cannot go untended here. For a considerable period of time, the person with substance use disorder is highly vulnerable to exacerbations of the disorder, and, in some respects, must be viewed with the considerable caution with which one treats the recently compensated person with psychosis.

Finally, after these priorities have been attended to, psychological conflicts that the patient must resolve, relative to his or her own growth, are considered. As the therapy continues, these come to assume a more prominent role. In the earlier phases, they are likely to reflect directly issues associated with the previous drug use. Later, however, as the issue of addiction becomes less compelling from day to day, the context of the treatment increasingly will come to resemble the traditional psychotherapeutic context. Given the optimism generated by an initial victory over the addictive process, the patient will be in an excellent position to move forward in therapy with a positive view of his or her future.

32.4 Twelve-Step Facilitation (TSF)

In addition to the NT approach described here, TSF can be employed by the treating clinician. TSF is designed to promote involvement in AA by engaging a patient in participating in the fellowship's first three steps. It was developed for alcohol use disorder, but it can be employed for other substances, as well. (A full description of TSF is available at https://pubs.niaaa.nih.gov.) It can be combined in practice with group therapeutic approaches [13].

Over the course of treatment, which can supplement Network sessions, the patient is encouraged to participate in AA, and his or her progress can be shared with Network members. The patient is expected to attend AA meetings weekly and discuss his or her experience with the treating clinician.

Step 1 of Alcoholics Anonymous reads as follows:
> We Admitted We Were Powerless Over Alcohol—
> That Our Lives Had Become Unmanageable

This entails the acceptance of personal limitation, in this case, involving the loss of control over drinking. Although some individuals apparently achieve this acceptance via a single leap of faith, it is also possible to think of acceptance as a process involving a series of stages. This can begin with "I have a problem with alcohol," followed by "Alcohol (drinking) is gradually mak-

ing my life more difficult and is causing problems for me," and "I have lost my ability to effectively control (limit) my use of alcohol."

This represents a statement of personal *limitation*. Accepting powerlessness over alcohol is much like having to accept any other personal limitation or handicap. Some people have a hard time relating to Step 1 as it is written. They can relate to it better if it is framed in terms of limitation.

Steps 2 and 3 are framed as such:
> Came to Believe That a Power Greater Than Ourselves Could Restore Us to Sanity.

> Made a Decision to Turn Our Will and Our Lives Over to the Care of God as We Understood Him.

Discussion with the patient focuses on issues like this: What does he or she believe in? Who are his or her heroes? What are his or her most cherished values? Of what religious background is the patient? Does he or she still practice? If not, when and why did he or she stop? What does the idea of "turning over" your will mean to patients? Has the patient ever followed someone else's advice, simply on the basis of trust and faith? If so, who and when? What about trusting the wisdom of AA based on faith? What resistance does the patient have to Turning It Over as opposed to "going it alone"?

32.4.1 General Approach

The clinician reviews with the patient on a weekly basis: What meetings were attended, and what were the patient's reactions to them? Reading: What did the patient read in the book, *Alcoholics Anonymous*, and what was his or her reaction?

Urges to drink are reviewed weekly: When and where? What did the patient do? How could the patient use AA to help with urges in the future?

It is emphasized that recovery comes only through active involvement in the 12-Step program as opposed to trying not to drink through solitary, white-knuckle determination or by simply attending but not participating in meetings. Attending meetings marks the start of establishing a new network of friends that will be critical to recovery. Patients are encouraged to get phone numbers of people whom they can call. Merely going to meetings without participating in them is not the same thing as working the 12-Step program and is not likely to be helpful to recovering patients when they have strong urges to drink or when they have a slip.

32.5 Research on Network Therapy

Network therapy is included under the American Psychiatric Association (APA) Practice Guidelines [3] for substance use disorders as an approach to facilitating adherence to a treatment plan. The Substance Abuse and Mental Health Services Administration (SAMHSA) includes a description of NT in its National Registry of Evidence-based Program and Practices [42] and NT is listed as one of its Treatment Improvement Protocol TIP 39 Substance Abuse Treatment and Family Therapy approaches [9]. To date, five studies have demonstrated their effectiveness in treatment and training. Each addressed the technique's validation from a different perspective: a trial in office management; studies of its effectiveness in the training of psychiatric residents and of counselors who work with people with cocaine use disorder; an evaluation of acceptance of the network approach in an Internet technology transfer course and a trial evaluating the impact of NT relative to medication management in heroin-addicted persons inducted on to buprenorphine. In addition, NT components that have been adapted and combined with other psychosocial treatments to treat patients with opioid or alcohol dependence are described later.

32.5.1 An Office-Based Clinical Trial

A chart review was conducted on a series of 60 substance-dependent patients, with follow-up appointments scheduled through the period of treatment and up to 1 year thereafter [18]. For 27 patients, the primary drug of dependence was alcohol; for 23, it was cocaine; for 6, it was opioids; for 3, it was marijuana; and for 1, it was nicotine. In all but eight of the patients, networks were fully established. Of the 60 patients, 46 experienced full improvement (i.e., abstinence for at least 6 months) or major improvement (i.e., a marked decline in drug use to nonproblematic levels). The study demonstrated the viability of establishing networks and applying them in the practitioner's treatment setting. It also served as a basis for the ensuing developmental research supported by the National Institute on Drug Abuse.

32.5.2 Treatment by Psychiatry Residents

We developed and implemented a network therapy training sequence in the New York University psychiatric residency program and then evaluated the clinical outcome of a group of cocaine-dependent patients treated by the residents. The psychiatric residency was chosen because of the growing importance of clinical training in the management of addiction in outpatient care in residency programs, in line with the standards set for specialty certification.

A training manual was prepared on the network technique, defining the specifics of the treatment in a manner allowing for uniformity in practice. It was developed for use as a training tool and then as a guide for the residents during the treatment phase. Network therapy tape segments drawn from a library of 130 videotaped sessions were used to illustrate typical therapy situations. A network therapy rating scale was developed to assess the technique's application, with items emphasizing key aspects of treatment [29]. The scale was evaluated for its reliability in distinguishing between two contrasting addiction therapies, network therapy and systemic family therapy, both presented to faculty and residents on videotape. The internal consistency of responses for each of the techniques was high for both the faculty and the resident samples, and both groups consistently distinguished the two modalities. The scale was then used by clinical supervisors as a didactic aid for training and to monitor therapist adherence to the study treatment manual.

We trained third-year psychiatry residents to apply the network therapy approach, with an emphasis placed on distinctions in technique between the treatment of addiction and of other major mental illness or personality disorder. The residents then worked with a sample of 47 patients with cocaine use disorder. Once treatment was initiated, 77% of the subjects established a network, that is, brought in at least one member for a network session. In fact, 1.47 collaterals on average attended any given network session, across all the subjects and sessions. This is notable, because compliance after initial screening was not necessarily assured. Almost all of those who completed a 24-week regimen (15 of 17) produced urines negative for cocaine in their last three toxicologies. On the other hand, only a minority of those who attended the first week but who did not complete the sequence (4 of 18) met this outcome criterion [20]. The residents, inexperienced in drug treatment, achieved results similar to those reported for experienced professionals [8, 25]. These comparisons supported the feasibility of successful training of psychiatry residents naive to addiction treatment and the efficacy of the treatment in their hands.

To better understand the role of therapeutic alliance in NT, Glazer et al. [22] reviewed videotaped network sessions on 21 out of the 47 patients with cocaine use disorder and rated them on level of patient–therapist alliance using the PENN Helping Alliance Rating Scale and the Working Alliance Inventory. The tapes that were selected to be rated were those that represented the participants' first videotaped NT session. Results showed a significant positive correlation between therapeutic alliance and outcomes as measured by the percentage of cocaine-free urine toxicology screens and by eight consecutive cocaine-free urines.

32.5.3 Treatment by Addiction Counselors

This study was conducted in a community-based addictions treatment clinic, and the network therapy training sequence was essentially the same as the one applied to the psychiatry residents [28]. A cohort of 10 cocaine-dependent patients received treatment at the community program with a format that included network therapy, along with the clinic's usual package of modalities, and an additional 20 cocaine-dependent patients received treatment as usual and served as control subjects. The network therapy was found to enhance the outcome of the experimental patients. Of 107 urinalyses conducted on the network therapy patients, 88% were negative, but only 66% of the 82 urine samples from the control subjects were negative, a significantly lower proportion. The mean retention in treatment was 13.9 weeks for the network patients, reflecting a trend toward greater retention than the 10.7 weeks for control subjects.

The results of this study supported the feasibility of transferring the network technology into community-based settings with the potential for enhancing outcomes. Addiction counselors working in a typical outpatient rehabilitation setting were able to learn and then incorporate network therapy into their largely Twelve-Step-oriented treatment regimens without undue difficulty and with improved outcome.

32.5.4 Use of the Internet

We studied ways in which psychiatrists and other professionals could be offered training by a distance-learning method using the Internet, a medium that offers the advantage of not being fixed in either time or location. An advertisement was placed in *Psychiatric News*, the newspaper of the American Psychiatric Association, offering an Internet course combining network therapy with the use of naltrexone for the treatment of alcoholism.

The sequence of material presented on the Internet was divided into three didactic "sessions," followed by a set of questions, with a hypertext link to download relevant references and a certificate of completion. The course took about 2 hours for the student to complete. Our assessment was based on 679 sequential counts, representing 240 unique respondents who went beyond the introductory web page [21]. Of these respondents, 154 were psychiatrists, who responded positively to the course. A majority responded "a good deal" or "very much" (a score of 3 or 4 on a 4-point scale) to the following statements: "It helped me understand the management of alcoholism treatment" (56%); "It helped me learn to use family or friends in network treatment for alcoholism" (75%); and "It improved my ability to use naltrexone in treating alcoholism" (64%). The four studies described in this section support the use of network therapy as an effective treatment for addictive disorders. They are especially encouraging given the relative ease with which different types of clinicians were engaged and trained in the network approach. Because the approach combines a number of well-established clinical techniques that can be adapted to delivery in typical clinical settings, it is apparently suitable for use by general clinicians and addiction specialists.

32.5.5 Network Therapy in Buprenorphine Maintenance

Galanter et al. [19] evaluated the impact of NT relative to a control condition (medical management, MM) among 66 patients who were inducted on to buprenorphine for 16 weeks and then tapered to zero dose. Network Therapy resulted in a greater percentage of opioid-free urines than did MM (65% vs. 45%). By the end of treatment, NT patients were more likely to experience a positive outcome relative to secondary heroin use (50% vs. 23%). The use of NT in office practice may enhance the effectiveness of eliminating secondary heroin use during buprenorphine maintenance.

32.5.6 Use of Alcoholics Anonymous and Other Self-Help Groups

This approach involves the option for use of Twelve Step facilitation concomitant with Network Therapy. TS involves the following points:

1. Patients should be expected to go to meetings of AA or related groups at least two to three times, with follow-up discussion in therapy.
2. If patients have reservations about these meetings, the therapist should try to help them understand how to deal with those reservations. Issues such as social anxiety should be explored if they make a patient reluctant to participate. Generally, resistance to AA can be related to other areas of inhibition in a person's life, as well as to the denial of addiction.
3. As with other spiritually oriented involvements, it is important to explore the patient's orientation toward this issue.
4. Be prepared to listen.

32.6 Adaptations of Network Therapy Treatment

Rothenberg et al. [41] adapted NT and combined it with relapse prevention and a voucher reinforcement system in the treatment of opioid-dependent patients who were enrolled in a 6-month course of treatment with naltrexone referred to as behavioral naltrexone therapy (BNT). The NT component involved one significant other who could monitor adherence to naltrexone. In addition to the patient receiving vouchers for each day of abstinence and each pill taken, the network member was reinforced with a voucher for each pill recorded as monitored. The primary treatment outcome was retention in treatment. Patients who used methadone at baseline did more poorly than those using only heroin as demonstrated in the retention rates: 39% vs. 65%, and 0% vs. 31%, respectively, at 1 month and 6 months.

Copello et al. [10] combined elements of NT with social aspects of the community reinforcement approach and relapse prevention referred to as social behavior and network therapy (SBNT) in the treatment of persons with alcohol drinking problems. A number of social skills training strategies are incorporated into the treatment especially those involving social competence in relation to the development of positive social support for change in alcohol use. Every individual involved in treatment is considered a client in his or her own right and the person with alcohol problems is referred to as the focal client. The core element of the approach is mobilizing the support of the network even though this may involve network sessions that are conducted in the absence of the focal client. In their initial feasibility study with 33 clients, there were two cases in which sessions were held with network members in the absence of the focal client and in both cases reengagement of the focal client in treatment was achieved. Out of the 33 clients enrolled in the study, 23 formed a network with the mean number of network members = 1.82 and the mean number of network sessions = 5.24. In a multisite, randomized, controlled trial of 742 clients with alcohol problems, the UKATT Research Team [45] compared SBNT to motivational enhancement therapy (MET). Both treatment groups exhibited similar reductions in alcohol consumption and alcohol-related problems and improvement in mental functioning over a 12-month period. Attending more sessions was associated with a better outcome, and SBNT patients with greater motivation to change and those with more negative short-term expectancies were more likely to attend [12].

Additional studies involving the UKATT study sample were conducted assessing (1) cost-effectiveness [46], (2) client-treatment matching effects [47], (3) clients' perceptions of change in alcohol drinking behaviors [40], and drinking goal preference [1]. The UKATT team evaluated the cost-effectiveness of SBNT relative to motivational enhancement therapy. SBNT resulted in a fivefold cost savings in health, social, and criminal justice service expenditures and was similar to cost-effectiveness estimates obtained for motivational enhancement therapy. The UKATT Research Team [47] tested a priori hypotheses concerning client-treatment matching effects similar to those tested in Project MATCH. The findings were consistent with Project MATCH in that no hypothesized matching effects were significant. Orford et al. [40] interviewed a subset of clients ($n = 397$) who participated in this trial to assess their views concerning whether any positive changes in drink-

ing behavior had occurred and to what they attributed those changes. At 3 months after randomization to treatment, SBNT clients made more social attributions (e.g., involvement of others in supporting behavioral change) and MET clients made more motivational attributions (e.g., awareness of the consequences of drinking). Patients who initially stated a preference for abstinence showed a better outcome than those stating a preference for nonabstinence. This was true at both 3-month and 12-month follow-ups [1].

Copello et al. [11] adapted SBNT for persons presenting with drug problems. Of 31 clients enrolled in the study, 23 received SBNT and had outcomes data available at 3-month follow-up. Reductions in the amount of heroin used per day and increases in family cohesion and family satisfaction were documented. Open-ended interviews with clients, network members, and therapists were conducted in a qualitative investigation of respondents' perceptions of SBNT [49]. Major themes that emerged from analysis of the interview responses included the value of SBNT in (1) increasing network support for reducing drug use, (2) promoting open and honest communication between clients and network members about drug use, and (3) increasing network members' understanding of drugs and the focal person's behavior. Williamson et al. [49] suggest that these features of SBNT may be more prominent when the problem is one of illicit drug use than when the problem involves the alcohol use.

32.7 Principles of Network Treatment

32.7.1 Start a Network as Soon as Possible

1. It is important to see the alcohol or drug abuser promptly, because the window of opportunity for openness to treatment is generally brief. A week's delay can result in a person's reverting back to drunkenness or losing motivation.

2. If the person is married, engage the spouse early on, preferably at the time of the first

phone call. Point out that substance use disorder is a family problem. For most drugs, you can enlist the spouse in assuring that the patient arrives at your office with a day's sobriety.

3. In the initial interview, frame the exchange so that a good case is built for the grave consequences of the patient's substance use disorder, and do this before the patient can introduce his or her system of denial. That way you are not putting the spouse or other network members in the awkward position of having to contradict a close relation.

4. Then make clear that the patient needs to be abstinent, starting now. (A tapered detoxification may be necessary sometimes, as with depressant pills.)

5. When seeing a patient with alcohol use disorder for the first time, start the patient on disulfiram treatment as soon as possible, in the office if you can. Have the patient continue taking disulfiram under observation of a network member.

6. Start arranging for a network to be assembled at the first session, generally involving a number of the patient's family or close friends.

7. From the very first meeting you should consider how to ensure sobriety till the next meeting, and plan that with the network. Initially, their immediate company, a plan for daily AA attendance, and planned activities may all be necessary.

32.7.2 Manage the Network With Care

1. Include people who are close to the patient, have a long-standing relationship with the patient, and are trusted. Avoid members with substance problems, because they will let you down when you need their unbiased support. Avoid superiors and subordinates at work, because they have an overriding relationship with the patient independent of friendship.

2. Get a balanced group. Avoid a network composed solely of the parental generation, or of younger people, or of people of the opposite sex. Sometimes a nascent network selects itself for a consultation if the patient is reluctant to address his or her own problem. Such a group will later supportively engage the patient in the network, with your careful guidance.

3. Make sure that the mood of meetings is trusting and free of recrimination. Avoid letting the patient or the network members feel guilty or angry in meetings. Explain issues of conflict in terms of the problems presented by substance use disorder; do not get into personality conflicts.

4. The tone should be directive. That is to say, give explicit instructions to support and ensure abstinence. A feeling of teamwork should be promoted, with no psychologizing or impugning members' motives.

5. Meet as frequently as necessary to ensure abstinence, perhaps once a week for a month, every other week for the next few months, and every month or two by the end of a year.

6. The network should have no agenda other than to support the patient's abstinence. But as abstinence is stabilized, the network can help the patient plan for a new drug-free adaptation. It is not there to work on family relations or help other members with their problems, although it may do this indirectly.

32.7.3 Keep the Network's Agenda Focused

1. Maintaining abstinence. The patient and the network members should report at the outset of each session any exposure of the patient to alcohol and drugs. The patient and network members should be instructed on the nature of relapse and plan with the therapist how to sustain abstinence. Cues to conditioned drug-seeking should be examined.

2. Supporting the network's integrity. Everyone has a role in this. The patient is expected to make sure that network members keep their meeting appointments and stay involved with the treatment. The therapist sets meeting times and summons the network for any emergency,

such as relapse; the therapist does whatever is necessary to secure stability of the membership if the patient is having trouble doing so. Network members' responsibility is to attend network sessions, although they may be asked to undertake other supportive activity with the patient.

3. Securing future behavior. The therapist should combine any and all modalities necessary to ensure the patient's stability, such as a stable, drug-free residence; the avoidance of substance-abusing friends; attendance at Twelve-Step meetings; medications such as disulfiram or blocking agents; observed urinalysis; and ancillary psychiatric care. Written agreements may be handy, such as a mutually acceptable contingency contract with penalties for violation of understandings.

References

1. Adamson S, Heather N, Morton V, Raistrick D. Initial preference for drinking goal in the treatment of alcohol problems: II. Treatment outcomes. Alcohol Alcohol. 2010;45:136–42.
2. American Psychiatric Association. Diagnostic and statistical manual of mental disorders (DSM-IV-TR). 4th ed. Washington, D.C.: American Psychiatric Press; 1997.
3. American Psychiatric Association. Practice guidelines for the treatment of patients with substance use disorders: alcohol, cocaine, opioids. Am J Psychiatry. 1995;152:1.
4. Azrin NH, Sisson RW, Meyers R. Alcoholism treatment by disulfiram and community reinforcement therapy. J Behav Ther Psychiatry. 1982a;13:105–12.
5. Azrin NH, Sisson RW, Meyers R, Godley M. Alcoholism treatment by disulfiram and community reinforcement therapy. J Behav Therapy Exp Psychiatry. 1982b;13:105–12.
6. Beckman LJ, Amaro H. Personal and social difficulties faced by women and men entering alcoholism treatment. J Stud Alcohol. 1986;47:135–45.
7. Carroll KM. A cognitive-behavioral approach: treating cocaine addiction. Rockville: National Institute on Drug Abuse; 1998.
8. Carroll KM, Rounsaville BJ, Gordon LT, et al. Psychotherapy and pharmacotherapy for ambulatory cocaine abusers. Arch Gen Psychiatry. 1994;51:177–87.
9. Center for Substance Abuse Treatment. Substance abuse treatment and family therapy. Treatment Improvement Protocol (TIP) series, No. 39. DHHS Publication No. (SMA) 05-4006. Rockville: Substance Abuse and Mental Health Services Administration; 2004.
10. Copello A, Orford J, Hodgson R, et al. Social behaviour and network therapy: basic principles and early experiences. Addict Behav. 2002;27:345–66.
11. Copello A, Williamson E, Orford J, Day E. Implementing and evaluating social behaviour and network therapy in drug treatment practice in the UK: a feasibility study. Addict Behav. 2006;31:802–10.
12. Dale V, Coulton S, Godfrey C, et al. Exploring treatment attendance and its relationship to outcome in a randomized controlled trial of treatment for alcohol problems: secondary analysis of the UK alcohol treatment trial (UKATT). Alcohol Alcohol. 2011;46:592–9.
13. Daley DC, Baker S, Donanvan DM, et al. A combined group and individual 12-step facilitative intervention targeting stimulant abuse in the NIDA clinical trials network: STAGE-12. J Groups Addict Recover. 2011;6:228–44.
14. Fals-Stewart W, O'Farrell TJ, Feehan M, et al. Behavioral couples therapy versus individual-based treatment for male substance-abusing patients. J Subst Abuse Treat. 2000;18:249–54.
15. Fuller R, Branchey L, Brightwell DR, et al. Disulfiram treatment of alcoholism. A veterans administration cooperative study. JAMA. 1986;256:1449–55.
16. Galanter M. Cognitive labeling: psychotherapy for alcohol and drug abuse: an approach based on learning theory. J Psychiatr Treat Eval. 1983;5:551–6.
17. Galanter M. Network therapy for addiction: a model for office practice. Am J Psychiatry. 1993a;150:28–36.
18. Galanter M. Network therapy for substance abuse: a clinical trial. Psychotherapy. 1993b;30:251–8.
19. Galanter M, Dermatis H, Glickman L, et al. Network therapy: decreased secondary opioid use during buprenorphine maintenance. J Subst Abuse Treat. 2004;26:313–8.
20. Galanter M, Dermatis H, Keller D, et al. Network therapy for cocaine abuse: use of family and peer supports. Am J Addict. 2002;11:161–6.
21. Galanter M, Keller DS, Dermatis H. Using the internet for clinical training: a course on network therapy. Psychiatr Serv. 1997;48:999. Available at: http://mednyu/substanceabuse/course.
22. Glazer SS, Galanter M, Megwinoff O, et al. The role of therapeutic alliance in network therapy: a family and peer support-based treatment for cocaine abuse. Subst Abuse. 2003;24(2):93–100.
23. Gitlow SE, Peyser HS, editors. Alcoholism: a practical treatment guide. New York: Grune & Stratton; 1980.
24. Helzer JE, Robins LN, Taylor JR, et al. The extent of long-term drinking among alcoholics discharged from medical and psychiatric facilities. N Engl J Med. 1985;312:1678–82.
25. Higgins ST, Budney AJ, Bickel WK, et al. Achieving cocaine abstinence with a behavioral approach. Am J Psychiatry. 1993;150:763–9.

26. Jellinek EM. The disease concept of alcoholism. Hillhouse: New Haven; 1963.

27. Johnson VE. Intervention: how to help someone who doesn't want help. Minneapolis: Johnson Institute; 1986.

28. Keller D, Galanter M, Dermatis H. Technology transfer of network therapy to community-based addiction counselors. J Subst Abuse Treat. 1999;16:183–9.

29. Keller D, Galanter M, Weinberg S. Validation of a scale for network therapy: a technique for systematic use of peer and family support in addiction treatment. Am J Drug Alcohol Abuse. 1997;23:115–27.

30. Khantzian EJ. The primary care therapist and patient needs in substance abuse treatment. Am J Drug Alcohol Abuse. 1988;14:159–67.

31. Kirby KC, Marlowe DB, Festinger DS, et al. Community reinforcement training for family and significant others of drug abusers: a unilateral intervention to increase treatment entry of drug users. Drug Alcohol Depend. 1999;56:85–96.

32. Landau J, Stanton DM, Brinkman-Sull D, et al. Outcomes with the ARISE approach to engaging reluctant drug- and alcohol-dependent individuals in treatment. Am J Drug Alcohol Abuse. 2004;30(4):711–48.

33. McCrady BS, Stout R, Noel N, et al. Effectiveness of three types of spouse-involved behavioral alcoholism treatment. Br J Addict. 1991;86:1415–24.

34. Mee-Lee D, Gastfriend DR. Patient placement criteria, Chapter 8. In: Galanter M, Kleber HD, Brady KT, editors. Textbook of substance abuse treatment. 5th ed. Washington, D.C.: American Psychiatric Publishing; 2015. p. 111–28.

35. Meyers RJ, Miller WR, Smith JE, Tonigan JS. A randomized trial of two methods for engaging treatment-refusing drug users through concerned significant others. J Consult Clin Psychol. 2002;70:1182–5.

36. Meyers RJ, Smith JE, Lash DN. The community reinforcement approach. Recent Dev Alcohol. 2003;16:183–95.

37. Miller WF, Rollnick S. Motivational interviewing: helping people change (applications of motivational interviewing). 3rd ed. New York: Guildford Publications; 2013.

38. Morgenstern J, Longabaugh R. Cognitive-behavioral treatment for alcohol dependence: a review of the evidence for its hypothesized mechanisms of action. Addiction. 2000;95:1475–90.

39. O'Farrell TJ. Marital therapy in the treatment of alcoholism. In: Jacobson NS, Gurman AS, editors. Clinical handbook of marital therapy. New York: Guilford Press; 1986. p. 513–35.

40. Orford J, Hodgson R, Copello A, et al. To what factors do clients attribute change? Content analysis of follow-up interview with clients of the UK alcohol treatment trial. J Subst Abuse Treat. 2009;36:49–58.

41. Rothenberg JL, Sullivan MA, Church SH, et al. Behavioral naltrexone therapy: an integrated treatment for opiate dependence. J Subst Abuse Treat. 2002;23:351–60.

42. SAMHSA's National registry of evidence-based programs and practices. Network Therapy Review. Available at: http://www.nrepp.samhsa.gov/porgram-fulldetails.asp?PROGRAM_ID=61. Review conducted Feb 2007.

43. Speck R. Psychotherapy of the social network of a schizophrenic family. Fam Process. 1967;6:208.

44. Stephens RS, Babor TF, Kadden R, et al. The marijuana treatment project: rationale, design, and participant characteristics. Addiction. 2002;94:109–24.

45. UKATT Research Team. Cost effectiveness of treatment for alcohol problems: findings of the randomised UK alcohol treatment trial (UKATT). BMJ. 2005a;331:544–9.

46. UKATT Research Team. Effectiveness of treatment for alcohol problems: findings of the randomised UK alcohol treatment trial (UKATT). BMJ. 2005b;331:541–3.

47. UKATT Research Team. UK alcohol treatment trial: client-treatment matching effects. Addiction. 2008;103:228–38.

48. Wikler A. Dynamics of drug dependence: implications of a conditioning theory for research and treatment. Arch Gen Psychiatry. 1973;28:611–6.

49. Williamson E, Smith M, Orford J, et al. Social behavior and network therapy for drug problems: evidence of benefits and challenges. Addict Disord Treat. 2007;6:167–79.

50. Zywiak WH, Wirtz PW. Decomposing the relationships between pretreatment social network characteristics and alcohol treatment outcome. J Stud Alcohol. 2002;63(1):114–21.

CRA and CRAFT: Behavioral Treatments for Both Motivated and Unmotivated Substance-Abusing Individuals and Their Family Members

33

Hendrik G. Roozen and Jane Ellen Smith

Contents

Abstract

The Community Reinforcement Approach (CRA) is a behavioral treatment for individuals with substance-use problems. It is predicated upon the belief that a non-drinking/non-using lifestyle must be experienced by individuals as rewarding in order for them to choose it consistently over substance use. As part of CRA, the client's "community" (e.g., family, friends, colleagues, organizations, work) is explored to find new areas of potential reinforcement that can compete with substance use. CRA therapists work with clients to decide on which goals they want to pursue in life, and they then teach these clients the skills required to achieve these goals. An adaptation of CRA is the Adolescent Community Reinforcement Approach (A-CRA), which is geared specifically toward the treatment of adolescents, young adults, and their parents or caregivers. Community Reinforcement and Family Training (CRAFT) is a treatment for the family members or close friends (Concerned Significant Others, CSOs) of unmotivated, treatment-refusing substance abusers (Identified Patients, IPs). CRAFT therapists work with CSOs in an attempt to change the home environment of the unmotivated IPs such that a healthy and enjoyable lifestyle is supported over one dominated by substance use. CRAFT goals include getting IPs to seek treatment and reducing IP substance use, and also having CSOs increase

H. G. Roozen
University of New Mexico, Albuquerque, NM, USA

J. E. Smith (✉)
Department of Psychology, University of New Mexico, Albuquerque, NM, USA
e-mail: janellen@unm.edu

© Springer Nature Switzerland AG 2021
N. el-Guebaly et al. (eds.), *Textbook of Addiction Treatment*,
https://doi.org/10.1007/978-3-030-36391-8_33

their own happiness regardless. CRA, A-CRA, and CRAFT have solid empirical support, and each has been used successfully with diverse populations and various drugs of choice.

33.1 Introduction

The Community Reinforcement Approach (CRA) is built upon the Skinnerian principles of behavioral modification. The rationale is that desired behaviors are considered malleable by their consequences and will most likely occur when they are systematically reinforced. Skinner's colleague, Nathan Azrin, tested and applied this perspective in clinical practice to treat various mental health problems, including addictions [7, 11, 44]. Given the scientific, theoretically driven background of operant conditioning, it is not surprising that CRA has proven to be efficacious in routine clinical practice. This same operant behavioral foundation has been considered the lynchpin of the Token Economy [5] and Contingency Management (CM) [42].

Azrin believed that individuals' physical environment (their "community"), including their family, work, recreational activities, and social life, could be rearranged such that they received more powerful reinforcement from the community for sober behavior versus substance-using behavior. As part of this strategy, CRA assists clients to sample enjoyable pro-social activities that are unrelated to alcohol and/or drugs. Importantly, experimental research on instrumental learning has shown that new learning is context dependent [16, 17]. Thus, behavioral modifications to prevent relapse should eventually take place in clients' own communities. Furthermore, an important aspect of CRA is that it teaches clients new skills to make their reinforcers more accessible, and to help them to cope with obstacles and potential high-risk situations. As such, CRA involves a variety of techniques, including the training of communication skills, alcohol and/or drugs refusal skills, problem solving, behavioral partner relationship therapy, procedures to support medication compliance, and career counsel-

ing for the unemployed. CRA makes extensive use of modeling, role-playing, and shaping.

Two offshoots of CRA, the Adolescent Community Reinforcement Approach (A-CRA) and Community Reinforcement and Family Training (CRAFT) were created to prioritize family members or even target them directly by unilateral therapy (i.e., CRAFT). These will be discussed in this chapter as well.

33.2 Understanding and Using CRA, A-CRA, and CRAFT

33.2.1 CRA Procedures

33.2.1.1 CRA Functional Analyses

One of the first CRA procedures conducted by a clinician is the functional analysis (FA) of substance-using behavior. This semi-structured interview (see [58]) allows the clinician *and* the client to clearly see the events that set the stage for a common substance-use episode, as well as the positive and negative consequences that follow. The clinician first works with the client to identify external (people, places, times) and internal (thoughts, feelings) triggers. This information is later used to determine how to alter or effectively cope with triggers that have led to substance use in the past. The second part of the FA involves the clinician gathering more information about how the substance of choice is used, such as how much is consumed and over what period of time. These details can be useful in quantitatively gauging progress as therapy proceeds.

Finally, the clinician uses the FA to explore both the positive and negative consequences associated with substance use. Discussing the positive consequences is critical, because they represent the motives that sustain the substance use. For example, a client may state that he enjoys drinking because it allows him to avoid dealing with all his negative thoughts about work and finances. Once these drinking-related "rewards" (positive consequences) are identified, the clinician can help the client generate non-drinking alternatives either for avoiding the negative thoughts, or for solving the work and finance problems themselves. The negative consequences of substance use are broken down into multiple domains, such as interpersonal, physical, emotional, legal, job, and financial.

The CRA program's second type of FA is for healthy, pro-social behaviors (e.g., going for a walk with a friend). The objective is to work with the client to *increase* these behaviors so that they can compete with substance use. A better understanding of the antecedents and consequences surrounding these behaviors helps the clinician see why a pro-social behavior is sometimes chosen over a substance-using one (and vice versa) and identify possible mechanisms for getting the client to select the healthy alternative more often.

33.2.1.2 Sobriety Sampling

Sobriety sampling is a method for encouraging clients to "sample" a time-limited period of sobriety. A "trial period" of sobriety is experienced by clients as more attainable than a demand for a life-long commitment to abstinence. Sobriety sampling is used regardless of whether the final treatment goal is abstinence, moderation, or even harm reduction. If the goal is abstinence, small, manageable periods of sobriety are linked together over time. If the client hopes to become a moderate drinker/substance user, the clinician still asks for the client to start treatment by sampling a period of sobriety. Some of the benefits of sobriety sampling, which are discussed with the client, include providing an opportunity to experiment with new coping strategies, and increasing self-efficacy through goal attainment.

Once the client has agreed to sample sobriety, the length of the trial period must be negotiated. The client's motivators for abstinence are linked to the goal. For example, a clinician might state, "You said that your next review at your job is 6 weeks away, and that your boss has already expressed some concern about your work performance. I bet if you were totally sober for the next 6 weeks your behavior at work would improve, and it would be obvious to your boss. That might be a good reason to shoot for 6 weeks of sobriety. What do you think?" If the client is unwilling or

feels unable to agree to the suggested period of sobriety, the clinician will negotiate with the client to reach a mutually agreed-upon goal.

The final part of sobriety sampling entails setting up a plan such that the client can actively work to achieve the goal. Using information collected during the FA for substance use, the client is encouraged to identify alternatives to substance use and to develop plans for handling common triggers. It is often helpful to identify and problem solve any upcoming high-risk situation and to develop specific backup plans.

33.2.1.3 CRA Treatment Plan: Happiness Scale and Goals of Counseling

The CRA treatment plan is built around the Happiness Scale and the Goals of Counseling forms. The Happiness Scale is a multi-item questionnaire that asks clients to rate their happiness on a 10-point scale (where 10 indicates "completely happy") in each of the following areas: substance use, job or educational progress, money management, social life, personal habits, marriage/family relationships, legal issues, emotional life, communication, spirituality, and general happiness (see [58]). Information regarding the client's happiness in each of these categories helps set the stage for developing the goals of treatment. For example, the clinician might say, "I see that you've rated your 'personal habits' a '4.' What would have to change in order for you to be able to rate 'personal habits' a '5' or '6'?" The Happiness Scale also can be readministered throughout therapy to track progress in specific domains.

The same domains from the Happiness Scale are listed on the Goals of Counseling form, where the clinician works with the client to set goals that are positive (what the client *wants* as opposed to what he/she does not want anymore), specific, measurable, realistic, and under the client's control. In addition to setting specific goals, the clinician and client work together to identify the necessary steps needed to accomplish each goal. A representative goal in the personal habits area might be to eat at least two fruits and vegetables every day. The initial steps toward attaining that goal might be to identify a conveniently located store that carries good fruits/vegetables, and to sample a new fruit and vegetable in the upcoming week. These weekly steps toward a goal are essentially the homework assignment. Importantly, the clinician checks on progress toward completing the homework weekly and discusses any barriers that have appeared.

Establishing and working on goals to improve various areas of the client's life is fundamental to the CRA approach, given that the overall objective is to increase sources of substance-free reinforcement for the client. Many of these goals, and the strategies (steps) for attaining them, require specific behavioral skills training. The CRA program offers skills training in such areas as communication, problem solving, and drink/drug refusal.

33.2.1.4 Positive Communication Skills

CRA emphasizes the importance of positive communication training, in part because many individuals who abuse substances report that problematic interactions serve as relapse triggers. Furthermore, effective communication paves the way for the successful implementation of goal-related tasks, such as interviewing for jobs, asking teachers for extra help, and talking with a partner about relationship struggles. CRA clinicians present the rationale for focusing on communication training, and then offer several communication guidelines for starting a difficult conversation (see full list in [58]): (1) label your feeling: "I feel ___"?, (2) give an understanding statement, (3) take partial responsibility, and (4) offer to help. Assume, for example, that an adolescent male who has been grounded for 4 weeks would like to attend a school social event. The clinician would work with the client to develop the beginning of a conversation with his mother that sounded somewhat similar to: "Mom, I feel a bit disappointed (*label your feeling*), but can totally see why you'd want me to finish out this last week of being grounded (*understanding statement*). I know I screwed up, and that's what got me grounded in the first place (*partial respon-*

sibility statement). But I haven't gotten into any trouble the last 3 weeks. Is there anything else I could do to make up for cutting the full 4 weeks a few days short in order to attend the school event?" (*offer to help*).

Clients report that when they start a conversation with these communication components, they typically are met with less defensiveness from the listener. The message being conveyed is that more than one person contributes to interpersonal problems, and the communicator is willing to take an active role in improving the situation. Clinicians teach these skills by providing relevant examples and engaging the client in role-plays.

33.2.1.5 Problem-Solving Skills

Many individuals who abuse substances report that they resort to alcohol or drugs as their strategy for dealing with problems that seem unsolvable (or that at least generate considerable stress). CRA's problem-solving skills training module, which is based on the work by D'Zurilla and Goldfried [20], outlines seven main steps: (1) narrowly define the problem, (2) generate potential solutions (brainstorm), (3) eliminate undesired suggestions, (4) select one potential solution, (5) generate possible obstacles, (6) address these obstacles, and (7) assign the specific task (i.e., the homework). As with all homework assignments, the clinician carefully evaluates the outcome of the task at the start of the next therapy session.

This problem-solving procedure allows clients to break down problems into manageable steps, to think creatively about possible solutions, and to realistically assess the likelihood that the proposed solution will work. Once clients have put their proposed solution into action, they are taught to critically evaluate the outcome. If the proposed solution did not meet their needs, they are encouraged either to modify the attempted solution or to select a different solution generated during step #2. Some of the common types of problems for which this exercise is conducted include finding new non-drinking friends, developing healthy sleep routines, dealing with cravings, and managing stress.

33.2.1.6 Drink and Drug Refusal Skills

CRA encourages clients to create social environments that are supportive of sobriety, and nonetheless clients will find themselves periodically in situations that require them to assertively refuse offers of alcohol or drugs. CRA's drink/drug refusal skills training starts with helping clients anticipate and prepare for high-risk situations, and identifying supportive individuals who can be available in the event that a client is struggling in one of these situations. Information gathered during the FA can be extremely useful when helping the client identify personally relevant high-risk situations. Assertive communication skills are then taught and practiced with the client in role-plays.

Oftentimes clients are overly confident that they will be able to walk into these situations and "simply not drink" (and not use other substances). Despite this confidence, refusal is often much more difficult than anticipated, and thus clients are encouraged to practice refusing offers assertively. Clients first are asked to identify verbal responses or behaviors that have helped them successfully reject offers of substances in the past. These suggestions are supplemented with additional ideas, such as: (1) simply saying "no, thanks" without feeling guilty, (2) using appropriate body language (good eye contact, a firm stance, etc.), (3) suggesting alternatives ("No, thanks, but I'll take a coffee"), (4) changing the subject ("Did you see that game last night? Unbelievable!"), (5) directly addressing the aggressor about the issue if needed ("I'm definitely not interested in smoking. Why is it important to *you* that I smoke?"), and (6) leaving the situation. Clients are asked to generate their own assertive response style and are coached in its implementation.

33.2.1.7 Job-Finding Skills

An important component of reinforcement for many individuals is a job that they value. Meaningful employment can compete with time otherwise left idle for substance use, and can provide a boost to self-esteem, enjoyable social relationships, and of course—money. Relying on the work outlined by Azrin and Besalel in their Job Club Counselor's Manual [8], CRA offers a step-by-step approach to obtaining a satisfying job and keeping it. The procedure begins by asking clients to carefully consider the types of jobs for which they are best suited, such as ones that are unlikely to contribute to relapse. A system is established for tracking contacts with potential employers, and clients are assisted with developing resumes and completing job applications in a manner that highlights their strengths. Role-plays are conducted to provide practice in calling potential employers and going on job interviews. With respect to keeping a job, clinicians help clients anticipate difficult work situations based on previous job problems, and problem-solving skills are used to generate potential solutions.

33.2.1.8 Social/Recreational Counseling

Prior to treatment, clients' social and recreational environments are strongly associated with substance use, and consequently identifying enjoyable substance-free social activities often is a difficult task. Clinicians ideally should attempt to identify at least some activities that occur during high-risk times (e.g., weekends, evenings) and thereby directly compete with substance use. CRA offers several methods for developing ideas and specific plans for increasing healthy social activities, including the use of problem solving, or setting goals and strategies as part of the Goals of Counseling procedure. Additionally, the FA for pro-social, healthy behaviors (see Sect. 33.2.1.1) can be conducted. Instruments such as the Pleasant Activities List (PAL; [72]) or Social Circle [93] can be employed as well. Once an activity is identified, a homework assignment is made to sample the activity, and, as usual, potential barriers (e.g., transportation, money, fear of rejection) are discussed.

Periodically clinicians are skeptical about a client following through and sampling a new activity despite being motivated to do so. In these cases, clinicians utilize Systematic Encouragement to increase the likelihood that the client will successfully complete that homework assignment in the upcoming week. Systematic Encouragement involves helping the client take the first step toward engaging in the new activity before leaving the session. For example, assume a client is interested in learning how to do woodworking, but appears unlikely to make any progress toward pursuing that goal without assistance. The clinician would help the client search for relevant information about woodworking courses or workshops online, and then would ask the client to register right in the session. Potential obstacles would be addressed in the process, such as whether the client had sufficient money for the course, and if transportation was available. The clinician would start the next session by reviewing the client's woodworking assignment, primarily to determine whether the experience had been enjoyable.

33.2.1.9 Relapse Prevention

CRA has multiple procedures that can be used to address relapses. For example, the FA can be readministered, but with a focus on the specific relapse episode. The clinician takes a solution-oriented approach to highlighting what triggered the relapse and to identifying alternatives to substance use in that particular situation. CRA clinicians also can borrow from the relapse literature more generally by drawing and labeling a behavioral "chain" to illustrate the events that led to the relapse. Clients are shown how a number of small and seemingly unrelated decisions throughout the day led them down the path to a relapse. Clinicians work with the clients to help them generate different decisions at multiple points along the chain—decisions that ultimately would not result in a relapse. Finally, CRA relapse prevention may include the Early Warning System, which entails clients setting up a plan for enlisting the support of a concerned family member or friend in the event that a relapse appears imminent.

33.2.1.10 Medication Monitoring

CRA's medication monitoring procedure is used with clients who have difficulty taking their prescribed medication. The procedure originally was developed for clients who were taking disulfiram (Antabuse), a medication that causes individuals to become very ill if they ingest alcohol. This "deterrent" to drinking is sometimes introduced to clients who repeatedly are unsuccessful at achieving even short periods of abstinence or who face serious consequences if they drink. But in order for disulfiram to be effective, it must be taken several days per week, and therefore, it is important to incorporate a medication monitoring component. The "monitor," a concerned individual who has daily contact with the client, attends a session with the client in order to learn positive communication skills for administering the disulfiram. For example, the monitor rehearses a conversation such as, "I appreciate you taking your pill today. This shows how hard you're trying, and how much you care about our family." In addition to teaching the monitor to express support and appreciation for the client's efforts, a plan is developed (with the client's consent) regarding the steps to take if the client refuses to take his or her medication (e.g., call the therapist). Although initially introduced to monitor disulfiram administration, more recently the medication monitoring procedure has been used to monitor a variety of other kinds of medication, such as for attention deficit hyperactivity disorder (ADHD), bipolar disorder, and depression.

33.2.1.11 Relationship Therapy

Improving interactions with a romantic partner can be another powerful source of reinforcement. CRA's relationship therapy highlights the importance of having communication and problem-solving skills, and teaches couples how to request and negotiate reasonable goals. The couple begins by completing the Relationship Happiness Scale, a tool similar to the original Happiness Scale. However, each individual rates his/her happiness with the *partner* on a 10-point scale across ten domains: household responsibilities, raising the children, social activities, money management, communication, sex and affection, job or school, emotional support, partner's independence, and general happiness. Each partner is asked to write down what he/she would like the partner to do in several of the ten domains while utilizing the guidelines for specifying goals and strategies (see Sect. 33.2.1.3), including being positive, specific, and using measurable terms.

They then are taught to use positive communication skills to make the request verbally. Homework assignments are made to tackle the negotiated goals. As part of the "Daily Reminder to be Nice" exercise, each partner commits to increasing at least one of seven partner-pleasing behaviors (e.g., expressing appreciation, giving a pleasant surprise) on a daily basis in an effort to reinstate positive behaviors that were more frequent at the beginning of the relationship. In subsequent sessions, the partners report on any barriers to completing their goals for the week and identify future goals.

33.2.2 CRA Scientific Support

For almost half a century, CRA has been accruing evidence of its efficacy and effectiveness in treating alcohol and drug problems. It is even viewed as one of the earliest evidence-based treatment methods [64]. The seminal CRA studies were conducted with inpatients on alcohol wards [7, 44]. In both studies, CRA did significantly better than standard treatment, which at the time was participation in a hospital's Alcoholics Anonymous program. Specifically, at 6-month follow-up, CRA participants had less drinking days and institutionalization and more days working compared to those in standard treatment. The second of these studies introduced several new procedures to the original CRA protocol, most notably a disulfiram (Antabuse) compliance monitoring program [7].

The third CRA study was the first one to use an outpatient population of problem drinkers [9]. The researchers contrasted three treatments: traditional (12-step) treatment with a disulfiram prescription, traditional treatment with the disulfiram compliance program, and CRA with the disulfiram compliance program. The compliance program included not only monitoring of the daily disulfiram use by a significant other (e.g., a spouse), but also training in positive communication skills. As expected, the conditions that included the disulfiram compliance component had the highest abstinence rates, with the CRA program outperforming the traditional program overall at 6 months.

A much larger study ($N = 237$) with an ethnically diverse population was conducted, which extended the design of the first outpatient study by examining whether one's willingness to take disulfiram affected the findings [62]. Although the study revealed less robust results, CRA still showed an advantage over traditional treatment on several outcome measures. The CRA program was modified in another study to make it applicable to a day treatment program for homeless alcohol-dependent individuals [87]. As predicted, CRA (conducted in groups) was proven to be more effective than the standard treatment offered at that particular homeless shelter in terms of drinking outcomes.

Although originally developed as a treatment for individuals with alcohol problems, CRA has proven to be promising for other types of substance use, including cocaine [6], tobacco [71], and opioids (e.g., [1, 12, 70]). Bickel and colleagues determined that a computerized version of CRA for opioid-dependent individuals that were on buprenorphine maintenance did as well as a therapist-delivered version of CRA, both of which did significantly better than standard treatment [13].

One hallmark of CRA is the clinical application of the CRA Happiness Scale (CRA-HS; [44, 58]). As noted, it serves as a compass for tracking satisfaction with life across multiple domains, and can be used to evaluate treatment outcome by repeatedly assessing changes that occur during treatment. It also is used as the basis for setting treatment goals. The shared decision-making involved in this process was already launched in the seminal studies and nowadays is considered critical in the recovery movement [4]. In a recent Dutch CRA study [73], it was shown that patients with high baseline levels of psychiatric symptoms reported relatively lower baseline and follow-up scores on the CRA-HS than patients with low initial levels of psychiatric symptoms. Interestingly, although patients with high levels of psychiatric symptoms on admission were relatively disadvantaged in terms of CRA-HS outcomes both at pre- and post-measurement, they showed a stronger and more remarkable improvement on this measure during the course of treatment [73].

Originally, the CRA-HS was based on the 10-item Marital Happiness Scale [10]. This scale was modified by Azrin [7] in order to be applicable to individual clients, and was coined the CRA-HS. About 20 years later, Meyers and Smith [58] published a version that contained a few modified life domains (see, [60], p 383). This scale was further expanded in the Netherlands by including several new items (see [77]), yet recent psychometric work in the Netherlands reduced the measure to 12 "core" items (with 6 additional optional items and 1 open-ended item; [15]). The newest studies also have confirmed the strong psychometric properties of the CRA-HS, and have focused on measurement invariance in cross-cultural non-clinical populations [75] and external validity in a clinical population [46].

33.2.2.1 CRA and Contingency Management

Contingency Management (CM), a behavioral program for substance-abusing individuals, has been among the highest-ranked treatments in several meta-analyses [25, 52, 68]. To date, almost 500 empirical CM studies have been conducted, with a large majority of them demonstrating the efficacy of CM [21]. CM has been extensively applied in concert with CRA [22]. For cocaine-dependent clients treated with CRA, the addition of CM was found to yield better results in Spain [26, 42, 81, 82, 83]. Even the efficacy of CRA and CM was shown in pregnant women or women with young children [80]. Over the years a series of studies that have examined cocaine-dependent individuals treated with a combination of CRA and CM (vouchers) for clean urines has found highly favorable results when contrasted with standard treatment (e.g., [27]; see [40]).

In an effort to identify patterns among CRA study results, Roozen and colleagues conducted a systematic review of 11 randomized controlled trials. They discovered strong evidence that CRA with vouchers was more effective than usual care in achieving cocaine abstinence and more effective than CRA alone. However, there was evidence that the effect of the vouchers dissipated over time after their discontinuation [69].

Interestingly, one study clearly determined that the addition of CRA to CM improved alcohol and employment outcomes compared to vouchers alone in cocaine-addicted individuals [41].

33.2.2.2 International Considerations

CRA has gained international recognition in more recent years. Besides the USA, the Netherlands, and Spain, a pilot study of CRA with substance-abusing individuals in Mexico detected highly promising findings [92]. Furthermore, the National Drugs Strategy of Ireland has acknowledged CRA as an effective evidence-based approach that can be used as an adjunct to services delivered within the rehabilitation pillar, and Germany has already sponsored a CRA conference. In Australia, an Aboriginal version of CRA has been created [78]. The CRA trainers' manual, "Clinical Guide to Alcohol Treatment: The Community Reinforcement Approach" [58], has been translated into German, Japanese, and Dutch. Based on its strong scientific support, CRA has been increasingly spread in Europe during the last decade. Groups have been trained in Ireland, Wales, Scotland, Sweden, Japan, Germany, and the Netherlands.

In the Netherlands, CRA is established as a mainstream treatment delivery system, whereby more than 2000 health professionals in addiction care and (forensic) psychiatry have been trained in CRA. Both outpatient and inpatient teams have successfully implemented CRA within the forensic psychiatry system [38]. Furthermore, several Dutch addiction treatment institutes are actively participating in trajectories to improve CRA treatment fidelity by having their clinicians' CRA sessions digitally recorded and then rated by CRA supervisors using a CRA coding system. Thus far at least 100 therapists have been successfully certified using this process. To further ensure treatment fidelity, a Dutch CRA therapist manual was developed, which describes the clinical CRA procedures in detail [77]. This manual has been translated into Japanese recently (2019). In summary, although the dissemination of CRA is moving forward rapidly in several countries, the number of European studies that report on outcomes of CRA-based treatment programs fall short and efforts are needed to increase future research output.

33.2.3 A-CRA Procedures

33.2.3.1 Additional or Modified Procedures

When the substance-using client is an adolescent, the adolescent version of CRA (A-CRA) can be used (see [31, 36]). A-CRA comprises both an extension and adaption of CRA. For the most part this entails relying on age-modified questionnaires, and additional procedures such as anger management and the inclusion of sessions for the caregivers (e.g., parents, grandparents), both alone and with the adolescent client.

The sessions with just the caregiver(s) focus on discussing basic parenting practices that support the adolescent's sobriety, and teaching CRA communication and problem-solving skills. The "family" sessions that include the adolescent are similar in structure to the relationship therapy sessions, in that they emphasize the negotiation of goals and the establishment of clear strategies for obtaining the goals.

33.2.4 A-CRA Scientific Support

Multiple randomized clinical trials of A-CRA have been published in the past two decades. A-CRA was one of the treatments in the national Cannabis Youth Treatment Study. Similar to other treatments, A-CRA demonstrated significant pre–post improvements in days of abstinence and days in recovery (i.e., no substance-use problems and not institutionalized) *and* was the most cost-effective treatment [23]. Slesnick et al. [85] showed that A-CRA was more effective than usual care for homeless adolescents who used drugs. Specifically, the Community Reinforcement program resulted in less substance abuse (37% vs. 17% decrease), less depression (40% vs. 23%), and more increased social reliance (58% vs. 13%) than usual care. Moreover, early results from a multi-site study with over 2000

adolescents showed that A-CRA was equally effective across ethnic groups [30].

Additional randomized clinical trials have shown A-CRA to be effective for youth with juvenile justice involvement [39] and as a continuing care approach for adolescents after residential treatment [32, 33]. Secondary evaluation studies suggest that A-CRA shows potential to be an effective transdiagnostic treatment for adolescents with co-occurring psychiatric disorders [35], adolescents with forensic problems [45], and youth with opioid use problems [37].

Similar to adult CRA, clinicians decide which A-CRA procedures to use on the basis of individual client needs. Consequently, some clients may receive certain procedures multiple times (e.g., problem solving or communication skills) but never receive other procedures (e.g., anger management; [28]). Importantly, receiving ten or more unique procedures during a treatment episode has been found to maximize client outcomes [29]. The ratings of therapist fidelity have been based on an A-CRA coding manual [89] that used specific, behaviorally anchored items [88]. Using this rating system it was determined that the more competent the therapist was in delivering A-CRA, the better the adolescent did in treatment [18]. Also, a paper is available that addresses successful A-CRA dissemination and implementation in a national study [34].

33.2.4.1 International Considerations

In the USA, the practice of A-CRA has become mainstream, as it is offered in almost 100 different locations throughout the USA. Several A-CRA books [36] and manuals [31] have become available, and they have been translated into Portuguese and Dutch.

33.2.5 CRAFT Procedures

33.2.5.1 Enhancement of the Concerned Significant Other's Motivation

CRAFT does not work directly with the individual with the substance-use problem (Identified

Patient; IP), but with a concerned significant other (CSO). CRAFT teaches the CSO new behaviors and strategies to try out at home with the IP, with the overall goal of getting this treatment-refusing individual to seek treatment. CSOs' motivation to fully engage in CRAFT is enhanced when they are told that their wealth of knowledge about the IP's substance use, and their degree of contact with the IP, allows CSOs to make powerful changes in their IP's environment. The initial part of this foundational session begins by asking CSOs to describe the negative consequences they and their IP have experienced as a result of the substance use. Any past successful attempts to influence the IP's behavior are reviewed. Clinicians establish positive expectancies by reporting that CRAFT is highly effective in helping IPs engage in treatment (nearly seven out of ten times) and in decreasing the distress experienced by the CSO regardless of whether the IP enters treatment. Additionally, clinicians emphasize that CRAFT is effective across a wide variety of CSO–IP relationships (e.g., spouse, friend, parent), ethnicities, and substances. The clinician then outlines CRAFT's three main goals: (1) decrease the IP's substance use, (2) get the IP to enter treatment, and (3) increase the CSO's happiness (see [86]).

33.2.5.2 Functional Analysis of IP's Substance-Using Behavior

A functional analysis (FA) quite similar to the one completed with the substance-using individual during CRA is completed as part of CRAFT as well, but with the *CSO* providing the information about the IP. A common using episode is identified, and both the triggers and consequences (positive and negative) of the use are delineated. The CSO's challenge is to influence/change the IP's environment so that the IP responds in a healthier manner to triggers. Importantly, this new IP behavior must allow the IP to experience some of the positive consequences (and none of the negative consequences) that have been associated with substance use, or it will not be maintained over time. For example, assume the IP has gotten into a routine of starting to drink as soon as she arrives home from work, and then continuing this

throughout the dinner preparation and well into the evening. Her partner (CSO) believes that the IP has resorted to alcohol as a way to alleviate stress. The CSO could develop a plan to help the IP deal with her stress in healthier ways, such as by hooking up a sound system in the kitchen for her so that she can listen to soothing music (a reinforcer for the IP) while cooking. Another option would be for the CSO to urge the IP to meet with her friend for a walk right after work, and then for the CSO to join the IP in the kitchen to prepare dinner together (like they used to enjoy doing). Ideally, the exercise and the conversation during the walk would alleviate some of the IP's stress, and would help the IP reestablish connections with non-drinking friends. As far as the CSO joining the IP in the kitchen, it would be necessary to establish that this still would be viewed by the IP as a rewarding activity.

As CSOs start attempting these "homework" assignments, it is worthwhile for CRAFT clinicians to help CSOs understand that simply making one change in behavior will not suddenly solve the IP's substance-use problem. Instead, CSOs typically need to introduce a number of changes (as outlined in the remaining CRAFT procedures below) before their IP decides to seek treatment.

33.2.5.3 Domestic Violence Precautions

CRAFT teaches CSOs how to modify their own behavior such that only substance-free IP behaviors are "rewarded," and how to allow IPs to experience the natural negative consequences of their substance use (see Sect. 33.2.5.6). However, before CSOs attempt to modify any behavior at home, domestic violence precautions must be discussed. IPs routinely are *not* pleased with these CSO behavior changes, and a high correlation already exists between domestic violence and substance use [2]. Thus, CRAFT clinicians always assess the risk for domestic violence, either through standard assessment instruments, or through a functional analysis for domestic violence (see [86]). If any doubt remains regarding whether a CSO will be safe while participating in CRAFT, the CSO will be referred to another program.

33.2.5.4 Communication Skills

Positive communication skills are essential for several CRAFT procedures, including the ultimate invitation for the IP to enter treatment. In the earlier stages of treatment, CSOs' reliance upon positive communication can help minimize IP defensiveness and anger when explaining the rationale behind the CSO's own behavior change, and when requesting changes in the IP's behavior. The basic components of positive communication for CRAFT essentially are the same as those introduced for CRA: offer an understanding statement, accept partial responsibility, and offer to help. Assume that a mother (CSO) is trying to get her 17-year-old daughter (IP), who recently was caught with marijuana at school, to check out a new substance-free music establishment with a non-using friend on a Saturday night. The CSO might be encouraged to say, "I'm guessing you might be reluctant to try out this new place. After all, we haven't heard much about it yet, and maybe you're worried that some of your friends won't think it's 'cool' (*understanding statement*). And maybe I shouldn't have dumped the idea on you so 'enthusiastically' yesterday when I first brought it up (*partial responsibility statement*). But I know you love getting out and listening to music with people your age. What about giving it a try? I'll even pay for a ride for you if you want to go (*offer to help*)." As noted previously, communication skills are taught through repeated practice in the context of role-plays.

33.2.5.5 Positive Reinforcement for Clean and Sober IP Behavior

CRAFT helps CSOs understand that individuals are more likely to repeat behaviors that are reinforced (rewarded), and so when CSOs actively reward *sober* behaviors, they increase the likelihood that those sober behaviors will be repeated. CSOs also are taught the distinction between CRAFT's positive reinforcement (which increases the likelihood of clean/sober behaviors) and "enabling," which unintentionally increases the likelihood of substance use. Once the idea of rewarding sober behavior is explained, clinicians assist CSOs in developing a plan for administering reasonable rewards for the most appropriate times and occasions. The rewards themselves should be inexpensive, but the type of reward varies based on the CSO–IP relationship, the personal preferences of the IP (i.e., what the IP really enjoys), and what the CSO feels comfortable offering. Common examples include CSOs doing a favor for the IP, offering a compliment, giving a hug, or spending pleasant time with the IP.

Since it is imperative that the rewards follow sober behavior, CSOs sometimes require training in discerning whether or not the IP has engaged in substance use recently. Also, if CSOs are interested in explaining *why* they are giving a reward to their IP, positive communication skills (noted above) are rehearsed. For example, a CSO might say to the IP, "I know you really like it when I go antiquing with you on Saturdays (*understanding statement*), and I haven't been making the time to do that lately (*partial responsibility statement*). I'll happily go with you tomorrow, and I'll even pack a lunch like I used to (*offer to help*), but only if you don't get high. You're really a lot of fun to be with when you're not using." The importance of the CSO leaving the situation (but without any "drama") if the IP ended up smoking would be stressed.

33.2.5.6 Negative Consequences for Substance-Using Behavior

Just as a behavior is likely to be repeated if it is rewarded, a behavior is less likely to be repeated if it is followed by a decrease in rewards or an increase in negative consequences. Oftentimes CSOs can play an active role in reducing the IP's substance use by withdrawing the same rewards mentioned above (or additional ones) when the IP has been using substances. CSOs typically feel more comfortable removing rewards if they have discussed the rationale for needing to do so with the IP in advance. Again, positive communication is essential, and the risk for a violent IP reaction is discussed.

Since CSOs tend to care deeply about the well-being of their IP, they find themselves engaging in certain behaviors that inadvertently interfere with the natural, negative consequences of their IP's substance use. For example, by preparing something for the IP to eat when he comes home late and has missed dinner due to drinking, the CSO is preventing the IP from experiencing the full natural (negative) consequences of the decision to use substances. Clinicians discuss the potential ramifications of CSOs changing their own behavior (i.e., not getting the IP something to eat), including whether it would create more problems than it would solve. For example, an IP might lose a job and thus financially damage the entire family if the CSO did not call in sick for a hungover IP. But if deemed an appropriate behavior to target, a specific plan for changing the CSO's behavior would be developed. If the CSO wanted to explain the plan to the IP, the conversation would be rehearsed.

33.2.5.7 Helping CSOs Improve Their Own Lives

Most CSOs present to treatment in a state of distress, often in the form of anxiety, depression, or physical symptoms [67]. One of the primary goals of CRAFT is to help CSOs improve their own lives, regardless of whether the IP enters treatment. CSOs complete the Happiness Scale (from the CRA protocol) so that their degree of satisfaction across a variety of life domains can be assessed and goals can be set. For example, assume a CSO has elected not to pursue additional schooling, due to concerns about needing to be home to address any IP-related problem that arises. If this CSO rated "Job/Education" a "4," the clinician would work with the CSO to create a plan that would result in a higher rating in a few weeks. For instance, the CSO might decide to investigate online coursework, or to make an appointment with a college advisor about degree requirements and paths. As always, potential obstacles would be anticipated and addressed, including a possible negative reaction from the IP.

33.2.5.8 Inviting the IP to Sample Treatment

CRAFT clinicians urge CSOs to spend time learning the necessary skills prior to inviting their IP to enter treatment. This includes practicing

and implementing the CRAFT procedures just outlined, such as rewarding non-using IP behavior, introducing negative consequences for IP substance use, and relying on positive communication skills throughout. Not surprisingly, CSOs often report that their IP's substance use has decreased somewhat prior to the IP agreeing to seek treatment. In addition to allowing time for the CRAFT procedures to have an effect on the IP, CSOs need to learn the communication skills required for extending the invitation, and to identify the ideal time to have that conversation. Regarding the latter, CSOs are taught to extend the invitation at a time when the IP is most likely to be willing to sample treatment. These "windows of opportunity" may occur when the IP is inquiring about what the CSO is addressing in treatment, is questioning why the CSO's behavior has changed (in reference to rewarding and withdrawing rewards for different behaviors), or is remorseful about a salient substance-related negative consequence.

"Motivational hooks" are incorporated into the treatment invitation, such as pointing out that IPs can have their own therapist (separate from the CSO's clinician), highlighting that therapy can help the IP in non-substance use domains as well (e.g., finding a job, decreasing anxiety or depression), and suggesting that the IP sample a session or two without making a full commitment to therapy. CSOs are taught that if their IP initially declines the invitation, they should continue engaging in their new CRAFT-consistent behaviors in order to increase the likelihood of treatment engagement in the near future. Importantly, clinicians need to do preparatory work to ensure that a therapist is available to see the IP without delay as soon as the IP agrees to sample treatment. Furthermore, the IP's therapist should have a theoretical approach consistent with CRAFT, such as a behavioral or cognitive behavioral orientation.

33.2.6 CRAFT Scientific Support

Data show that many individuals with substance-use disorders (SUDs) are treatment resistant [19].

For individuals with alcohol-use disorders, evidence suggests a large treatment gap, which is defined as the difference between the number of people who need care and those who actually receive it [51]. Although a relatively smaller treatment gap than previously reported has been observed recently, it still has been estimated that one-quarter of the people with alcohol-use disorders do not receive treatment [94].

Prior to the development of CRAFT, only a limited number of traditional programs were available for CSOs of treatment-refusing individuals (Identified Patients; IPs) with substance-use problems: Al-Anon/Nar-Anon [3] and the Johnson Institute Intervention (JII; [47]). Unilateral Family Therapy (UFT) was introduced as a format for involving individuals other than the IP. Thomas and colleagues conducted several studies with UFT and found promising results, but the studies tended to be small and lacked controls (e.g., [90, 91]).

In the tradition of UFT, CRAFT was created. Originally called CRT—Community Reinforcement Training—the first small study was conducted by Sisson and Azrin [84]. Twelve female CSOs were randomly assigned into either CRT ($n = 7$) or individual counseling + Al-Anon referrals ($n = 5$). Six of the seven women in the CRT group (86%) were able to get their problem-drinking IPs into treatment compared to none of the IPs in the comparison group.

The second CRAFT study that focused on IPs with alcohol problems was a large NIAAA-funded project that randomly assigned 130 CSOs into one of the three treatment groups: CRAFT, Al-Anon Facilitation Therapy (an individual therapy version of Al-Anon; [66]), or the JII. Results indicated that CRAFT-trained CSOs were significantly more effective in engaging unmotivated problem drinkers in treatment (64%) as compared with the CSOs in Al-Anon (13%) and JII (30%, [61]). Interestingly, CSOs improved in their own functioning independent of treatment condition and whether their IP entered treatment. For those IPs who entered treatment, they did so with their CSOs receiving an average of only 4.7 CRAFT or Al-Anon sessions and 5.7 Johnson Institute sessions.

The success of CRAFT also has been established for treatment-refusing IPs with illicit drug problems. In a pilot project, 62 CSOs from diverse ethnic backgrounds received CRAFT. As expected, these CSOs were able to get a high percentage of IPs (74%) into treatment very quickly (less than five CSO sessions) while also reducing the CSOs' own levels of depression, anxiety, and anger [56].

Kirby and colleagues conducted a CRAFT study in which 32 CSOs were randomly assigned to either CRAFT or 12-step meetings. Engagement rates were 64% for the CRAFT-trained CSOs and 17% for CSOs in the 12-step condition [48]. A large NIDA-funded study was conducted next in which 90 CSOs of illicit drug-using IPs were randomly assigned to CRAFT, CRAFT + Aftercare, or Al-Anon/Nar-Anon Facilitation Therapy. An aftercare component was added to one of the CRAFT conditions to mimic the availability of ongoing aftercare groups within the 12-step model. The results demonstrated that the combined CRAFT conditions' engagement rates (67%) were significantly higher than the Al-Anon/Nar-Anon rates (29%), but there were no significant engagement differences between the two CRAFT conditions [57]. More recently, an effectiveness study demonstrated that CRAFT could be successfully transferred from a controlled research setting to a community treatment agency, while maintaining levels of engagement quite similar to previous controlled studies [24]. CRAFT's success with adults was tested with adolescents in an uncontrolled trial that recruited the parents of 42 drug-abusing, treatment-refusing adolescents [95]. A total of 71 of the parents engaged their adolescents into treatment using CRAFT, and the parents overall experienced a significant reduction in negative symptoms. A recent project has focused on training parents in CRAFT in order to facilitate their treatment-resistant adolescent's treatment entry, and to manage their child after entry into community-based treatment [50].

A meta-analysis has confirmed the effectiveness of CRAFT [76]. It was demonstrated that CRAFT produced three times more IP engagement than Al-Anon/Nar-Anon and twice the engagement of the Johnson Institute intervention. Furthermore, CSOs' mental health and family function improved, irrespective of IPs' successful treatment engagement.

A unique application of the CRAFT protocol was a study that delivered CRAFT in a group treatment format [54]. Participants were randomly assigned to a CRAFT group or to self-directed CRAFT, with the latter receiving the CRAFT self-help book [59]. The intent-to-treat analysis contrasted the CRAFT group engagement rate (60%) with the self-directed CRAFT rate (40%) and detected no statistically significant difference. However, for those CSOs assigned to the CRAFT group condition who attended at least one session, 71% engaged their IP into treatment. The implication is that CRAFT delivered in groups can be a cost-effective method of getting treatment-refusing IPs into treatment.

In summary, CRAFT has been found superior in engaging treatment-refusing substance-abusing individuals compared with traditional programs. CRAFT has been shown effective across ethnicities, different types of CSO–IP relationships, and various kinds of drugs of abuse. Furthermore, CRAFT works in less than five CSO sessions on average, and CSOs report psychological improvement regardless of the outcome of their engagement efforts.

33.2.6.1 International Considerations

Outside the USA, favorable results for CRAFT have been observed when compared to a waiting list [14]. The use of CRAFT recently has been expanded to target new populations, such as family members of already treatment-engaged substance-abusing individuals [55], parents of individuals with autism-spectrum disorders [96, 97], and family members of hikikomori individuals [79]. CRAFT has shown potential in forensic settings as well [63, 74]. Furthermore, CRAFT component analyses have been conducted to identify main components that facilitate treatment entry [49]. Three studies have now investigated using CRAFT with the CSOs of problem gamblers [43, 53, 65].

The CRAFT training manual, "Motivating Substance Abusers to Enter Treatment: Working with Family Members" [86], has been translated into German, Korean, Finnish, and Japanese to date. The self-help version [59] is available in Dutch, Finnish, Japanese, and Spanish. Therapists have been trained in CRAFT across the world, including the USA, Australia, Ireland, Wales, Scotland, the Netherlands, Sweden, Finland, Germany, Japan, and Canada.

33.2.7 Conclusion

The CRA/CRAFT "family" comprises a comprehensive and complementary treatment modality aimed at both individuals with substance-use problems and their family members. As noted, evidence has supported the efficacy and effectiveness of CRA/CRAFT in a wide variety of diagnostic and ethnic populations, as well as different age groups. Since the treatment does not exclusively reduce substance abuse but also addresses psychiatric and forensic problems, it has transdiagnostic potential. Furthermore, it has shown efficacy in both in- and outpatient facilities and outreach teams. Fortunately, the dissemination of these treatment packages is moving forward in many places throughout the world.

References

1. Abbott PJ, Weller SB, Delaney HD, Moore BA. Community reinforcement approach in the treatment of opiate addicts. Am J Drug Alcohol Abuse. 1998;24:17–30.
2. Afifi TO, Henriksen CA, Asmundson GJ, Sareen J. Victimization and perpetration of intimate partner violence and substance use disorders in a nationally representative sample. J Nerv Ment Dis. 2012;200:684–91.
3. Al-Anon Family Groups. Al-Anon faces alcoholism. New York: Author; 1984.
4. Anthony WA. Recovery from mental illness: the guiding vision of the mental health service system in the 1990s. Psychosoc Rehabil J. 1993;16:11–23.
5. Ayllon T, Azrin NH. The token economy: a motivational system for therapy and rehabilitation. New York: Appleton Century Crofts; 1968.

6. Azrin NH, Acierno R, Kogan ES, Donohue B, Besalel VA, McMahon PT. Follow-up results of supportive versus behavioral therapy for illicit drug use. Behav Res Ther. 1996;34:41–6.

7. Azrin NH. Improvements in the community-reinforcement approach to alcoholism. Behav Res Ther. 1976;14:339–48.

8. Azrin NH, Besalel VA. Job club counselor's manual. Baltimore: University Press; 1980.

9. Azrin NH, Sisson RW, Meyers R, Godley M. Alcoholism treatment by disulfiram and community reinforcement therapy. J Behav Ther Exp Psychiatry. 1982;13:105–12.

10. Azrin NH, Naster BJ, Jones R. Reciprocity counseling: a rapid learning-based procedure for marital counseling. Behav Res Ther. 1973;11(4):365–82.

11. Azrin NH. A strategy for applied research. Learning based but outcome oriented. Am Psychol. 1977;32(2):140–9.

12. Bickel WK, Amass L, Higgins ST, Badger GJ, Esch RA. Effects of adding behavioral treatment to opioid detoxification with buprenorphine. J Consult Clin Psychol. 1997;65:803–10.

13. Bickel WK, Marsch LA, Buchhalter AR, Badger GJ. Computerized behavior therapy for opioid-dependent outpatients: a randomized controlled trial. Exp Clin Psychopharmacol. 2008;16:132–43.

14. Bischof G, Iwen J, Freyer-Adam J, Rumpf HJ. Efficacy of the community reinforcement and family training for concerned significant others of treatment-refusing individuals with alcohol dependence: a randomized controlled trial. Drug Alcohol Depend. 2016;163:179–85.

15. Bouten C, Roozen HG, Greeven PGJ. Verbeteren van kwaliteit van leven bij verslaafden: een psychometrische analyse van de CRA-TvL. Gedragstherapie. 2017;50(2):123–36. [Dutch].

16. Bouton ME, Winterbauer NE, Todd TP. Relapse processes after the extinction of instrumental learning: renewal, resurgence, and reacquisition. Behav Process. 2012;90(1):130–41.

17. Bouton ME. Context and behavioral processes in extinction. Learn Mem. 2004;11:485–94.

18. Campos-Melady M, Smith JE, Meyers RJ, Godley SH, Godley MD. The effect of therapists' adherence and competence in delivering the adolescent community reinforcement approach on client outcomes. Psychol Addict Behav. 2017;31:117–29.

19. Compton WM, Thomas YF, Stinson FS, Grant BF. Prevalence, correlates, disability, and comorbidity of DSM-IV drug abuse and dependence in the United States: results from the national epidemiologic survey on alcohol and related conditions. Arch Gen Psychiatry. 2007;64(5):566–76.

20. D'Zurilla T, Goldfried M. Problem solving and behavior modification. J Abnorm Psychol. 1971;78:107–26.

21. Davis DR, Kurti A, Redner R, White T, Higgins ST. A review of the literature on contingency management in the treatment of substance use disorders, 2009–2015. Prev Med. 2016;92:36–46.

22. DeFuentes-Merillas L, Roozen H. Community Reinforcement Approach en Contingency Management. In: Schippers GM, Smeerdijk M, Merkx MJM, editors. Handboek cognitieve gedragstherapie bij stoornissen in het gebruik van middelen en gedragsverslaving. Utrecht: Resultaten Scoren, Perpectief Uitgeverijen; 2014. p. 377–93. [Dutch].

23. Dennis ML, Godley SH, Diamond G, Tims FM, Babor T, Donaldson J, Liddle H, Titus JC, Kaminer Y, Webb C, Hamilton N, Funk RR. The Cannabis youth treatment (CYT) study: main findings from two randomized trials. J Subst Abuse Treat. 2004;27:197–213.

24. Dutcher LW, Anderson R, Moore M, Luna-Anderson C, Meyers RJ, Delaney HD, Smith JE. Community Reinforcement and Family Training (CRAFT): An effectiveness study. Journal of Behavior Analysis in Health, Sports, Fitness and Medicine. 2009;2(1):80–90.

25. Dutra L, Stathopoulou G, Basden SL, Leyro TM, Powers MB, Otto MW. A meta analytic review of psychosocial interventions for substance use disorders. Am J Psychiatr. 2008;165:179–87.

26. García-Fernández G, Secades-Villa R, García-Rodríguez O, Peña-Suárez E, Sánchez-Hervás E. Contingency management improves outcomes in cocaine-dependent outpatients with depressive symptoms. Exp Clin Psychopharmacol. 2013;21(6):482–9.

27. Garcia-Rodriguez O, Secades-Villa R, Higgins ST, Fernandez-Hermida JR, Carballo JL, Errasti Perez JM, Al-halabi Diaz S. Effects of voucher-based intervention on abstinence and retention in an outpatient treatment for cocaine addiction: a randomized controlled trial. Exp Clin Psychopharmacol. 2009;17:131–8.

28. Garner BR, Hunter SB, Funk RR, Griffin BA, Godley SH. Toward evidence-based measures of implementation: examining the relationship between implementation outcomes and client outcomes. J Subst Abuse Treat. 2016;67:15–21.

29. Garner BR, Godley SH, Funk RR, Dennis ML, Smith JE, Godley MD. Exposure to adolescent community reinforcement approach treatment procedures as a mediator of the relationship between adolescent substance abuse treatment retention and outcome. J Subst Abuse Treat. 2009;36:252–64.

30. Godley SH, Hedges K, Hunter B. Gender and racial differences in treatment process and outcome among participants in the adolescent community reinforcement approach. Psychol Addict Behav. 2011a;25:143–54.

31. Godley SH, Meyers RJ, Smith JE, Godley MD, Titus JC, Karvinen T, Dent G, Passetti LL, Kelberg P. The adolescent community reinforcement approach (A-CRA) for adolescent cannabis users (DHHS publication no. SMA 01-3489), Cannabis youth treatment (CYT) manual series, vol 4, Center for Substance Abuse Treatment. Rockville: Substance Abuse and Mental Health Services Administration; 2001.

32. Godley MD, Godley SH, Dennis ML, Funk RR, Passetti LL, Petry NM. A randomized trial of assertive continuing care and contingency management for

adolescents with substance use disorders. J Consult Clin Psychol. 2014a;82(1):40–51.

33. Godley MD, Godley SH, Dennis ML, Funk RR, Passetti LL. The effectiveness of assertive continuing care on continuing care linkage, adherence, and abstinence following residential treatment for substance use disorders in adolescents. Addiction. 2007;102:81–93.

34. Godley SH, Garner BR, Smith JE, Meyers RJ, Godley MD. A large-scale dissemination and implementation model. Clin Psychol Sci Pract. 2011b;18:67–83.

35. Godley SH, Smith JE, Passetti LL, Subramanian G. The adolescent community reinforcement approach (A-CRA) as a model paradigm for the management of adolescents with substance use disorders and co-occurring psychiatric disorders. Subst Abuse. 2014b;35:352–63.

36. Godley SH, Smith JE, Meyers RJ, Godley MD. The adolescent community reinforcement approach: a clinical guide for treating substance use disorders. Normal: Chestnut Health Systems; 2016.

37. Godley MD, Passetti LL, Subramaniam GA, Funk RR, Smith JE, Meyers RJ. Adolescent Community Reinforcement Approach implementation and treatment outcomes for youth with opioid problem use. Drug Alcohol Depend. 2017;174:9–16.

38. Greeven PGJ, Roozen HG. Der Community Reinforcement Approach aus forensisch psychiatrischer und psychotherapeutischer Perspektive. Forensische Psychiatrie und Psychotherapie. 2019;26(1):40–56. [German].

39. Henderson CE, Wevodau AL, Henderson SE, Colbourn SL, Gharagozloo L, North LW, Lotts VA. An independent replication of the adolescent community reinforcement approach with justice-involved youth. Am J Addict. 2016;25:233–40.

40. Higgins ST, Abbott PJ. CRA and treatment of cocaine and opioid dependence. In: Meyers RJ, Miller WR, editors. A community reinforcement approach to addiction treatment. Cambridge: Cambridge University Press; 2001. p. 123–46.

41. Higgins ST, Sigmon SC, Wong CJ, Heil SH, Badger GJ, Donham R, Dantona RL, Anthony S. Community reinforcement therapy for cocaine-dependent outpatients. Arch Gen Psychiatry. 2003;60:1043–52.

42. Higgins ST, Silverman K, Heil SH. Contingency management in substance abuse. New York: Guilford Publications; 2007.

43. Hodgins DC, Toneatto T, Makarchuk K, Skinner W, Vincent S. Minimal treatment approaches for concerned significant others of problem gamblers: a randomized controlled trial. J Gambl Stud. 2007;23:215–30.

44. Hunt GM, Azrin NH. A community-reinforcement approach to alcoholism. Behav Res Ther. 1973;11:91–104.

45. Hunter BD, Godley SH, Hesson-McInnis MS, Roozen HG. Longitudinal change mechanisms for substance use and illegal activity for adolescents in treatment. Psychol Addict Behav. 2014;28(2):507–15.

46. Irsel van MAHM, DeFuentes-Merillas L, Walhout S, Roozen HG. Reliability and validity of the Dutch version of the community reinforcement approach happiness scale (Submitted).

47. Johnson VE. Intervention: how to help those who don't want help. Minneapolis: Johnson Institute; 1986.

48. Kirby KC, Marlowe DB, Festinger DS, Garvey KA, LaMonaca V. Community reinforcement training for family and significant others of drug abusers: a unilateral intervention to increase treatment entry of drug users. Drug Alcohol Depend. 1999;56:85–96.

49. Kirby KC, Benishek LA, Kerwin ME, Dugosh KL, Carpenedo CM, Bresani E, Haugh JA, Washio Y, Meyers RJ. Analyzing components of community reinforcement and family training (CRAFT): is treatment entry training sufficient? Psychol Addict Behav. 2017;31(7):818–27.

50. Kirby KC, Versek B, Kerwin ME, et al. Developing Community Reinforcement and Family Training (CRAFT) for Parents of Treatment-Resistant Adolescents. J Child Adolesc Subst Abuse. 2015;24(3):155–65.

51. Kohn R, Saxena S, Levav I, Saraceno B. The treatment gap in mental health care. Bull World Health Organ. 2004;82(11):858–66.

52. Lussier JP, Heil SH, Mongeon JA, Badger GJ, Higgins ST. A meta-analysis of voucher based reinforcement therapy for substance use disorders. Addiction. 2006;101:192–203.

53. Makarchuk K, Hodgins DC, Peden N. Development of a brief intervention for concerned significant others of problem gamblers. Addict Disord Treat. 2002;1:126–34.

54. Manuel JK, Austin JL, Miller WR, McCrady BS, Tonigan JS, Meyers RJ, Smith JE, Bogenschutz MP. Community reinforcement and family training: a pilot comparison of group and self-directed delivery. J Subst Abuse Treat. 2012;43:129–36.

55. Markus, Ormskerk W, Schoen R, Roozen HG. CRAFT: improvements in quality of life of concerned significant others of treatment seeking individuals with substance use disorders (in preparation).

56. Meyers RJ, Miller WR, Hill DE, Tonigan JS. Community reinforcement and family training (CRAFT): engaging unmotivated drug users in treatment. J Subst Abuse. 1999;10:291–308.

57. Meyers RJ, Miller WR, Smith JE, Tonigan JS. A randomized trial of two methods for engaging treatment-refusing drug users through concerned significant others. J Consult Clin Psychol. 2002;70:1182–5.

58. Meyers RJ, Smith JE. Clinical guide to alcohol treatment: the community reinforcement approach. New York: Guilford Press; 1995.

59. Meyers RJ, Wolfe BL. Get your loved one sober: alternatives to nagging, pleading, and threatening. Center City: Hazelden; 2004.

60. Meyers RJ, Roozen HG, Smith JE. The community reinforcement approach: an update of the evidence. Alcohol Res Health. 2011;33(4):380–8.

61. Miller WR, Meyers RJ, Tonigan JS. Engaging the unmotivated in treatment for alcohol problems: a comparison of three strategies for intervention through family members. J Consult Clin Psychol. 1999;67:688–97.

62. Miller WR, Meyers RJ, Tonigan JS, Grant KA. Community reinforcement and traditional approaches: findings of a controlled trial. In: Meyers RJ, Miller WR, editors. A community reinforcement approach to addiction treatment. Cambridge: Cambridge University Press; 2001. p. 79–103.

63. Miller JM, Miller HV, Barnes JC. Outcome evaluation of a family-based jail reentry program for substance abusing offenders. Prison J. 2016;96(1):53–78.

64. Miller WR, Forcehimes AA, Zweben A. Treating addiction: a guide for professionals. New York: The Guilford Press; 2011.

65. Nayoski N, Hodgins DC. The efficacy of individual community reinforcement and family training (CRAFT) for concerned significant others of problem gamblers. J Gambl Issues. 2016;33:189–212.

66. Nowinski J, Baker S, Carroll K. 12-step facilitation therapist manual: a clinical research guide for therapists treating individuals with alcohol abuse and dependence, vol 1, Project MATCH monograph series. Rockville: National Institute on Alcohol Abuse and Alcoholism; 1992.

67. Orford J, Natera G, Copello A, Atkinson C, Mora J, Velleman R, et al. Coping with alcohol and drug problems: the experiences of family members in three contrasting cultures. London: Brunner-Routledge; 2005.

68. Prendergast M, Podus D, Finney J, Greenwell L, Roll J. Contingency management for treatment of substance use disorders: a meta-analysis. Addiction. 2006;101:1546–60.

69. Roozen HG, Boulogne JJ, van Tulder MW, van den Brink W, De Jong CA, Kerkhof AJ. A systematic review of the effectiveness of the community reinforcement approach in alcohol, cocaine and opioid addiction. Drug Alcohol Depend. 2004;74:1–13.

70. Roozen HG, Kerkhof AJ, van den Brink W. Experiences with an out-patient relapse program (community reinforcement approach) combined with naltrexone in the treatment of opioid-dependence: effect on addictive behaviors and the predictive value of psychiatric comorbidity. Eur Addict Res. 2003;9:53–8.

71. Roozen HG, van Beers SE, Weevers HJ, Breteler MH, Willemsen MC, Postmus PE, Kerkhof AJ. Effects on smoking cessation: naltrexone combined with a cognitive behavioral treatment based on the community reinforcement approach. Subst Use Misuse. 2006;41:45–60.

72. Roozen HG, Wiersema H, Strietman M, Feij JA, Lewinsohn PM, Meyers RJ, Koks M, Vingerhoets JJ. Development and psychometric evaluation of the pleasant activities list. Am J Addict. 2008;17(5):422–35.

73. Roozen HG, Greeven P, Dijkstra B, Bischof G. Verbesserung bei patienten durch den community reinforcement approach: effecte auf zufriedenheid and psychiatrische symptom. Suchttherapie. 2013;14:72–7.

74. Roozen HG, Blaauw E, Meyers RJ. Advances in management of alcohol use disorders and intimate partner violence: community reinforcement and family training. Psychiatry Psychol Law. 2009;16(1):74–80.

75. Roozen HG, Bravo AJ, Pilatti A, Mezquita L, Vingerhoets A, Cross-cultural Addictions Study Team. Cross-cultural examination of the community reinforcement approach happiness scale (CRA-HS): testing measurement invariance in five countries Current Psychology. (in press).

76. Roozen HG, de Waart R, van der Kroft P. Community reinforcement and family training: an effective option to engage treatment-resistant substance-abusing individuals in treatment. Addiction. 2010;105:1729–38.

77. Roozen HG, Meyers RJ, Smith JE. Community Reinforcement Approach: Klinische procedures voor de behandeling van alcohol- en drugverslaving. Utrecht: Bohn Stafleu & van Loghum; 2013. [Dutch].

78. Rose M, Calabria B, Allan J, Clifford A, Shakeshaft AP. Aboriginal-specific community reinforcement approach (CRA) training manual. Sydney: National Drug and Alcohol Research Centre, University of New South Wales; 2014.

79. Sakai M, Hirakawa S, Nonaka S, Okazaki T, Seo K, Yokose Y, Inahata Y, Ushio M, Mizoguchi A. Effectiveness of community reinforcement and family training (CRAFT) for parents of individuals with "Hikikomori". Jpn J Behav Ther. 2015;41(3):167–78.

80. Schottenfeld RS, Moore B, Pantalon MV. Contingency management with community reinforcement approach or twelve-step facilitation drug counseling for cocaine dependent pregnant women or women with young children. Drug Alcohol Depend. 2011;118(1):48–55.

81. Secades-Villa R, Sanchez-Hervas E, Zacares-Romaguera F, Garcıa-Rodrıguez O, Santonja-Gomez FJ, Garcia-Fernandez G. Community reinforcement approach (CRA) for cocaine dependence in the Spanish public health system: 1 year outcome. Drug Alcohol Rev. 2011;30:606–12.

82. Secades-Villa R, García-Rodríguez O, Higgins ST, Fernández-Hermida JR, Carballo JL. Community reinforcement approach plus vouchers for cocaine dependence in a community setting in Spain: six-month outcomes. J Subst Abuse Treat. 2008;34(2):202–7.

83. Secades-Villa R, García-Fernández G, Peña-Suárez E, García-Rodríguez O, Sánchez-Hervás E, Fernández-Hermida JR. Contingency management is effective across cocaine-dependent outpatients with different socioeconomic status. J Subst Abuse Treat. 2013;44(3):349–54.

84. Sisson RW, Azrin NH. The use of systematic encouragement and community access procedures to increase attendance at alcoholics anonymous and Al-Anon meetings. Am J Drug Alcohol Abuse. 1986;8:371–6.

85. Slesnick N, Prestopnik JL, Meyers RJ, Glassman M. Treatment outcome for street-living, homeless youth. Addict Behav. 2007;32:1237–51.

86. Smith JE, Meyers RJ. Motivating substance abusers to enter treatment: working with family members. New York: Guilford Press; 2004.

87. Smith JE, Meyers RJ, Delaney HD. The community reinforcement approach with homeless alcohol-dependent individuals. J Consult Clin Psychol. 1998;66:541–8.

88. Smith JE, Gianini LM, Garner BR, Malek KL, Godley SH. A behaviorally-anchored rating system to monitor treatment integrity for clinicians using the A-CRA approach. J Child Adolesc Subst Abuse. 2014;23(3):185–99.

89. Smith JE, Lundy SL, Gianini L. Community reinforcement approach (CRA) and adolescent community reinforcement approach (A-CRA) therapist coding manual. Bloomington: Chestnut Health Systems; 2007.

90. Thomas EJ, Ager RD. Unilateral family therapy with the spouses of uncooperative alcohol abusers. In: O'Farrell TJ, editor. Treating alcohol problems: marital and family interventions. New York: Guilford Press; 1993. p. 3–33.

91. Thomas EJ, Santa C, Bronson D, Oyserman D. Unilateral family therapy with spouses of alcoholics. J Soc Serv Res. 1987;10:145–63.

92. Torres LB, Vazquez JG, Medina-Mora ME, Velazquez HA. Adaptation of a model of cognitive-behavioral intervention for dependent users of alcohol and other drugs in Mexico: a preliminary study. Salud Mental. 2005;28:61–71.

93. Tracy E, Whittaker J. The social network map: assessing social support in clinical practice. Fam Soc. 1990;71:461–70.

94. Tuithof M, Ten Have M, van den Brink W, Vollebergh W, de Graaf R. Treatment seeking for alcohol use disorders: treatment gap or adequate self-selection? Eur Addict Res. 2016;22(5):277–85.

95. Waldron HB, Kern-Jones S, Turner CW, Peterson TR, Ozechowski TJ. Engaging resistant adolescents in drug abuse treatment. J Subst Abuse Treat. 2007;32:133–42.

96. Yamamoto A, Murohashi M. CRAFT application in an intervention program for hikikomori cases with (suspected) autism spectrum disorder: program description and retrospective analysis of 30 cases. Jpn J Child Adolesc Psychiatry. 2014;55(3):280–94.

97. Yamamoto A, Roozen HG. A CRAFT parent support program focused on supporting children with autism spectrum disorder and other neurodevelopmental problems: a pilot study. Adv Neurodev Disord. 2020;4:15–9.

Exercise for Substance Use Disorders

34

Larissa J. Mooney and Richard A. Rawson

Contents

Abstract

This chapter provides an overview of the rationale and evidence for exercise as a treatment intervention for substance use disorders.

L. J. Mooney (✉)
Department of Psychiatry and Biobehavioral Sciences, University of California Los Angeles (UCLA), Los Angeles, CA, USA

VA Greater Los Angeles Healthcare System, Los Angeles, CA, USA
e-mail: lmooney@mednet.ucla.edu

R. A. Rawson
Department of Psychiatry and Biobehavioral Sciences, University of California Los Angeles (UCLA), Los Angeles, CA, USA

Vermont Center for Behavior and Health, University of Vermont, Burlington, VT, USA

The benefits of exercise on physical health, including weight management and cardiovascular outcomes, are well documented. Research has also demonstrated positive effects of exercise in reducing depression and anxiety and improving sleep and cognitive function. Negative affect states, such as depression and anxiety, are commonly associated with substance use and are risk factors for relapse. Exercise may facilitate abstinence by ameliorating negative affect via effects on the endogenous opioid system and potentiation of dopaminergic transmission. Recent clinical trials have demonstrated benefits of exercise as a treatment intervention for methamphetamine, alcohol, and other substance use disorders. Engagement in activities such as exercise may provide a reinforcing alternative behavior that is complementary to other treatment interventions while promoting health and facilitating treatment goals.

Keywords

Exercise · Substance use disorders · Treatment · Methamphetamine · Depression · Anxiety

34.1 Exercise Is Effective for Medical Conditions and Symptoms

The U.S. Department of Health and Human Services' updated *Physical Activity Guidelines for Americans* [91] provide a comprehensive review of the literature and document strong evidence for the general health benefits of physical activity. For adults, improvements ensuing from regular exercise at moderate levels include lower risk of early death, heart disease, stroke, diabetes, high blood pressure, adverse blood lipid profile, metabolic syndrome, and colon and breast cancers. Exercise is helpful for the prevention of weight gain and weight loss, particularly when combined with a lower caloric diet, and is also associated with improved cardiorespiratory and muscular fitness, reduced depression and anxiety risk, and better sleep and cognitive function.

Exercise has been shown to reduce fatigue in individuals with multiple medical conditions, including fibromyalgia [36] and ankylosing spondylitis [25]. The benefits of exercise in reducing chronic pain have also been extensively documented in the literature [29], including reductions in lower back pain and functional improvements from prescribed aerobic [55] and resistance [81] exercise programs. Although the overall quality of evidence is low due to sample sizes and issues with study design, improvements have been demonstrated in chronic pain severity, physical function, and quality of life [29].

34.2 Exercise Is Effective for Psychiatric Conditions and Symptoms

Substance use disorders (SUDs) are associated with elevated rates of comorbid psychiatric disorders, particularly depressive and anxiety disorders (e.g., [31, 40]). Severity of psychiatric symptoms has been associated with poorer treatment outcomes in multiple prior studies (e.g., [15, 30]). Upon cessation of substance use, withdrawal and abstinence syndromes comprising prominent psychiatric features may emerge (e.g., [56]). Syndromes may be characterized by drug cravings, coupled with marked depressive symptoms, including anhedonia, dysphoria, irritability, poor concentration, hypersomnia, low energy, and even suicidality [60]. The contribution of emotional stress to drug use and relapse has been well documented (e.g., [27, 83, 87]), and considerable evidence is accumulating to suggest that substance users exhibit deficits in their ability to process and regulate such stress.

Aerobic and resistance exercise interventions are useful for a wide range of psychiatric conditions, including anxiety and depression [79, 93]. The majority of studies have demonstrated efficacy of exercise in reducing symptoms of depression in both inpatient [54] and outpatient (e.g., [58]) settings; favorable results have been highlighted in several review articles (e.g., [6, 53]) and meta-analyses [20, 65]. Exercise has been shown to reduce depressive symptoms in medically compromised populations, including cardiac [69] and cancer [57] patients. The benefits of exercise relative to psychotropic medication [8] and psychotherapy [28, 33, 42] have also been investigated; equivalent benefits have been found comparing exercise with medication, time-limited or time-unlimited psychotherapy, group therapy, and cognitive–behavioral therapy.

State anxiety has been shown to acutely diminish after individual episodes of exercise [73], and aerobic exercise may confer significant benefit in the treatment of adults with moderate to severe panic disorder [12, 85] and obsessive–compulsive disorder [1]. The majority of studies have suggested efficacy of exercise in mitigating stress-related symptoms across a variety of study populations, including nonclinical [5, 9, 47], clinical [1], and medically compromised [72] adults. In a study of adults with significant anxiety sensitivity, a 2-week exercise intervention significantly reduced anxiety sensitivity relative to a no-treatment control [84], an effect that mediated the benefits of exercise on negative affect states, including anxious and depressed mood.

34.3 Exercise Improves Cognition

Cognitive deficits have been observed in long-term users of various substances. Chronic opioid use, for example, is associated with deficits in attention, processing speed, working memory, and executive functions [61], which can negatively impact methadone treatment response [21]. Methamphetamine users suffer from cognitive impairments during initial months of abstinence, including working memory, selective attention [82], learning [32], and decision making (e.g., [7, 68]). Deficits in multiple cognitive domains have been observed in alcohol-dependent individuals, including impairment in visuospatial and perceptuomotor functions, executive functions, and short-term memory, in addition to dementia and Korsakoff syndrome [43].

Meta-analyses of randomized, controlled trials confirm that normal and cognitively impaired adults derive cognitive benefits from physical exercise [4, 17, 26, 38]. Improvements are the greatest for executive control processes (e.g., planning, scheduling, working memory, dealing with distraction, multitasking), for participants in combined strength and aerobic training regimens, and when exercise duration is greater than 30 minutes [17]. Angevaren et al. [4] found the largest effects of aerobic exercise on motor and auditory function, and moderate effects on cognitive speed and visual attention. Executive and other cognitive functions have been shown to improve after acute bouts of resistance exercise in middle-aged adults [16].

34.4 Exercise and Substance Use Disorders

34.4.1 Neurobiology of Exercise and Substance Use Disorders

Exercise may hasten or improve recovery from SUDs by modifying underlying neurobiological processes, such as dopamine activity [77]. A study demonstrated reversal of methamphetamine-induced striatal dopamine transporter and tyrosine hydroxylase damage after exercise in rodents [67]. In addition, neurotrophic proteins may be regulated in part by exercise and play an important role in regulating neuronal function in the brain and help to sustain normal cognitive, emotional, and behavioral functioning. Brain-derived neurotrophic factor (BDNF), the most widely expressed neurotrophin in the brain, supports synaptic plasticity, facilitates neurogenesis, and modulates neurotransmission [22].

An emerging literature suggests that BDNF may have a role in the pathogenesis of addictive disorders [37]. Treatment interventions that affect BDNF production may mediate synaptic plasticity and neuroprotection, which could, in turn, ameliorate negative affective symptoms, impulsivity, and other cognitive deficits associated with ongoing drug use and relapse risk. Exercise, for example, has been shown in preclinical [78, 80] and human [70] studies to enhance the BDNF release in the brain. This is potentially significant because of the purported benefits of exercise on cognitive functioning [64]; cognitive deficits have been observed in chronic substance users as evidenced by poor performance on memory, attention tasks, and learning deficits [74]. Substance use disorders are also associated with poor impulse control and selective processing [49]. In addition, exercise has been shown to ameliorate negative mood states that may contribute to substance relapse, and prior literature has suggested that low BDNF levels in individuals with SUDs may predispose individuals to higher rates of psychiatric comorbidity [3].

34.4.2 Exercise for Reducing Substance Use and Preventing Relapse

An emerging literature on exercise-based interventions for SUDs provides preliminary evidence in support of this approach. In a study of cocaine-addicted rodents, rats given access to aerobic activity demonstrated reduction in cocaine-seeking, relative to those that did not have access to such activity [50]. The majority of clinical research has focused on aerobic exercise as a potential intervention to aid smoking cessation and has shown mixed effects of exercise on smoking abstinence [90]; more consistent positive effects on cigarette cravings, withdrawal symptoms, and smoking-related behaviors after exercise sessions have been demonstrated [88]. In an investigation of women enrolled in a 12-week cognitive–behavioral smoking-cessation program, subjects were randomized to receive either vigorous aerobic exercise or health education three times a week [10]. Those who participated in the exercise group evidenced significant reductions in cigarette craving, negative affect, and nicotine withdrawal during most weeks of the program.

More recent studies have suggested a preliminary positive effect of exercise in facilitating alcohol use reduction in individuals with alcohol use disorder [51] and in reducing substance use in both treatment-engaged substance users [13] and in non-treatment-seeking cannabis users [14]. In the treatment-engaged population, it was noted that substance use outcomes were significantly better among substance users who attended at least 75% of exercise sessions [13]. An 8- to 9-week structured exercise program has also demonstrated efficacy in adolescents enrolled in drug-treatment programs; adolescents who improved in self-concept, anxiety, and depression risk factors reported reduced substance use relative to those who did not improve on similar measures [18]. Similarly, a prospective investigation of more than 4000 twins revealed lower rates of illicit drug use and alcohol-use consequences in adulthood among physically active adolescents, supporting prior work suggesting a rela-

tionship between low physical activity in adolescents and drug use [44].

There have been a number of recent reviews and meta-analyses on the role of exercise in treating patients with SUDs. Hallgren et al. [35] reviewed 22 studies on the efficacy of exercise to reduce alcohol use. Although the evidence did not support the efficacy of exercise to directly reduce alcohol use, exercise did provide benefits in reducing symptoms of depression and improving physical fitness. These conclusions were supported by Stoutenberg et al. [86], who emphasized that while exercise appeared to produce significant positive benefits to individuals in treatment for alcohol use disorders (e.g., reduced anxiety, depression, and impulsivity, and improved self-efficacy), the evidence for exercise in reducing alcohol use was very limited. Linke and colleagues [46] reviewed the impact of exercise on a heterogeneous set of patients with SUDs. Although they concluded that exercise might be a potentially useful intervention that warranted further research, they noted that in many trials, adherence to exercise protocols is poor and, therefore, results are difficult to interpret. Finally, Morris et al. [62] reviewed the literature on the role of exercise in improving outcomes and quality of life for individuals who had been previous users of methamphetamine. The results from this literature review support other findings that exercise can reduce anxiety and depression and improve numerous medical measures and quality of life in this population of former drug users.

34.5 Study of Exercise as an Intervention for Methamphetamine Use Disorder

A multisite study was conducted in the United States by the Clinical Trials Network (CTN), funded by the National Institute on Drug Abuse (NIDA), investigating the benefits of an exercise component added to residential programs addressing stimulant use disorders. The Stimulant Reduction Intervention using Dosed Exercise (STRIDE) study was a randomized controlled trial that tested the effectiveness of the addition of exercise versus the addition of health education to treatment as usual in improving drug treatment outcomes in 302 participants with diagnostic and statistical manual of mental disorders, fourth edition (*DSM-IV*)-diagnosed stimulant abuse or dependence (e.g., cocaine, methamphetamine, and amphetamine) and receiving treatment initially in residential settings and then transitioning to outpatient settings; participants were randomized to receive either a dosed exercise intervention plus usual care or a health education intervention control plus usual care. Although the primary outcome of percentage of abstinent days did not show a significant treatment effect between groups, post hoc analyses controlling for treatment adherence and baseline stimulant use demonstrated greater stimulant abstinence rates among exercise-adherent participants [89].

From 2010 to 2015, the chapter authors (Mooney and Rawson) led a research team in conducting a NIDA-funded evaluation of exercise as a therapeutic intervention for methamphetamine users in early abstinence. The study examined the utility and efficacy of an 8-week, evidence-based aerobic and resistance exercise intervention to promote improved treatment outcomes for a sample of 150 individuals in residential treatment for methamphetamine use disorder. The study examined medical, psychiatric, neurocognitive, and behavioral benefits that may accrue during participation in an 8-week exercise intervention, as well as possible sustained beneficial impacts on drug use following completion of the exercise protocol and discharge from the residential treatment program. The project also included a brain imaging component to collect data leading to an improved understanding of the mechanisms that may underlie observed effects on treatment outcomes and symptom remediation associated with the exercise intervention.

DSM-IV-diagnosed methamphetamine-dependent individuals were screened to determine eligibility, and those randomized to the exercise intervention participated in supervised progressive endurance and resistance training three times per week for 8 weeks (24 sessions),

consistent with current guidelines for comprehensive exercise programs (American College of Sports Medicine [ACSM], [2]). Each session consisted of a 5-minute warm-up, 30 minutes of aerobic activity on a treadmill, 15 minutes of resistance training, and a 5-minute cool-down with stretching and light calisthenics. The goal of the aerobic training was to accumulate at least 30 minutes of continuous aerobic exercise at a target intensity set by data derived from maximal incremental exercise testing (XT), as described later. Information derived from the incremental testing was also used to define a safe ceiling for exercise intensity for each participant. The goal of the resistance training was to develop adaptations in muscle strength and body composition to complement the aerobic training program. A total of nine exercises involving the major muscle groups were performed each day.

Participants randomized to the control condition participated in a health and wellness education session three times a week for 45 minutes. A counselor provided informational materials, facilitated discussion of educational content, monitored attendance, and documented participants' involvement. Sessions consisted of an integrated multimedia educational program addressing a variety of health, wellness, and lifestyle topics such as nutrition, dental care, acupressure, sleep hygiene, and health screening, adapted from a previously implemented wellness manual used by Kinnunen et al. [41].

All study participants completed a maximal incremental exercise test (XT) on a treadmill ergometer using a symptom-limited incremental protocol with linear increases in the work rate with respect to time [19]. This test occurred three times during participation—at baseline, study week 5, and immediately following the intervention phase or upon intervention termination. Aerobic capacity ($\dot{V}O_2$ max) and the metabolic or lactate threshold ($\dot{V}O_2 \theta$), which is the level of oxygen uptake that defines one's ability to perform prolonged work, were measured using indirect calorimetry with an automated metabolic measurement system. The $\dot{V}O_2$ max and $\dot{V}O_2 \theta$ were used as baseline markers of aerobic fitness as well as for objective indices of each individual's tailored aerobic exercise intervention.

Participants underwent further fitness assessments to determine baseline body composition (skinfolds), muscle strength by 1-repetition maximum (1-RM) for leg press and chest press, and muscle endurance (repetitions to failure using 85% of their leg press and chest press 1-RM values). The 1-RM represents the maximum weight that can be lifted only once through a complete range of motion. The 1-RM and muscle endurance test data were used to establish baseline values of muscle strength and endurance in the study population and to help guide the development of the individually tailored resistance training exercise program (National Strength and Conditioning Association [NSCA], [63]). This test was administered at baseline, week 5, and upon intervention termination. Data obtained from the body composition analysis enabled tracking of changes in fat mass and, importantly, changes in the fat-free mass and skeletal muscle mass. These data were obtained using standard skinfold and girth measurement techniques [48] and calculated using the Jackson and Pollack equation [39] and magnetic resonance imaging (MRI)-validated equations, respectively [45].

A subset of consenting participants (15 from each condition) underwent two positron emission tomography (PET) sessions and two magnetic resonance imaging (MRI) sessions before commencement of the experimental condition and again after the 8 weeks of intervention. Brain region volumes were determined for subcortical regions, including the caudate, putamen, and nucleus accumbens. Dopamine D_2/D_3 receptor availability was calculated as binding potential (BP_{ND}) using the D2/D3 ligand [(18)F] fallypride. The MRI scan was used to confirm the absence of structural brain lesions and to aid in localization of volumes of interest.

34.5.1 Results from the Exercise Study

Methamphetamine users over the course of the 8-week trial were able to safely engage in exercise and derived significant health benefits over a

short period. Data from the first 29 study completers, randomized to either exercise (EX, $n = 15$) or health education (ED, $n = 14$), were analyzed to evaluate exercise-related physical outcomes, including aerobic fitness, body composition, and muscle strength. EX subjects significantly improved maximum oxygen uptake by 0.63 ± 0.22 L/min (21%), leg press (LP) strength improved by 24.4 ± 5.6 kg (40%), and chest press (CP) strength by 20.6 ± 5.7 kg (49%). For EX subjects, LP and CP endurance improved by ten repetitions (120%) and seven repetitions (96%), respectively, and these changes were significantly greater than those seen in the ED group. Changes in body composition for EX subjects included significant reductions in body weight (average 1.7 ± 2.4 kg, 2%), percentage of relative body fat (2.8 ± 1.3%, 15%), and fat weight (2.8 ± 1.8 kg, 18%). None of these variables changed significantly in participants receiving ED [24].

Preliminary data collected from 50 study participants revealed diminished heart-rate variability (HRV) relative to age-matched, drug-free controls. HRV reflects the ability of the autonomic nervous system (ANS) to adapt quickly to stress and changes in the environment [23]. At the end of the 8-week study, HRV increased in individuals who participated in the exercise program, but no significant change was observed relative to baseline in individuals randomized to the health education control group, suggesting that physical activity improved balance in autonomic tone in MA users. In addition, results from the PET and MRI neuroimaging examination of a subset of participants suggest improvement in striatal dopamine receptor binding after participation in the exercise program. Study participants in the EX condition ($n = 10$) demonstrated improvement in striatal D2/D3 binding after 8 weeks of exercise according to analysis of PET (using ^{18}F-fallypride), whereas those in the ED condition ($n = 9$) did not [77], suggesting that exercise is an intervention that may ameliorate dopaminergic deficits in individuals with methamphetamine use disorder.

Although differences in relapse rates post discharge from residential treatment did not differ between 135 individuals randomized to the 8-week EX condition versus ED at 1, 3, and

6 months, when groups were analyzed based on the severity of methamphetamine use at baseline, a significant difference in relapse rates was observed in the lower severity users (as defined by use up to 18 days in the month prior to admission). Lower severity users (45.2% of the sample) were less likely to relapse to methamphetamine use at all three time points than higher severity users (54.8% of the sample), as measured by self-report and urine drug screen results [76]. Participants randomized to the EX intervention were more likely to experience reduction in depression and anxiety symptom severity than those in the ED group, and a dose effect was observed whereby attending more EX sessions was associated with greater reduction in symptoms [75]; furthermore, those with more severe medical, psychiatric, and SUDs were most likely to derive benefit in reduction of depressive symptoms from the EX intervention [34].

34.6 Summary/Conclusion

Exercise may be a useful approach to aiding individuals with SUDs in their efforts to avoid relapse after they have achieved abstinence via treatment. The addition of a new, non-drug-related activity could provide a reinforcing alternative behavior that may be effective in facilitating abstinence by enhancing positive mood states via the effects of exercise on the endogenous opioid system and potentiation of dopaminergic transmission [59]. Prior literature demonstrates that exercise can improve anxiety and depression, symptoms that are often associated with initial phases of abstinence after cessation of drug use. Such conditions predispose individuals to relapse and predict poorer treatment outcomes (e.g., [66, 71]). Exercise also improves sleep [92] and performance on cognitive tasks, which may be impaired in chronic substance users. In light of the documented associations between stress, negative affect, and substance relapse in addicted populations [11, 52], together with evidence demonstrating stress regulation deficits in substance users, the development of interventions to ameliorate symptoms of depression and anxiety and improve affect regulation may help to reduce relapse risk in this population. Relief of distressing psychological symptoms may serve to complement relapse prevention skills taught in common therapy approaches for substance users and to promote health and positive behavioral changes consistent with treatment goals.

Key Points
- Exercise is associated with numerous physical health benefits, including improved strength, cardiovascular fitness, weight management, and cognitive function.
- Emerging evidence demonstrates improvements in mental health symptoms associated with exercise, including reduction in depression and anxiety and improved sleep.
- Emerging evidence suggests beneficial effects of exercise as a treatment intervention for substance use disorders.
- Negative affects states, such as anxiety and depression, are common effects of substance use and are risk factors for relapse.
- Exercise may facilitate abstinence from substances by ameliorating negative affect via effects on the endogenous opioid system and dopaminergic transmission.

References

1. Abrantes AM, Strong DR, Cohn A, Cameron AY, Greenberg BD, Mancebo MC, et al. Acute changes in obsessions and compulsions following moderate-intensity aerobic exercise among patients with obsessive-compulsive disorder. J Anxiety Disord. 2009;23(7):923927. https://doi.org/10.1016/j.janxdis.2009.06.008.
2. American College of Sports Medicine. ACSM's guidelines for exercise testing and prescription. 6th ed. Baltimore: Lippincott Williams & Wilkins; 2000.
3. Angelucci F, Ricci V, Pomponi M, Conte G, Mathe AA, Tonali PA, et al. Chronic heroin and cocaine abuse is associated with decreased serum concentrations

of the nerve growth factor and brain-derived neurotrophic factor. J Psychopharmacol. 2007;21(8):820–5. https://doi.org/10.1177/0269881107078491.

4. Angevaren M, Aufdemkampe G, Verhaar HJ, Aleman A, Vanhees L. Physical activity and enhanced fitness to improve cognitive function in older people without known cognitive impairment. Cochrane Database Syst Rev. 2008;16(3):CD005381. https://doi.org/10.1002/14651858.CD005381.pub3.

5. Bahrke M, Morgan W. Anxiety reduction following exercise and meditation. Cogn Ther Res. 1978;2(4):323–33. https://doi.org/10.1007/BF01172650.

6. Barbour KA, Edenfield TM, Blumenthal JA. Exercise as a treatment for depression and other psychiatric disorders: a review. J Cardiopulm Rehabil Prev. 2007;27(6):359–67. https://doi.org/10.1097/01.HCR.0000300262.69645.95.

7. Bechara A, Damasio H. Decision-making and addiction (part I): impaired activation of somatic states in substance dependent individuals when pondering decisions with negative future consequences. Neuropsychologia. 2002;40(10):1675–89. https://doi.org/10.1016/S0028-3932(02)00015-5.

8. Blumenthal J, Babyak M, Moore K, Craighead WE, Herman S, Khatri P, et al. Effects of exercise training on older patients with major depression. Arch Intern Med. 1999;159(19):2349–56. https://doi.org/10.1001/archinte.159.19.2349.

9. Blumenthal JA, Williams RS, Wallace AG, Williams RB Jr, Needles TL. Physiological and psychological variables predict compliance to prescribed exercise therapy in patients recovering from myocardial infarction. Psychosom Med. 1982;44(6):519–27. https://insights.ovid.com/pubmed?pmid=7163455.

10. Bock BC, Marcus BH, King T, Borrelli B, Roberts MR. Exercise effects on withdrawal and mood among women attempting smoking cessation. Addict Behav. 1999;24(3):399–410. https://doi.org/10.1016/S0306-4603(98)00088-4.

11. Breslin FC, Zack M, McMain S. An information-processing analysis of mindfulness: implications for relapse prevention in the treatment of substance abuse. Clin Psychol Sci Pract. 2002;9(3):275–99. https://doi.org/10.1093/clipsy/9.3.275.

12. Broocks A, Bandelow B, Pekrun G, George A, Meyer T, Bartmann U, et al. Comparison of aerobic exercise, clomipramine, and placebo in the treatment of panic disorder. Am J Psychiatr. 1998;155(5):603–9. https://doi.org/10.1176/ajp.155.5.603.

13. Brown RA, Abrantes AM, Read JP, Marcus BH, Jakicic J, Strong DR, et al. A pilot study of aerobic exercise as an adjunctive treatment for drug dependence. Ment Health Phys Act. 2010;3(1):27–34. https://doi.org/10.1016/j.mhpa.2010.03.001.

14. Buchowski MS, Meade NN, Charboneau E, Park S, Dietrich MS, Cowan RL, et al. Aerobic exercise training reduces cannabis craving and use in nontreatment seeking cannabis-dependent adults. PLoS One.

2011;6(3):e17465. https://doi.org/10.1371/journal.pone.0017465.

15. Cacciola JS, Alterman AI, Rutherford MJ, McKay JR, Mulvaney FD. The relationship of psychiatric comorbidity to treatment outcomes in methadone maintained patients. Drug Alcohol Depend. 2001;61(3):271–80. https://doi.org/10.1016/S0376-8716(00)00148-4.

16. Chang YK, Tsai CL, Huang CC, Wang CC, Chu IH. Effects of acute resistance exercise on cognition in late middle-aged adults: general or specific cognitive improvement? J Sci Med Sport. 2014;17(1):51–5. https://doi.org/10.1016/j.jsams.2013.02.007.

17. Colcombe SJ, Kramer AF. Fitness effects on the cognitive function of older adults: a meta-analytic study. Psychol Sci. 2003;14(2):125–30. https://doi.org/10.1111/1467-9280.t01-1-01430.

18. Collingwood TR, Reynolds R, Kohl HW, Smith W, Sloan S. Physical fitness effects on substance abuse risk factors and use patterns. J Drug Educ. 1991;21(1):73–84. https://doi.org/10.2190/HV5J-4EYN-GPP7-Y3QG.

19. Cooper CB. Exercise in chronic pulmonary disease: aerobic exercise prescription. Med Sci Sports Exerc. 2001;33(Suppl. 7):S671–9. https://insights.ovid.com/pubmed?pmid=11462076.

20. Craft LL, Landers DM. The effect of exercise on clinical depression and depression resulting from mental illness: a metaanalysis. J Sport Exerc Psychol. 1998;20:339–57. https://doi.org/10.1123/jsep.20.4.339.

21. Davis PE, Liddiard H, McMillan TM. Neuropsychological deficits and opiate abuse. Drug Alcohol Depend. 2002;67(1):105–8. https://doi.org/10.1016/S0376-8716(02)00012-1.

22. de Cid R, Fonseca F, Gratacos M, Gutierrez F, Martin-Santos R, Estivill X, et al. BDNF variability in opioid addicts and response to methadone treatment: preliminary findings. Genes Brain Behav. 2008;7(5):515–22. https://doi.org/10.1111/j.1601-183X.2007.00386.x.

23. Dolezal BA, Chudzynski J, Dickerson D, Mooney L, Rawson RA, Garfinkel A, et al. Exercise training improves heart rate variability after methamphetamine dependency. Med Sci Sports Exerc. 2014;46(6):1057–66. https://doi.org/10.1249/MSS.0000000000000201.

24. Dolezal BA, Chudzynski J, Storer TW, Abrazado M, Penate J, Mooney L, et al. Eight weeks of exercise training improves fitness measures in methamphetamine-dependent individuals in residential treatment. J Addict Med. 2013;7(2):122–8. https://doi.org/10.1097/ADM.0b013e318282475e.

25. Durmuş D, Alayli G, Uzun O, Tander B, Cantürk F, Bek Y, et al. Effects of two exercise interventions on pulmonary functions in the patients with ankylosing spondylitis. Joint Bone Spine. 2009;76(2):150–5. https://doi.org/10.1016/j.jbspin.2008.06.013. Epub 2008 Dec 11.

26. Etnier JL, Nowell PM, Landers DM, Sibley BA. A meta-regression to examine the relationship between aerobic fitness and cognitive performance. Brain Res

Rev. 2006;52(1):119–30. https://doi.org/10.1016/j.brainresrev.2006.01.002.

27. Fox HC, Bergquist KL, Hong KI, Sinha R. Stress-induced and alcohol cue-induced craving in recently abstinent alcohol-dependent individuals. Alcohol Clin Exp Res. 2007;31(3):395–403. https://doi.org/10.1111/j.1530-0277.2006.00320.x.

28. Fremont J, Craighead LW. Aerobic exercise and cognitive therapy in the treatment of dysphoric moods. Cogn Ther Res. 1987;11:241–51. https://doi.org/10.1007/BF01183268.

29. Geneen LJ, Moore RA, Clarke C, Martin D, Colvin LA, Smith BH. Physical activity and exercise for chronic pain in adults: an overview of Cochrane Reviews. Cochrane Database Syst Rev. 2017;14(4):CD011279. https://doi.org/10.1002/14651858.CD011279.pub2.

30. Glasner-Edwards S, Mooney LJ, Marinelli-Casey P, Hillhouse M, Ang A, Rawson RA, et al. Psychopathology in methamphetamine dependent adults 3 years after treatment. Drug Alcohol Rev. 2009;29:12–20. https://doi.org/10.1111/j.1465-3362.2009.00081.x.

31. Glasner-Edwards S, Mooney LJ, Marinelli-Casey P, Hillhouse M, Ang A, Rawson R, et al. Identifying methamphetamine users at risk for major depressive disorder: findings from the methamphetamine treatment project at three-year follow-up. Am J Addict. 2008;17(2):99–102. https://doi.org/10.1080/10550490701861110.

32. Gonzalez R, Rippeth JD, Carey CL, Heaton RK, Moore DJ, Schweinsburg BC, et al. Neurocognitive performance of methamphetamine users discordant for history of marijuana exposure. Drug Alcohol Depend. 2004;76(2):181–90. https://doi.org/10.1016/j.drugalcdep.2004.04.014.

33. Greist JH, Klein MH, Eischens RR, Faris J, Gurman AS, Morgan WP. Running as treatment for depression. Compr Psychiatry. 1979;20:41–54. https://doi.org/10.1016/0010-440X(79)90058-0.

34. Haglund M, Ang A, Mooney L, Gonzalez R, Chudzynski J, Cooper CB, et al. Predictors of depression outcomes among abstinent methamphetamine-dependent individuals exposed to an exercise intervention. Am J Addict. 2015;24(3):246–51. https://doi.org/10.1111/ajad.12175.

35. Hallgren M, Vancampfort D, Giesen ES, Lundin A, Stubbs B. Exercise as treatment for alcohol use disorders: systematic review and meta-analysis. Br J Sports Med. 2017;51(14):1058–64. https://doi.org/10.1136/bjsports-2016-096814. Epub 2017 Jan 13.

36. Häuser W, Klose P, Langhorst J, Moradi B, Steinbach M, Schiltenwolf M, et al. Efficacy of different types of aerobic exercise in fibromyalgia syndrome: a systematic review and meta-analysis of randomized controlled trials. Arthritis Res Ther. 2010;12(3):R79. https://doi.org/10.1186/ar3002.

37. Heberlein A, Dürsteler-MacFarland KM, Lenz B, Frieling H, Grösch M, Bönsch D, et al. Serum levels of BDNF are associated with craving in opiate-dependent patients. J Psychopharmacol. 2011;25(11):1480–4. https://doi.org/10.1177/0269881111411332.

38. Heyn P, Abreu BC, Ottenbacher KJ. The effects of exercise training on elderly persons with cognitive impairment and dementia: a meta-analysis. Arch Phys Med Rehabil. 2004;85(10):1694–704. https://doi.org/10.1016/j.apmr.2004.03.019.

39. Jackson AS, Pollock ML. Generalized equations for predicting body density of men. Br J Nutr. 1978;40(3):497–504. https://doi.org/10.1079/bjn19780152.

40. Kingston REF, Marcel C, Mills KL. A systematic review of the prevalence of comorbid mental health disorders in people presenting for substance use treatment in Australia. Drug Alcohol Rev. 2017;36(4):527–39. https://doi.org/10.1111/dar.12448.

41. Kinnunen T, Leeman RF, Korhonen T, Quiles ZN, Terwal DM, Garvey AJ, et al. Exercise as an adjunct to nicotine gum in treating tobacco dependence among women. Nicotine Tob Res. 2008;10(4):689–703. https://doi.org/10.1080/14622200801979043.

42. Klein MH, Greist JH, Gurman AS, Neimeyer RA, Lesser DP, Bushnell NJ, et al. A comparative outcome study of group psychotherapy vs. exercise treatments for depression. Int J Ment Health. 1985;13:148–76. https://doi.org/10.1080/00207411.1984.11448982.

43. Kopera M, Wojnar M, Brower K, Glass J, Nowosad I, Gmaj B, et al. Cognitive functions in abstinent alcohol-dependent patients. Alcohol. 2012;46(7):665–71. https://doi.org/10.1016/j.alcohol.2012.04.005.

44. Korhonen T, Kujala UM, Rose RJ, Kaprio J. Physical activity in adolescence as a predictor of alcohol and illicit drug use in early adulthood: a longitudinal population-based twin study. Twin Res Hum Genet. 2009;12(3):261–8. https://doi.org/10.1375/twin.12.3.261.

45. Lee RC, Wang Z, Heo M, Ross R, Janssen I, Heymsfield SB. Total-body skeletal muscle mass: development and cross-validation of anthropometric prediction models1–3. Am J Clin Nutr. 2000;72(3):796–803. https://doi.org/10.1093/ajcn/72.3.796.

46. Linke SE, Ussher M. Exercise-based treatments for substance use disorders: evidence, theory, and practicality. Am J Drug Alcohol Abuse. 2015;41(1):7–15. https://doi.org/10.3109/00952990.2014.976708.

47. Lion LS. Psychological effects of jogging: a preliminary study. Percept Mot Skills. 1978;47:1215–8. https://doi.org/10.2466/pms.1978.47.3f.1215.

48. Lohman TG, Roche AF, Martorell R, editors. Anthropometric standardization reference manual. Champaign: Human Kinetics Books; 1991.

49. Lundqvist T. Cognitive consequences of cannabis use: comparison with abuse of stimulants and heroin with regard to attention, memory and executive functions. Pharmacol Biochem Behav. 2005;81(2):319–30. https://doi.org/10.1016/j.pbb.2005.02.017.

50. Lynch WJ, Piehl KB, Acosta G, Peterson AB, Hemby SE. Aerobic exercise attenuates reinstatement of cocaine-seeking behavior and associated neuroad-

aptations in the prefrontal cortex. Biol Psychiatry. 2010;68(8):774–7. https://doi.org/10.1016/j.biopsych.2010.06.022. Epub 2010 Aug 8.

51. Manthou E, Georgakouli K, Fatouros IG, Gianoulakis C, Theodorakis Y, Jamurtas AZ. Role of exercise in the treatment of alcohol use disorders. Biomed Rep. 2016;4(5):535–45. https://doi.org/10.3892/br.2016.626.

52. Marlatt GA. Taxonomy of high-risk situations for alcohol relapse: evolution and development of a cognitive-behavioral model. Addiction. 1996;91(12 Suppl 1):S37–49. https://doi.org/10.1046/j.1360-0443.91.12s1.15.x.

53. Martinsen EW. Physical activity in the prevention and treatment of anxiety and depression. Nord J Psychiatry. 2008;62(Suppl 47):25–9. https://doi.org/10.1080/08039480802315640.

54. Martinsen EW, Medhus A, Sandvik L. Effects of aerobic exercise on depression: a controlled study. Br Med J (Clinical Research Edition). 1985;291(6488):109. https://doi.org/10.1136/bmj.291.6488.109.

55. McDonough SM, Tully MA, O'Connor SR, Boyd A, Kerr DP, O'Neill SM, et al. The back 2 activity trial: education and advice versus education and advice plus a structured walking programme for chronic low back pain. BMC Musculoskelet Disord. 2010;11:163. https://doi.org/10.1186/1471-2474-11-163.

56. McGregor C, Srisurapanont M, Jittiwutikarn J, Laobhripatr S, Wongtan T, White JM. The nature, time course and severity of methamphetamine withdrawal. Addiction. 2005;100(9):1320–9. https://doi.org/10.1111/j.1360-0443.2005.01160.x.

57. McLellan R. Exercise programs for patients with cancer improve physical functioning and quality of life. J Physiother. 2013;59(1):57. https://doi.org/10.1016/S1836-9553(13)70150-4.

58. McNeil JK, LeBlanc EM, Joyner M. The effect of exercise on depressive symptoms in the moderately depressed elderly. Psychol Aging. 1991;6(3):487–8. https://doi.org/10.1037/0882-7974.6.3.487.

59. Meeusen R. Exercise and the brain: insight in new therapeutic modalities. Ann Transplant. 2005;10(4):49–51. PMID:17037089.

60. Meredith C, Jaffe C, Ang-Lee K, Saxon A. Implications of chronic methamphetamine use: a literature review. Harv Rev Psychiatry. 2005;13(3):141–54. https://doi.org/10.1080/10673220591003605.

61. Mintzer MZ, Stitzer ML. Cognitive impairment in methadone maintenance patients. Drug Alcohol Depend. 2002;67(1):41–51. https://doi.org/10.1016/S0376-8716(02)00013-3.

62. Morris L, Stander J, Ebrahim W, Eksteen S, Meaden OA, Ras A, et al. Effect of exercise versus cognitive behavioural therapy or no intervention on anxiety, depression, fitness and quality of life in adults with previous methamphetamine dependency: a systematic review. Addict Sci Clin Pract. 2018;13:4. https://doi.org/10.1186/s13722-018-0106-4.

63. National Strength and Conditioning Association (NSCA). Strength and conditioning professional standards and guidelines. Colorado Springs: Author; 2010. Available at http://www.nsca-lift.org/publications/SCStandards.pdf.

64. Neeper SA, Gomez-Pinilla F, Choi J, Cotman C. Exercise and brain neurotrophins. Nature. 1995;373(6510):109. https://doi.org/10.1038/373109a0.

65. North TC, McCullagh P, Tran ZV. Effects of exercise on depression. Exerc Sport Sci Rev. 1990;18:379–415. PMID2141567.

66. Nunes EV, Levin FR. Treatment of depression in patients with alcohol or other drug dependence: a meta-analysis. JAMA. 2004;291(15):1887–96. https://doi.org/10.1001/jama.291.15.1887.

67. O'Dell SJ, Galvez BA, Ball AJ, Marshall JF. Running wheel exercise ameliorates methamphetamine-induced damage to dopamine and serotonin terminals. Synapse. 2012;66(1):71–80. https://doi.org/10.1002/syn.20989.

68. Paulus MP, Hozack N, Frank L, Brown GG, Schuckit MA. Decision making by methamphetamine-dependent subjects is associated with error-rate-independent decrease in prefrontal and parietal activation. Biol Psychiatry. 2003;53(1):65–74. https://doi.org/10.1016/S0006-3223(02)01442-7.

69. Pinto BM, Dunsiger SI, Farrell N, Marcus BH, Todaro JF. Psychosocial outcomes of an exercise maintenance intervention after phase II cardiac rehabilitation. J Cardiopulm Rehabil Prev. 2013;33(2):91–8. https://doi.org/10.1097/HCR.0b013e3182825531.

70. Ploughman M. Exercise is brain food: the effects of physical activity on cognitive function. Dev Neurorehabil. 2008;11(3):236–40. https://doi.org/10.1080/17518420801997007.

71. Poling J, Kosten TR, Sofuoglu M. Treatment outcome predictors for cocaine dependence. Am J Drug Alcohol Abuse. 2007;33(2):191–206. https://doi.org/10.1080/00952990701199416.

72. Prosser G, Carson P, Phillips R, Gelson A, Buch N, Tucker H, et al. Morale in coronary patients following an exercise programme. J Psychosom Res. 1981;25(6):587–93. https://doi.org/10.1016/0022-3999(81)90114-8.

73. Raglin JS, Morgan WP. Influence of exercise and quiet rest on state anxiety and blood pressure. Med Sci Sports Exerc. 1987;19:456–63. PMID:3316903.

74. Ramey T, Regier PS. Cognitive impairment in substance use disorders. CNS Spectr. 2018;28:1–12. [Epub ahead of print]. https://doi.org/10.1017/S1092852918001426.

75. Rawson RA, Chudzynski J, Gonzales R, Mooney L, Dickerson D, Ang A, et al. The impact of exercise on depression and anxiety symptoms among abstinent methamphetamine-dependent individuals in a residential treatment setting. J Subst Abus Treat. 2015a;57:36–40. https://doi.org/10.1016/j.jsat.2015.04.007.

76. Rawson RA, Chudzynski J, Mooney L, Gonzales R, Ang A, Dickerson D, et al. Impact of an exercise intervention on methamphetamine use out-

comes post-residential treatment care. Drug Alcohol Depend. 2015b;156:21–8. https://doi.org/10.1016/j.drugalcdep.2015.08.029.

77. Robertson CL, Ishibashi K, Chudzynski J, Mooney LJ, Rawson RA, Dolezal BA, et al. Effect of exercise training on striatal dopamine D2/D3 receptors in methamphetamine users during behavioral treatment. Neuropsychopharmacology. 2016;41(6):1629–36. https://doi.org/10.1038/npp.2015.331.

78. Russo-Neustadt AA, Beard RC, Huang YM, Cotman CW. Physical activity and antidepressant treatment potentiate the expression of specific brain-derived neurotrophic factor transcripts in the rat hippocampus. Neuroscience. 2000;101(2):305–12. https://doi.org/10.1016/s0306-4522(00)00349-3.

79. Saeed SA, Cunningham K, Bloch RM. Depression and anxiety disorders: benefits of exercise, yoga and meditation. Am Fam Physician. 2019;99(10):620–7. PMID:31083878.

80. Seifert T, Brassard P, Wissenberg M, Rasmussen P, Nordby P, Stallknecht B, et al. Endurance training enhances BDNF release from the human brain. Am J Physiol Regul Integr Comp Physiol. 2010;298:R372–7. https://doi.org/10.1152/ajpregu.00525.2009.

81. Shirado O, Doi T, Akai M, Hoshino Y, Fujino K, Hayashi K, et al. Multicenter randomized controlled trial to evaluate the effect of home-based exercise on patients with chronic low back pain: the Japan low back pain exercise therapy study. Spine. 2010;35(17):E811–9. https://doi.org/10.1097/BRS.0b013e3181d7a4d2.

82. Simon SL, Domier CP, Sim T, Richardson K, Rawson RA, Ling W. Cognitive performance of current methamphetamine and cocaine abusers. J Addict Dis. 2002;21(1):61–74. PMID:11831501.

83. Sinha R, Garcia M, Paliwal P, Kreek MJ, Rounsaville BJ. Stress-induced cocaine craving and hypothalamic-pituitary-adrenal responses are predictive of cocaine relapse outcomes. Arch Gen Psychiatry. 2006;63(3):324–31. https://doi.org/10.1001/archpsyc.63.3.324.

84. Smits JA, Berry AC, Rosenfield D, Powers MB, Behar E, Otto MW. Reducing anxiety sensitivity with exercise. Depress Anxiety. 2008;25(8):689–99. https://doi.org/10.1002/da.20411.

85. Ströhle A, Graetz B, Scheel M, Wittmann A, Feller C, Heinz A, et al. The acute antipanic and anxiolytic activity of aerobic exercise in patients with panic disorder and healthy control subjects. J Psychiatr Res. 2009;43(12):1013–7. https://doi.org/10.1016/j.jpsychires.2009.02.004.

86. Stoutenberg M, Rethorst CD, Lawson O, Read JP. Exercise training—A beneficial intervention in the treatment of alcohol use disorders? Drug Alcohol Depend. 2016;160:2–11. https://doi.org/10.1016/j.drugalcdep.2015.11.019.

87. Tate SR, Wu J, McQuaid JR, Cummins K, Shriver C, Krenek M, et al. Comorbidity of substance dependence and depression: role of life stress and self-efficacy in sustaining abstinence. Psychol Addict Behav. 2008;22(1):47–57. https://doi.org/10.1037/0893-164X.22.1.47.

88. Taylor RS, Unal B, Critchley JA, Capewell S. Mortality reductions in patients receiving exercise-based cardiac rehabilitation: how much can be attributed to cardiovascular risk factor improvements? Eur J Cardiovasc Prev Rehabil. 2006;13(3):369–74. https://doi.org/10.1097/01.hjr.0000199492.00967.11.

89. Trivedi MH, Greer TL, Rethorst CD, Carmody T, Grannemann BD, Walker R, et al. Randomized controlled trial comparing exercise to health education for stimulant use disorder: results from the CTN-0037 stimulant reduction intervention using dosed exercise (STRIDE) study. J Clin Psychiatry. 2017;78(8):1075–82. https://doi.org/10.4088/JCP.15m10591.

90. Ussher MH, Taylor AH, Faulkner GE. Exercise interventions for smoking cessation. Cochrane Database Syst Rev. 2014;29(8):CD002295. https://doi.org/10.1002/14651858.CD002295.pub5.

91. U.S. Department of Health and Human Services. Physical activity guidelines for Americans. 2nd ed. Washington, DC: U.S. Department of Health and Human Services; 2018.

92. Youngstedt SD. Effects of exercise on sleep. Clin Sports Med. 2005;24:355–65. https://doi.org/10.1016/j.csm.2004.12.003.

93. Zschucke E, Gaudlitz K, Ströhle A. Exercise and physical activity in mental disorders: clinical and experimental evidence. J Prev Med Public Health. 2013;46:S12–21. https://doi.org/10.3961/jpmph.2013.46.S.S12.

Towards Addiction Treatment: Technological Advances & Applying Technology

35

Shea M. Lemley and Lisa A. Marsch

Contents

Abstract

Digital health, broadly defined as applying technology to better understand health behavior and offer healthcare resources, has shown promise in improving the treatment of substance use disorders (SUDs) worldwide. Relatively few individuals seek and receive SUD treatment due to factors such as lack of access and stigma; however, digital health interventions may help address these limitations. Digital health treatments have been shown to be effective when integrated into traditional care, as well as offered as standalone interventions outside of traditional care settings. Future efforts in the field of digital health for SUD treatment will need to address barriers such as consumer engagement and privacy issues.

Keywords

Addiction treatment · Digital technology · Substance use disorder · Digital health · Digital therapeutics

S. M. Lemley · L. A. Marsch (✉)
Geisel School of Medicine at Dartmouth,
Lebanon, NH, USA
e-mail: lisa.a.marsch@dartmouth.edu

© Springer Nature Switzerland AG 2021
N. el-Guebaly et al. (eds.), *Textbook of Addiction Treatment*,
https://doi.org/10.1007/978-3-030-36391-8_35

35.1   Introduction

In this chapter, we review applications of digital technology to substance use disorder (SUD) treatment. We provide an overview of the clinical utility of digital therapeutics for patients and providers and a review of technology-based treatments that are integrated within traditional care models and others that are standalone. We also discuss various limitations and constraints on the use of digital health in the treatment of substance use disorders. The goal of this chapter is to introduce clinicians to recent advances in the application of digital technology to substance use disorder care.

35.2   How Is Technology Relevant for Substance Use Disorder Treatment?

Digital technology has become increasingly pervasive in modern life, and access continues to spread across both geographic and demographic boundaries. From 2008 to 2018, the percentage of the world's population with internet access more than doubled, from an estimated 23.1–51.7% [1]. Much of this growth comes from less-developed countries, with internet use rates among the least developed countries more than tripling in this 10-year span, growth that was more than nine times that of developed countries [1]. And, within developed countries, under-served populations increasingly have access to the internet. In the United States, for example, internet access rates among those with low incomes increased from 54% to 81% during the period from 2008 to 2018 [2]. Not only is technology reaching more people, but novel applications of technology in everyday life have fundamentally changed areas as diverse as commerce, education, and communication. Although some of the most profound changes have been seen in these areas, digital technology also shows promise for improving health care [3].

Applications of digital technology to health care, broadly called digital health, have created new opportunities across the healthcare sector,

changing how providers communicate with patients; create, maintain, and share medical records; and even receive training [4]. Advances in telehealth, for example, permit providers to work with patients remotely or receive training from experts in other locations [4]. Implementing electronic health and medical records (EHR/EMR) increases standardization, improves accuracy, and permits easier sharing of information across providers [5].

Growing numbers of digital health applications have been paralleled by increasing research that systematically seeks to evaluate the effectiveness and utility of digital health tools and interventions. There has been dramatic growth in recent decades in the number of publications on applications of digital technology to healthcare. Figure 35.1 illustrates the marked growth in published research containing the terms eHealth, digital health, mHealth, and digital therapeutics between 1995 and 2018.

In addition to research on digital health more broadly, researchers have examined applications of technology to substance use disorder (SUD) care. Because a thorough discussion of all areas of digital health for SUD is beyond the scope of this chapter, the chapter focuses on digital interventions to improve patient outcomes for substance use treatment. And, specifically, the chapter provides an overview of treatments for SUDs with empirical support from randomized controlled trials (RCTs), even though other promising technology-based treatments for SUD may be in earlier stages of research and development.

Moreover, various other stakeholders are interested in the potential applications of digital technology to health, including providers, countries, and international organizations [6, 7]. For example, the World Health Organization (WHO) and European Parliament have directed resources toward examining and addressing the use of digital health [6, 7]. Recognizing the growing prevalence and potential of digital health to address treatment needs, groups such as the WHO have also prepared and published plans and guidance on using and implementing digital health [7]. In addition to this national and international inter-

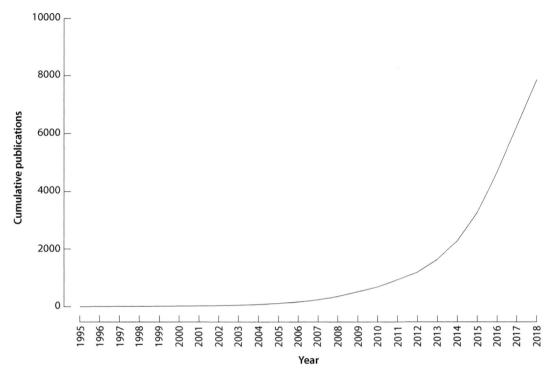

Fig. 35.1 Cumulative publications by year in eHealth, mHealth, "digital health," or "digital therapeutics" from Web of Science search for these terms spanning the years 1995–2018

est, digital health offers several advantages for providers and their patients.

35.3 Why Should SUD Providers Care?

Even the most effective healthcare providers can only help those who are receiving treatment. Unfortunately, only 7% of individuals with SUD seek and receive minimally adequate treatment [8]. Such low rates of seeking and receiving treatment are influenced by myriad patient-centered barriers, such as a lack of financial resources, few available providers, or a perception that treatment is unnecessary or will not be effective [8]. Two of the most common barriers that can prevent individuals from accessing needed services, however, are geographic isolation and stigma surrounding SUD and SUD treatment [9]. Importantly, digital interventions can extend access to care to reduce

the impact of geographic and stigmatization barriers on treatment utilization. For example, individuals in rural and underserved settings may need to travel to see treatment providers, but digital interventions can reduce the burden of a provider visit by offering treatment in the patient's home. Similarly, individuals whose work schedules or other commitments prevent visiting a clinic during normal hours may benefit from the increased convenience of interventions that can be accessed remotely. When it comes to sensitive issues such as substance use, individuals—including those with SUD—are often more comfortable disclosing to a computer than to another person [10].

Not only do digital therapeutics demonstrate potential to reach individuals who would not otherwise receive care, they also have the advantage of providing more treatment to those already receiving services. Even when engaged in care, individuals typically receive relatively limited therapy time; the vast majority of a person's life—approximately 5000 hours per year—is spent outside of treatment [11]. Thus, most of a person's experiences and decisions are occurring outside of the care setting. When it comes to this 5000-hour problem, digital treatments can help address this barrier by increasing time in treatment. For example, web-delivered treatment can effectively replace more than 80% of in-person therapy, such that a patient may only see a clinician twice a month [12]. Other exciting developments in digital health may also help extend treatment into individual's daily lives. One such development, ecological momentary interventions (EMI) use mobile digital technology to provide an intervention in "real time" and in real-world settings, increasing its temporal proximity to behaviors as they occur. For example, text messages have been used to deliver in-the-moment implementation intentions, which help patients link common substance use situations with alternative, non-substance-use behaviors [13]. Further, advances in mobile technology and passive sensing may provide promising extensions of SUD treatment into daily life. Such technology harnesses recent advances in GPS and biometric sensing to determine an individual's location and context using smartphones and wearable devices. Such tools can facilitate delivery of an intervention at the times and locations where it may be most likely to have an effect for that individual. These just-in-time adaptive interventions (JITAIs) are currently being developed to passively monitor an individual's context and behavior and then deliver appropriate interventions at precisely the time they are most needed [14].

Individuals with SUD are a heterogeneous population with varied demographic characteristics, in addition to various personal factors that may influence response to treatment. This heterogeneity may limit the effectiveness of standardized or "one-size-fits-all" treatments. Fortunately, many digital interventions provide individualized feedback based on a patient's current substance use or treatment progress. Others incorporate self-pacing of psychoeducational content and mastery-based progression through skill acquisition-based intervention components [12].

Such individualization allows for treatment success with varied substances of abuse and individuals from various walks of life, including youths and adults, individuals from lower socioeconomic status backgrounds, those with lower cognitive functioning, comorbid mental health and SUD, and polysubstance use [15–17].

Although a primary advantage of digital treatments is how they improve patient care, other advantages more directly benefit providers. Although a shortage of trained mental health providers is a global issue, this shortfall is worse in low- and middle-income countries [18]. Adding digital interventions as a supplement to in-person therapy can reduce the amount of time the provider spends with each patient, increasing the number of patients the provider can treat [19], as well as potentially improving cost-effectiveness [20]. Because providers can access more patient information to support data-based decisions, digital interventions may also improve clinical decision making [5]. Moreover, because intervention components are delivered in a pre-programmed manner, implementation can occur with greater fidelity [21].

35.4 How Are Digital Therapeutics Being Used in Substance Use Disorder Treatment?

Interventions have been developed and implemented across a range of modalities and platforms, including computer or web-based [19]; short message service (SMS) or text messaging [22]; and mobile applications (apps) [23]. Today, distinguishing between digital health modalities is of less concern, as digital health interventions increasingly operate across platforms. For example, after an in-person motivational interviewing session (i.e., brief personalized intervention to promote change in substance use; MI), the HealthCall intervention used daily calls to help reduce alcohol and drug use among participants with HIV, but a mobile app has been developed as a replacement for the daily phone calls [24]. Similarly, the Alcohol eCheckUp to Go (e-CHUG) is a web-based intervention, but the addition of a text messaging component showed greater reductions in drinking than the web-based intervention alone [25].

Digital health interventions have been utilized throughout the care continuum, from prevention, screening, and assessment, through treatment and recovery. Computerized prevention interventions, for example, may target communication or self-efficacy skills in adolescents or their parents [26]. Digital screening and assessment tools for SUDs are available to aid in the identification of problematic substance use. For example, computerized substance use screening tools have been successfully implemented in primary care settings, permitting identification of problematic substance use among individuals who are not presenting for SUD treatment [27]. More intensive digital health interventions may be incorporated alongside traditional treatment models or offered as standalone treatments.

35.4.1 Digital Treatments Integrated with Traditional Care

Many examples of digital health tools for substance use have been integrated into existing care models. Such tools may be offered as a supplement to existing treatment or used to replace a portion of usual care.

35.4.1.1 Intensive Digital Interventions Alongside Care

Digital therapeutics offered alongside clinical care offer advantages over traditional therapy alone. Adding a digital health component improves treatment retention and abstinence rates over office-based therapy alone, often at only modest per-patient cost increases [12, 20]. Further, by replacing a portion of treatment with digital therapy, a provider may be able to see more patients by reducing face time per patient. Rigorous evaluation through randomized controlled trials (RCTs) has demonstrated the clinical efficacy and effectiveness of a number of these therapeutics for supplementing traditional office-based therapy.

The Therapeutic Education System (TES) is a customizable, web-based intervention based on the community reinforcement approach (CRA) that incorporates contingency management (i.e., incentives provided for objectively verified abstinence; CM) [12, 19]. Up to 65 interactive modules cover content such as psychosocial skills and risk reduction, and TES includes several modalities of instruction, including therapeutic content presented as text or audio, quizzing to fluency, and modeling and role play of real-world scenarios. Evaluations of TES have shown it effectively replaces up to 80% of in-person therapy, results in cocaine and opioid abstinence outcomes that exceed those of care as usual, and improves treatment retention (e.g. [12, 19],). TES has been evaluated and shown to be effective with several demographic groups, including those currently using substances when they started the intervention and those with poorer cognitive functioning [15, 19].

The TES has been adapted into a 12-week web-based intervention for cannabis use. The intervention incorporated components of cognitive behavioral therapy (CBT) and motivational enhancement therapy (i.e., interventions based on motivational interviewing; MET), along with CM, or incentives for providing cannabis-free urine samples. This web-based MET/CBT/CM intervention had nine computer-based sessions with three short, supportive therapist sessions [28]. In an RCT, participants were randomized to one of three conditions: a computer-based cMET/CBT/CM intervention with incentives for cannabis-free urine samples, an entirely therapist-delivered MET/CBT/CM treatment with incentives for cannabis-free urine samples, and a brief, two-session MI-based intervention with incentives just for providing urine samples, whether or not they were positive for cannabis use. The MET/CBT/CM treatment packages—whether delivered by therapist or computer—produced similar rates of abstinence, which were greater than those produced by the brief intervention.

The Computer-Based Training for Cognitive Behavioral Therapy (CBT4CBT) digital health intervention provides computer-based CBT in conjunction with office-based therapy [29], though emerging evidence suggests it may also be effective as a standalone treatment [30]. The CBT4CBT program addresses topics such as cravings, problem solving, and decision making in six modules. Relative to treatment as usual, the addition of CBT4CBT has been shown to reduce days of substance use and increase continuous abstinence among participants with cocaine, opioid, marijuana, and alcohol dependence [29].

The Self-Help Alcohol and other drug use and Depression (SHADE) program is a computer-delivered intervention incorporating components from CBT and MI to target comorbid depression and substance use [17]. The SHADE program features nine weekly computerized sessions followed by a brief follow-up with a therapist. An RCT comparing the SHADE program, a therapist-delivered CBT/MI intervention, and a person-centered therapy control condition in Australian adults found that both the SHADE program and therapist-delivered CBT/MI intervention reduced depression and alcohol use more than person-centered therapy at three-month follow-up [17]. For depression, there were no differences between the SHADE program and the therapist-delivered CBT/MI intervention, but those in the SHADE program had greater reductions in alcohol use than those in either therapist-delivered intervention.

An app-based treatment for those leaving residential treatment, the Addiction-Comprehensive Health Enhancement Support System (A-CHESS) uses a smartphone app to provide information, adherence strategies, decision-making tools, and social support for adults with alcohol dependence who are transitioning out of inpatient treatment [23]. The A-CHESS app also includes a risk assessment component to deliver targeted messages and social support, as needed. Relative to usual continuing care, patients randomized to receive A-CHESS had fewer self-reported risky drinking days (i.e., >3/>4 drinks for women/men) in an RCT.

To address the limited availability of mental health services in Asian countries, the S-Health China app was developed for smart phone [31]. S-Health China incorporates cognitive-behavioral elements, such as trigger recognition, coping, and

self-management. In a pilot study with participants who used heroin or other drugs, users of the app reported fewer drug use days relative to an educational text-messaging control condition, but there were no between-group differences in positive urine samples at the weekly drug screens during the four-week intervention period.

A web-based treatment for cannabis use, Can Reduce incorporates elements of CBT and MI and features eight online modules plus access to a therapist [32]. An RCT compared Can Reduce with and without the inclusion of up to two counselor chat sessions with a control condition, and results suggested that the availability of the chat component was necessary for reductions in cannabis use at three-month follow-up, even if participants did not take advantage of the chat sessions.

Other treatment approaches have used new technology to remotely verify abstinence and deliver incentives. For example, a secure website and webcams were used to video record participants' breath carbon monoxide (CO) samples and readings because breath CO provides an objective measure of smoking [33]. In a 6-week RCT, rural participants were randomized to an intervention in which they received monetary incentives contingent on providing CO samples below an abstinence threshold or to a control condition in which participants provided CO samples on video but received noncontingent incentives. Participants receiving the incentives contingent on abstinence were more likely to provide CO samples that were negative for smoking and had greater levels of continuous abstinence.

35.4.1.2 Digital Health Following Brief In-person Interventions

Other digital interventions have been designed to follow in-person brief interventions to enhance or extend their effects. For example, the HealthCall intervention was developed to reduce drug and alcohol use among persons living with HIV, though not all studies have shown evidence of clinical effects. After a single session of in-person MI, the HealthCall intervention featured automated daily calls that incorporated elements of MI, self-monitoring, and personalized feedback.

An RCT showed that MI + HealthCall—but not MI alone—reduced alcohol use more than an educational control condition, and among alcohol-dependent patients, MI + HealthCall reduced alcohol use relative to both MI alone and control [34]. However, challenges were identified with the repetitive nature of the calls and engagement with HealthCall. More recently, a pilot study tested the efficacy of a smartphone app to replace the automated daily phone calls [24]. The app-based intervention included more interactive content, such as videos, and resulted in improved engagement relative to the phone calls. The app-based HealthCall intervention significantly reduced drug use, but not alcohol use, relative to motivational interviewing alone.

The MOMENT intervention follows two in-person sessions of motivational enhancement therapy (MET) to target adolescents' cannabis use [35]. Designed as an ecological momentary intervention (EMI), MOMENT features momentary assessment of cannabis use followed by support and coping strategies delivered through text messaging. Relative to MET alone, the MOMENT intervention demonstrated reductions in cannabis desire and cannabis use following targeted contexts or events.

35.4.2 Standalone Digital Treatments

Digital health interventions provided outside of traditional care have the potential to reach populations unlikely to present for treatment in standard clinical settings. Because major barriers to SUD treatment involve treatment availability and stigma [8], online interventions accessible outside of traditional care models can fill an unmet need. For example, the Can Reduce intervention for cannabis use identified key differences between users of its online, self-directed intervention and traditional clinic-based therapy [32]. Namely, the Can Reduce users were older and reported more cannabis use days. Similarly, the treatment-seeking population of cocaine users recruited into an RCT to evaluate Snow Control was older and more educated than individuals

typically entering outpatient treatment for cocaine use disorder [36].

35.4.2.1 Brief Standalone Digital Interventions

Although digital screening and assessment tools may focus solely on identification of substance use problems [27], several direct-to-consumer digital tools include screening and brief treatment components that are available in one or more brief, online sessions. These brief interventions typically assess an individual's use patterns and then provide personalized feedback addressing topics such as social norms and the health and financial consequences of substance use. Brief online interventions often target alcohol use by college students, with findings generally supporting short-term efficacy for reducing alcohol consumption (e.g., [25]). A one-session online brief intervention called Drinker's Check-up has been tested in adults and has produced short-term reductions in alcohol use, consistent with those produced by in-person brief motivational interventions [37]. A brief online intervention has also been developed to reduce cannabis use among college students, but the intervention resulted only in changes to perceptions about cannabis but not use [38].

Relatively few brief interventions address substance use beyond alcohol or cannabis, but the Motivational Enhancement System (MES) has been used to target multiple substances in a single session, computer-delivered brief intervention that incorporates elements of MI [39]. Developed for use in perinatal women, MES features three components: assessment and feedback, advantages and disadvantages of changing substance use, and a summary of the individual's interest in change and optional goal setting. Although the effects of the intervention do not seem to maintain long term, MES has produced short-term reductions in use of most drugs in RCTs [39].

35.4.2.2 Intensive Standalone Digital Interventions

Intensive standalone digital interventions are designed to deliver treatment spanning several weeks but outside of traditional care settings. These interventions feature multiple sessions or modules focusing on skill development and coping skills and behavior change strategies. Other components may include social support or progress tracking. Many of these intensive digital interventions have been developed for alcohol and tobacco, although some programs target cannabis, cocaine, or amphetamine-type stimulant (ATS) use.

Some online digital interventions feature multiple self-directed modules designed to be accessed over the course of several weeks. The DEpression-ALcohol Project (DEAL Project) is a four-week, web-based intervention for young adults with depression symptomology and hazardous alcohol used [16]. Based on the SHADE program, the intervention features four modules covering topics such as assessment and goal setting, behavioral activation, cognitive restructuring, and mindfulness. In an RCT, Australian young adults were randomized to the DEAL Project intervention or to view a website featuring informational health modules. Relative to the health information website, those receiving the DEAL Project intervention showed reductions in alcohol use and depression symptoms post-treatment. These reductions were maintained up to 6-months post-treatment, but differences between the intervention and control group were no longer significant, limiting conclusions that can be made about longer-term effects.

For treatment to decrease cannabis use, Reduce Your Use delivers six modules of a web-based intervention based on MI and CBT that includes motivational feedback, goal setting, and skill development focused around urges, withdrawal, and expectancies [40]. In an RCT comparing Reduce Your Use with web-based educational information, Reduce Your Use resulted in lower cannabis use at six-week follow-up and fewer, less-severe cannabis dependence symptoms at three-month follow-up.

Web-based interventions have also been developed for treatment of cocaine and stimulant use, but to date, their effects have been limited. Snow Control is a 6-week, internet-based, pro-gram to reduce hazardous and harmful cocaine use with techniques from MI and CBT [36]. In an RCT, the eight Snow Control modules were no more effective than an informational website at reducing cocaine use among Swiss participants. Breakingtheice is a web-based program with three modules that incorporates elements of both MI and CBT to reduce amphetamine-type stimulant (ATS) use [41]. An RCT comparing Breakingtheice to a waitlist control group showed Breakingtheice increased help seeking and reduced days out of role but did not reduce ATS use among Australian adults.

35.4.2.3 EMI

Some standalone treatments leverage the unique accessibility provided by mobile devices to provide treatments in the patient's daily life in real time. These EMIs show promise as a method to encourage use of new skills in the times and places where they are most needed. Some EMIs include both in-the-moment intervention and other components. For example, the Location-Based Monitoring and Intervention for Alcohol Use Disorders (LBMI-A) is a standalone smart phone intervention using techniques from CBT-based treatments for alcohol use disorders [42]. The app featured seven psychoeducational models, progress tracking, and tools that could be accessed in the moment, such as coping strategies. In a pilot study comparing LBMI-A to brief MI with bibliotherapy, participants receiving LBMI-A increased their percent of days abstinent over the course of 6 weeks. Moreover, greater use of LBMI-A in a given week was associated with fewer drinks per week and lower percent heavy drinking days.

Other EMIs focus solely on a text-messaging component without additional modules. For example, Riordan and colleagues examined an EMI that used SMS messages to describe the negative consequences of alcohol consumption on heavy drinking days during a college orientation week in New Zealand [22]. In an RCT, students in one of two colleges at a university showed reduced drinking during orientation week and across the academic year, but significant differences were not obtained at the other college [22]. Although such EMI messages may show promise for reducing alcohol use, the discrepant results suggest that variables such as context and demographics need to be further examined. By contrast, another EMI study used implementation intentions, which focus on prompting non-substance use alternative behaviors in the presence of substance use contexts [13]. In an evaluation of this implementation intentions EMI, adults with alcohol use disorder were randomized to receive text messages of their pre-specified implementation intentions, which linked high-risk drinking situations with alternative responses or a control condition in which these situations and responses were not linked. At the end of the two-week intervention, participants in the implementation intentions condition reduced their number of drinks per occasion more than those in the control condition, but these effects did not maintain at a one-month follow-up. Although EMIs generally show promise for producing short-term reductions in alcohol use, the relatively early nature of this type of intervention calls for more research to determine how frequency, content, and demographic variables influence responses to these interventions.

Several text messaging interventions have targeted tobacco cessation. For example, the Happy Quit text messaging intervention examined frequency of CBT-based text messages to promote smoking cessation among a sample of adults throughout China [43]. The text messages focused on motivational messages and behavior change techniques, and participants could text to request additional supportive messages. In a 12-week RCT, participants were assigned to a high-frequency messaging group (three to five messages per day), a low-frequency messaging group (three to five messages per week), and a control group that received a single message each week featuring study information but no cessation-related content. Participants in both the high- and low-frequency text messaging groups were more likely to be abstinent than control participants at 12-week follow-up, but there were no differences in abstinence between the high-frequency and low-frequency groups.

35.4.2.4 Gaming Elements

Other digital interventions have begun to incorporate game-like elements [44, 45]. One game-based intervention, Alcohol Alert, features three sessions of a web-based game in which adolescents navigate role-play situations dealing with the negative consequences of binge drinking [44]. Adolescents receive personalized feedback for their in-game responses, as well as advice about real-world drinking situations. Among Dutch adolescents recruited from schools, Alcohol Alert showed potential to reduce short- and long-term binge drinking relative to a no-intervention control, but issues with attrition limit conclusions about the intervention. The QuitIt Coping Skills Game gives patients who smoke the opportunity to role-play coping strategies in situations that are relevant to smoking relapse [45]. Tobacco-dependent cancer patients scheduled for surgery were recruited for an RCT. Although more participants who played the game were abstinent relative to those in a standard care control group, the small sample size and issues with retention limit the generality of these findings. Game-based interventions show promise for reducing use of alcohol and tobacco, but the small size of the pilot studies to date limits the conclusions and generality of these findings to broader populations.

35.5 What Can Help Guide the Use of Digital Therapeutics?

The rapid growth in technology and its reach have been accompanied by growth in digital health applications. Although digital health shows promise for improving aspects of SUD treatment, several concerns associated with digital health applications merit consideration prior to adoption for SUD treatment. For providers, general guidelines for digital health, though not focused on substance use, can help guide and inform considerations for use of digital health tools. For example, the WHO's Report on Monitoring and Evaluating Digital Health provides guidance for monitoring processes and evaluating outcomes when implementing and scaling up digital health [7]. Such reports can inform practical considerations for implementation, but such guidelines do not replace research- and evidence-based best practice.

One example of regulating and disseminating digital interventions comes from the Food and Drug Administration (FDA) in the United States, which recently launched an authorization program for prescription digital therapeutics that directly treat a disease [46]. This program offers a certification framework for digital health interventions that have demonstrated safety and efficacy via RCTs. The FDA authorization process situates these products into existing prescription and reimbursement structures, offering greater potential to promote use of digital therapeutics among providers and their patients. Because digital therapeutics will need to demonstrate clinical efficacy through a rigorous investigation process to receive authorization, this program is an important step in offering both providers and consumers an avenue to verify safety and efficacy of digital treatments. Unfortunately, because few individuals with SUD go to a provider for treatment [8], prescription digital therapeutics may still leave unmet need among those individuals who do not seek professional help. Researchers and developers should continue to consider other flexible models of deployment for their digital health treatments.

The wide availability of technology and the increasing penetration of smartphones may increase the likelihood that individuals seek self-help solutions through commercial outlets, such as the Apple App Store or Google Play. Although some apps available through such sources can be helpful, recent reviews of apps targeting smoking and alcohol use suggest the quality and content of available apps can vary dramatically, with only 5% of smoking cessation apps being judged as high quality using the Mobile App Rating Scale [47]. In 2018, the American Psychiatric Association published guidelines specifically for providers seeking to evaluate mobile phone mental health apps for their clients [48]. These recommendations include considerations about privacy and security; the evidence for the tool; its

ease of use; and its interoperability with clinical care. Although helpful, these recommendations may change over time as new research becomes available and technology continues to advance, introducing new concerns.

35.6 What Are Concerns and Limitations of Digital Therapeutics?

Although digital health shows promise for the treatment of SUDs, limitations should be considered with use of these technologies. One major concern involves equity in access to digital interventions. Data suggest that more than half of the world's population are internet users, but internet access rates of the most developed nations are approximately four times those of the least-developed countries [1]. Most digital health interventions for substance use have been evaluated with participants in a single, developed country, though some have recruited participants internationally [40]. The generality of such findings to contexts that differ in financial resources and culture remains underexamined.

Within developed and developing countries, economic inequality represents one of the greatest barriers to internet access. Although the introduction of smartphones has extended internet access to more individuals and groups, within both developing and developed countries [1, 2], an internet access divide still exists. For example, in the United States, 98% of people with high incomes use the internet, compared to only 82% of those with low incomes [2]. Although growing internet access rates across groups are promising, lingering differences in internet access may contribute to inequity in digital treatment availability. Even with internet access, however, individuals vary in their comfort using technology and have differing skillsets that may be necessary to access some digital health treatments, such as numeracy or literacy. Some digital interventions present treatment content as text (e.g., [43]), meaning that individuals need a minimum level of literacy to use such interventions. Although past research has suggested that individuals with varied skillsets can successfully navigate and benefit from digital health treatments, user skillsets need to be considered before incorporating digital health interventions. Particularly relevant are questions relating to comfort navigating technology and skills required to benefit from a selected intervention. Providers may consider selecting digital interventions that have options to improve accessibility, such as larger text size or content presented in audio or video formats. Other options improving access might involve additional trainings and supports, either within the digital intervention or as an adjunct to treatment.

Other considerations involve the use and implementation of digital interventions outside research settings. Problems with engagement and attrition have been identified with digital health interventions [49]. Specifically, engagement with digital interventions may be limited or start high but fall over time, whereas attrition issues may manifest as high study dropout rates from baseline to follow-up [49]. Attrition can not only make it difficult to assess the effectiveness of an intervention but may also suggest limited generality of the treatment to non-research contexts. Although strategies that may improve engagement have been proposed, more research needs to be done to determine their effectiveness. Incorporating provider contact may reduce attrition in digital health studies [50], and incorporating social aspects into treatments may enhance their effects. Some interventions have shown improved efficacy with some provider contact or the option for therapist contact [32], whereas other interventions have included social components, such as peer contact and support [23]. The relative contribution of these social aspects to SUD treatment effectiveness remains underexamined. Another major consideration is how to transition digital health interventions to broader implementation. In a UN Parliament survey of European experts in the field of SUDs, 64.4% indicated that they never or rarely use technology-based interventions for SUDs, broadly defined to include telehealth, online therapy, and self-help interventions [6].

Other limitations are related to privacy and security of the technologies themselves [50].

Well-publicized breaches of both commercial and healthcare data highlight the very real security and privacy concerns inherent to use of any digital health application. Those who develop technology will continue to grapple with improving the privacy and security of their applications, but providers using digital health technology will need to evaluate the risks and benefits of a given intervention, keeping issues of security in mind. Acquisition of samples for biochemical verification of abstinence may also raise privacy issues. Although the entire process of obtaining a breath CO sample to verify smoking abstinence can be video-recorded to ensure the sample was given reliably and by the appropriate individual [33], other objective measures of abstinence cannot be remotely verified due to privacy concerns.

35.7 Conclusion

Applications of technology to health care, broadly called digital health, show promise in promoting access to and availability of SUD treatment. Digital treatments for SUDs have been developed for various digital platforms and treatment settings, and these treatments have been demonstrated to be effective through RCTs across substances and demographic groups. Technological innovation is enabling novel, promising treatment approaches, such as JITAI and EMI, that can extend treatment into patients' everyday lives. Despite these intriguing advances in digital health for SUD, barriers to use and adoption of digital treatments, such as privacy issues, remain. Despite these barriers, digital health treatments for SUD show promise for increasing the availability of effective SUD treatment.

References

1. International Telecommunication Union. Key 2005–2018 ICT Data. 2018. Retrieved from: https://www.itu.int/en/ITU-D/Statistics/Pages/stat/default.aspx.
2. Pew Research Center. Internet/broadband fact sheet. 2018. Retrieved from https://www.pewinternet.org/fact-sheet/internet-broadband/.

3. Moerenhout T, Devisch I, Cornelis GC. E-health beyond technology: analyzing the paradigm shift that lies beneath. Med Health Care Philos. 2018;21(1):31–41. https://doi.org/10.1007/s11019-017-9780-3.

4. Imison C, Castle-Clarke S, Watson R, Edwards N. Delivering the benefits of digital health care. London: Nuffield Trust; 2016.

5. Bell D, Gachuhi N, Assefi N. Dynamic clinical algorithms: digital technology can transform health care decision-making. Am Soc Trop Med Hyg. 2018;98(1):9–14. https://doi.org/10.4269/ajtmh.17-0477.

6. Quaglio G, Esposito G. Technological innovation strategies in substance use disorders. Brussels: European Union: European Parliament; 2017.

7. World Health Organization. Monitoring and evaluating digital health interventions: a practical guide to conducting research and assessment. (978-92-4-151176-6). Geneva: World Health Organization; 2016.

8. Degenhardt L, Glantz M, Evans-Lacko S, Sadikova E, Sampson N, Thornicroft G, et al. Estimating treatment coverage for people with substance use disorders: an analysis of data from the World Mental Health Surveys. World Psychiatry. 2017;16(3):299–307. https://doi.org/10.1002/wps.20457.

9. Priester MA, Browne T, Iachini A, Clone S, DeHart D, Seay KD. Treatment access barriers and disparities among individuals with co-occurring mental health and substance use disorders: an integrative literature review. J Subst Abus Treat. 2016;61:47–59. https://doi.org/10.1016/j.jsat.2015.09.006.

10. Butler SF, Villapiano A, Malinow A. The effect of computer-mediated administration on self-disclosure of problems on the addiction severity index. J Addict Med. 2009;3(4):194–203. https://doi.org/10.1097/ADM.0b013e3181902844.

11. Asch DA, Muller RW, Volpp KG. Automated hovering in health care--watching over the 5000 hours. N Engl J Med. 2012;367(1):1–3. https://doi.org/10.1056/NEJMp1203869.

12. Bickel WK, Marsch LA, Buchhalter AR, Badger GJ. Computerized behavior therapy for opioid-dependent outpatients: a randomized controlled trial. Exp Clin Psychopharmacol. 2008;16(2):132–43.

13. Moody LN, Tegge AN, Poe LM, Koffarnus MK, Bickel WK. To drink or to drink less? Distinguishing between effects of implementationintentions on decisions to drink and how much to drink in treatment-seeking individuals with alcohol use disorder. Addict Behav. 2018;83:64–71. https://doi.org/10.1016/j.addbeh.2017.11.010.

14. Nahum-Shani I, Smith SN, Spring BJ, Collins LM, Witkiewitz K, Tewari A, Murphy SA. Just-in-Time Adaptive Interventions (JITAIs) in mobile health: key components and design principles for ongoing health behavior support. Ann Behav Med. 2018;52:446–62. https://doi.org/10.1007/s12160-016-9830-8.

15. Acosta MC, Marsch LA, Xie H, Guarino H, Aponte-Melendez Y. A web-based behavior therapy program

influences the association between cognitive functioning and retention and abstinence in clients receiving methadone maintenance treatment. J Dual Diagn. 2012;8(4):283–93. https://doi.org/10.1080/15504263.2012.723317.

16. Deady M, Mills K, Teesson M, Kay-Lambkin F. An online intervention for co-occurring depression and problematic alcohol use in young people: primary outcomes from a randomized controlled trial. J Med Internet Res. 2016;18(3):e71. https://doi.org/10.2196/jmir.5178.

17. Kay-Lambkin F, Baker A, Kelly B, Lewin T. Clinician-assisted computerised versus therapist-delivered treatment for depressive and addictive disorders: a randomised controlled trial. Med J Aust. 2011;195(3):S44–50.

18. Bruckner TA, Scheffler RM, Shen G, Yoon J, Chisholm D, Morris J, et al. The mental health workforce gap in low- and middle-income countries: a needs-based approach. Bull World Health Organ. 2011;89:184–94. https://doi.org/10.2471/BLT.10.082784.

19. Campbell AN, Nunes EV, Matthews AG, Stitzer M, Miele GM, Polsky D, et al. Internet-delivered treatment for substance abuse: a multisite randomized controlled trial. Am J Psychiatr. 2014;171(6):683–90. https://doi.org/10.1176/appi.ajp.2014.13081055.

20. Olmstead TA, Ostrow CD, Carroll KM. Cost-effectiveness of computer-assisted training in cognitive-behavioral therapy as an adjunct to standard care for addiction. Drug Alcohol Depend. 2010;110(3):200–7. https://doi.org/10.1016/j.drugalcdep.2010.02.022.

21. Miller W, Rollnick S. The effectiveness and ineffectiveness of complex behavioral interventions: impact of treatment fidelity. Contemp Clin Trials. 2014;37(2):234–41. https://doi.org/10.1016/j.cct.2014.01.005.

22. Riordan BC, Conner TS, Flett JA, Scarf D. A text message intervention to reduce first year university students' alcohol use: a pilot experimental study. Digital Health. 2017;3:1–10. https://doi.org/10.1177/2055207617707627.

23. Gustafson DH, McTavish FM, Chih MY, Atwood AK, Johnson RA, Boyle MG, et al. A smartphone application to support recovery from alcoholism: a randomized clinical trial. JAMA Psychiat. 2014;71(5):566–72. https://doi.org/10.1001/jamapsychiatry.2013.4642.

24. Aharonovich E, Stohl M, Cannizzaro D, Hasin D. HealthCall delivered via smartphone to reduce co-occurring drug and alcohol use in HIV-infected adults: a randomized pilot trial. J Subst Abus Treat. 2017;83:15–26. https://doi.org/10.1016/j.jsat.2017.09.013.

25. Tahaney K, Palfai T. Text messaging as an adjunct to a web-based intervention for college student alcohol use: a preliminary study. Addict Behav. 2017;73:63–6. https://doi.org/10.1016/j.addbeh.2017.04.018.

26. Ismayilova L, Terlikbayeva A. Building competencies to prevent youth substance use in Kazakhstan: mixed methods findings from a pilot family-focused multi-

media trial. J Adolesc Health. 2018;63(3):301–12. https://doi.org/10.1016/j.jadohealth.2018.04.005.

27. McNeely J, Wu LT, Subramaniam G, Sharma G, Cathers LA, Svikis D, et al. Performance of the tobacco, alcohol, prescription medication, and other substance use (TAPS) tool for substance use screening in primary care patients. Ann Intern Med. 2016;165(10):690–9. https://doi.org/10.7326/M16-0317.

28. Budney AJ, Stanger C, Tilford JM, Scherer EB, Brown PC, Li Z, et al. Computer-assisted behavioral therapy and contingency management for cannabis use disorder. Psychol Addict Behav. 2015;29(3):501–11. https://doi.org/10.1037/adb0000078.

29. Carroll KM, Kiluk BD, Nich C, Gordon MA, Portnoy GA, Marino DR, Ball SA. Computer-assisted delivery of cognitive-behavioral therapy: efficacy and durability of CBT4CBT among cocaine-dependent individuals maintained on methadone. Am J Psychiatr. 2014;171(4):436–44. https://doi.org/10.1176/appi.ajp.2013.13070987.

30. Kiluk BD, Devore KA, Buck MB, Nich C, Frankforter TL, LaPaglia DM, et al. Randomized trial of computerized cognitive behavioral therapy for alcohol use disorders: efficacy as a virtual stand-alone and treatment add-on compared with standard outpatient treatment. Alcohol Clin Exp Res. 2016;40(9):1991–2000. https://doi.org/10.1111/acer.13162.

31. Liang D, Han H, Du J, Zhao M, Hser Y-I. A pilot study of a smartphone application supporting recovery from drug addiction. J Subst Abus Treat. 2018;88:51–8. https://doi.org/10.1016/j.jsat.2018.02.006.

32. Schaub MP, Haug S, Wenger A, Berg O, Sullivan R, Beck T, Stark L. Can reduce – the effects of chat-counseling and web-based self-help, web-based self-help alone and a waiting list control program on cannabis use in problematic cannabis users: a randomized controlled trial. BMC Psychiatry. 2013;13(1):305. https://doi.org/10.1186/1471-244X-13-305.

33. Stoops W, Dallery J, Fields N, Nuzzo P, Schoenberg N, Martin C, et al. An internet-based abstinence reinforcement smoking cessation intervention in rural smokers. Drug Alcohol Depend. 2009;105(1–2):56–62. https://doi.org/10.1016/j.drugalcdep.2009.06.010.

34. Hasin DS, Aharonovich E, O'Leary A, Greenstein E, Pavlicova M, Arunajadai S, et al. Reducing heavy drinking in HIV primary care: a randomized trial of brief intervention, with and without technological. Addiction. 2013;108(7):1230–40. https://doi.org/10.1111/add.12127.

35. Shrier LA, Burke PJ, Kells M, Scherer EA, Sarda V, Jonestrask C, et al. Pilot randomized trial of MOMENT, a motivational counseling-plus-ecological momentary intervention to reduce marijuana use in youth. mHealth. 2018;4:29. https://doi.org/10.21037/mhealth.2018.07.04.

36. Schaub M, Sullivan R, Haug S, Stark L. Web-based cognitive behavioral self-help intervention to reduce cocaine consumption in problematic cocaine users:

randomized controlled trial. J Med Internet Res. 2012;14(6):e166. https://doi.org/10.2196/jmir.2244.

37. Hester RK, Squires DD, Delaney HD. The Drinker's check-up: 12-month outcomes of a controlled clinical trial of a stand-alone software program for problem drinkers. J Subst Abus Treat. 2005;28(2):159–69. https://doi.org/10.1016/j.jsat.2004.12.002.

38. Palfai TP, Saitz R, Winter M, Brown TA, Kypri K, Goodness TM, et al. Web-based screening and brief intervention for student marijuana use in a university health center: pilot study to examine the implementation of eCHECKUP TO GO in different contexts. Addict Behav. 2014;39(9):1346–52. https://doi.org/10.1016/j.addbeh.2014.04.025.

39. Ondersma S, Svikis D, Thacker L, Beatty J, Lockhart N. Computer-delivered screening and brief intervention (e-SBI) for postpartum drug use: a randomized trial. J Subst Abus Treat. 2014;46(1):52–9. https://doi.org/10.1016/j.jsat.2013.07.013.

40. Rooke S, Copeland J, Norberg M, Hine D, McCambridge J. Effectiveness of a self-guided web-based cannabis treatment program: randomized controlled trial. J Med Internet Res. 2013;15(2):e26. https://doi.org/10.2196/jmir.2256.

41. Tait R, McKetin R, Kay-Lambkin F, Carron-Arthur B, Bennett A, Bennett K, et al. A web-based intervention for users of amphetamine-type stimulants: 3-month outcomes of a randomized controlled trial. J Med Internet Res. 2014;1(1):e1. https://doi.org/10.2196/mental.3278.

42. Gonzalez V, Dulin P. Comparison of a smartphone app for alcohol use disorders with an internet-based intervention plus bibliotherapy: a pilot study. J Consult Clin Psychol. 2015;83(2):335–45. https://doi.org/10.1037/a0038620.

43. Liao Y, Wu Q, Kelly BC, Zhang F, Tang Y-Y, Wang Q, et al. Effectiveness of a text-messaging-based smoking cessation intervention ("Happy Quit") for smoking cessation in China: a randomized controlled trial. PLoS Med. 2018;15(12):e1002713. https://doi.org/10.1371/journal.pmed.1002713.

44. Jander A, Crutzen R, Mercken L, Candel M, Vries HD. Effects of a web-based computer-tailored game to reduce binge drinking among Dutch adolescents: a cluster randomized controlled trial. J Med Internet Res. 2016;18(2):e29. https://doi.org/10.2196/jmir.4708.

45. Krebs P, Burkhalter J, Fiske J, Snow H, Schofield E, Iocolano M, et al. The QuitIT coping skills game for promoting tobacco cessation among smokers diagnosed with cancer: pilot randomized controlled trial. JMIR Mhealth Uhealth. 2019;7(1):e10071. https://doi.org/10.2196/mhealth.10071.

46. U.S. Food and Drug Administration. Digital Health Software Precertification (Pre-Cert) Program. 2017. Retrieved from https://www.fda.gov/MedicalDevices/DigitalHealth/DigitalHealthPreCertProgram/default.htm Archived at: http://www.webcitation.org/6wQGHE27Z.

47. Thornton L, Quinn C, Birrell L, Guillaumier A, Shaw B, Forbes E, et al. Free smoking cessation mobile apps available in Australia: a quality review and content analysis. Aust N Z J Public Health. 2017;41(6):625–30. https://doi.org/10.1111/1753-6405.12688.

48. American Psychiatric Association. App evaluation model. 2018. Retrieved from https://www.psychiatry.org/psychiatrists/practice/mental-health-apps/app-evaluation-model. Archived at: http://www.webcitation.org/6wQH7bzmT.

49. Kazemi DM, Borsari B, Levine MJ, Li S, Lamberson KA, Matta LA. A systematic review of the mHealth interventions to prevent alcohol and substance abuse. J Health Commun. 2017;22(5) https://doi.org/10.1080/10810730.2017.1303556.

50. Muench F. The promises and pitfalls of digital technology in its application to alcohol treatment. Alcohol Res. 2014;36(1):131–42.

Cultural Adaptation of Empirically Validated Therapies for Treating Drug Dependence: International Considerations

36

Felipe González Castro, Manuel Barrera Jr, and Flavio F. Marsiglia

Contents

F. G. Castro (✉)
Edson College of Nursing and Health Innovation,
Arizona State University, Phoenix, AZ, USA
e-mail: felipe.castro@asu.edu

M. Barrera Jr
Department of Psychology, Arizona State University,
Tempe, AZ, USA

F. F. Marsiglia
School of Social Work, Arizona State University,
Phoenix, AZ, USA

© Springer Nature Switzerland AG 2021
N. el-Guebaly et al. (eds.), *Textbook of Addiction Treatment*,
https://doi.org/10.1007/978-3-030-36391-8_36

Abstract

This chapter examines issues and challenges in the local and cultural adaptation of evidence-based interventions (EBIs) and empirically validated treatments (EVTs). We examined the prior Fidelity-Adaptation Dilemma from the contemporary perspective that regards both *fidelity* and *adaptation* as equally important intervention imperatives. This approach involves implementation fidelity in congruence with the theory-based and empirically validated core therapeutic thrust of the intervention, while also exercising flexibility in conducting planned adaptations that are responsive to the "real world," needs of diverse cultural subgroups of clients. The need to develop pretreatment "integrative modules" is described as an innovative feature of contemporary EBI design, to aid in integrating the EBI for effective "function and fit" within various communities and health service delivery settings. The goal is to facilitate EBI widespread dissemination and implementation to thus improve the health and well-being of diverse clients and community residents. The implications for international dissemination and implementation across nations, cultures, and among diverse clients are described.

Keywords

Cultural adaptations · Evidence-based interventions · Empirically validated treatments · Integrative modules · Fidelity · Adaptation

36.1   Introduction

36.1.1 The Case for the Cultural Adaptation of Drug Abuse Treatments

Interest in the *adaptation* of model treatments—*evidence-based interventions* (EBIs) and *empirically validated therapies* (EVTs)—has increased in recent years [7, 13]. This chapter examines issues, perspectives, and approaches in the cultural adaptation of original EBIs or EVTs, respectively, as examined within two research areas: (a) prevention interventions with adolescents and (b) drug abuse treatments with young adult and middle-aged clients. It also examines (c) issues of intervention "fit and function" within a community or health service agency seeking to adopt that EBI.

The strategy of adapting a validated model treatment, as opposed to its delivery with total fidelity and thus without adjustment [18], has emerged as a significant and controversial approach. Some research investigators have argued that evidence-based interventions (EBIs) and evidence-based treatments (EVTs) [7] should be disseminated widely to diverse client groups, and when implemented with high fidelity should work as designed, thus obviating any need for adaptation. By contrast, evidence from a study of school-based drug abuse prevention curricula [40] reveals that classroom teachers who administered manualized model prevention interventions frequently modified the original intervention because they saw significant limitations in the original model intervention. These teachers generally sought to modify the original EBI to make it more culturally relevant for their adolescent students. Similarly, among drug abuse counselors and therapists, fidelity in the delivery of original and validated EVTs has also been remarkably low [7].

Regarding efforts at local adaptation, teachers from schools populated by high percentages of racial/ethnic minority students have been most active in making relevant adaptations. These adaptations have focused on three major content areas: (a) adding content on preventing youth violence, (b) accommodating limited English proficiency students, and (c) addressing issues relevant for racial and ethnic minority students [40]. Although this issue relates to substance use preventive interventions for adolescents within the United States, these adaptation issues parallel similar concerns in the adaptation of drug abuse treatments within the United States, as implemented with major racial/ethnic minority populations—African Americans, Hispanics/Latinos, Asian Americans, and Native Americans.

Furthermore, adaptations conducted not only to accommodate cultural variations within nations but also conducted to make interventions developed in one nation more suitable for use in other countries [27]. The complexities of international adaptations will also be discussed later in this chapter.

36.1.2 Issues Involving Fidelity and Adaptation

Fidelity refers to the extent to which a treatment is delivered as originally developed and implemented by the treatment's manualized procedures that have been validated within one or more randomized controlled trials [19]. By contrast, the *adaptation* of a model treatment refers to modifications in one or more treatment components or activities to increase treatment *relevance* and *effectiveness* for a specific cultural subgroup of clients [9]. Such modifications often focus on treatment contents, activities, or forms of implementation that neglect or conflict with the needs of a cultural subgroup of clients. Ideally, such adaptations will increase intervention *reach, participant engagement*, as well as intervention *efficacy*, and *sustainability* [1]. Presently, this Fidelity-Adaptation Dilemma [13] has been reframed from the original polarized perspective that pitted fidelity against adaptation, to an integrative perspective that acknowledges the importance of both approaches. This reframed view asserts that implementation fidelity to the theoretical foundations of the intervention is important, yet so it well planned flexibility to adapt certain aspects of the EBI to respond to "real-world" issues, particularly in response to issues central to the lives of individuals from culturally diverse populations.

In principle, each EBI should be broadly disseminated, thus making that treatment readily available to many communities and consumers [44]. Nonetheless, and as noted, in practice this broad-based dissemination and implementation have not been fully realized [7]. Since the emergence of fidelity-adaptation controversies, efforts to adapt model treatments have become "the rule rather than the exception" [40]. This suggests that there may exist few truly "universal" or "one-size-fits all" interventions that work well for nearly everyone, and thus not in need of local adaptations. This universality appears to diminish when treating more complex health and mental heathy problem, such as obesity reduction or the treatment of post-traumatic stress disorder. A more realistic scenario is that some form of *local adaptation* will be necessary, at least in the form of a linguistic translation, although it is likely that other cultural modifications will likely be necessary.

36.1.3 Lessons Learned From the Clinical Trials Network

Regarding efficacious outcomes from drug abuse treatments, Carroll and collaborators summarized the lessons learned from 10 years of research from the National Institute on Drug Abuse Clinical Trials Network [7]. Regarding emergent issues that affect empirically validated therapies (EVTs) for drug abuse treatment, these investigators noted that (a) retention in treatment remains a major problem in substance abuse treatment, since treatment retention is critical to treatment success; (b) EVTs are still not broadly implemented in practice, (c) when implemented are often delivered with low fidelity; and (d) at the agency level, effort, support, and commitment are essential factors for adopting and sustaining an EVT, given the costs of implementation, staff training, and supervision [7]. Given the importance of client retention, along with the problem of low utilization of EVTs, these issues should be addressed in the design of future EVTs to promote client retention by enhancing the treatment's cultural relevance as this can increase client engagement [26].

36.1.4 Intervention Dissemination and Implementation Within Diverse Settings

A major problem that has limited the widespread dissemination and implementation of evidence-based interventions (EBIs) is that despite their established effectiveness, these EBIs have attained limited adoption and utilization within various community and healthcare service settings [25]. Thus, the design of future EBIs could benefit from the addition of a preintervention "integration module," for effectively "grounding" the EBI within any of several service delivery settings. This integration module would focus not on intervention *content*, but instead on the intervention's *structural features* to promote a seamless "fit and function" within a given setting [20], by integrating the EBI in congruence with the structure and operations of a local community or service agency.

This integration module may also enhance the EBI's *acceptability* among the local community of consumers, while also enhancing the interventions capacity for *engagement* among these consumers, across the various forms of engagement: attendance, enrollment retention, consumer satisfaction, in-session participation, and home practice [1]. This integration module could build upon and operate as an abbreviated form of the *Planned Intervention Adaptation Framework* that involves conducting one or more preintervention studies to inform forthcoming adaptation activities [46]. The difference would be that these integration modules would aim to promote EBI fit and function within a short period of time thus preparing the EBI and the agency (intervention-setting congruence) for the EBI's effective implementation within as short a time as possible.

Generally, this integration module would be designed to align with: (a) the *interventions of structural characteristics*, for example, adaptability, design quality and packaging, cost, etc.; (b) the healthcare treatment setting's *inner setting characteristics*, that is, structural characteristics, communication networks, institutional culture, implementation climate, readiness for implementation; and (c) the *characteristics of participating individuals*, for example, their knowledge and beliefs about the intervention, self-efficacy, individual stage of change, among other relevant personal characteristics [15].

In summary, the issue of significant limitations in EBI dissemination and implementation into "real-world" community and healthcare delivery settings, as has occurred within the United States, may be regarded as a subset of the larger and more complex issue that involves the dissemination and implementation of EBIs across diverse nations, cultures, and settings worldwide. This emerging challenge can be addressed with the use of the community participatory approach to organize stakeholders from the nation or community interested in adopting a specific EBI, in collaboration with stakeholders from the United States (or another nation) that has developed the original EBI. Much interesting and greatly needed research and planning can be conducted in developing these preintervention "integration modules," for improving the widespread dissemination, implementation, adoption, utilization, and sustainability of these EBIs, thus to hasten their availability for prevention and treatment to improve health outcomes worldwide.

36.1.5 Cultural Considerations in Drug Abuse Treatment

In 1999, the National Institute on Drug Abuse (NIDA) published *NIDA's 13 Principles of Drug Addiction Treatment* [34]. It is noteworthy that none of these 13 principles directly addressed issues of *culture* in the treatment of drug-dependent clients [12]. A few years earlier, issues of culture and ethnicity have been recognized as important for the complete and culturally sensitive treatment of many clients, and primarily for those from racial/ethnic backgrounds [24, 47]. Terrell [47] discussed several strategies for the design and implementation of efficacious alcohol and drug abuse treatments for racial/ethnic minority clients. These strategies include (a) assessing the client's immigration and acculturation experiences including *acculturation stress*, as a factor that can erode the protective effects of the client's traditional or native culture, (b) assessing a client's experiences with *discrimination*, and (c) developing *culturally responsive* treatment interventions [47]. Today, the contextual factors of race, ethnicity, gender, sexual orientation, and other cultural factors or contextual factors are important for a more complete treatment of diverse drug-dependent clients [10, 12, 46].

Beyond cultural issues, some of these 13 principles may be regarded as elements of a drug abuse treatment that can operate as core treatment components. The multiplicity of these NIDA principles also underscores the complexities inherent in the delivery of a comprehensive drug abuse treatment. Such treatment also includes the need for ongoing monitoring of client progress, and the ongoing clinical need to make relevant adjustments to optimize treatment by tailoring it to the client's needs [6].

36.2 Description of Approach

36.2.1 Exemplar of a Tested and Effective Drug Abuse Treatment Program

The Matrix Model is a manualized multicomponent model treatment. In its basic form, the Matrix Model consists of a 16-week program delivered in 3 sessions per week for a total of 48 sessions [35]. The Matrix Model treatment includes (a) 12 family therapy sessions, (b) 4 social support group sessions, (c) 4 individual treatment sessions, and (d) a weekly breath alcohol testing and urine testing protocol. This treatment is nonjudgmental and nonconfrontational and includes positive reinforcement from therapists and peers for appropriate behavior change [23, 38].

The Matrix Model was developed from the integration of empirically based interventions and "grassroots" clinical experiences [38]. This manualized treatment includes patient handouts and a patient workbook that introduce evidence-based recovery activities as developed from the integration of five theory-based treatment approaches: (a) motivational interviewing, (b) early recovery phase treatment activities, (c) cognitive-behavioral therapy (CBT) including contingency management, (d) family therapy, and (e) 12-step facilitation [35]. As developed from these five treatment approaches, the formal *core components* of the Matrix Model consist of (a) early recovery phase treatment activities, (b) individual sessions, (c) urine testing, (d) family and conjoint sessions, (e) family education groups, (f) social support groups, (g) relapse analysis, and (h) relapse prevention training.

The Matrix Model is guided by eight *treatment principles*: (a) create explicit structure and expectations; (b) establish a positive collaborative relationship with the client; (c) teach information and cognitive-behavioral concepts; (d) reinforce positive behavior change; (e) provide corrective feedback when necessary; (f) educate the family regarding stimulant/drug abuse recovery; (g) introduce and encourage self-participation; (h) use urinalysis to monitor drug use ([38]; J. Obert, personal communication, April 2, 2013).

36.2.2 Cultural Adaptation of the Matrix Model

In principle, the cultural adaptation of the Matrix Model or any EVT begins by identifying problems in treatment implementation, and also by identifying sources of client-treatment mismatches (non-fit) [9]. This is followed by making planned adaptations in treatment content, activities, or forms of delivery, as recommended by consumer feedback from key informants, stakeholders, and as reviewed by a Cultural Advisory Committee. These adaptations would be accomplished: (a) while seeking to maintain identified core treatment components (essential program activities); (b) increasing the cultural relevance of the treatment for local consumers (clients and subcultural groups); (c) increasing client motivation, engagement and treatment involvement; (d) sustaining the efficacy of the treatment effect (i.e., maintaining the "effect size" on targeted outcomes); and (e) ideally increasing the treatment's "effect size" [8], that is, producing a greater and clinically significant magnitude of improvement on targeted outcome variables.

Moreover, effective cultural adaptation can ideally advance "beyond the black box," meaning that these adaptations would introduce: (a) a greater understanding of how cognitive-behavioral theory or the treatment's *logic model* produces therapeutic improvements on targeted outcome variables, and (b) greater knowledge of how cultural treatment factors improve the treatment's relevance for addressing client needs, while also increasing the treatment's effect size.

Reducing client-treatment mismatches Conceptually, the greater the gap or *mismatch* between the EBI's core concepts and activities, and the needs and preferences of a clients, the greater the adaptive changes necessary to fit the needs of a targeted group of clients. For implementation in international venues, a relevant question is, "In what ways should an original EVT developed for American drug dependent clients be modified for application with specific groups of clients from another country?" In this regard, within the United States, certain "mainstream treatments," which were designed for middle class White American clients, have been shown to be insensitive to the needs of many low-income African American and other racial/ethnic minority clients [5, 10]. This observation led to calls not only for *cultural sensitivity* in treatment development [45] but also for greater *cultural competence* [41] among the counselors or therapists who would deliver these treatments. Such observations ultimately prompted the development of stage models for adapting model treatments (an original EBI) to better fit the needs of specific cultural subgroups [3].

Need for gender sensitivity Historically, one example regerding the need to adapt prior drug abuse treatments is that they were originally developed for treating drug dependent *male* clients, thus inadvertently insensitive to the needs of many *female* drug dependent clients [22]. Such treatments did little to address certain critical

issues affecting drug-dependent women, such as their victimization from domestic violence. Thus, gender-sensitive programs were developed for delivery to drug-dependent women. Unfortunately, these treatments, when compared with conventional mixed-gender treatments, in randomized controlled trials have *not* been shown to be more effective in promoting recovery among drug-dependent women. Nonetheless, these gender-sensitive treatments have shown greater acceptability in addressing the common needs of drug-dependent women [22].

36.3 Evidence to Support the Approach

36.3.1 Evidence Regarding the Effects of Core Components

In principle, intervention activities and procedures that constitute a treatment's "core components" are based on theory and on clinical procedures shown empirically to produce desired therapeutic effects. For example, a treatment that utilizes principles from Social Cognitive Theory and cognitive-behavioral procedures, for example, contingency management, might exhibit near-universal effects on human behavior, and thus generally applicable for treating clients from many parts of the world [25].

Given that the Matrix Model is based on Social Cognitive Theory, as well as on principles from cognitive-behavioral therapy (CBT) and family systems therapies, its major core components are (a) family sessions, (b) enhancing social supports, (c) individual treatment sessions, and (d) breathalyzer and urine testing. Furthermore, in principle, within an adapted version of this model treatment, none of these core treatment components should be eliminated or modified. For example, the Matrix Model treatment might lose some of its treatment effectiveness if breathalyzer and urine testing were eliminated within a culturally adapted version of the original Matrix Model.

36.3.2 Evidence on the Need for Assessing Cultural Factors

A study in Belgium illustrates several core issues were examined in an international setting regarding the role of cultural factors in drug abuse treatment. That study conducted a qualitative analysis using in-depth interviews with drug treatment center staff and clients [48]. First, these investigators reported on problems emerging from the existing treatment system's client database it did not distinguish the construct of "ethnicity" from "nationality." This omission lacked information on ethnic issues, as these were conflated with very different issues that involve clients' nationality. From ethnic themes emerging from these interviews, ethnic clients complained that the drug treatment lacked cultural responsiveness. Another theme involved cultural barriers in communication with the therapist, as these barriers became detrimental to progress in treatment. Other barriers included clients' perceptions that their own treatment needs conflicted with their therapist's Westernized world views.

Ironically, most of these clients and therapists recommended that developing a separate ethnic-specific treatment program would *not* be useful. Clients recommended retaining the conventional treatment, although supplemented with attention to cultural factors and issues [48]. This outcome underscores the need to base drug abuse treatment on established scientific principles of recovery from addiction, while also attending to issues of culture and local client needs. Such cultural issues can be addressed without replacing the treatment in its entirety, by adding one or more modules to the original treatment, to address specific cultural issues. Although data are limited, evidence exists that adaptations that are additions to core components are associated with positive intervention outcomes, but changes to components and their deletions are not [1].

36.3.3 Evidence Regarding Engagement and Retention

Issues in reducing the number of sessions As noted previously, in drug abuse treatment, several challenges exist involving client engagement and retention [7]. One approach to increase treatment engagement and retention among youth and families is to reduce the total number of program sessions, for example, from 12 to 8 sessions. However, some evidence indicates that reduction in sessions can also diminish program effectiveness [26], as clients retain less essential knowledge and skills due to this reduction in sessions.

Indices of treatment outcome Based on research conducted with the Matrix Model, major indicators of client retention are (a) *engagement*—staying in treatment as assessed at the 2-week and 1-month observations; (b) *retention*—staying in treatment as measured by the number of weeks remaining in treatment, with a maximum of 16 weeks, and also as measured by staying in treatment for 90 days or more, versus less than 90 days; (c) *abstinence*—as indicated by the average number of drug-free urinalysis tests collected during treatment, and the occurrence of three consecutive drug-free urine analyses during treatment; and (d) *completion*—the completion of the 16-week Matrix Model treatment with no more than two consecutive missed weeks of treatment versus noncompletion of this 16-week program [23]. These indices of client treatment participation are likely correlated, although each provides slightly different indicators of treatment effects.

36.4 International Considerations

36.4.1 General Considerations in Dissemination and Implementation

A major Matrix Model treatment goal involves its broad dissemination to enhance the availability for treating drug-dependent clients [43]. The successful dissemination and implementation of evidence-based interventions (EBIs) and of empirically validated therapies (EVTs) offer great potential for enhancing public health and well-being [44]. This approach, identified as "Type 2 translation research," involves generating scientific evidence on best approaches for (a) building community and agency infrastructures to deliver EVTs and EBIs, (b) creating practitioner-scientist partnerships, and (c) establishing effective implementation procedures for adopting, implementing, and sustaining EBIs and EVTs within diverse community settings [44].

As an exemplar of this pursuit, the Matrix Model has been translated into nine languages, and disseminated to over 6000 therapists or counselors in the United States and internationally, as taught by 320 key supervisors. These supervisors have conducted Matrix Model training in 21 countries and in all 50 of states of the United States, resulting in staff training conducted in over 2500 treatment agencies (J. Obert, personal communication, April 2, 2013).

Based on challenges from Matrix Model dissemination efforts as conducted in Thailand, Mexico, and in other countries worldwide, the developers of the Matrix Model offer several observations to guide future dissemination and implementation efforts. First, despite the availability of a published Matrix Model treatment manual, this treatment cannot be delivered effectively from this manual alone; formal training of Matrix Model implementers is necessary. Second, at the organizational and community levels, agency and civic leaders must understand fundamental aspects of drug abuse treatment, to provide appropriate support that ensures correct treatment implementation, and avoids administrative decisions that conflict with or that undermine Matrix Model principles and activities (J. Obert, personal communication, April 2, 2013). Third, dissemination efforts are best guided by a clear dissemination plan that is monitored for quality and professionalism in its implementation. Based on prior difficulties encountered in initial dissemination efforts, the developers of the Matrix Model also designed a certification program to ensure quality in training of Matrix Model therapists and counselors. The aim is to implement this treatment with requisite fidelity and with treatment insights regarding fidelity of implementation and/or adaptation planning when encountering problems in the implementation of the Matrix Model (J. Obert, personal communication, April 2, 2013).

36.4.2 General Considerations in International Adaptations

The world is a diverse place in which cultural diversity is expressed in a multiplicity of spoken languages, variations in literacy levels, diversity of religious and cultural systems of beliefs, and a multiplicity of sociocultural attitudes, values, and norms as exhibited across nations, and even within nation (REF). Within this context, worldwide there exists a dynamic tension between the sociocultural forces of *modernization* and quests for change, versus *traditionalism* and quests for the preservation of tradition and a resistance to change [42]. Factors that promote modernism, such as international globalization, emphasize growth and standardization, and operate as forces that tend to homogenize cultural practices. By contrast, factors that promote traditionalism and its indigenous perspectives [37] tend to diversify whole populations into distinct cultural subgroups, emphasizing the retention of unique cultural and local identities and lifeways. These broad cultural influences provide a systemic context against which to consider the cultural adaptation of EBIs and EVTs.

36.4.3 Stage Models of Adaptation and Applications Across Cultures

Within the past decade, several stage models have been developed to guide the cultural adaptation of prevention and treatment interventions [2, 16, 27, 49]. Several of those models were developed for the adaptation of treatments developed initially for majority middle-class populations within the United States, as these original EBIs or EVTs could be modified for greater relevance as delivered to member of the major US subcultural groups, that is, African Americans, Hispanics/Latinos, Asian Americans, Native Americans. However, with a few exceptions [27, 49], cultural adaptation models have *not* been developed for international applications in which EVTs and EBIs created in one country have been adapted culturally for use in another country.

Segmentation: Beyond "country" or "nationality" as the unit of analysis One important way to reframe the approach to cultural adaptation is to avoid a one-size-fits all approach, such as planning to adapt the Matrix Model to be equally effective across the entire country of Mexico. A more useful approach is to consider adaptation for a *local community* or *region* of a country, given the remarkable within-country heterogeneity that exists within most countries worldwide. In other words, sensibly adapting an original EVT "for Mexico" requires a more refined approach to adaptation, one that considers a *smaller unit of analysis* rather than adaptation for an entire nation. Adaptation to a local region or to a local community is critically important. This more *micro-level* approach advances beyond an "ethnic gloss" that occurs under a more *macro-level* of analysis, that is, the nation, given that a macro-approach often glosses over important within-country variations.

For example, in considering the cultural adaptation of the Matrix Model for use "in the country of Mexico," besides a translation from English to Spanish, this adaptation would also require variations for its use within large urban and lower- and middle-class environments, such as within Mexico City and Guadalajara. By contrast, a second modified and adapted version may be needed for use with residents from rural and indigenous communities, such as with residents from rural communities from the Mexican states of Chiapas and Yucatan. For example, within indigenous Mexico, some local residents have very low literacy levels, and may not communicate well in Spanish, with some who do not speak Spanish as their preferred language. Thus, a linguistic adaptation of the Matrix Model to Spanish could render this adapted version culturally relevant only in part, when administered with an indigenous cultural subgroup from the region of rural Chiapas, Mexico. Moreover, such a linguistic adaptation alone would not address long standing cultural traditions, thus also highlighting the need for a local or regional cultural adaptation. Some rural indigenous males from this region of Mexico may also have culturally based *macho*

gender role norms and expectations that confer them with considerable male authority and privilege over their family and within their community. Such traditions and cultural practices must be addressed if this treatment is to engage such clients in culturally relevant activities, and operate effectively with the male residents of this local community.

36.4.4 Approaches to International Adaptation

Planning for the cultural adaptation of an intervention A recent article has presented an international model of intervention adaptations, an approach titled, *Planned Intervention Adaptation* (PIA) [46]. The authors described PIA as a synthesis of several models that outline stages or conceptual frameworks for systematically adapting interventions for applications in new cultural contexts [46]. PIA consists of two broad phases that were inspired by Resnicow and colleagues, who distinguished between the concepts of "deep structure" elements of an intervention, from "surface structure" elements [39].

In reality, PIA is not fundamentally different than other cultural adaptation stage models (see Barrera et al. [3]). However, it does distinguish itself from others in the detail of its recommendations. For example, PIA specifies a time period for the initial adaptation stages and a sampling strategy for formative studies. Phase 1 of PIA consists roughly of a 1.5–2 year period when intervention developers and stakeholders (agency staff, potential consumers) agree to collaborate on five preliminary steps that are summarized in a table and detailed in text (e.g., language translations, tests of translated materials, focus group checks on the cultural appropriateness of intervention materials and activities). These preliminary steps help to shape the adapted intervention.

In Phase 2 of PIA, the authors recommend conducting a three-arm effectiveness study which would consist of (a) a minimally adapted intervention (solely surface structure changes such as language translation), (b) a fully adapted intervention (both surface and deep structure changes), and (c) a control condition. However, even for this recommendation, given the complexities in conducting *conceptually equivalent* linguistic translations, a linguistic translation itself may actually involve more than just surface changes. The PIA also recommends the inclusion of appropriate measures and data analytic procedures to identify possible mediators and moderators of intervention effects [30]. Unfortunately, based on Sundell et al.'s [46] article, it is not certain that the PIA framework actually has been used in the international adaptation of an original EVT intervention.

Undoubtedly, the best examples of international adaptations involve studies of the Strengthening Families Program (SFP), a family skills intervention for the prevention of youth substance abuse [27]. SFP was initially developed and tested in the United States, and subsequently has been adapted for applications in Australia, Canada, Central America, Europe, South America, and Southeast Asia. The results of that work have been summarized with the following statement ([28], p. 176).

> Replications of SFP in non-experimental and quasi-experimental studies in about 17 countries and randomized control trials (RCTs) in nine countries (United States, Canada, Australia, UK, Sweden, Netherlands, Spain, Italy, and Thailand) with different cultural groups by independent evaluators have found SFP to be an effective program in reducing multiple risk factors for later alcohol and drug abuse, mental health problems and delinquency by increasing family strengths, children's social competencies and improving parent's parenting skills.

Kumpfer and her colleagues [29] details 10 steps that should be followed in creating an international adaptation of SFP, and perhaps for other evidence-based programs. Table 36.1 summarizes these 10 steps. Kumpfer et al. [27] illustrated the steps with examples from their extensive experience in many countries. This article contains guidance and best practices for those who are planning international adaptations of evidence-based interventions.

A case analysis of the cultural adaptation of a preventive intervention for Mexico An efficacious prevention intervention originally designed and tested in the Southwest United States was culturally adapted with and for Mexico youth. The intervention's name is *keepin' it REAL (kiR)*, a widely used prevention program in the United States with some localized cultural adaptations in Mexico [31]. This more comprehensive adaptation effort includes the three largest cities in Mexico; NIDA/NIH funded the study.

To learn from the end users what was in need of adaptation, one school in each city implemented the linguistic adapted version of the intervention. The research team collected data regarding cultural adaptation through (a) *focus groups with students:* More than 100 students participated in 21 focus groups; 73 students from 7th grade and 30 from 9th grade; (b) *focus groups with teachers:* At each site, three teachers who implemented *kiR* discussed their curriculum reactions in a focus group format; (c) *lesson fidelity observations:* The team conducted 47 classroom fidelity observations; (d) *teacher reflection forms and notes:* At the end of each lesson, all implementing teachers ($n = 9$) completed a reflection form assessing cultural appropriateness of the lessons; (e) *external Expert Reviews:* The study team sought input and feedback from five external expert reviewers to ensure the adaptations were appropriate and representative of the study sites.

The team developed a coding system and process to establish consistent meanings among the coders [33]. Six research team members—three bilingual coders from U.S. and three from Mexico conducted coding independently. By employing multiple data sources and relying on Mexican partners in this adaptation process, the surface and deep structure adaptations made to the *kiR* curriculum increased the chances that *kiR* will be successful in Mexico and provide an opportunity to extend knowledge and expertise to create a national substance use prevention programming for Mexico. This process enabled the team to preserve the core elements of the curriculum while making the necessary adaptations to enhance cultural fit across diverse settings. As a result, other researchers can employ this approach to develop culturally relevant and scientifically sound prevention interventions.

Table 36.1 Two systematic approaches to cultural adaptation

Step	Action (from Ref. [28])	Stage	Action
1	*Needs Assessment*—Collect needs assessment information from new or existing data to determine major family risk and protective factors for child developmental problems	1	*Information Gathering*—Review of the current drug treatment literature and a screening of client-treatment mismatches
2	*Literature Review*—Collect information from research literature or websites on appropriate family skills. Select the best program for age, ethnicity and risk level of families (e.g., universal, selective, or indicated prevention approaches)		
3	*Cultural Adaptation Team*—Create a cultural adaptation team including family members and the original program developer	2	*Preliminary Adaptation Design*—Propose adapted modifications of specific mismatched content or activities for the original model treatment
4	*Linguistic Translation*—Translate into local language and do minor cultural adaptations		
5	*Initial Implementation*—Implement "as is" with minimal adaptation at first	3	*Preliminary Adaptation Test*—Test this pilot adaptation to assess how well it works with clients from the targeted subcultural client group
6	*Implementation of Initial Changes*—Have implementers from local culture make gradual changes based on what works (culturally appropriate language, stories, and songs)		
7	*Ongoing Cultural Adaptations*—Continuously make additional cultural adaptations and add to curriculum with the program developer's approval	4	*Adaptation Refinement*—Using client feedback from the prior stage, make adjustments on revisions to refine the emerging adapted model treatment
8	*Ongoing Evaluation*—Continuously conduct pre-and post-test evaluations on each family group to measure if the local cultural adaptations are making the program better or worse	5	*Cultural Adaptation Test*—As viable, conduct a small scale or ideally a large scale randomized controlled trial to formally assess the efficacy of the adapted model treatment, as compared with the original model treatment, and ideally also against a treatment as usual (TAU) control group
9	*Add or Drop Adaptations*—Make adjustments to add or drop new cultural adaptations		
10	*Dissemination to Similar Groups*—Disseminate the culturally adapted version to similar cultural groups if effective		

36.5 Conducting a Streamlined Cultural Adaptation: A Five-Stage Model

We recognize that many drug abuse treatment programs in the United States, and in various communities worldwide are delivered within medical centers and in a variety of community-based agencies, large and small. These professional settings often lack the requisite research infrastructure (the program evaluation or research staff, the funding and time, and other research or evaluation resources) to conduct a formalized and months-long randomized controlled clinical trial to test the efficacy of an EVT adaptation as described by Sundell and colleagues and by Kumpfer and colleagues.

36.5.1 A Practical Approach to the Cross-Cultural Adaptation of a Treatment Program

How then might a treatment center or community-based agency conduct a cost-effective, culturally responsive, and scientifically defensible cultural adaptation of an original EVT? Within such an abbreviated cultural adaptation effort, to avoid engaging in misadaptation, we encourage rigor in the application of scientific and community-based participatory research procedures (CBPR) [32]. This abbreviated approach would aim to achieve, and perhaps enhance, certain targeted treatment outcomes: (a) treatment engagement, (b) retention in treatment, (c) abstinence from drug use, and (d) program completion [23]. In addition, as noted, another goal is to avoid introducing iatrogenic effects as consequences of misadaptation.

36.5.2 General Strategy and Procedures for a Streamlined Intervention Adaptation

An initial assessment step in the cultural adaptation of an original EVT is to establish a Cultural Advisory Committee to identify and address cultural and other forms of local problems in treatment implementation and in client-treatment mismatches. Such culturally incongruous contents or activities refer to treatment elements that are confusing, objectionable (low acceptability), or culturally offensive to members of a targeted subcultural client group. Under a community-based participatory research approach (CBPR), these forms of mismatch are identified by conducting *focus groups, key advisor, (key informant) interviews,* and interviews with *stakeholders,* as well as with individuals who represent future recipients of this treatment [36]. It would also be important to conduct interviews with agency therapists or counselors. The identification and assessment of cultural mismatches would reveal significant problems in EVT implementation within the agency or setting, as well as approaches for correcting them. If not identified and addressed initially, such sources of "cultural non-fit" can alienate members of a targeted client group and could induce them to drop out of treatment.

Castro, Barrera and Martinez [9] outlined three major dimensions of model treatment adaptation. These three major dimensions are (a) *cognitive-information processing* characteristics such as language and age/developmental or literacy levels; (b) *affective-motivational* characteristics, including gender, racial/ethnic identity and background, religious background, socioeconomic status, as these factors can influence clients' comfort in accepting the EVT's messages and activities; and (c) *environmental* characteristics, including ecological aspects of the client's local community.

Cognitive-informational adaptation This involves modifying program contents or activities so that clients can understand them. In international adaptations, this would involve a linguistic translation for equivalence in meaning (conceptual equivalence), and not in a word-for-word translation [21]. This should consider the literacy level of members of the targeted subcultural group.

Affective-motivational adaptation This involves modifications of program content or activities that can induce *cultural conflict* or that *prompt reactance* (behavioral resistance). An example might be a Westernized cultural approach requiring male clients to publicly disclose their drug dependence or to discuss sexual issues in the presence of certain family members. Without understanding the possible cultural implications, that practice might be perceived by traditional culture males as inappropriate, feeling stigmatized and resisting participation in an important treatment activity. Conversely, as a culturally modest adaptation, eliminating a discussion of stimulant use as a trigger for sexual arousal and behaviors could undermine drug treatment, given the association between stimulant use and sexual activity as a trigger of a relapse episode (J. Obert, personal communication, April 2, 2013). Thus, a discussion of benefits and liabilities from such adaptations is critical for making sound adaptation decisions that are both culturally sensitive and that also adhere to scientific principles of effective drug abuse treatment.

Environmental adaptation This involves therapeutic changes in a client's family system, in the living situation, and within the treatment agency, thus modifying local environment conditions to aid in the client's recovery. Within this domain, two basic forms of adaptation consist of (a) modifying *program content,* which relates to the environment, and (b) modifying the *form of program delivery.* Modification of content would include shallow or deep-structure changes. Changes in form of delivery would involve presenting the same treatment content, with changes in (a) *characteristics of delivery personnel*—lay health workers rather than health educators; (b) *channel of delivery*—internet delivery rather than a group session; or (c) *location of delivery*—improving access by delivering the program within a church setting, rather than within a drug treatment center.

36.5.3 Five Basic Stages in a Local or Cultural Adaptation

In a version that parallels Kumpfer's ten-step approach to cultural adaptations, the cultural or *local adaptation* of an original drug abuse model treatment (an empirically validated therapy—an EVT) can be conducted via a basic five-stage process [3]. Ideally, this five-stage process is conducted formally under a randomized controlled trial. In the absence of that option, four of these five stages can be conducted using a community-based participatory research (CBPR) approach as overseen by a well-informed Cultural Adaptation Committee (CAC). Accordingly, this adaptation effort as conducted by a drug treatment agency would be conducted: (a) with the aid and oversight of a Cultural Adaptation Committee, and (b) using CBPR procedures to facilitate input

from key advisors, stakeholders, and agency staff to review consumer feedback for a culturally sensitive and scientifically informed analysis of appropriate adaptations. The CBPR approach is a bidirectional approach involving a collective dialogue and group decisions for adapting an original EVT [17]. Table 36.1 presents these five stages as described by Barrera and colleagues [3]. Based in this framework and process, these five stages are as follows:

Information Gathering This involves qualitative research with potential participants and community experts who are familiar with working with targeted cultural groups; and review relevant drug treatment literature as background to identify implementation problems and sources of client-treatment mismatches, as linked to the three major dimensions of cultural adaptation assessment, along with proposed adaptive changes that consider (a) participant characteristics, (b) program delivery staff, and (c) administrative/community factors (see [9]).

Preliminary Adaptation Design *This involves integrating the information and data collected* by the Cultural Adaptation Committee which is staffed by (a) select stakeholders, (b) community experts, (c) developers of the model treatment, and (d) former drug treatment clients or their representatives (treatment insiders); and if needed, other important representatives from the local community or treatment center. A general aim will be to preserve the core interview components, unless there exists strong evidence that one or more aspects of a core component is detrimental to the well-being of clients from the targeted constituency.

Preliminary Adaptation Tests This involves conducting a pilot test of the preliminary adapted version of the original EVT. to assess (a) the elimination of prior implementation difficulties, (b) the emergence of problems with content or activities, (c) client satisfaction with treatment elements, and (d) planned adaptations for improving identified problems.

Adaptation Refinement This involves revising the adapted intervention. Then, if viable as a more formal adaptation activity, proceed to stage 5. That stage involves:

The Cultural Adaptation Trial Formally determine the efficacy of this adapted version by comparing it to a treatment as usual (TAU) control group, and ideally to the original EVT. It will also be important to assess the adapted version's improvements over the original EVT on indicators of client acceptability, engagement, attendance, treatment completion. Although seldom evaluated, within the cultural adaptation trial stage, intervention evaluators could also assess the effects of the adapted EVT on specified mediators and moderators [30]. For example, if a culturally adapted EVT adds a cultural pride component for a mediation analyses to determine whether the intervention was effective in enhancing cultural pride, and then if cultural pride enhancement exerts an effect in reducing drug use or in avoiding relapse. Similarly, moderator analyses could be examine if the culturally adapted EVT was differentially effective: (a) for men versus for women, (b) for clients high versus low in levels of acculturation, (c) among immigrants versus natives, or (d) for any other potential moderators of intervention efficacy [4].

Use of a mixed methods methodology This adaptation analysis could utilize a rigorous mixed methods research design [14], one that includes in-depth interviews with participants and interventionists, for an in-depth assessment of treatment outcomes that provides more complex information on intervention process, client responses to the intervention, and other aspects of this adapted version [11]. This mixed methods approach could provide a deep-structure analysis of client and therapist commentaries on factors that (a) may operate as new core treatment components, (b) may operate as sources of problems within treatment, and (c) worked very well and should be kept, along with (d) client feedback for enhancing the content or delivery of treatment

modes to aid in treatment revisions as incorporated into a future enhancement of adaptation.

36.6 Some Recommendations for Adaptation of Drug Abuse EVTs

From this analysis of the cultural adaptation of EVTs and EVIs and their international considerations, we offer a few observations and recommendations.

1. *Identifying robust principles and guidelines for effective cultural adaptations.* There exists the need to identify a few principles and guidelines, such as the principle of "knowing the theories and goals at the core of each intervention component, to avoid changing the core approach when making an adaptation to address participants' cultural or other needs and preferences."

2. *Increasing treatment relevance and "fit and function" with clients and within the treatment setting.* A treatment that not designed for the needs of a specific cultural subgroup may exhibit insensitivity to that group's needs and preferences. EBI implementers can assess aspects of a treatment that lack relevance to the needs of a local group of participants, thus to consider adaptations to address those needs, while still maintaining fidelity to the EBI's major therapeutic thrusts.

3. *Recognizing the importance of cultural factors.* Recent studies have highlighted the importance of considering various cultural factors and contextual influences. These factors include gender, racial or ethnic identity, sexual orientation, levels of acculturation as influences on recovery from drug dependence. Drug abuse treatments can be enhanced by infusing cultural sensitivity and relevant cultural contents and activities to promote full recovery among diverse drug-dependent clients and to avoid relapse [12].

4. *Increasing cultural relevance without reconstructing a treatment.* Increasing an existing EBI's cultural relevance need not involve a

complete reconstruction of an existing EBI. Adding a relevant treatment module or culturally relevant content and activities may be sufficient to enhance treatment relevance and client-treatment fit.

5. *Enhancing client engagement and intervention acceptability*. Client engagement in treatment is important to promote client retention and treatment completion. Low engagement can affect treatment efficacy and the benefits that can be derived from that treatment [7]. It is thus essential that newly developed, adapted, or refined EBIs increase their capacity for client engagement.

6. *Cultural adaptation as a systematic and team effort*. The effective adaptation of an EBI benefits from a planned and systematic team effort that involves a scientist-provider partnership between the developers of the treatment and other stakeholders [17]. Organized agency structures can facilitate this partnership to promote well-planned and executed treatment adaptations. This also includes sustainability plans to fund and maintain the treatment well into the future.

References

1. Barrera M, Berkel C, Castro FG. Directions for the advancement of culturally adapted preventive interventions: local adaptations, engagement, and sustainability. Prev Sci. 2017;18:640–8. https://doi.org/10.1007/s11121-016-075-9.
2. Barrera M Jr, Castro FG. A heuristic framework for the cultural adaptation of interventions. Clin Psychol Sci Pract. 2006;13:311–6.
3. Barrera M Jr, Castro FG, Strycker LA, Toobert DJ. Cultural adaptation of behavioral health interventions: a progress report. J Consult Clin Psychol. 2013;81:196–205. https://doi.org/10.1037/a0027085.
4. Barrera M Jr, Toobert DJ, Strycker LA, Osuna D. Effects of acculturation on a culturally-adapted diabetes intervention for Latinas. Health Psychol. 2012;31:51–4. https://doi.org/10.1037/a0025205.
5. Bernal G, Adames C. Cultural adaptations: conceptual, ethical, contextual, and methodological issues for working with ethnocultural and majority-world populations. Prev Sci. 2017;18:681–8. https://doi.org/10.1007/s11121-017-0806-0.
6. Bernal G, Jimenez-Chafey MI, Domenech Rodriguez MM. Cultural adaptation of treatments: a resource for considering culture in evidence-based practice. Prof Psychol Res Pract. 2009;40:361–8.
7. Carroll KM, Ball SA, Jackson R, Martino S, Petry NM, Stitzer ML, et al. Ten take home lessons from the first 10 years of the CTN and 10 recommendations for the future. Am J Drug Alcohol Abuse. 2011;37:275–82.
8. Castro FG, Barrera M Jr, Holleran Steiker LK. Issues and challenges in the design of culturally adapted evidence-based interventions. Annu Rev Clin Psychol. 2010;6:213–39.
9. Castro FG, Barrera M Jr, Martinez CR. The cultural adaptation of prevention interventions: resolving tensions between fidelity and fit. Prev Sci. 2004;5:41–5.
10. Castro FG, Hernández-Alarcón E. Integrating cultural factors into drug abuse prevention and treatment with racial/ethnic minorities. J Drug Issues. 2002;32:783–810.
11. Castro FG, Morera OF, Kellison JG, Aguirre KM. Mixed methods research design for prevention science: methods, critiques and recommendations. In: Sloboda Z, Petras H, editors. Defining prevention science. New York: Springer; 2014. p. 453–90.
12. Castro FG, Nichols E, Kater K. Relapse prevention with Hispanic and other racial/ethnic populations: can cultural resilience promote relapse prevention? In: Witkiewitz K, Marlatt GA, editors. A therapist's guide to evidence-based relapse prevention. Boston: Academic Press; 2007. p. 259–92.
13. Castro FG, Yasui M. Advances in EBI development for diverse populations: towards a science of intervention adaptation. Prev Sci. 2017;18:623–9. https://doi.org/10.1007/s11121-017-0809-x.
14. Creswell JW, Creswell JD. Research design: qualitative, quantitative, and mixed methods approaches. Thousand Oaks: Sage; 2018.
15. Damschrader LJ, Hagedorn HJ. A guiding framework and approach for implementation research in substance use disorder treatment. Psychol Addict Behav. 2011;23(2):194–205.
16. Domenech-Rodriguez M, Wieling E. Developing culturally appropriate, evidence-based treatments for interventions with ethnic minority populations. In: Rastogi M, Wieling E, editors. Voices of color: first-person accounts of ethnic minority therapists. Thousand Oaks, CA: Sage. 2004; pp. 313–33.
17. Donovan DM, Daley DC, Brigham GS, Hodgkins CC, Perl H, Floyd AS. How practice and science are balanced and blended in the NIDA Clinical Trials Network: the bidirectional process in the development of the STAGE-12 protocol as an example. Am J Drug Alcohol Abuse. 2011;37:408–16.
18. Elliot DS, Mihalic S. Issues in disseminating and replicating effective prevention programs. Prev Sci. 2004;5:47–53.
19. Flay BR, Biglan A, Boruch RF, Castro FG, Gottfredson D, Kellum S, et al. Standards of evidence: criteria for efficacy, effectiveness and dissemination. Prev Sci. 2005;6(3):151–75. https://doi.org/10.1007/s11121-005-5553-y.
20. Gonzales NA. Expanding the cultural adaptation framework for population-level impact. Prev Sci. 2017;18:689–93.

21. Gonzalez VM, Stewart A, Ritter PL, Lorig K. Translation and validation of arthritis outcome measures into Spanish. Arthritis Rheum. 1995;38:1429–46.

22. Greenfield SF, Brooks AJ, Gordon SM, Green CA, Kropp F, McHugh RK, et al. Substance abuse treatment entry, retention, and outcome in women: a review of the literature. Drug Alcohol Depend. 2007;86:1–21.

23. Hillhouse MP, Martinelli-Casey P, Gonzales R, Ang A, Rawson RA. Predicting in-treatment performance and post-treatment outcomes in methamphetamine users. Addiction. 2007;102(Suppl. 1):84–95.

24. Ja D, Aoki B. Substance use treatment: cultural barriers in the Asian American community. J Psychoactive Drugs. 1993;25:61–71.

25. Karlin BE, Cross G. From the laboratory to the therapy room: national dissemination and implementation of evidence-based psychotherapies in the U.S. Department of Veterans Affairs health care system. Am Psychol. 2014;69(1):19–33.

26. Kumpfer KL, Alvarado R, Smith P, Bellamy N. Cultural sensitivity in universal family-based prevention interventions. Prev Sci. 2002;3:241–4.

27. Kumpfer KL, Pinyuchon M, de Melo A, Whiteside HO. Cultural adaptation process for international dissemination of the strengthening families program (SFP). Eval Health Prof. 2008;33(2):226–39.

28. Kumpfer KL, Xie J, O'Driscoll R. Effectiveness of a culturally adapted strengthening families program 12–16 years for high-risk Irish families. Child Youth Care Forum. 2012;41:173–95.

29. Kumpfer K, Magalhaes C, Xie J. Cultural adaptation of implementation of family evidence-based interventions with diverse populations. Prev Sci. 2017;18:649–659.

30. MacKinnon DP. Introduction to statistical mediation analysis. New York: Lawrence Erlbaum; 2008.

31. Marsiglia FF, Kulis S, Booth JM, Nuño-Gutiérrez BL, Robbins DE. Long-term effects of the *keepin'it REAL* model program in Mexico: substance use trajectories of Guadalajara middle school students. J Prim Prev. 2015;36:93–104.

32. Minkler M, Wallerstein N, Wilson N. Improving health through community organization and community building. In: Glanz K, Rimer BK, Viswanath K, editors. Health behavior and health education: theory, research and practice. 4th ed. San Francisco: Jossey-Bass; 2008. p. 287–312.

33. Morse JM. Critical analysis of strategies for determining rigor in qualitative inquiry. Qual Health Res. 2015;25:1212–22.

34. National Institute on Drug Abuse. Principles of drug addiction treatment: a research-based guide. NIH Publication No. 99-4180. Rockville: National Institute on Drug Abuse; 1999.

35. Obert JL, McCann MJ, Martinelli-Casey P, Weiner A, Minsky S, Brethen P, et al. The matrix model of out-patient stimulant abuse treatment: history and description. J Psychoactive Drugs. 2000;32:157–64.

36. Parsai MB, Castro FG, Marsiglia FF, Harthun M, Valdez H. Using community based participatory research to create a culturally grounded intervention for parents and youth to prevent risky behaviors. Prev Sci. 2011;12:34–47.

37. Ramirez M. Multicultural psychotherapy: an approach to individual and cultural differences. 2nd ed. Boston: Allyn & Bacon; 1999.

38. Rawson RA, Shoptaw SJ, Obert JL, McCann MJ, Hasson AL, Martinelli-Casey PJ, et al. An intensive approach to cocaine abuse treatment. J Subst Abuse Treat. 1995;12:117–27.

39. Resnicow K, Soler R, Braithwait RL, Ahluwalia JS, Butler J. Cultural sensitivity in substance abuse prevention. J Community Psychol. 2000;28:271–90.

40. Ringwald CL, Vincus A, Ennett S, Johnson R, Rohrbach LA. Reasons for teachers' adaptation of substance use prevention curricula in schools with non-white student populations. Prev Sci. 2004;5:61–7.

41. Schwartz A, Domenech Rodriguez MM, Santiago-Rivera AL, Arredondo P, Field LD. Cultural and linguistic competence: welcome challenges from successful diversification. Prof Psychol Res Pract. 2010;41:210–20.

42. Shiraev EB, Levy DA. Cross-cultural psychology: critical thinking and contemporary applications. Boston: Allyn & Bacon; 2010.

43. Shoptaw S, Rawson RA, McCann MJ, Obert JL. The matrix model of outpatient stimulant abuse treatment: evidence of efficacy. J Addict Dis. 1994;13(4):129–41.

44. Spoth R, Rohrbach LA, Greenberg M, Leif P, Brown H, Fagan A, et al. Addressing core challenges for the next generation of type 2 translation research and systems: the translation science to population impact (TSci Impact) framework. Prev Sci. 2013;14:319–51. https://doi.org/10.1007/s11121-012-0362-6.

45. Sue DW, Sue D. Counseling the culturally different: theory and practice. 3rd ed. New York: Wiley; 1999.

46. Sundell K, Ferrer-Wreder L, Fraser MW. Going global: a model for evaluating empirically supported family-based interventions in new contexts. Eval Health Prof. 2014;37(2):203–30. https://doi.org/10.1177/0163278712469813.

47. Terrell MD. Ethnocultural factors and substance abuse towards culturally sensitive treatment models. Psychol Addict Behav. 1993;7:162–7.

48. Vandevelde S, Vanderplasschen W, Broekaert E. Cultural responsiveness in substance-abuse treatment: a qualitative study using professionals and clients perspectives. Int J Soc Welf. 2003;12:221–8.

49. Wingood GM, DiClemente RJ. The ADAPT-ITT model: a novel method of adapting evidence-based HIV interventions. J Acquir Immune Defic Syndr. 2008;47:S40–6. https://doi.org/10.1097/QAI.0b013e3181605df1.

Multidisciplinary Management of Acute and Chronic Pain in the Presence of Substance Use Disorder (SUD)

37

Daniel L. Krashin, Natalia Murinova, and Jane Ballantyne

Contents

Abstract

The management of pain is greatly complicated by comorbid substance use disorder (SUD), particularly opioid use disorder. Patient with SUD may have more difficulty coping with pain, decreased response to analgesics, and higher rates of complications with pain treatment. Multimodal therapy that is personalized to the patient is much more effective for acute pain. Chronic pain treatment in the setting of SUD is particularly challenging. Chronic opioid therapy is now known to be riskier and less effective than was previously thought. Tapering high-dose opioids reduces risk and may improve functioning for some patients. Others respond poorly to taper and may respond better to buprenorphine substitution.

D. L. Krashin (✉) · N. Murinova · J. Ballantyne
University of Washington, Seattle, WA, USA
e-mail: krashind@uw.edu

© Springer Nature Switzerland AG 2021
N. el-Guebaly et al. (eds.), *Textbook of Addiction Treatment*,
https://doi.org/10.1007/978-3-030-36391-8_37

Keywords

Pain · Opioids · Substance · Addiction ·
Tapering · Buprenorphine

37.1   Introduction

Substance abuse and addiction have created crises in many countries, rich and poor, in many areas but particularly affecting healthcare. Addiction has continued to be a highly significant public health issue for decades, while the specific drugs of abuse have changed over time. In rich countries, prescription drug addiction has become a particularly challenging issue and area of rapid growth. This development has particularly effected prescription opioids in North America, as they are prescribed in greater amounts to more patients there than anywhere else in the world, particularly for non-cancer pain. The increase in the frequency and dosage of opioid prescribing in the USA was dramatic and has only recently begun to trail off [7]. The opioid crisis in the USA became obvious and severe in part due to prescription opioid misuse [35]. Unfortunately, the high levels of morbidity, mortality, and social chaos resulting from this crisis have continued even as prescription opioid prescribing has declined [19].

The practice of pain medicine has been significantly complicated and strained by this public health crisis. While fewer chronic pain patients are being started on high daily doses of opioids, a cohort of patients on these high doses continues, sometimes known as "legacy patients," and there is no clear consensus on the best path forward for these patients' pain care. The 2016 Center for Disease Control (CDC) guidelines for opioid treatment in chronic pain were very influential in encouraging tapers of opioid medication to lower doses [14, 15]. Concerns have been raised that many patients have been tapered involuntarily and quickly in order to meet this pressure, regardless of their clinical status or whether they had shown any signs of opioid misuse. Opioid prescribers felt considerable pressure in this regard, not only from

the CDC but also from state and national regulators and insurance companies. There were plentiful reports of patients suffering severe loss of function, worsening depression and suicidality, and even completed suicides [31]. At the time of this writing, the authors of the original CDC guidelines had issued a clarification stressing that the recommended ceiling dose should not be taken as a mandate for all patients, especially those legacy patients who had been functioning well on higher doses of medication [16].

The other face of pain crisis is the large population of patients who suffer from both opioid use disorder (OUD) and pain. Patients with opioid use disorder who are physiologically dependent on opioids present multiple obstacles to acute and chronic pain treatment, including lower pain thresholds and high opioid tolerance. Comorbid use of other illicit substances is also common. Patients with OUD who are in medication-assisted treatment pose other treatment challenges. In addition to these OUD patients, there are other patients for whom opioid prescribing is problematic, including patients who sell or otherwise divert their prescriptions. There are as well a large number of pain patients that have developed aberrant use of their chronically prescribed opioids. Some of these patients improve dramatically after opioid taper, but many seem to do even worse, becoming more aberrant in their medication use, more distressed, less active, and less functional in everyday activities.

37.2   Substance Use Disorder Complicates the Treatment of Pain

The argument for opioid analgesia for cancer pain remains strong, and this is the most common use of opioids worldwide, although there are some regions with significant access issues to this class of medications and subsequent undertreatment of pain. The best practices of opioid prescribing for chronic non-cancer pain are much less clear. While higher doses and longer duration of prescription are both associated with increased mortality, there does not appear a perfectly safe dosage of opioids [45]. Mounting evidence suggests that receiving opioids after surgery for any length of time raises the risk of opioid misuse or OUD [25].

The interaction between pain treatment and substance use disorder can be complex and hazardous. Treatment of pain with opioids raises iatrogenic addiction risk [4]. In the USA, illicit drug use was estimated by government survey to be almost 9% [53]. While some subgroups of prescription opioid abusers, such as youth, are clinically similar to other substance abusers [8], there is a wide spectrum of illness, and many of the older pain patients who develop problems with opioids have significant physical and psychiatric comorbidities, particularly females [11]. National survey data from 2015 and 2016 suggest that of the 89 million Americans using opioids, almost 4 million (4.4%) engage in prescription opioid misuse, which frequently co-occurs with illicit opioid use, illicit benzodiazepine use, and psychological distress [39].

Patients with substance use disorders are more challenging and risky to treat for pain for multiple reasons. For patients who are actively using, there is naturally a high risk that the opioids will simply add into the mix of drugs that are being abused, with potentially lethal results, particularly in the presence of sedatives or alcohol. Active substance use also decreases adherence to treatments, and these patients are more likely to be lost to follow-up.

For patients whose substance use disorder is in remission, reexposure opioids may be a trigger for relapse in their drug of choice, and they are at increased risk of iatrogenic opioid use disorder.

37.3 Diagnosis and Assessment of Addiction in the Pain Treatment Setting

The diagnosis of addiction in psychiatry has been complicated by a distinction between substance abuse and substance dependence. This has always been a poor fit for the particulars of opioids, which cause a withdrawal syndrome in everyone who takes them chronically, regardless of addiction issues. In the DSM-5, the categories of sub-

stance abuse and substance dependence have been collapsed into substance use disorder [44]. Both the DSM-5 criteria for substance use disorder and the ASAM-APS-AAPM criteria for addiction address similar symptoms of impaired control over use or compulsive use, continued use despite harm, and preoccupation with use or cravings [23]. The DSM-5 criteria for opioid use disorder specifically exclude consideration of opioid tolerance and withdrawal, since these will develop in all patients who take opioids chronically [1]. The DSM-5 also specifically excludes this diagnosis in patients who are only taking their prescribed opioid medication, which provides diagnostic clarity but may result in underdiagnosis of patients with iatrogenic OUD.

Addiction can be challenging to recognize in many settings but is particularly difficult in pain clinics, where the majority of patients are in some degree of emotional distress; there is high psychiatric comorbidity with depression and anxiety, frequent occupational and interpersonal problems, and many patients are seeking or are already prescribed habit-forming medications. Studies suggest that clinicians may overestimate their ability to recognize substance abusers "by feel" and that they are prone to fall into prejudicial misapprehension, overestimating prevalence of substance abuse in minority patients and failing to detect it in other population groups. The use of best practices for safe opioid prescribing has risen from a low baseline in an uneven manner, for example, laws have been passed in many states mandating that opioid prescribers check the prescription monitoring program report before writing a new prescription, but the actual adoption of this evidence-based practice has varied [52].

However clinicians can reliably observe two important sets of clues to addiction: risk factors

Table 37.1 Opioid aberrancies

Escalation of medication dosage
Requesting early refills
Doctor-shopping
Losing prescription medications
Tampering with prescriptions

and aberrancies. Aberrancies cover a wide spectrum of undesirable, unsafe, or boundary-transgressing patient behavior (see Table 37.1). The use of prescription monitoring programs and urine drug screenings can also be very helpful in identifying aberrant behavior. Once identified, whether by a physician, support staff, or lab, it is important to consider the anomalies in context of the clinical picture. The differential for addiction includes major mental disorders, delirium, misunderstanding, and interference by family members, roommates, or romantic partners.

Risk factors can be obtained from the patient, his other providers, and family. Several standardized questionnaires, such as the SOAPP and ORT, allow providers to identify known risk factors for addiction by self-report at time of intake.

It is important not only to make an accurate pain diagnosis and detect substance abuse in patients but also identify any other psychiatric comorbidities they may have. Once a patient has been identified as having a complex pain problem with addiction or dual diagnosis issues, they need to be evaluated more thoroughly to develop a good understanding of their psychosocial situation, their social and other resources, and significantly their limitations and challenges, including limited resources, legal issues, and family problems [12].

37.4   Acute Pain in Addicted Patients

The evidence suggests that nonaddicted patients in acute pain who have not had opioids before are at low risk for developing addiction during a short course of treatment with low-potency opioids [50]. However, brain changes of unclear significance are observable after as little as a month of treatment with opioids [56]. Clinical observations suggest that it is quite difficult for patients to discontinue opioids after 90 days of continuous treatment, which is also the threshold for pain conditions to be considered chronic. It is not unusual in academic pain centers to encounter patients who have undergone procedures and been prescribed pain medication for 1, 2, or even 3 months before they are referred to the pain service for a subacute problem which is rapidly

becoming a chronic condition. Particularly when discharge is looming, the patient may not be safe to be discharged on high doses of opioids, but abrupt taper prior to discharge may result in a crisis and failure of disposition planning.

This situation requires close assessment to determine what is happening, as this clinical picture may represent reactivation of addiction and medication overuse, an inadequately treated pain condition, or diversion. Ideally, in the case of elective procedures, these issues can be identified beforehand and incorporated into treatment planning; however, a significant proportion of acute pain patients, particularly those with substance abuse issues, will present with pain secondary to trauma occurring due to assault, injury, or motor vehicle collision with no advance warning. When these issues are identified, they should be incorporated into treatment planning for their care of that acute pain episode and beyond. This can also be an excellent time for substance abuse interventions, particularly if the patient's injury was related in some way to their addiction, as this provides a clear adverse consequence to use as a platform for motivational interviewing or other interventional techniques. Motivational interviewing (MI) has been beneficial for preventing alcohol-related reinjury [18] and for increasing exercise in fibromyalgia patients [3], but there is no solid evidence for MI-based interventions for opioid dependence at this time. At the same time, further psychiatric assessment may be indicated, particularly if there is concern for suicidality prior to hospitalization or during the hospital stay. Some hospitals will have 12 step-based program meeting on their grounds, and this may also be an option for motivated and mobile patients to attend.

For pain specialists, the greatest challenge in acute pain in patients with substance use is finding safe and adequate treatments in patients who may have elevated opioid tolerance, lower pain threshold, and difficulty coping with stress and discomfort. Perioperative management must take into account patients' use of prescribed opioids, illicit opioids such as heroin, and potentially patients on chronic buprenorphine or methadone for opioid dependence who will have high tolerance and, in the case of the buprenorphine patient, some initial difficulty in getting adequate analgesia due to the partial antagonism of the buprenorphine [38]. The provider must also be watchful for signs of other substance toxicity or withdrawal, such as stimulant-inducted psychosis or benzodiazepine withdrawal.

For the pain relief provider, it is important to determine, or at least estimate, their baseline opioid dosage and then maintain them on a regimen of opioids close to this in potency, with additional opioids available as needed for the acute pain. This may require conversion to parenteral opioids, and frequently the use of IV PCA analgesia is the safest and most effective strategy for managing their acute pain needs. In cases of thoracic or abdominal surgery or trauma, neuraxial anesthesia using epidural catheters to deliver local anesthetics or opioids can be very effective. Epidural morphine, for example, is ten times more potent than systemic morphine. Where the pain has a focal source, particularly in an extremity, regional anesthesia, such as using nerve catheters, can block much of the nociception from the injury and thus reduce the need for opioids overall as well as improve perfusion and recovery time. When patients with extremely high opioid tolerance require systemic opioids, a switch to methadone can often allow a decrease of overall dose. Very high doses of opioids raise the risk of respiratory depression and opioid-induced hyperalgesia, a condition characterized by whole-body pain that only worsens with increased opioid dosing.

37.5 Treating Chronic Pain with Opioids

Chronic pain is a highly significant and growing problem as the world's population gets older and more people are surviving significant illness or injury. Addicts are more likely to have all kinds of comorbidities, psychiatric and physical, and have a higher rate of physical injury and chronic pain as well [29]. The phenomenon of so-called self-medication for chronic pain is another mechanism by which patients may be exposed to these medications and develop addiction [46]. Chronic pain has been defined variously as pain lasting

more than 3 or more than 6 months; for our purposes, the ASA description of chronic pain as pain lasting longer than "the expected temporal boundary of tissue injury and normal healing and adversely affecting the function or well-being of the individual" is most germane [2]. Perhaps the most important fact about chronic pain is that it is chronic; in other words, it should be managed without the expectation of complete resolution, a quick return to premorbid function, or a short horizon for treatment. The effectiveness of chronic pain treatments is also less than those for acute pain, with average effect size of 40–50% and a substantial minority of patients who receive no benefit from treatment. Any treatments offered for chronic pain should be safe and sustainable in terms of availability and affordability.

The most vexing question in the treatment of chronic pain, particularly chronic pain in addicts, is that of chronic opioid therapy. Patients prescribed opioids for pain are also likely to use opioids nonmedically. This finding has been seen in military veterans and in the general population [5, 17]. A history of substance use disorder makes it less likely that primary care patients will have good relief after 12 months of treatment for musculoskeletal pain including opioids [42]. Some systematic reviews of chronic opioid therapy for non-cancer pain have failed to present strong evidence for the effectiveness of chronic opioid therapy [9].

"Adverse selection" is the phenomenon of the sickest and highest-risk patients receiving more opioids for longer and often receiving the bulk of opioid prescriptions in any given population. This phenomenon has been demonstrated in multiple settings [54]. Similar findings have also been reported among US military veterans and HIV patients [41, 48].

The APS-AAPM guidelines published in 2009 for treatment of non-cancer chronic pain may be helpful in guiding treatment, although they are not specifically focused on substance abuse patients [10]. These patients are often more complex, with layered conditions including substance use disorders, one or more primary pain conditions, and frequently psychiatric comorbidities as well. Although these complex pain patients have been shown to respond better to intensive treatment, the healthcare system rarely allows them to receive it [43]. Interdisciplinary pain care, which includes treatment by allied professionals and mental health, is rarely available in the USA due to coverage and access issues. The more recent and conservative CDC guidelines for opioids in chronic pain are also helpful and recommend low doses of opioids on a trial basis, with a ceiling dosage of 40 mg morphine equivalents [14, 15].

37.6 Treating Chronic Pain in the Setting of Substance Use Disorder

In this patient population, opioids should be prescribed cautiously if at all, in the knowledge that this is intrinsically risky, and more as a last resort than a first step. Providers without the requisite training or experience, or who do not have adequate support, are recommended to avoid opioid prescribing entirely in this population. If the patient is enrolled in substance treatment, or about to enter treatment, opioids may be incompatible and actually sabotage the patient's placement in a treatment program and should be avoided. These patients should first have the benefit of alternative treatment methods to the greatest extent possible, including non-opioid pain medications, nerve medications that are not addictive, behavioral interventions, and physical interventions such as physical therapy, TENS units, and injections where appropriate.

The initial intake for pain treatment should routinely include risk assessment, and this should be repeated regularly during treatment. Once risk factors such as a past history of SUD have been identified, or current aberrancies suggestive of SUD are seen, the decision must be made how to respond. Seeing potential problems of this nature or taking no action is not ethical or professionally advisable for the prescriber; in an older study of disciplinary actions taken against physicians related to opioid prescribing, 12% of the charged physicians had recognized SUD issues in their patients and continued prescribing without taking any action.

If opioids are felt to be a necessary part of pain treatment, they should be prescribed at the lowest dose possible. Many experts recommend short-acting opioids used on a schedule. If the patient is converted to a longer-acting opioid, it is recommended that they are not also prescribed short-acting opioids on an as-needed basis. This practice of treating "breakthrough pain," while very helpful in cancer pain, often results in patients taking both their scheduled and as-needed medications daily to the maximum extent possible, increasing risks and total opioid dosage [33]. It is predictable that some patients will overuse or misuse their medications. Many patients, after an initial good response, will quickly develop tolerance to at least part of the analgesic effect of the opioids and will escalate use on their own or request dosage increases. Increasing opioid doses tends to be a temporary solution only and increases morbidity and mortality risks.

Treatment should be individualized; however, there are many best practices that should be routinely followed in pain treatment, particularly as these risk factors and aberrancies may not be identified initially. Patients with fewer risk factors and less severe aberrancy may not require specific changes in treatment beyond closer monitoring. For high-risk patients and those whose aberrancy is more concerning, practices including a written, explicit treatment agreement, compliance checklists, and randomized urine drug screens may be helpful and should be used in every case. Early intervention with behavioral treatments may also be helpful [27], but there is little strong evidence to guide treatment in these high-risk patients. For patients with ongoing substance use issues or serious aberrancies, such as obtaining opioids from multiple prescribers for routine care or diversion, there may be no better option than stopping the opioids entirely. A taper should be done if safety allows, possibly with referral for consideration of medication-assisted treatment.

37.7 Problems with Tapering and Stopping Opioids

When opioid therapy is tapered or discontinued in patients who have been on opioids chronically, patients often experience at least transitory distress and increase of pain symptoms. Patients with comorbid depression or anxiety may have exacerbations of these symptoms. A particularly challenging constellation of symptoms occurs in those pain patients who have been on chronic opioids for some time and have developed aberrancies or behavioral complications, which only seem to worsen when the opioid dosage is decreased. At worst, this can lead to a catastrophic scenario where the patient's distress becomes uncontrollable, placing patient and provider in a dilemma as neither further taper nor return to high-dose opioids seems a workable option [34]. This is hypothesized to result from physiological changes in the nervous system with prolonged opioid which make the patient unable to tolerate opioid tapering. This has been called "complex persistent dependence" and has been observed to respond well to buprenorphine therapy. In the USA, this treatment may be difficult to access, particularly if the patient does not meet formal criteria for OUD; some patients are also understandably resistant to this diagnosis, which is highly stigmatized and may have negative impacts on their employment and access to health insurance. In addition, relatively few pain specialists prescribe buprenorphine, and most addiction treatment programs do not feel comfortable addressing pain in addition to SUD.

If not treated with buprenorphine or methadone, chronic pain patients with SUD histories are more likely to relapse, particularly those with OUD [24]. A manualized treatment program emphasizing behavioral treatment including cognitive-behavioral therapy and acceptance and commitment therapy has been developed for veterans with comorbid pain and SUD [26]. Some patients in this position will complain that they are being driven to seek illicit drugs. For ethical and professional reasons, it is recommended to continue to offer these patients the full panoply of non-opioid pain treatments to the extent that they are appropriate.

lems associated with life-threatening illness [47]. In this specialized arena of healthcare, the mandate to provide comfort may take precedence over concerns about addiction. While it is rare for patients in this clinical context to develop new addiction issues, preexisting psychiatric and addiction issues may be reactivated or worsen under the stresses of serious illness and may go unrecognized by providers. Untreated alcohol dependence, for example, is linked to other substance misuse and worse outcomes in pain patients [13]. Some cancer patients are provided with pain medications in larger quantities and dosages toward the end of life than any other types of patient. In addition to addiction, misuse or simple incorrect use due to misunderstanding can put patients at risk. These patients, who may be dependent on others for the management and administration of their medications, are also more vulnerable to diversion of medications by people near them. At the same time, many cancer patients do not receive adequate pain treatment due to access to care issues and also due to patient reluctance to use these medications for fear of addiction [49].

Following best practices in these patients can help track their medication use and identify aberrancies earlier. Close monitoring of symptoms and more frequent dispensing of opioids can be useful in harm reduction approaches. In larger, well-staffed cancer care centers, even daily dispensation of pain medications may be a useful intervention for selected patients. Pill safes and enlisting family members to dispense daily dosages can also improve safety and reduce the risk of misuse/overuse/diversion. In many cases, the medication misuse is also being driven by complex physical and emotional distress, with combined factors of depression, anxiety, worry about the future, impending death, being a burden on family, how family will fare after the patient's death, and non-pain forms of suffering such as dyspnea, fatigue, constipation, or immobility [32].

37.8 Palliative Care in Addicted Patients

Palliative care was defined by the WHO as an approach to treatment which improves the quality of life of patients and their families facing the prob-

37.9 Best Practices for Risk Management

All patients may be potentially at risk for addiction, and current approaches to risk stratification are very limited. For example, there is consensus that there is a large genetic component in predisposition to addiction, with abnormalities of the endogenous opioid system in particular being linked to increased risk of opioid abuse. However, no standard, evidence-based genetic testing protocol has been introduced. While family history may provide some clues to genetic predisposition, addiction is well known to "skip generations" and is often not openly discussed within families, so that the patient may not be aware of relevant history.

Therefore, the concept of universal screening in pain medicine, similar to the use of universal precautions for infection control, is becoming more popular [20]. This universal approach may also serve to reduce stigma and improve the detection of misuse. For example, opioid dependence is more likely to be overlooked in older adults and in Whites [6, 55]. This screening and risk stratification may also help use scarce community mental health, pain management, and substance abuse treatment resources more effectively, as low-risk patients remain in the primary care setting as long as they are doing well, while riskier patients are able to access more specialized and interdisciplinary care. Patients with serious psychiatric issues, substance dependence, or both should generally be seen in a setting with the availability of mental health consultation. This model tends to apply most to large cities and areas near academic medical centers; however, telemedicine applications may extend the reach of these specialties into rural areas and isolated regions [36].

Several useful screening tools for determining risk factors for patients include the COMM, SOAPP, and ORT. These are all brief, self-administered tests. The COMM has 17 items, while the ORT 8 and the SOAPP come in a full 24-item version and briefer versions [37]. The full version of the SOAPP may be the most effective at predicting future aberrancy [40]. Note that even a high score does not automatically translate into "do not prescribe opioids"; these tests must always be interpreted using clinical judgment. Since they are self-reported screens and do not attempt to conceal the nature of the assessment, they may underestimate risks in patients who are unreliable historians or deliberately deceitful.

The use of an opioid treatment agreement is also widespread, although there is very little evidence to support its efficacy. The greatest usefulness of this measure is to provide a transparent means of disclosing treatment policy to patients in advance. It is important to discuss the agreement with patients, along with obtaining fully informed consent for any treatments and documenting same. Since the risks of opioid therapy are much better appreciated now than they were even a decade ago, it is not safe to assume that a patient who is seen already on chronic opioids has full understanding of the implications and risks of this treatment. Any specific policies regarding prescription monitoring, pill counts, and urine drug screens should also be discussed at this time.

Urine drug testing (UDT) offers the promise of letting the prescriber know what the patient is exactly taking. Simple immunoassays have high false-positive and false-negative rates and should be followed up with confirmatory gas chromatography/mass spectrometry testing. Since even monotherapy with some opioids may result in numerous metabolites, these results should be reviewed with an expert, such as a pain specialist, pharmacist, or pathologist, before taking clinical action. UDT is most helpful in demonstrating that patients are not taking prescribed medications or taking additional, non-prescribed medications or illicit drugs. A policy should be developed to guide providers consistently on what actions to take in the event of an unexpected UDT result. Some studies have shown that even when UDT is obtained and shows unexpected results, prescribers continue to prescribe opioids [21]. In some states, where state law recognizes a role for medical marijuana, providers may choose to obtain UDT without checking routinely for THC. UDT is not able to reliably determine whether a patient is taking the full dose of their prescribed medication. These limitations aside, UDT helps providers recognize aberrancy that would not be identified by behavioral monitoring [30]. In the USA, many health insurances will not cover the cost of UDT, so providers must make smart choices about when and how often to order them. Systematic reviews suggest that the benefit for patients of standard UDT policies is modest [51].

37.10 Cooperation with Allied Providers

Primary care providers and pain specialists cannot be expected to master the fields of psychiatry and addiction but must understand enough to recognize patients with these issues, make appropriate referrals, and collaborate with the appropriate allied providers. It is important to provide solid information to colleagues about the nature of the patient's pain diagnoses and their treatment. For patients with addiction issues, some medications such as benzodiazepines and opioids may be both inadvisable and incompatible with their addiction treatment. In this case, prescribing these medications for the patient may unknowingly sabotage their addiction treatment or provoke relapse.

In patients who have been diagnosed with opioid dependence, a possible option for them may be opioid agonist therapy, namely, methadone or buprenorphine. In the USA, methadone may be prescribed freely for pain but only prescribed for the treatment of addiction by federally recognized methadone clinics. In addition, methadone clinics provide patients with a single larger daily dose of methadone, rather than dosing three times a day as is done for pain. Buprenorphine, in the form of Suboxone, may be prescribed for opioid dependence and (off-label) for pain. Buprenorphine is also available without the combination of naloxone and as a long-acting transdermal patch, Butrans. Both of these forms are more prone to abuse. Since buprenorphine is a partial opioid agonist, it may be less prone to abuse than other opioids, and it is also not suitable for combining with other opioids and may precipitate withdrawal in a patient who has been taking other opioids chronically. Bupropion treatment has been shown to be an effective treatment of opioid dependence and also reduces the rush experienced by patients who do relapse and use other opioids on top of the buprenorphine [28]. Naltrexone is also effective for OUD but has no analgesic effect and may worsen mood disorders; this medication, particularly in its long-acting injectable form, will complicate acute pain treatment due to the opioid blockade. A recent review by Harrison et al. provides an excellent overview of perioperative care in patients receiving medication-assisted treatment [22].

37.11 Conclusion

Substance dependence is a large and growing problem in developed countries. Prescription opioid misuse appears to have crested as a public health problem but remains significant, and the wider opioid crisis continues unabated as of this writing. Pain medicine has become intimately involved with this opioid crisis. Many pain patients have comorbid conditions including depression, anxiety, and SUD which complicate their treatment and worsen their prognosis. These patients should be offered the full range of pain management services, with particular emphasis on behavioral interventions; opioids should only be considered, if at all, after reasonable trials of other, safer treatment approaches. Early recognition of the patients by identifying their high-risk status and detecting aberrancies can help with early referrals to mental health and substance abuse providers and cautious, closely monitored prescribing practices. Many patients fall into this overlap between disorders, and there is an acute need for providers who are able to manage these challenging conditions. Specifically, a subset of patients who seem unable to tolerate opioid weaning and discontinuation has been identified. While they may not meet formal criteria for OUD, they may respond to behavioral treatment and buprenorphine.

References

1. American Psychiatric Association. Diagnostic and statistical manual of mental disorders: DSM-5. Arlington: American Psychiatric Association; 2013.
2. American Society of Anesthesiologists Task Force on Chronic Pain Management, American Society of Regional Anesthesia and Pain Medicine. Practice guidelines for chronic pain management: an updated report by the American Society of Anesthesiologists Task Force on Chronic Pain Management and the American Society of Regional Anesthesia and Pain Medicine. Anesthesiology. 2010;112(4):810–33. Retrieved from http://www.ncbi.nlm.nih.

gov/pubmed/20124882. https://doi.org/10.1097/ALN.0b013e3181c43103.

3. Ang D, Kesavalu R, Lydon JR, Lane KA, Bigatti S. Exercise-based motivational interviewing for female patients with fibromyalgia: a case series. Clin Rheumatol. 2007;26(11):1843–9. Retrieved from http://www.ncbi.nlm.nih.gov/pubmed/17310268. https://doi.org/10.1007/s10067-007-0587-0.

4. Ballantyne JC, LaForge KS. Opioid dependence and addiction during opioid treatment of chronic pain. Pain. 2007;129(3):235–55. Retrieved from http://www.ncbi.nlm.nih.gov/pubmed/17482363. https://doi.org/10.1016/j.pain.2007.03.028.

5. Barry DT, Goulet JL, Kerns RK, Becker WC, Gordon AJ, Justice AC, Fiellin DA. Nonmedical use of prescription opioids and pain in veterans with and without HIV. Pain. 2011;152(5):1133–8. Retrieved from <Go to ISI>://WOS:000289507500027. https://doi.org/10.1016/j.pain.2011.01.038.

6. Becker WC, Starrels JL, Heo M, Li X, Weiner MG, Turner BJ. Racial differences in primary care opioid risk reduction strategies. Ann Fam Med. 2011;9(3):219–25. Retrieved from <Go to ISI>://WOS:000291284200007. https://doi.org/10.1370/afm.1242.

7. Boudreau D, Von Korff M, Rutter CM, Saunders K, Ray GT, Sullivan MD, et al. Trends in long-term opioid therapy for chronic non-cancer pain. Pharmacoepidemiol Drug Saf. 2009;18(12):1166–75. Retrieved from http://www.ncbi.nlm.nih.gov/entrez/query.fcgi?cmd=Retrieve&db=PubMed&dopt=Citation&list_uids=19718704. https://doi.org/10.1002/pds.1833.

8. Catalano RF, White HR, Fleming CB, Haggerty KP. Is nonmedical prescription opiate use a unique form of illicit drug use? Addict Behav. 2011;36(1–2):79–86. Retrieved from <Go to ISI>://WOS:000285326900012. https://doi.org/10.1016/j.addbeh.2010.08.028.

9. Chan BK, Tam LK, Wat CY, Chung YF, Tsui SL, Cheung CW. Opioids in chronic non-cancer pain. Expert Opin Pharmacother. 2011;12(5):705–20. Retrieved from http://www.ncbi.nlm.nih.gov/pubmed/21254859. https://doi.org/10.1517/14656566.2011.536335.

10. Chou R, Ballantyne J, Fanciullo G, Fine P, Miaskowski C. Research gaps on use of opioids for chronic non-cancer pain: findings from a review of the evidence for an American Pain Society and American Academy of Pain Medicine clinical practice guideline. J Pain. 2009;10(2):147–59. Retrieved from http://www.ncbi.nlm.nih.gov/entrez/query.fcgi?cmd=Retrieve&db=PubMed&dopt=Citation&list_uids=19187891. doi: S1526-5900(08)00830-4 [pii]. https://doi.org/10.1016/j.jpain.2008.10.007.

11. Cicero TJ, Surratt HL, Kurtz S, Ellis MS, Inciardi JA. Patterns of prescription opioid abuse and comorbidity in an aging treatment population. J Subst Abuse Treat. 2012;42(1):87–94. Retrieved from http://www.ncbi.nlm.nih.gov/pubmed/21831562. https://doi.org/10.1016/j.jsat.2011.07.003.

12. Clark MR, Treisman GJ. Optimizing treatment with opioids and beyond. In: Clark MR, Treisman GJ, editors. Chronic pain and addiction, vol. 30. Karger, Basel, Switzerland; 2011. p. 92–112.

13. Dev R, Parsons HA, Palla S, Palmer JL, Del Fabbro E, Bruera E. Undocumented alcoholism and its correlation with tobacco and illegal drug use in advanced cancer patients. Cancer. 2011;117(19):4551–6. Retrieved from http://www.ncbi.nlm.nih.gov/pubmed/21446042. https://doi.org/10.1002/cncr.26082.

14. Dowell D, Haegerich TM, Chou R. CDC guideline for prescribing opioids for chronic pain - United States, 2016. MMWR Recomm Rep. 2016a;65(1):1–49. Retrieved from https://www.ncbi.nlm.nih.gov/pubmed/26987082. https://doi.org/10.15585/mmwr.rr6501e1.

15. Dowell D, Haegerich TM, Chou R. CDC guideline for prescribing opioids for chronic pain—United States, 2016. JAMA. 2016b;315(15):1624–45.

16. Dowell D, Haegerich T, Chou R. No shortcuts to safer opioid prescribing. N Engl J Med. 2019;380:2285.

17. Edlund MJ, Martin BC, Fan MY, Devries A, Braden JB, Sullivan MD. Risks for opioid abuse and dependence among recipients of chronic opioid therapy: results from the TROUP study. Drug Alcohol Depend. 2010;112(1–2):90–8. Retrieved from http://www.ncbi.nlm.nih.gov/pubmed/20634006. doi: S0376-8716(10)00204-8 [pii]. https://doi.org/10.1016/j.drugalcdep.2010.05.017.

18. Gentilello LM, Rivara FP, Donovan DM, Jurkovich GJ, Daranciang E, Dunn CW, et al. Alcohol interventions in a trauma center as a means of reducing the risk of injury recurrence. Ann Surg. 1999;230(4):473–80; discussion 480–473. Retrieved from http://www.ncbi.nlm.nih.gov/pubmed/10522717.

19. Gomes T, Tadrous M, Mamdani MM, Paterson JM, Juurlink DN. The burden of opioid-related mortality in the United States. JAMA Netw Open. 2018;1(2):e180217.

20. Gourlay DL, Heit HA, Almahrezi A. Universal precautions in pain medicine: a rational approach to the treatment of chronic pain. Pain Med. 2005;6(2):107–12. Retrieved from http://www.ncbi.nlm.nih.gov/pubmed/15773874. https://doi.org/10.1111/j.1526-4637.2005.05031.x.

21. Gupta A, Patton C, Diskina D, Cheatle M. Retrospective review of physician opioid prescribing practices in patients with aberrant behaviors. Pain Physician. 2011;14(4):383–9. Retrieved from <Go to ISI>://WOS:000295613500012.

22. Harrison TK, Kornfeld H, Aggarwal AK, Lembke A. Perioperative considerations for the patient with opioid use disorder on buprenorphine, methadone, or naltrexone maintenance therapy. Anesthesiol Clin. 2018;36(3):345–59.

23. Heit HA. Addiction, physical dependence, and tolerance: precise definitions to help clinicians evaluate and treat chronic pain patients. J Pain Palliat Care Pharmacother. 2003;17(1):15–29. Retrieved from http://www.ncbi.nlm.nih.gov/pubmed/14640337.

24. Heiwe S, Lonnquist I, Kallmen H. Potential risk factors associated with risk for drop-out and relapse during and following withdrawal of opioid prescription medication. Eur J Pain. 2011;15(9):966–70. Retrieved from http://www.ncbi.nlm.nih.gov/pubmed/21546290. https://doi.org/10.1016/j.ejpain.2011.03.006.

25. Higgins C, Smith B, Matthews K. Incidence of iatrogenic opioid dependence or abuse in patients with pain who were exposed to opioid analgesic therapy: a systematic review and meta-analysis. Br J Anaesth. 2018;120(6):1335–44.

26. Ilgen MA, Haas E, Czyz E, Webster L, Sorrell JT, Chermack S. Treating chronic pain in veterans presenting to an addictions treatment program. Cogn Behav Neurol. 2011;18(1):149–60. Retrieved from <Go to ISI>://WOS:000286648400017. https://doi.org/10.1016/j.cbpra.2010.05.002.

27. Jamison RN, Ross EL, Michna E, Chen LQ, Holcomb C, Wasan AD. Substance misuse treatment for high-risk chronic pain patients on opioid therapy: a randomized trial. Pain. 2010;150(3):390–400. Retrieved from http://www.ncbi.nlm.nih.gov/pubmed/20334973. https://doi.org/10.1016/j.pain.2010.02.033.

28. Jones JD, Sullivan MA, Manubay J, Vosburg SK, Comer SD. The subjective, reinforcing, and analgesic effects of oxycodone in patients with chronic, non-malignant pain who are maintained on sublingual buprenorphine/naloxone. Neuropsychopharmacology. 2011;36(2):411–22. Retrieved from http://www.ncbi.nlm.nih.gov/pubmed/20980992. https://doi.org/10.1038/npp.2010.172.

29. Karasz A, Zallman L, Berg K, Gourevitch M, Selwyn P, Arnsten JH. The experience of chronic severe pain in patients undergoing methadone maintenance treatment. J Pain Symptom Manage. 2004;28(5):517–25. Retrieved from http://www.ncbi.nlm.nih.gov/pubmed/15504628. https://doi.org/10.1016/j.jpainsymman.2004.02.025.

30. Katz NP, Sherburne S, Beach M, Rose RJ, Vielguth J, Bradley J, Fanciullo GJ. Behavioral monitoring and urine toxicology testing in patients receiving long-term opioid therapy. Anesth Analg. 2003;97(4):1097–102, table of contents. Retrieved from http://www.ncbi.nlm.nih.gov/pubmed/14500164.

31. Kertesz SG. Turning the tide or riptide? The changing opioid epidemic. Subst Abus. 2017;38(1):3–8.

32. Kircher S, Zacny J, Apfelbaum SM, Passik S, Kirsch K, Burbage M, Lofwall M. Understanding and treating opioid addiction in a patient with cancer pain. J Pain. 2011;12(10):1025–31. Retrieved from http://www.ncbi.nlm.nih.gov/pubmed/21968264. https://doi.org/10.1016/j.jpain.2011.07.006.

33. Manchikanti L, Singh V, Caraway DL, Benyamin RM. Breakthrough pain in chronic non-cancer pain: fact, fiction, or abuse. Pain Physician. 2011;14(2):E103–17. Retrieved from http://www.ncbi.nlm.nih.gov/pubmed/21412376

34. Manhapra A, Arias AJ, Ballantyne JC. The conundrum of opioid tapering in long-term opioid therapy for chronic pain: a commentary. Subst Abus. 2018;39(2):152–61.

35. Maxwell JC. The prescription drug epidemic in the United States: a perfect storm. Drug Alcohol Rev. 2011;30(3):264–70. Retrieved from http://www.ncbi.nlm.nih.gov/pubmed/21545556. https://doi.org/10.1111/j.1465-3362.2011.00291.x.

36. McGeary DD, McGeary CA, Gatchel RJ. A comprehensive review of telehealth for pain management: where we are and the way ahead. Pain Pract. 2012;12:570. Retrieved from http://www.ncbi.nlm.nih.gov/pubmed/22303839. https://doi.org/10.1111/j.1533-2500.2012.00534.x.

37. Meltzer EC, Rybin D, Saitz R, Samet JH, Schwartz SL, Butler SF, Liebschutz JM. Identifying prescription opioid use disorder in primary care: diagnostic characteristics of the Current Opioid Misuse Measure (COMM). Pain. 2011;152(2):397–402. Retrieved from http://www.ncbi.nlm.nih.gov/pubmed/21177035. https://doi.org/10.1016/j.pain.2010.11.006.

38. Mitra S, Sinatra RS. Perioperative management of acute pain in the opioid-dependent patient. Anesthesiology. 2004;101(1):212–27. Retrieved from http://www.ncbi.nlm.nih.gov/pubmed/15220793.

39. Mojtabai R, Amin-Esmaeili M, Nejat E, Olfson M. Misuse of prescribed opioids in the United States. Pharmacoepidemiol Drug Saf. 2019;28(3):345–53.

40. Moore T, Jones T, Browder J, Daffron S, Passik S. A comparison of common screening methods for predicting aberrant drug-related behavior among patients receiving opioids for chronic pain management. Pain Med. 2009;10(8):1426–33. Retrieved from http://www.ncbi.nlm.nih.gov/entrez/query.fcgi?cmd=Retrieve&db=PubMed&dopt=Citation&list_uids=20021601. PME743 [pii]. https://doi.org/10.1111/j.1526-4637.2009.00743.x.

41. Morasco BJ, Duckart JP, Carr TP, Deyo RA, Dobscha SK. Clinical characteristics of veterans prescribed high doses of opioid medications for chronic non-cancer pain. Pain. 2010;151(3):625–32. Retrieved from http://www.ncbi.nlm.nih.gov/pubmed/20801580. doi: S0304-3959(10)00469-0 [pii]. https://doi.org/10.1016/j.pain.2010.08.002.

42. Morasco BJ, Corson K, Turk DC, Dobscha SK. Association between substance use disorder status and pain-related function following 12 months of treatment in primary care patients with musculoskeletal pain. J Pain. 2011a;12(3):352–9. Retrieved from http://www.ncbi.nlm.nih.gov/pubmed/20851057. https://doi.org/10.1016/j.jpain.2010.07.010.

43. Morasco BJ, Duckart JP, Dobscha SK. Adherence to clinical guidelines for opioid therapy for chronic pain in patients with substance use disorder. J Gen Intern Med. 2011b;26(9):965–71. Retrieved from http://www.ncbi.nlm.nih.gov/pubmed/21562923. https://doi.org/10.1007/s11606-011-1734-5.

44. O'Brien C. Addiction and dependence in DSM-V. Addiction. 2011;106(5):866–7. Retrieved from <Go to ISI>://WOS:000289296900002. https://doi.org/10.1111/j.1360-0443.2010.03144.x.

45. Paulozzi LJ, Kilbourne EM, Shah NG, Nolte KB, Desai HA, Landen MG, et al. A history of being prescribed controlled substances and risk of drug overdose death. Pain Med. 2012;13(1):87–95. Retrieved from http://www.ncbi.nlm.nih.gov/pubmed/22026451. https://doi.org/10.1111/j.1526-4637.2011.01260.x.

46. Rosenblum A, Joseph H, Fong C, Kipnis S, Cleland C, Portenoy RK. Prevalence and characteristics of chronic pain among chemically dependent patients in methadone maintenance and residential treatment facilities. JAMA. 2003;289(18):2370–8. Retrieved from http://www.ncbi.nlm.nih.gov/pubmed/12746360. https://doi.org/10.1001/jama.289.18.2370.

47. Sepulveda C, Marlin A, Yoshida T, Ullrich A. Palliative care: the World Health Organization's global perspective. J Pain Symptom Manage. 2002;24(2):91–6. Retrieved from http://www.ncbi.nlm.nih.gov/pubmed/12231124

48. Silverberg MJ, Ray GT, Saunders K, Rutter CM, Campbell CI, Merrill JO, et al. Prescription long-term opioid use in HIV-infected patients. Clin J Pain. 2012;28(1):39–46. Retrieved from http://www.ncbi.nlm.nih.gov/pubmed/21677568. https://doi.org/10.1097/AJP.0b013e3182201a0f.

49. Simone CB 2nd, Vapiwala N, Hampshire MK, Metz JM. Cancer patient attitudes toward analgesic usage and pain intervention. Clin J Pain. 2012;28(2):157–62. Retrieved from http://www.ncbi.nlm.nih.gov/pubmed/21705874. https://doi.org/10.1097/AJP.0b013e318223be30.

50. Skurtveit S, Furu K, Borchgrevink P, Handal M, Fredheim O. To what extent does a cohort of new users of weak opioids develop persistent or probable problematic opioid use? Pain. 2011;152(7):1555–61. Retrieved from http://www.ncbi.nlm.nih.gov/pubmed/21450405. https://doi.org/10.1016/j.pain.2011.02.045.

51. Starrels JL, Becker WC, Alford DP, Kapoor A, Williams AR, Turner BJ. Systematic review: treatment agreements and urine drug testing to reduce opioid misuse in patients with chronic pain. Ann Intern Med. 2010;152(11):712–20. Retrieved from http://www.ncbi.nlm.nih.gov/pubmed/20513829. https://doi.org/10.1059/0003-4819-152-11-201006010-00004.

52. Strickler GK, Zhang K, Halpin JM, Bohnert AS, Baldwin G, Kreiner PW. Effects of mandatory prescription drug monitoring program (PDMP) use laws on prescriber registration and use and on risky prescribing. Drug Alcohol Depend. 2019;199:1.

53. Substance Abuse and Mental Health Services Administration. Results from the 2010 National Survey on Drug Use and Health: summary of national findings. Rockville: SAMHSA; 2011.

54. Sullivan MD, Edlund MJ, Fan MY, Devries A, Brennan Braden J, Martin BC. Risks for possible and probable opioid misuse among recipients of chronic opioid therapy in commercial and medicaid insurance plans: the TROUP study. Pain. 2010;150(2):332–9. Retrieved from http://www.ncbi.nlm.nih.gov/pubmed/20554392. https://doi.org/10.1016/j.pain.2010.05.020.

55. Vijayaraghavan M, Penko J, Guzman D, Miaskowski C, Kushel MB. Primary care providers' judgments of opioid analgesic misuse in a community-based cohort of HIV-infected indigent adults. J Gen Intern Med. 2011;26(4):412–8. Retrieved from http://www.ncbi.nlm.nih.gov/pubmed/21061084. https://doi.org/10.1007/s11606-010-1555-y.

56. Younger JW, Chu LF, D'Arcy NT, Trott KE, Jastrzab LE, Mackey SC. Prescription opioid analgesics rapidly change the human brain. Pain. 2011;152(8):1803–10. Retrieved from <Go to ISI>://WOS:000292862400020. https://doi.org/10.1016/j.pain.2011.03.028.

Part IV

Main Systems Components in Addictions Treatment

Ambros Uchtenhagen and Giuseppe Carrà

Main Elements of a Systems Approach to Addiction Treatment: An Introduction

38

Ambros Uchtenhagen and Giuseppe Carrà

Abstract

The focus of this section is mainly on the treatment system and on the community, at a regional or national level, as a comprehensive network of different approaches, services, and actors, covering all types of addictive behaviors. This implies the preference for a public health perspective, combining the care for the individual patients in their diversity with the intention to cover the treatment needs in a specific catchment area and for a given population. In addition, there are some chapters focusing on diagnostic issues and reviews of specific therapeutic approaches.

This aim has to consider the availability, affordability, and accessibility of appropriate and qualified treatment. It has to build on effective treatment, provided in an efficient and cost-effective way. It has to stress connections among services, shared concepts of different indications, and routine rules for patient pathways through treatment phases, ranging from first contact, screening, and assessment to treatment planning and monitoring, rehabilitation, and aftercare. Pathways may also follow models of stepped care in an attempt to avoid misplacement of patients and to make best use of the available human and financial resources. Quality of intervention is embedded in evidence based also in the field of drug addiction treatment.

A comprehensive network goes beyond formal therapeutic regimes, by including low-threshold approaches for establishing contact by outreach activities and by harm reduction interventions in support of those still actively engaging in addictive behavior. This includes measures to reduce the risks of injecting, of acquiring blood-borne infectious diseases, and of overdose-related mortality. Such interventions are not in contradiction to others offering a structured regime of substitution medication (e.g., for opiates or nicotine) or even aiming at abstinence from substance use and full recovery. The system has to integrate all these approaches in order to best meet the needs and preferences of the equally diverse people with substance use disorders. Everyone should be able to find what is appropriate and suits him or her best under present conditions.

Such a comprehensive network is work in progress, as addictive behaviors and treatment populations change over time. New therapeutic methods and instruments also ask for adaptation

A. Uchtenhagen (✉)
Swiss Research Foundation for Public Health and Addiction, Zurich University, Zurich, Switzerland
e-mail: ambros.uchtenhagen@isgf.uzh.ch

G. Carrà
Mental Health Department, University of Milano-Bicocca, Monza, Italy
e-mail: giuseppe.carra@unimib.it

© Springer Nature Switzerland AG 2021
N. el-Guebaly et al. (eds.), *Textbook of Addiction Treatment*,
https://doi.org/10.1007/978-3-030-36391-8_38

and suited implementation at the system level. Where no such network is in place, the relevant steps for building up a system responding to the needs are recommended. All this goes not without a political support to provide adequate and sustainable resources, in the framework of a treatment policy which is in line with an overall drug policy.

The structure of this section in its revised format can be divided into two parts: The first is about the principles and aspects of the systems approach to addiction treatment, presented in the text above. In the second part, the reader will find information on the individual chapters in this section. This is presented in the following text.

Chapter 39 by Babor TF, "Treatment Systems for Population Management of Substance Use Disorders: Requirements and Priorities from a Public Health Perspective," is a systematic analysis of what has to be considered in a treatment system, in order to best serve all in need of treatment in a given population. *Method:* It is based on relevant previous publications by the author and others, providing additional information on the various aspects, also in a historical perspective. The *Text* focuses on concepts, requirements, and priorities recommended for building up an adequate treatment system, starting out with definitions and rationale, going on to conceptual developments, and finally listing priorities. The *Conclusions* ask for an appropriate resource allocation if the treatment system should allow to cover the treatment needs, including good service quality and access to care.

Chapter 40 by Saunders JB and Latt NC, "Screening, Early Detection, and Brief Intervention for Alcohol Use Disorders," starts out from the observation that alcohol problems are frequently diagnosed too late before becoming chronic and disabling conditions. Therefore, secondary interventions such as providing help for self-recognition, early diagnosis, self-management of use, and therapeutic approaches to change behavior are essential. *Method:* The aim is to provide screening instruments and information on their usefulness, with bibliographic details, rather than a systematic literature search. *Text:* Besides providing evidence for the observations made, the focus is how to implement the use of screening instruments and of brief intervention techniques into clinical practice, including Internet and mobile phone techniques for interactive support.

Chapter 41 by Bobes-Bascaràn T et al., "Clinical Assessment of Alcohol Use Disorders," describes how to evaluate the type and extent of alcohol use and the type and extent of psychiatric comorbidities, of neuropsychological performance, and of psychosocial functioning and quality of life. *Text:* Besides reviewing the necessary elements of a comprehensive clinical procedure, a description of the most relevant psychometric instruments is provided, covering symptomatology; legal, economic, and occupational problems; coping behaviors; and readiness to change.

Chapter 42 by Wurst FM et al., "Biological State Marker for Alcohol Consumption," has a strong focus on the various direct ethanol metabolites and the use of their measurement, adding an overview of the traditional biological markers on consumption. *Method:* systematic description of the various biomarkers and their advantages and limitations. *Text:* Epidemiological data justify the need for better implementation of how to assess alcohol consumption by using biological markers. The main part is a detailed, literature-based description of direct ethanol metabolites and their assessment and value for clinical use. *Conclusion:* advancements in diagnosis and therapy, new perspectives for prevention, and interdisciplinary cooperation due to extended use of direct biomarkers.

Chapter 43 by Assanangkornchai S and Edwards G, "Clinical Screening for Illegal and Prescription Drug Misuse and Nicotine Use," covers screening instruments used in detecting substance use in medical, psychiatric, and forensic services, with a view of providing subsequent treatment. Specific tests utilized are discussed, along with their psychometric properties, intended screening populations and validity, as well as the importance of proper and ethical use. Conclusion: Despite its limitations, screening is a first, small step toward providing successful treatment outcomes.

Chapter 44 by Tremonti C, "Drug Testing in Addiction Medicine," explains in detail how a range of psychoactive substances can be detected in body fluids and tissues for medical and legal purposes, how findings are interpreted on the basis of appropriate knowledge about pharmacokinetics, and characteristics of the various samples to be analyzed. *Method:* Technologies and their applicability are described on the basis of best known standard procedures. *Text:* Drug screening is explained in a range of different contexts, such as hospital toxicology, workplace drug testing, forensic toxicology, postmortem toxicology, sports toxicology, and drugs of abuse testing. *Conclusion:* Close collaboration with laboratory specialists is essential for obtaining adequate results.

Chapter 45 by Harland J, Henry-Edwards S, Gowing L, and Ali R, "Brief Interventions for Illicit Drug Users," focuses on brief interventions as an effective and targeted tool, in the interest of the individual and of public health. *Method:* extended use of updated literature. *Text:* concise description of the nature and the effectiveness of brief interventions, for both legal and illegal substances of abuse, adding specificities of working with illicit drug users and the key principles to be followed. Settings for brief interventions are described. *Conclusion:* Including knowledge and training of brief interventions in medical school and nursing schools, as well as continued education later on, is considered a must.

Chapter 46 by Rush B, "Screening and Assessment of People with Substance Use Disorders: A Focus on Developed Countries," is about best practice procedures including a staged approach and subsequent monitoring of outcome, in order to maximize efficiency. *Method:* selected essential literature. *Text:* Various collaborative models in screening and assessment facilitate such procedures early in contact of persons with psychiatric and especially substance use problems with the treatment system. Best practices are based on an individual's needs and strengths, adhering to a bio- and psychosocial model of understanding disorders, cultural differences and characteristics of a given service, and research evidence of usefulness. *Conclusion:* A more pro-

active concerted effort to screening for mental health problems and at-risk consumption of alcohol and other drugs is recommended.

Chapter 47 by Uchtenhagen A, "Stepped Care in Addiction Treatment," deals with models and procedures on how treatment intensity can be determined by a systematic screening of patient characteristics, in order to make best use of available human and financial resources in a given treatment system. *Method:* Available literature describes and compares two models. *Text:* Procedures to start out with the least intensive intervention, progressing to more intensive ones if ineffective, are known from psychiatry and other medical disciplines. In the case of addiction treatment, two outstanding models have been developed, one by the American Society of Addiction Medicine ASAM and the other by a Dutch group as a national project MATE (Measurements in the Addictions for Triage and Evaluation). The first developed special models for adolescents and patients with psychiatric comorbidity and the later for patients with legal problems. The implementation meets some resistance from services used to take on patients even if those do not need this type of service. *Conclusion:* Further use and development of stepped care models needs political support.

Chapter 48 by De Leon G et al., "Therapeutic Communities for Addictions: Essential Elements and Cultural and Current Issues," describes community as a method, its various applications worldwide, its outcomes according to research, and challenges and how to meet those. *Method:* based on the extensive knowledge of the authors. *Text:* Besides the explanation of the TC model and its unique role in the treatment system as a recovery-oriented therapeutic method, available knowledge on its effectiveness and adaptations and modifications for special populations and settings are presented. Details on implementing a TC include funding, workforce, duration of treatment, research, challenges, and fidelity to treatment. *Conclusion:* defending the TC model and its unique mission for a recovery-oriented treatment.

Chapter 49 by Galanter M, "Spiritual Aspects of the Twelve-Step Method in Addiction," is directed at defining the nature of spirituality and its relationship to empirical research and clinical practice. *Method: based* on the extensive knowledge of the author. Text: Diverse theoretical and empirically grounded sources provide an initial understanding of spirituality. More concretely, the movement of Alcoholics Anonymous illustrates the impact of spirituality on addiction in different cultural and clinical settings. Subjective spiritual experience can be assessed systematically by employing empirical techniques, thereby studying an important aspect of recovery. *Conclusion:* more integration into professional treatment needed.

Chapter 50 by Best D and Hamer R, "Addiction Recovery in Services and Policy: An International Overview," emphasizes the growing role of recovery as a treatment goal and a policy vision, aiming at healthy lifestyle and good quality of life. *Method*: based on the authors' knowledge of relevant literature. *Text:* Addiction is a chronic condition, and recovery needs a continuing care approach. Emerging service models and peer-driven recovery supports are described. The aim goes beyond changes in addictive behaviors, to improved overall functioning of the person and his/her quality of life. *Conclusion:* strategies recommended for medical professionals on how to promote recovery in substance-using patients.

Chapter 51 by Smith DE and Davidson LD, "Strategies of Drug Prevention in the Workplace: An International Perspective on Drug Testing and Employee Assistance Programmes (EAPS)," describes the diverse regulation mechanisms and instances for drug testing in the workplace, in the USA and Europe, especially for improving workplace safety by preventing or reducing substance use in staff. *Method:* based on the authors' knowledge of relevant literature. *Text:* A detailed and extensive description of regulation diversity and practices, including statistical information on findings from workplace testing, is provided, as well as much background information in graphs and figures. Same for employee assistance programs. *Conclusion:* The advantages of employee assistance programs for employers and employees are highlighted.

Chapter 52 by Hedrich D and Hartnoll R, "Harm Reduction Interventions, Policies, Settings, and Challenges," is a comprehensive description of all approaches to minimize the impact and negative consequences of substance use in persons unable to quit their substance use or having no access to effective treatment. *Method:* based on the authors' knowledge of relevant literature. Bibliography includes recommendations for further reading. *Text:* Main types of drug use-related interventions to reduce harm are described in detail. Best policy favors combination interventions, illustrated by integrated approaches at the local level. Further topics are enabling environments, prison settings, and ways to overcome barriers. *Conclusion:* Single interventions have best outcomes if they are part of a comprehensive policy to reduce harm from substance use and other addictive behaviors.

Treatment Systems for Population Management of Substance Use Disorders: Requirements and Priorities from a Public Health Perspective

39

Thomas F. Babor

Contents

Abstract

This chapter describes the requirements and priorities of service systems designed to treat persons with substance use disorders. Research and theory are reviewed to inform policymakers, program administrators, and treatment providers about the best ways to organize or to expand treatment services using a public health systems approach, which is concerned primarily with how services contribute to the health and welfare of a population. The requirements of a service system include sound policies (especially stable financing); appropriate structural features, such as facilities and trained personnel; and services that are effective, accessible, affordable, and integrated. The priorities for establishing such a system will depend on the assessment of population needs, as well as needs-based planning and the support of mutual help organizations. It is concluded that a public health approach to the development of treatment systems provides a useful way of responding to the changing needs of the population in relation to substance use disorders.

Keywords

Treatment · Systems · Alcohol · Drugs · Public health

39.1 Introduction

At the time when health-care delivery is changing rapidly throughout the world and new substance abuse treatment services are being developed, it is

T. F. Babor (✉)
Department of Public Health Sciences, University of Connecticut School of Medicine,
Farmington, CT, USA
e-mail: Babor@uchc.edu

© Springer Nature Switzerland AG 2021
N. el-Guebaly et al. (eds.), *Textbook of Addiction Treatment*,
https://doi.org/10.1007/978-3-030-36391-8_39

critical that services for persons with alcohol and drug problems be delivered in the most effective as well as in the most efficient manner. The focus on treatment system issues represented in the title of this chapter is designed to direct attention at the growing body of research and theory that can be used to inform treatment planning and quality improvement at the community and national levels. The development of an effective treatment system is a crucial part of a country's public health response to the problems associated with substance use disorders. Although a great amount of research has been conducted on treatment of substance use disorders, most of it deals with clinical issues, such as the efficacy of different psychotherapies or pharmacotherapies, rather than the larger treatment service issues that often result from tradition, budget constraints, procurement procedures, or political decisions. As described in a conceptual paper by Babor et al. [8], what is now needed is a comparable effort to use systems-level research to inform policymakers and program administrators about the best ways to configure and expand their treatment services to maximize their impact at the population level.

This chapter deals with the requirements and priorities of the treatment system, which are approached from a public health perspective. The requirements of a service system include sound policies (especially stable financing); appropriate structural features, such as facilities and trained personnel; and services that are effective, accessible, affordable, and integrated. The priorities of such a system include the accurate estimation of population needs through service mapping and needs assessment, as well as rational service planning that includes an emphasis on community support networks such as mutual help organizations.

39.2 Concepts, Requirements, and Priorities

39.2.1 Definitions and Rationale

A treatment system for persons with substance use disorders is an arrangement of facilities, programs, and personnel that is designed to function in a coordinated way. Such an arrangement includes linkages between specialized care and other types of services, such as mental health, primary health care, social welfare, criminal justice, and mutual help organizations [8]. The focus on the arrangement and coordination of services, rather than just the personnel, programs, and therapeutic aspects of treatment, raises a new set of questions for clinicians, program administrators, and policymakers. Can systems concepts help to reduce the gap between population needs and the current availability of substance abuse services? How can treatment services be made more accessible to those in need? Are the needs of affected populations being met by the current array of services? Are services being distributed and accessed appropriately? Are screening and referral conducted at gateway institutions, such as primary health care, schools, and employment settings? Are there appropriate diagnostic capabilities? What are the most effective administrative linkages between substance abuse services and criminal justice, mental health, primary care, and other human services? Are specialized services coordinated in a continuum of care? Are evidence-based services available and relevant? What is the policy support for integrated structures? What can be done to build stronger community support networks (e.g., Alcoholics Anonymous (AA), family social clubs)? To what extent can mental health and general medical services be better integrated with addiction treatment? Are there advantages to having separate systems for substance abuse, or should they be integrated administratively with mental health care or services for other health conditions or social problems?

These questions define issues that can be addressed by a public health systems perspective, which is concerned primarily with how services contribute to the health and welfare of a population. Services for substance use disorders expanded dramatically in developed countries in the 1970s but often in a fragmented and arbitrary way. Resource allocation decisions and treatment policies have a major effect on the development of services for persons with substance use disorders, but there is little research to guide service planning or to indicate whether services achieve their public health objectives. Low- and middle-income countries are now investing in services as substance use prevalence rates increase with new epidemics or rising national incomes, but there is little systematic knowledge to guide the development of service systems that would best address the needs of their populations.

39.2.2 History and Conceptual Developments

Conceptual, theoretical, and empirical work on treatment systems is a recent development, but substance abuse treatment has a long history that can be traced back at least 200 years in some countries [55, 63]. A rudimentary set of treatment services, mostly specialized residential programs, emerged from the nineteenth-century asylum movement originally designed for mental patients but which also served large numbers of alcoholics [63]. Since the 1960s in the industrialized countries, there has been a steady growth of specialized medical, psychiatric, and social services for individuals with substance use disorders [32]. Although each country developed a different mix of services and administrative structures, there were some commonalities across national systems in the types of service settings (residential, detoxification, and outpatient) and therapeutic approaches [25]. As treatment services became more numerous and specialized, new concepts were developed to describe how they related to the different types of population needs. These concepts include the continuum of care, broadening the base of treatment, the chronic care model, and service system levels.

The *continuum of care* concept, as described by Rush et al. [49], refers to the mix of services available to patients and the way patients are expected to pass through it. The services are generally arranged sequentially beginning with screening and diagnostic assessment. Patients are then assigned to different settings and services depending on acuity, severity, and complexity. The main services that have been incorporated into the systems framework in most countries are withdrawal management (including detoxification), residential rehabilitation, outpatient counseling, continuing care, harm reduction programs, and community support networks such as Alcoholics Anonymous. Variations of the continuum of care concept are the core-shell model and the stepped-care approach. In the core-shell model, core functions, such as intake assessment and treatment assignment to the most appropriate type of care (the shell), are facilitated by case management [15]. In the stepped-care approach, patients are assigned to the least intensive level of care initially. If outcomes are not optimal, they can be "stepped up" to a more intensive level, and if outcomes are positive, they can be "stepped down" to appropriate continuing services.

Another innovation that has contributed to the systems concept is SBIRT, which refers to screening, brief intervention, and referral to treatment, typically in the context of early intervention in primary health-care settings [5–7]. The SBIRT model grew out of a seminal report issued by the US Institute of Medicine [23], called *Broadening the Base of Treatment for Alcohol Problems*. SBIRT is a comprehensive and integrated approach to the delivery of early intervention and treatment services through universal screening for persons with substance use disorders and those at risk. Beginning in the 1980s, concerted efforts were made by the World Health Organization (WHO) to provide an evidence base for alcohol screening and brief intervention in primary health-care settings, in order to *broaden the base of treatment* in countries where specialized services were unavailable. With the development of reliable and accurate screening tests for alcohol, more than a hundred clinical trials were conducted to evaluate the efficacy and cost-effectiveness of alcohol screening and brief intervention in primary care, emergency departments, and trauma centers [5–7, 24].

Just as SBIRT attempts to integrate specialized substance abuse treatment services with outreach to the general health-care system, the *chronic care model* addresses the needs of more serious cases of substance dependence by coordinating specialized services over time under the assumption that once substance dependence has developed, there is a need for continuing care and management, as is done with chronic conditions like diabetes and hypertension. The chronic care model has been adapted to substance abuse by

Rush [48, 49] who has defined a series of "tiers" that constitute the most important elements of a continuum of services for the management of chronic substance users (see also Rush and Urbanoski [50]). Five tiers are defined on the basis of their functions, which are higher-order groupings of similar services or interventions, such as early intervention, detoxification, outpatient counseling, and residential programs. Tier 1 refers to health promotion and prevention functions targeted at the general population. This tier recognizes the likelihood that public policies, the regulatory environment, and lifestyle factors contribute to the risk of substance abuse and the need for treatment. Tier 2 consists of early intervention and self-management functions directed at persons at risk. This incorporates the SBIRT activities that have provided an important link to other health-care settings. Tier 3 consists of treatment planning, crisis management, and support functions for persons with identified substance-related problems. Tier 4 includes specialized care for people in need of more intensive services, such as residential programs, outpatient counseling, and pharmacotherapy. Finally, Tier 5 comprises highly specialized care functions for individuals with complex problems, such as inpatient withdrawal management, forensic services, and long-term psychiatric care. The tiered framework is designed to be used as a planning tool for the development of an integrated system of service functions for substance abuse, mental disorders, and gambling problems that takes into account problem severity and complexity.

Despite the growth of treatment services and systems of care in many countries, the services in most parts of the world are fragmentary and lack coordination. Four development levels have been proposed to account for the range of systems that have evolved in different countries [3]. Level I refers to services that are "minimal" in relation to population needs. If they exist at all, services tend to be fragmentary, with rudimentary care available in some settings (e.g., emergency departments or psychiatric wards) and perhaps specialized services in medical and psychiatric settings where a residential unit might provide care for a limited number of patients.

Level II is described as "limited" in terms of systems development, with some specialized services in medical and psychiatric settings. Level III refers to a "modest" level of development where a variety of services are delivered in most settings and there is some regional coordination and planning. Level IV refers to "mature" systems, with a variety of integrated services in a range of settings and stable financing for these services. The specification of these levels is useful for suggesting ways in which a system at a particular level of development can be improved and for monitoring changes in systems development over time.

39.2.3 Requirements of an Optimal Treatment System

Babor et al. [3, 8] have described the components and dynamics of an optimal treatment system from a public health perspective. These are the basic "building blocks" of a service system [22]. As illustrated in Fig. 39.1, the first requirement is a set of policies that make the governance of the service system and its constituent parts possible. The second component is the system's structural resources, including infrastructure, technologies, personnel, programs, and facilities. The third component consists of system qualities, such as accessibility, economy, and efficiency, which contribute to the smooth functioning of the service system.

According to this model, the policies, resources, and qualities of the system should not only translate into the effectiveness of services on individuals exposed to them, it should also contribute to population health through reductions in death, disease, and disability.

The components of this model and the research supporting it are discussed in the remainder of this section in order to indicate how a systems model might best contribute to population health.

39.2.3.1 Policies
The first requirement of an effective treatment system is appropriate treatment policies that provide a statutory basis for designing treat-

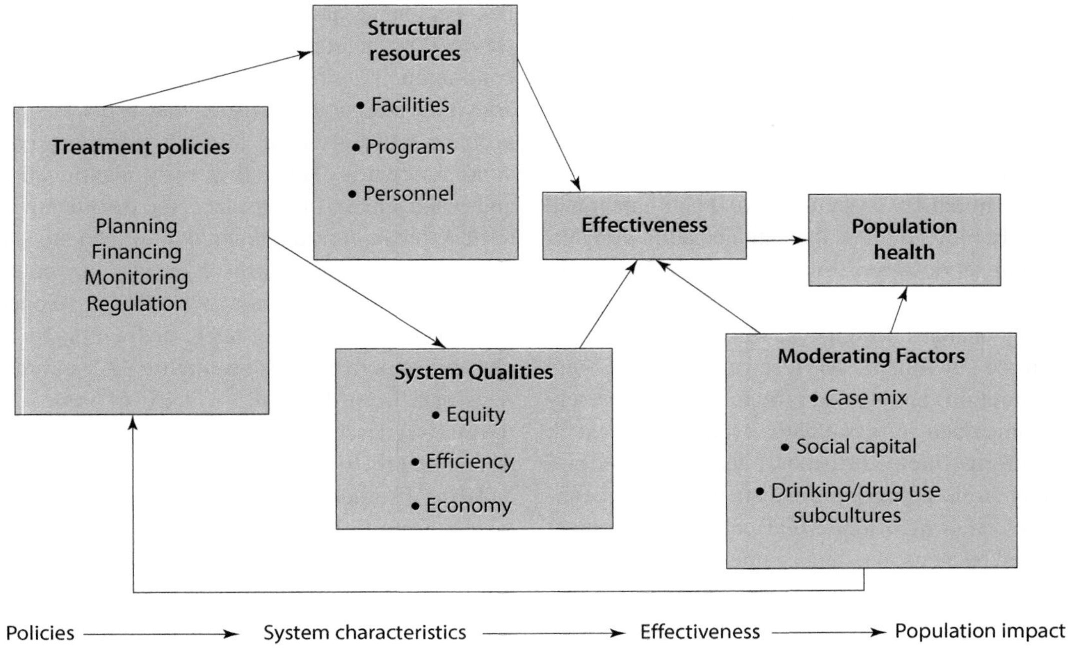

Policies ──────────→ System characteristics ──────────→ Effectiveness ──────────→ Population impact

Fig. 39.1 Conceptual model of service system policies, resources, and qualities and their potential impact on population health. (Source: Adapted from Babor et al. [8])

ment programs, licensing of treatment providers, and funding for programs and personnel. Policies determine the size, the administrative location, and the organization of the treatment system. They provide a framework for the allocation of resources. There is a great deal of legislation for the treatment and rehabilitation of persons with substance use disorders, but much of the legislation is concerned with provisions for compulsory treatment or for treatment in lieu of jail [46]. Other kinds of policy include national standards for clinical practices and licensing requirements for treatment personnel.

According to a survey conducted by the World Health Organization [64], 66.2% of the 145 countries surveyed have a government unit or government official responsible for treatment services for substance use disorders, but fewer than half of these countries have a specific budget line for these services. Financing mechanisms vary but most countries use tax revenues, user fees, and private insurance to pay for alcohol and drug services. User-based funding models depend

on private financing for services or insurance coverage. Population-based financing relies on public funding of services and is typified by the inclusion of addiction treatment in the social welfare systems of the Nordic countries.

Resource allocation and financing decisions have had a major effect on the development of these services. For example, the number and variety of services increased dramatically in the United States when the US Public Health Service invested in treatment services as part of a broader public health approach to reduce the burden of disease, disability, and social problems that accompany substance use [63]. The rapid development of federally supported residential and outpatient treatment programs, along with an expansion of insurance coverage for private programs, established the feasibility of serving large numbers of alcohol- and drug-dependent patients within a specialized set of services.

Treatment policies and financing mechanisms affect the degree of centralized management of treatment services and their incorporation into other human service areas, such as social welfare, mental health, general medicine, and criminal justice. In Denmark, policies were used to decentralize treatment services, whereas in Norway, they moved the system toward a more centralized, medically oriented structure [57]. In Canada and the Netherlands, mental health and substance abuse treatment systems have been integrated [48]. In Finland, mental health and addiction outpatient services were merged, and patients were also managed in primary care [29]. Although policy changes designed to reform the organization of treatment services may have sound assumptions and a good rationale, they are rarely accompanied by systematic evaluation research to inform future decisions. One exception is a study of marketization trends in the Nordic countries [58], which found that public procurement guided by a business management model may not be appropriate for addiction services.

39.2.3.2   Structural Resources
The next requirement of an effective treatment system is to have sufficient resources to meet population needs and the demand for treatment services. The core structural elements are facili-

ties, personnel, and programs. Alcohol and drug services in "mature" treatment systems form a continuum ranging from primary prevention activities designed to ensure that a disorder or problem will not occur, through secondary prevention activities (including early identification and management of substance use disorders), to tertiary prevention activities that aim to stop or retard the progress of a disorder. In many countries, these services have generally developed separately and are rarely integrated within a single service delivery system. Figure 39.2 summarizes data from the WHO *ATLAS on Substance Abuse* [64] describing the most common settings throughout the world for the treatment of alcohol and drug disorders. In the plurality of the responding countries (39.8%), mental health services are the most common treatment setting for alcohol use disorders, whereas the main setting for the treatment of drug use disorders (51.5%) is specialized treatment services.

Approximately 10% of the countries reported primary health care to be the most commonly used setting for treating alcohol and drug use disorders.

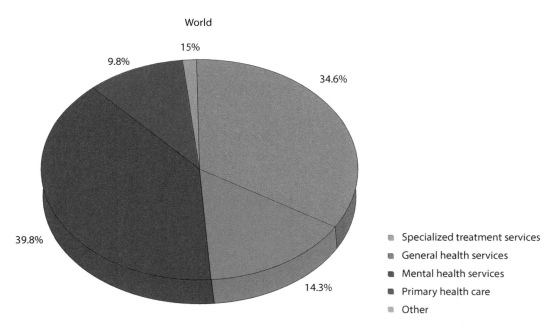

Fig. 39.2 Most common settings for treatment of alcohol and drug disorders in WHO member states. (Source: WHO ATLAS on Substance Abuse)

Another structural resource is the capacity of the system in terms of the number of beds and length of stay. The median number of beds for alcohol and drug use disorders globally was 1.7 per 100,000 population (range 0–52) [64]. The lowest number of beds was reported in the African regions, whereas the highest number was reported from countries in the European Region (10.3 beds per 100,000 population). Median length of stay for drug and alcohol detoxification was found to be 14.0 and 10.3 days, respectively, with low-income countries reporting a longer median length of stay than high-income countries.

Finally, treatment personnel have become a central feature of a country's treatment infrastructure. Among the various health professions involved in treating substance use disorders, the majority of countries reporting in the WHO ATLAS include psychiatrists, general practitioners, and narcologists as the most important [64]. That situation may be changing in the high-income countries of Europe and North America with the growth of specialized study programs for addiction treatment specialists, who are being trained at the bachelor, master, and doctoral levels to deliver services and manage programs [41, 42]. In addition to these professional addiction specialist groups, nonprofessional organizations have emerged as a critical part of the workforce in the formation of self-help organizations. Former alcoholics and drug addicts play an important role in providing community support services in many countries [64].

39.2.3.3 System Qualities

Over time, the collection of services used to manage persons with substance use disorders takes on the characteristics of a system, with unique configurations emerging not only in terms of policies and structural resources but also in terms of system qualities that characterize the functioning of a system. According to the model in Fig. 39.1, these qualities can be described in terms of equity, efficiency, and integration.

Equity refers to the extent to which services are equally available and accessible to all population groups. In South Africa, a study found inequitable access to substance abuse treatment services among the poor, with non-need factors, such as gender, mainly determining utilization [38]. Access to treatment may be as important as the type of treatment. Findings from large-scale treatment matching studies indicate that the decision to enter treatment is associated with considerable reductions in drinking, but once someone is admitted to a particular program, they do equally well regardless of the type of psychotherapy they receive [2].

Research [13] suggests that the key ingredient of the success of any therapy may be its ability to attract clients and generate enthusiasm among therapists. Instead of distinct nonoverlapping elements, different types of therapy may work through common mechanisms, such as empathy, an effective therapist-client alliance, a desire to change, ability to mobilize the client's inner resources, the creation of a supportive social network, and the provision of a culturally appropriate solution to a socially defined problem. Thus, the more that treatment services are made available to all population segments, the greater the system's effectiveness is likely to be.

Some therapeutic interventions are more cost-effective than others, suggesting that resources could be allocated more efficiently and economically without compromising effectiveness. One way to improve the efficiency of treatment is to organize treatment teams or sites to work together for a 12- to 24-month period with the aim of improving a specific area of care. This "improvement collaborative" approach combines traditional quality improvement methods of teamwork, process analysis, adoption of standards, training, and coaching. In a study by Gustafson et al. [16], the use of collaborative methods, especially coaching, was found to decrease waiting time, improve treatment retention, and increase recruitment of new patients. Humphreys and McLellan [21] found that process improvements can change the efficiency of treatment programs, but the link to better outcomes is weak, in part because outcomes are mainly influenced by environmental factors and life events outside of formal treatment.

System integration is a term that refers to the amount of interconnectedness among the organizations in a network. Research suggests several ways to improve system integration: drug courts, SBIRT, integrated treatment programs for pregnant drug users, managed care, case management, and New Public Management (NPM), a market-oriented approach used in the Nordic countries to improve efficiency and lower costs [27]. There is some evidence to suggest that drug courts can increase social controls, lengthen the duration of treatment, reduce criminal behavior, and lower rates of recidivism [14]. The elements of SBIRT have been evaluated in clinical trials and found to be effective [5] to such an extent that programs have been initiated in large population areas of several countries, including Finland [53], Norway [1], Denmark [10], South Africa [52], Brazil [56], and the United States [31]. Despite some successes in primary health care [56], the results of programs relying on the training of physicians and other health personnel without adequate logistical support have not been encouraging.

In the United States, a large-scale program operating in 27 states since 2005 [6, 7] has been found to enhance the states' continuum of care to include universal, adult SBIRT services in primary care and other community settings (e.g., health centers, nursing homes, university health centers, hospitals, emergency departments, and military). In an evaluation of SBIRT's system effects, the program filled gaps in services for substance users in both the medical and specialty treatment systems of care. It was also associated with improved system equity (i.e., equal access to all population groups) and efficiency by extending services to underserved populations, expanding services within facilities and across tasks, and improving system linkages [6, 7].

Another way to improve system integration is through integrated treatment programs. Examples include treatment of pregnant women who have substance use disorders and the delivery of mental health services to patients with co-occurring mental disorders. Integrated women's programs providing pregnancy and parenting services have been associated with improvements in child development [39]. To the extent that clients with co-occurring disorders tend to have a more severe course of illness, more severe health and social consequences, more difficulties in treatment, and worse treatment outcomes than clients with a single disorder, research suggests that these outcomes might be improved when treatment modalities are offered in combination within an integrated treatment plan that simultaneously addresses substance abuse and psychiatric problems [36].

39.2.3.4 Effectiveness and Population Impact

When the requirements for an optimal treatment system are met, treatment services are available, affordable, and accessible. Under these conditions, the system should not only deliver effective services, it should also have a population impact. Effectiveness means the extent to which one or more services are responsible for positive changes in substance use and substance-related problems. Effective services should promote abstinence (or at least reduce substance use), prevent relapse, and address such substance-related problems as unemployment and marital adjustment. As suggested in Fig. 39.1, the impact of these services should translate into population health benefits, such as reduced mortality and alcohol-related disease rates, as well as benefits to social welfare, such as reduced unemployment, disability, crime, suicide, and health-care costs. One way this may happen is through the rapid diffusion of innovation within and across systems. To the extent that a new treatment innovation is perceived as being consistent with existing values, past experiences, and the needs of the country, the treatment system's communication processes may facilitate the transfer of evidence-based approaches [27].

Can the integrative effects of prevention, early intervention, and treatment systems reduce population rates of alcohol and drug problems? This issue has not been investigated extensively. There is suggestive evidence for such an effect with treatment services but not for screening and brief intervention [17]. For example, growth in the availability of opioid maintenance treatment is associated with reductions in illicit opiate use, crime, and HIV risk behaviors in the United Kingdom, France, Norway, and the United States [12, 34]. Increases in the proportion of alcoholics in treatment have been linked to decreases in liver cirrhosis morbidity [19, 33], and increases in AA membership and amount of treatment linked to decreased alcohol problems [54].

Given the possibility that policies, resources, and system qualities, as core requirements, can be used to provide a more effective set of services and contribute to the system's public health impact, the next section of this chapter considers the main priorities for developing such a system.

39.2.4 Priorities

Substance use services have traditionally been established without the benefit of a comprehensive, quantitative planning process that is aligned with population needs. Priorities for developing an optimal treatment service system will vary according to a country's current level of services, as well as the nature of their alcohol and drug problems. Among the highest priorities are service mapping, needs assessment, and service planning. Another priority that is often neglected despite its recognized effectiveness is the establishment and support of mutual help organizations that provide a critical community resource for the initiation and maintenance of recovery.

39.2.4.1 Service Mapping

Treatment service mapping involves the documentation and description of system structures and qualities. Treatment mapping research has been conducted in Hungary, Poland, the Russian Federation, France, Switzerland, Germany, the United Kingdom of Great Britain and Northern Ireland, the United States of America, Finland, Sweden, and a variety of other countries [25, 26, 28]. Data collection tools have been developed for treatment mapping purposes, but most of these instruments do not examine the treatment system components described in this chapter.

To promote the orderly planning and dissemination of evidence-based addiction treatment within national health-care systems, the World Health Organization has designed a procedure for assessing, monitoring, and evaluating treatment systems for substance use disorders, in relation to population needs [3]. The WHO Substance Abuse Instrument for Mapping Services (WHO-SAIMS) was developed to provide information on prevention and treatment services that can be used for policy planning, service design, and service improvement. In its present form, the WHO-SAIMS has a primarily descriptive function that identifies gaps in service delivery and areas for system improvement. The primary purpose of the WHO-SAIMS is to examine the structure and functioning of alcohol and drug service systems in terms of resources, facilities, personnel, and programs. It can also be used at the national and subnational levels for monitoring and process evaluation to identify changes in the system over time and to assess the extent to which system improvement strategies have been implemented. The scope and configuration of the instrument are described in Table 39.1.

Table 39.1 Scope and configuration of the World Health Organization's Substance Abuse Instrument for Mapping Services (WHO-SAIMS)

Policy and legislative domain: This includes items about national alcohol and drug policies; legislation governing drug control, prevention, and treatment; strategic plans that address substance use disorders, workforce development for substance abuse professionals, and resource allocation to and the financing of alcohol and drug services
The substance abuse situation and current alcohol and drug service needs: This section is designed to (1) help identify whether current services match needs and (2) estimate service coverage of the current alcohol and drug treatment system. This domain described the type and mix of services provided, service integration, and system complexity
The alcohol and drug services domain. This section covers (1) other residential services for alcohol and drug problems such as halfway houses and sober living environments; (2) alcohol and drug services provided by other sectors such as mental health facilities, primary health-care services, and the criminal justice sector; (3) the linkages between these services; (4) the availability of psychosocial treatments and psychotropic medications; and (5) drug substitution therapies and harm reduction services for opioid users
The primary care domain. Items in this category refer to interventions used in primary care settings. The human resource domain. This describes the quantity of human resources as well as human resource development, including mutual help organizations and recovering communities such as AA and NA

Source: Babor and Poznyak [3]

39.2.4.2 Estimating Demand for Treatment and Treatment Needs

Demand for treatment refers to the number of people who want to access treatment, including those who receive treatment (met demand) and those who want treatment but cannot access it (unmet demand). Unmet demand may exist because services do not exist, are not available, are too expensive, or are inaccessible [44, 45]. Need for treatment refers to the number of people in a geographic region who meet the criteria for dependence or harmful use and who would benefit from treatment but do not access it. Some of these people want treatment but cannot access it (for the above reasons), while others do not want treatment nor do they seek it [44, 45]. The numbers of "unmet need" are likely to be greater than the numbers of "demand for treatment" because "unmet need" includes those people who do not perceive the need for or do not desire any treatment.

There are several methods to identify unmet treatment need, some involving primary data collection and others relying on secondary analysis of existing data sources. The simplest procedure is to use population surveys to estimate the number of people in need of treatment (see [43–45, 61]). If the rates of dependence and harmful use are used, these can translate into the potential demand for specialized services (residential and outpatient) as well as early intervention services in other health-care settings. These services can be directed at patients with dependence and harmful use, respectively. Because of the limitations of using survey measures of diagnostic criteria, population survey data should be supplemented by obtaining prevalence estimates from settings where substance users are likely to be encountered, such as prisons, emergency departments, and HIV clinics. The need for substance abuse services among the general population can also be estimated through the use of health and social indicators, such as substance-related mortality, morbidity, social problem statistics, and expert opinion on treatment needs. A major difficulty in using population data to estimate treatment need is the occurrence of "sponta-

neous remission," which refers to the changes in substance use that occur without treatment. Because of these problems, some experts suggest focusing on treatment demand, which can be measured through self-reported intentions to seek treatment or client perceptions of the need for treatment [44, 45]. Another option is to use waiting list data. If these data are not available or are difficult to obtain, harm indicators derived from administrative databases can be used as well. For alcohol, the harm indicators that have been used include arrests for alcohol-impaired driving and alcohol-related morbidity rates for different diseases and conditions. Although these indicators of treatment need or demand have limitations, a combined approach is sometimes used to provide greater confidence in the estimates [61] and to help direct resources to those services that conform best to the various indicators of severity (e.g., opiate withdrawal) and complexity (e.g., psychiatric co-morbidity).

39.2.4.3 Needs-Based Planning

For service systems at a modest (Level III) or mature (Level IV) stage of development, it may be more fruitful to use the "needs-based planning" approach described in Fig. 39.3. This model uses population prevalence data to estimate the types of treatment services to be received by subgroups in the population. As such, it is more advanced than the SAIMS methods because it takes into account different types of treatment and respective "need" by treatment type.

In the "Rush model," help-seeking populations are allocated across three treatment service categories: withdrawal management, community services and supports, and residential treatment services. Projections of need and required service capacity for Canadian health planning regions were derived by synthetic estimation according to age and gender. The model and gap analysis was piloted in nine regions of Canada, producing the following national distribution of need across the five categories: Tier 1, 80.7%; Tier 2, 10.4%; Tier 3, 6.1%; Tier 4, 2.6%; and Tier 5, 0.2%.

The "Rush model," initially developed in the early 1990s [47] to estimate treatment needs in Ontario, Canada, has been followed by similar

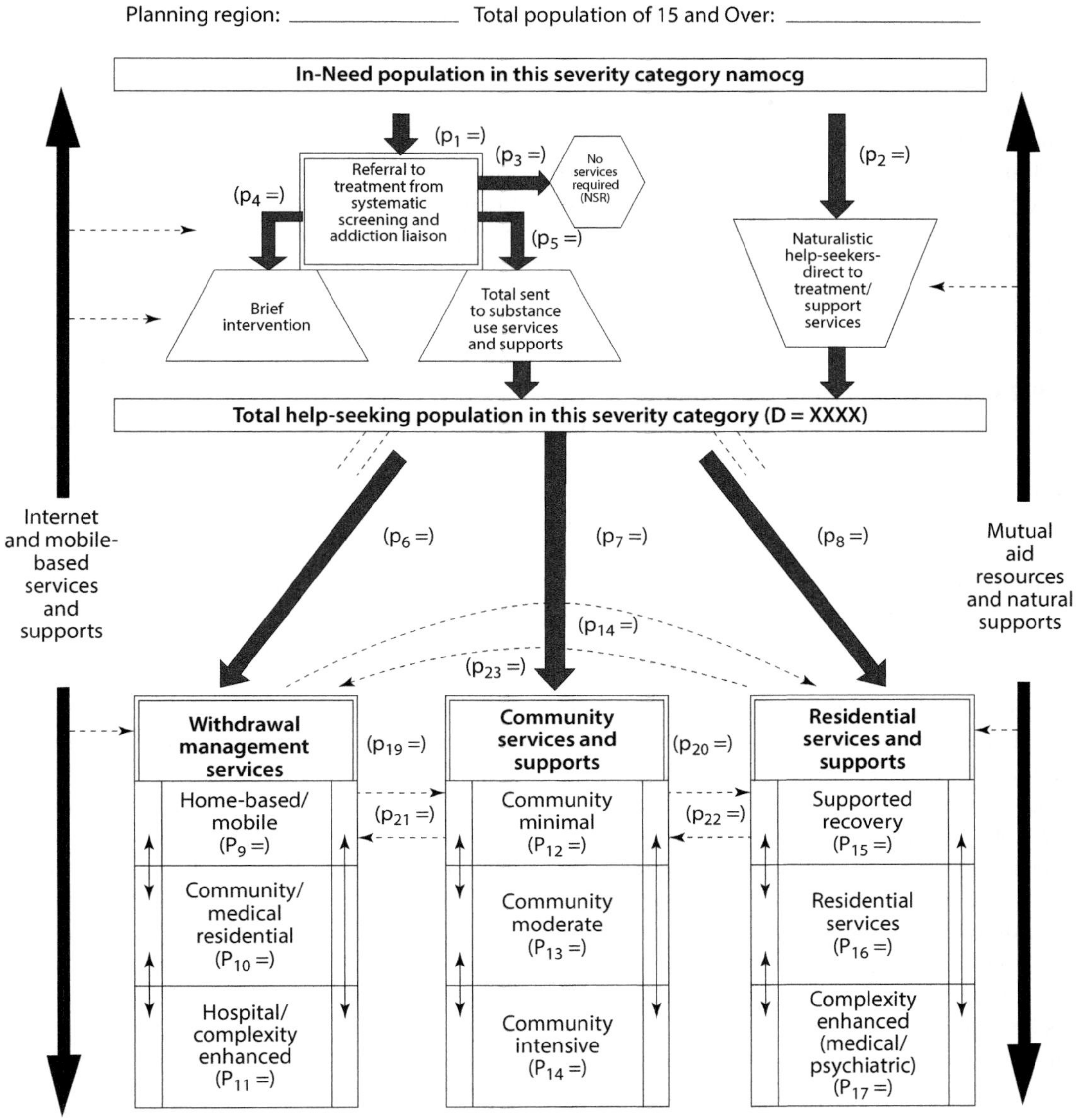

Planning region: _____   Total population of 15 and Over: _____

In-Need population in this severity category namocg

$(p_1 =)$
$(p_3 =)$ No services required (NSR)
$(p_2 =)$

$(p_4 =)$
Referral to treatment from systematic screening and addiction liaison

$(p_5 =)$

Naturalistic help-seekers-direct to treatment/support services

Brief intervention

Total sent to substance use services and supports

Total help-seeking population in this severity category (D = XXXX)

Internet and mobile-based services and supports

$(p_6 =)$ $(p_7 =)$ $(p_8 =)$

Mutual aid resources and natural supports

$(p_{14} =)$

$(p_{23} =)$

Withdrawal management services	$(p_{19} =)$	Community services and supports	$(p_{20} =)$	Residential services and supports
Home-based/ mobile ($P_9 =$)	$(p_{21} =)$	Community minimal ($P_{12} =$)	$(p_{22} =)$	Supported recovery ($P_{15} =$)
Community/ medical residential ($P_{10} =$)		Community moderate ($P_{13} =$)		Residential services ($P_{16} =$)
Hospital/ complexity enhanced ($P_{11} =$)		Community intensive ($P_{14} =$)		Complexity enhanced (medical/ psychiatric) ($P_{17} =$)

Fig. 39.3 Schematic diagram of needs-based planning model for substance use services and supports. (Source: Rush et al. [51])

approaches in Australia [44, 45]; the UK [11]; Brazil [37]; and Quebec, Canada [60]. As noted by Babor et al. [9], these initiatives differ in key features such as the substances of concern, populations of interest, criteria to define need for treatment, as well as methodological details. Nevertheless, they share several common features, such as the use of epidemiological measures of need and help-seeking to estimate the demand for treatment and postulating an "ideal" system design composed of evidence-based interventions.

Another commonality is the assumption that "treatment need" and the "treatment gap" should be estimated at the level of different services and client characteristics, rather than reported only as an undifferentiated measure of overall treatment coverage. In the past, diagnostic criteria derived from health statistics or epidemiological surveys have typically been used as an indicator of the "treatment gap." In some cases, the estimates are so crudely constructed that they grossly overestimate total need without specifying how those estimates map on to specific service components and population groups [9]. An example is the use of the AUDIT and AUDIT-C that are sometimes used to estimate the need for early intervention services despite the number of false positives that can be included in such estimates [18].

39.2.4.4 Mutual Help Organizations

Alcoholics Anonymous and other mutual help organizations represent a critical resource both in countries with mature systems and in those with limited resources. Not only do these approaches provide continued support in the community, they do so at minimal cost. A variety of mutual help models have been developed throughout the world [20], many of them seemingly capable of managing some of the most difficult cases of drug and alcohol dependence. With an estimated 2.2 million members affiliated with more than 125,000 groups in 180 countries, AA is by far the most widely utilized source of help for drinking problems in the world [20, 30]. And the AA recovery program has been applied to a variety of other addictive behaviors, including drug use and problem gambling [30].

Although it is regarded as one of the most useful resources for recovering alcoholics, the research literature supporting the efficacy of AA is limited [35]. Attendance at AA tends to be correlated with long-term abstinence [20, 59], but this may reflect motivation for recovery. Several large-scale, well-designed studies [40, 62] suggest that AA can have an incremental effect when combined with formal treatment, and AA attendance alone may be better than no intervention. When AA is combined with a 12-week individual therapy called Twelve-Step Facilitation (TSF), one study [2] found that TSF not only increased affiliation with AA, it also had a demonstrable effect on clients whose social networks contained many drinking companions. This study suggested that AA is effective because it helps to change the drinker's social environment rather than through some form of spiritual conversion.

Similar mutual help organizations have been developed in a number of other countries, such as Danshukai in Japan, Kreuzbund in Germany, Croix d'Or and Vie Libre in France, Abstainers Clubs in Poland, Family Clubs in Italy, Links in the Scandinavian countries, Pui Hong self-help organizations in Hong Kong, Oxford House in North America and Australia, and Narcotics Anonymous worldwide [4, 20, 63].

39.3 Conclusion

Treatment systems for substance use disorders are a significant part of national responses to the burden of disease and disability resulting from substance abuse. In well-resourced countries, a relatively integrated system of services has been developed in response to population needs. In less-resourced countries, treatment services are often inadequate and fragmentary. Regardless of development level, appropriate population health-care management requires the allocation of resources to preventive, curative, restorative, and rehabilitative services, using the most effective and efficient evidence-based practices. By organizing service providers into networks, it should be possible to shift utilization to lower cost settings or the most appropriate level of care.

Despite the lack of systems research in low- and middle-income countries, some progress has also been reported in emerging economies where treatment services are expanding. For example, the implementation of needs assessment and performance measurement protocols has been found to be feasible and helpful for treatment systems planning in countries like Brazil and South Africa [9, 37]. These developments suggest a shift in the ability of governments and public health authorities to estimate need and plan services in countries where the epidemiological tools and the necessary service elements already exist.

A system-wide holistic approach to the planning and coordination of services for substance use disorders is more than the mere sum of gains attributable to discrete interventions and technologies, such as new screening tools, better diagnostic instruments, improved intervention techniques, and more numerous services. The systems approach goes beyond capacity building and technical innovation. It is designed to coordinate services so that they are capable of responding to the changing needs of the population.

References

1. Aasland OG, Johannesen A. Screening and brief intervention for alcohol problems in Norway. Not a big hit among general practitioners. Nordic Stud Alcohol Drugs. 2008;25:515–22.
2. Babor TF, Del Boca FK, editors. Treatment matching in alcoholism. Cambridge, UK: Cambridge University Press; 2003.
3. Babor TF, Poznyak V. The World Health Organization substance abuse instrument for mapping services. Rationale, structure and functions. Nordic Stud Alcohol Drugs. 2010;27:703–11.
4. Babor T, Caulkins J, Edwards G, Fischer B, Foxcroft D, Humphreys K, et al. Drug policy and the public good. Oxford: Oxford University Press; 2010.
5. Babor TF, McRee B, Kassebaum P, Grimaldi P, Ahmed K, Bray J. Screening, brief intervention, and referral to treatment (SBIRT): toward a public health approach to the management of substance abuse. Subst Abus. 2007;28:7–30.
6. Babor TF, DelBoca F, Bray J. Screening, brief Intervention and referral to treatment: implications of SAMHSA's SBIRT initiative for substance abuse policy and practice. Addiction. 2017;112(S2):110–7. https://doi.org/10.1111/add.13675.
7. Babor TF, Robaina K, Noel J. Enhancing access to alcohol screening, brief intervention, and referral to treatment to better serve individuals and populations. In: Giesbrecht N, Bosma L, editors. Preventing alcohol-related problems: evidence and community-based initiatives. Washington, DC: APHA Press; 2017.
8. Babor TF, Stenius K, Romelsjo A. Alcohol and drug treatment systems in public health perspective: mediators and moderators of population effects. Int J Methods Psychiatr Res. 2008;17(S1):S50–9.
9. Babor TF, Rush B, Tremblay J. Needs-based planning for substance use treatment systems: progress, prospects, and the search for a new perspective. J Stud Alcohol Drugs Suppl. 2019;18:154–60.
10. Barfod S. A GP's reflections on brief intervention in primary health care in Denmark. Nordic Stud Alcohol Drugs. 2008;25:523–8.
11. Brennan A, McManus D, Stone T, et al. Modeling the potential impact of changing access rates to specialist treatment for alcohol dependence for local authorities in England: the specialist treatment for alcohol model (stream). J Stud Alcohol Drugs Suppl. 2019;18:96–109.
12. Bukten A, Skurtveit S, Gossop M, et al. Engagement with opioid maintenance treatment and reductions in crime: a longitudinal national cohort study. Addiction. 2012;107:393–9.
13. Cooney NL, Babor TF, DiClemente CC, Del Boca FK. Clinical and scientific implications of project MATCH. In: Babor TF, Del Boca FK, editors. Treatment matching in alcoholism. Cambridge, UK: Cambridge University Press; 2003. p. 222–37.
14. Eibner C, Morral A, Pacula RL, MacDonald J. Is the drug court model exportable? An examination of the cost-effectiveness of a Los Angeles-based DUI court. J Subst Abuse Treat. 2006;31(1):75–85.
15. Glaser FB, Greenberg SW, Barrett M. A systems approach to alcohol treatment. Toronto: Alcohol Research Foundation; 1978.
16. Gustafson DH, Quanbeck AR, Robinson JM, et al. Which elements of improvement collaboratives are most effective? A cluster-randomized trial. Addiction. 2013;108:1145–57.
17. Heather N. Can screening and brief intervention lead to population-level reductions in alcohol-related harm? Addict Sci Clin Pract. 2012;7:15.
18. Higgins-Biddle JC, Babor TF. A review of the alcohol use disorders identification test (AUDIT), AUDIT-C, and USAUDIT for screening in the United States: past issues and future directions. Am J Drug Alcohol Abuse. 2018;44(6):578–86.
19. Holder H, Parker RN. Effect of alcoholism treatment on cirrhosis mortality: a 20-year multivariate time series analysis. Br J Addict. 1992;87:1263–74.
20. Humphreys K. Circles of recovery: self-help organizations for addictions. Cambridge, UK: Cambridge University Press; 2004.
21. Humphreys K, McLellan T. A policy-oriented review of strategies for improving the outcomes of services for substance use disorder patients. Addiction. 2011;106:2058–66.
22. Huntington D, Banzon E, Recidoro Z. A system approach to improving maternal health in the Philippines. Bull World Health Organ. 2012;90:104–10.
23. Institute of Medicine. Broadening the base of treatment for alcohol problems. Washington, DC: National Academy Press; 1990.
24. Kaner EFS, Beyer FR, Muirhead C, Campbell F, Pienaar ED, Bertholet N, Daeppen JB, Saunders JB, Burnand B. Effectiveness of brief alcohol interventions in primary care populations. Cochrane Database Syst Rev. 2018(2). Art. No.: CD004148. https://doi.org/10.1002/14651858.CD004148.pub4.
25. Klingemann H, Hunt G, editors. Treatment systems in an international perspective: drugs, demons and delinquents. Thousand Oaks/London/New Delhi: SAGE Publications; 1998. p. 3–19.
26. Klingemann H, Takala JP, Hunt G. Cure, care or control: alcoholism treatment in sixteen countries. Albany: State University of New York Press; 1992.
27. Klingemann H, Storbjörk J. The treatment response: systemic features, paradigms and socio-cultural

frameworks. In: Kolind T, Thom B, Hunt G, editors. The SAGE handbook of drug and alcohol studies. London: SAGE; 2016. p. 260–86.

28. Klingemann H, Takala JP, Hunt G. The development of alcohol treatment systems: an international perspective. Alcohol Health Res World. 1993;3:221–7.

29. Kuussaari K, Partanen A. Administrative challenges in the Finnish alcohol and drug treatment system. Nordic Stud Alcohol Drugs. 2010;27:667–84.

30. Laudet AB. The impact of alcoholics anonymous on other substance abuse-related twelve-step programs. Recent Dev Alcohol. 2008;18:71–89.

31. Madras B, Compton W, Avulac D, Stegbauerc T, Steinc J, Clark HW. Screening, brief interventions, referral to treatment (SBIRT) for illicit drug and alcohol use at multiple healthcare sites: comparison at intake and 6 months later. Drug Alcohol Depend. 2009;99:280–95.

32. Mäkelä K, Room R, Single E, Sulkunen P, Walsh B. Alcohol, society, and the state. A comparative study of alcohol control, vol. 1. Toronto: Alcohol Research Foundation; 1981.

33. Mann RE, Smart R, Anglin L, Rush B. Are decreases in liver cirrhosis rates a result of increased treatment for alcoholism. Br J Addict. 1988;83:683–8.

34. Marsch L. The efficacy of methadone maintenance interventions in reducing illicit opiate use, HIV risk behavior and criminality: a meta-analysis. Addiction. 1998;93:515–32.

35. McCrady B, Miller W. Research on alcoholic anonymous. Opportunities and alternatives. New Brunswick: Rutgers Center of Alcohol Studies; 1993.

36. Morisano D, Babor T, Robaina K. Co-occurrence of substance use disorders with other psychiatric disorders: implications for treatment services. Nordic Stud Alcohol Drugs. 2014;31(1):5–25. https://doi.org/10.2478/nsad-2014-0002.

37. Mota D, Silveira C, Siu E, et al. Estimating service needs for alcohol and other drug users according to a tiered framework: the case of the São Paulo, Brazil, Metropolitan Area. J Stud Alcohol Drugs Suppl. 2019;18:87–95.

38. Myers B, Louw J, Pasche S. Gender differences in barriers to alcohol and other drug treatment in Cape Town, South Africa. Afr J Psychiatry (South Afr). 2011;14:146–53.

39. Niccols A, Milligan K, Smith A, et al. Integrated programs for mothers with substance abuse issues and their children: a systematic review of studies reporting on child outcomes. Child Abuse Negl. 2012;36:308–22.

40. Ouimette PC, Finney JW, Gima K, Moos RH. A comparative evaluation of substance abuse treatment: examining mechanisms underlying patient-treatment matching hypotheses for 12-step and cognitive-behavioral treatments for substance abuse. Alcohol Clin Exp Res. 1999;23:545–51.

41. Pavlovská A, Miovsky M, Babor TF, Gabrhelik R. Overview of the European university-based study programmes in the addictions field. Drug Educ Prev Policy. 2017;24(6):485–91. https://doi.org/10.1080/09687637.2016.1223603.

42. Pavlovská A, Peters RH, Gabrhelík R, Sloboda Z, Babor TF, Miovský M. A survey of addiction studies programs in North American universities. J Subst Abus. 2019;24(910):55–60. https://doi.org/10.1080/14659891.2018.1505970.

43. Ritter A, Berends L, Clemens C, Devaney M, Bowen K, Tiffen R. Pathways: a review of the Victorian drug treatment service system. Final report. Melbourne: Turning Point Alcohol and Drug Centre; 2003.

44. Ritter A, Mellor R, Chalmers J, Sunderland M, Lancaster K. Key considerations in planning for substance use treatment: estimating treatment need and demand. J Stud Alcohol Drugs. 2019;Supplement No. 19:S42–50.

45. Ritter A, Gomez M, Chalmers J. Measuring unmet demand for alcohol and other treatment: the application of an Australian population based planning model. J Stud Alcohol Drugs. 2019;Supplement No. 19:S42–50.

46. Room R. Alcohol and drug treatment systems: what is meant, and what determines their development. Nordic Stud Alcohol Drugs. 2010;27:575–9.

47. Rush B. A systems approach to estimating the required capacity of alcohol treatment services. Br J Addict. 1990;85(1):49–59.

48. Rush B. Tiered frameworks for planning substance use service delivery systems: origins and key principles. Nordic Stud Alcohol Drugs. 2010;27:617–36.

49. Rush B, Tremblay J, Fougere C, Perez W, Fineczko J. Development of a needs-based planning model for substance use services and supports in Canada: final report. Toronto: Centre for Addiction and Mental Health; 2013.

50. Rush B, Urbanoski K. Seven core principles of substance use treatment system design to aid in identifying strengths, gaps, and required enhancements. J Stud Alcohol Drugs Suppl. 2019;18:9–21.

51. Rush B, et al. Development of a needs-based planning model to estimate required capacity of a substance use treatment system. J Stud Alcohol Drugs Suppl. 2019;Supplement 18:51–63.

52. Seale JP, Monteiro M. The dissemination of screening and brief intervention for alcohol problems in developing countries: lessons from Brazil and South Africa. Nordic Stud Alcohol Drugs. 2008;25:565–77.

53. Seppa K, Kuokkanen M. Implementing brief alcohol intervention in primary and occupational health care. Reflections on two Finnish projects. Nordic Stud Alcohol Drugs. 2008;25:505–14.

54. Smart RG, Mann RE. The impact of programs for high-risk drinkers on population levels of alcohol problems. Addiction. 2000;95:37–52.

55. Souria JC. A history of alcoholism. Oxford: Basil Blackwell; 1990.

56. Souza-Formigoni M, Boerngen-Lacerda R, Vianna VP. Implementing screening and brief intervention in primary care units in two Brazilian states: a case study. Nordic Stud Alcohol Drugs. 2008;25:553–64.

57. Stenius K, Witbrodt J, Engdahl B, Weisner C. For the marginalized, or for the integrated? A comparative study of the treatment systems in Sweden and the US. Contemp Drug Probl. 2010;37:417–48.

58. Storbjörk J, Stenius K. Why research should pay attention to effects of marketization of addiction treatment systems. J Stud Alcohol Drugs Suppl. 2019;18(s18):31–9.

59. Timko C, Moos RH, Finney JW, Lesar MD. Long-term outcomes of alcohol use disorders: comparing untreated individuals with those in alcoholics anonymous and formal treatment. J Stud Alcohol. 2000;61:529–38.

60. Tremblay J, Bertrand K, Blanchette N, et al. Estimation of needs for addiction services: a youth

model. J Stud Alcohol Drugs Suppl. 2019;18:64–75.

61. Ungemack J, Babor TF, Bidiorini A. Connecticut compendium on substance abuse treatment need. Hartford: Department of Mental Health and Addiction Services; 2001.

62. Walsh DC, Hingson RW, Merrigan DM, Levenson SM, Cupples LA, Heeren T, et al. A randomized trial of treatment options for alcohol-abusing workers. N Engl J Med. 1991;325:775–81.

63. White W. Slaying the dragon: the history of addiction treatment and recovery in America. Bloomington: Chestnut Health Systems; 1998.

64. World Health Organization. ATLAS on substance use: resources for the prevention and treatment of substance use disorders. France: WHO; 2010.

Screening, Early Detection, and Brief Intervention of Alcohol Use Disorders

40

John B. Saunders and Noeline C. Latt

Contents

J. B. Saunders (✉)
National Centre for Youth Substance Use Research,
University of Queensland, St Lucia, QLD, Australia

Formerly Disciplines of Psychiatry and Addiction
Medicine, Faculty of Medicine, University of Sydney,
Camperdown, NSW, Australia
e-mail: mail@jbsaunders.net

N. C. Latt
Disciplines of Psychiatry and Addiction Medicine,
Faculty of Medicine, University of Sydney,
Camperdown, NSW, Australia

Formerly Northern Area Drug and Alcohol Service,
Royal North Shore Hospital,
St Leonards, NSW, Australia
e-mail: noelinelatt@bigpond.com

© Springer Nature Switzerland AG 2021
N. el-Guebaly et al. (eds.), *Textbook of Addiction Treatment*,
https://doi.org/10.1007/978-3-030-36391-8_40

Abstract

Self-recognition of an alcohol use disorder is often late in the natural history of this condition. Because of this and the limited impact of treatment for patients with late-stage complications of their alcohol problem, there has been considerable effort made to identify alcohol consumption where it has reached a hazardous or risky stage or is starting to cause problems, before dependence becomes entrenched and complications irreversible. The approach of screening and brief intervention represents a secondary intervention approach, which aims to help people reduce their alcohol consumption to low-risk levels and thereby avoid progression to dependence and the development of harmful physical and mental sequelae and social problems. This chapter describes the development of screening instruments such as the Alcohol Use Disorders Identification Test (AUDIT) and several derivatives and alternatives. The performance and applicability of these screening instrument is reviewed. Following this, there is an account of brief intervention approaches which aim to provide succinct information on alcohol use and risks to the individual, often combined with brief motivational and behavioral strategies. There is considerable evidence from scores of randomized controlled trials and meta-analyses for the effectiveness of brief interventions in reducing hazardous alcohol consumption and alcohol-related problems. In the long-term follow-up studies, there is also evidence for reduced rates of hospitalization and mortality. The latest developments in screening and brief intervention are their presentation in various electronic formats. Online screening with feedback and brief intervention has shown to be efficacious and has the potential to be accessible to a greater section of the general population than face-to-face interventions in healthcare settings.

Keywords

Hazardous alcohol use · Harmful alcohol use · Alcohol dependence · Alcohol use disorders · Screening instruments · Early intervention · Brief intervention · Electronic screening · e-SBI

40.1 Broadening the Spectrum of Intervention for Alcohol Use Disorders

Self-recognition of an alcohol use disorder is often late in the natural history of the condition. Frequently, patients seen in healthcare services have well-established alcohol dependence and often physical, neurocognitive, psychiatric, and social complications when they present for treatment. At this stage, the road back to reasonable health and well-being is a long and sometimes uncertain one, requiring considerable personal resources and involvement in treatment, support, and lifestyle changes.

An important movement in recent years has been to broaden the spectrum of responses so that people with hazardous, harmful (or unhealthy) alcohol consumption and those with less severe alcohol use disorders, as well as those with alcohol dependence, have an opportunity to be alerted to the risks of their drinking and to change their consumption patterns in a healthy direction. Screening and brief intervention has its origins in the work of a World Health Organization (WHO) Expert Committee in the late 1970s. In its report, the Expert Committee recommended "the development of methods for identifying and modifying potentially harmful patterns of alcohol consumption before dependence developed and disease was entrenched."

Arising from this report was a WHO program of work on development of techniques for early detection and intervention for hazardous and harmful alcohol consumption. Parallel work in the area was undertaken by pioneers such as Kristenson [41] and Heather [33]. Since those early days, there has been a substantial effort to develop screening instruments, such as the Alcohol Use Disorders Identification Test (AUDIT) [67], and brief structured therapies designed to be used at the time hazardous and harmful alcohol use is identified.

This approach has been endorsed by many authorities. In 1990 an influential report from the US Institute of Medicine [35] recommended that healthcare responses should extend beyond the provision of treatment for people with established alcohol dependence (or "alcoholism") to encompass early detection and treatments in primary care and in other nonspecialist settings. It noted the evidence accumulating for the effectiveness of opportunistic screening and brief intervention for hazardous and harmful alcohol consumption. Since that time, a national alcohol screening day has been introduced in the USA, and screening and brief intervention is identified as an essential approach for primary healthcare services. The US National Institute on Alcohol Abuse and Alcoholism (NIAAA) has issued a clinician's guide on "Helping patients who drink too much" [52]. The UK's National Institute for Health and Care Excellence's (NICE) guideline on the prevention of alcohol use disorders [53] and the World Health Organization's intervention guide for mental, neurological, and substance use disorders [80] support the widespread screening and implementation of brief intervention approaches in people with nondependent hazardous and harmful drinking.

Screening and brief intervention is analogous to screening for asymptomatic hypertension, hyperlipidemia, and a range of medical, mental, and social disorders. It is predicated on the basis that early detection and treatment of a disorder in its developmental stage has advantages over treatment of severe alcohol use disorder or dependence disorder in terms of reduced morbidity, better and more guaranteed response to treatment, and the avoidance of the costs of treating the advanced disorder and prevention of premature mortality.

This present chapter will (1) review the current criteria for nondependent hazardous/ unhealthy alcohol consumption, harmful alcohol consumption, and mild alcohol dependence/ mild alcohol use disorder, (2) examine the available screening instruments (focusing on instruments specifically derived to screen for a range of hazardous consumption and alcohol use disorders), (3) review the evidence for the effectiveness of brief alcohol interventions, (4) review the key therapeutic components of brief interventions, (5) examine the implementations of such interventions in healthcare systems, and (6) examine electronic screening and brief intervention approaches which have been developed to further broaden the access of people with hazardous or unhealthy patterns of alcohol consumption to information and advice, who otherwise might not be engaged in the healthcare system.

40.2 The Spectrum of Nondependent Alcohol Use Disorders

Alcohol use and misuse exists as a continuum, and an important realization is that harm can occur at many points along this continuum. Excess alcohol use is a significant cause of morbidity, mortality, and social problems. Accidents can occur due to a single episode of excessive consumption; they are more likely to occur with repeated bouts of drinking; social problems can arise due to intoxicated behaviors, and acute medical disorders may also arise from periodic binges. Many chronic disease states are linked to regular consumption of alcohol that may not reflect alcohol dependence. Although the risks of all these are multiplied in people who have alcohol dependence, and it is right that much attention be paid to this group, it is important to capture a broad range of consumption patterns and alcohol disorders.

Alcohol consumption may be facilitated by external factors such as cultural norms and practices, peer pressure, work culture, and work pressure or internal factors such as the person's feelings and mental state or desire to experience the euphoria and state of intoxication that alcohol can cause.

Fig. 40.1 The spectrum
of alcohol use disorders

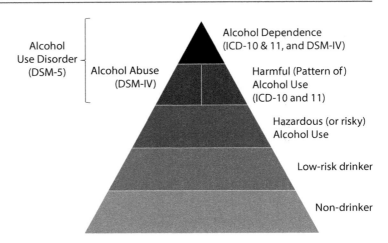

Nondependent alcohol use disorders include the following diagnostic terms from the World Health Organization's International Classification of Diseases (ICD) system: hazardous alcohol use [79], harmful alcohol use [78], and harmful pattern of alcohol use [79]. The American Psychiatric Association's Diagnostic and Statistical Manual of Mental Disorders (DSM) includes alcohol abuse [1] and mild alcohol use disorder [2]. "Unhealthy alcohol use" is an umbrella term referring to that spectrum of alcohol use that can result in health consequences and broadly covers hazardous use, harmful use, and alcohol abuse and dependence and all grade of alcohol use disorder [64, 65] (See Fig. 40.1).

40.2.1 Hazardous Alcohol Use (ICD-11)

Hazardous alcohol use is defined as a pattern of alcohol use that appreciably increases the risk of harmful physical or mental consequences to the drinker or to others [79]. Hazardous use has not yet reached the level of having caused harm. "Risky use" is similarly defined as alcohol consumption in amounts that increase the likelihood of health consequences, e.g., injury, interpersonal problems, and medical consequences [64, 65].

The risk of harm is related to the level of alcohol consumption and the frequency and duration of consumption. In addition, psychosocial, envi-

ronmental, and genetic influences may play a role [69, 72, 73]. Examples of national criteria for hazardous or risky alcohol use are as follows:

(a) *USA*: for women and men aged 65 years and older, drinking more than 7 drinks in a week or more than 3 drinks per day; for men under age 65 years, drinking more than 14 drinks in a week or more than 4 drinks in a day (1 drink being approximately 12–14 g of alcohol) [50, 52].

(b) *UK*: regular drinking of more than 14 units a week but less than 35 units a week for women; drinking more than 14 units a week but less than 50 units for men (1 unit is approximately 8 g or 10 ml of ethanol). Regular drinkers are advised to spread the amount evenly over 3 days or more, with some alcohol-free days per week [53]. In the UK risky drinking is sometimes graded as low risk, increasing risk, or higher risk. A single episode of heavy drinking, e.g., five to seven units in a 3–6-hour period (binge), increases the risk of accidents and injury two to five times [75].

(c) *Australia:* more than two standard drinks on any day (for both men and women) or more than four standard drinks on a single occasion (one standard drink being approximately 10 g of alcohol). For those under the age of 16 years or if a woman is pregnant or planning to become pregnant or breastfeeding, the safest option is not to drink alcohol [51].

Hazardous drinking includes any use of alcohol in pregnancy, when driving or working with machinery, when taking medications that interact with alcohol, and in certain medical conditions, e.g., chronic hepatitis C. Women should be warned that consumption of alcohol in early pregnancy carries the risk of fetal alcohol spectrum disorder (FASD) [68].

40.2.2 Harmful Alcohol Use (ICD-10) or Harmful Pattern of Alcohol Use (ICD-11)

Harmful (pattern of) alcohol use is a repetitive pattern of use at levels which have caused damage to a person's physical or mental health or resulted in behavior leading to harm to the health of others but does not fulfill the criteria for dependence of alcohol [78, 79]. The harmful effects may be acute (e.g., trauma) or chronic (e.g., alcoholic liver disease, depression). An episode of harmful alcohol use is a new ICD-11 diagnostic term for situations where harm has resulted from drinking, without information on whether the consumption represents a pattern of repeated use or a one-off episode [23, 29, 78, 79]. In DSM-IV TR, the term "alcohol abuse" is defined as a maladaptive pattern of alcohol use over a 12-month period leading to clinically significant failure to fulfill major obligations at work, school, or home and legal problems or interpersonal problems or which is physically hazardous [1].

40.2.3 Alcohol Use Disorder: Mild (DSM-V)

The DSM-V replaced the terms alcohol abuse and alcohol dependence under a broad term "alcohol use disorder." It is defined as a cluster of cognitive, behavioral, and physiological symptoms following a problematic pattern of alcohol use leading to clinically significant impairment or distress, manifested by at least 2 of 11 criteria within a 12-month period. The severity of the disorder is graded on the number of criteria met, viz., mild, two to three; moderate, three to four;

or severe, six or more [2]. Nondependent alcohol use disorder lies in the lower end of this spectrum.

40.3 Alcohol Dependence (ICD-10, ICD-11, DSM-IV TR)

The DSM-V moderate to severe range of alcohol use disorder may conveniently be considered a counterpart to the ICD-10, ICD-11, and DSM-IV TR definition of alcohol dependence. Alcohol dependence is defined as a cluster of behavioral, cognitive, and physiological phenomena that develop after repeated alcohol use which tends to be self-perpetuating. The psychobiological syndrome is best understood as a disorder where there is impaired control over alcohol use and a persistent internal drive to consume alcohol such that alcohol increasing takes "center stage" or priority in the person's life and other enjoyments, activities, and responsibilities are pushed to the periphery. It reflects enduring changes in key neurocircuits that subserve reward, alertness, response control, and salience in the ventral tegmental area of the midbrain, the nucleus accumbens, and related structures of the lower forebrain and with projections to and from the prefrontal gyrus and the circulate gyrus of the cortex. It is more "disease-like" than any other form of repetitive alcohol use and tends to be self-perpetuating and to run true when active at different periods in the person's life. Physiological features indicative of neuroadaptation are manifested by tolerance, withdrawal symptoms following cessation or reduction of drinking, repeated use to prevent or alleviate withdrawal symptoms, and continued use despite harmful consequences.

Once alcohol dependence sets in, the patient may require prolonged treatment in a continuing care program. This includes inpatient or ambulatory detoxification followed by a comprehensive relapse-prevention program involving pharmacotherapy, a variety of psychosocial interventions, as well as self-help and mutual aid group therapy and family therapy. Where medical, psychiatric, or social complications have arisen, referral to appropriate specialties is required. In severe cases, the patient may eventually require long-term residential or inpatient treatment.

There are more people with nondependent hazardous or harmful alcohol consumption than those with established alcohol dependence/moderate to severe alcohol use disorder. Approximately 15–20% of adults consume alcohol in a hazardous/harmful manner and 5% have alcohol dependence [68]. In England, alcohol dependence affects 2% of women and 6% of men, while over 24% of the English population consume alcohol in a way that is potentially harmful or actually harmful to their health and well-being [54] (see Fig. 40.1). Because of the greater prevalence of hazardous and harmful alcohol use in the population, more alcohol-related problems are attributable to hazardous and harmful alcohol use than to alcohol dependence. Screening and identification of nondependent hazardous and harmful drinking and provision of brief intervention are effective and cost-effective preventative approaches in preventing progression to more severe alcohol dependence, other alcohol-related harm, and death [31, 68].

40.4 Screening

For the spectrum of nondependent hazardous alcohol use, harmful alcohol use, and mild alcohol use disorder, there is a need for reliable methods of screening and brief intervention. Screening and early detection can also be applied to alcohol dependence, and brief interventions can be adapted and used in therapy at the start of treatment for persons with alcohol dependence. The 10-question Alcohol Use Disorders Identification Test (AUDIT) is a useful screening instrument in differentiating alcohol dependence from nondependent hazardous or harmful alcohol use: A score of 8 or more is associated with hazardous or harmful drinking, while a score of 15 or more is likely to indicate alcohol dependence [5, 7, 15, 18, 67, 68].

40.5 Development of the AUDIT

The modern era of screening for hazardous and harmful alcohol consumption and alcohol use disorders began with the development of the AUDIT [4, 5, 66, 67]. Prior to this, alcohol screening instruments focused on the detection of alcoholism. They were not designed to detect the range of alcohol use disorders or hazardous/unhealthy alcohol consumption, the reason being that these concepts had not gained general acceptance at the time the older instruments were introduced. These older instruments include the Michigan Alcoholism Screening Test (MAST), developed in 1971 which exists in several versions including brief ones, and the four-item CAGE, this being an acronym of Cut down, Annoyed, Guilty, and Eye-opener [30, 46]. The T-ACE is a variant of CAGE with guilt being replaced by tolerance (Tolerance, Annoyed, Cut down, Eye-opener), to identify excess drinking during pregnancy [71].

Given the increasing focus on identifying hazardous and harmful alcohol use before dependence has become entrenched, the MAST and the CAGE have become less widely used as they perform poorly as screens for less severe unhealthy hazardous or harmful drinking.

The AUDIT has its origins in the WHO collaborative work that was initiated by the Expert Committee and was derived from findings in a World Health Organization Collaborative Study [66, 67, 4, 5]. The AUDIT was developed from the empirical selection of items contained in a WHO assessment instrument, comprising more than 150 questions. Participating centers from six countries around the world (which represented different cultures, healthcare systems, stages of economic development and political systems) were involved. The 10 items which formed the AUDIT were those which had the following characteristics:

1. They had the highest or comparably high item-total correlations with the domains they represented.
2. Individually and collectively they had the greatest discriminatory value between patients who had hazardous or harmful consumption and/or alcohol use disorders and those who did not.
3. The questions not only conformed to the then bidimensional concept of alcohol dependence

and its consequences but extended it to a tridimensional concept of (i) intake measures, (ii) measures of the urge or drive to consume alcohol (and putative dependence), and (iii) direct or proxy measures of alcohol-related consequences.

4. The sensitivity and specificity and positive and negative predictive values for the AUDIT in clinical and also general populations indicated a high degree of accuracy of classification and therefore practical utility.

5. Likewise the sensitivity and specificity of questions in the three individual domains were psychometrically acceptable.

6. The questionnaire as a whole and questions within the three domains had acceptable psychometric performance as judged by measures such as Cronbach's alpha coefficient.

7. Each individual question had high-face validity, the meaning of the question was clear, and it explicitly mentioned the link with alcohol consumption.

8. Each question was suitable in providing a means of exploring further the patient's experiences with alcohol, and the questionnaire as a whole was suitable as a framework for intervention.

9. The individual questions could be translated readily and accurately (both grammatically and idiomatically) into major world languages.

Subsequent studies showed that the AUDIT:

1. Performed as well as a stand-alone questionnaire as it did when the questions were embedded in a general health screening instrument.

2. Had high acceptance among populations being screened.

3. It could be adapted easily to an electronic format including interactive media where feedback on the AUDIT score and on responses to individual questions could be provided.

The AUDIT questionnaire offers a simple and systematic way of assessing alcohol intake (Questions 1–3), alcohol dependence (Questions 4–6), and alcohol-related harm (Questions 7–10). The questionnaire may be self-administered while the patient is awaiting the consultation or may be used by the clinician during the assessment. Responses in the AUDIT are quantified from 0 (far left column) through to 4 (far right column) for Questions 1–8 and 0, 2, and 4 for Questions 9–10. The AUDIT score may range from 0 (for an abstainer of alcohol) to 40. A presumptive diagnosis of hazardous or harmful consumption is made if the AUDIT score is 8 or above. More severe harm and dependence is likely when the score is 15 or more and to be extremely likely if the score is 20 or more. The scores on the AUDIT can also point to the intervention required, if any. Scores of 0 and 1–7 may result in some feedback but otherwise no specific intervention. A score of 8 or more merits a brief intervention, with scores of 15 or more (and certainly 20 or more) alerting the clinician to the need for detoxification and referral for specialist treatment. Assessment by completion of the AUDIT questionnaire itself is reported to reduce hazardous drinking [42].

AUDIT screening for early diagnosis of hazardous and harmful alcohol use is recommended as part of a routine examination in the Accident and Emergency Department, during pregnancy, prior to prescribing medication that interacts with alcohol and where there is evidence of alcohol-related harm, e.g., cardiac arrhythmia, dyspepsia, liver disease, hypertension, depression, anxiety, insomnia, and trauma [13, 54].

40.6 Derivatives of the AUDIT and Alternative Screening Instruments

Several derivatives of the AUDIT have been published over the years. The most popular of these is the AUDIT-C, a three-item questionnaire which comprises simply the first three questions of the AUDIT consumption measures. The AUDIT-C and the single-item AUDIT-3 (which comprises the third question on heavy episodic drinking alone) have been shown to be more convenient, brief, and effective instruments for diagnosing alcohol use disorders in a primary care setting [15, 19, 70].

40.6.1 AUDIT-C

1. How often do you have a drink containing alcohol?
2. How many standard drinks containing alcohol do you have on a typical drinking day?
3. How often do you have four drinks (women) and six drinks (men) or more on one occasion?

A score of 3 or more in women and 4 or more in men has a sensitivity of 73% and 86% and a specificity of 91% and 89%, respectively [16]. A score of 7–10 or more suggests there may be alcohol dependence [60].

The Fast Alcohol Screening Test (FAST), a four-item questionnaire based on the AUDIT, is another useful screening tool. The first question is, "How often do you have eight (for men) or six (for women) or more standard drinks on one occasion?" A response of monthly or more is considered a positive answer. Three further questions make up the FAST [34] with a score of 3 or more indicating hazardous alcohol drinking.

The WHO Alcohol, Smoking and Substance Involvement Screening Test (ASSIST) is a combined screen for drug and alcohol misuse and is available for self-completion while the patient is in the waiting room or hospital clinic. It is designed to inquire about alcohol use in context of health enquiries to detect problem or risky alcohol and other substance use in primary healthcare. It is linked to a brief intervention based on the acronym FRAMES (Feedback, Responsibility, Advice, Menu, Empathetic interviewing and Self-efficacy) and incorporates motivational interviewing [57, 77].

40.6.2 Screening in Special Populations

Some alcohol screening instruments have been developed to identify hazardous consumption and alcohol use disorders within specific populations such as pregnant women, youth and adolescents, ethnic minorities, and the elderly. These include the TWEAK, a quick five-item screening and assessment tool for alcohol use during pregnancy [62, 63] and an acronym of Tolerance, Worried, Eye-opener, Amnesia and Cut down (K). A review of alcohol screening in women suggests that the TWEAK appears to be the optimal screening questionnaire for identifying women with excess alcohol use in racially mixed populations with the AUDIT as a reasonable alternative [14].

The CRAFFT, a six-item screening tool and an acronym for Car, Relax, Alone, Family, Friends, and Trouble, was developed specifically to screen for problematic substance use in teens [40] and found to be a suitable alternative to AUDIT in adolescents and young adults, with excellent sensitivity and no gender-based or race-based differences [22]. Another questionnaire for adolescents called the POSIT (an acronym for Problem-Oriented Screening Instrument for Teenagers and a lengthy 16-item screening questionnaire) was found to perform better than the CRAFFT [61]. The MAST-G, an "elderly-specific" questionnaire, and the CAGE were reported to be better than the AUDIT in a study of elderly male veterans [48]. The MAST-G and the CAGE are appropriate screening instruments for alcohol abuse and dependence in the elderly [10]. The CAGE is reported to be superior to the MAST in the elderly [6]. However, the AUDIT remains a more useful tool for identifying nondependent hazardous and harmful alcohol use in the elderly.

40.7 Brief Interventions: Background and Evidence

Once a person has been identified, through screening or clinical enquiry, as having unhealthy alcohol use, a brief, focused form of therapy is beneficial. The usual term to describe this is "brief alcohol intervention." As described above, brief intervention aims to engage with people who have hazardous or harmful alcohol consumption and offer simple advice on the harmful physical, mental, and social consequences of excess alcohol. In the ICD system, this means people with hazardous alcohol use (use which confers the risk of future harm) or harmful alcohol use (use which has already caused physical, mental, or behavioral problems). In DSM-5, the nearest counterpart would be mild alcohol use disorder. The focused advice and therapy is provided before the person has developed a more severe alcohol use disorder or more severe physical, mental, or personal harm.

Brief intervention is therefore a proactive strategy comprising of provision of brief advice on the consequences of hazardous/harmful drinking or alcohol use disorder feedback of harm and relating this to the patient's excess drinking, setting goals for safe levels of drinking, outlining benefits obtained from cutting down drinking, and setting strategies to overcome "at-risk" times. The intervention may take only 4–5 minutes. If a structured brief intervention does not lead to reduction of hazardous or harmful drinking, it may be extended to 30–40 minutes to include motivational interviewing techniques [17, 47, 54].

While there is limited evidence on the effectiveness of brief interventions for young people under the age of 16 years [54], there is a wealth of evidence attesting to the effectiveness of brief alcohol interventions in reducing alcohol intake and alcohol-related problems in adults with alcohol use disorders. Approximately 50 randomized controlled trials of various forms of brief intervention compared with no intervention or an alternative form of intervention have been published. Furthermore, several meta-analyses have been published since the early 2000s.

Systematic reviews have shown that brief intervention reduces mortality over a 10-year follow-up, with a relative risk of 0.47 (95% CI 0.25–0.89) [24, 76].

Systematic reviews and meta-analysis confirm the effectiveness of brief intervention in reducing excess alcohol consumption and alcohol-related harm in a primary care setting [8, 58]. In a UK multicenter SIPS (Screening and Intervention Program for Sensible drinking) trial, 3562 primary care patients were screened for hazardous/harmful drinking using either the FAST or the single alcohol screening questionnaire. Patients randomized to three interventions were compared, each of which built on the previous one, namely, (i) a patient information leaflet control group, (ii) 5 minutes of structured brief advice, and (iii) 20 minutes of brief lifestyle counseling linked to motivational interviewing. The WHO screening instrument AUDIT (score of <8) was used as a primary outcome measure at 6 months. There was no difference in benefit between the three arms although patients in the 20-minute intervention reported greater satisfaction with treatment. The authors concluded that screening followed by simple feedback and written information may be the most appropriate strategy to reduce hazardous and harmful drinking in a primary care setting [27, 28, 39].

Meta-analysis of 22 randomized clinical trials of 5800 participants not seeking help for alcohol problems in a primary care setting showed that brief intervention was effective in reducing alcohol consumption in men with hazardous and harmful alcohol consumption but unproven in women [37]. Further supportive evidence was provided in a more recently updated Cochrane collaboration systematic review of 69 studies on a total of 33,642 participants with primary meta-analysis of 34 trials of 15,197 participants in general practices or emergency care. Brief intervention reduced alcohol consumption in hazardous and harmful drinkers compared to minimal or no intervention in both men and women, compared to controls after 1 year [11, 38].

Brief interventions, typically lasting 5–15 minutes (and no longer than 30 minutes), included feedback on alcohol use and health-related harms, identification of high-risk situations for heavy drinking, simple advice about how to cut down drinking, strategies to increase motivation to change drinking behavior, and the development of a personal plan to cut down drinking. Short advice-based intervention is as effective as extended counseling-based intervention [11, 37, 38, 49].

The efficiency of screening and brief intervention will vary according to the prevalence of hazardous alcohol consumption in general practice. A degree of effort is required to provide brief intervention in practice although information on alcohol consumption is relevant to much of the healthcare when other issues such as the potential for interactions with medications and advice needed for pregnant women and people with a range of chronic medical disorders are taken into consideration.

40.8 Implementation of Screening and Brief Intervention in Clinical Practice

There is a wealth of evidence that demonstrates that brief interventions reduce hazardous and harmful alcohol consumption, as judged by overall alcohol consumption, reduced frequency of binge drinking, alcohol-related problems, and various secondary measures such as healthcare utilization. Some of the findings vary from study to study and among the meta-analyses. However, the overall message is clear that for these interventions benefits are clear and the strength of the evidence would suggest that their general availability in the healthcare system should be assured. The reality is somewhat different.

Brief interventions are some of the most consistently effective and potent interventions directed at individuals, and considerable effort is being made to incorporate them into the healthcare system. This is proven to be more difficult than originally anticipated. Very often screening and brief intervention can be established as a brief project, but it tends not to be continued in systematic way when external support and interest ceases.

It is fair to say that screening and brief intervention remains under utilized. Certainly systematic screening in primary care and the delivery when appropriate of a brief therapy remain unusual, even in healthcare systems that

have a strong primary prevention and population health orientation. Various barriers to implementation have been reported by health professionals and include (i) reluctance to inquire about alcohol consumption, (ii) poor role adequacy, (iii) inadequate resources to address alcohol use and problems, and (iv) poor role support [56]. There remain significant issues regarding training and confidence in providing brief interventions, issues of remuneration, and competition for the time of medical practitioners and other health professionals given their overall responsibilities. Ethical considerations have also been raised as to the appropriateness of introducing a health issue which is not on the patient's agenda when he/she booked the consultation. More broadly there is debate about which healthcare professionals have the capacity to provide these interventions.

Detection and diagnosis of alcohol use disorders remains low, and it is estimated that of the 15–30% of patients in primary care or hospital settings who have an alcohol use disorder, in only one-third of the cases is it diagnosed. It must be emphasis that screening and early detection therefore has a greater role than leading to a brief intervention. Early detection can often result in the correct diagnosis being expedited, with the patient being spared unnecessary investigations. Equally importantly, knowledge of the alcohol use disorder may prevent months or indeed years of inappropriate or ineffective treatment for patients who have disorders that may be related to alcohol consumption, such as hypertension, esophagitis and gastritis, anxiety, depression, and recurrent headache. It can also often provide an answer for patients who have multiple nonspecific and seemingly unconnected symptoms.

Examples of policy recommendations and directives include the expectation that screening and brief intervention will be provided in all healthcare settings in the recommendations of the US Preventive Services Task Force [50], the guidelines published by the UK National Institute of Clinical Excellence [53] and the British Medical Association (BMJ) Best Practice

Alcohol Use Disorder Guidelines [13], and the National Preventative Health Taskforce, Australia [55].

Opportunities for screening, early detection, and brief intervention for unhealthy alcohol use exist in many settings. These include general medical/family medical practice, other primary care settings (nurse, psychologist, social worker delivered), emergency departments and acute care clinics, student health services, work place health programs, and also certain public areas such as shopping centers.

In addition to these primary care or community contact settings, brief interventions can be offered in hospital wards (general and psychiatric) and in a range of specialist services such as diabetes, hypertension, and liver clinics. A large number of hospital outpatients who are not seeking treatment for their drinking could benefit from early intervention [36]. There is mixed evidence for the effectiveness of brief intervention in hospital wards, while significant reduction in alcohol consumption and less likelihood of alcohol-related injury have been reported following screening and brief intervention for alcohol use disorders in the emergency department [26, 32, 45].

These settings are of course quite diverse, and the extent to which a person can be engaged in any alcohol intervention will vary according to the primary task of a particular setting. Still, given that few people specifically request treatment and assistance in an alcohol use disorder, any attempt to identify these and to place alcohol on the healthcare agenda is to be welcomed.

Throughout this period, there has been a tendency for patients who have actual alcohol use disorders to present for care at an earlier stage than was the case a generation ago. Furthermore, developments in general practice mean that questions on alcohol as well as cigarette smoking are more commonly part of the routine enquiry when patients attend primary care for the first time or are part of a periodic annual or biannual assessment. Even though the systematic approach of

brief intervention may be less common than had been anticipated by those working in the area, nonetheless in various areas of the world it is more common for inquiry about alcohol use to be made.

In addition to screening instruments, good history taking, physical examination, and laboratory tests help to provide useful diagnostic information. This includes measurement of alcohol levels in the breath or blood, full blood count (macrocytosis), and liver function tests: GGT (gamma-glutamyl transpeptidase), ALT (alanine aminotransferase), AST (aspartate aminotransferase), and CDT (carbohydrate-deficient transferase) [21].

40.9 Brief Intervention in Practice: The Techniques

Brief intervention techniques vary widely in content and duration [12, 52, 65]. A structured brief intervention begins with personalized feedback regarding a person's alcohol intake and/or experience of problems and an indication that the level of consumption puts them at risk of future harm and/or that problems have arisen due to their alcohol intake. This is followed by recommendation for behavior change and advice to reduce consumption to approved guidelines for low-risk intake. These latter vary from country to country but typically would be under 20 g daily for men and 10–20 g daily for women Finally, negotiation and confirmation of goals and arrangement for follow up is made. This information and advice is typically conveyed to the patient over 5 minutes.

Many brief interventions incorporate other strategies. They include:

– Normative feedback, in which the person's alcohol intake is compared to that of the population at large and the risk levels and harmful effects of excess alcohol
– Brief motivational enhancement approaches, which may employ techniques of empathic feedback and cognitive dissonance

– Strategies for limiting alcohol consumption which are typically brief, cognitive behavioral interventions and may focus on avoiding high-risk situations for drinking and managing emotions such as frustration and boredom
– Measures aimed at moderated or controlled drinking such as always eating some food before any alcohol consumption, spacing drinks and extending the interval between drinks and counting drinks, and having alternate alcoholic and nonalcoholic drinks.

Based on motivational interviewing techniques [47], two popular approaches to brief intervention are set out below.

The first, FLAGS, an acronym for Feedback, Listen, Advice, Goals, and Strategies [68], is derived from the intervention developed from the WHO brief intervention collaborative study [3, 5].

FLAGS

Feedback: Problems experienced or likely to occur and link this with unhealthy drinking

Listen: Listen to the patient's response and assess his/her readiness to change (use motivational interviewing techniques as required [59])

Advice: Give clear advice to change and/or reduce unhealthy levels of drinking; list the benefits of change

Goals: Negotiate goals to reduce drinking to recommended limits

Strategies: Discuss practical methods and strategies, for example, how to determine at-risk times, and develop coping strategies

---

The second, FRAMES, an acronym for Feedback, Responsibility, Advice, Menu, Empathetic interviewing and Self-efficacy, is an intervention which has a major component of motivational interviewing and enhancement. It is derived from the work of Miller and colleagues and is an abbreviated form of a more extended intervention which has been developed for psychological practice [68].

FRAMES: (brief intervention with motivational interviewing)

Feedback: about personal risk and impairment

Responsibility: emphasis on personal responsibility for change

Advice: to cut down, abstain if indicated, because of severe dependence or harm

Menu: of alternative options for changing drinking pattern and, jointly with the patient, setting a target; intermediate goals of reduction can be a start

Empathic interviewing: listening reflectively without cajoling or confronting, exploring with patients the reasons for change as they see their situation

Self-efficacy: an interviewing style which enhances peoples' belief in their ability to change
[12]

40.10 Electronic Screening and Brief Intervention

Worldwide, 70% of the adult population has ready access to the Internet typically through smartphones or numerous other electronic devices. In some countries, the coverage of the Internet reaches 98% of the population. Communication of information is easier than ever before. In addition, the interactivity that is possible electronically means that intervention can be offered in real time. In many areas of healthcare, this technology has been put to use for the provision of screening and assessment and the provision of relevant information and advice. Screening and brief intervention for alcohol use has been part of this.

Electronic screening and brief intervention (e-SBI) has its origins in the late 1990s when the potential of the technology became apparent and also when there was interest in the widespread dissemination of health advice about alcohol. Soon, pioneering efforts in the provision of alcohol screening and brief intervention were made, and the first systematic studies appeared in the early 2000s. A series of controlled studies in student populations, both in individual campuses and national studies, have shown significant effect sizes on measures of overall alcohol consumption, binge drinking, alcohol-related problems, measures of academic performance, and healthcare utilization. The effect size does appear to be slightly less for electronic interventions than that seen for clinician-provided interventions [44]. In several other populations controlled trials have since shown electronic screening and brief intervention to result in significant changes in alcohol consumption and associated problems [25, 43]. However, given the high acceptability of electronic interventions and the potential reach to the at-risk population, electronic interventions have far greater capacity to be disseminated universally than could be achieved realistically through the dissemination of clinician-provided interventions.

Screening and brief intervention have high levels of acceptability particularly among populations (such as young people) who are electronically literate. Studies among university and college students show acceptability levels exceeding 80%, and receiving information electronically is preferred among young people to receiving such information from a health professional. A pilot project has shown that while implementation of self-administered electronic screening and brief intervention is acceptable and feasible in primary care practices, its use is rather limited without human support. This could be improved by training of desk personnel or practice nurses [9].

Based on evidence from a systematic review of 31 studies showing the effectiveness of electronic screening and brief intervention in reducing excessive alcohol consumption and alcohol-related problems [20, 74], the use of electronic devices (computers, telephones, or mobile devices) is recommended to facilitate screening and personalized feedback about the risks of excessive drinking. However, a randomized double blind controlled study of e-SBI to adults with hazardous and harmful drinking was not found to be effective in a hospital outpatient setting [36].

More broadly, screening and brief intervention including its electronic forms offers the prospect of reducing alcohol-related harm at a population level as an alternative to primary prevention approaches based on control of per capita alcohol consumption. These latter approaches, although empirically sound, are difficult for governments to enact into effective policy as they impact on the availability and access to alcohol of the entire population and not just those whose drinking is hazardous and causing problems. In the modern world, governments have been reticent to impose tax imposts and restrictive legislation on alcohol consumption generally for fear of electoral unpopularity and economic considerations, particularly in those countries where the production of alcohol drinks is a significant part of the national economy. Screening and brief intervention therefore offers a population-wide and more politically acceptable approach to reducing harm from alcohol in the population at large. Both clinician-provided and electronic interventions have important roles to offer in the fulfillment of this goal.

Acknowledgments We thank Corinne Lim for her expert contribution to the literature and cross-checking of the citations to the literature.

Resources

https://www.auditscreen.org. This website provides an electronic version of the AUDIT, with immediate feedback based on the score. Translations into 50 languages are available.

References

1. American Psychiatric Association (APA). Diagnostic and statistical manual of mental disorders, text revision IV (DSM IV TR). Washington, D.C: American Psychiatric Association; 2000.

2. American Psychiatric Association (APA). The diagnostic and statistical manual of mental disorders, 5th edition (DSM-5). Washington, D.C: American Psychiatric Association; 2013.

3. Babor TF, Acuda W, Campillo C, Del Boca FK, et al. A cross-national trial of brief interventions with heavy drinkers. Am J Public Health. 1996;86:948–55.

4. Babor TF, de la Fuente JR, Saunders JB, Grant M. AUDIT. The alcohol use disorders identification test: guidelines for use in primary health care. Geneva: World Health Organization (WHO); 1992.

5. Babor TF, Higgins-Biddle JC, Saunders JB, et al. The alcohol use disorders identification test- guidelines for use in primary care. 2nd ed. Geneva: Department of Mental Health and Substance Dependence, World Health Organization (WHO); 2001. Retrieved from https://apps.who.int/iris/handle/10665/67205.

6. Berks J, McCormick R. Screening for alcohol misuse in elderly primary care patients: a systematic literature review. Int Psychogeriatr. 2008;20(6):1090–103. https://doi.org/10.1017/S1041610208007497.

7. Berner MM, Kriston L, Bentelo M, et al. The alcohol use disorders test for detecting at risk drinking: a systematic review and meta-analysis. J Stud Alcohol Drugs. 2007;68:461–73.

8. Bertholet N, Daeppen JB, Wietlisbach V, et al. Reduction of alcohol consumption by brief alcohol intervention in primary care: systematic review and meta-analysis. Arch Intern Med. 2005;165:986–95.

9. Bertholet N, Cunningham JA, Adam A, et al. Electronic screening and brief intervention for unhealthy alcohol use in primary care waiting rooms - a pilot project. Subst Abus. 2019;31:1–9. https://doi.org/10.1080/08897077.2019.1635963.

10. Beullens J, Aertgeerts B. Screening for alcohol abuse and dependence in older people using DSM criteria: a review. Aging Ment Health. 2004;8:76–82. https://doi.org/10.1080/13607860310001613365.

11. Beyer FR, Campbell F, Bertholet N, Daeppen JB, Saunders JB, et al. The Cochrane 2018 review on brief interventions in primary care for hazardous and harmful alcohol consumption: a distillation for clinicians and policy makers. Alcohol Alcohol. 2019;54:417–27.

12. Bien TH, Miller WR, Tonigan JS. Brief interventions for alcohol problems: a review. Addiction. 1993;88:315–35.

13. BMJ Best Practice. Alcohol Use Disorder. BMJ best practice. London: BMJ Publishing Group; 2018, Updated June. Retrieved from http://bestpractice.bmj.com/topics/en-gb/198.

14. Bradley KA, Boyd-Wickizer J, Powell SH, et al. Alcohol screening questionnaires in women: a critical review. JAMA. 1998;280:166–71.

15. Bradley KA, Bush KR, Epler AJ, et al. Two brief alcohol-screening tests from the alcohol use identification test (AUDIT): validation in female veterans affairs patient population. Arch Intern Med. 2003;163:821–9.

16. Bradley KA, DeBenedetti AF, Volk RJ, et al. AUDIT C as a brief screen for alcohol misuse in primary care. Alcohol Clin Exp Res. 2007;31:1208.

17. Brown M, Masterson C, Latchford G, et al. Therapist-client interactions in motivational interviewing: the effect of therapists' utterances on client change talk. Alcohol Alcohol. 2018;53(4):408–11.

18. Bohn MJ, Babor TF, Kranzler HR. The alcohol use disorders identification test (AUDIT): validation of a screening instrument for use in medical settings. J Stud Alcohol. 1995;56(4):423–32.

19. Bush K, Kivlahan DR, McDonell MB, et al. The AUDIT alcohol consumption questions (AUDIT-C): an effective brief screening test for problem drinking. Arch Intern Med. 1998;158:1789–95.

20. Community Preventive Services Task Force (CPSTF). Alcohol electronic screening and brief intervention: recommendation of the community preventive services task force. Am J Prev Med. 2016;51(5):812–3.

21. Conigrave KM, Davies P, Haber P, Whitfield J. Traditional markers of excessive alcohol use. Addiction. 2003;98(suppl 2):31–43.

22. Cook RL, Chung T, Kelly TM, Clark DB. Alcohol screening in young persons attending a sexually transmitted disease clinic: comparison of AUDIT, CRAFFT, and CAGE instruments. J Gen Intern Med. 2005;20:1–6.

23. Cottler LB, Grant BF, Blaine J, et al. Concordance of DSM-IV alcohol and drug use disorder criteria and diagnoses as measured by AUDADIS-ADR, CIDI and SCAN. Drug Alcohol Depend. 1997;47:195–205.

24. Cuijpers P, Riper H, Lemmers L. The effects on mortality of brief interventions for problem drinking: a meta-analysis. Addiction. 2004;99:839–45.

25. Donnoghue K, Patton R, Phillips T, et al. The effectiveness of electronic screening and brief intervention for reducing levels of alcohol consumption: a systematic review and meta-analysis. J Med Internet Res. 2014;16:e142.

26. D'Onofrio G, Fiellin DA, Pantalon MV, et al. A brief intervention reduces hazardous and harmful drinking in emergency department patients. Ann Emerg Med. 2012;60:181–92.

27. Drummond C, Coulton S, James D, et al. Effectiveness and cost effectiveness of a stepped care intervention for alcohol use disorders in primary care: pilot study. Br J Psychiatry. 2009;195:448–56.

28. Drummond C, Deluca P, Coulton S, Bland M, Cassidy P, et al. The effectiveness of alcohol screening and brief intervention in emergency departments: a multicentre pragmatic cluster randomized controlled trial. PLoS One. 2014;9:e99463. https://doi.org/10.1371/journal.pone.0099463.

29. Ducci F, Goldman D. The genetic basis of addictive disorders. Psychiatr Clin North Am. 2012;35: 495–519.

30. Ewing J. Detecting alcoholism (the CAGE questionnaire). J Am Med Assoc. 1984;252:11905–7.

31. Geijer-Simpson E, McGovern R, Kaner E. Alcohol prevention and treatment: interventions for hazardous, harmful, and dependent drinkers. In: Hilliard ME, Riekert KA, Ockene JK, Pbert L, editors. The handbook of health behavior change. 5th ed. New York: Springer Publishing Company; 2018. p. 223.

32. Havard A, et al. Systematic review and meta-analysis of strategies targeting alcohol problems in emergency department: interventions reduce alcohol related injuries. Addiction. 2008;103:368–76.

33. Heather N, Campion PD, Neville RG, Maccabe D. Evaluation of a controlled drinking minimal intervention for problem drinkers in general practice (the DRAMS scheme). J R Coll Gen Pract. 1987;37:358–63.

34. Hodgson R, Alwyn T, John B, et al. The FAST alcohol screening test. Alcohol Alcohol. 2002;37:61–6.

35. Institute of Medicine. Broadening the base of treatment for alcohol problems. Washington, D.C.: The National Academies Press; 1990. https://doi.org/10.17226/1341.

36. Johnson NA, Kypri K, Saunders JB, et al. Effect of electronic screening and brief intervention on hazardous and harmful drinking among adults in the hospital outpatient setting: a randomised double blind controlled trial. Drug Alcohol Depend. 2018;191(2018):78–85.

37. Kaner EF, Dickinson HO, Beyer F, Pienaar E, et al. The effectiveness of brief alcohol interventions in primary care settings: a systematic review. Drug Alcohol Rev. 2009;28:301–23.

38. Kaner EF, Beyer FR, Muirhead C, et al. Effectiveness of brief alcohol interventions in primary care populations. Cochrane Database Syst Rev. 2018;2:CD004148.

39. Kaner E, Bland M, Cassidy P, et al. Effectiveness of screening and brief alcohol intervention in primary care (SIPD trial): pragmatic cluster randomized controlled trial. BMJ. 2013;346:e8015. https://doi.org/10.1136/bmj.e8501.

40. Knight JR, Sherritt L, Harris SK, Gates EC, Chang G. Validity of brief alcohol screening tests among adolescents: a comparison of the AUDIT, POSIT, CAGE, and CRAFFT. Alcohol Clin Exp Res. 2003;27:67–73.

41. Kristenson H, Öhlin H, Hultén-Nosslin M, Trell E, Hood B. Identification and intervention of heavy drinking in middle-aged men: results and follow-up of 24–60 months of long-term study with randomized controls. Alcohol Clin Exp Res. 1983;7:203–9.

42. Kypri K, Langley JD, Saunders JB, et al. Assessment may conceal therapeutic benefit: findings from a randomized controlled trial for hazardous drinking. Addiction. 2007;102:62–70.

43. Kypri K, Langley JD, Saunders JB, et al. Randomised controlled trial of web-based alcohol screening and brief intervention in primary care. Arch Intern Med. 2008;168:530–6.

44. Kypri K, Saunders JB, Williams SM, et al. Web-based screening and brief intervention for hazardous drinking: a double-blind randomized controlled trial. Addiction. 2004;99(11):1410–7.

45. Landy MS, Davey CJ, Quintero D, et al. A systematic review on the effectiveness of brief interventions foe alcohol misuse among adults in emergency departments. J Subst Abus Treat. 2016;61:1–12.

46. Mayfield D, McLeod G, Hall P. The CAGE questionnaire: validation of a new alcoholism screening instrument. Am J Psychiatry. 1974;131:1121–3.

47. Miller WR, Rollnick S. Motivational interviewing: helping people change. 3rd ed. New York: Guilford Press; 2013.

48. Morton JL, Jones TV, Manganaro MM. Performance of alcoholism screening questionnaires in elderly veterans. Am J Med. 1996;101:153–9.

49. Moyer A, Finney JW, Swearingen CE, Vergun P. Brief interventions for alcohol problems: a meta-analytic review of controlled investigations in treatment-seeking and non-treatment-seeking populations. Addiction. 2002;2002(97):279–92.

50. Moyer VA, on behalf of the U.S. Preventive Services Task Force. Screening and behavioral counseling interventions in primary care to reduce alcohol misuse: U.S. preventive services task force recommendation statement. Ann Intern Med. 2013;159:210–8.

51. National Health and Medical Research Council (NHMRC). Australian guidelines to reduce health risks from drinking alcohol 2009. 2009. Retrieved from https://www.nhmrc.gov.au/health-advice/alcohol.

52. National Institutes of Health (NIH), National Institute on Alcohol Abuse and Alcoholism (NIAAA). Helping patients who drink too much: a clinician's guide. Bethesda: NIH/NIAAA; 2005. Retrieved from https://www.niaaa.nih.gov/guide. Updated June 2019.

53. National Institute for Health and Care Excellence (NICE). Alcohol use disorders: prevention; public health guideline (PH24). London: National Institute for Health and Care Excellence; 2010. Retrieved from https://www.nice.org.uk/guidance/ph24.

54. National Institute for Health and Care Excellence (NICE). Alcohol use disorders: diagnosis, assessment and management of harmful drinking (high-risk drinking) and alcohol dependence; clinical guidelines (CG115). London: National Institute for Health and Care Excellence; 2011. Retrieved from https://www.nice.org.uk/guidance/cg115.

55. National Preventative Health Taskforce, the Alcohol Working Group. Australia: the healthiest country by 2020, preventing alcohol-related harm in Australia: a window of opportunity: including addendum for October 2008 to June 2009. Canberra: Australian Government; 2009.

56. Nilsen P. Brief alcohol intervention – where to from here? Challenges remain for research and practice. Addiction. 2010;105:954–9.

57. Newcombe D, Humeniuk RE, Ali R. Validation of the WHO alcohol, smoking and substance involvement screening test (ASSIST): report of results from the Australian site phase 11 study. Drug Alcohol Rev. 2005;23:217–26.

58. O'Donnell A, Anderson P, Newbury-Birch D, et al. The impact of brief alcohol interventions in primary healthcare: a systematic review of reviews. Alcohol Alcohol. 2014;49:66–78.

59. Prochaska JO, DiClemente CC, Norcross JC. In search of how people change. Applications to addictive behaviours. Am Psychol. 1992;47:1102–14.

60. Rubinsky AD, Kivlahan DR, Volk RJ, Maynard C, Bradley KA. Estimating risk of alcohol dependence using alcohol screening scores. Drug Alcohol Depend. 2010;108(1–2):29–36. https://doi.org/10.1016/j.drugalcdep.2009.11.009.

61. Rumpf HJ, Wohlert T, Freyer-Adam J, Grothues J, Bischof G. Screening questionnaires for problem drinking in adolescents: performance of AUDIT, AUDIT-C, CRAFFT and POSIT. Eur Addict Res. 2013;19:121–7.

62. Russell M. New assessment tools for drinking in pregnancy. Alcohol Health Res World. 1994;18:55–61.

63. Russell M, Martier SS, Sokol RJ, et al. Screening for pregnancy risk-drinking: TWEAKING the tests. Alcohol Clin Exp Res. 1991;15:368.

64. Saitz R. Unhealthy alcohol use. N Engl J Med. 2005;352:596–607.

65. Saitz R. Screening for unhealthy use of alcohol and other drugs in primary care. Waltham: UpToDate Inc; 2018. Retrieved from https://www.uptodate.com/home/content.

66. Saunders JB, Aasland OG, World Health Organization, Division of Mental Health. WHO collaborative project on the identification and treatment of persons with harmful alcohol consumption, Report on phase I: the development of a screening instrument. Geneva: World Health Organization; 1987. Retrieved from https://apps.who.int/iris/handle/10665/62031.

67. Saunders JB, Aasland OG, Babor TF, et al. Development of the alcohol use disorders identification test (AUDIT): WHO collaborative project on early detection of persons with harmful alcohol consumption II. Addiction. 1993;88:791–804.

68. Saunders JB, Conigrave KM, Latt NC, Nutt DJ, Marshall EJ, Ling W, Higuchi S. Addiction medicine. 2nd ed. Oxford: Oxford University Press; 2016. ISBN: 978-0-19-871475-0.

69. Schuckit MA. An overview of genetic influences in alcoholism. J Subst Abus Treat. 2009;36:S5–14.

70. Smith PC, Schmidt SM, Allensworth-Davies D, Saitz R. Primary care validation of a single-question alcohol screening test. J Gen Intern Med. 2009;24:783–8.

71. Sokol RJ, Martier SS, Ager JW. The T-ACE questions: practical prenatal detection of risk drinking. Am J Obstet Gynecol. 1989;160:863–70.

72. Stickel F, Hampe J. Genetic determinants of alcoholic liver disease. Gut. 2012;61:150–9.

73. Swift RM. Drug therapy for alcohol dependence. N Engl J Med. 1999;340:1482–90.

74. Tansil KA, Esser MB, Sandhu P, et al. Alcohol electronic screening and brief intervention: a community guide systematic review. Am J Prev Med. 2016;51:801–11.

75. UK Chief Medical Officers' low risk drinking guidelines. London: Department of Health and Social Care; 2016. Retrieved from https://www.gov.uk/government/publications/alcohol-consumption-advice-on-low-risk-drinking.

76. Wutzke SE, Conigrave KM, Saunders JB, et al. The long-term effectiveness of brief interventions for unsafe alcohol consumptions: a 10-year follow-up. Addiction. 2002;97:665–75.

77. WHO ASSIST Working Group. The alcohol, smoking and substance involvement screening test (ASSIST): development, reliability and feasibility. Addiction. 2002;97:1183–94.

78. World Health Organization (WHO). The ICD-10 classification of mental and behavioural disorders: clinical descriptions and diagnostic guidelines. Geneva: World Health Organization; 1992.

79. World Health Organization (WHO). International classification of diseases 11th revision (ICD-11). Geneva: World Health Organization; 2019. Retrieved from via https://icd.who.int/en/.

80. World Health Organization (WHO). mhGAP Intervention Guide - Version 2.0 for mental, neurological and substance use disorders in non-specialized health settings. Geneva: World Health Organization; 2016. Retrieved via https://www.who.int/mental_health/mhgap/mhGAP_intervention_guide_02/en/.

Clinical Assessment of Alcohol Use Disorders

41

M. Teresa Bobes-Bascarán, M. Teresa Bascarán,
M. Paz García-Portilla, and Julio Bobes

Contents

M. T. Bobes-Bascarán
Servicio de Salud Del Principado de Asturias
(SESPA), Oviedo, Spain

Department of Psychology, University of Oviedo,
Oviedo, Spain

INEUROPA-ISPA, Oviedo, Spain

CIBERSAM, Oviedo, Spain

M. T. Bascarán
INEUROPA-ISPA, Oviedo, Spain

CIBERSAM, Oviedo, Spain

M. P. García-Portilla · J. Bobes (✉)
INEUROPA-ISPA, Oviedo, Spain

CIBERSAM, Oviedo, Spain

Department of Psychiatry, University of Oviedo,
Oviedo, Spain
e-mail: bobes@uniovi.es

Abstract

Alcohol use disorder assessment needs different strategies depending on whether screening/early use or severity and depth of the condition is yielded. The former implies the simpler and agile instruments while the latter complex and sophisticated instruments that usually require specific training. An efficacious clinical treatment starts with an integrative comprehension of the individual. Ongoing assessment and monitoring are crucial because clients' symptoms and functioning may change throughout treatment and so do priorities and targets of intervention. Alcohol use is known to interfere with neuropsychological performance, psychiatric symptomatology,

© Springer Nature Switzerland AG 2021
N. el-Guebaly et al. (eds.), *Textbook of Addiction Treatment*,
https://doi.org/10.1007/978-3-030-36391-8_41

and social and personal functioning, so it is strongly recommended to conduct multiple evaluations to determine a better approach of patient's genuine mental health and cognitive performance. An all-embracing assessment should appraise multiple domains of need and delve into the following areas: historical and recent patterns of drinking, dependence and withdrawal symptomatology, alcohol craving and impulsiveness, alcohol-related problems (i.e., legal, economic, occupational), self-efficacy and confidence in relapse prevention, readiness to change, other drug misuse including prescribed and under-the-counter medication, comorbid mental health disorders, comorbid physical health conditions, neurocognitive performance, social and personal functioning, quality of life, and disability. This information may be obtained by a precise clinical interview, but standardized tools and measures should be administered as well. This chapter will enumerate and briefly describe the most relevant psychometric instruments to evaluate alcohol use disorders and related problems, psychiatric comorbid symptomology, neurocognitive performance, and social functioning and quality of life issues.

Keywords

Alcohol assessment · Alcohol clinical assessment · Alcohol screening test · Alcohol use detection · Alcohol evaluation · Clinical evaluation of alcohol use

Screening and early detection of alcohol use disorders should be the initial step in the process of identifying possible conditions (see Chap. 40). After a person has been detected and diagnosed, an in-depth assessment, which involves both integrative comprehension of the patient and monitoring of patient's progress, is needed. Ongoing assessment and monitoring is important because clients' symptoms and functioning may change throughout treatment and so do priorities and targets of intervention. For instance, a patient may report anxiety symptoms or dysphoric mood upon

treatment intake and have these symptoms attenuated after achieving abstinence. By the same token, another person could enter treatment with apparently no mental health symptomatology but develop them after a period of reduced use, if self-medication with alcohol existed [18]. At the same time, it should be noted that recent alcohol abuse may influence neuropsychological performance, psychiatric symptomatology, and social and personal functioning, so it is strongly recommended to conduct further evaluations to determine a better approach of patient's genuine mental health and cognitive performance. It is fundamental to bear in mind that the primary benefit of assessment is not only to accurately and efficiently determine the treatment needs of the patient but to build rapport. For this reason, it is the heart of the assessment to avoid confrontative approaches and adopt a motivational one instead (see Chap. 24).

An all-embracing evaluation should appraise multiple domains of need and delve into the following areas:

- Alcohol consumption:
  - Historical and recent patterns of drinking
  - Dependence and withdrawal symptomatology
  - Alcohol craving and impulsiveness
  - Alcohol-related problems (i.e., legal, economic, occupational)
  - Self-efficacy and confidence in relapse prevention
  - Readiness to change
- Other drug misuse, including prescribed and under-the-counter medication
- Comorbid mental health disorders
- Comorbid physical health conditions
- Neurocognitive performance
- Social and personal functioning
- Quality of life and disability

This information may be obtained by a precise clinical interview, but standardized tools and measures should be administered as well (see Table 41.1).

This chapter will enumerate and briefly describe the most relevant psychometric instruments to evaluate alcohol use disorders and related problems, psy-

Table 41.1 Distinctive features in instrument selection

Feature	Characteristics
Clinical utility	Screening
	Diagnosis
	Assessment of drinking behavior
	Treatment planning
	Intervention monitoring
	Outcome appraisal
Time frame	Recent/short-term/current use vs. chronic/long-term/lifetime use
Specific subgroup	Adolescent, adult, elderly
	Women (pregnant)
	Imprisoned
	Homeless
	Inpatient vs. outpatient
	Cultural issues/ethnicity
Sensitivity/ positive predictive value (PPV)	Proportion of patients with the condition correctly classified as "diseased"
Specificity/ negative predictive value (NPV)	Proportion of individuals without the condition who are correctly classified as "disease-free"
Validity (test measures what is intended to measure)	Content (comprehensiveness)
	Construct (conceptual components, internal structure)
	Convergent (similar to other tests to assess that construct)
	Discriminant (different to tests that assess other constructs)
	Criterion (correlation with gold standard measures)
	Concurrent (similar measures obtained to comparative tests at same time frame)
	Predictive (ability to predict future outcome)
Reliability (accuracy of assessment)	Test-retest (correlation at two different time points)
	Inter-rater (degree of agreement by different raters)
	Internal consistency (items of test measure same aspect)

chiatric comorbid symptomology, neurocognitive performance, and social functioning and quality of life issues. Chapter 40 on Screening, Early Detection & Brief Intervention for AUD and Laboratory Tests for Alcohol Chap. 42. Biological State Marker for Alcohol Consumption may be searched through for further information. Regarding physical and mental health comorbidities, Part VIII is an exhausted revision on Medical Disorders, Complications of Alcohol and Others, and Pain Section, and Part IX addresses Psychiatric Comorbidities and Complications of Alcohol and Other Drugs.

41.1 Evaluation of Alcohol Use

There are no specific instruments to diagnose alcohol misuse, so fundamental diagnostic methods consist of an accurate anamnesis and a meticulous clinical exam. Albeit this fact, psychometric tools are of considerable aid to appraise addictive disorders when used by trained specialists.

41.1.1 Clinical Severity of Addiction

- Addiction Severity Index [45]. The ASI is a semi-structured interview designed to address seven potential impairments and problem areas in substance-abusing patients: medical conditions, employment and support, drug use, alcohol use, legal issues, family/social relationships, and psychiatric disorders. It consists of 200 items, which gather information on recent (past 30 days) and lifetime problems in all of the problem areas. Last version (ASI 6.0) [13, 44] is composed of 15 scales: 9 primary scales (related to main problem areas) and 6 secondary scales (perceived support and conflicts with partner, family, and friends). There is a follow-up version (ASI-FU follow-up) designed to monitor patients' evolution and treatment outcomes and several adaptations to adolescent population: Teen-ASI [36], T-ASI-2 [11].
- Alcohol Use Inventory [35]. The AUI is a self-administered instrument which includes 24 scales that intend to describe different ways in which individuals use alcohol, benefits and negative consequences derived from such use, and awareness and readiness for help. It consists of 228 items grouped in primary scales regarding benefits, styles, consequences and concerns and acknowledgments of alcohol use, and other second-order factor scales.
- Comprehensive Drinker Profile [48]. The CDP is a structured interview that contains 88 questions inquiring different areas of interest: alcohol use, everyday problems, most common drinking settings, people with whom they drink, beverage preferences, reasons for drinking, effects and life problems related to alco-

hol use, and patient's concerns and issues. Three instruments were derived from the CDP: the Brief Drinker Profile (BDP), the Follow-up Drinker Profile (FDP), and the Collateral Interview Form (CIF).

41.1.2 Dependence/Withdrawal Symptoms

- Severity of Alcohol Dependence Questionnaire [69]. The SADQ is a self-administered questionnaire designed to measure severity of dependence. There are four items in each of the five scales that gather information on a 6-month time frame: physical withdrawal, affective withdrawal, withdrawal relief drinking, alcohol consumption, and rapidity of reinstatement. Scores range between 0 and 60 points, and scores greater than 30 are suggestive of severe alcohol dependence. It has demonstrated adequate content and criterion (predictive) validity and test-retest reliability.
- Alcohol Dependence Scale [66, 67]. The ADS consists of 25 items that interrogate alcohol withdrawal symptoms, impaired self-control over drinking, awareness of compulsive drinking, tolerance to alcohol, and salience of drink-seeking behavior. It has shown good predictive value, content and construct validity, and test-retest and internal consistency reliabilities. A computerized version is also available. It is an adequate instrument for clinical and research purposes.
- Short Alcohol Dependence Data [59]. This 15-item instrument was derived from the Alcohol Dependence Data (ADD) in order to accomplish an easier and faster measure profitable for seeking-help patients, current state dependence assessment, sensitive to change over time, and cultural-free influenced. It can be self- or hetero-administered in about 2–5 minutes and has provided good reliability and validity parameters.
- Clinical Institute Withdrawal Assessment [70]. The CIWA-AD is an eight-item scale for clinical quantification of the severity of the alcohol withdrawal syndrome. It is useful to monitor patients undergoing alcohol withdrawal as it focuses on both intensity and severity of symptoms. Scores over 20 indicate a severe withdrawal syndrome, and inpatient detoxification is strongly recommended.

41.1.3 Craving/Impulsiveness

- The Obsessive Compulsive Drinking Scale [4]. The OCDS is a 14-item scale developed to reflect obsession and compulsion related to craving and drinking behavior such as drinking-related thoughts and urges to drink and the ability to resist those thoughts and urges. The OCDS has been shown to be a reliable and sensitive monitoring tool and has proven content and predictive validity for relapse drinking. There is an adolescent version, the A-OCDS [19], which discriminates between problem drinkers and experimenters and detects functional impairment associated with alcohol abuse.
- Penn Alcohol Craving Scale [27]. The PACS is a five-item self-administered instrument for assessing frequency, intensity, and duration of thoughts about drinking and the ability to resist drinking. Although it was intended for adults, it may be used in adolescent population. Good reliability and validity measures have been obtained.
- Alcohol Craving Questionnaire [64]. The ACQ-NOW is a 47-item self-administered, multidimensional state measure of acute alcohol craving. It measures four dimensions: emotionality, purposefulness, compulsivity, and expectancy. There is a 12-item short form, the ACQ-SF-R. It has demonstrated adequate reliability and is sensitive to change.
- Impulsive Behavior Scale [76]. The UPPS is a 45-item scale designed to measure impulsivity across dimensions of the five-factor model of personality. It measures four domains: premeditation, urgency, sensation seeking, and perseverance. The revised version, UPPS-P, consists of 59 items and assesses an additional personality pathway to impulsive behavior, positive urgency [17].

- Barratt Impulsiveness Scale [5, 57]. The BIS is one of the oldest and most widely used measures of impulsive personality traits. The last version, BIS-11, contains 30 items grouped in 3 subscales: attentional impulsiveness, motor impulsiveness, and non-planning impulsiveness. This scale is intended to measure six factors: attention, motor impulsiveness, self-control, cognitive complexity, perseverance, and cognitive instability.

41.1.4 Self-Efficacy and Expectancy

- Alcohol Abstinence Self-Efficacy Scale [23]. The AASE was designed to evaluate self-efficacy in 20 situations that represent typical drinking cues associated to negative affect; social/positive, physical, and other concerns; and withdrawal and urges. It may be also used to assess an individual's temptation to drink. It has shown great utility to intervene over relapse potential situations, monitor progress in treatment, and assess outcomes.
- Drinking Refusal Self-Efficacy Questionnaire [81]. The DRSEQ is a 31-item measure of drinking-related self-efficacy. It is grouped in three factors: drinking in situations characterized by social pressure, opportunistic drinking, and emotional relief. Adequate reliability and validity have been analyzed.
- Alcohol Expectancy Questionnaire [12]. The AEQ is an empirically derived self-report form designed to assess the domain of alcohol reinforcement expectancies. It consists of six subscales: positive global changes in experience, sexual enhancement, social and physical pleasure, assertiveness, relaxation/tension reduction, and arousal/interpersonal power. Total scores are predictive of current and future drinking practices, persistence and participation in treatment, and relapse following treatment.
- Negative Alcohol Expectancy Questionnaire [46, 47]. The NAEQ is a 60-item questionnaire that assesses the extent to which negative consequences are expected to occur if that person were to "go for a drink now." The expected negative consequences are held to

represent motivation to stop drinking. There are three different time frames: same-day, next-day, and long-term expected consequences. Responses are measured in terms of how likely it is that a person would expect them to occur and are measured on a five-point Likert scale. A short version composed of 22 items is also available. This instrument is very useful at intake and during treatment to intervene over motivational factors during therapeutic process.

41.1.5 Motivation to Change

- University of Rhode Island Change Assessment [43]. The URICA is a 32-item self-report measure used to assess motivation for change that includes four subscales: precontemplation, contemplation, action, and maintenance. These subscales can be combined in order to yield a second-order continuous readiness to change score (C + A + M-PC). It has demonstrated adequate internal consistency as well as content and criterion validity.
- Readiness to Change Questionnaire [63]. The RCQ is comprised of 12 items and focuses on readiness to change drinking behavior. It is based on the URICA questionnaire and is founded on Prochaska and DiClemente's theory on stages of change. It is clustered into three factors: precontemplation, contemplation, and action. It has good psychometric properties, including predictive validity. There is a treatment version, the RCQ (TV), for use in patients at treatment settings.
- Stages of Change Readiness and Treatment Eagerness Scale [49]. The SOCRATES consists of 40 items grouped into 5 stages of change: precontemplation, contemplation, determination/preparation, action, and maintenance. The SOCRATES 8A is a 19-item version that yields 3 factorial-derived scale scores: recognition, ambivalence, and taking steps. There are available other forms of the SOCRATES: 8D, a 19-item drug/alcohol questionnaire for clients; 7A-SO-M, a 32-item alcohol questionnaire for significant others of males; 7A-SO-F, a 32-item alcohol questionnaire for SOs of females;

7D-SO-F, a 32-item drug/alcohol questionnaire for SOs of females; and the 7D-SO-M, a 32-item drug/alcohol questionnaire for SOs of males. These SO forms are intended to measure motivation for change of significant others (rather than patient's motivation).

41.2 Psychiatric Comorbidity Assessment

Individuals with alcohol use disorders often suffer from one (comorbid) or more (multimorbidity) psychiatric disorders. This frequent phenomenon indicates the necessity of specific assessment and treatment in the field of addictive behaviors, which has been historically narrowed and focused to the addiction per se. This section yields over basic instruments to assess psychiatric comorbidity in patients with alcohol problems (see Table 41.2). For further information on psy-

chiatric comorbidity, consult Part IX of this book, Psychiatric Comorbidities and Complications of Alcohol and Other Drugs.

41.3 Neuropsychological Performance

Scientific literature has well established that excessive alcohol use is associated to damage and impairment of brain structure and function, yielding to poor cognitive performance and behavior disturbances. Assessment and intervention over neuropsychological performance is fundamental as it involves assimilation and understanding of information, reasoning, and problem-solving in order to prevent oneself from relapse, to develop mnesic capacity to remember therapeutic guidelines, to learn new skills and maintain abstinence, and to develop more adaptable behaviors. This section enumerates the most

Table 41.2 Psychometric instruments to evaluate psychiatric comorbidity

Construct	Instrument	Author
Psychiatric comorbidity	Psychiatric Research Interview for Substance and Mental Disorders (PRISM)	[34]
	Composite International Diagnostic Interview (CIDI)	[78]
General symptoms	Symptom Checklist- 90- Revised (SCL 90-R)	[21]
	Minnesota Multiphasic Personality Inventory (MMPI-2)	[42]
Affective symptoms	Hamilton Depression Rating Scale (HDRS)	[33]
	Beck Depression Inventory-II (BDI-II)	[8]
	Young Mania Rating Scale (YMRS)	[80]
Autolytic risk	Scale for Suicidal Ideation (SSI)	[7]
	Hopelessness Scale (HS)	[9]
Anxiety	Hamilton Anxiety Rating Scale (HARS)	[32]
	State Trait Anxiety Inventory (STAI)	[68]
	Yale-Brown Obsessive Compulsive Scale (Y-BOCS)	[31]
	Clinician Administered PTSD Scale (CAPS)	[10]
Psychotic spectrum	Brief Psychiatric Rating Scale (BPRS)	[56]
	Positive and Negative Syndrome Scale (PANSS)	[38]
Personality	International Personality Disorder Examination (IPDE)	[41]
	Eysenck Personality Questionnaire-Revised (EPQ-R)	[25, 26]
	Millon Clinical Multiaxial Inventory-III (MCMI-III)	[50, 51]
Eating behavior disorders	Eating Disorders Inventory (EDI)	[29]
	Eating Disorder Examination (EDE)	[16]
Sexual dysfunction	Changes in Sexual Functioning Questionnaire (CSFQ)	[14]
	Derogatis Interview for Sexual Functioning-Self-Report (DISF-SR)	[20, 22]
ADHD	Conners' Adult ADHD Rating Scales	[15]
	The World Health Organization Adult ADHD Self-Report Scale (ASRS)	[39]

Table 41.3 Tests to assess neuropsychological performance

Function	Subcomponent	Instrument	Author
General mental function		Mini Mental State Examination (Mini-Mental)	[28]
Attention	Span and control	Digit span (WAIS-IV)	[72, 74]
		Mental control test	[72, 74]
	Sustained or vigilance	Visual Cancellation Test	[75]
	Selective	Stroop Color and Word Test	[30]
	Alternating	Trail Making Test- – Part B (TMT-B)	[60]
Executive function	Disexecutive syndrome	Behavioural Assessment of the Dysexecutive Syndrome	[77]
	Fluency	Verbal fluency	[40]
	Working memory	Letter-Number (WAIS-IV)	[72, 74]
	Flexibility and analogic reasoning	Wisconsin Card Sorting Test (WCST)	[53]
	Interference and inhibitory control	Go/No- Go Task	
	Planning	Key Search and Zoo Map (BADS) Plan	[77]
	Decision-making	Iowa Gambling Task (IGT)	[6]
Memory	Broad function	Wechsler Memory Scale (WMS-III)	[71, 73]
	Short-term/working memory	Letter-Number, Arithmetic, and Digit Span (WMS-III)	[71, 73]
	Episodic long-term	Rey Auditory Verbal Learning Test (R-AVLT)	[62]
	Semantic long-term	Boston Naming Test	[37]
	Procedural	Rivermead Behavioural Memory Test (RBMT)	[1]
Visuospatial and perceptual abilities		Rey-Osterrieth Complex Figure	[61]
Language and communication skills		Information and Comprehension (WAIS-IV)	[72, 74]
Premorbid and morbid intelligence		Wechsler Adult Intelligence Scale-IV (WAIS-IV)	[72, 74]
		National Adult Reading Test (NART)	[54, 55]

relevant tests to evaluate neuropsychological performance (see Table 41.3).

41.4 Psychosocial Functioning and Quality of Life

Alcohol and other drug use disorders are increasingly viewed as chronic conditions. This approach addresses the impact of disorder and resources on patient's overall well-being. From this perspective, integrative intervention in addictive behaviors should aim for the broad goal of recovery, which is defined as abstinence plus improved quality of life and psychosocial functioning. These social markers are essential in treatment planning and outcome assessment as they represent the abilities and skills of the individual to function independently in the community.

41.4.1 Disability

- Disability Assessment Schedule 2.0 [79]. The WHODAS 2.0 was developed through a collaborative international approach, with the aim of developing a single generic instrument for assessing health status and disability across different cultures and settings. It is short, simple, and easy to administer, and one first-level general disability factor and six second-level standardized domains may be obtained: cognition, mobility, self-care, getting along, life activities, and participation.

41.4.2 Quality of Life

- Quality of Life Enjoyment and Satisfaction Questionnaire [24]. The Q-LES-Q is a self-administered scale of 93 items designed to measure satisfaction and enjoyment in various domains of functioning: physical health and activities, mood state, work, household duties, academic/occupational activities, leisure and hobbies, social relationships, and general activities. There are various short forms available.

- World Health Organization Quality of Life Assessment [58]. The WHOQOL-100 includes 24 facets relating to quality of life, which are grouped into 4 larger domains: physical, psychological, social relationships, and environment. It also includes one facet examining overall quality of life and general health perceptions. There is an abbreviated, self-administered, 26-item version, the WHOQOL-BREF [65], which produces only domain scores.

41.4.3 Functioning

- Global Assessment of Function [2, 3]. The GAF is a 100-point tool rating overall psychological, social, and occupational functioning of people over 18 years of age and older. It excludes physical and environmental impairment. Scores range from 100 (extremely high functioning) to 1 (severely impaired). It has been replaced in the fifth edition of the Diagnostic and Statistical Manual for Mental Disorders (DSM-5) with the WHO Disability Assessment Schedule (WHODAS) which is supposed to be more detailed and objective than this brief global impression.
- Personal and Social Performance Scale [52]. The PSP is a global measure of personal and social functioning based on four domains of function: self-care, socially useful activities, personal and social relationships, and disturbing and aggressive behavior. Scores may vary from 0 to 100, with a higher score indicating a higher level of social and personal functioning.

References

1. Aldrich FK, Wilson B. Rivermead behavioural memory test for children (RBMT-C): a preliminary evaluation. Br J Clin Psychol. 1991;30(Pt 2):161–8.
2. American Psychiatric Association. Diagnostic and statistical manual of mental disorders. 4th ed. Washington, D.C.: American Psychiatric Association; 1994.
3. American Psychiatric Association. Diagnostic and statistical manual of mental disorders. 5th ed. Arlington: American Psychiatric Association; 2013.
4. Anton RF, Moak DH, Latham P. The obsessive compulsive drinking scale: a self-rated instrument for the quantification of thoughts about alcohol and drinking behavior. Alcohol Clin Exp Res. 1995;19:92–9.
5. Barratt ES. Anxiety and impulsiveness related to psychomotor efficiency. Percept Mot Skills. 1959;9(2):191–8.
6. Bechara A, Damasio A, Tranel D, Anderson S. Insensitivity to future consequences following damage to human prefrontal cortex. Cognition. 1994;50:7–15.
7. Beck AT, Kovacs M, Weissman A. Assessment of suicidal intention: the scale for suicide ideation. J Consult Clin Psychol. 1979;47(2):343–52.
8. Beck AT, Steer RA, Ball R, Ranieri W. Comparison of Beck Depression Inventories -IA and -II in psychiatric outpatients. J Pers Assess. 1996;67(3):588–97. https://doi.org/10.1207/s15327752jpa6703_13.
9. Beck AT, Weissman A, Lester D, Trexler L. The measurement of pessimism: the hopelessness scale. J Consult Clin Psychol. 1974;42(6):861–5.
10. Blake DD, Weathers FW, Nagy LM, Kaloupek DG, Gusman FD, Charney DS, Keane TM. The development of a clinician-administered PTSD scale. J Trauma Stress. 1995;8(1):75–90.
11. Brodey BB, McMullin D, Kaminer Y, Winters KC, Mosshart E, Rosen CS, Brodey IS. Psychometric characteristics of the teen addiction severity index-two (T-ASI-2). Subst Abus. 2008;29(2):19–32. https://doi.org/10.1080/08897070802092942.
12. Brown SA, Christiansen BA, Goldaman MS. The alcohol expectancy questionnaire: an instrument for the assessment of adolescent and adult alcohol expectancies. J Stud Alcohol. 1987;48:483–91.
13. Cacciola JS, Alterman AI, Habing B, McLellan AT. Recent status scores for version 6 of the Addiction Severity Index (ASI-6). Addiction. 2011;106(9):1588–602. https://doi.org/10.1111/j.1360-0443.2011.03482.x.
14. Clayton AH, McGarvey EL, Clavet GJ. The changes in sexual functioning questionnaire (CSFQ): development, reliability, and validity. Psychopharmacol Bull. 1997;33(4):731–45.
15. Conners CK, Erhardt D, Sparrow E. Conners' adult ADHD rating scales. North Tonawanda: Multi-Health Systems; 1999.
16. Cooper Z, Cooper PJ, Fairburn CG. The validity of the eating disorder examination and its subscales. Br J Psychiatry. 1989;154:807–12.
17. Cyders MA, Smith GT, Spillane NS, Fischer S, Annus AM, Peterson C. Integration of impulsivity and positive mood to predict risky behavior: development and validation of a measure of positive urgency. Psychol

Assess. 2007;19(1):107–18. doi: 2007-03014-009 [pii]. https://doi.org/10.1037/1040-3590.19.1.107.

18. Deady M. A review of screening, assessment and outcome measures for drug and alcohol settings. Woolloomooloo: Network of Alcohol & other Drug Agencies; 2009.

19. Deas D, Roberts J, Randall C, Anton R. Adolescent obsessive-compulsive drinking scale: an assessment tool for problem drinking. J Natl Med Assoc. 2001;93(3):92–103.

20. Derogatis LR. The Derogatis interview for sexual functioning (DISF/DISF-SR): an introductory report. J Sex Marital Ther. 1997;23(4):291–304. https://doi.org/10.1080/00926239708403933.

21. Derogatis LR, Cleary PA. Factorial invariance across gender for the primary symptom dimensions of the SCL-90. Br J Soc Clin Psychol. 1977;16(4):347–56.

22. Derogatis LR, Melisaratos N. The DSFI: a multidimensional measure of sexual functioning. J Sex Marital Ther. 1979;5(3):244–81. https://doi.org/10.1080/00926237908403732.

23. DiClemente CC, Carbonari JP, Montgomery RPG, Hughes SO. The alcohol abstinence self-efficacy scale. J Stud Alcohol. 1994;55:141–8.

24. Endicott J, Nee J, Harrison W, Blumenthal R. Quality of life enjoyment and satisfaction questionnaire: a new measure. Psychopharmacol Bull. 1993;29(2):321–6.

25. Eysenck HJ, Eysenck SBG. Manual of the Eysenck personality questionnaire. Londres: Hodder and Stoughton; 1975.

26. Eysenck SBG, Eysenck HJ, Barrett P. A revised version of the psychoticism scale. Personal Individ Differ. 1985;6(1):21–9.

27. Flannery BA, Volpicelli JR, Pettinati HM. Psychometric properties of the Penn alcohol craving scale. Alcohol Clin Exp Res. 1999;23(8):1289–95. doi: 00000374-199908000-00001 [pii].

28. Folstein MF, Robins LN, Helzer JE. The minimental state examination. Arch Gen Psychiatry. 1983;40(7):812.

29. Garner DM, Olmsted MP. Scoring the eating disorder inventory. Am J Psychiatry. 1986;143(5):680–1.

30. Golden CJ. Identification of brain disorders by the Stroop color and word test. J Clin Psychol. 1976;32(3):654–8.

31. Goodman WK, Price LH, Rasmussen SA, Mazure C, Fleischmann RL, Hill CL, et al. The Yale-Brown obsessive compulsive scale. I. Development, use, and reliability. Arch Gen Psychiatry. 1989;46(11):1006–11.

32. Hamilton M. The assessment of anxiety states by rating. Br J Med Psychol. 1959;32(1):50–5.

33. Hamilton M. A rating scale for depression. J Neurol Neurosurg Psychiatry. 1960;23:56–62.

34. Hasin DS, Trautman KD, Miele GM, Samet S, Smith M, Endicott J. Psychiatric research interview for substance and mental disorders (PRISM): reliability for substance abusers. Am J Psychiatry. 1996;153(9):1195–201.

35. Horn JL, Wanberg KW, Foster FM. Guide to the alcohol use inventory (AUI). Minneapolis: National Computer Systems; 1987.

36. Kaminer Y, Bukstein O, Tarter R. Teen addiction severity index (T-ASI): clinical and research implications: a preliminary report. NIDA Res Monogr. 1989;95:363.

37. Kaplan E, Goodglass H, Weintraub S. Boston naming test. Philadelphia: Lea & Febiger; 1983.

38. Kay SR, Fiszbein A, Opler LA. The positive and negative syndrome scale (PANSS) for schizophrenia. Schizophr Bull. 1987;13(2):261–76.

39. Kessler RC, Adler L, Ames M, Demler O, Faraone S, Hiripi E, et al. The World Health Organization adult ADHD self-report scale (ASRS): a short screening scale for use in the general population. Psychol Med. 2005;35(2):245–56.

40. Lezak MD. Neuropsychological assessment. New York: Oxford University Press; 1995.

41. Loranger AW. Personality disorder examination. Yonkers: DV Communications; 1988.

42. Mc Kinley JC, Hathaway SR, Meehl PE. The Minnesota multiphasic personality inventory; the K scale. J Consult Psychol. 1948;12(1):20–31.

43. McConnaughy EA, Prochaska JO, Velicer WF. Stages of change in psychotherapy: measurement and sample profiles. Psychother Theor Res Pract. 1983;20:368–75.

44. McLellan AT, Cacciola JC, Alterman AI, Rikoon SH, Carise D. The addiction severity index at 25: origins, contributions and transitions. Am J Addict. 2006;15(2):113–24. doi: H541367070207315 [pii]. https://doi.org/10.1080/10550490500528316.

45. McLellan AT, Luborsky L, Woody GE, O'Brien CP. An improved diagnostic evaluation instrument for substance abuse patients. The Addiction Severity Index. J Nerv Ment Dis. 1980;168(1):26–33.

46. McMahon J, Jones BT. The negative alcohol expectancy questionnaire. J Assoc Nurses Substance Abuse. 1993a;12:17.

47. McMahon J, Jones BT. Negative expectancy and motivation. Addict Res. 1993b;1:145–55.

48. Miller WR, Marlatt GA. Comprehensive drinker profile. Odessa: Psychological Assessment Resources Inc.; 1984.

49. Miller WR, Tonigan JS. Assessing drinkers' motivations for change: the stages of change readiness and treatment eagerness scale (SOCRATES). Psychol Addict Behav. 1996;10(2):81–9.

50. Millon T. Millon clinical multiaxial inventory manual. Minneapolis: National Computer Systems; 1983.

51. Millon T, Millon C, Davis R. Millon clinical multiaxial inventory - III manual. Minneapolis: National Computer Systems; 2004.

52. Morosini PL, Magliano L, Brambilla L, Ugolini S, Pioli R. Development, reliability and acceptability of a new version of the DSM-IV social and occupational functioning assessment scale (SOFAS) to assess routine social functioning. Acta Psychiatr Scand. 2000;101(4):323–9.

53. Nelson HE. A modified card sorting test sensitive to frontal lobe defects. Cortex. 1976;12(4):313–24.

54. Nelson HE. National adult reading test. Windsor: NFER-Nelson; 1982.

55. Nelson HE, Willison JR. The revised national adult reading test- test manual. Windsor: NFER-Nelson; 1991.

56. Overall JE, Gorham DR. The brief psychiatric rating scale. Psychol Rep. 1962;10:790–812.

57. Patton JH, Stanford MS, Barratt ES. Factor structure of the Barratt impulsiveness scale. J Clin Psychol. 1995;51(6):768–74.

58. Power M, Harper A, Bullinger M. The World Health Organization WHOQOL-100: tests of the universality of quality of life in 15 different cultural groups worldwide. Health Psychol. 1999;18(5):495–505.

59. Raistrick DS, Dunbar G, Davidson RJ. Development of a questionnaire to measure alcohol dependence. Br J Addict. 1983;78:89–95.

60. Reitan RM. The relation of the trail making test to organic brain damage. J Consult Psychol. 1955;19(5):393–4.

61. Rey A. L'examen psychologique dans le cas d'encephalopathie traumatique. Arch Psychol. 1942;28:286–340.

62. Rey A. L'examen clinique en Psychologia. Paris: Pressee Universitaires de France; 1964.

63. Rollnick S, Heather N, Gold R, Hall W. Development of a short 'readiness to change' questionnaire for use in brief, opportunistic interventions among excessive drinkers. Br J Addict. 1992;87(5):743–54.

64. Singleton EG, Tiffany ST, Henningfield JE. Development and validation of a new questionnaire to assess craving for alcohol. In: Paper presented at the 56th Annual Meeting: The College on Problems of Drug Dependence; 1995.

65. Skevington SM, Lotfy M, O'Connell KA. The World Health Organization's WHOQOL-BREF quality of life assessment: psychometric properties and results of the international field trial. A report from the WHOQOL group. Qual Life Res. 2004;13(2):299–310.

66. Skinner HA, Allen BA. Alcohol dependence syndrome: measurements and validation. J Abnorm Psychol. 1982;91:199–209.

67. Skinner HA, Horn JL. Alcohol dependence scale: users guide. Toronto: Addiction Research Foundation; 1984.

68. Spielberger CD, Gorsuch RL, Lushene R, Vagg PR, Jacobs GA. State-trait anxiety inventory. Menlo Park: Mind Garden Inc.; 1970.

69. Stockwell T, Hodgson R, Edwards G, Taylor C, Rankin H. The development of a questionnaire to measure severity of alcohol dependence. Br J Addict Alcohol Other Drugs. 1979;74(1):79–87.

70. Sullivan JT, Sykora K, Schneiderman J, Naranjo CA, Sellers EM. Assessment of alcohol withdrawal: the revised clinical institute withdrawal assessment for alcohol scale (CIWA-Ar). Br J Addict. 1989;84(11):1353–7.

71. Wechsler D. Wechsler memory scale. San Antonio: Psychological Corporation; 1945.

72. Wechsler D. Wechsler adult intelligence scale. Oxford: Psychological Corp; 1955.

73. Wechsler D. Wechsler memory scale- third edition (WMS-III). Londres: The Psychological Corporation; 1998.

74. Wechsler D. Wechsler adult intelligence scale-fourth edition (WAIS-IV). San Antonio: Psychological Corp; 2008.

75. Weintraub S, Mesulam MM. Visual hemispatial inattention: stimulus parameters and exploratory strategies. J Neurol Neurosurg Psychiatry. 1988;51(12):1481–8.

76. Whiteside SP, Lynam DR. The five factor model and impulsivity: using a structural model of personality to understand impulsivity. Personal Individ Differ. 2001;30(4):669–89.

77. Wilson BA, Alderman N, Burgess PW, Emslie H, Evans JJ. Behavioural assessment of the dysexecutive syndrome. Edmunds: Thames Valley Test Company; 1996.

78. World Health Organization. Composite international diagnostic interview (CIDI). Geneva: World Health Organisation; 1990.

79. World Health Organization. World Health Organization disability assessment scale 2.0 (WHODAS 2.0). Geneva: WHO; 2010.

80. Young RC, Biggs JT, Ziegler VE, Meyer DA. A rating scale for mania: reliability, validity and sensitivity. Br J Psychiatry. 1978;133:429–35.

81. Young RS, Oei TP. Development of a drinking self efficacy scale. J Psychopathol Behav Assess. 1991;13(1):1–15.

Biological State Marker for Alcohol Consumption

42

Friedrich Martin Wurst, Pablo Barrio, Antoni Gual,
Natasha Thon, Wolfgang Weinmann,
Frederike Stöth, Michel Yegles, Jessica Wong,
and Ulrich W. Preuss

Contents

F. M. Wurst (✉)
Medical Faculty, University of Basel,
Basel, Switzerland

Psychiatric University Hospital Basel,
Basel, Switzerland

P. Barrio
Addictions Unit, Department of Psychiatry,
University of Catalonia, Barcelona, Spain

A. Gual
Addictions Unit, Department of Psychiatry,
University of Catalonia, Barcelona, Spain

Neurosciences Institute, Hospital Clínic,
IDIBAPS, Barcelona, Spain

N. Thon
IDIBAPS Neurosciences Institute, Barcelona, Spain

W. Weinmann · F. Stöth
Institute of Legal Forensic Medicine, University of
Bern, Bern, Switzerland

M. Yegles
Laboratoire National de Santé, Forensic Toxicology,
Dudelange, Luxemburg

J. Wong
Klinik am Homberg, Bad Wildungen, Germany

U. W. Preuss
Vitos Hospital for Psychiatry and Psychotherapy,
Kassel, Germany

Department for Psychiatry, Psychotherapy and
Psychosomatic Medicine, University of Halle,
Halle, Germany

© Springer Nature Switzerland AG 2021
N. el-Guebaly et al. (eds.), *Textbook of Addiction Treatment*,
https://doi.org/10.1007/978-3-030-36391-8_42

Abstract

Alcohol-related disorders are common, expensive in their entire course, and often underdiagnosed. To facilitate early diagnosis and therapy of alcohol-related disorders and thus prevent later complications, questionnaires and biomarkers are useful. Indirect state markers such as gamma-glutamyl transpeptidase (GGT), mean corpuscular volume (MCV), and carbohydrate deficiency transferrin (CDT) are influenced by age, gender, various substances, and nonalcohol-related illnesses and do not cover the entire timeline for alcohol consumption. Direct state markers such as ethyl glucuronide (EtG), phosphatidylethanol (PEth), and fatty acid ethyl esters (FAEEs) have gained enormous interest in the last decades, as they are metabolites of alcohol becoming only positive in the presence of alcohol. As biomarkers with high sensitivity and specificity covering the complimentary timeline, they are already routinely in use and contribute to new perspectives in prevention, interdisciplinary cooperation, diagnosis, and therapy of alcohol-related disorders.

Keywords

Alcohol biomarker · Ethanol metabolites · Traditional biomarkers · Ethyl glucuronide · Phosphatidylethanol · Gamma-glutamyl transferase

Introductory Paragraph
Alcohol biomarkers offer the opportunity to objectively assess alcohol intake. According to their specific characteristics, they provide different types of information: from abstinence monitoring to heavy use over time. If appropriately applied and used in conjunction with self-reports and questionnaires, they become an indispensable tool in the assessment and treatment of many conditions, such as alcohol use disorders, evaluation of liver transplant candidates, forensic evaluations, and others.

42.1 Introduction

Alcohol-related disorders are in the top ten of the most common diseases worldwide. The point prevalence for alcohol dependence in Germany, as in other comparable countries, is 5%, and the lifetime prevalence is 10%. Worldwide, approximately 4% of deaths are attributable to alcohol, greater than deaths caused by HIV, violence, or tuberculosis [1]. The yearly costs attributable to alcohol in Europe are approximately 270 billion €. Costs produced by alcohol include both direct costs (i.e., costs in which goods or services are being used or delivered such as medical care) and indirect costs (those stemming from lost productivity due to illness, death, or accidents). Another relevant source of costs attributable to alcohol is intangible costs (costs which are not related to any material loss: e.g., emotional suffering). Importantly, many of these costs are borne not only by the individual drinking alcohol but by society as a whole (the so-called social costs) [2].

Of all alcohol-dependent individuals, it is estimated that only about 10% receive specific treatment, most of them by their general practitioner (about 80%) and only a minority in specialized settings or general hospitals [3].

Thus, alcohol-related disorders are common, expensive in their entire course, and often underdiagnosed.

To facilitate early diagnosis and therapy of alcohol-related disorders and thus prevent later complications, questionnaires such as the CAGE questionnaire or the Alcohol Use Disorders Identification Test (AUDIT) are useful. Biomarkers also play an important role in many of the stages of alcohol use disorders, from screening and early detection to treatment monitoring, especially in abstinence-oriented settings [4, 5].

Indirect state markers as well as direct state markers are routinely used to detect alcohol. The indirect state markers such as gamma-glutamyl transpeptidase (GGT), mean corpuscular volume (MCV), and carbohydrate deficiency transferrin (CDT) are influenced by age, gender, various substances, and nonalcohol-related illnesses and do not cover the entire timeline for alcohol consumption, meaning that they need prolonged ingestion of relatively high amounts of alcohol to become elevated [6].

On the other hand, direct state markers have gained enormous interest in the last decades as they are metabolites of alcohol becoming only positive in the presence of alcohol. As biomarkers with high sensitivity and specificity covering the complimentary timeline, they are already routinely in use and contribute to new perspectives in prevention, interdisciplinary cooperation, diagnosis, and therapy of alcohol-related disorders.

42.1.1 Direct Ethanol Metabolites

Routinely used direct ethanol metabolites are as follows:

- Ethyl glucuronide (EtG) in serum, urine, and hair
- Ethyl sulfate (EtS) in urine and serum
- Phosphatidylethanol (PEth) in whole blood
- Fatty acid ethyl ester (FAEEs) especially in hair

Ethanol metabolites are detectable in serum for hours, in urine for up to 7 days, in whole blood over 2 weeks, and in hair over months.

42.2　Ethyl Glucuronide

Ethyl glucuronide (EtG) is a phase II metabolite of ethanol and has a molecular weight of 222 g/mol. It is metabolized by the UDP-glucuronosyltransferase.

Only about 0.5% of all the ethanol ingested undergoes this degradation pathway, but it can function as a biomarker as it is only detectable in the presence of ethanol. Moreover, EtG is non-volatile, water-soluble, and stable in storage and can, depending on the amount consumed and time spent for consumption, still be detectable in the body long after completion of alcohol elimination [7]. It can be detected of up to 90 hours in urine. There is no difference regarding the elimination rate between a healthy population and heavy alcohol consumers at the beginning of detoxification treatment [8]. Ethyl glucuronide can also be detected in postmortem body fluids and tissues such as the gluteal and abdominal fat, liver, brain, and cerebrospinal fluid and even in the bone marrow and muscle tissue.

Compared to traditional biomarkers, ethyl glucuronide displays a high sensitivity. Even small amounts like 0.1 L champagne can be detected up to 27 hours with this biomarker. Experiments with 1 g ethanol (champagne, whisky) as well as the use of mouthwash and hand sanitizer gels might yield positive ethyl glucuronide concentrations, usually with values of less than 1 mg/L in urine [9]. Measurable concentrations in urine can be found up to 11 hours after ingestion.

This aspect is of relevance regarding unintentional exposure of alcohol: Pralines, nonalcoholic beer, pharmaceutical products, fruit juice, sauerkraut, mouthwash products, and hand sanitizer gels may contain small amounts of alcohol. Even the intake of 21–42 g yeast with approximately 50 g sugar leads to measurable EtG and EtS concentrations in the urine.

Therefore, a patients' claim not having consumed alcohol may be the truth even when EtG is detectable in the urine. Since patients in withdrawal treatment should avoid even the smallest amount of alcohol, they have to be informed of such hidden sources of ethanol to avoid unintentional alcohol intake. A differential cutoff of 0.1 mg/L in cases where total abstinence is the goal and 1.0 mg/L if small amounts of alcohol intake are tolerated have been recommended for practical reasons. Applying these cutoffs, the probability of false-positive results is very low [10].

> Sometimes a positive ethyl glucuronide in the urine will be a true laboratory positive, but a false clinical positive, meaning that the patient has not intentionally ingested significant amounts of ethanol. However, using appropriate cutoffs, this would be a low probability situation.

42.2.1　Selected Applications for the Use of EtG

1. Outpatient addiction treatment programs

   Regular alcohol screening is a frequent intervention in many outpatient addiction treatment settings. Urine ethyl glucuronide has shown a higher sensitivity compared to traditional screening methods in this population, providing a more accurate feedback to both patients and professionals. In a former study, the percentage of urine positive samples screened with ethanol was less than 2%, whereas the same samples screened positive for ethyl glucuronide in almost 22% of the cases [11].

2. Specific high-risk group

   Many patients in opioid-maintenance therapy suffer from hepatitis C (HCV) infection. Alcohol consumption especially in large amounts leads to the progression of cirrhosis. Previous studies showed the usefulness and necessity of the determination of ethyl glucuronide in patients in opioid-maintenance therapy. For example, one study showed that, of all EtG positive patients, 42% ($n = 8$ of 19) would have not reported the alcohol consumption [12]. The use of direct ethanol metabolites in high-risk groups therefore allows more possibilities for therapeutic interventions, consequently leading to improvement in the quality of life.

3. Monitoring programs

One example for using ethyl glucuronide successfully in monitoring programs is the physician health programs in the USA which provide a non-disciplinary therapeutic program for physicians with potentially impairing health conditions as, for example, substance-related disorders. Being in the monitoring program, physicians with substance-related disorders are allowed to keep on working provided a regularly proof of abstinence has to be shown. Measuring EtG in urine, Skipper and colleagues showed that of 100 random samples collected, no sample was positive for alcohol using standard testing; however, seven were positive for EtG (0.5–196 mg/l), suggesting recent alcohol use. EtG testing can provide additional information and consequently may lead to further treatment and improvement for the patient [13].

4. Pharmacotherapeutic studies

As an objective outcome parameter, EtG testing has shown to be useful in pharmacotherapeutic studies [14].

5. Liver transplantation

Up to 30% of liver transplantations are related to alcohol. Postoperatively, 20–25% of patients lapse or relapse to alcohol intake. In 18 patients with ALD (alcohol liver disease), Erim et al. found no self-report of alcohol consumption. One out of 127 tests for breath alcohol was positive, whereas 24 of 49 urine samples were positive for EtG. Comparable results were reported by another study which found self-reported alcohol consumption in 3% in contrast to 20% positive urine EtG and EtS tests [15].

6. Pregnant women

Alcohol intake during pregnancy is a well-established risk factor for developmental impairments, especially fetal alcohol spectrum disorders (FASD). It is also known that a relevant proportion of pregnant women drink alcohol. Therefore, alcohol screening during pregnancy should be routinely conducted. Alcohol intake during pregnancy can be investigated in maternal (including hair, blood, urine) and fetal specimens (meconium). Similarly to other groups, self-reports and other questionnaires tend to underestimate alcohol intake. Ethyl glucuronide both in urine and meconium has been shown to improve the detection of drinking [16].

The above mentioned applications show that ethyl glucuronide tests are complementary to self-reports and questionnaires, yielding valuable information on alcohol consumption which is relevant to diagnosis and therapy.

> Irrespective of the setting and population where it is applied, ethyl glucuronide always displays a significantly greater sensitivity for the detection of alcohol drinking when compared to questionnaires, self-reports, and traditional biomarkers. However, the information it provides must always be considered as complementary to that obtained from other sources.

42.2.2 Methodological Aspects

The gold standard for the detection of ethyl glucuronide is liquid chromatography-tandem mass spectrometry (LC/MS-MS), and it remains the only valid method of analysis in enquiries with medicolegal relevance [17]. However, availability and cost issues prevent this method to become ubiquitous.

Fortunately, a DRI ethyl glucuronide enzyme immunoassay ([DRI-EtG EIA) became commercially available a decade ago. It is a semiquantitative method with a clinical cutoff of 500 ng/ml. It also offers a low and clinically relevant analytical range (15.3–2000 ng/ml). Its validity is very similar to that of the gold standard.

The last available method of analysis has been the appearance of point-of-care EtG immunoassay dipcards, which are commercially available at a very low cost. A recent study suggests the validity of the method to be high [18].

42.2.3 Limitations

A potential problem with EtG is the potential false-negative results produced by urinary tract infections, especially *E. coli*, which is able to degrade EtG. That, however, does not happen with ethyl sulfate, which remains stable in spite of the infection. This leads some authors to recommend simultaneous analysis of both biomarkers when a false-negative result is suspected for EtG. Interestingly, a recent study reported that the bacterial degradation of EtG by *E. coli* can be prevented by the use of dried urine on filter paper.

Given the impact alcohol has on liver function, it is important to remark that liver disease does not influence on the validity of EtG, as has been shown in studies conducted in patients with liver disease, including cirrhosis. Similarly, previous studies also suggest that race, nicotine consumption, body mass index, and body water content do not influence EtG concentrations. Conversely, reduced renal function seems to prolong the elimination time of EtG. Other potential factors affecting EtG levels are age, gender, and cannabis consumption.

42.2.4 Clinical Impact of Ethyl Glucuronide

Traditional biomarker validation studies rely on cross-sectional designs where sensitivity and specificity are the cornerstone of the evidence-gathering process. Accordingly, EtG has shown a high sensitivity and also high predictive values, both positive and negative, both in experimental and clinical settings.

However, cross-sectional validation prevents linking biomarker properties to patient outcomes on a longitudinal basis. A recent publication of a diagnostic randomized clinical trial where ethyl glucuronide was compared to ethanol in a randomized design [19] enabled the connection of biomarker properties and diagnostic performance to patient outcomes, demonstrating that implementing ethyl glucuronide in the routine screening of alcohol-dependent outpatients leads to

decreased drinking and increased rates of abstinence over time.

> Recent evidence suggest that the application of a highly sensitive biomarker such as ethyl glucuronide has therapeutic properties, leading to reduced drinking and increased abstinence rates, probably due to increased feedback to both professionals and patients about their drinking.

42.3 Ethyl Sulfate

Ethyl sulfate (EtS) presents a secondary elimination pathway for alcohol and is usually detectable in varying interindividual concentrations. An immunochemical detection test is currently not commercially available for EtS. For combined detection of EtS and EtG, the use of rapid LC/MS-MS procedures is routinely applied. It is normally measured in urine, although it can also be assessed in plasma.

The formation is effected by sulfonyl transferase and the breakdown by sulfatases. The molecular weight is 126 g/mol and the molecular formula $C_2H_5SO_4H$.

Currently, a LC/MS-MS method with pentadeuterium EtS as internal standard and two ion transitions can be used in forensic and medicolegal cases as well as in clinical routine. The fact that its formation route is different to that of EtG offers the opportunity of increased sensitivity when analyzing the two biomarkers together. However, the discrepancies between the two are usually low [20].

In summary, a cutoff of 0.05 mg/l for repeated alcohol intake has been suggested. As for ethyl glucuronide, there is evidence of prolonged elimination in reduced renal function. Importantly, bacterial degradation of EtS has not been described. Therefore, EtS should be analyzed in conjunction with EtG when degradation of this biomarker is suspected, in order to prevent the appearance of a false-negative result.

Ethyl sulfate is seldom analyzed alone. Usually, both EtG and EtS are assessed, in order to complement each other's information. EtS might help prevent false-negative results due to bacterial degradation of EtG, especially by *E. coli*, and it might also increase the sensitivity of EtG alone.

42.4 Fatty Acid Ethyl Esters

In recent years, the existence of fatty acid ethyl esters and non-oxidative metabolic products of ethanol in the blood and various organs with reduced or deficient capacity to oxidize ethanol after consumption has been proven. Since these esters were proven to cause damage to subcellular structures, they were postulated to be mediators of organ damage.

Two enzymes catalyze the formation of FAEE: acyl coenzyme a-ethanol o-acyltransferase (AEAT) and fatty acid ethyl ester-synthase. FAEE-synthase can be isolated from the rabbit myocardium, human brain, and rat fat tissue. Two of these FAEE-synthases were shown to be identical to rat liver carboxyl esterase. Furthermore, pancreatic lipase, lipoprotein lipase, and glutathione transferase were shown to possess FAEE-synthase activity.

Fatty acid ethyl esters are formed in the presence of ethanol from free fatty acids, triglycerides, lipoproteins, or phospholipids affected by specific cytosolic or microsomal FAEE-synthases or through acyl coenzyme a-ethanol o-acyltransferase. Detectable levels are found in the blood shortly after alcohol consumption and remain positive for more than 24 hours.

Of 15 different FAEEs in hair, the sum of four of these (ethyl stearate, ethyl oleate, ethyl myristat, and ethyl palmitate) is shown to function as a marker in hair analysis. With a cutoff of 0.5 ng/ml, a sensitivity and a specificity of 90% were reported. A differentiation between abstinent, social, and excessive drinkers appears possible [21]. However, the complex GC/MS method lacks practicability for routine use.

42.5 Phosphatidylethanol

Phosphatidylethanol is an abnormal phospholipid formed in the presence of alcohol via the action of phospholipase D. The precursor is the naturally existing lipid-phosphatidylcholine. PEth consists of glycerol which is substituted at positions sn1 and sn2 by fatty acids and a phosphate group at position sn3 esterified with ethanol. Due to the variations of the fatty acids, various analogs of PEth can be detected. The PEth analogs 16:0/18:1 and 16:0/18:2 are most prevalent, and their combined sum correlates better with PEth than PEth 16:0/18:1 or PEth 16:0/18:2 alone.

Using the original HPLC methods, repeated consumption of more than 50 g alcohol over 2–3 weeks yielded positive results, lately even with daily consumption over 40 g [22].

A drinking experiment [23] with healthy persons with a target blood ethanol concentration of 1 g/kg (1 per mille) once on each of 5 consecutive days yielded PEth values up to 237 ng/ml. Measurements were performed with LC/MS-MS. In contrast to alcohol-dependent patients, the values were reported to be up to 213,000 ng/ml [24].

Various studies found no false-positive results. A linear relationship between consumed amounts of alcohol with phosphatidylethanol values has been described [22].

Interestingly, and thanks to constant refinements in analytical methods, the sensitivity and specificity of current PEth analysis seem to be extremely high [25]. Also relevant is the fact that, besides its already known potential for abstinence monitoring, current evidence suggests PEth could be a suitable biomarker for the differentiation between light and heavy drinking, a feature that is lacking in other direct alcohol biomarkers [26].

Importantly, PEth values seem not to be influenced by liver diseases and hypertension [27].

Among the new direct alcohol biomarkers, PEth seems to be the only one capable of assessing abstinence and also differentiating between light, moderate, and heavy drinking.

42.5.1 Methodological Aspects

The current approach for PEth determination is LC/MS and LC/MS-MS methods. These methods facilitate detection and quantification of single analogs, if a reference is available.

For everyday practical use, the use of dried blood spots may be of significant relevance. This method is suggested to have results similar to whole-blood measures. Furthermore, there is no difference between venous or capillary blood collection [28]. Sampling is simplified as nonmedical staff can obtain capillary blood, the risks for HIV and hepatitis C infections are decreased, and storage and transport are simplified.

42.5.2 Clinical Applications

Similar to what has been described with ethyl glucuronide, phosphatidylethanol has shown a high degree of sensitivity and specificity for the detection of alcohol drinking. It has been applied to different populations and clinical settings, such as HIV populations, pregnant women, and alcohol-dependent patients [29].

Interestingly, it seems like PEth shows good correlations with AUDIT-C scores [30]. Therefore, PEth might be a potential biomarker of heavy alcohol consumption over time.

Finally, some authors suggest that PEth might have a role in patients who are tested for EtG and EtS, have low positive values, and deny alcohol consumption, as a further evaluation with an even more sensitive biomarker.

42.5.3 Limitations

In blood and tissues containing ethanol, the formation of PEth under certain conditions may be feasible. Without influencing the PEth levels, whole-blood samples can be stored frozen at −80 °C [31], and DBS can be stored for at least 30 days at −20 °C [32].

In vitro formation of PEth in erythrocytes has been reported after addition of ethanol. Further experimental studies in rats showed that ceramide is able to block the activity of phospholipase D and inhibits the synthesis of PEth.

42.6 Hair Analyses

Hair analysis has been established to assess ethanol intake. FAEE and ethyl glucuronide (EtG), two metabolic by-products of ethanol, are gaining attention as alcohol markers in the hair.

The time frame for the detection of alcohol consumption is longer in the hair compared to blood or urine. Due to head hair growth of 1 cm per month, depending on the hair length, evidence of alcohol consumption can be found for the respective time period. The deposit of lipophilic FAEE in the hair occurs in sebum, whereas hydrophilic EtG is incorporated through perspiration and/or from blood.

Measurement of FAEE and EtG allows differentiation between chronic excessive and moderate alcohol consumption as well as abstinence or very low levels of alcohol consumption.

In a last consensus from the Society of Hair Testing, an essential change of the consensus was accepted for the FAEEs, where the concentration of ethyl palmitate (EtPa) can be used autonomously for interpretation instead of the concentration sum (ΣFAEE) of the four esters ethyl myristate, ethyl palmitate, ethyl oleate, and ethyl stearate, as previously applied [33]. The EtPa cutoff for abstinence assessment was defined at 0.12 ng/mg for the 0–3 cm segment and at 0.15 ng/mg for the 0–6 cm segment. The cutoff for chronic excessive drinking was fixed at 0.35 ng/mg for the 0–3 cm segment and at 0.45 ng/mg for the 0–6 cm segment. The use of EtPa with these cutoffs in place of ΣFAEE for alcohol intake assessment produces only a minor loss in discrimination power, leads to no essential difference in the interpretation concerning chronic excessive alcohol consumption, and is suitable to confirm EtG results in abstinence assessment.

An EtG concentration of over 30 pg/mg hair is interpreted as definite evidence for excessive and regular alcohol consumption (>60 g EtOH per day), whereas an EtG concentration of more than 7 pg/mg is a marker of frequent alcohol use. If samples less than 3 cm or greater than 6 cm are used, the results should be interpreted with caution. The analysis of FAEEs alone is not recommended to determine abstinence from ethanol.

For abstinence assessment, EtG should be the first choice, and the analysis of FAEEs alone is not recommended to determine abstinence from ethanol. A positive FAEE result combined with an EtG below 7 pg/mg does not clearly disprove abstinence but indicates the need for further monitoring. The combined use of FAEE and EtG can be recommended to increase the validity of hair analysis [34].

In an alcohol drinking experiment, 32 women who consumed 16 g alcohol per day had EtG values of less than 7 pg in their scalp hair [27]. These divergent results may be explained by the fact that EtG values lower than 7 pg/mg do not exclude alcohol ingestion. Furthermore, scalp hair was pre-analytically cut in this study, while previous studies pulverized the specimen: The preparation pre-analytically has been reported to influence the results significantly [35].

42.6.1 Other Influencing Factors

Whereas only in one case a false-positive result for EtG in the hair after use of EtG containing shampoo has been reported, regular use of alcohol-containing hair tonic can lead to false-positive FAEE results. No such false-positive results are reported for EtG. Impaired kidney function may lead to higher EtG levels, as preliminary results indicate. BMI showed to have also an influence on EtG concentration in the hair.

False-negative results for both alcohol markers can also be caused by the use of hair cosmetics, such as alkaline hair cosmetics for FAEE [36] or oxidative treatment for EtG and hair straightening for EtG. Cleansing shampoos may also alter EtG and FAEE concentrations in hair.

The hair color and melanin content in hair play no role, in contrast to drugs and medications. In segmental investigations of hair samples, a chronological correlation to drink or abstinent phase with FAEE is not possible, but for EtG, two studies have shown this to be feasible.

Altogether, hair analysis for FAEE or EtG is currently a sensible tool to clarify past alcohol consumption, as demonstrated in many studies.

42.6.2 Practical Use

Hair analysis for FSEE or EtG is applicable in several contexts including judging driving ability and forensic psychiatry. Another clinical use of alcohol metabolite measures is the screening for alcohol use in medication- assisted treatment of opioid-dependent subjects as mentioned above

42.7 Summary

In summary, specific ethanol metabolites are available which can detect the spectrum between short-term intake of small amounts and long-term use of large amounts of alcohol (s. Table 42.1). Cutoff values and influencing factors are summarized in Tables 42.2 and 42.3. Appropriate methods of analysis and pre-analytics are crucial for a valid and reliable detection of markers. For ethyl glucuronide (EtG), the most frequently used marker, the best method for detection is chromatographic approach which is considered a standard method especially in forensic cases. A commercial test

Table 42.1 Clinically relevant options for determination of direct biomarkers, with respect to amount and duration of alcohol intake

Duration of consumption	Amount of consumption	
	>1 g/d	>40–60 g/d
<1 day	Serum, urine: EtOH, EtG, EtS	Serum and urine: EtOH, EtG, EtS; PEth in whole blood and dried blood spots (LC/MS-MS)
>1 day	Serum, urine: EtOH, EtG, EtS	Serum and urine: EtOH, EtG, EtS; PEth in whole blood and dried blood spots (LC/MS-MS)
>14 days	Serum, urine: EtOH, EtG, EtS	Serum and urine: EtOH, EtG, EtS; PEth in whole blood and dried blood spots (HPLC LC/MS-MS)
Weeks to months	Serum, urine: EtOH, EtG, EtS	Serum and urine: EtOH, EtG, EtS; PEth in whole blood and dried blood spots (HPLC LC/MS-MS), EtG and FAEEs in hair

Modified according to Thon et al. [37]
EtOH ethanol, *EtG* ethyl glucuronide, *EtS* ethyl sulfate, *PEth* phosphatidylethanol, *FAEE* fatty -acid ethyl esters

Table 42.2 Clinically relevant options for determination of direct biomarkers, with respect to amount and duration of alcohol intake

Biomarkers	Amount of consumption	Cutoff
EtG in hair	Abstinence and low intake (<10 g alc/d)	<7 pg/mg
	Social consumption (20–40 g/d)	7–30 pg/mg
	Excessive drinking (>60 g/d)	>30 pg/mg
FAEEs in hair	Repeated alcohol intake	≥200 pg/mg
	Excessive intake	≥500 pg/mg
EtG in urine	Total abstinence	0.1 mg/L
	Unintentional intake Recent alcohol use Longer back-dated alcohol intake in larger amounts	0.1 mg/l–0.5 mg/L
	Unintentional intake unlikely, but possible, active alcohol intake probable	0.5–1 mg/L
EtS in urine	Total abstinence	0.05 mg/L
PEth	>40 g/d, more than 2 weeks alcohol intake at least once with 1‰ detectable	HPLC, 0.22 μM; LC/MS-MS, 20/30 ng/ml; PEth, 16:0/18:1 or 0.05 μM

Modified according to Thon et al. [37]

EtG ethyl glucuronide, *FAEEs* fatty -acid ethyl esters in hair, *EtS* ethyl sulfate, *PEth* phosphatidylethanol

Table 42.3 Detection of direct biomarker, with respect to amount and duration of alcohol intake

Direct biomarkers	Potential influencing factor	Influence
EtG in urine	*E. coli*, dried urine spots	No
	Grade of liver disease, smoking, BMI, body water content, reduced kidney function	No
EtS in urine	*E. coli*, dried urine spots	No
PEth	Liver disease	No
	Hypertension	No
	Storage of ethanol blood samples Refrigerator temperature, −80 °C	No
EtG in hair	Hairsprays with ethanol, hair color, melanin content, age, gender, BMI	No
Direct biomarkers	**Potential influencing factor**	**Type of influence**
EtG in urine	*E. coli, C. sordellii*	Decrease
	Reduced kidney function	Longer detection
	Chloral hydrate	False positives
EtS in urine	Reduced kidney function	Longer detection
	Closed Bottle Test (OECD 301 D) Manometer Respiratory Test (MRT)	28 days' stable detection, depletion after 6 days
FAEEs in hair	Aggressive alkaline hairsprays	False negative
	Hairsprays with ethanol	False positives
PEth	Ethanol-containing blood samples, storage of ethanol blood samples at RT and − 20 °C	Increase
EtG in hair	Hairspray with EtG	Increase
	Reduced kidney function	Increase
	Bleaching, hairstyling products	False negative

Modified according to Thon et al. [37]

EtG ethyl glucuronide, *FAEE* fatty -acid ethyl esters, *EtS* ethyl sulfate, *PEth* phosphatidylethanol, *BMI* body – mass index, *RT* room ambient temperature, *E. coli Escherichia coli*, *C. sordellii Clostridium sordellii*

kit is available and contributed to wide distribution of the test. Of course, lab values always require critical reappraisal. However, EtG is detectable in urine using LC/MS-MS even after an ingestion of low amounts of alcohol (1 g), which also occurs in some food, drugs, and disinfectants. Individuals with the motivation to or obligation for abstinence have to be informed about these "hidden contents" to avoid involuntary intake of alcohol. For forensic purposes, the current cutoff value of 0.1 mg/L should be adapted to exclude cases of involuntary alcohol use. With respect to differences in formation and degradation, EtG and ethyl sulfate (EtS) should be analyzed together, if possible. In the absence of known influencing factors, EtG in the hair can be recommended as a marker for alcohol intake for the last 3 months. Further, guidelines for interpretations of values from international society (SOHT) are available. While positive urine values of EtG and EtS can be in accord with innocent/unintentional alcohol intake, positive values of PEth are related to previous intoxications of 0.5‰ and more. The use of "dried blood spots" is promising and may facilitate sample taking, storage, distribution, and decrease of infection risk.

42.8 Traditional Biomarkers for Alcohol Consumption

Many clinical-chemical parameters show pathological changes as evidence of the biochemical burden of ethanol metabolism. None of these conventional indicators show 100% sensitivity or specificity. Nonetheless, evidence of long-term alcohol consumption can be obtained from these state markers, especially a combination of several individual indicators. The currently used and potential alcohol biomarkers are shown in Table 42.4.

Table 42.4 Diagnostic characteristics of several conventional and potential alcohol biomarkers

Alcohol biomarker (abbreviation)	Window of assessment	Specificity/ sensitivity	Type of alcohol consumption	Application	Specific comments
Conventional alcohol biomarkers					
Ethanol (EtOH)	6 hours	High/high	Recent alcohol consumption/ alcohol intoxication	In traffic safety/ emergency department	In combination with clinical observations – monitoring alcohol habits
Gamma-glutamyl transferase (GGT)	2–8 weeks	Moderate/ moderate	Chronic, heavy	Screening/ monitoring	More specific for alcoholics ages 30–50 years
Aminotransferase ratio AST/ALT ≥ 2	Unknown	High/low	Heavy	Alcoholic hepatitis/ relapse	Less frequently used than GGT for screening heavy alcoholics
Mean corpuscular volume (MCV)	Up to several months	Moderate to high/low	Chronic	Screening/fetal alcohol effects	Show dose-dependent response to the intensity of alcohol intake
Carbohydrate-deficient transferrin (CDT)	2–3 weeks	High/ moderate	Heavy	Screening/ monitoring/ relapse	No elevation in single episodes of acute alcohol intoxication
GGT-CDT	2–3 necks	High-high	Heavy	Abstinence/ relapse	Useful for diagnostic alcohol-liver damage due to excessive and prolonged intake
Potential alcohol biomarkers and devices					
Ethyl glucuronide (EtG) and ethyl sulfate (EtS)	Several days	High/high	Recent alcohol consumption	Abstinence/ relapse	High inter-individual variations

(continued)

Table 42.4 (continued)

Alcohol biomarker (abbreviation)	Window of assessment	Specificity/ sensitivity	Type of alcohol consumption	Application	Specific comments
Phosphatidylinositol (PEth)	1–2 necks	Unknown/ high	Heavy	Screening/ relapse	Promising in differentiating alcohol – from non-alcohol-induced liver disease
Fatty acid ethyl esters (FAEEs)	24 hours (after ingestion)/99 hours (heavy drinking)	High/high	Recent heavy	Distinguishing social drinkers from heavy	Combination of FAEE and EtG in meconium – markers for fetal alcohol exposure
Whole blood-associated acetaldehyde assay (WBAA)	Unknown	High/high	Chronic/heavy	Monitoring abstinence	IgAs against acetaldehyde protein adducts – promising in differentiating alcohol – from non-alcohol- induced liver disease
Total sialic acid (TSA)	Unknown	Between GGT and ALT	Chronic, heavy	Relapse	Increased in high alcohol consumption and reduced during abstinence, especially among women
5-HTOL/5-HIAA	1 day	High/high	Recent alcohol consumption	Evaluation of treatment/ relapse	5-HTOL/5-HIAA > 20 marker of recent drinking
Transdermal devices (SCRAM, WrisTAS)	–	High/high	Record continuous alcohol consumption	By court monitoring of abstinence	Need product improvements

From Topic and Djukic [38]

42.8.1 Blood Alcohol Content Calculation

A mathematical estimation of blood alcohol content is useful when blood alcohol is not currently detectable or for prediction of alcohol level. While there are several ways to calculate it, the simplest is Widmark's equation: $Co = A/[p \times r]$, where Co is the theoretical maximum concentration of alcohol in the blood (mg/g), A is the amount of alcohol in the body (g), p is the body weight (kg), r is the correction factor corresponding to the ratio of total body water and blood water (0.6 for females and 0.7 for males).

Gender plays an important role in the total amount of water in the body. In general, men have less fatty tissue and higher percentage of water (58%) than women (49%); thus, volume of distribution (Vd) for ethanol is higher in men. According to its partition coefficient (Poct/water is 0.1), ethanol is ten times more soluble in water than in lipids. Thus, upon ingestion of the same amount of ethanol, the BAC will be higher in females than in males. The Widmark's equation has been improved subsequently by introducing individual r, based on the multiple linear regression equations:

$$For\ females: r\mathrm{FI} = 0.31223 - 0.006446$$
$$\times body\ weight(kg) + 0.004466$$
$$\times body\ height(cm)$$

$$For\ males: r\mathrm{MI} = 0.31608 - 0.004821$$
$$\times body\ weight(kg) + 0.004632$$
$$\times body\ height(cm)$$

There is no absolute accurate blood alcohol calculator because numerous factors influence the BAC, such as gender (male/female), rate of metabolism/elimination, health status, medications that might be taken, drinking frequency, amount and the type of food in the stomach and small intestine, time when food was eaten, and others [38].

42.9 Gamma-Glutamyl Transferase (γ-GT)

γ-GT is a membrane-bound glycoprotein enzyme which occurs ubiquitous in the organism but mainly in the liver, pancreas, and renal proximal tubules. γ-GT detectable in serum arises mainly from the liver so that an increase in serum enzyme activity would be a sensitive indicator for hepatobiliary diseases. Chronic alcohol consumption induces an increase in enzyme synthesis and, through direct activation of the enzyme from membrane binding, leads to increase of γ-GT in serum. The release of enzymes through liver parenchymal damage also presents a secondary mechanism in chronic alcoholic hepatitis. To exceed the normal values (4–18 U/l in women and 6–28 U/l in men) requires the chronic, daily alcohol intake over at least 4–6 weeks. A short-term, higher alcohol burden causes no such increase. Nevertheless, drinking intensity has more influence on γ-GT than drinking frequency. In absolute alcohol abstinence, normalization of the values occurs within 3 weeks to 60 days.

The sensitivity of γ-GT varies, according to age, gender, and body weight, from 35% to 85%. γ-GT increases with age in heavy alcohol drinkers as well as moderate drinkers. Contrarily, in young adults less than 30 years, even when these are alcohol dependent, the sensitivity of the markers is very low. In addition, the higher vulnerability of women to alcohol-associated liver diseases is well known. Other studies have shown that the relationship between overweight (BMI > 25) and an increase in γ-GT [39] is related. γ-GT levels can also be increased by various other causes, for example, the effects of medication and teratogens, adiposities, diabetes,

cholestasis, or inflammatory liver diseases. Accordingly, the specificity of 63–85% is only satisfactory, and γ-GT, in spite of its practicability as solitary indicator of chronic alcohol misuse and current liver diseases, is deemed unsuitable [40].

42.10 Mean Corpuscular Erythrocyte Volume (MCV)

Measurements of MCV are common in standard investigations; an increase occurs in 4% of the general population and in 40–60% of patients with alcohol misuse. Koivisto et al. [41] reported definite evidence of marked dose-dependent relationship between MCV and the intensity of alcohol consumption. Increase in MCV is to be expected in long-term alcohol consumption; by contrast, the values normalize slowly during abstinence over a period of 2–4 months. Compared to γ-GT, the sensitivity of MCV in screening as evidence of alcohol misuse, at least in men, is inferior. In interpreting MCV values, other causes such as vitamin B12 or folic deficiency, nonalcoholic liver diseases, reticulocytosis, and hematologic diseases should be considered.

The mechanism responsible for increasing MCV is hitherto unclear, and direct hematotoxic damage or interaction of ethanol and its metabolites, especially acetaldehyde, with erythrocyte membrane has been suggested [42].

42.11 Carbohydrate-Deficient Transferrin (CDT)

Transferrin is the most important iron transport molecule in humans, and its synthesis and glycolization occur in hepatocytes. Depending on the iron load as well as the number and breakdown of carbohydrate chains, different isoforms can be detected. Differentiation occurs through measurements of isoelectric points (pl), whose values depend on the load of bound iron ions and number of sialic acid residues in carbohydrate chains. Abnormal isoforms with much increased pl-values over 5.65 in the liquor and serum of alcohol-dependent patients were found and were traced back to small levels of bound sialic acid residues. In subsequent investigations, more precise differentiation in mono-, di-, and asialotransferrin was feasible, and all abnormal isoforms were subgrouped under CDT [43]. All abnormal transferrin molecules increase in chronic alcohol consumption. Measurements with HPLC showed that increased alcohol consumption leads to increased disialotransferrins, while increases in asialotransferrin occur in chronic increased alcohol consumption only. A variety of methods and respective reference levels for the detection of CDT are available. Hitherto, measurements of CDT using HPLC is the reference standard, with routine measurements of various enzyme immunoassays in use. For confirmation analyses, immune electrophoresis is employed, while direct CDT detection method using specific antibodies is still under development [44].

The underlying pathomechanism for CDT development is not exactly known. Inhibition of intracellular transmission of carbohydrates to change through toxic effects from ethanol or acetaldehyde is presumed. Ethanol's influence on the activities of membrane-bound sialine transferases and plasma sialidases in hepatocytes has been discussed, in which an imbalance in favor of sialine acid reduction enzymes occurred.

There has been no agreement in previous studies concerning the correlation between CDT concentrations in serum and the absorbed alcohol amounts. Though an increase in CDT with daily consumption of 60–80 g alcohol over 7 days has been shown, other studies have reported contradicting results. Additionally, contradicting results on the effect of moderate drinking (<40 g alcohol) are found. In alcohol-dependent patients, it is, however, sensitive enough for detecting relapses and monitoring sobriety [45].

The clinical strengths of CDT as a biomarker vary depending on gender, BMI, age, nicotine abuse, and anorexia [46]. Previous studies showed that CDT in men is a more sensitive indicator of alcohol-related diseases compared to women. CDT values in women might be increased under natural conditions but not much in increased alcohol use. Furthermore, hormonal factors appear to play a role – CDT values are definitely increased in pregnant women but reduced in postmenopausal women. Obviously in the female gender, differences in CDT serum activity depend on age as well.

Among the various conventional alcohol markers, CDT is currently considered the most useful and significant indicator [47]. Information on sensitivity and specificity varies, since no methodical standardization exists. Further, the heterogeneity of test populations concerning age, gender, alcohol consumption, duration of abstinence before serum extraction, as well as current liver diseases makes the comparison with other traditional markers difficult. In selected clinical patient groups, various test methods with specificity between 90% and 100% with high sensitivity (50–90%) have been reported.

In WHO/ISBRA study, the sensitivity of CDT with 60% in men was slightly less than that of γ-GT, and in women the sensitivity reached only 29% [6]. False-positive increased CDT values can occur in biliary cirrhotic, autoimmune hepatitis, genetically determined transferrin variants, or the autosomal recessive inherited CDG syndrome. Most patients with liver diseases have insignificantly increased CDT values so that the specificity, especially in comparison with other state markers, must be stated exceptionally high and usually reach at least 90%. Thus, CDT could be used for detection of chronic alcohol consumption and changes in drinking patterns in these patients. With a half-life of 14 days and normalization of CDT values in abstinence, evidence of drinking relapses in the post-acute phase after alcohol withdrawal treatment can be obtained.

42.12　Serum Transaminases (ASAT/ALAT)

Increases of aspartate aminotransferase (ASAT) and alanine aminotransferase (ALAT) in serum are unspecific signs of hepatocellular damage. While ASAT is produced in the liver, skeleton, and cardiac muscle tissues, ALAT is a liver-specific enzyme. Thus, an increase in ALAT practically indicates liver diseases (fatty degeneration, tumors, metastases, cirrhosis, cholangitis). By contrast, measurements of ASAT must differentiate between alcohol-sensitive, mitochondrial (m-ASAT), and cytoplasmic isoform (c-ASAT). Conclusions on an alcohol-induced liver damage can only be drawn from increased m-ASAT/c-ASAT quotients. Increased ASAT values would be found in alcohol-dependent patients from 39% to 47%. In the WHO/ISBRA study, sensitivity of ASAT between 23% and 45% (women vs. men) could be found. The toxic effects of ethanol on mitochondria lead to increased release of ASAT compared to ALAT. Thus, measurements of de-Ritis-Quotient (ASAT/ALAT) increase the alcohol specificity of both markers – a quotient over 1 and even 2 would offer strong indications for an ethyl toxic etiology.

In summary, the sensitivity and specificity of both enzymes as indicators for alcohol misuse are considered variable so that an interpretation of an increased serum activity is mainly meaningful in the context of other liver values (bilirubin, alkaline phosphatase, γ-GT).

42.13 HDL Cholesterine and Apolipoprotein

Increases in HDL cholesterol and apoprotein I/II are described in many studies as specific and sensitive indicators of chronic alcohol strain; by contrast, triglycerides and total cholesterine are nutritionally influenced. Alcohol leads to an increase in the concentrations of cholesterol and phospholipids within the HDL particles and causes a shift to bigger portions of phospholipids in richer, larger HDL_2 particles [48].

Studies showed this phenomenon to be the basic principle for the observed cardioprotective character of moderate alcohol consumption [49]. Chronic alcohol load causes an increase in HDL over 50 mg/dl, and after withdrawal and with continuing abstinence, the values normalize within 1–4 weeks. The pathogenic cause of alcohol-related HDL and apoprotein increases is postulated to be an enzyme induction as well as increased lipoprotein lipase activity.

Increased HDL levels without alcohol can occur under the influence of medication (seda-tives, lovastatin), pronounced underweight, and physical strain. Still, the specificity of this marker is highly esteemed. Moreover, it proved itself to be practicable. Particularly in patients without liver damage, HDL and apoprotein I/II can be used for monitoring abstinence since changes in alcohol consumption would be accurately reflected.

42.14 Cholesteryl Ester Transfer Protein (CETP)

Cholesteryl ester transfer protein is a glycoprotein synthesized in the liver and catalyzed out of HDL particles through lipid diffusion into LDL particles. Through alcohol consumption, the plasma concentration and activity of CETP are reduced, thereby increasing HDL concentration. Moderate drinking, by contrast, hardly influences CETP activity. The sensitivity and specificity of CETP as an alcohol marker can be compared to those of MCV, γ-GT, ASAT, and ALAT. Nonetheless, the use of CETP as an indicator for alcohol misuse is limited by the complex measurement method and by the influence of drugs and various diseases.

42.15 β-Hexosaminidase

β-Hexosaminidase is a lysosomal liver enzyme detected in serum or urine using spectrometric methods. Higher serum activity of this glycoprotein was reported in alcohol-dependent patients. A daily consumption of 60 g alcohol leads to significant serum increases; even short-term alcohol load is reflected in alcohol patients by its low half-life and resulting limited normalization in values (<6, 2 U/l) 2–4 days later. The pathological mechanism in rats is the reduction in biliary elimination of the enzyme in chronic ethanol intake. The specificity of β-hexosaminidase in serum is stated to be 91–98%, and the sensitivity is 69–94%. β-Hexosaminidase activity reflects recent alcohol consumption, while β-hexosaminidase in urine remains increased for longer periods after alcohol consumption (Fig. 42.1).

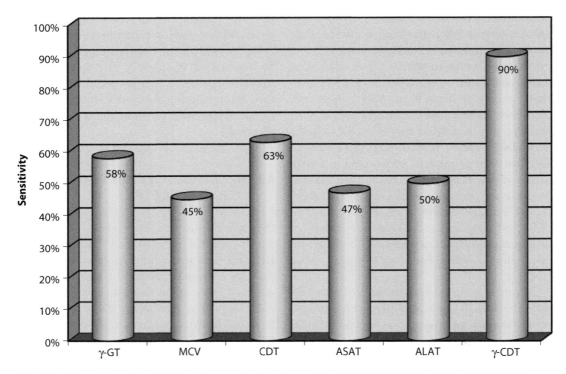

Fig. 42.1 Comparison of sensitivities of conventional markers with γ-CDT. (Modified from Niemelä [50]) [15]

42.16 Methanol (MeOH)

Methanol is a monovalent alcohol produced endogenously; under physiological conditions, the concentration in serum is between 0.5 and 1.0 mg/l. Methanol can be ingested exogenously through alcoholic drinks, fruit juice, and pectin-containing fruits (e.g., bananas or apples). The metabolism of methanol occurs in the liver through alcohol dehydrogenase (ADH), which shows a manifold increased affinity to ethanol compared to methanol even without alcohol ingestion. That being so, in the presence of ethanol in concentrations over 0.2–0.5%, a competitive inhibition of methanol breakdown occurs, which, in continuing ethanol availability, leads to accumulation of endogenous methanol. Should the ingested alcohol also contains methanol (e.g., fruit-flavored gin, whisky), the blood levels would be potentiated even more by endogenous accumulation. The methanol levels normalize itself in alcohol abstinence within several hours to several days. Early evidence of increased

blood methanol levels after longer drinking periods was reported in the 1970s, among others. In numerous studies, a coincidence between increased methanol levels and blood alcohol levels has been found. Consequently, methanol values >10 mg/l, which were not caused by normal and short term, even high alcohol load over 1.5–2.0%, were estimated and considered as an indicator for recent alcohol misuse or longer alcohol consumption phase. Despite its high specificity, methanol is only suitable as a short-term state marker because it is rapidly normalized. Its significance lies primarily in screening alcohol misuse in clinical as well as forensic cases.

42.17 Acetone and Isopropanol

Physiologic levels of isopropanol in blood are up to 0.1 mg/l and acetone up to 7 mg/l. Both substances are not found in alcoholic drinks. Isopropanol and acetone are in reciprocal biotransformation process, meaning isopropanol is reduced to acetone and formed, through oxidehydration, from acetone. Both processes occur via alcohol dehydrogenase. Alcohol load causes an increase in isopropanol in blood; conversely during withdrawal, acetone is increased. Higher isopropanol and acetone levels occur mainly in alcohol-dependent patients with concurrent eating disorders or reduced nutritional intake. It is established practice to pool both substances in serum concentration, and a level of 9 mg/l has been recommended. Still, isopropanol and acetone appear less convincing than methanol as alcohol markers because increased acetone levels also result from metabolic disorders such as ketosis in hunger, diabetes, cooling, and heavy physical strain (Fig. 42.2).

42.18 Combination of Individual State Markers

Since individual conventional alcohol markers were found to be insufficiently sensitive and/or specific for the recognition of alcohol misuse, several important parameters in varying combinations were investigated. The better known combinations comprised of CDT, γ-GT, MCV, and ASAT.

42.19 Gamma-Glutamyl Transferase and Carbohydrate-Deficient Transferrin

Some studies showed that the combined use of γ-GT and CDT resulted in higher sensitivity and specificity compared to use of either one alone. Sillanaukee et al. [52] reported a sensitivity of 75% and specificity of 93% for γ-CDT from 257 alcohol-dependent patients and 362 occasional drinkers. γ-CDT is estimated using the formula $[γ\text{-}CDT = 0.8 \ln(γ\text{-}GT) + 1.3 \ln(CDT)]$. Compared to CDT and γ-GT alone, ASAT, ALAT, or MCV showed the logarithmic transformation from γ-GT and CDT to have the best predictive value to differentiate between alcohol-dependent patients and occasional drinkers. Values for γ-CDT correlate to current amounts of consumption, regardless of whether a heavy alcohol-dependent individual or an occasional drinker was tested. γ-CDT can thus be used to monitor abstinence, though in continuing abstinence the values normalize within 2–3 weeks. Considering the cost efficiency and simple application, γ-CDT appears to be a suitable indicator in clinical routine work.

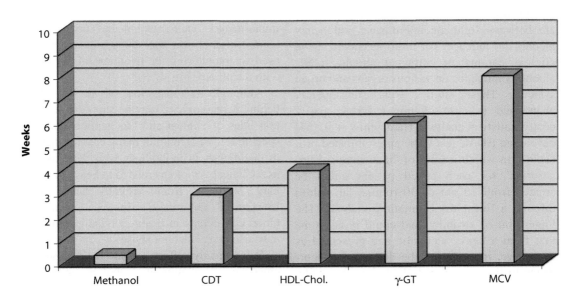

Fig. 42.2 Depiction of alcohol markers in appropriate time lines. (Modified from Gilg [51])

42.20 Alc Index

By combining methanol, acetone/isopropanol, γ-GT, and CDT in a logistic regression formula, Brinkmann et al. [53] developed the so-called Alc index to differentiate between alcohol-dependent patients and nondrinkers. The basic principle for the investigations was the hypothesis that each of these alcohol markers shows overlap in values in the collective with none or low alcohol consumption and alcoholics. From the results, an Alc index of 1.7 as cutoff was defined with a specificity of 100% and a sensitivity of 90% to differentiate between alcohol-dependent and nonalcohol-dependent individuals. The advantage of this index is the single cutoff point instead of four for individual markers, through which it can prevent false conclusions with raised values of an isolated marker.

42.21 Early Detection of Alcohol Consumption (EDAC) Test

EDAC uses results from a series of routine lab parameters to identify heavy drinkers and light drinkers in study groups. Already in the 1980s, attempts have been made, through multivariate statistical analysis with blood samples from conspicuous patients with alcohol, to differentiate between light alcohol misuse and heavy alcohol dependence. The multiple chemical and clinical parameters extracted should reflect alcohol's influence on various organs and organ systems. These studies were subsequently abandoned because of impracticable, partly costly statistical analysis. Harasymiw et al. [54] developed EDAC test to be an established procedure, in which a form of "mathematical fingerprint" for each tested patient could be created from 10 out of 30 routine lab values through a linear discrimination analysis. The fingerprint of an individual could possibly be that from a heavy alcoholic and presented as P-positive, representing the degree of concordance to the stereotyped alcoholic lab profile. In general, a P-positive value over 50% showed current heavy alcohol consumption, whereas values below or equal to 50% showed evidence of light alcohol misuse. The EDAC test was successfully used as screening for alcohol misuse and to identify heavy or risky alcohol consumption in various studies on different study populations. A higher sensitivity of 34–65% (women/men) for EDAC test compared to 23–30% for γ-GT in a population of 1605 heavy drinkers or probands with risky alcohol consumption has been reported. The specificity is 89% (men) and 98% (women). Sensitivity and specificity over 80% each was reported in the identification of alcohol misuse in heavy male and female drinkers. Considering these results, EDAC test in primary care can establish itself as a suitable procedure for use in routine blood tests, its cost efficiency through freely optional lab values, as well as the availability of an electronic version with automatic statistical analysis from certain providers.

42.22 GGT-ALT Combination

Another combination of enzymes, GGT-ALT (alkaline phosphatase), can also be useful for clinical diagnostic validation of liver damage related to excessive and prolonged intake of alcohol. If the ratio of GGT-ALT exceeds the value 1.4, there is a probability of 78% that the liver impairment is due to alcoholism. This particular combination shown was not a biomarker when used for monitoring the treatment of alcoholics with disulfiram (Fig. 42.3).

Although the suspicion of alcohol abuse behind hepatotoxicity may be supported by several lines of clinical and biochemical data, the specific role of alcohol in many cases is difficult to distinguish in individuals who deny alcohol use. Clinical symptoms related to heavy drinking may originate from virtually any tissue. Unexpected abnormalities in liver enzymes or blood cell counts in health screening programs may also reveal alcohol abuse.

Subsequently, efforts should be focused on objective confirmation of alcohol use and to rule out other etiologies. Nonalcoholic fatty liver disease (NAFLD) is the most common nonalcoholic

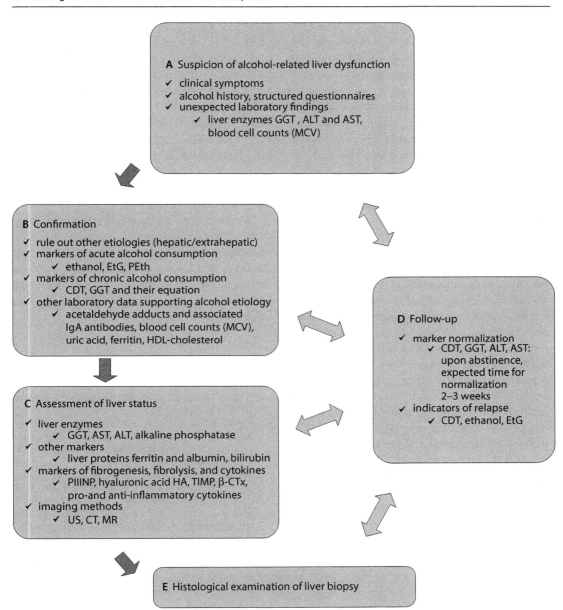

Fig. 42.3 Schematic representation of the clinical assessment of liver dysfunction in alcohol consumers. (Niemela and Alatalo [55])

etiology behind liver dysfunction, and the workup should consist of evaluating metabolic comorbidities with measurements of body mass index, waist circumference, and oral glucose tolerance. Specific tests are available to rule out viral hepatitis and several genetic diseases, such as hemochromatosis. In alcohol consumers, ethanol may be present even at the time of the clinic visit.

Measurements of ethanol metabolites or other laboratory parameters sensitive to ethanol may provide confirmatory data. Liver enzymes give information on the nature of the liver pathology. An isolated abnormality in GGT is usually reversible and related to increased oxidative stress burden. Increased ALT is commonly a result of fat deposition in the liver and can be reversible.

Elevated ferritin and albumin may occur in early phases of liver disease, whereas in patients with advanced alcoholic liver disease (ALD), the rates of albumin synthesis decrease and correlate with poor prognosis. ALD status is also associated with both the collagen and cytokine markers. Markers of collagen synthesis and degradation as well as pro- and anti-inflammatory cytokines may follow inverse kinetics, which may help to differentiate alcoholics at risk for cirrhosis. US (ultrasonography), CT, computed tomography, MRI, and proton magnetic resonance spectroscopy are commonly suggested. Follow-up of laboratory values is an integral part of the comprehensive assessment and treatment of patients with signs of liver dysfunction. If excess alcohol consumption (or obesity) is suspected, normalization during abstinence (or weight loss) is confirmatory. If initial GGT levels return to normal after abstention, and the patient is likely to have recovered from liver disease. Liver enzyme activities repeatedly above twice the upper reference limit are used as decision-making point for liver biopsy to rule out severe liver diseases and to distinguish patients needing the closest monitoring. Follow-up by markers of ethanol consumption, such as CDT, can be used to assess the degree of alcohol dependence and to detect relapses, which increase the probability of subsequent severe liver problems. Current clinical gold standard for the diagnosis and grading of hepatic disease is liver biopsy. It is, however, an invasive procedure with sampling variability and therefore is not suitable for screening or repeated measurements.

42.23 Conclusion

Biomarkers, as additions to self-reports, are important in the diagnosis and therapy of alcohol-related disorders. The traditional biomarkers have varying other limitations besides practicability and cost efficiency.

In summary, especially regarding traditional biomarkers, a combination of various lab parameters (e.g., CDT and γ-GT) allows sufficient inference on regular and even longer-term (days, weeks) alcohol consumption The diagnostic sensitivity of individual parameters, such as ASAT or ALAT, is low, and the specificity is moderately high, with the exception of CDT which shows moderate sensitivity and high specificity to differentiate between alcohol-dependent individuals and control persons. The strengths of these traditional markers lie in their practicability and, except for CDT, cost efficiency in clinical routine. Normalization of this marker occurs only after weeks or months of abstinence so that inference of current or short-term recent alcohol consumption can be made.

In comparison, direct ethanol metabolites are highly sensitive and specific, covering the complimentary period between consumption and detection, and are routinely used. Thus, they open new perspectives in the prevention, interdisciplinary cooperation, diagnosis, and therapy of alcohol-related disorders.

References

1. WHO | Global status report on alcohol and health 2014. WHO; 2016.
2. Barrio P, Reynolds J, García-Altés A, Gual A, Anderson P. Social costs of illegal drugs, alcohol and tobacco in the European Union: a systematic review. Drug Alcohol Rev. 2017;36:578.
3. Kohn R, Saxena S, Levav I, Saraceno B. The treatment gap in mental health care. Bull World Health Organ [Internet]. 2004 [cited 2014 Sept 17];82(11):858–66. Available from: http://www.pubmedcentral.nih.gov/articlerender.fcgi?artid=2623050&tool=pmcentrez&rendertype=abstract.
4. Mann K, Batra A, Hoch E, Karl Mann R, Gerhard Reymann P, Lorenz G, et al. Screening, diagnose und Behandlung alkoholbezogener Störungen [Internet]. [cited 2019 Jun 4]. Available from: https://www.awmf.org/uploads/tx_szleitlinien/076-0011_S3-Leitlinie_Alkohol_2016-02.pdf.
5. Mann K, Batra A, Fauth-Bühler M, Hoch E, and the Guideline Group. German guidelines on screening, diagnosis and treatment of alcohol use disorders. Eur Addict Res [Internet]. 2017 [cited 2019 Jun 4];23(1):45–60. Available from: http://www.ncbi.nlm.nih.gov/pubmed/28178695.
6. Conigrave KM, Degenhardt LJ, Whitfield JB, Saunders JB, Helander A, Tabakoff B, et al. CDT, GGT, and AST as markers of alcohol use: the WHO/ISBRA collaborative project. Alcohol Clin Exp Res [Internet]. 2002 [cited 2019 Feb 12];26(3):332–9. Available from: http://www.ncbi.nlm.nih.gov/pubmed/11923585.

7. Wurst FM, Wiesbeck GA, Metzger JW, Weinmann W. On sensitivity, specificity, and the influence of various parameters on ethyl glucuronide levels in urine--results from the WHO/ISBRA study. Alcohol Clin Exp Res [Internet]. 2004 [cited 2015 Sept 30];28(8):1220–8. Available from: http://www.ncbi.nlm.nih.gov/pubmed/15318121.

8. Høiseth G, Morini L, Polettini A, Christophersen A, Mørland J. Blood kinetics of ethyl glucuronide and ethyl sulphate in heavy drinkers during alcohol detoxification. Forensic Sci Int [Internet]. 2009 [cited 2019 Jan 31];188(1–3):52–6. Available from: http://www.ncbi.nlm.nih.gov/pubmed/19395207.

9. Thierauf A, Halter CC, Rana S, Auwaerter V, Wohlfarth A, Wurst FM, et al. Urine tested positive for ethyl glucuronide after trace amounts of ethanol. Addiction [Internet]. 2009 [cited 2019 Apr 23];104(12):2007–12. Available from: http://www.ncbi.nlm.nih.gov/pubmed/19922567.

10. Musshoff F, Albermann E, Madea B. Ethyl glucuronide and ethyl sulfate in urine after consumption of various beverages and foods--misleading results? Int J Legal Med [Internet]. 2010 [cited 2015 Apr 1];124(6):623–30. Available from: http://www.ncbi.nlm.nih.gov/pubmed/20838803.

11. Barrio P, Teixidor L, Rico N, Bruguera P, Ortega L, Bedini JL, et al. Urine ethyl glucuronide unraveling the reality of abstinence monitoring in a routine outpatient setting: a cross-sectional comparison with ethanol, self report and clinical judgment. Eur Addict Res [Internet]. 2016 [cited 2016 Jun 20];22(5):243–8. Available from: http://www.ncbi.nlm.nih.gov/pubmed/27220985.

12. Wurst FM, Haber PS, Wiesbeck G, Watson B, Wallace C, Whitfield JB, et al. Assessment of alcohol consumption among hepatitis C-positive people receiving opioid maintenance treatment using direct ethanol metabolites and self-report: a pilot study. Addict Biol [Internet]. 2008 [cited 2015 Apr 1];13(3–4):416–22. Available from: http://www.ncbi.nlm.nih.gov/pubmed/17711559.

13. Skipper GE, Weinmann W, Thierauf A, Schaefer P, Wiesbeck G, Allen JP, et al. Ethyl glucuronide: a biomarker to identify alcohol use by health professionals recovering from substance use disorders. Alcohol Alcohol [Internet]. Jan [cited 2015 Apr 1];39(5):445–9. Available from: http://www.ncbi.nlm.nih.gov/pubmed/15289206.

14. Dahl H, Hammarberg A, Franck J, Helander A. Urinary ethyl glucuronide and ethyl sulfate testing for recent drinking in alcohol-dependent outpatients treated with acamprosate or placebo. Alcohol Alcohol [Internet]. 2011 [cited 2015 Apr 1];46(5):553–7. Available from: http://www.ncbi.nlm.nih.gov/pubmed/21616946.

15. Erim Y, Böttcher M, Dahmen U, Beck O, Broelsch CE, Helander A. Urinary ethyl glucuronide testing detects alcohol consumption in alcoholic liver disease patients awaiting liver transplantation. Liver Transplant [Internet]. 2007 [cited 2019 Apr 23];13(5):757–61. Available from: http://www.ncbi.nlm.nih.gov/pubmed/17457868.

16. Graham AE, Beatty JR, Rosano TG, Sokol RJ, Ondersma SJ. Utility of Commercial Ethyl Glucuronide (EtG) and Ethyl Sulfate (EtS) testing for detection of lighter drinking among women of childbearing years. J Stud Alcohol Drugs [Internet]. 2017 [cited 2019 Apr 23];78(6):945–8. Available from: http://www.ncbi.nlm.nih.gov/pubmed/29087831.

17. Weinmann W, Schaefer P, Thierauf A, Schreiber A, Wurst FM. Confirmatory analysis of ethylglucuronide in urine by liquid-chromatography/electrospray ionization/tandem mass spectrometry according to forensic guidelines. J Am Soc Mass Spectrom [Internet]. 2004 [cited 2019 Jan 31];15(2):188–93. Available from: http://www.ncbi.nlm.nih.gov/pubmed/14766286.

18. Leickly E, Skalisky J, McPherson S, Orr MF, McDonell MG. High agreement between benchtop and point-of-care dipcard tests for ethyl glucuronide. Ther Drug Monit [Internet]. 2017 [cited 2019 Feb 1];39(4):461–2. Available from: http://insights.ovid.com/crossref?an=00007691-201708000-00025.

19. Barrio P, Teixidor L, Ortega L, Lligoña A, Rico N, Bedini JL, et al. Filling the gap between lab and clinical impact: an open randomized diagnostic trial comparing urinary ethylglucuronide and ethanol in alcohol dependent outpatients. Drug Alcohol Depend [Internet]. 2018 [cited 2018 Mar 27];183:225–30. Available from: http://www.ncbi.nlm.nih.gov/pubmed/29291550.

20. Jatlow PI, Agro A, Wu R, Nadim H, Toll BA, Ralevski E, et al. Ethyl glucuronide and ethyl sulfate assays in clinical trials, interpretation, and limitations: results of a dose ranging alcohol challenge study and 2 clinical trials. Alcohol Clin Exp Res [Internet]. 2014 [cited 2015 Apr 1];38(7):2056–65. Available from: http://www.ncbi.nlm.nih.gov/pubmed/24773137.

21. Yegles M, Labarthe A, Auwärter V, Hartwig S, Vater H, Wennig R, et al. Comparison of ethyl glucuronide and fatty acid ethyl ester concentrations in hair of alcoholics, social drinkers and teetotallers. Forensic Sci Int [Internet]. 2004 [cited 2019 Feb 4];145(2–3):167–73. Available from: http://linkinghub.elsevier.com/retrieve/pii/S0379073804002476.

22. Aradottir S, Asanovska G, Gjerss S, Hansson P, Alling C. Phosphatidylethanol (PEth) concentrations in blood are correlated to reported alcohol intake in alcohol-dependent patients. Alcohol Alcohol [Internet]. 2006 [cited 2019 Apr 23];41(4):431–7. Available from: http://www.ncbi.nlm.nih.gov/pubmed/16624837.

23. Schröck A, Thierauf-Emberger A, Schürch S, Weinmann W. Phosphatidylethanol (PEth) detected in blood for 3 to 12 days after single consumption of alcohol-a drinking study with 16 volunteers. Int J Legal Med [Internet]. 2017 [cited 2019 Feb 1];131(1):153–60. Available from: http://link.springer.com/10.1007/s00414-016-1445-x.

24. Faller A, Richter B, Kluge M, Koenig P, Seitz HK, Thierauf A, et al. LC-MS/MS analysis of phosphati-

dylethanol in dried blood spots versus conventional blood specimens. Anal Bioanal Chem [Internet]. 2011 [cited 2017 Feb 2];401(4):1163–6. Available from: http://www.ncbi.nlm.nih.gov/pubmed/21743983.

25. Wurst FM, Thon N, Aradottir S, Hartmann S, Wiesbeck GA, Lesch O, et al. Phosphatidylethanol: normalization during detoxification, gender aspects and correlation with other biomarkers and self-reports. Addict Biol [Internet]. 2010 [cited 2019 Feb 1];15(1):88–95. Available from: http://www.ncbi.nlm.nih.gov/pubmed/20002024.

26. Viel G, Boscolo-Berto R, Cecchetto G, Fais P, Nalesso A, Ferrara S. Phosphatidylethanol in blood as a marker of chronic alcohol use: a systematic review and meta-analysis. Int J Mol Sci [Internet]. 2012 [cited 2019 Jan 31];13(12):14788–812. Available from: http://www.ncbi.nlm.nih.gov/pubmed/23203094.

27. Stewart SH, Reuben A, Brzezinski WA, Koch DG, Basile J, Randall PK, et al. Preliminary evaluation of phosphatidylethanol and alcohol consumption in patients with liver disease and hypertension. Alcohol Alcohol [Internet]. 2009 [cited 2019 Feb 13];44(5):464–7. Available from: https://academic.oup.com/alcalc/article-lookup/doi/10.1093/alcalc/agp039.

28. Luginbühl M, Weinmann W, Butzke I, Pfeifer P. Monitoring of direct alcohol markers in alcohol use disorder patients during withdrawal treatment and successive rehabilitation. Drug Test Anal [Internet]. 2019 [cited 2019 May 16]; Available from: http://doi.wiley.com/10.1002/dta.2567.

29. Viel G, Boscolo-Berto R, Cecchetto G, Fais P, Nalesso A, Ferrara SD. Phosphatidylethanol in blood as a marker of chronic alcohol use: a systematic review and meta-analysis. Int J Mol Sci [Internet]. 2012 [cited 2019 Feb 1];13(11):14788–812. Available from: http://www.mdpi.com/1422-0067/13/11/14788.

30. Schröck A, Wurst FM, Thon N, Weinmann W. Assessing phosphatidylethanol (PEth) levels reflecting different drinking habits in comparison to the alcohol use disorders identification test – C (AUDIT-C). Drug Alcohol Depend [Internet]. 2017 [cited 2019 Jan 31];178:80–6. Available from: http://www.ncbi.nlm.nih.gov/pubmed/28645063.

31. Nguyen VL, Fitzpatrick M. Should phosphatidylethanol be currently analysed using whole blood, dried blood spots or both? Clin Chem Lab Med [Internet]. 2019 [cited 2019 May 16];57(5):617–22. Available from: http://www.degruyter.com/view/j/cclm.ahead-of-print/cclm-2018-0667/cclm-2018-0667.xml.

32. Faller A, Richter B, Kluge M, Koenig P, Seitz HK, Skopp G. Stability of phosphatidylethanol species in spiked and authentic whole blood and matching dried blood spots. Int J Legal Med [Internet]. 2013 [cited 2019 Feb 1];127(3):603–10. Available from: http://link.springer.com/10.1007/s00414-012-0799-y.

33. 2016 consensus for the use of alcohol markers in hair for assessment of both abstinence and chronic excessive alcohol consumption [Internet]. [cited 2019 May 13]. Available from: https://www.soht.org/images/pdf/Revision2016_Alcoholmarkers.pdf.

34. Suesse S, Pragst F, Mieczkowski T, Selavka CM, Elian A, Sachs H, et al. Practical experiences in application of hair fatty acid ethyl esters and ethyl glucuronide for detection of chronic alcohol abuse in forensic cases. Forensic Sci Int [Internet]. 2012 [cited 2019 Feb 4];218(1–3):82–91. Available from: https://linkinghub.elsevier.com/retrieve/pii/S0379073811004816.

35. Kummer N, Wille SMR, Di Fazio V, Ramírez Fernández MDM, Yegles M, Lambert WEE, et al. Impact of the grinding process on the quantification of ethyl glucuronide in hair using a validated UPLC-ESI-MS-MS method. J Anal Toxicol [Internet]. 2015 [cited 2019 Feb 4];39(1):17–23. Available from: http://academic.oup.com/jat/article/39/1/17/2797999/Impact-of-the-Grinding-Process-on-the.

36. Hartwig S, Auwärter V, Pragst F. Effect of hair care and hair cosmetics on the concentrations of fatty acid ethyl esters in hair as markers of chronically elevated alcohol consumption. Forensic Sci Int. 2003;131(2–3):90–7. https://doi.org/10.1016/s0379-0738(02)00412-7.

37. Thon N, Weinmann W, Yegles M, Preuss U, Wurst FM. Direct metabolites of ethanol as biological markers of alcohol use: basic aspects and applications. Fortschr Neurol Psychiatr [Internet]. 2013 [cited 2019 Apr 24];81(9):493–502. Available from: http://www.thieme-connect.de/DOI/DOI?10.1055/s-0033-1335586.

38. Topic A, Djukic M. Diagnostic characteristics and application of alcohol biomarkers. Clin Lab [Internet]. 2013 [cited 2019 May 13];59(3–4):233–45. Available from: http://www.ncbi.nlm.nih.gov/pubmed/23724610.

39. Puukka K, Hietala J, Koivisto H, Anttila P, Bloigu R, Niemelä O. Additive effects of moderate drinking and obesity on serum-glutamyl transferase activity 1–3 [Internet]. Am J Clin Nutr. 2006 [cited 2019 May 13]; 83. Available from: http://citeseerx.ist.psu.edu/viewdoc/download?doi=10.1.1.1033.9468&rep=rep1&type=pdf.

40. Neumann T, Spies C. Use of biomarkers for alcohol use disorders in clinical practice. Addiction [Internet]. 2003 [cited 2019 May 13];98 Suppl 2:81–91. Available from: http://www.ncbi.nlm.nih.gov/pubmed/14984245.

41. Koivisto H, Hietala J, Anttila P, Parkkila S, Niemelä O. Long-term ethanol consumption and macrocytosis: diagnostic and pathogenic implications. J Lab Clin Med [Internet]. 2006 [cited 2019 May 13];147(4):191–6. Available from: https://linkinghub.elsevier.com/retrieve/pii/S0022214305004142.

42. Allen JP, Marques P, Wurst F. Biomarkers of alcohol use: their nature, strengths, and limitations. Mil Med [Internet]. 2008 [cited 2019 May 13];173(8):v–viii. Available from: http://www.ncbi.nlm.nih.gov/pubmed/18751582.

43. Koch H, Meerkerk G-J, Zaat JOM, Ham MF, Scholten RJPM, Assendelft WJJ. Accuracy of carbohydrate-deficient transferrin in the detection of excessive alcohol consumption: a systematic review. Alcohol Alcohol [Internet]. 2004 [cited 2019 May 16];39(2):75–85. Available from: http://www.ncbi.nlm.nih.gov/pubmed/14998820.

44. Hackler R, Arndt T, Helwig-Rolig A, Kropf J, Steinmetz A, Schaefer JR. Investigation by isoelectric focusing of the initial carbohydrate-deficient transferrin (CDT) and non-CDT transferrin isoform fractionation step involved in determination of CDT by the ChronAlcoI.D. assay. Clin Chem [Internet]. 2000 [cited 2019 May 16];46(4):483–92. Available from: http://www.ncbi.nlm.nih.gov/pubmed/10759472.

45. Niemelä O. Biomarker-based approaches for assessing alcohol use disorders. Int J Environ Res Public Health [Internet]. 2016 [cited 2019 May 13];13(2):166. Available from: http://www.ncbi.nlm.nih.gov/pubmed/26828506.

46. Fleming MF, Anton RF, Spies CD. A review of genetic, biological, pharmacological, and clinical factors that affect carbohydrate-deficient transferrin levels. Alcohol Clin Exp Res [Internet]. 2004 [cited 2019 May 13];28(9):1347–55. Available from: http://www.ncbi.nlm.nih.gov/pubmed/15365305.

47. Bortolotti F, De Paoli G, Tagliaro F. Carbohydrate-deficient transferrin (CDT) as a marker of alcohol abuse: a critical review of the literature 2001–2005. J Chromatogr B [Internet]. 2006 [cited 2019 May 13];841(1–2):96–109. Available from: http://www.ncbi.nlm.nih.gov/pubmed/16725384.

48. Lucas DL, Brown RA, Wassef M, Giles TD. Alcohol and the cardiovascular system. J Am Coll Cardiol [Internet]. 2005 [cited 2019 May 16];45(12):1916–

24. Available from: http://www.ncbi.nlm.nih.gov/pubmed/15963387.

49. Moore RD, Pearson TA. Moderate alcohol consumption and coronary artery disease. A review. Medicine (Baltimore) [Internet]. 1986 [cited 2019 May 16];65(4):242–67. Available from: http://www.ncbi.nlm.nih.gov/pubmed/3523113.

50. Niemelä O. Biomarkers in alcoholism. Clin Chim Acta. 2007;377(1–2):39–49.

51. Gilg T. Rechtsmedizinische Aspekte von Alkohol und Alkoholismus. In: Singer MV, Teyssen S (Eds.) Alkohol und Alkoholfolgekrankheiten. Springer Berlin, Heidelberg, 1995. pp. 526–51.

52. Sillanaukee P, Strid N, Allen JP, Litten RZ. Possible reasons why heavy drinking increases carbohydrate-deficient transferrin. Alcohol Clin Exp Res. 2001;25(1):34–40.

53. Brinkmann B, Köhler H, Banaschak S, Berg A, Eikelmann B, West A, et al. ROC analysis of alcoholism markers--100% specificity. Int J Legal Med [Internet]. 2000 [cited 2019 May 13];113(5):293–9. Available from: http://www.ncbi.nlm.nih.gov/pubmed/11009066.

54. Harasymiw J, Seaberg J, Bean P. Detection of alcohol misuse using a routine test panel: the early detection of alcohol consumption (EDAC) test. Alcohol Alcohol [Internet]. 2004 [cited 2019 May 16];39(4):329–35. Available from: https://academic.oup.com/alcalc/article-lookup/doi/10.1093/alcalc/agh061.

55. Niemelä O, Alatalo P. Biomarkers of alcohol consumption and related liver disease. Scand J Clin Lab Invest [Internet]. 2010 [cited 2019 May 16];70(5):305–12. Available from: http://www.ncbi.nlm.nih.gov/pubmed/20470213.

Clinical Screening for Illegal Drug Use, Prescription Drug Misuse and Tobacco Use

43

Sawitri Assanangkornchai and J. Guy Edwards

Contents

Abstract

Screening aims at detecting substance use (ideally at an early stage) with a view of providing subsequent treatment if required. It is most productively employed in populations in whom there is a high prevalence of use, such as general and emergency medical patients and those attending clinics for pain or sexually transmitted disorders. It is of less value in well-staffed facilities that already routinely inquire about substance use during comprehensive clinical assessments. Screening may also be helpful in people who have come into conflict with the law.

Numerous screening instruments have been designed, but few have satisfactory psychometric properties, and none has been

S. Assanangkornchai (✉)
Epidemiology Unit, Faculty of Medicine,
Prince of Songkla University, Songkhla, Thailand
e-mail: savitree.a@psu.ac.th

J. G. Edwards
Formerly of Southampton University Hospitals,
Southampton, UK

© Springer Nature Switzerland AG 2021
N. el-Guebaly et al. (eds.), *Textbook of Addiction Treatment*,
https://doi.org/10.1007/978-3-030-36391-8_43

shown to produce a better long-term outcome in the real world of clinical psychiatry than asking brief questions about substance use followed by referral for specialist treatment and rehabilitation when required.

Examples of the more widely used instruments are the Alcohol, Smoking and Substance Involvement Screening Test (ASSIST), CAGE-AID (mnemonic for items Cut down, Annoyed, Guilty, Eye-opener, -Adapted to Include Drugs), Drug Abuse Screening Test, and Fagerström Test for Nicotine Dependence. The choice of an instrument should depend on its psychometric properties, the population being screened, availability of staff to use it properly, and practicality of introducing it into the facility.

Ethical aspects of the use of the instruments are important. Outside purely clinical or sociological research screening is likely to have limited value unless follow-on treatment is available and offered to the substance misuser, and he/she is encouraged to accept it and adhere to it. The best test of the real value of screening will be a clear demonstration that it prevents longer-term medical and psychosocial consequences of substance misuse.

43.1   Introduction

Screening for substance misuse and use disorders aims at helping to identify people who have suffered the consequences of using one or more substances or are at risk of future harm if they continue to use the substance(s). Ideally this should be at an early stage and should be followed by treatment if indicated. Included among the WHO's recommended indications for screening in general are the seriousness of the effect the medical condition has on the health and well-being of the individual and the community and the availability of a suitable, reasonably priced screening test and effective treatment for patients screened positive. It is accepted that early recognition of the disorder followed by intervention

leads to a more favorable outcome. Based on these indications, screening for misuse of psychoactive drugs is clearly indicated [5].

Screening instruments for drug misuse have been designed for use in the community and healthcare facilities and to help in medicolegal assessments. Cross-sectional and longitudinal screening for drug use is of value in research into medical treatment and academic sociological research.

43.2   Screening in Different Settings

43.2.1 Healthcare Facilities

Screening may be undertaken in primary care; general and emergency medical, psychiatric, and other specialized facilities (e.g., HIV/AIDS clinics or obstetric units); and community hostels. Some instruments are self-administered, whereas others are administered by staff of various disciplines. Studies have shown benefits of screening for drug use in healthcare settings using the Screening, Brief Interventions, Referral for Treatment (SBIRT). This is employed in an integrated, public health approach to the management of people at risk of adverse consequences of alcohol and other drug use and probable drug use disorders (DUD) [6]. Various factors militate against the implementation of SBIRT, the main ones being underfunding, understaffing, and competing priorities.

43.2.1.1   Primary Care
Primary care deals with a wide range of people and an equally wide range of lifestyles and disorders, including substance use disorders. Its workers are usually seen as trustworthy, and it provides an excellent opportunity for screening for drug misuse as a routine part of healthcare. Patients with problems related to drug misuse are likely to have frequent consultations. Screening in primary care may identify nondependent individuals who use drugs in a harmful way and respond well to intervention. Drug misuse may worsen concomitant health problems, so screening pro-

vides an opportunity to educate patients about this risk. We therefore endorse WHO recommendations on screening in general practice, with consideration given to the use of the Alcohol, Smoking, Substance Involvement Screening Test (ASSIST) or one of its modified versions [59].

However, the workload in primary care is usually stretched to capacity, so screening may only be carried out with great difficulty (or not at all) without extra resources. An example of this is seen in the UK where the current government underfunds the National Health Service (NHS) to such a degree that clinics typically have to ration time to only 10 minutes per symptom or problem per appointment. And that harsh rationing even applies to elderly patients with multiple pathologies.

If that is the situation in the fifth richest country in the world, it is not difficult to imagine the situation in the most deprived, poorest countries where even 10 minutes might be considered a luxury.

43.2.1.2   Secondary Care

General Medicine

There is a high prevalence of substance use among general medical patients. Hospitals are therefore important places in which to screen patients, hoping that any substance misusers identified will accept treatment. In hospitals there is more time for screening than in most other medical settings and also more time to educate the patient about the relationship between substances misused and his/her medical condition [41].

Emergency Medicine

Drug misusers often attend accident and emergency (A&E) departments with substance-related medical or surgical problems, notably toxic or withdrawal states, trauma due to accidents, deliberate self-injury, or injury caused by others. Thus, emergency departments too are appropriate facilities to screen, especially for the benefit of people who have less access to alternative healthcare. Screening instruments that rapidly identify patients who require further diagnostic evalua-

tion and/or brief intervention are important. A systematic review identified 11 instruments that have been used in youngsters under 21 attending A&E and recommended asking just one question to detect cannabis use disorder – "In the past year, how often have you used cannabis?" – with the response categories, "Once or less" or "Two or more times" (sensitivity, 0.96; specificity, 0.86) [43].

To illustrate the problems faced by A&E departments, let us again consider the situation of the British NHS. Just as the government's gross underfunding has an adverse effect on patient care in other key services like general practice, so it affects overworked A&E departments. As a result, severely ill patients often have to wait for hours in ambulances and/or lay on trollies in corridors waiting to be assessed, and some patients needing admission may have a further wait for an inpatient bed to be found for them. So it is not difficult to understand why A&E staff, however much they would like to help in screening for drugs, may simply not have time to do so.

Services for Youngsters

Early to late adolescence is a critical risk period for starting to use substances, which peaks between the ages of 18 and 25 [58]. The American Academy of Pediatrics [1] therefore recommends screening of every pediatric patient aged 12 or over, whether or not they are reported as having used drugs.

The screening can be undertaken in healthcare facilities, schools, child welfare facilities, and the juvenile justice system. It should be carried out with a valid, sensitive instrument, and, when the results suggest there is cause for concern, youngster should be referred for a comprehensive clinical assessment. At all stages of the process, care should be taken to ensure that no vulnerable young person is unjustifiably labeled as a drug misuser.

The easy availability of cannabis, coupled with the erroneous idea that it rarely causes harm, makes this drug one of the most common substances initiated in adolescence [58]. So screening adolescents for its use is particularly important.

Validated screening tools available for substance use disorder (SUD) among adolescents aged 12–17 in primary care are the Brief Screener for Alcohol, Tobacco and other Drugs (BSTAD) and Screening to Brief Intervention (S2BI) [42].

Services for the Elderly

During recent years, there has been mounting concern over substance misuse in the elderly. There are many explanations for this. They include the 1946–1964 baby boom effect, with children born during this time reaching adolescence at a time of escalating substance use worldwide, and people then continuing to misuse substances throughout midlife until old age. During this period, there was also an increase in life expectancy. Increasing age was accompanied by multiple pathology, increased misuse of over-the-counter and illegal drugs, and increased prescription of drugs with addiction potential, notably benzodiazepines and opioids [58].

In addition to these trends, there has been a relaxation of enforcement of laws on cannabis possession (with some countries and states legalizing it) and latterly a relaxation of legislation of the use of cannabis for therapeutic purposes.

For these reasons, older adults should be sensitively but routinely screened for alcohol and other drug use, despite difficulties arising from similarities between the symptoms of drug misuse and those of some of the common illnesses of later life and lack of a specific screening instrument for the elderly.

Pain Clinics

Pain can be associated with drug misuse in several ways: there may be an underlying condition contributing to both the severity of the pain and the drug misuse (e.g., a depressive disorder); patients may become dependent on their prescribed analgesics (therapeutic dependence); and substance misusers with pain of organic origin, or with exaggerated or simulated pain, may try to manipulate their doctors into prescribing more addictive substances than are clinically needed – for themselves and/or to give or sell to other substance misusers. Whatever the relationship, screening patients attending pain clinics for the

inappropriate use of prescribed or illegal drugs is important. During recent years, there has been a dramatic increase in the use of opioids for treating pain and a corresponding escalation in the number of deaths from overdoses of opioids at great human and economic cost [58].

Attempts to understand and tackle these increases are hampered by difficulty in diagnosing dependence in patients prescribed opioids [24]. If it is so difficult to make a valid diagnosis, it is not surprising that it is also difficult to create a valid screening instrument for opioid dependence, and we have to place much reliance on the clinical assessment.

The US National Institute of Drug Abuse (NIDA) recommends supplementing this by screening patients for opioid misuse on their initial clinic visit and prior to prescribing any opioids for pain, using the Opioid Risk Tool (ORT) [42, 60].

Psychiatric Units

There is evidence to suggest that the prevalence of tobacco and other substance misuse in patients with some disorders is higher than in others, but substance misuse and psychiatric comorbidity in general occurs so often that it is essential that a history of misuse is taken routinely in all psychiatric patients. In fact, failure to do so in some patients can be a serious omission, sometimes even bordering on negligence. Tiet et al. [56] in their review concluded that there are no currently available instruments that have particular advantages in psychiatric patients, while the lengthier, more complicated ones can be confusing for those with severe illnesses – particularly when administered in addition to a thorough psychiatric assessment.

Antenatal Care

Universal screening of pregnant women for substance misuse has been recommended [62]. It should be performed as early as possible in pregnancy and at every subsequent antenatal visit so that clinicians are aware of their patient's substance use, can make better informed decisions about drug treatment and prenatal care, and can minimize the time the fetus is exposed to the drug(s).

Screening during pregnancy is especially important in those with a previous history of drug misuse, prenatal and/or birth complications, delays in accessing prenatal care, or frequently missing prenatal appointments. Some screening instruments have been specifically designed for pregnant women, e.g., 4P's Plus [18], the Substance Use Risk Profile-Pregnancy (SURP-P) scale [63], and Wayne Indirect Drug Use Screener (WIDUS) [45].

43.2.2 Medicolegal Practice

43.2.2.1 Criminal Justice System

There is a high prevalence of substance misuse also in people who come into conflict with the law, especially those whose crimes have been carried out to acquire money for drugs. So here too there is fertile ground for screening – by personnel within the criminal justice system or by colleagues working in associated medical services, like prison medical officers or staff working in court diversion schemes. An aim of screening, in addition to providing treatment for those in immediate need, is to help interrupt the cycle of addiction and drug-related crime, with benefits to society as well as to the drug misuser.

Although drug-using offenders are mostly abstinent while in custody or prison, when released many resume their previous patterns of drug and alcohol use, placing them at risk of rearrest and increased health problems, including HIV. Thus, there is need for intervention to help reduce risky behaviors and encourage treatment.

During detention, people are at a "teachable moment" for screening and intervention. They have just been arrested and may want to avoid further conflict with the law. Initially, they may be distressed or simply just want "something to do" by way of distraction. That in itself does not mean the subject is well motivated for treatment, but in this teachable moment better motivation could follow [47].

Screening should begin with simple questions regarding substance misuse asked by the arresting police officer. Following this, there are several other opportunities for screening as the accused moves through the justice system: in the police station and prison and during pretrial investigations, meetings between prosecuting and defense council, and social assessments conducted by probation officers. The UNCOPE is a valid, brief six-item screen used for identifying substance use disorders among prisoners [48].

43.3 Some General Considerations

43.3.1 Ethics

There are many ethical as well as legal and social issues to be considered when deciding whether and how to screen patients. Screening is generally accepted as being harmless so long as the patient is fully informed of its purpose, permission is given, and any appropriate follow-up treatment required is provided.

Even when using a simple screening instrument, it is important that we remain aware of the concerns and sensitivities of our patients/clients, concerns such as embarrassment at succumbing to their "weakness" in taking drugs, believing there is no point in screening as there is no "cure" for their "addiction," or fear of the legal and social consequences of drug use, including stigmatization. As in all good medical practice, we should also ensure that honesty and transparency are central to our dealings with patients.

We can go some way toward allaying patient's anxieties by emphasizing that the decision to reveal information in response to questions asked by an instrument is theirs and theirs alone and assuring them that anything revealed will be treated in strict confidence and not disclosed to others without their permission. Doing this is particularly important in medicolegal work (whether in civil or criminal cases), especially when dealing with delinquent youngsters, to help gain their trust, confidence, and cooperation.

It should also be made clear to the patient that screening instruments do not possess "magical" properties; they simply comprise a set of questions that are asked regularly in a clinical assessment and contain no questions that attempt to "catch them out" – which we have no right to ask. Any attempt to do so would be dishonest and, like failing to observe the fundamental principles of confidentiality, a breach of professional ethics.

43.3.2 Psychometric Properties

It is important to confirm that all instruments were properly constructed to begin with, properly evaluated subsequently, and then properly administered to the right person or population in the right way. Even when these principles have been conscientiously adhered to, there remains the glaring uncertainty as to whether the instrument measures what it sets out to measure. And, of course, what a person says he does is not necessarily the same as what he actually does.

43.3.3 Main Aims of Screening

While it is of interest academically to elicit data on all substance use, as clinicians we are less interested in people who occasionally take substances "recreationally," especially if conforming with the behavior of their peers or take them only in certain situations, like clubs or raves. Similarly, we are less interested in those who take substances for clearly defined, short periods, as during their university days, or for specific purposes like attempting to increase their sexual excitement.

We are prepared to advise all people of the dangers of such sporadic or short periods of drug-taking, but our main concern is for those who take drugs for longer periods. This is especially the case when they are dependent on one or more substance, have already experienced adverse medical or psychosocial consequences, or are exposed to the risk of these problems in the future.

Several familiar words and terms are used in the field of substance use, and there are debates on what is normal as opposed to abnormal use; differences between use, misuse, and abuse; when psychological and/or physical dependence

begins; the difference between these conditions; and the question, "What is a disorder?" These are of theoretical and practical interest but matter less at the screening stage than later in assessment. The main aim at this stage is to identify people who have or are at risk of substance-related problems and may therefore benefit from advice and/or intervention regardless of what provisional labels are applied to them.

Having done the screening, the clinician, aided by the data elicited by the screening instrument, may then complete the assessment, sharpen up on the diagnosis, and provide the appropriate intervention.

43.4 Screening Instruments for Substance Use

There are available screening instruments for single or multiple substance use, problems caused by the substances, and comorbidity (Table 43.1). Some of these have been created for particular patient groups. We summarize below their main characteristics and uses of the most commonly used instruments.

43.4.1 Instruments Inquiring about the Use of One or More Drugs

ASSIST The ASSIST has high construct and concurrent validity [28] and is currently the most extensively studied and widely used instrument. It was developed by a group of WHO researchers to help detect substance use and related problems in primary and general medical care and assess the level of risk for each substance identified. It seeks information on the use of all types of psychoactive substances, including tobacco, alcohol, cannabis, cocaine, amphetamine-type stimulants, sedatives, hallucinogens, inhalants, and opioids. It asks if any of these have ever been used and, if so, the frequency of use during the past 3 months; if the respondents have had a strong desire or urge to use the substance; the frequency of any problems they have had; if the substance has interfered with their responsibilities; if anyone

Table 43.1 Screening instruments for drug use and drug use disorders

(a) Instruments inquiring about one or more drugs

Instrument	Full name	Reference	Population studied	Time frame	No. of items	Administered by	Approx. time required	Responses/scores
ASSIST	Alcohol, smoking and substance involvement screening test	[61]	Adults	Lifetime Past 3 months	8 items	Clinician interviewed, computer administered, self-administered	10 min for administration, 5 min for scoring	0–3: low risk – no intervention (0–10 for alcohol) 4–26: moderate risk – brief intervention (11–26 for alcohol) 27+: high risk – more intensive intervention
DHQ PDHQ	Drug history questionnaire Psychoactive drug history questionnaire	[54]	Adults	Lifetime Past 6 months	5 items	Self-administered	5–10 min	No specific cutoff
S2BI	Screening to brief intervention	[36]	Adolescents 12–17 years	Past 12 months	8 items	Computerized self-administered	2 min	Answer "use" to each drug type
BSTAD	Brief screener for alcohol, tobacco, and other drugs	[31]	Adolescents 12–17 years	Past 12 months	3 + 2 items	Computerized self-administered	2 min	Answer "use" to individual drug and then continue to more drugs
SUBS	Substance use brief screen	[39]	Adult primary care patients	Past 12 months	4 items	Computerized self-administered	5–10 min	Answer "use 1–2 days in the past 12 months" to individual drug
TAPS	Tobacco, alcohol, prescription medication, and other substance use	[38, 40]	Adult primary care patients	Past 12 months and 3 months	4 + 25 items	Computerized self-administered and clinician interviewed	5–10 min	TAPS-1: Positive = use that substance and then continue to TABS-2 items specific to that substance class

(continued)

Table 43.1 (continued)

Instrument	Full name	Reference	Population studied	Time frame	No. of items	Administered by	Approx. time required	Responses/scores
CAGE-AID	Cut down, annoyed, guilty, eye-opener-adapted to include drugs	[13]	Adolescent; patients with comorbidity; adults	Lifetime	4 items	Self-administered	5 min	Range: 0–4 Cutoff score 1 or more for drug dependence
CRAFFT RAFFT	Car, relax, alone, forget, friends, trouble	[32]	Adolescents American Indian/native Alaskans	Lifetime past year	6 items	Clinician-interviewed, self-administered, computerized	5 min	Range: 0–6 Cutoff score of >2 for risky use
DAST	Drug abuse screening test. Adolescent version (DAST-A) available	[53]	Adults College students; pregnant women	Lifetime	10, 20, 28 items	Self-administered	5–10 min	Range: 0–10, 20, 28 DAST-28: Cutoff 6 DAST-20: Cutoff 6 DAST-10: Cutoff 2
DAP quick screen DAP-4	Drug and alcohol problem quick screen	[51]	Adolescents	Lifetime	30 items and 4 items	Self-administered	<10 minutes	Range: 0–30 Score of >6 considered high risk for "red flag" behaviors
DUDIT	Drug use disorder identification test	[10]	Adults	Lifetime past year	11 items	Self-administered	5–10 min	Range: 0–44 Cutoff score of 25 suggestive of substance dependence Cutoff score of 8 or less severe drug abuse
SACS	Substances and choice scale	[19]	Adolescents	Past month	10 items	Self-administered	5–10 min	Each item scores 0, 1, 2 for not true, somewhat true, certainly true Range:0–20 Cutoff: 2

SSI-SA	[17]	Simple screening instrument for substance abuse	Adults; law-enforced treatment programs for patients with comorbidity; adolescent medical patients	Lifetime	16 items	Clinician- interviewed, Self-administered	10 min	0–1: No/low risk 2–3: Minimal risk 4+: Moderate/high risk
TICS	[12]	Two item conjoint screen for alcohol and other drug problems	Adults	Past year	2 items	Self-administered	<5 min	Cutoff: 1
UNICOPE	[27]	Use, neglected, cut down, objection, preoccupied, emotional discomfort	Adults	Lifetime Past year	6 items	Interviewer administered	5–10 min	Cutoff: 2
(b) Instruments specific to one drug								
CAST	[35]	Cannabis abuse screening test	Adolescents	Lifetime	6 items	Self-administered	< 5 min	Range: 0–6 Score > 4: Problematic cannabis use
CUDIT CUDIT-R	[2]	Cannabis use disorders identification test	Adults; adolescents	Past 6 months Current	10 items 5-point Likert scale	Self-administered	5–10 min	Range: 0–40 Cutoff:8
CUPIT	[8]	Cannabis use problems identification test	Adolescents; adults	Lifetime Past 12 months	16 items	Self- administered	5 min	Range: 0–82 Cutoff:12
MSI	[3]	Marijuana screening inventory	Adults	Lifetime Past year	31 items	Self- administered	5–10 min	Range: 0–31 Cutoff:3

(continued)

Table 43.1 (continued)

Instrument	Full name	Reference	Population studied	Time frame	No. of items	Administered by	Approx. time required	Responses/scores
PUM	Problematic use of marijuana	[44]	General adult population	Lifetime	8 items	Self- administered		Range: 0–8 Cutoff:2
CDS-12 CDS-5	Cigarette dependence scale	[23]	Adults adolescents	Lifetime Current	12 & 5 items	Self- administered	10 min	Range: CDS-12: 12–60; CDS-5: 5–25
FTND FTQ m-FTND	Fagerstrom test for nicotine dependence	[26]	Adults adolescents college students	Lifetime	6 items	Clinician-interviewed; self-administered	<5 min	Range: 0–2 cutoff: 6
TDS	Tobacco dependence screener	[30]	Adults; smokers	Lifetime	10 items	Self- administered	5 min	Range: 0–10 Cutoff:
COMM	Current opioid misuse measure (for opioid medication misuse)	[15]	Adult patients with chronic non-cancer pain	Current past 30 days	17 items	Self- administered	5–10 min	Cutoff: 9
ORT	Opioid risk tool	[60]	Adult patients prescribed opioids for chronic pain	Lifetime	5 items	Patient-completed (PC-ORT) clinician-completed (CC-ORT)	5 min	Range: 0–16 Cutoff: 0–3 low risk, 4–7 moderate risk > 8 high risk
SOAPP	Screener and opioid assessment for patients with pain	[14]	Adult patients taking opioids for chronic pain	Lifetime	5, 14, or 24 items	Self-administered	5–10 min	Cutoff: >7

PDUQ	Prescription drug use questionnaire, -patient version	[21, 22]	Patients with chronic non-malignant pain and on opioid therapy	Current	42 & 31 items	Clinician-interviewed (PDUQ), self-administered (PDUQp)	20 min	Cutoff: 10

(c) Instruments inquiring about multiple problems, including dual diagnosis

CODSI-MD CODSI-SMD	Co-occurring disorder screening instrument	[50]	Offenders	Past 12 months	6-item version (CODSI-MD) screens for any mental disorder 3-item version (CODSI-SMD) screens for severe mental disorder	Self-administered	5–10 min	CODSI-MD Range:0–6 Cutoff: >3 CODSI-SMD Range: 0–3 Cutoff: >2
DUSI[a]	Drug use screening inventory-revised	[55]	Adults; adolescents	Current status	159 items	Self-administered computer-based available	20–40 min	Range: 0–100% No cutoff specified in documents
PL	DrugCheck problem list	[29]	Adolescents, adults, co-occurring clients	Past 3 months	12 item	Clinician-interviewed	5–10 min	Range:0–12 Cutoff: >2
POSIT	Problem-oriented screening instrument for teenagers	[16]	Adolescents	Lifetime	139 items, 10 problem areas	Self-administered	20–30 min	Cutoff scores indicating low, medium, or high risk for each of the ten problem areas

[a]Fee required for use; other instruments free in public domain

has expressed concern about their substance use; if they have tried to decrease or discontinue use; and if they have ever used any substance by injection. Linked with brief intervention, the ASSIST can help a person explore options for addressing their substance use [59].

There are modified forms of the ASSIST – the NM-ASSIST (NIDA-modified ASSIST) [42]; ASSIST-Lite (ultrarapid ASSIST) [4]; ASSIST-Y for use in children and adolescents aged 10–17 years [59]; "ASSIST on ICE," which is the instructional video and manual of the ASSIST and brief intervention specific for methamphetamine use [25]; and the ASSIST Checkup, which is a free downloadable app for use on a mobile device and gives instant feedback and tips on how to cut back or stop substance use. It also provides information on where to seek help. Electronic versions of the ASSIST (eASSIST) and ASSIST-Lite (eASSIST-Lite) are also available. The ASSIST and its modified forms have been translated into several languages, including Arabic, Chinese, French, German, Spanish, and Thai [59].

In addition to the clinician interview version, self-report, paper-based [7], and computer-based (ASSISTc) [20] formats of the ASSIST were developed for use in university students and a self-administered audio computer-assisted, self-interview (ACASI-ASSIST) format for primary care [38, 40]. Both formats are comparable to the clinician interview format but have the apparent advantages of not requiring an interviewer, facilitating screening and assessment in college students and busy healthcare settings, and reducing costs.

Substance Use Brief Screen & Tobacco, Alcohol, Prescription medication and other Substance use (SUBS & TAPS) Based on the NM-ASSIST, the Substance Use Brief Screen (SUBS), a four-item computerized, self-administered screening instrument [39], and the Tobacco, Alcohol, Prescription medication, and other Substance use (TAPS) tool, a two-step screening and brief assessment instrument, were developed [38, 40]. They both seek information on the frequency of use of tobacco,

four or more alcoholic drinks per day, illicit drugs including cannabis, and the inappropriate use of prescription drugs during the past 12 months. The TAPS consists of two parts: a four-item screen (TAPS-1) and a substance-specific assessment of risk tool (TAPS-2) for individuals who screen positive on TAPS-1. Both instruments performed well in primary care, and they have the advantages of being brief and self-administered, using a tablet computer or online tool [52].

Examples of instruments that inquire about any drug use and their adverse effects are CAGE-AID [13] and CRAFFT/RAFFT [32]. The CAGE Adapted to Include Drugs (*CAGE-AID*) is a modification of CAGE – a mnemonic based on Cut down, Annoyed, Guilty, Eye-opener – which has been used in screening for alcohol misuse since the mid-1970s [37].

CRAFFT is a mnemonic, based on its individual items: Car, Relax, Alone, Forget, Friends, Trouble [32]. It is the most well-studied instrument for screening for alcohol and drug use and related problems in adolescents and adults. Its six items are preceded by three preliminary questions that ask about the use of alcohol, cannabis, and other drugs. It asks about specific lifetime events and behaviors, irrespective of when they occurred.

The instrument was found to be suitable for distinguishing between alcohol and other substance use, problem use, abuse, and dependence. Although the CRAFFT was designed for clinical use, it is also suitable for large-scale surveys in other settings and provides a measure of severity but not frequency of use in adolescents [11].

Drug Abuse Screening Test (DAST) The DAST-28 is a research instrument used to screen and assess the effectiveness of treatment [53]. It provides a measure of the severity of drug-related and other problems experienced during the respondent's lifetime. It has been found most useful in people who do not seek treatment. The DAST cannot distinguish between active or inactive drug use or abstinence and low-risk use, abuse, or dependence.

Alternative versions of the DAST-28 have been developed – the DAST-20, DAST-10, and DAST-A (for adolescents). DAST has moderate to high reliability and validity, depending on the group studied [64]. Most recently, a two-item brief DAST (DAST-2) has been developed. The questions asked are "How many days in the past 12 months have you felt bad or guilty about your drug use?" and "How many days in the past 12 months have you used drugs other than those required for medical reasons?" A response of 1 or more days to each question was considered to meet the DAST criteria for drug use disorder (DUD) and negative consequences of drug use [57].

Screening questionnaires of this type are not only quick to administer, but they also have the advantage that people who use multiple substances may be more likely to respond positively to a question about drugs in general than to questions about specific drugs. However, they have some disadvantages. For example, they may not detect specific substances, and someone who uses only alcohol may not respond positively to a question that refers to "drugs."

43.4.2 Instruments that Ask about the Use of Single Drugs

Apart from instruments used to screen for alcohol, there are also instruments that screen for individual drugs.

43.4.2.1 Cannabis

Short instruments designed specifically for cannabis screening that have satisfactory psychometric properties and have been used in various populations include the Cannabis Abuse Screening Test (CAST) [35], Cannabis Use Disorders Identification Test (CUDIT) [2], and Problematic Use of Marijuana (PUM) [46].

43.4.2.2 Opioids

Because of the widespread increase in prescription of opioids, several instruments have been developed to detect prescription opioid misuse in various clinical settings, including A&E departments, pain clinics, and pharmacies. Examples of these include the Prescription Drug Use Questionnaire (PDUQ) [21], Opioid Risk Tool (ORT) [60], and Current Opioid Misuse Measure (COMM) [15].

The Opioid Risk Tool (ORT) is a brief, self-report, screening tool designed for use in adults in primary care to assess the risk of opioid abuse among individuals prescribed these drugs for chronic pain. It can be administered and scored in less than 1 minute and has been validated in men and women treated for pain [60].

Prescription Drug Use Questionnaire (PDUQ)

The 42-item Prescription Drug Use Questionnaire (PDUQ), clinician interview version [21], and its 31-item self-report patient version (PDUQp) [22] have been validated to detect "problematic opioid medication use" in patients with chronic pain. It has domains of pain, opioid use patterns, social/family factors, and substance use history and can be self-administered in a busy clinical setting. The PDUQp has been shown to perform well in screening for prescription opioid misuse and use disorder among older adults in emergency setting [9].

43.4.2.3 Nicotine

The Fagerström Test for Nicotine (or Cigarette) Dependence (FTND) is a revision of the Fagerström Tolerance Questionnaire (FTQ) [26] and is the instrument most widely used to screen for nicotine use. The FTND was designed to provide an ordinal measure of nicotine dependence. It contains six items that seek information on the number of cigarettes smoked, compulsion to smoke, and dependence. It provides a rating of severity that can be used to help plan treatment and assess the prognosis. Its brevity and ease of scoring make it an efficient way of obtaining clinically meaningful information. It can be incorporated into general health and lifestyle screening questionnaires in clinical and nonclinical settings.

A modified version of the scale (modified Fagerström Tolerance Questionnaire, mFTQ) has been adapted for use in adolescents, which shows acceptable internal consistency and validity across countries [49].

Other available instruments are the Tobacco Dependence Screener (TDS) [30] and Cigarette Dependence Scale (CDS) [23].

43.4.3 Instruments that Inquire about Multiple Drug-Related Problems and Comorbidity

These instruments help identify drug-related problems in mental and physical health, relationships, and adjustment at school or work. They may locate areas in need of further assessment and suggest services required. Examples include the Drug Use Screening Inventory-Revised (DUSI-R) [55], Problem-Oriented Screening Instrument for Teenagers (POSIT) [16], Co-occurring Disorder Screening Instrument (CODSI) [50], and DrugCheck Problem List (PL) [29].

Problem-Oriented Screening Instrument for Teenagers (POSIT) The POSIT is a self-administered 139-item questionnaire, with fixed "yes/no" responses, designed for use in adolescents aged 12 to 19 [16]. It identifies problems in ten domains that require further assessment and might need intervention – substance use/abuse, mental and physical health, family and peer relations, vocation, and special education. The instrument can be used by school personnel, juvenile and family court personnel, medical and mental healthcare staff, and staff working in substance use disorder treatment programs. The POSIT has been found to have strong internal consistency in several of its subscales and good test-retest reliability and overall validity ([33], [34]).

43.5 Conclusion

Because of the high and increasing prevalence of substance use disorders and its consequences, screening for substance use is important in medical, psychiatric, and forensic services. There is a higher prevalence of use in some groups than others, such as those attending A&E departments and pain clinics and those who come into conflict with the law.

Numerous screening instruments have been designed and validated. Factors that determine the choice of an instrument are not only its psychometric properties but also the practicality of employing it. The enormous pressures of working in a busy clinical unit often preclude screening without special assistance.

Screening is only the first step on a very long journey toward providing a successful treatment and rehabilitation outcome. It is of limited value without the provision of treatment opportunities and encouraging substance users to accept and then adhere to any treatment offered. Finally, it is important to determine the success rate of screening in terms of discontinuation or at least decreased use of substances compared with standard practice and to assess what effect it has in reducing complications.

References

1. Committee on Substance Abuse, Levy SJ, Kokotailo PK. Substance use screening, brief intervention, and referral to treatment for pediatricians. Pediatrics. 2011;128(5):e1330–40.
2. Adamson SJ, Sellman JD. A prototype screening instrument for cannabis use disorder: the Cannabis use disorders identification test (CUDIT) in an alcohol-dependent clinical sample. Drug Alcohol Rev. 2003;22(3):309–15.
3. Alexander D. A marijuana screening inventory (experimental version): description and preliminary psychometric properties. Am J Drug Alcohol Abuse. 2003;29(3):619–46.
4. Ali R, Meena S, Eastwood B, Richards I, Marsden J. Ultra-rapid screening for substance-use disorders: the alcohol, smoking and substance involvement screening test (ASSIST-lite). Drug Alcohol Depend. 2013;132(1–2):352–61.
5. Andermann A, Blancquaert I, Beauchamp S, Dery V. Revisiting Wilson and Jungner in the genomic age: a review of screening criteria over the past 40 years. Bull World Health Organ. 2008;86(4):317–9.
6. Babor TF, Del Boca F, Bray JW. Screening, Brief Intervention and Referral to Treatment: implications of SAMHSA's SBIRT initiative for substance abuse policy and practice. Addiction. 2017;112(Suppl 2):110–7.
7. Barreto HA, de Oliveira Christoff A, Boerngen-Lacerda R. Development of a self-report format of ASSIST with university students. Addict Behav. 2014;39(7):1152–8.
8. Bashford J, Flett R, Copeland J. The Cannabis use problems identification test (CUPIT): development, reliability, concurrent and predictive valid-

ity among adolescents and adults. Addiction. 2010;105(4):615–25.

9. Beaudoin FL, Merchant RC, Clark MA. Prevalence and detection of prescription opioid misuse and prescription opioid use disorder among emergency department patients 50 years of age and older: performance of the prescription drug use questionnaire, patient version. Am J Geriatr Psychiatry. 2016;24(8):627–36.

10. Berman, A., H. Bergman, T. Palmstierna and F. Schlyter. DUDIT, The drug use disorders identification test: manul. 2003. Retrieved 9 Jan 2019, from https://www.scribd.com/document/206439188/Dudit-Manual.

11. Boston Children's Hospital & Harvard Medical School Teaching Hospital. CRAFFT. 2018. Retrieved 7 Jan 2019, from http://crafft.org.

12. Brown RL, Leonard T, Saunders LA, Papasouliotis O. A two-item conjoint screen for alcohol and other drug problems. J Am Board Fam Pract. 2001;14(2):95–106.

13. Brown RL, Rounds LA. Conjoint screening questionnaires for alcohol and other drug abuse: criterion validity in a primary care practice. Wis Med J. 1995;94(3):135–40.

14. Butler SF, Budman SH, Fernandez K, Jamison RN. Validation of a screener and opioid assessment measure for patients with chronic pain. Pain. 2004;112(1–2):65–75.

15. Butler SF, Budman SH, Fernandez KC, Houle B, Benoit C, Katz N, Jamison RN. Development and validation of the current opioid misuse measure. Pain. 2007;130(1–2):144–56.

16. Center for Substance Abuse Treatment. A guide to substance abuse services for primary care clinicians. Rockville (MD): Substance Abuse and Mental Health Services Administration (US); 1997. (Treatment Improvement Protocol (TIP) Series, No. 24.) [Table, Problem Oriented Screening Instrument for Teenagers (POSIT)]. 1997. Retrieved 9 Jan 2019, from https://www.ncbi.nlm.nih.gov/books/NBK64829/table/A46035/.

17. Center for Substance Abuse Treatment. Substance abuse treatment for persons with co-occurring disorders. (Treatment Improvement Protocol (TIP) Series, No. 42.) Appendix H: Screening Instruments. 2005. Retrieved 9 Jan 2019, from http://www.ncbi.nlm.nih.gov/books/NBK64187/.

18. Chasnoff IJ, Wells AM, McGourty RF, Bailey LK. Validation of the 4P's plus screen for substance use in pregnancy validation of the 4P's plus. J Perinatol. 2007;27(12):744–8.

19. Christie G, Marsh R, Sheridan J, Wheeler A, Suaalii-Sauni T, Black S, Butler R. The substances and choices scale (SACS)–the development and testing of a new alcohol and other drug screening and outcome measurement instrument for young people. Addiction. 2007;102(9):1390–8.

20. Christoff AO, Barreto HG, Boerngen-Lacerda R. Development of a computer-based format for the alcohol, smoking, and substance involvement screening test (ASSIST) with university students. Subst Use Misuse. 2016;51(9):1207–17.

21. Compton P, Darakjian J, Miotto K. Screening for addiction in patients with chronic pain and "problematic" substance use: evaluation of a pilot assessment tool. JPSM. 1998;16(6):355–63.

22. Compton PA, Wu SM, Schieffer B, Pham Q, Naliboff BD. Introduction of a self-report version of the prescription drug use questionnaire and relationship to medication agreement noncompliance. JPSM. 2008;36(4):383–95.

23. Etter J-F, Le Houezec J, Perneger TV. A self-administered questionnaire to measure dependence on cigarettes: the cigarette dependence scale. Neuropsychopharmacology. 2003;28(2):359–70.

24. Gorfinkel L, Voon P, Wood E, Klimas J. Diagnosing opioid addiction in people with chronic pain. BMJ. 2018;362:k3949.

25. Harland, J. and R. Ali. ASSIST on Ice: The alcohol, smoking and substance involvement screening test and brief intervention for methamphetamine use. Adelaide, DASSA-WHO Collaborating Centre, University of Adelaide, Australia. 2017.

26. Heatherton TF, Kozlowski LT, Frecker RC, Fagerstrom KO. The Fagerstrom test for nicotine dependence: a revision of the Fagerstrom tolerance questionnaire. Br J Addict. 1991;86(9):1119–27.

27. Hoffmann NG, Hunt DE, Rhodes WM, Riley KJ. UNCOPE: a brief substance dependence screen for use with arrestees. J Drug Issues. 2003;33(1):29–44.

28. Humeniuk R, Ali R, Babor TF, Farrell M, Formigoni ML, Jittiwutikarn J, de Lacerda RB, Ling W, Marsden J, Monteiro M, Nhiwatiwa S, Pal H, Poznyak V, Simon S. Validation of the alcohol, smoking and substance involvement screening test (ASSIST). Addiction. 2008;103(6):1039–47.

29. Kavanagh DJ, Trembath M, Shockley N, Connolly J, White A, Isailovic A, Young RM, Saunders JB, Byrne GJ, Connor J. The DrugCheck problem list: a new screen for substance use disorders in people with psychosis. Addict Behav. 2011;36(9):927–32.

30. Kawakami N, Takatsuka N, Inaba S, Shimizu H. Development of a screening questionnaire for tobacco/nicotine dependence according to ICD-10, DSM-III-R, and DSM-IV. Addict Behav. 1999;24(2):155–66.

31. Kelly SM, Gryczynski J, Mitchell SG, Kirk A, O'Grady KE, Schwartz RP. Validity of brief screening instrument for adolescent tobacco, alcohol, and drug use. Pediatrics. 2014;133(5):819–26.

32. Knight J, Shrier L, Bravender T, Farrell M, Vander Bilt J, Shaffer H. A new brief screen for adolescent substance abuse. Arch Pediatr Adolesc Med. 1999;153(6):591–6.

33. Knight JR, Goodman E, Pulerwitz T, DuRant RH. Reliability of the problem oriented screening instrument for teenagers (POSIT) in adolescent medical practice. J Adolesc Health. 2001;29(2):125–30.

34. Knight JR, Sherritt L, Harris SK, Gates EC, Chang G. Validity of brief alcohol screening tests among adolescents: a comparison of the AUDIT, POSIT, CAGE, and CRAFFT. Alcohol Clin Exp Res. 2003;27(1):67–73.

35. Legleye S, Karila L, Beck F, Reynaud M. Validation of the CAST, a general population Cannabis abuse screening test. J Subst Use. 2007;12(4):233–42.

36. Levy S, Weiss R, Sherritt L, Ziemnik R, Spalding A, Van Hook S, Shrier LA. An electronic screen for triaging adolescent substance use by risk levels. JAMA Pediatr. 2014;168(9):822–8.

37. Mayfield D, McLeod G, Hall P. The CAGE questionnaire: validation of a new alcoholism screening instrument. Am J Psychiatry. 1974;131(10):1121–3.

38. McNeely J, Strauss SM, Rotrosen J, Ramautar A, Gourevitch MN. Validation of an audio computer-assisted self-interview (ACASI) version of the alcohol, smoking and substance involvement screening test (ASSIST) in primary care patients. Addiction. 2016a;111(2):233–44.

39. McNeely J, Strauss SM, Saitz R, Cleland CM, Palamar JJ, Rotrosen J, Gourevitch MN. A brief patient self-administered substance use screening tool for primary care: two-site validation study of the Substance Use Brief Screen (SUBS). Am J Med. 2015;128(7):784. e9–19.

40. McNeely J, Wu LT, Subramaniam G, Sharma G, Cathers LA, Svikis D, Sleiter L, Russell L, Nordeck C, Sharma A, O'Grady KE, Bouk LB, Cushing C, King J, Wahle A, Schwartz RP. Performance of the tobacco, alcohol, prescription medication, and other substance use (TAPS) tool for substance use screening in primary care patients. Ann Intern Med. 2016b;165(10):690–9.

41. Mdege ND, Lang J. Screening instruments for detecting illicit drug use/abuse that could be useful in general hospital wards: a systematic review. Addict Behav. 2011;36(12):1111–9.

42. National Institute on Drug Abuse. Drug screening and assessment resources. 2018. Retrieved 7 Jan 2019, from https://www.drugabuse.gov/nidamed-medical-health-professionals/tool-resources-your-practice/additional-screening-resources.

43. Newton AS, Gokiert R, Mabood N, Ata N, Dong K, Ali S, Vandermeer B, Tjosvold L, Hartling L, Wild TC. Instruments to detect alcohol and other drug misuse in the emergency department: a systematic review. Pediatrics. 2011;128(1):e180–92.

44. Okulicz-Kozaryn K, Sierosławski J. Validation of the "problematic use of narcotics" (PUN) screening test for drug using adolescents. Addict Behav. 2007;32(3):640–6.

45. Ondersma SJ, Svikis DS, LeBreton JM, Streiner DL, Grekin ER, Lam PK, Connors-Burge V. Development and preliminary validation of an indirect screener for drug use in the perinatal period. Addiction. 2012;107(12):2099–106.

46. Piontek D, Kraus L, Klempova D. Short scales to assess cannabis-related problems: a review of psy-chometric properties. Subst Abuse Treat Prev Policy. 2008;3:25.

47. Prendergast M, Cartier J, Lee AB. Considerations for introducing SBIRT into a jail setting. Offender Programs Rep. 2014;17(6):81–6.

48. Proctor SL, Hoffmann NG. The UNCOPE: an effective brief screen for DSM-5 substance use disorders in correctional settings. Psychol Addict Behav. 2016;30(5):613–8.

49. Prokhorov AV, Khalil GE, Foster DW, Marani SK, Guindani M, Espada JP, Gonzalvez MT, Idrisov B, Galimov A, Arora M, Tewari A, Isralowitz R, Lapvongwatana P, Chansatitporn N, Chen X, Zheng H, Sussman S. Testing the nicotine dependence measure mFTQ for adolescent smokers: a multinational investigation. Am J Addict. 2017;26(7):689–96.

50. Sacks S, Melnick G, Coen C, Banks S, Friedmann PD, Grella C, Knight K, Zlotnick C. CJDATS co-occurring disorders screening instrument for mental disorders: a validation study. Crim Justice Behav. 2007;34(9):1198–215.

51. Schwartz RH, Wirtz PW. Potential substance abuse: detection among adolescent patients using the drug and alcohol problem (DAP) quick screen, a 30-item questionnaire. Clin Pediatr. 1990;29(1):38–43.

52. Schwartz RP, McNeely J, Wu LT, Sharma G, Wahle A, Cushing C, Nordeck CD, Sharma A, O'Grady KE, Gryczynski J, Mitchell SG, Ali RL, Marsden J, Subramaniam GA. Identifying substance misuse in primary care: TAPS tool compared to the WHO ASSIST. J Subst Abus Treat. 2017;76:69–76.

53. Skinner HA. The drug abuse screening test. Addict Behav. 1982;7(4):363–71.

54. Sobell LC, Kwan E, Sobell MB. Reliability of a drug history questionnaire (DHQ). Addict Behav. 1995;20(2):233–41.

55. Tarter RE, Kirisci L. The drug use screening inventory for adults: psychometric structure and discriminative sensitivity. Am J Drug Alcohol Abuse. 1997;23(2):207–19.

56. Tiet QQ, Finney JW, Moos RH. Screening psychiatric patients for illicit drug use disorders and problems. Clin Psychol Rev. 2008;28(4):578–91.

57. Tiet QQ, Leyva YE, Moos RH, Smith B. Diagnostic accuracy of a two-item drug abuse screening test (DAST-2). Addict Behav. 2017;74:112–7.

58. United Nations Office on Drugs and Crime. World drug report 2018 (United Nations publication, Sales No. E.18.XI.9). Vienna, Division for Policy Analysis and Public Affairs United Nations Office on Drugs and Crime. 2018.

59. University of Adelaide. ASSIST portal. 2018. Retrieved 29 Dec 2018, from https://assistportal.com.au.

60. Webster LR, Webster RM. Predicting aberrant behaviors in opioid-treated patients: preliminary validation of the opioid risk tool. Pain Med. 2005;6(6):432–42.

61. WHO ASSIST Working Group. The alcohol, smoking and substance involvement screening test (ASSIST): development, reliability and feasibility. Addiction. 2002;97(9):1183–94.

62. World Health Organization. Guidelines for the identification and management of substance use and substance use disorders in pregnancy. Geneva: World Health Organization; 2014.

63. Yonkers KA, Gotman N, Kershaw T, Forray A, Howell HB, Rounsaville BJ. Screening for prenatal substance use: development of the substance use risk profile-pregnancy scale. Obstet Gynecol. 2010;116(4):827–33.

64. Yudko E, Lozhkina O, Fouts A. A comprehensive review of the psychometric properties of the drug abuse screening test. J Subst Abus Treat. 2007;32(2):189–98.

Drug Testing in Addiction Medicine

44

Christopher Tremonti and Paul S. Haber

Contents

C. Tremonti (✉)
Sydney Local Health District,
Camperdown, NSW, Australia
e-mail: chris.tremonti@health.nsw.gov.au

P. S. Haber (✉)
Drug Health Services, Sydney Local Health District,
The University of Sydney Central Clinical School,
Sydney, NSW, Australia
e-mail: paul.haber@sydney.edu.au

© Springer Nature Switzerland AG 2021
N. el-Guebaly et al. (eds.), *Textbook of Addiction Treatment*,
https://doi.org/10.1007/978-3-030-36391-8_44

Abstract

Drug testing in addiction medicine is typically carried out via either immunoassay, such as in urine drug screens, or gas chromatography mass spectrometry (GCMS). Immunoassays are prone to false positives, and where there is conjecture, should be confirmed with GCMS. Guidelines, such as AS/NZS 4308:2008 in Australia, currently dictate the levels at which a test is considered positive in order to avoid false positives caused by such situations as passive cannabis inhalation or poppy seed ingestion. Most tests typically utilize urine, though other matrixes can be tested including saliva, blood, and hair. Amphetamine immunoassays in particular are prone to a high number of false positives due to their cross-reactivity with other medications. Cocaine, on the other hand, is typically fairly specific for its metabolite benzoylecgonine. Urine drug screens usually screen for non-synthetic opioids only: morphine, codeine, and heroin. While 6-monoacetylmorphine is pathognomonic for heroin use, this is often not present, and it can be challenging to determine the true source when opioids are detected in urine. Methadone metabolite EDDP can be tested via immunoassay; however, buprenorphine requires being sent to a laboratory that can perform GCMS. Chronic cannabis use can result in a positive immunoassay for weeks following cessation of use. Benzodiazepines have a complex metabolic pathway, and as such it is normal for patients on diazepam to test positive for temazepam or oxazepam. The increasing use of synthetic cannabis and cathinones presents a challenge for diagnostic testing, as there are vast numbers of new products entering the market regularly and diagnostics cannot maintain pace with production.

Keywords

Urine drug screen · Gas chromatography mass spectrometry (GCMS) · Illicit drugs · Immunoassay · Opioids · Benzodiazepines

Drug testing involves the analysis of urine or other bodily fluids for the presence of prescription drugs, illicit substances, and/or their metabolites. Drug testing is done in several contexts: clinical toxicology in emergency departments and clinics including addiction treatment, workplace drug testing, postmortem toxicology forensic toxicology including drug-facilitated sexual assault, and sports toxicology. Each setting adopts different approaches and technologies to detect the relevant drugs of abuse. This chapter primarily focuses on clinical issues relevant to addiction specialists. Testing for alcohol and its metabolites is considered in Chap. 10. Therapeutic drug monitoring is not considered here, with the exception of methadone blood levels to monitor agonist treatment.

44.1   Introduction

Self-report generally provides valid information concerning drug use, but valid and independent information about substance exposure is often very valuable. Laboratory methods may be employed to determine the substances used, the timing, and the amount of use. A range of bodily fluids or tissues can be assayed for the presence of drugs of abuse, including urine, blood, oral fluid, sweat, meconium, vitreous humor, and hair. Each has its own advantages and disadvantages. With some exceptions, the results are qualitative rather than quantitative and provide only limited specificity concerning time of use.

Urine is the most commonly used matrix as it tends to offer a longer detection window compared to blood and oral fluid and can be obtained via relatively noninvasive means. The convenience of urine, however, is weighed against the risk of adulteration or substitution by the patient.

At this point, it is worth noting the medicolegal status of the tests done in addiction medicine. There are standards, such as AS/NZS 4308:2008 in Australia, that specify how samples need to be collected and tested in order to satisfy regulatory requirements for medicolegal testing (Table 44.1). Most hospital laboratories do not document chain of custody of sample nor adhere to the rigorous practice demanded for medicolegal testing. Thus, testing that is done for "clinical purposes" may not satisfy the regulatory requirements applied to medicolegal testing, depending on local policy. It is important to understand the testing procedures in the local setting and to discuss this with patients when doing drug testing.

Nonetheless, there are steps the addiction specialist can take to ensure a more reliable test. Collection should be done in an area without access to water and ideally where a dye has been added to cistern water. The temperature of the urine should be tested immediately after collection to determine that the sample has been freshly voided. The creatinine concentration, the pH, and the presence of oxidizing agents should also be tested to determine dilution or adulteration that can interfere with drug detection.

Table 44.1 Overview of standards for drug testing (Australian AS/NZS 4308:2008)

Collection site	Privacy Security and access Chain of custody
Integrity and identify of specimen	Precautions to prevent dilution Collection procedure Preparation for dispatch Transportation to laboratory
Laboratory requirements	Security Specimen reception Specimen integrity testing (measure creatinine) Specimen storage
Testing procedures	Use of immunoassay Personnel Quality control Cutoff levels (see Table 44.2) Confirmatory testing Reporting Record keeping

It is also worth noting that no single assay technology or assay strategy will detect all drugs of possible interest. Should a patient present appearing intoxicated, there is no specific test that will reliably identify the substance that has caused the reduction in consciousness. Comprehensive broad-spectrum analyses for all intoxicating drugs are labor intensive, and so most clinical laboratories that perform drug testing adopt a limited testing strategy to satisfy specific clinical situations and with varying degrees of success.

44.2 Drug Screening and Limitations of Testing

There are some important principles that apply to the use of drug testing in addiction medicine, namely, the concept of *screening tests*, *confirmatory tests*, *false positives*, and *false negatives*.

The most common test undertaken in addiction medicine, the urine drug screen, is an excellent example of a screening test, used to identify the most commonly abused substances. Most drug-screening tests use immunoassay technology, which use antibodies to detect the metabolites of drugs [1]. Because of cross-reactivity with other drugs, and because the cutoffs for screening tests are usually set very low in order to not miss positive results, there is a low specificity and high sensitivity. This will result in a higher number of false positives.

Most confirmatory testing for drugs, including those of dependence, is done via specific chromatography, typically gas chromatography mass spectrometry (GCMS) [2]. These tests are much more complicated and typically require being sent to a specific lab with specific conditions under which the tests are performed in accordance with relevant standards [3]. As these tests are more specific, they do not produce as many false positives. If there is discordance between the clinical situation and the result of a screening test, the sample should be sent for confirmatory testing with GCMS. The key practice point is that an aliquot from the *same sample* must be sent because drug(s) present in the first sample may no longer be present in a sample obtained days or weeks later. Consequently, results must be reviewed and supplementary tests correctly ordered before the sample is discarded. This requires effective collaboration between clinical services and laboratories.

On top of this, it is important to appreciate that all laboratory testing, screening, or confirmatory, has cutoff values in order to avoid false positives. Part of the reason for this is that testing often occurs in the workplace, and a false-positive result can have significant consequences for an employee. A commonly used example is of poppy seeds causing positive opioid results [4, 5]. As such, the levels at which a test is deemed positive has been set for each illicit substance, be that opioid, amphetamine, or cannabis, by the particular standards of each country, such as AS/NZS 4308:2008 in Australia and New Zealand [3]. A negative result does not mean that the drug is absent, rather that the concentration in the matrix is less than the threshold concentration and, even if positive, considered unlikely to be of practical importance (a potential false negative). Cutoffs for immunoassay testing of common drugs of abuse according to AS/NZS 4308:2008 are shown below (Table 44.2).

As such we can see that all testing needs to serve the clinical context. A positive urinary drug screen should be sent for confirmation to ensure it is not a false positive particularly if significant action may follow from a positive result. On the other hand, when there is a high clinical suspicion for drug misuse, but a negative urinary drug screen, the sample should be sent for GCMS testing specific for the agent of concern.

This chapter will provide common false positives for each drug of abuse, but it is worth noting that circumstances can be highly variable. The strongest evidence of a legitimate false positive

would be to have a patient produce a negative urine drug test, witness them take the suspected interfering drug, and send their urine for testing that shows positive immunoassay and negative GCMS. The weakest would be a case of a person denying use of an illicit substances and claiming use of an interfering substance [6].

There are other limitations on testing. Designer drugs, such as synthetic cannabis or cathinones ("bath salts"), are so new that specific assays are not available to test for these. Urinary drug screens are limited by time and as such cannot assess patterns of use and burden of dependence [7]. Furthermore, there are literature reports of passive inhalation of particular substances of abuse yielding a positive result [1].

44.3   Clinical Role of Drug Testing in Addiction Practice

The main role for drug testing is to detect the use of drugs not reported by the patient. Drug tests are no substitute for a good clinical history. There have been studies questioning the validity of self-reporting as a screening tool [8–10]. However it is worth noting that even within these studies, the sensitivity and negative predictive value of self-reporting remain quite high [8]. Furthermore, it appears that in patients seeking treatment – the very patients we work with in addiction medicine practice – the sensitivity and negative predictive value of self-reporting increase [11, 12]. Some papers also show that the bigger shortfall in self-reporting is *overstating* use, rather than under-stating [7, 13], and this may be because patients feel they need to overstate their dependence issue in order to receive treatment. Interestingly, Digiusto et al. looked at the urinary drug screens and self-reporting of 341 patients attempting to enter methadone treatment and found that while most drug use was overreported, especially in patients who had been treated before, the major drug underreported was methadone itself. This suggests patients are desperate for treatment, but may have already started medicating themselves illicitly, and fear the consequences of this being detected by the clinical team [13]. In short, uri-

Table 44.2 Cutoff levels for drug detection. (Reproduced from Australian Standard AS/NZS 4308:2008)

Class of drug	Cutoff level (ug/L)
Amphetamine type substances	300
Benzodiazepines	200
Cannabis metabolites	50
Cocaine metabolites	300
Opiates	300

nary drug screens should be an adjunct to clinical history but not a substitute. Typically, the patient will be more likely to report drug use if there is a strong therapeutic relationship and if there are no adverse consequences of reporting recent use. In this setting, self-report will provide details of quantity and frequency that laboratory testing is unable to match, such that self-reports are more useful than laboratory data. For the patient who does not appear intoxicated and who reports no recent drug use, periodic urine drug screening can be worthwhile. Indeed, the main clinical use of a positive urine drug test is to encourage more forthright and detailed self-reporting in this context.

In the addiction setting, there are a number of situations where drug testing can be useful, such as monitoring the use of prescribed benzodiazepines, ensuring that takeaway doses are being used by the patient and not diverted, and when there is concern around concomitant use of sedatives, in particular opioids and benzodiazepines. Even in these situations, an honest, nonjudgmental conversation about what substances the patient is using will supplant urine drug testing. For example, if a patient on a methadone program admits to using heroin, there is little benefit in testing for heroin on a urine drug screen particularly as most tests cannot detect heroin. Again, we emphasize the importance of clinical acumen and good rapport with a patient more than relying on regimented testing.

44.4 Dealing with a Positive Test Result

Discussing a positive test result with a patient can be confronting. It is therefore important to explain to patients in a clear and nonjudgmental manner prior to testing the reasons for performing drug screening. This will alleviate many of the anxieties around a positive result. Should a patient return an unexpected positive specimen, the clinician should undertake the following steps [14]:

– Review the patient's medications for possible false positives.

– Confirm the result with GCMS on the same sample if clinically indicated.
– Present the result to the patient in a clear and nonjudgmental manner.

Test results should only be interpreted by a suitably skilled clinician with knowledge of the patient and the testing process. The authors have experience of community workers removing children from their mothers because of false-positive urine tests as just one example.

44.5 Testing in the Emergency Department

The question of whether to use urine drug screens on patients in the emergency department is a vexed one. Some authors have suggested utilizing the UDS in order to diagnose substance abuse disorders and provide primary care [14]. However, there is no clear evidence to suggest this is useful. A literature review from Tenenbein of over 6000 patients presenting to the emergency department concluded that A UDS was unlikely to significantly impact upon management of the patient in the emergency department [15]. While this review focused primarily on immediate management outcomes, such as time in the emergency department, and procedures the patient received, others have suggested limited utility beyond this time frame. Riccoboni retrospectively reviewed over 200 psychiatric admissions, comparing those that had UDS to those who did not, and found it made little difference in management of their psychiatric illness [16]. This is supported by other studies in psychiatric patients that emphasize the urine drug screen should not trump good clinical history [17, 18]. The authors would suggest that urine drug testing in the emergency department should be performed in order to confirm a suspected diagnosis related to substance abuse when the patient's history does not corroborate. Furthermore, the information should only be presented to the patient when confirmed via GCMS and as a means of helping the patient seek appropriate treatment of a potential substance dependence.

44.6 Point-of-Care Testing

There are a variety of new point-of-care tests entering the market, including dipsticks, breath tests, cassettes, and urine drug cups, which integrate the testing strip with the collection cup [14, 19].

Point-of-care devices have the benefit of fast results and appear to have low rates of false positives and false negatives [14]. However, it is worth looking at devices that have been externally validated in studies and noting the cutoffs used by the particular test. Ultimately, they cannot replace GCMS for performance.

44.7 Saliva/Oral Fluid/Mobile Drug Testing

Mobile drug testing is now being utilized in the USA, Europe, and Australia for the detection of cannabis, cocaine, and MDMA in drivers [20–22]. These have many of the same advantages and disadvantages with other point-of-care tests listed above [2]. Saliva typically remains positive for 12–24 hours after drug use, though potentially longer in chronic users [22]. It is also worth noting a few idiosyncrasies to the testing of saliva. Cannabis has been shown to be more difficult to detect [22, 23], while drug deposits in the mouth can cause increased levels in quantitative testing when done in the immediate period after use [24].

Despite these shortcomings, saliva testing has the advantage of limited opportunity for adulteration [2, 22].

44.8 Detection Times

An often-asked question is how long a test will remain positive for, to which there is no hard and fast answer. One can expect a test to remain positive for around five half-lives of the drug, as this is the time taken to excrete around 97% of the drug. However, duration of positivity is determined by many pharmacological factors, including body weight and composition, half-life of the drug, dose, duration of use, volume of distribution, bioavailability of the drug, and the half-lives

of metabolites [1, 2, 25]. Nonetheless, this chapter will attempt to provide a guide for each substance of abuse around how long a test will remain positive.

44.9 Drug Testing Technologies

44.9.1 Immunoassay

Most clinical laboratories use immunoassay on high-capacity automated analyzers as first-line screening. All immunoassays are based on an antibody directed against either the drug of interest or a metabolite of the drug of interest. An example would be the immunoassay screen for cocaine, which has an antibody against benzoylecgonine.

Cloned enzyme donor immunoassay is the most commonly used assay in Australasian laboratories. The process involves mixing the patient's sample with an assay kit. The kit will contain an antibody against the metabolite of the drug being tested for and also the antigen of the drug being tested for tagged with an enzyme, such as glucose-6-phosphate dehydrogenase [26]. This enzyme converts NAD to NADH. If there is no drug present in the patient's simple, then the antibody from the kit will bind the antigen from the kit, and no enzymatic reaction will occur. However, if there is drug present in the patient's sample, then these metabolites will bind the antibody of the kit, leaving the antigen from the kit free and thus able to complete its reaction. The product of the reaction, in this case NADH, can then be tested for.

Because of cross-reaction of different substances for the antibody in the assay kit, one can easily see how false positives and false negatives can occur frequently. This is a major limitation of immunoassays in drug testing.

44.9.2 Chromatography and Mass Spectrometry

Chromatography is a process whereby individual components of a complex mixture are physically separated and identified. There are three techniques that can be used to separate and identify drugs in a body fluid such as urine: thin-layer chromatography (TLC), gas chromatography (GC), and liquid chromatography (LC). All these techniques involve a stationary phase and a mobile phase. For example, in GC the stationary phase is a polymer that coats the inner wall of a silica capillary tube. The mobile phase is an inert gas, such as helium. As in all forms of chromatography, the separation is achieved by allowing the drug to bind to the stationary phase and passing the mobile phase through so as to progressively remove the drug.

The identification of the drug eluted into the mobile phase uses a variety of techniques and requires comparison of the test sample with known pure standards. In TLC, drugs are detected by direct visualization, requiring the interpreter of the test to have knowledge of the various patterns that may be formed. GC and LC, however, use instrumental techniques of analysis, and while there are several different detectors that can be used to distinguish the presence of a drug, the preferred detectors in drug analysis are mass spectrometers.

Mass spectrometry involves the formation of charged ion(s) from the drug molecule. These charged ions can be sorted in the mass spectrometer and the mass of each ion determined. Different drugs give rise to a distinctive ion "fingerprint."

44.10 Detecting Specific Drug Classes

It is worth looking at each drug individually, focusing on the metabolism of the drug and the metabolites being test, the expected duration the test will remain positive, common cross-reactions, and, for certain drugs, whether passive inhalation can cause positive results.

44.10.1 Amphetamines

It is important to appreciate that the term "amphetamine" refers specifically to 1-phenylpropan-2-amine. There are, however, many other compounds structurally related to amphetamine that are often categorized under the broad umbrella of "amphetamines": methamphetamine ("crystal meth" or "ice"), methylenedioxyamphetamine (MDA), and methylenedioxymethylamphetamine (MDMA or "ecstasy"). The different assays used in urinary drug screens vary in reactivity for the various types of amphetamine.

Amphetamines are typically detectable in urine for around 48 hours after administration of the drug, though this can vary [27]. Amphetamines are typically basic, and consequently the rate of renal excretion of the unchanged drug is dependent on urine pH. Acidic urine gives amphetamine a charge that promotes excretion because the ionized form of amphetamine is poorly reabsorbed across the distal convoluted tubule of the kidney. Therefore by acidifying urine, such as with high doses of vitamin C, one can theoretically excrete amphetamine quicker. The half-life of amphetamines can be as short as 4 hours with acidic urine, as opposed to 12 hours with uncontrolled urinary pH, theoretically dropping the excretion time to less than 24 hours.

While there have been some concerns around immunoassay detection of amphetamines at low doses [28], GCMS is around 90% sensitive for detection even in doses as low as 10 mg [27]. It would not be unusual for a patient abusing amphetamines to be using far higher doses [25]. At the same time, patients that use medicinal amphetamines, particularly lisdexamfetamine for ADHD, would be expected to test positive as this is a prodrug converted in vivo to amphetamine.

As already mentioned, amphetamines have a vast number of cross-reactivities. This stems largely from the simplicity of the molecule, making it difficult to develop specific antibodies, and the high number of structurally similar sympathomimetics [6]. The most common source of a false-positive test is cold medicines such as pseudoephedrine. Promethazine [29], labetalol [30], ofloxacin [31], and bupropion [32] have all been shown to cause false-positive results for methamphetamines.

Furthermore methamphetamine is a chiral molecule. Typically, the illicit form is dextrorotary (d-form) or a racemic mixture of levorotary (l-form) and d-form. L-form methamphetamine is also a metabolite of selegiline and Vicks VapoRub and thus these can cause false positives [33].

There is no evidence that passive inhalation of methamphetamines can cause false-positive urine drug tests [34].

Designer amphetamines and synthetic cathinones, such as mephedrone or methcathinone, present a new challenge for drug testing, due to the number of different chemical structures that exist among these drugs [35]. Furthermore, new designer drugs are being introduced into the market regularly, making it difficult to produce immunoassays for each drug. Nonetheless, there is at least one immunoassay on the market, validated for mephedrone, methcathinone, methylenedioxypyrovalerone (MDPV), and 3′,4′-methylenedioxy-α-pyrrolidinobutiophenone (MDPBP) [36]. Many other established cathinones can also be detected via GCMS [35].

44.10.2 Benzodiazepines

Benzodiazepines have a variety of metabolic pathways, which can complicate testing.

There is almost no excretion of unconjugated parent benzodiazepines, and only three are excreted following glucuronidation alone: oxazepam, temazepam, and lorazepam. However, these three drugs show the complexity of testing for benzodiazepines, as the immunoassays will not detect their glucuronide conjugates unless the urine was treated with β-glucuronidase before testing, a practice not commonly done.

The metabolism of diazepam also warrants specific discussion. Diazepam can be demethylated to form nordiazepam or hydroxylated to form temazepam. Both these metabolites can form oxazepam. When taken orally, temazepam itself is demethylated to oxazepam. As such, benzodiazepine assays typically look for oxazepam and nordiazepam, as they are common metabolites in benzodiazepine metabolism. However, they may miss other commonly abused benzodiazepines, such as alprazolam, whose main metabolites are α-hydroxyalprazolam and 4-hydroxyalprazolam [37]. Clonazepam is converted to 7-aminoclonazepam, and flunitrazepam, metabolized to 7-aminoflunitrazepam. Lorazepam is excreted as an inactive glucuronide (Fig. 44.1).

Given the above, if monitoring use of prescribed benzodiazepines in an addiction setting, a simple immunoassay will not suffice, and the urine should be sent for formal GCMS.

Interpretation of results is a key issue. A patient may be prescribed diazepam, and urine testing may reveal diazepam, nordiazepam, oxazepam, and temazepam. This result reflects normal drug metabolism and does not signify nonprescribed use of the latter two drugs.

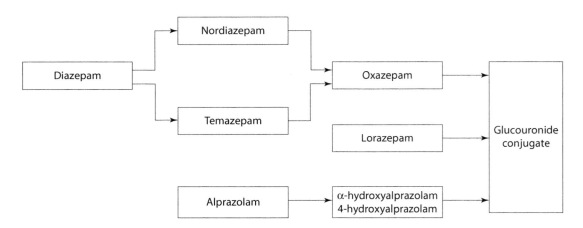

Fig. 44.1 Interconversion of commonly used benzodiazepines. (Adapted from Moeller 2016)

Detection times for benzodiazepines vary depending on duration of action. Diazepam, a long-acting benzodiazepine, can be detected for up to a week even after a single dose [26], while the metabolite nordiazepam can be detected for up to 3 weeks [38]. Short-acting benzodiazepines, such as alprazolam, temazepam, and oxazepam, may only be detectable for around 24 hours, while intermediate acting benzodiazepines, such as lorazepam, can be detected for up to 12 days [14]. Having said this, chronic use of benzodiazepines can result in a positive test for up to a month following cessation [14]. Flunitrazepam has received a lot of attention due to reports of it being used in cases of date-rape and is detectable after acute dosing for at least 48 hours using GCMS [39].

There is strong evidence that efavirenz [40], an antiviral used for HIV, and sertraline [41] both cause false positives in urine drug testing for benzodiazepines, while there has been a case report of oxaprozin, a nonsteroidal anti-inflammatory, causing a false positive [42].

44.10.3 Cannabis

Tetrahydrocannabinol (THC), the main psychoactive component of the hemp plant cannabis sativa, undergoes a complex metabolism to carboxy-THC. Carboxy-THC is not psychoactive and is extensively conjugated with glucuronic acid before excretion into urine.

The current cutoff concentration for immunoassay of cannabis metabolites has been set at 50 µg/L in the Australasian standard AS/NZS 4308:2008 because of concerns around passive smoking. There have been several studies that have looked at passive smoking, and the consensus is that passive smoking is unlikely to result in a urinary concentration of cannabis metabolites that exceeds 50 µg/L.

Carboxy-THC has an elimination half-life of around 6 days. However, THC is lipophilic and has a high volume of distribution, meaning chronic users of cannabis establish a significant reservoir of carboxy-THC in adipose tissue. The time taken for carboxy-THC to fall back to below the cutoff concentration in urine therefore depends on the amount of THC stored in tissue lipids, which in itself depends on duration and amount of exposure.

Following a single occasion of cannabis use, GCMS will typically be positive for 72 hours. Moderate users of cannabis, using four times per week, will typically have a negative test in 5–7 days after stopping the drug. Daily users will typically test positive for about 12 days post ceasing use, but chronic users may have a positive test for more than 30 days [43].

Given the extended duration of detection of carboxy-THC in the urine of long-term heavy users of the drug, it can make ongoing detection post cessation challenging. One approach is to determine a carboxy-THC: creatinine ratio for urine samples collected at different times. A comparison of these two ratios allows for assessment of continued use.

Detection of synthetic cannabinoids is difficult for many reasons. Typically, they are highly potent, so only a small dose is required, and metabolized quickly [44, 45]. Furthermore, there are over 800 different types of synthetic cannabinoids, making it difficult to produce immunoassays to detect all types and to keep up with the new drugs being introduced into the illicit market [44]. Despite the challenges, there are some immunoassay kits available for detection of synthetic cannabinoids, including DrugCheck K2/Spice Test, DrugSmart Cassette, and RapiCard InstaTest [45].

Clinicians should also be aware that dronabinol, a synthetic form of THC approved for use in spasticity in multiple sclerosis, will test positive on urine drug screens, though nabilone, approved in some countries for use in nausea during chemotherapy, will not [46, 47]. While both are synthetic cannabinoids, nabilone is a synthetic derivative [48] and has enough difference in structure to test negative.

Proton pump inhibitors have been shown to cause false positives both in case reports and formalized testing [49, 50]. The urinary metabolite of Efavirenz, 8-ether-glucoronide, cross-reacts with cannabinoid immunoassays [51, 52]. Naproxen and ibuprofen also have a small possibility of false-positive results on immunoassay, and as such, confirmatory testing with GCMS is warranted should this occur [53]. Certain baby wash products can also produce a false positive on immunoassay, which is important in the setting of neonatal drug testing [54].

44.10.4 Opioids

An understanding of opioid metabolism is critical when interpreting urine drug tests. It is important to note that morphine, codeine, and heroin (diacetylmorphine) are the only fully natural opioids, and most immunoassays are directed at these three substances and their metabolites. Synthetic opioids, such as fentanyl, methadone, buprenorphine, pethidine, oxycodone, and oxymorphone, are structurally different enough to natural opioids that they will not be detected by these immunoassays and require either specific assays directed at their metabolites or GCMS [14]. Thus, a patient using illicit fentanyl or prescribed buprenorphine will typically have a negative urine drug screen, and further testing is required in order to show use of synthetic opioids.

44.10.5 Morphine, Codeine, and Heroin

Heroin is rapidly metabolized to both 3-monoacetylmorphine, which is inactive, and 6-monoacetylmorphine (6-MAM), which is rapidly deacetylated to morphine, and has a half-life of about 5 minutes. 6-Acetylcodeine is an impurity often found in illicit heroin, and this can be metabolized to codeine also [55, 56].

Morphine is mostly metabolized to 3-glucuronide and 6-glucuronide, though it has a number of minor metabolic pathways, including to form normorphine and hydromorphone [55, 57].

Codeine is O-demethylated to yield morphine via the actions of CYP2D6 in the liver. However, a large portion of codeine is excreted as codeine 6-glucouronide, while it may also be metabolized to norcodeine and hydrocodone [55, 57, 58] (Fig. 44.2).

Urine immunoassay will not distinguish between codeine, morphine, and heroin. If there is conjecture over which opioid the patient took, the sample needs to be sent for GCMS. Detection of 6-MAM is pathognomonic for heroin use; however, it is usually only detectable for a few hours because of its short half-life (20 minutes) [6–8]. This will often leave the clinician with a

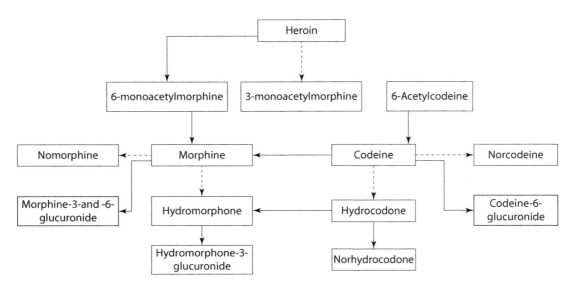

Fig. 44.2 Interconversion of commonly used opioids. (Adapted from French [55])

test that is positive for morphine, codeine, or both, which presents an interesting challenge. Codeine may arise from prescribed analgesics or, as mentioned above, from an impurity in heroin. Morphine may also be derived from codeine, from a prescription for the medication, or from heroin. Furthermore the patient may have used multiple opioids, further complicating the picture [59]. The codeine/morphine ratio may help in this situation. Several studies in both urine and blood have shown that when patients have used heroin, confirmed by the presence of 6-MAM, morphine levels will be greater than codeine [56, 59, 60]. Furthermore, when healthy volunteers take codeine alone, the level of morphine metabolites in urine will typically be lower than codeine, even though codeine is metabolized in part to morphine [59, 61, 62]. This has even been observed in the blood of rapid codeine metabolizers [63]. The following has therefore been suggested: A urine morphine/codeine ratio greater than 2 and total morphine >200 ng/ml suggests morphine or heroin use, while a morphine/codeine ratio less than 2 and total morphine <200 ng/ml suggests codeine use alone [60, 64] (Table 44.3).

Furthermore, current Australian guidelines dictated by AS/NZS 4308:2008 prescribes an opioid cutoff of 300 µg/L for immunoassay screening. This can still result in false positives caused by the ingestion of poppy seeds. In the USA, the Substance Abuse and Mental Health Services Administration (SAMHSA) changed this cutoff to >2000 µg/L in order to exclude poppy seeds as a potential cause of a positive opiate immunoassay. This cutoff, however, may miss true positives.

Several non-opiate drugs may cause false positive tests including the quinolone antibiotic gatifloxacin [65], ofloxacin [66], rifampin, and rifampicin [67, 68].

Table 44.3 Urine findings after use of morphine or codeine. (Adapted from Stefanidou [64])

Morphine/codeine ratio	Total morphine	Suggests
>2	>200 ng/ml	Morphine or heroin use
<2	<200 ng/ml	Codeine use

44.10.6 Methadone

Methadone immunoassays can test for either methadone itself or the inactive metabolite 2-ethylidene-1,5-dimethyl-3,3-diphenylpyrrolidene (EDDP) [1]. The latter is preferred for testing as patients can spike their urine with methadone in order to avoid detection of diversion of methadone doses. Methadone typically remains positive in urine for around 2–4 days, though it can be positive for up to 11 days [14, 69].

Quetiapine [70, 71] and verapamil [72] have both been demonstrated to cause false positives on methadone immunoassays.

The role of monitoring methadone serum levels during methadone treatment warrants some discussion. Currently, there is no recommendation to perform routine methadone levels in patients on methadone treatment. Currently, clinicians in NSW, Australia, only require a trough methadone level in order to apply to prescribe beyond 200 mg/day [73]. This is thought to identify patients that may be rapid metabolizers of methadone and thus require higher doses. At this stage, however, there is no clear plasma level at which methadone dosing is considered "effective." Trough levels tend to sit between 200 and 400 ng/ml [74, 75]. There have been a number of studies evaluating the relationship between methadone dose and plasma concentration, with some suggesting a strong relationship [76], some suggesting a poor relationship [77], while another has shown a strong relationship that only exists at doses less than 80 mg [78]. Further research is still required in this area. Specific stereoisomer testing for R- and S-methadone may improve the relevance of blood levels, but the assay is not widely available [79–81]. Serial measures of methadone levels may be helpful to detect rapid metabolizers but require patient attendance for many hours for multiple blood tests. This may be further complicated by often poor venous access, making this approach impractical for routine care.

44.10.7 Fentanyl

The main metabolite of fentanyl is norfentanyl [82, 83]. Because of its potency, estimated as

50–100 times that of morphine [84], only small concentrations are found in urine following prescribed or illicit use. Detection requires sophisticated techniques and sensitive analyzers that will not be available in many laboratories. Nonetheless, laboratories are improving their ability to detect fentanyl at smaller doses via GCMS and, with a smaller sample of matrix, even as low as 0.175 ml of serum [85]. Furthermore, new assays are now available for use in detecting fentanyl [86, 87], though these are not part of a standard urine drug screen.

Risperidone has been shown to cross-react with at least one fentanyl immunoassay [88]. Fentanyl metabolites are detectable via GCMS for at least 24 hours in urine following a single intravenous dose [84].

Street heroin has been found to be laced with fentanyl and its synthetic analogs, which can have potentially catastrophic consequences given its potency. The use of fentanyl testing in urine may therefore have a public health benefit as a warning to other users, though widespread use for this is not currently done [89].

44.10.8 Buprenorphine

Buprenorphine, widely used in opioid treatment programs, is not typically part of a standard urine drug screen panel, though it can be tested via immunoassay or GCMS [90, 91].

It is important to monitor the use of buprenorphine in patients on opioid treatment, especially those on takeaway dosing, as diversion of doses remains a risk [92]. Buprenorphine is dealkylated to form norbuprenorphine [90]. Both buprenorphine and norbuprenorphine can be glucuronidated, leaving four main metabolites in urine: buprenorphine, norbuprenorphine, buprenorphine-glucuronide, and norbuprenorphine-glucuronide [90, 93].

The laboratory may help with the detection of patients who spike their urines with their own supply of buprenorphine to give the impression that they are using the drug, when in fact they are diverting it [94]. The concentration of parent buprenorphine is typically lower than the other metabolites [95]. Therefore, norbuprenorphine/buprenorphine ratios are a good way to detect for spiked urines. In theory, all patients taking buprenorphine orally should have a norbuprenorphine/buprenorphine ratio greater than 1, and any ratio < 0.02 is considered to be spiked [90, 94]. One study has also suggested that norbuprenorphine levels may be able to estimate and guide the patient's dose of buprenorphine, though this is not validated or routine practice [96].

There are case reports that amisulpride [97], and high-dose morphine [98] can cause false-positive buprenorphine immunoassay results. The window of detection for buprenorphine is 4 days with a cutoff of 0.5 ng/ml [14].

44.10.9 Cocaine

The major metabolite of cocaine is benzoylecgonine, with around 45% of the dose excreted in the urine as such. Standard immunoassays show good reaction to benzoylecgonine, limited reaction to cocaine, and virtually no reaction to other metabolites. After use of 1.5 mg/kg intranasally, GCMS and immunoassay both appear to remain positive for around 2–3 days [99]. Interestingly, after administration of 20 mg of intravenous cocaine, immunoassays remain positive for only 2 days [100].

It is also worth noting that cocaine is still used as a vasoconstrictor and topical anesthetic for nasal surgery and that urines will test positive for similar timeframes as for illicit use [101]. Furthermore, passive inhalation of cocaine when smoked does not appear to cause false positives [34].

44.10.10 GHB

Gamma-hydroxybutyric acid (GHB) is particularly difficult to pick up on urine testing due to its short half-life and because it requires GCMS for detection, not immunoassay [14]. Furthermore, GHB is produced endogenously, and because of this, it has been suggested that 10 μg/ml is the cutoff for urine testing [25]. A 100 mg/kg dose of

GHB is undetectable in urine 12 hours later [102]. It is not routinely tested in the addiction medicine field.

44.10.11 Nitrous Oxide

The use of nitrous oxide among recreational drug users appears to be increasing, with around one quarter of ecstasy users admitting use in their lifetime [103, 104]. Subacute combined degeneration of the cord (SCID) has become a serious health issue in these patients [105]. While nitrous oxide is not tested in urine or other matrices, it is important for the addiction physician to be aware of the appropriate serum tests should a patient admit to using nitrous oxide recreationally. A normal B12 level is not reassuring because nitrous oxide inactivates B12, but it does not reduce serum levels, so serum B12 is often normal. Physicians should instead test for homocysteine levels. Vitamin B12 is important for the conversion of homocysteine to methionine, an important element for myelin production. An elevated homocysteine level suggests reduced levels of active B12, and potential risk of subacute combined degeneration of the cord [106, 107].

44.10.12 Ketamine and Phencyclidine

Ketamine has two major metabolites, norketamine and dehydronorketamine [108], which, along with ketamine itself, can all be tested via GCMS [109]. While not part of a typical urine drug screen, specific immunoassays are becoming increasingly available for ketamine as well [110, 111]. Ketamine is typically detectable for 3 days by GCMS when taken orally; however, dehydronorketamine can be detected for up to 10 days [112]. Quetiapine has been reported in two case reports to cause false positives on ketamine immunoassay [110].

Phencyclidine is now available on some urine drug screen panels, such as the Medtox Diagnostics EZ screen. Urine drug tests can detect PCP for up to 10 days post use. Ibuprofen, dextromethorphan, and metamizole have all been

shown in both case reports and in spiked urine testing to cause false positives [113]. Venlafaxine has also caused false positives in both of these circumstances [114], while there has been a case report of desvenlafaxine doing likewise [115]. There have been cases reports of tramadol causing positive PCP result on immunoassay, though this appears to occur more readily at supratherapeutic doses [116, 117].

44.10.13 Lysergic Acid Diethylamide (LSD)

LSD is converted to a number of different metabolites, and only around 1% of the drug is excreted unchanged [118]. Despite this, most immunoassays are still directed at LSD itself [119], and these are typically positive for around 24 hours, though there has been a report of detection 80 hours post use [25].

Ritter et al. found 71 false-positive LSD results from immunoassay testing of almost 1900 positive samples [120]. Potential causative drugs included amitriptyline, bupropion, metoclopramide, labetalol, and calcium channel blockers; however, no confirmatory testing has been undertaken to prove which agents truly cross-react with the immunoassay. Ambroxol, however, has been seen in both case report and spiked urine testing to cause false-positive immunoassay results [121].

References

1. Moeller KE, Kissack JC, Atayee RS, Lee KC. Clinical interpretation of urine drug tests: what clinicians need to know about urine drug screens. Mayo Clin Proc England. 2017;92(5):774–96.
2. Jaffe A, Molnar S, Williams N, Wong E, Todd T, Caputo C, et al. Review and recommendations for drug testing in substance use treatment contexts. J Reward Defic Syndr Addict Sci. 2016;2(1):28–45.
3. Australian/New Zealand Standard. Procedures for specimen collection and the detection and quantitation of drugs of abuse in urine. 2008;1–41.
4. Narcessian EJ, Yoon HJ. False-positive urine drug screen: beware the poppy seed bagel. J Pain Symptom Manag. 1997;14(5):261–3.
5. Pearson ACS, Eldrige JS, Hooten WM. Interpreting urine drug screen results in the context of poppy seed

use. Mayo Clin Proc. 2015;90(12):1734–5. https://doi.org/10.1016/j.mayocp.2015.08.011.

6. Park H-D, Fitzgerald RL, Saitman A. False-positive interferences of common urine drug screen immunoassays: a review. J Anal Toxicol. 2014;38(7):387–96. https://doi.org/10.1093/jat/bku075.

7. Darke S. Self-report among injecting drug users: a review. Drug Alcohol Depend Ireland. 1998;51(3):253–8.

8. Magura S, Goldsmith D, Casriel C, Goldstein PJ, Lipton DS. The validity of methadone clients' self-reported drug use. Int J Addict. 1987;22(8):727–49.

9. Akinci IH, Tarter RE, Kirisci L. Concordance between verbal report and urine screen of recent marijuana use in adolescents. Addict Behav. 2001;26(4):613–9. Available from: https://www.sciencedirect.com/science/article/abs/pii/S0306460300001465?via%3Dihub.

10. Marques PR, Tippetts AS, Branch DG. Cocaine in the hair of mother-infant pairs: quantitative analysis and correlations with urine measures and self-report. Am J Drug Alcohol Abuse. 1993;19(2):159–75.

11. Sherman MF, Bigelow GE. Validity of patients' self-reported drug use as a function of treatment status. Drug Alcohol Depend. 1992;30(1):1–11. Available from: http://www.sciencedirect.com/science/article/pii/037687169290030G.

12. Solbergsdottir E, Bjornsson G, Gudmundsson LS, Tyrfingsson T, Kristinsson J. Validity of self-reports and drug use among young people seeking treatment for substance abuse or dependence. J Addict Dis. 2004;23(1):29–38. https://doi.org/10.1300/J069v23n01_03.

13. Digiusto E, Seres V, Bibby A, Batey R. Concordance between urinalysis results and self-reported drug use by applicants for methadone maintenance in Australia. Addict Behav. 1996;21(3):319–29.

14. SAMHSA. Clinical drug testing in primary care [Internet]. Technical Assistance Publication (TAP) 32. 2012. Available from: www.samsah.gov.

15. Tenenbein M. Do you really need that emergency drug screen? Clin Toxicol. 2009;47(4):286–91.

16. Riccoboni ST, Darracq MA. Does the U stand for useless? The urine drug screen and emergency department psychiatric patients. J Emerg Med. 2018;54(4):500–6.

17. Akosile W, McDermott BM. Use of the urine drug screen in psychiatry emergency service. Australas Psychiatry. 2015;23(2):128–31. https://doi.org/10.1177/1039856214568213.

18. Perrone J, De Roos F, Jayaraman S, Hollander JE. Drug screening versus history in detection of substance use in ED psychiatric patients. Am J Emerg Med. 2001;19(1):49–51. Available from: http://www.sciencedirect.com/science/article/pii/S0735675701899964.

19. Lin C-N, Nelson GJ, McMillin GA. Evaluation of the NexScreen and DrugCheck waive RT urine drug detection cups. J Anal Toxicol. 2012;37(1):30–6. https://doi.org/10.1093/jat/bks087.

20. Veitenheimer AM, Wagner JR. Evaluation of oral fluid as a specimen for DUID. J Anal Toxicol. 2017;41(6):517–22.

21. Van der Linden T, Wille SMR, Ramirez-Fernandez M, Verstraete AG, Samyn N. Roadside drug testing: comparison of two legal approaches in Belgium. Forensic Sci Int. 2015;249:148–55.

22. Rouen D, Dolan K, Kimber J. A review of drug detection testing and an examination of urine, hair, saliva and sweat [Internet]. Sydney; 2001. Available from: http://www.sciencedirect.com/science/article/pii/S0002937805019174.

23. Menkes DB, Howard RC, Spears GF, Cairns ER. Salivary THC following cannabis smoking correlates with subjective intoxication and heart rate. Psychopharmacology. 1991;103(2):277–9.

24. Cone EJ. Saliva testing for drugs of abuse. Ann N Y Acad Sci. 1993;694:91–127.

25. Verstraete AG. Detection times of drugs of abuse in blood, urine, and oral fluid. Ther Drug Monit. 2004;26(2):200–5.

26. Johnson-Davis KL, Thompson CD, Clark CJ, McMillin GA, Lehman CM. Method comparison of the ortho vitros fusion 5,1 chemistry analyzer and the roche COBAS integra 400 for urine drug screen testing in the emergency department. J Anal Toxicol. 2012;36(5):345–8. https://doi.org/10.1093/jat/bks028.

27. Oyler JM, Cone EJ, Joseph REJ, Moolchan ET, Huestis MA. Duration of detectable methamphetamine and amphetamine excretion in urine after controlled oral administration of methamphetamine to humans. Clin Chem. 2002;48(10):1703–14.

28. Poklis A, Still J, Slattum PW, Edinboro LF, Saady JJ, Costantino A. Urinary excretion of d-amphetamine following oral doses in humans: implications for urine drug testing. J Anal Toxicol. 1998;22(6):481–6.

29. Melanson SEF, Lee-Lewandrowski E, Griggs DA, Long WH, Flood JG. Reduced interference by phenothiazines in amphetamine drug of abuse immunoassays. Arch Pathol Lab Med. 2006;130(12):1834–8.

30. Yee LM, Wu D. False-positive amphetamine toxicology screen results in three pregnant women using labetalol. Obstet Gynecol. 2011;117(2):503–6.

31. Nomier MA, Al-Huseini HK. False-positive TDxFLx® urine amphetamine/metamphetamine II assay from ofloxacin. Saudi Pharmaceutical Journal. 2004;12:42–6.

32. Casey ER, Scott MG, Tang S, Mullins ME. Frequency of false positive amphetamine screens due to bupropion using the Syva EMIT II immunoassay. J Med Toxicol. 2011;7(2):105–8.

33. West R, Pesce A, West C, Mikel C, Velasco J, Gonzales E, et al. Differentiating medicinal from illicit use in positive methamphetamine results in a pain population. J Anal Toxicol. 2013;37(2):83–9.

34. elSohly MA, Jones AB. Drug testing in the workplace: could a positive test for one of the mandated drugs be for reasons other than illicit use of the drug? J Anal Toxicol. 1995;19(6):450–8.

35. Neifeld JR, Regester LE, Holler JM, Vorce SP, Magluilo J Jr, Ramos G, et al. Ultrafast screening of synthetic cannabinoids and synthetic cathinones in urine by RapidFire-tandem mass spectrometry. J Anal Toxicol. 2016;40(5):379–87.

36. Ellefsen KN, Anizan S, Castaneto MS, Desrosiers NA, Martin TM, Klette KL, et al. Validation of the only commercially available immunoassay for synthetic cathinones in urine: randox drugs of abuse V biochip Array technology. Drug Test Anal 2014;6(7–8):728–38.

37. Laloup M, Fernandez M, Wood M, Maes V, De Boeck G, Vanbeckevoort Y, et al. Detection of diazepam in urine, hair and preserved oral fluid samples with LC-MS-MS after single and repeated administration of myolastan (R) and valium (R). Anal Bioanal Chem. 2007;388:1545–56.

38. SAMHSA. Clinical drug testing in primary care. Tech Assist Publ 32 [Internet]. 2012; Available from: www.samsah.gov.

39. Kintz P, Villain M, Cirimele V, Goulle J, Ludes B. Usage criminel de substances psycho-actives: le probleme de la duree de detection. Acta Clin Belg. 2002;57(Suppl 1):24–30.

40. Blank A, Hellstern V, Schuster D, Hartmann M, Matthee AK, Burhenne J, et al. Efavirenz treatment and false-positive results in benzodiazepine screening tests. Clin Infect Dis. 2009;48(12):1787–9.

41. Nasky KM, Cowan GL, Knittel DR. False-positive urine screening for benzodiazepines: an association with sertraline?: a two-year retrospective chart analysis. Psychiatry (Edgmont). 2009;6(7):36–9. Available from: https://www.ncbi.nlm.nih.gov/pubmed/19724768.

42. Pulini M. False-positive benzodiazepine urine test due to oxaprozin. JAMA. 1995;273(24):1905. https://doi.org/10.1001/jama.1995.03520480023025.

43. Dackis CA, Pottash AL, Annitto W, Gold MS. Persistence of urinary marijuana levels after supervised abstinence. Am J Psychiatry. 1982;139(9):1196–8.

44. Diao X, Huestis MA. Approaches, challenges, and advances in metabolism of new synthetic cannabinoids and identification of optimal urinary marker metabolites. Clin Pharmacol Ther. 2017;101(2):239–53.

45. Namera A, Kawamura M, Nakamoto A, Saito T, Nagao M. Comprehensive review of the detection methods for synthetic cannabinoids and cathinones. Forensic Toxicol. 2015;33(2):175–94. https://doi.org/10.1007/s11419-015-0270-0.

46. Kulig K. Interpretation of workplace tests for cannabinoids. J Med Toxicol. 2017;13(1):106–10. Available from: https://www.ncbi.nlm.nih.gov/pubmed/27686239.

47. Fraser A, Meatherall R. Lack of interference by nabilone in the EMIT(R) d.a.u. cannabinoid assay, Abbott TDx(R) cannabinoid assay, and a sensitive TLC assay for 9-THC-Carboxylic acid. J Anal Toxicol. 1989;13:240.

48. Murnion B. Medicinal cannabis. Aust Prescr. 2015;38(6):212–5. Available from: https://www.ncbi.nlm.nih.gov/pubmed/26843715.

49. Gomila I, Barcelo B, Rosell A, Avella S, Sahuquillo L, Dastis M. Cross-reactivity of pantoprazole with three commercial cannabinoids immunoassays in urine. J Anal Toxicol. 2017;41(9):760–4.

50. Felton D, Zitomersky N, Manzi S, Lightdale JR. 13-year-old girl with recurrent, episodic, persistent vomiting: out of the pot and into the fire. Pediatrics. 2015;135(4):e1060–3.

51. Rossi S, Yaksh T, Bentley H, van den Brande G, Grant I, Ellis R. Characterization of interference with 6 commercial Δ9-tetrahydrocannabinol immunoassays by efavirenz (Glucuronide) in urine. Clin Chem. 2006;52(5):896–7. Available from: http://clinchem.aaccjnls.org/content/52/5/896.abstract.

52. Oosthuizen NM, Laurens JB. Efavirenz interference in urine screening immunoassays for tetrahydrocannabinol. Ann Clin Biochem. 2012;49(2):194–6. Available from: https://journals.sagepub.com/doi/abs/10.1258/acb.2011.011118.

53. Rollins DE, Jennison TA, Jones G. Investigation of interference by nonsteroidal anti-inflammatory drugs in urine tests for abused drugs. Clin Chem. 1990;36(4):602–6. Available from: http://clinchem.aaccjnls.org/content/36/4/602.abstract.

54. Cotten SW, Duncan DL, Burch EA, Seashore CJ, Hammett-Stabler CA. Unexpected interference of baby wash products with a cannabinoid (THC) immunoassay. Clin Biochem. 2012;45(9):605–9.

55. French D. The challenges of LC-MS/MS analysis of opiates and opioids in urine. Bioanalysis. 2013;5(22):2803–20.

56. Ceder G, Jones AW. Concentration ratios of morphine to codeine in blood of impaired drivers as evidence of heroin use and not medication with codeine. Clin Chem. 2001;47(11):1980–4.

57. Smith HS. Opioid metabolism. Mayo Clin Proc. 2009;84(7):613–24. Available from: https://www.ncbi.nlm.nih.gov/pubmed/19567715.

58. Oyler JM, Cone EJ, Joseph REJ, Huestis MA. Identification of hydrocodone in human urine following controlled codeine administration. J Anal Toxicol. 2000 Oct;24(7):530–5.

59. Kronstrand R, Jones AW. Concentration ratios of codeine-to-morphine in plasma after a single oral dose (100 mg) of codeine phosphate. J Anal Toxicol. 2001;25(6):486–7.

60. Moriya F, Chan KM, Hashimoto Y. Concentrations of morphine and codeine in urine of heroin abusers. Leg Med (Tokyo). 1999;1(3):140–4.

61. Lafolie P, Beck O, Lin Z, Albertioni F, Boreus L. Urine and plasma pharmacokinetics of codeine in healthy volunteers: implications for drugs-of-abuse testing. J Anal Toxicol. 1996;20(7):541–6.

62. Shah JC, Mason WD. Plasma codeine and morphine concentrations after a single oral dose of codeine phosphate. J Clin Pharmacol. 1990;30(8):764–6.

63. He YJ, Brockmoller J, Schmidt H, Roots I, Kirchheiner J. CYP2D6 ultrarapid metabolism and morphine/codeine ratios in blood: was it codeine or heroin? J Anal Toxicol. 2008;32(2):178–82.

64. Stefanidou M, Athanaselis S, Spiliopoulou C, Dona A, Maravelias C. Biomarkers of opiate use. Int J Clin Pract. 2010;64(12):1712–8.

65. Straley CM, Cecil EJ, Herriman MP. Gatifloxacin interference with opiate urine drug screen. Pharmacotherapy. 2006;26(3):435–9.

66. Meatherall R, Dai J. False-positive EMIT II opiates from ofloxacin. Ther Drug Monit. 1997;19(1):98–9.

67. Daher R, Haidar JH, Al-Amin H. Rifampin interference with opiate immunoassays. Clin Chem. 2002;48(1):203–4. Available from: http://clinchem.aaccjnls.org/content/48/1/203.abstract.

68. de Paula M, Saiz LC, Gonzalez-Revalderia J, Pascual T, Alberola C, Miravalles E. Rifampicin causes false-positive immunoassay results for urine opiates. Clin Chem Lab Med. 1998;36(4):241–3.

69. Cone EJ. New developments in biological measures of drug prevalence. NIDA Res Monogr. 1997;167:108–29.

70. Lasić D, Uglešić B, Žuljan-Cvitanović M, Šupe-Domić D, Uglešić L. False-positive methadone urine drug screen in a patient treated with quetiapine. Acta Clin Croat. 2012;51(2):269–72.

71. Cherwinski K, Petti TA, Jekelis A. False methadone-positive urine drug screens in patients treated with quetiapine. J Am Acad Child Adolesc Psychiatry. 2007;46:435–6.

72. Lichtenwalner MR, Mencken T, Tully R, Petosa M. False-positive immunochemical screen for methadone attributable to metabolites of verapamil. Clin Chem. 1998;44(5):1039–41. Available from: http://clinchem.aaccjnls.org/content/44/5/1039.abstract.

73. NSW Health. NSW clinical guidelines: treatment of opioid dependence – 2018 [Internet]. 2018. Available from: https://www1.health.nsw.gov.au/pds/ActivePDSDocuments/GL2018_019.pdf.

74. Jiang H, Hillhouse M, Du J, Pan S, Alfonso A, Wang J, et al. Dose, plasma level, and treatment outcome among methadone patients in Shanghai, China. Neurosci Bull. 2016;32(6):538–44. Available from: https://www.ncbi.nlm.nih.gov/pubmed/27612968.

75. Mohamad N, Mohd R, Ghazali B, Abu Bakar NH, Musa N, Abdulkarim M, et al. Plasma methadone level monitoring in methadone maintenance therapy: a personalised methadone therapy. In: New insights into toxicity and drug testing. 2013.

76. Wolff K, Rostami-Hodjegan A, Hay AW, Raistrick D, Tucker G. Population-based pharmacokinetic approach for methadone monitoring of opiate addicts: potential clinical utility. Addiction. 2000;95:1771–83.

77. Charlier C, Dessalles MC, Plomteux G. Methadone maintenance treatment: is it possible to adapt the daily doses to the metabolic activity of the patient? Ther Drug Monit. 2001;23(1):1–3.

78. Okruhlica L, Valentova J, Devinsky F, Formakova S, Klempova D. Methadone serum concentration and its relationship to methadone dose revisited. Heroin Addict Relat Clin Probl. 2005;7(4):49–57.

79. Souverain S, Eap C, Veuthey J-L, Rudaz S. Automated LC-MS method for the fast stereoselective determination of methadone in plasma. Clin Chem Lab Med. 2003;41(12):1615–21.

80. Chang Y, Fang WB, Lin S, Moody DE. Stereoselective metabolism of methadone by human liver microsomes and cDNA-expressed cytochrome P450s: a reconciliation. Basic Clin Pharmacol Toxicol. 2010;108:55–62.

81. Rodriguez-Rosas ME, Medrano JG, Epstein DH, Moolchan ET, Preston KL, Wainer IW. Determination of total and free concentrations of the enantiomers of methadone and its metabolite (2-ethylidene-1,5-dimethyl-3,3-diphenyl-pyrrolidine) in human plasma by enantioselective liquid chromatography with mass spectrometric detection. J Chromatogr A. 2005;1073(1–2):237–48.

82. Labroo RB, Paine MF, Thummel KE, Kharasch ED. Fentanyl metabolism by human hepatic and intestinal cytochrome P450 3A4: implications for interindividual variability in disposition, efficacy, and drug interactions. Drug Metab Dispos. 1997;25(9):1072–80.

83. Feierman DE, Lasker JM. Metabolism of fentanyl, a synthetic opioid analgesic, by human liver microsomes. Role of CYP3A4. Drug Metab Dispos. 1996;24(9):932–9.

84. Mahlke NS, Ziesenitz V, Mikus G, Skopp G. Quantitative low-volume assay for simultaneous determination of fentanyl, norfentanyl, and minor metabolites in human plasma and urine by liquid chromatography—tandem mass spectrometry (LC-MS/MS). Int J Legal Med. 2014;128(5):771–8. https://doi.org/10.1007/s00414-014-1040-y.

85. Swaminathan SK, Fisher J, Kandimalla KK. Sensitive determination of fentanyl in low-volume serum samples by LC-MS/MS. AAPS PharmSciTech. 2018;19(7):2812–7.

86. Wang G, Huynh K, Barhate R, Rodrigues W, Moore C, Coulter C, et al. Development of a homogeneous immunoassay for the detection of fentanyl in urine. Forensic Sci Int. 2011;206(1–3):127–31.

87. Snyder ML, Jarolim P, Melanson SEF, Flood JG. A new highly specific buprenorphine immunoassay for monitoring buprenorphine compliance and abuse. J Anal Toxicol. 2012;36(3):201–6. https://doi.org/10.1093/jat/bks003.

88. Wang B-T, Colby JM, Wu AHB, Lynch KL. Cross-reactivity of acetylfentanyl and risperidone with a fentanyl immunoassay. J Anal Toxicol. 2014;38(9):672–5. https://doi.org/10.1093/jat/bku103.

89. Barratt MJ, Latimer J, Jauncey M, Tay E, Nielsen S. Urine drug screening for early detection of unwitting use of fentanyl and its analogues among people

who inject heroin in Sydney, Australia. Drug Alcohol Rev. 2018;37(7):847–50.

90. Hull MJ, Bierer MF, Griggs DA, Long WH, Nixon AL, Flood JG. Urinary buprenorphine concentrations in patients treated with Suboxone as determined by liquid chromatography-mass spectrometry and CEDIA immunoassay. J Anal Toxicol. 2008;32(7):516–21.

91. Hand CW, Ryan KE, Dutt SK, Moore RA, O'Connor J, Talbot D, et al. Radioimmunoassay of buprenorphine in urine: studies in patients and in a drug clinic. J Anal Toxicol. 1989;13(2):100–4.

92. Yokell MA, Zaller ND, Green TC, Rich JD. Buprenorphine and buprenorphine/naloxone diversion, misuse, and illicit use: an international review. Curr Drug Abus Rev. 2012;4(1):28–41.

93. Cone EJ, Gorodetzky CW, Yousefnejad D, Buchwald WF, Johnson RE. The metabolism and excretion of buprenorphine in humans. Drug Metab Dispos. 1984;12(5):577–81.

94. Suzuki J, Zinser J, Issa M, Rodriguez C. Quantitative testing of buprenorphine and norbuprenorphine to identify urine sample spiking during office-based opioid treatment. Subst Abus. 2017;38(4):504–7.

95. Tzatzarakis MN, Vakonaki E, Kovatsi L, Belivanis S, Mantsi M, Alegakis A, et al. Determination of buprenorphine, norbuprenorphine and naloxone in fingernail clippings and urine of patients under opioid substitution therapy. J Anal Toxicol. 2015;39(4):313–20.

96. Fareed A. Factors affecting norbuprenorphine level in monitoring clinical outcome for buprenorphine-maintained patients. Addict Disord Treat. 2013;12:167–74.

97. Birch MA, Couchman L, Pietromartire S, Karna T, Paton C, McAllister R, et al. False-positive buprenorphine by CEDIA in patients prescribed amisulpride or sulpiride. J Anal Toxicol. 2013;37(4):233–6.

98. Tenore PL. False-positive buprenorphine EIA urine toxicology results due to high dose morphine: a case report. J Addict Dis. 2012;31(4):329–31.

99. Hamilton HE, Wallace JE, Shimek ELJ, Land P, Harris SC, Christenson JG. Cocaine and benzoylecgonine excretion in humans. J Forensic Sci. 1977;22(4):697–707.

100. Cone EJ, Menchen SL, Paul BD, Mell LD, Mitchell J. Validity testing of commercial urine cocaine metabolite assays: I. assay detection times, individual excretion patterns, and kinetics after cocaine administration to humans. J Forensic Sci. 1989;34(1):15–31.

101. Reichman OS, Otto RA. Effect of intranasal cocaine on the urine drug screen for benzoylecgonine. Otolaryngol Head Neck Surg. 1992;106(3):223–5.

102. Hoes MJ, Vree TB, Guelen P. Gamma-hydroxybutyric acid as hypnotic. Clinical and pharmacokinetic evaluation of gamma-hydroxybutyric acid as hypnotic in man. L'Encéphale. 1980;6:93–9.

103. Kaar SJ, Ferris J, Waldron J, Devaney M, Ramsey J, Winstock AR. Up: the rise of nitrous oxide abuse. An international survey of contemporary nitrous oxide use. J Psychopharmacol. 2016;30(4):395–401.

104. National Drug and Alcohol Research Centre. Australian drug trends 2013, findings from the Ecstasy and Related Drugs Reporting System (EDRS); Key findings, drug trends conference handout [Internet]. 2013. Available from: https://ndarc. med.unsw.edu.au/sites/default/files/ndarc/resources/ Conference handout_National 2013 EDRS findings. pdf.

105. Yuan JL, Wang SK, Jiang T, Hu WL. Nitrous oxide induced subacute combined degeneration with longitudinally extensive myelopathy with inverted V-sign on spinal MRI: a case report and literature review. BMC Neurol. 2017;17(1):222.

106. Stabler SP. Vitamin B12 Deficiency. N Engl J Med. 2013;368(2):149–60. Available from: http://www. nejm.org/doi/10.1056/NEJMcp1113996.

107. Hathout L, El-Saden S. Nitrous oxide-induced B(1) (2) deficiency myelopathy: perspectives on the clinical biochemistry of vitamin B(1)(2). J Neurol Sci. 2011;301(1–2):1–8.

108. Li J-H, Vicknasingam B, Cheung Y-W, Wang Z, Nurhidayat AW, Des Jarlais DC, et al. To use or not to use: an update on licit and illicit ketamine use. Subst Abus Rehabil. 2011;2:11–20.

109. Cheng P-S, Fu C-Y, Lee C-H, Liu C, Chien C-S. GC-MS quantification of ketamine, norketamine, and dehydronorketamine in urine specimens and comparative study using ELISA as the preliminary test methodology. J Chromatogr B Anal Technol Biomed Life Sci. 2007;852(1–2):443–9.

110. Liu CH, Wang HY, Shen SH, Chiu YW. False positive ketamine urine immunoassay screen result induced by quetiapine: a case report. J Formos Med Assoc. 2017;116(9):720–2. Available from: https:// www.sciencedirect.com/science/article/pii/S092966 4616303795?via%3Dihub.

111. Huang M-H, Wu M-Y, Wu C-H, Tsai J-L, Lee H-H, Liu RH. Performance characteristics of ELISAs for monitoring ketamine exposure. Clin Chim Acta. 2007;379(1–2):59–65.

112. Parkin MC, Turfus SC, Smith NW, Halket JM, Braithwaite RA, Elliott SP, et al. Detection of ketamine and its metabolites in urine by ultra high pressure liquid chromatography-tandem mass spectrometry. J Chromatogr B Anal Technol Biomed Life Sci. 2008;876(1):137–42.

113. Marchei E, Pellegrini M, Pichini S, Martin I, Garcia-Algar O, Vall O. Are false-positive phencyclidine immunoassay instant-view multi-test results caused by overdose concentrations of ibuprofen, metamizol, and dextromethorphan? Ther Drug Monit. 2007;29:671–3.

114. Sena SF, Kazimi S, Wu AHB. False-positive phencyclidine immunoassay results caused by venlafaxine and O-desmethylvenlafaxine. Clin Chem. 2002;48:676–7.

115. Farley TM, Anderson EN, Feller JN. False-positive phencyclidine (PCP) on urine drug screen attrib-

uted to desvenlafaxine (Pristiq) use. BMJ Case Rep. 2017;2017:bcr-2017-222106. Available from: http://casereports.bmj.com/content/2017/bcr-2017-222106.abstract.

116. Hull MJ, Griggs D, Knoepp SM, Smogorzewska A, Nixon A, Flood JG. Postmortem urine immunoassay showing false-positive phencyclidine reactivity in a case of fatal tramadol overdose. Am J Forensic Med Pathol. 2006;27(4):359–62.

117. Ly BT, Thornton SL, Buono C, Stone JA, Wu AHB. False-positive urine phencyclidine immunoassay screen result caused by interference by tramadol and its metabolites. Ann Emerg Med. 2012;59(6):545–7. Available from: http://

www.sciencedirect.com/science/article/pii/S0196064411015368.

118. Dolder PC, Schmid Y, Haschke M, Rentsch KM, Liechti ME. Pharmacokinetics and concentration-effect relationship of oral LSD in humans. Int J Neuropsychopharmacol. 2016;19(1):1–7.

119. CEDIA. LSD Assay. Vol. 1732137.

120. Ritter D, Cortese CM, Edwards LC, Barr JL, Chung HD, Long C. Interference with testing for lysergic acid diethylamide. Clin Chem. 1997;43(4):635–7.

121. Röhrich J, Zörntlein S, Lotz J, Becker J, Kern T, Rittner C. False-positive LSD testing in urine samples from intensive care patients. J Anal Toxicol. 1998;22(5):393–5.

Brief Intervention for Illicit Drug Use

45

Jennifer Harland, Susan Henry-Edwards, Linda Gowing, and Robert Ali

Contents

Abstract

Approximately 29.5 million people, or 0.6% of the global adult population, have a drug use disorder (United Nations Office on Drugs and Crime (UNODC), World Drug Report (ISBN: 978–92–1-148291-1, eISBN: 978–92–1-060623-3, United Nations publication, Sales No. E.17.XI.6), 2017). People who use illicit drugs often do not disclose their drug use due to the illegality and stigma associated with that use. The opportunistic nature of brief interventions for illicit drug use makes therapeutic engagement critical to effectiveness. In many settings time will be limited so that brief interventions also need to be efficient.

This chapter focuses on opportunistic brief interventions with people who use illicit drugs and are not engaged in treatment for their drug use. In this context the aim of the brief intervention is to reduce substance use and associated risk behavior as well as to prevent the development of dependence or to motivate the individual to obtain more struc-

J. Harland (✉) · S. Henry-Edwards (✉)
L. Gowing (✉) · R. Ali (✉)
University of Adelaide, Adelaide, SA, Australia
e-mail: jennifer.harland@adelaide.edu.au; susan.henry-edwards@adelaide.edu.au; linda.gowing@adelaide.edu.au; robert.ali@adelaide.edu.au

© Springer Nature Switzerland AG 2021
N. el-Guebaly et al. (eds.), *Textbook of Addiction Treatment*,
https://doi.org/10.1007/978-3-030-36391-8_45

tured treatment for their drug use. The objective is to reduce the overall burden of drug-related harms in the community or in particular target groups by identifying individuals who are experiencing, or are at risk of developing, drug use problems, to raise awareness of potential drug-related harms, and to intervene early before problems have developed or become severe. Brief interventions are part of a public health approach to drug use problems [3, 21].

This chapter provides practical information on the conduct of effective brief interventions covering the general approach to brief interventions, responding to the stage of change, and assessing risk.

Keywords

Brief intervention · Screening · Illicit drugs
ASSIST · Stages of change · FRAMES model
SBIRT

45.1   Introduction

Substance use is one of the major preventable causes of disease and disability [31]. Alcohol and tobacco are by far the most prevalent substances used globally [26], but the prevalence of illicit drug use is still substantial. In 2015 an estimated quarter of a billion people, or around 5% of the global adult population, used illicit drugs at least once [31]. Cannabis was the most commonly used drug, with a reported 183 million users globally. Amphetamine and prescription stimulants were used by 37 million people, and 35 million people used illicit opioids [31].

The magnitude of harm caused by illicit drug use is substantial and has increased over the last decade. In 2015 an estimated 28 million years of "healthy" life (disability-adjusted life years (DALYs)) were lost worldwide as a result of premature death and disability caused by drug use. Of those years lost, 17 million were attributable solely to drug use disorders, across all drug types. Around 70% of the global burden of disease

caused by drug use disorders is attributable to opioid use [31], reflecting the high risk of overdose associated with opioid use and the transmission of blood-borne viruses (HIV and hepatitis C) through use by injection [11].

Treatment is effective in reducing illicit drug use, reducing risk behaviors and improving physical and mental well-being, but fewer than one in six persons with drug use disorders are provided with treatment each year. In part this reflects limited availability of and access to appropriate treatments [31], but it is also likely to reflect the hidden nature of illicit drug use.

The stigma associated with illicit drug use, and possible legal implications, means that people who use illicit drugs may be reluctant to disclose their use. They may not be aware of the risks of harm associated with their substance use and not see the connection to negative consequences. For all these reasons, people who use illicit drugs rarely seek treatment unless pushed by a crisis of some sort – legal, financial, family pressure, or acute health effects.

This is where brief interventions come in. Brief interventions have been used in a variety of ways, including as adjuncts to structured treatment for alcohol and other drug problems and to reduce risk behaviors in specific populations such as people with HIV. Brief interventions have also been used to structure brief conversations about healthcare in general [6]. In this chapter we are focusing on opportunistic brief interventions with people who use illicit drugs and are not engaged in treatment for their drug use. In this context the aim of the brief intervention is to reduce substance use and associated risk behavior as well as to prevent the development of dependence or to motivate the individual to obtain more structured treatment for their drug use. The objective is to reduce the overall burden of drug-related harms in the community or in particular target groups by identifying individuals who are experiencing, or are at risk of developing, drug use problems, to raise awareness of potential drug-related harms and to intervene early before problems have developed or become severe. Brief interventions are part of a public health approach to drug use problems [4, 21].

Brief interventions can take place in various settings, such as primary healthcare, and can be implemented by a variety of trained healthcare providers. They are low in cost and time efficient and can be effective across many levels of hazardous and harmful drug use. This makes brief interventions ideally suited for use as a method of health promotion and disease prevention with primary care patients [16, 34].

The opportunistic nature of brief interventions for illicit drug use makes therapeutic engagement critical to effectiveness. In many settings time will be limited so that brief interventions also need to be efficient.

Brief interventions are most useful for those who are at low to moderate risk of drug-related harm. They are not intended as a stand-alone treatment for people with significant drug use disorders although a brief intervention can increase the proportion of patients identified as high risk or dependent who subsequently attend their first appointment at a specialist drug and alcohol treatment facility [3, 18]. Hence it is important to tailor the intervention to the individual by reflecting the risk of drug-related harm. Another important aspect of tailoring the intervention to the individual is taking account of the person's current stage of behavioral change.

There is moderately good evidence for the effectiveness of brief interventions in primary care settings for alcohol and tobacco [22, 30] and growing evidence for other drugs.

Brief interventions consist of feedback about personal risk, explicit advice on change, and emphasis on individual responsibility for change and provide a variety of ways to effect change. Brief interventions in primary care can range from five minutes of brief advice to 15–30 minutes of brief counselling [24]. Shorter duration interventions are typically the requirement in acute care settings where time may be particularly limited.

This chapter provides practical information on the conduct of effective brief interventions covering the general approach to brief interventions (Sect. 45.2), responding to the stage of change (Sect. 45.3), and assessing risk (Sect. 45.4).

45.2 General Approach to Brief Interventions

The aim of a brief intervention is to help the person understand that their substance use is putting them at risk and to encourage them to reduce or give up their substance use. Brief interventions should be personalized and offered in a supportive, nonjudgmental manner. Brief intervention techniques include an empathetic style and support for the person's perception of self-efficacy or optimism that they can change [32].

A number of brief intervention models have been developed, based on principles of motivational interviewing. These include the Brief Negotiated Interview (BNI) [8]; "FLO" – Feedback, Listen, Options [12]; and the 5 As (ask, assess, advise, assist, and arrange follow-up) that are widely implemented for smoking cessation [29].

Experience and research into brief interventions for substance use have found that effective brief interventions comprise a number of consistent and recurring features. These features have been summarized using the acronym FRAMES: feedback, responsibility, advice, menu of options, empathy, and self-efficacy [25]. The FRAMES model is considered in detail here as it is used extensively in brief interventions for alcohol and other drug use and is the approach we recommend for people who use illicit drugs.

Feedback of Personal Status Relative to Norms

Feedback is the provision of personally relevant information which is pertinent to the individual and is delivered in a non-judgemental and objective way in the Spirit of Motivational Interviewing [25]. The provision of personally relevant feedback (as opposed to general feedback) is a key component of a brief intervention. This includes information about the individual's substance use, the level of risk associated with their use, and the benefits of reducing or stopping use.

Information about personal risks associated with current drug use patterns (e.g., low mood, anxiety, relationship problems, health problems) combined with general information about substance-related risks and harms comprises powerful feedback.

Responsibility for Personal Change

A key principle of an effective brief intervention is to acknowledge and accept that a person is responsible for their own behavior and will make choices about their substance use. Adopting phrases such as *"Are you interested in seeing how you scored on this questionnaire?"* and *"What you do with this information I'm giving you is up to you"* enables the person to retain control over their behavior and its consequences and the direction of the intervention. This sense of control has been found to be an important element in motivation for change [24]. Using language such as *"I think you should…"* may create resistance in the interaction and not be beneficial to behavior change.

Advice to Change

A central component of effective brief interventions is the provision of clear objective advice regarding how to reduce the harms associated with continued use. This needs to be delivered in a non-judgemental manner and in the Spirit of Motivational Interviewing. People may be unaware that their current pattern of substance use could lead to problems or make existing issues worse. Ask permission to give advice and then provide clear, objective information. Explain that cutting down or stopping substance use is the best way to reduce their risk of harms both now and in the future. This will increase their awareness of their personal risk and provide reasons to consider changing their behavior.

Advice can be summed up by delivering a simple statement such as *"the best way you can reduce your risk of* (e.g. depression, anxiety, injuries) *is to cut down or stop using."* This is best followed by an open-ended question to help explore the person's readiness to change. Once again, the language used to deliver this message is an important feature and comments such as *"I think you should stop using substances"* does not provide clear, objective advice nor promote further discussion.

Menu of Options from Which to Choose in Pursuing Change

Effective brief interventions provide the individual with a range or menu of options to cut down or stop their substance use in the pursuit of change. This allows the individual to choose the strategies which are most suitable for their situation and which they feel will be most helpful. Providing choices reinforces the sense of personal control and responsibility for making change and can help to strengthen the person's motivation for change.

Examples of options for clients to consider include

- Keeping a diary of substance use (where, when, how much used, how much spent, with whom, why)
- Identifying high-risk thoughts and beliefs and challenging them
- Identifying high-risk associates and situations and exploring alternate strategies
- Identifying other activities instead of drug use (constructive use of leisure)—education, volunteering, hobbies, sports, gym, etc.
- Identifying non-drug rewards and pleasurable activities
- Identifying people who could provide support and help for the changes they want to make
- Attending a self-help or peer support groups
- Putting aside the money they would normally spend on substances for something else
- Setting goals and working toward achieving them

You can also assist by

- Providing information about other self-help resources and written information
- Providing information about groups or programs that specialize in drug and alcohol issues

Empathic Counselor Style

Empathy is taking an active interest and effort to understand another's internal perspective, to see the world through their eyes. It does not mean sympathy, a feeling of pity, camaraderie, or identification with the person. Statements such as

"I've been there and know what you are experiencing, let me tell you my story" are not useful. The opposite of empathy is the imposition of one's own perspective, perhaps with the assumption that the other's views are irrelevant or misguided. Empathy is the ability to understand another's frame of reference and the conviction that it is worthwhile to do so [23].

In a brief intervention, empathy comprises an accepting, nonjudgmental approach that seeks to understand the individual's point of view. It is especially important to avoid confrontation and blaming or criticism of the individual. Adopting a position of *curious intrigue* is helpful. Skilful reflective listening which clarifies and amplifies the person's experience and meaning is a fundamental part of expressing empathy. The empathy and understanding of the professional are important contributors to how well the individual responds to the intervention [25].

Support for Self-Efficacy

The final component of effective brief interventions is to encourage the person's confidence that they are able to make changes in their substance use. Exploring other areas where the individual has made positive change is helpful. People who believe that they are likely to make positive changes are more likely to do so than those who feel powerless or helpless to change their behaviour. It is particularly helpful to elicit self-efficacy statements from individuals as they are likely to believe what they hear themselves say, and belief in the possibility of change is an important motivator.

45.3   Linking to Stage of Behavioral Change

Brief interventions are structured and personalized discussions which aim to motivate clients to undertake positive behavior change. The transtheoretical model of behavior change developed by Prochaska and DiClemente presents behavioral change as occurring in distinct stages [27]. The aim of intervention is to support people to move through the stages of change. While a person's stage of change may not be formally mea-

sured or assessed, interventions that are tailored to the likely stage of change may be more effective.

The transtheoretical model of behavior change proposes several stages (pre-contemplation, contemplation, preparation, action, and maintenance). The model identifies a number of stages which are commonly experienced during the process of adopting a new behavior. Progression is not necessarily linear, and the time spent in each stage is highly variable.

People in the *pre-contemplation* stage generally do not link their substance use to any problems. Commonly, they are unconcerned by their drug use or related consequences and are not yet considering a change or are unwilling to change. Motivational interviewing strategies are appropriate for this stage of change. Such strategies involve exploration of both the pros and cons of substance use and development of discrepancies between a client's current behaviors and future ambitions/goals.

In the *contemplation* stage, the person acknowledges concerns and is considering the possibility of change but is still ambivalent or uncertain about that change. Motivational interviewing is again appropriate, with the aim of normalizing feelings of ambivalence and helping the client to move toward change.

In the *preparation* stage, the balance has shifted. Change is seen as worthwhile, and the person is gaining confidence in their capacity to change. The person is preparing to take action by gathering information that will assist them. The negative consequences of drug use are now seen as outweighing the benefits. The focus should be on helping the person consider barriers to change and ways to overcome those barriers, exploring options, eliciting from the person what has worked in the past for them or others, and assisting the client to enlist social support.

In the *action* stage, the person is actively taking steps to change but has not yet reached a stable state. They are implementing strategies to change their drug use pattern. It is important to support their engagement in change, reinforce the importance of remaining committed, and help to find new reinforcers of positive change, including assessment of the strength of family and other social supports.

In the *maintenance* stage, the person has succeeded in stopping their harmful drug use and is concentrating on continuing that progress. The focus in this stage is on building resilience, self-monitoring, identifying high-risk situations, and developing appropriate coping skills. It is important to affirm the person's resolve and self-efficacy and review long-term goals. It is helpful to encourage them to articulate the positive reasons for maintaining change to reinforce their decisions and reaffirm relapse prevention approaches.

A *relapse* (or lapse – a one off or short period) is a return to the old behavior that was the focus of change. Most people who try to make changes in their substance use behavior may relapse to substance use, at least for a time. This should be viewed as a learning process rather than failure. Few people change on the first attempt, and relapse is an opportunity to help people review their action plan. A review should examine time frames, what strategies did actually work, and whether the strategies used were realistic. For many people, changing their substance use gets easier each time they try until they are eventually successful.

Most people identified opportunistically for brief interventions aimed at illicit drug use are likely to be mainly in the pre-contemplation stage, with some in contemplation. The aim of brief interventions for people engaged in the least amount of change is to help them understand that their drug use is putting them at risk and to develop ambivalence about their drug use that would then lead to them preparing to take action to change their drug use.

The principles outlined here can also be adapted for people preparing for change but who lack the confidence and knowledge and for clients who are in the action stage.

45.4 Assessing Level of Risk

A wide variety of standardized questionnaires and biological tests have been developed to detect psychoactive substance use [3]. Biological tests are generally not suitable for routine screening prior to brief intervention as they are costly, invasive, can only detect recent use, and results are not available immediately. A major shortcoming of biological screening is that biological tests fail to assess a person's pattern of use and level of risk of harm or dependence and so do not provide a foundation for brief intervention. Hence, assessing a person's level of risk to inform a brief intervention will generally involve use of a screening instrument.

Many of the available screening instruments are specific to alcohol (e.g., AUDIT) or tobacco (e.g., Fagerstrom). The Alcohol, Smoking and Substance Involvement Screening Test (ASSIST) was developed under the auspices of the World Health Organization (WHO) by an international group of specialist addiction researchers and clinicians in response to the overwhelming public health burden associated with psychoactive substance use worldwide [19] and offers the advantage of screening for alcohol, tobacco, illicit drugs, and the unsanctioned use of pharmaceutical drugs.

Other characteristics that should be considered when selecting a screening instrument to assess risk prior to a brief intervention include —

- Acceptability: The instrument should be acceptable to both health workers and those being screened in terms of safety, simplicity, and ease and time of administration.
- Reliability/repeatability: The instrument must give consistent results when repeated more than once on the same individual under the same conditions. It should also give consistent results when administered by different people (inter-rater reliability).
- Validity: The instrument must accurately measure what it purports to measure (construct validity) and accurately separate those who have the condition from those who do not (discriminant validity). Discriminant validity has two components, sensitivity and specificity.
  - Sensitivity is the ability of the instrument to identify correctly those who have the condition, that is, "true positives."
  - Specificity is the ability of the instrument to identify correctly those who do not have the condition, that is, "true negatives."

- In the context of brief interventions for illicit drug use, sensitivity should be emphasized over specificity so as to minimize the possibility of not identifying people at risk of harm from their drug use.
- Cost which will depend on whether the instrument is self-administered or administered by a health worker or clinician, how long it takes, and what special training (if any) is required.
- Non-judgemental and non-confrontational: This is important so that people feel able to report their drug use.
- Culturally neutral: A culturally neutral screening test will have wider acceptability with different populations both nationally and internationally.

45.4.1 The Alcohol, Smoking and Substance Involvement Screening Test (ASSIST)

The ASSIST V3.1 (Appendix A) is an eight-item questionnaire designed to be either self-administered or by a health worker. For most people, the ASSIST can be completed in about five minutes and can be incorporated into routine consultation. The ASSIST is available as a web-based version which can be self-administered or administered by a health worker and as a smartphone/tablet application for self-administration (https://assistportal.com.au/).

The ASSIST has been through rigorous scientific testing to ensure that it is a reliable and valid instrument in international settings and able to link into a brief intervention [20]. The ASSIST has shown good cross-cultural neutrality, has been validated for use in adult populations (between 18 and 60 years of age), and is appropriate for use with adolescents.

The ASSIST obtains information about lifetime and recent use (last three months) of the following substances:

- Tobacco
- Alcohol
- Cannabis
- Cocaine
- Amphetamine-type stimulants (ATS)

- Inhalants
- Sedatives and sleeping pills (benzodiazepines)
- Hallucinogens
- Inhalants
- Opioids
- "Other drugs"

"Other" drugs are those that do not readily belong in any of the other drug categories. This could include Kava, Datura, Khat, Kratom, gamma hydroxybutyrate (GHB), and any other drugs of concern in the local population. There may be other substances native to some regions which don't easily fit into any of the other substance classes and need to be put into this "other drugs" category.

The ASSIST can identify a range of issues related to substance use including the risks associated with acute intoxication, regular use, dependent or "high risk," use and injecting behavior. Taken together, these questions provide an indication of the level of risk associated with the person's substance use and whether use is hazardous and likely to be causing harm (now or in the future) if use continues.

The score obtained for each substance falls into a "low," "moderate," or "high' risk category. Scores in the mid-range on the ASSIST are likely to indicate hazardous or harmful substance use ("moderate risk"), and higher scores are likely to indicate substance dependence ("high risk"). The level of risk determines the most appropriate intervention for that level of use ("no treatment," "brief intervention," or "referral to specialist assessment and treatment," respectively).

45.4.2 Linking Assessed Risk to a Brief Intervention

The ASSIST-linked Brief Intervention was specifically designed for people who are at *moderate risk* from their substance use, according to their ASSIST scores, to provide them with a structured appropriate brief intervention depending on their stage of change, that is, people who are *not* dependent, but are using substances in a risky, hazardous, or harmful way that may be creating health, social, legal, occupational, or financial problems for the person or has the potential to create those problems should the substance use continue.

The ASSIST-linked Brief Intervention is based on the FRAMES model and motivational interviewing techniques. It follows ten main steps:

1. *Asking* if they are interested in seeing their questionnaire scores
2. Providing personalized *Feedback* to clients about their scores using the ASSIST Feedback Report Card
3. Giving *Advice* about how to reduce risk associated with substance use
4. Allowing people to take ultimate *Responsibility* for their choices
5. Asking how *Concerned* they are by their scores
6. Weighing up the *Good things* about using the substance against the
7. *Less good things* about using the substance
8. *Summarizing and Reflecting* on statements about their substance use with emphasis on the less good things
9. Asking how *Concerned* they are by the less good things
10. Giving clients *Take-home materials* to bolster the brief intervention

The suggested ten-step ASSIST-linked Brief Intervention is particularly appropriate for clients who are in the contemplation or pre-contemplation stage of change.

While the majority of people screened in primary care settings are likely to be at low to moderate risk of substance related harm, a proportion will be at high risk and may have a substance use disorder (including dependence). Brief interventions are not intended as a stand-alone intervention for people who are dependent or at "high risk" from their substance use. However, a brief intervention should be used to encourage such people to accept referral to specialized drug and alcohol assessment and treatment, either within a primary care setting or at a specialized alcohol and drug treatment agency.

45.4.3 The ASSIST-Lite

Translating the ASSIST into routine use in health services has proved problematic. Substance use disorders are not systematically screened, diagnosed, or treated in general medical settings, and time constraints on staff appear to be the main barrier [1]. In 2008, an American Preventive Service Task Force called for a research and development initiative to *provide questionnaires short enough to be potentially useful in the practice setting with acceptable accuracy and reliability*. The ASSIST-Lite was developed to address this need and is ideally suited for opportunistic and routine screening for substance use in primary, general medical, and welfare service settings [1].

The ASSIST-Lite is a short form of the ASSIST. The ASSIST-Lite screens for risk of harm from substance use, specifically, tobacco, alcohol, cannabis, stimulants including amphetamine-type stimulants, and cocaine, sedatives, and opioids including prescription opioids. There is also the opportunity to ask about any other psychoactive substance not listed. The ASSIST-Lite identifies which substances are of concern and gives an indication of the severity of substance-related risks and harms. Consequently, it can form a valuable part of a comprehensive health assessment.

The ASSIST-Lite risk score refers to risk of harm from current patterns of substance use. Harm is broadly defined and includes health, legal, social, financial, work, and family issues. The risk of harm score for each substance helps to initiate and frame a brief discussion with individuals about their substance use. Like the full ASSIST, the score obtained from the ASSIST-Lite for each substance falls into a "low," "moderate," or "high' risk category which determines the most appropriate linked brief intervention for that level of use.

A copy of the ASSIST-Lite is included in Appendix B. The ASSIST-Lite is available as a web-based platform and as a smartphone/tablet application for self-completion (available at https://assistportal.com.au/).

The ASSIST and ASSIST-Lite can be read-ministered after three months to monitor progress and changes over time. Interventions can be stepped up if the score has increased, and the Brief Intervention can be used to intervene early if it appears that other issues are developing.

45.5 Settings for Brief Intervention

Primary care settings such as general practice, community health centers, and other local health services are the first point of contact with the health system for most people. Primary care provides a wide range of services including health promotion, prevention and screening, early intervention, treatment, and management of a variety of chronic health conditions. This includes preventive activities such as immunization, as well as screening and early intervention for high blood pressure, obesity, high cholesterol, and other lifestyle risk factors. Screening and brief intervention for illicit drug use fit well with this role.

In the developed world, 85% of the population visit a primary healthcare clinician such as a general practitioner at least once a year [10], and there is evidence that people who have substance use-related problems have more frequent consultations [5, 17]. Widespread screening in primary care settings increases the likelihood of identifying and intervening with people who use illicit drugs. As a result of their position in the healthcare system, primary care clinicians are likely to see a wide cross-section of the community and hence are more likely to see people at an earlier stage in their drug use when risk and harm are lower. They have a unique opportunity to provide comprehensive, continuing, and person-centered healthcare as well as to link those in need to specialist services when required.

Primary care workers often have an ongoing relationship with clients of their service which enables them to develop rapport and demonstrate genuine concern for their welfare. People expect their primary care clinician to be involved in all aspects of their health and are likely to feel more comfortable about discussing sensitive issues such as drug use with someone they know and trust. The ongoing nature of the relationship means that such discussions can be spread out over time and form part of a number of consultations. Specialist drug and alcohol services may be associated with stigma which can deter some people from seeking assistance for substance use problems. Primary healthcare settings are not associated with this stigma making people more likely to attend a primary care service.

People who use alcohol and other drugs are also over represented in hospital emergency care presentations [14]. Australian research found that while alcohol is the most common substance used by intoxicated people who attend the emergency department, the contribution of other drugs is substantial [15].

Attendance at an emergency department is often a time of crisis when patients may be more willing to accept help and advice [8, 13, 33]. A brief intervention delivered in the context of presentation to a hospital emergency department can be used to help the patient gain insight into the consequences of their substance use and may be a motivating factor to encourage behavioral change [8] or engagement in structured treatment. Interventions in the emergency setting would have a public health aim [7], with those presenting in emergency department comprising a higher-risk population [28].

Providing brief interventions for substance use to people presenting to hospital emergency departments has the potential to facilitate management and discharge of some patients and may reduce the likelihood of repeat presentations [2, 9].

Screening and brief intervention can also be undertaken in specialist medical services such as mental health services and sexual health services where substance use is more prevalent than in the general population. A number of services worldwide have embedded the ASSIST and linked brief intervention into their routine practice demonstrating the feasibility of implementing brief interventions for illicit drug use in a wide range of contexts.

Appendix A: WHO - ASSIST V3.1

WHO - ASSIST V3.1

CLINICIAN NAME		CLINIC	
CLIENT ID OR NAME		DATE	

INTRODUCTION (Please read to client. Can be adapted for local circumstances)

The following questions ask about your experience of using alcohol, tobacco products and other drugs across your lifetime and in the past three months. These substances can be smoked, swallowed, snorted, inhaled or injected (show responsecard).

Some of the substances listed may be prescribed by a doctor (like amphetamines, sedatives, pain medications). For this interview, we will not record medications that are used as prescribed by your doctor. However, if you have taken such medications for reasons other than prescription, or taken them more frequently, at higher doses than prescribed or in ways in which it wasn't intended, please let me know.

While we are also interested in knowing about your use of various illicit drugs, please be assured that information on such use will be treated as strictly confidential.

NOTE: BEFORE ASKING QUESTIONS, GIVE ASSIST RESPONSE CARD TO CLIENT

Question 1 (please mark the response for each category of substance)

In your life, which of the following substances have you **ever used?** *(NON-MEDICAL USE ONLY)*	No	Yes
a. Tobacco products (cigarettes, chewing tobacco, cigars, etc.)	☐	☐
b. Alcoholic beverages (beer, wine, spirits, etc.)	☐	☐
c. Cannabis (marijuana, pot, grass, hash, etc.)	☐	☐
d. Cocaine (coke, crack, etc.)	☐	☐
e. Amphetamine type stimulants (speed, meth, ecstasy, etc.)	☐	☐
f. Inhalants (nitrous, glue, petrol, paint thinner, etc.)	☐	☐
g. Sedatives or Sleeping Pills (Diazepam, Alprazolam, Flunitrazepam, Midazolam etc.)	☐	☐
h. Hallucinogens (LSD, acid, mushrooms, trips, Ketamine, etc.)	☐	☐
i. Opioids (heroin, morphine, methadone, Buprenorphine, codeine, etc.)	☐	☐
j. Other - specify:	☐	☐

Probe if all answers are negative: **"Not even when you were in school?"**	*If "No" to all items, stop interview.* *If "Yes" to any of these items, ask Question 2 for each substance ever used.*

Question 2

In the past three months, how often have you used the substances you mentioned (FIRST DRUG, SECOND DRUG, ETC)?	Never	Once or Twice	Monthly	Weekly	Daily or Almost Daily
a. Tobacco products (cigarettes, chewing tobacco, cigars, etc.)	0	2	3	4	6
b. Alcoholic beverages (beer, wine, spirits, etc.)	0	2	3	4	6
c. Cannabis (marijuana, pot, grass, hash, etc.)	0	2	3	4	6
d. Cocaine (coke, crack, etc.)	0	2	3	4	6
e. Amphetamine type stimulants (speed, meth, ecstasy, etc.)	0	2	3	4	6
f. Inhalants (nitrous, glue, petrol, paint thinner, etc.)	0	2	3	4	6
g. Sedatives or Sleeping Pills (Diazepam, Alprazolam, Flunitrazepam, Midazolam etc.)	0	2	3	4	6
h. Hallucinogens (LSD, acid, mushrooms, trips, Ketamine, etc.)	0	2	3	4	6
i. Opioids (heroin, morphine, methadone, codeine, etc.)	0	2	3	4	6
j. Other - specify:	0	2	3	4	6

If "Never" to all items in Question 2, skip to Question 6.

If any substances in Question 2 were used in the previous three months, continue with Questions 3, 4 & 5 for each substance used.

Question 3

During the past three months, how often have you had a strong desire or urge to use (FIRST DRUG, SECOND DRUG, ETC)?	Never	Once or Twice	Monthly	Weekly	Daily or Almost Daily
a. Tobacco products (cigarettes, chewing tobacco, cigars, etc.)	0	3	4	5	6
b. Alcoholic beverages (beer, wine, spirits, etc.)	0	3	4	5	6
c. Cannabis (marijuana, pot, grass, hash, etc.)	0	3	4	5	6
d. Cocaine (coke, crack, etc.)	0	3	4	5	6
e. Amphetamine type stimulants (speed, meth, ecstasy, etc.)	0	3	4	5	6
f. Inhalants (nitrous, glue, petrol, paint thinner, etc.)	0	3	4	5	6
g. Sedatives or Sleeping Pills (Diazepam, Alprazolam, Flunitrazepam, Midazolam etc.)	0	3	4	5	6
h. Hallucinogens (LSD, acid, mushrooms, trips, Ketamine, etc.)	0	3	4	5	6
i. Opioids (heroin, morphine, methadone, codeine, etc.)	0	3	4	5	6
j. Other - specify:	0	3	4	5	6

Question 4

During the <u>past three months,</u> how often has your use of *(FIRST DRUG, SECOND DRUG, ETC)* led to health, social, legal or financial problems?	Never	Once or Twice	Monthly	Weekly	Daily or Almost Daily
a. Tobacco products (cigarettes, chewing tobacco, cigars, etc.)	0	4	5	6	7
b. Alcoholic beverages (beer, wine, spirits, etc.)	0	4	5	6	7
c. Cannabis (marijuana, pot, grass, hash, etc.)	0	4	5	6	7
d. Cocaine (coke, crack, etc.)	0	4	5	6	7
e. Amphetamine type stimulants (speed, meth, ecstasy, etc.)	0	4	5	6	7
f. Inhalants (nitrous, glue, petrol, paint thinner, etc.)	0	4	5	6	7
g. Sedatives or Sleeping Pills (Diazepam, Alprazolam, Flunitrazepam, Midazolam etc.)	0	4	5	6	7
h. Hallucinogens (LSD, acid, mushrooms, trips, Ketamine, etc.)	0	4	5	6	7
i. Opioids (heroin, morphine, methadone, codeine, etc.)	0	4	5	6	7
j. Other - specify:	0	4	5	6	7

Question 5

During the <u>past three months</u>, how often have you failed to do what was normally expected of you because of your use of *(FIRST DRUG, SECOND DRUG, ETC)*?	Never	Once or Twice	Monthly	Weekly	Daily or Almost Daily
a. Tobacco products	/////////	/////////	/////////	/////////	/////////
b. Alcoholic beverages (beer, wine, spirits, etc.)	0	5	6	7	8
c. Cannabis (marijuana, pot, grass, hash, etc.)	0	5	6	7	8
d. Cocaine (coke, crack, etc.)	0	5	6	7	8
e. Amphetamine type stimulants (speed, meth, ecstasy, etc.)	0	5	6	7	8
f. Inhalants (nitrous, glue, petrol, paint thinner, etc.)	0	5	6	7	8
g. Sedatives or Sleeping Pills (Diazepam, Alprazolam, Flunitrazepam, Midazolam etc.)	0	5	6	7	8
h. Hallucinogens (LSD, acid, mushrooms, trips, Ketamine, etc.)	0	5	6	7	8
i. Opioids (heroin, morphine, methadone, codeine, etc.)	0	5	6	7	8
j. Other - specify:	0	5	6	7	8

Ask Questions 6 & 7 for all substances ever used (i.e. those endorsed in Question 1)

Question 6

Has a friend or relative or anyone else <u>ever</u> expressed concern about your use of *(FIRST DRUG, SECOND DRUG, ETC.)?*	No, Never	Yes, in the past 3 months	Yes, but not in the past 3 months
a. Tobacco products (cigarettes, chewing tobacco, cigars, etc.)	0	6	3
b. Alcoholic beverages (beer, wine, spirits, etc.)	0	6	3
c. Cannabis (marijuana, pot, grass, hash, etc.)	0	6	3
d. Cocaine (coke, crack, etc.)	0	6	3
e. Amphetamine type stimulants (speed, meth, ecstasy, etc.)	0	6	3
f. Inhalants (nitrous, glue, petrol, paint thinner, etc.)	0	6	3
g. Sedatives or Sleeping Pills (Diazepam, Alprazolam, Flunitrazepam, Midazolam etc.)	0	6	3
h. Hallucinogens (LSD, acid, mushrooms, trips, Ketamine, etc.)	0	6	3
i. Opioids (heroin, morphine, methadone, codeine, etc.)	0	6	3
j. Other – specify:	0	6	3

Question 7

Have you <u>ever</u> tried to cut down on using *(FIRST DRUG, SECOND DRUG, ETC.)* but failed?	No, Never	Yes, in the past 3 months	Yes, but not in the past 3 months
a. Tobacco products (cigarettes, chewing tobacco, cigars, etc.)	0	6	3
b. Alcoholic beverages (beer, wine, spirits, etc.)	0	6	3
c. Cannabis (marijuana, pot, grass, hash, etc.)	0	6	3
d. Cocaine (coke, crack, etc.)	0	6	3
e. Amphetamine type stimulants (speed, meth, ecstasy, etc.)	0	6	3
f. Inhalants (nitrous, glue, petrol, paint thinner, etc.)	0	6	3
g. Sedatives or Sleeping Pills (Diazepam, Alprazolam, Flunitrazepam, Midazolam etc.)	0	6	3
h. Hallucinogens (LSD, acid, mushrooms, trips, Ketamine, etc.)	0	6	3
i. Opioids (heroin, morphine, methadone, codeine, etc.)	0	6	3
j. Other – specify:	0	6	3

Question 8 (please mark the response)

	No, Never	Yes, in the past 3 months	Yes, but not in the past 3 months
Have you **ever** used any drug by injection? *(NON-MEDICAL USE ONLY)*	☐	☐	☐

IMPORTANT NOTE:

Clients who have injected drugs in the last 3 months should be asked about their pattern of injecting during this period, to determine their risk levels and the best course of intervention.

PATTERN OF INJECTING   INTERVENTION GUIDELINES

4 days per month, on average, over the last 3 months or less	→	Brief Intervention including the "Risks of Injecting" card

More than 4 days per month, on average, over the last 3 months	→	Further assessment and more intensive treatment*

HOW TO CALCULATE A SPECIFIC SUBSTANCE INVOLVEMENT SCORE.

For each substance (labelled a. to j.) add up the scores received for questions 2 through 7 inclusive. Do not include the results from either Q1 or Q8 in this score. For example, a score for cannabis would be calculated r example, a score for cannabis would be calculated as: **Q2c + Q3c + Q4c + Q5c + Q6c + Q7c**

Note that Q5 for tobacco is not coded, and is calculated as: **Q2a + Q3a + Q4a + Q6a + Q7a**

THE TYPE OF INTERVENTION IS DETERMINED BY THE PATIENT'S SPECIFIC SUBSTANCE INVOLVEMENT SCORE

	Record specific substance score	no intervention	receive brief intervention	more intensive treatment *
a. tobacco		0 - 3	4 - 26	27+
b. alcohol		0 - 10	11 - 26	27+
c. cannabis		0 - 3	4 - 26	27+
d. cocaine		0 - 3	4 - 26	27+
e. amphetamine		0 - 3	4 - 26	27+
f. inhalants		0 - 3	4 - 26	27+
g. sedatives		0 - 3	4 - 26	27+
h. hallucinogens		0 - 3	4 - 26	27+
i. opioids		0 - 3	4 - 26	27+
j. other drugs		0 - 3	4 - 26	27+

Now use ASSIST FEEDBACK REPORT CARD to give client brief intervention.

Appendix B: ASSIST-Lite

Alcohol, Smoking and Substance Involvement Screening Test
ASSIST-Lite

Instructions

The questions ask about psychoactive substance use in the PAST 3 MONTHS ONLY.

Ask about each substance in order and only proceed to the supplementary questions if the person has used that substance.

On completion of all the questions, count the number of "yes" responses to obtain a score for each substance, and mark the risk category.

Provide a brief intervention relevant to the risk category.

In the past 3 months	YES	NO
1. Did you smoke a cigarette containing tobacco?	☐	☐
1a. Did you usually smoke more than 10 cigarettes each day?	☐	☐
1b. Did you usually smoke within 30 minutes after waking?	☐	☐
Score for tobacco (count "yes" answers)		
Risk category: ☐ Low (0) ☐ Moderate (1 or 2) ☐High (3)		
2. Did you have a drink containing alcohol?	☐	☐
2a. On any occasion, did you drink more than 4 standard drinks of alcohol?	☐	☐
2b. Have you tried and failed to control, cut down or stop drinking?	☐	☐
2c. Has anyone expressed concern about your drinking?	☐	☐
Score for alcohol (count "yes" answers)		
Risk category: ☐ Low (0 or 1) ☐Moderate (2)☐ High (3 or 4)		
3. Did you use cannabis?	☐	☐
3a. Have you had a strong desire or urge to use cannabis at least once a week or more often?	☐	☐
3b. Has anyone expressed concern about your use of cannabis?	☐	☐
Score for cannabis (count "yes" answers)		
Risk category: ☐ Low (0) ☐ Moderate (1 or 2) ☐High (3)		
4. Did you use an amphetamine-type stimulant, or cocaine, or a stimulant medication not as prescribed?	☐	☐
4a. Did you use a stimulant at least once each week or more often?	☐	☐
4b. Has anyone expressed concern about your use of a stimulant?	☐	☐
Score for stimulants (count "yes" answers)		
Risk category: ☐ Low (0) ☐ Moderate (1 or 2) ☐High (3)		
5. Did you use a sedative or sleeping medication not as prescribed?	☐	☐
5a. Have you had a strong desire or urge to use a sedative or sleeping medication at least once a week or more often?	☐	☐
5b. Has anyone expressed concern about your use of a sedative or sleeping medication?	☐	☐
Score for sedatives (count "yes" answers)		
Risk category: ☐ Low (0) ☐ Moderate (1 or 2) ☐High (3)		
6. Did you use a street opioid (e.g. heroin) or an opioid-containing medication not as prescribed?	☐	☐
6a. Have you tried and failed to control, cut down or stop using an opioid?	☐	☐
6b. Has anyone expressed concern about your use of an opioid?	☐	☐
Score for opioids (count "yes" answers)		
Risk category: ☐ Low (0) ☐ Moderate (1 or 2) ☐High (3)		
7. Did you use any other psychoactive substances?	☐	☐
If yes, what did you take?		
(Not scored, but prompts further assessment)		

Rapid guide to a Brief Intervention

Low risk: General health advice and encourage not to increase use.

Moderate risk: Provide a brief intervention using the FRAMES Model and offer take home information

High risk: Provide a brief intervention using the FRAMES Model and encourage further assessment by a specialist drug and alochol service. Facilitate referral and provide take home information.

Note: FRAMES - Feedback, Responsibility, Advice, Menu of options, Empathy, Self-efficacy.

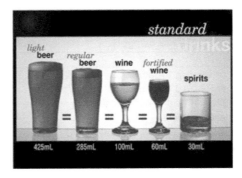

References

1. Ali R, Meena S, Eastwood B, Richards I, Marsden J. Ultra-rapid screening for substance use disorders: the alcohol, smoking and substance involvement screening test (ASSIST-lite). Drug Alcohol Depend. 2013;132:352–61.
2. Agerwala S, McCance-Katz E. Integrating screening, brief intervention, and referral to treatment (SBIRT) into clinical practice settings: a brief review. J Psychoactive Drugs. 2012;44(4):307–17.
3. Babor T, McRee B, Kassebaum P, Grimaldi P, Ahmed K, Bray J. Screening, brief intervention, and referral to treatment (SBIRT). Subst Abus. 2007;28(3):7–30. https://doi.org/10.1300/J465v28n03_03.
4. Babor T, Del Boca F, Bray J. Screening, brief intervention and referral to treatment: implications of SAMHSA's SBIRT initiative for substance abuse policy and practice. Addiction. 2017;112(Suppl. 2):110–7.
5. Buchan I, Buckley E, Deacon G, Irvine R, Ryan M. Problem drinkers and their problems. Journal of Royal College General Practitioners. 1981;31:151–3.
6. Center for Behavioral Health Statistics and Quality. Behavioral health trends in the United States: Results from the 2014 National Survey on Drug Use and Health (HHS Publication No. SMA 15-4927, NSDUH Series H-50). 2015.; Retrieved from http://www.samhsa.gov/data/.
7. Cunningham R, Bernstein S, Walton M, Broderick K, Vaca F, Woolard R, D'Onofrio G. Alcohol, tobacco, and other drugs: future directions for screening and intervention in the emergency department. Acad Emerg Med. 2009;16(11):1078–88. https://doi.org/10.1111/j.1553-2712.2009.00552.x.
8. D'Onofrio G. Screening and brief intervention for alcohol and other drug problems: what will it take? Acad Emerg Med. 2000;7(1):69–71.
9. D'Onofrio G, Degutis L. Preventive care in the emergency department: screening and brief intervention for alcohol problems in the emergency department: a systematic review. Acad Emerg Med. 2002;9(6):627–38.
10. Deeble J. Medical Services through Medicare, National Health Strategy Background. Department of Health, Housing and Community Services. Canberra. 1991.
11. Degenhardt L, Charlson F, Mathers B, Hall WD, Flaxman AD, Johns N, Vos T. The global epidemiology and burden of opioid dependence: results from the global burden of disease 2010 study. Addiction. 2014;109:1320–33.
12. Dunn C, Fields C. SBI training for trauma care, providers. Substance abuse and mental health services administration, CSAT. 2007; George Washington University, June 15, 2007.
13. European Monitoring Centre for Drugs and Drug Addiction. Emergency department-based brief interventions for individuals with substance-related problems: a review of effectiveness, Luxembourg. 2016.
14. Forsythe M, Lee G. The evidence for implementing alcohol screening and intervention in the emergency department – time to act. Int Emerg Nurs. 2012;20(3):167–72.
15. Government of South Australia. Royal adelaide hospital emergency department designer drug early warning system (D2EWS) 12-month technical report,

DASSA Research Monograph No.19 Research Series. 2005. https://www.sahealth.sa.gov.au.

16. Group WBIS. A randomised cross-national clinical trial of brief interventions with heavy drinkers. Am J Public Health. 1996;86(7):948–5.

17. Gruer L, Wilson P, Scott R. General practitioner centred scheme for treatment of opiate dependent drug injectors in Glasgow. Br Med J. 1997;314:1730–5.

18. Henry-Edwards S, Humeniuk R, Ali R, Monteiro M, Poznyak V. Brief intervention for substance use: a manual for use in primary care. Geneva: World Health Organization; 2003.

19. Humeniuk R, Ali R, Babor T, Farrell M, Formigoni M, Jittiwutikarn J, et al. Validation of the alcohol smoking and substance involvement screening test (ASSIST). Addiction. 2008;103(6):1039–47.

20. Humeniuk R, Dennington V, Ali R. The effectiveness of a brief intervention for illicit drugs linked to the ASSIST screening test in primary health care settings: a technical report of phase III findings of the WHO ASSIST randomised controlled trial. Geneva: World Health Organization; 2008.

21. Humeniuk R, Henry-Edwards S, Ali R, Poznyak V, Monteiro M. The ASSIST-linked brief intervention for hazardous and harmful substance use: manual for use in primary care. Geneva: World Health Organization; 2010.

22. Kaner E, Beyer F, Muirhead C, Campbell F, Pienaar ED, Bertholet N, et al. Effectiveness of brief alcohol interventions in primary care populations. Cochrane Database Syst Rev. 2018;2:CD004148. https://doi.org/10.1002/14651858.CD004148.pub4.

23. Mearns D, McLeod J. Person-Centred Counseling in action. 4th ed. London: Sage Publications; 2008.

24. Miller W, Rollnick S. Motivational interviewing – helping people change. 2nd ed. New York and London: Guilford Press; 2002.

25. Miller W, Rollnick S. Motivational interviewing – helping people change. 3nd ed. New York and London: Guilford Press; 2013.

26. Peacock A, Leung J, Larney S, Colledge S, Hickman M, Rehm J, et al. Global statistics on alcohol, tobacco and illicit drug use: 2017 status report. Addiction. 2018;113(10):1905–26. https://doi.org/10.1111/add.14234.

27. Prochaska J, DiClemente C, Norcross J. In search of how people change. Applications to addictive behaviour. Am Psychol. 1992;47:1102–14.

28. Roche A, Watt K, McClure R, Purdie D, Green D. Injury and alcohol: a hospital emergency department study. Drug Alcohol Rev. 2001;20(2):155–66.

29. Royal Australain College of General Practitioners. Supporting smoking cessation. A guide for health professionals. The 5 A's structure for smoking cessation. 2014. www.racgp.org.au. Accessed 07/06/2019.

30. Stead LF, Buitrago D, Preciado N, Sanchez G, Hartmann-Boyce J, Lancaster T. Physician advice for smoking cessation. Cochrane Database Syst Rev. 2013;5 https://doi.org/10.1002/14651858.CD000165.pub4.

31. United Nations Office on Drugs and Crime (UNODC), World Drug Report 2017 (ISBN: 978–92–1-148291-1, eISBN: 978–92–1-060623-3, United Nations publication, Sales No. E.17.XI.6).

32. Whitlock E, Orleans T, Pender N, Allan J. Evaluating primary care behavioral counseling interventions: an evidence-based approach. Am J Prev Med. 2002;22(4):267–84.

33. Woolard R, Cherpitel C, Thompson K. Brief intervention for emergency department patients with alcohol misuse: implications for current practice. Alcohol Treat Q. 2011;29(2):146–57. https://doi.org/10.1080/07347324.2011.557978.

34. Wutzke S, Shiell A, Gomel M, Conigrave K. Cost effectiveness of brief interventions for reducing alcohol consumption. Soc Sci Med. 2001;52(6):863–70.

Screening and Assessment for People with Substance Use Disorders: A Focus on Developed Countries

46

Brian Rush

Contents

Abstract

This chapter outlines the rationale for a more proactive concerted effort for screening and assessment of at-risk consumption, substance use disorders, and related comorbidity, with a special focus on a broad system approach that engages multiple services and sectors alongside specialist programs and providers. This aspect of clinical practice as well as treatment system development should be a priority given the strong evidence concerning under-detection in routine practice and the excellent performance of a host of screening and assessment tools and processes. When used for clinical decision making, best practice calls for a staged approach to maximize efficiency of the overall screening and assessment process and ensure a link to measurement-based care and subsequent outcome monitoring. Grounded in a conceptual framework that articulates this staged approach, several specific tools are highlighted. The essential principle for service and system planning is that these tools must be tailored to the setting and target population

B. Rush (✉)
Centre for Addiction and Mental Health,
Toronto, ON, Canada
e-mail: brian.rush@camh.ca

© Springer Nature Switzerland AG 2021
N. el-Guebaly et al. (eds.), *Textbook of Addiction Treatment*,
https://doi.org/10.1007/978-3-030-36391-8_46

for which they are being implemented. Whether working in generic settings such as primary care or specialized treatment settings, a collaborative approach, drawing upon multidisciplinary, multi-provider, and multi-sectoral expertise, is needed across the stages of screening and assessment. This approach also needs to be accompanied by a collaborative response protocol for level-of-care placement inclusive of adaptive treatment and support for smooth transitions. There are many challenges to implementing and evaluating the effectiveness of screening and assessment tools and processes, and more research is needed on the facilitators and barriers to implementation at both the level of the individual service provider and within collaborative, shared care arrangements.

Keywords

Screening · Assessment · Outcome monitoring Collaboration · Systems approach

46.1   Introduction

The purpose of this chapter is to provide an overview of screening and assessment tools and processes in the context of middle- to high-income (i.e., "developed") countries. In this context, there are important similarities but also differences in the many other books and practice guidelines synthesizing this work from various disciplinary perspectives (e.g., psychiatric [26], psychotherapy [35], behavioral [86], psychosocial [85], or social work perspectives [42]). Like previous work, there is an acknowledgement of important principles and practices that may be seen as universal in nature, for example, the need for an evidence-based approach grounded on a comprehensive bio-psycho-social-spiritual model; sensitivity to individual differences in culture, diversity, and developmental age; the critical importance of empathy, listening skills, and therapeutic alliance; and the appropriate involvement of family and significant others. These aspects are critical elements of the inter-

face between clinician and client. Such similarities notwithstanding, this chapter emphasizes more of a systems approach, recognizing that in so-called developed countries, the greater resource base offers an opportunity for a collaborative approach to engaging people in need, identifying and assessing their strengths and problem areas, offering a wide range of service options along a continuum of care, and adapting services based on measurement of outcomes. This collaborative approach may involve more than one professional, organization, and service delivery sector – a scenario that professionals working in low-income countries may only dream about in terms of collegial support for their work. Further, many screening and assessment tools that complement clinical skills and experience are not available and/or validated in many low-income countries. This is another advantage conferred on moderate- to high-income countries that have capacity for research and development.

In short, this chapter acknowledges screening and assessment as a core component of a broader "whole systems," public health approach to treatment and support for substance use, addictions, and co-occurring conditions [5, 76]. Given this foundation, this chapter is aimed at people working from a range of professional disciplines, for example, psychology, social work, nursing, family practice, psychiatry, and other medical and nonmedical specialists. Thus, some readers working from a particular disciplinary perspective may benefit from additional, reference texts such as those noted above.

Although there are many important intercountry differences in the capacity for screening and assessment, it is also important to recognize that many "developed" countries are far from homogenous in terms of community need and capacity to respond. Taking Canada as but one example, there is a tremendous range within the country in terms of rurality/urbanicity, multiculturalism, Indigenous versus non-Indigenous populations, and substance use patterns and related harms. These and many other factors all influence beliefs about substance use and addiction, the perceived value of treatment, help-seeking behavior, and no doubt cultural interpretation of concepts such as "assessment" or "treatment." There is also wide variation in availability and accessibility of options for treatment and support, an obvious factor critical to screening and assessment considerations.

46.2 Rationale for Screening and Assessment

It is widely recognized that only a small minority of people with mental health and substance use-related concerns seek help from either community professionals or less formal services and that, among that do, the largest proportion will access a primary healthcare provider or other health and social service professional [87, 88]. Although many people with mental health and substance use- related problems, or who are at risk of such problems, are in contact with various service providers, these risks or problems are often not identified [62]. These contacts are missed opportunities for offering advice, more extended consultation, or referral for additional support. This highlights the importance of broadening the base of treatment through a system-wide, public health response [5] with generic community services, including primary care, hospitals, social services, educational, and justice-related services, being proactive in asking questions about mental health, substance use, and addiction-related issues. The aim is to identify concerns, increase opportunities for early identification, provide access to more in-depth assessment and other services and supports, and link the person to more specialized services when needed. For people with low- to moderate risk, or less severe mental health and substance use problems, engaging in proactive, opportunistic screening and on-site, brief intervention is intended to reduce risks and harms. For those with higher risk, or more severe and complex problems, opportunistic screening is intended to open a pathway to more comprehensive assessment, an appropriate treatment and support response, and improved health outcomes. Savings are also anticipated in future medical-, social-, and criminal justice-related costs.

Service providers differ in their attitudes and beliefs about the role of systematic screening and assessment to support their work with people seeking help: beliefs that reflect personal experience, training, and organizational context. Some professionals rely on their training and experience to guide problem identification and client-focused decisions. Some may have philosophical and ethical concerns related to asking about mental health and substance use issues, considering it to be intrusive or possibly harmful due to potential stigmatization and labeling (e.g., in educational settings). Some may doubt the increased efficacy and efficiency of these tools over their routine decision-making processes, while others may be reluctant to engage in consistent, structured screening due to concerns that they do not have the expertise or resources to respond appropriately. Research, however, suggests that critically important mental health and substance use concerns are missed when clinicians do not use structured tools and processes to prompt thorough questioning [93].

Given the high level of heterogeneity in demographic, cultural, psychosocial, and clinical characteristics of people needing treatment and support for substance use problems, it is axiomatic that no approach will meet everyone's needs. This calls for a thorough investigation of needs and strengths and a co-constructed matching of this profile to available service options across a continuum of care. The focus on screening and assessment is intended to increase the efficiency of client intake and engagement, improve individual treatment outcomes, and minimize service delivery costs across the system as a whole [40]. Best practices for treatment and support of people with co-occurring disorders who are already engaged with specialized services also call for more proactive screening of these co-occurring problem areas [71]. This includes screening for mental health problems among people seeking substance use treatment, as well as screening for high-risk/hazardous substance use and addiction-related problems among people seeking mental health treatment and support [70].

Research also shows that screening is most effective when combined with other staged investigations and matched therapeutic and motivation-based interventions [32]. Collaborative approaches can serve to mitigate the reluctance of professionals to use formal screening techniques by bringing together complementary services and resources, ultimately building capacity for improved service to individuals who come to them for assistance.

46.3 Collaborative Models for Screening and Assessment

Many service providers external to the specialized mental health and substance use treatment sector do not have the expertise and resources to identify mental health, substance use, and co-occurring concerns. Further, most specialist service providers do not have the resources to respond to the breadth of complex issues and problems that are identified through many screening tools. Collaborative care models provide the opportunity for various providers to bring together their collective strengths and capabilities to construct a system whereby individuals are screened and can receive required services in a seamless manner [2]. As such, screening processes must be connected to well-articulated response protocols in order to be useful and effective. These protocols should describe required actions among all partners based on positive results on screening tools, including recommendations for more in-depth screening and assessment, and follow-up consultation and referrals.

There are various models of collaboration that can incorporate screening, assessment, and referral protocols, and these include

- Single-site assessment process incorporating multidisciplinary teams – Single assessment processes reduce the number of assessments between mental health, addictions, and various health and social service professionals in order to enable a seamless care process [61].
- Integrated treatment and support for people with co-occurring disorders, whereby competencies and processes related to screening and assessment are key criteria for defining integrated programs as "concurrent disorder capable" [54].
- Centralized access point to care – This approach aims to reduce the number of points of entry of care for users, in some cases to a single-access point in order to reduce the number of professionals and organizations prospective to whom clients and their families have to tell their story [74].
- Network model with distributed common tools – Rather than a single point of access, this approach uses common screening and assessment tools across a network of providers and with electronic sharing of the information and joint treatment and support planning.
- Screening, brief intervention, and referral to treatment (SBIRT) – This approach requires health and social service professionals to use brief screening instruments to identify people at risk of, or experiencing, mental health and/or substance use problems and who then receive brief intervention on treatment on-site or who are proactively linked to specialist providers depending on severity [7].
- Co-located substance use specialists in generic settings – This involves either assigning/hiring a substance use worker to perform in-house screening and brief assessment or co-locating a worker from a specialized substance use service into the nonspecialized setting, for example, an emergency department [13]

46.4 Best Practices for Screening and Assessment

Through a treatment system lens, there are many disciplines and service delivery settings potentially involved in the screening and assessment process. An individual situation may require input from a medical, psychiatric, nursing, psychological, psychosocial rehabilitation, social work, and/or spiritual perspective. A collaborative approach to screening and assessment requires mutual interprofessional respect for the unique contributions that each has to offer to a client- and family-centered approach. The uniqueness of the various perspectives notwithstanding common principles include

- A "whole-person perspective" on strengths and needs
- Close engagement of family and other loved ones, while respecting client's preferences for privacy of information

– A sensitivity to diversity and related health equity issues
– A strong emphasis on creating a welcoming, motivation-based, therapeutic interface
– Adherence to an evidence-based approach

An evidence-based approach encompasses several factors including clinician expertise, exploration of person characteristics and contextual variables using psychometrically sound tools, critical thinking skills, personal and collateral input, and knowledge of evidence-informed interventions [42]. Screening and assessment must be seen as a process that continues over time as more information is shared and therapeutic relationships strengthen. A collaborative, longitudinal approach is particularly critical for the assessment of complex, co-occurring disorders given the need to disentangle etiological sequencing (e.g., depressive symptoms induced by heavy alcohol use). In a collaborative approach to screening and assessment, the sharing of infor-

mation across service providers is also critical. If possible, this should be done through e-health technology but minimally through telephone, email, or written communication.

Best practice entails a staged approach that links screening, assessment, and outcome monitoring with a family of tools and related decision-making processes that are developmentally appropriate and delivered through a diversity-based approach to ensure equitable access and subsequent assessment and treatment. This approach is articulated in the conceptual framework for screening and assessment described below (see Fig. 46.1). The framework can assist in choosing the "right" tools and using them with the "right" people at the "right" time. It is recommended that in order to effectively apply the framework, it be considered in the context of a multi-sectoral continuum of care and the specific collaborative models and service delivery settings under consideration. Thus, application of the framework is very context-specific. For example,

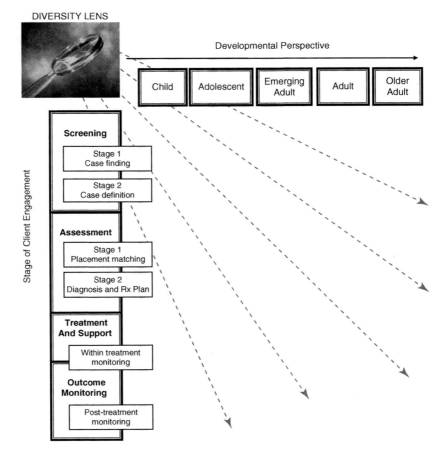

Fig. 46.1 Conceptual framework for screening and assessment. (Adapted from Rush and Castel [70])

the required level of treatment and support may not be readily available due to waiting time or the lack of service availability within the jurisdiction or via realistic distance/travel time. Collaborative arrangements with existing services may be required in order to offer the best service available at that point in time and to maintain client engagement. In the case of people with co-occurring disorders, provision of mental health services will often reduce substance use and ameliorate substance use-related problems [27]. Evidence reviewed by these same authors also suggests the reverse to be true for the provision of substance use treatment and consequent reduction of many mental health-related symptoms and improved functioning. Parikh [67] discusses several evidence-based mental health interventions that can be delivered in substance use services.

In short, it is important to work with local resources as best as possible while advocating for additional resources with a need-based planning model [75]. Alternative therapist-assisted and/or self-management tools delivered through the Internet or mobile-based technology are also increasingly available.

46.4.1 Diversity Lens

Every individual has a unique and complex set of strengths, circumstances, and challenges shaped in large part by the social determinants of health and including, for example, gender, sexual orientation, culture, ethnicity, social location, geography, political views, and religious/spiritual affiliation. As such, each component of this framework must be considered through a "diversity lens" when implementing tools, interpreting the results, and providing feedback to individuals in the context of day-to-day service delivery.

46.4.2 Developmental Perspective

The horizontal axis of the framework articulates the developmental trajectory across the life span as a frame of reference to also guide the choice of screening and assessment tools and processes. At

each stage of this trajectory, there are specific developmental tasks and challenges that an individual must navigate, further complicated by the diversity lens noted above. Importantly, most tools are validated for use with groups of individuals defined by age rather than stage. For example, some emerging adults in the 18–24 range may be well-served by screening and assessment with adult measures and being treated in the adult sector, while others with adolescent measures and corresponding services in the youth sector. Therefore, tools and services that can be applied differentially to match developmental stage, rather than being bound by strict age boundaries, are preferred. The GAIN-Short Screener [21] is appropriate for use from age 10 to older adulthood and is, therefore, particularly helpful for collaborative, system-level application [52].

Developmental stage and consideration of service delivery settings that may be unique to specific stages are also important considerations for determining when during the engagement, treatment, and support process to ask different types of screening questions. For example, for young people being seen on an outreach basis in their school or street environment, it would not be appropriate to begin asking screening questions about sensitive topics such as high-risk sexual behavior, trauma experiences, or illegal behavior before a trusting relationship has been initiated. This will also be the case for many other settings and populations, especially those impacted by trauma. Interpretation and action in response to screening results also need to be developmentally informed. Considerable attention has been paid to this issue with respect to children, adolescents, and adults, but much attention has gone to further articulating the role of developmental stages in service transitions for transitional-aged youth and older adults.

46.4.3 Screening

In the context of substance use and addictions, and the broader field of mental health, screening is a relatively brief process designed to identify individuals who are at risk of having particular problems or diagnosable disorders that warrant immediate attention, intervention, or more comprehensive review. The organizational context and population served will dictate whether screening will start at Stage 1 or 2, as further described below.

46.4.3.1 Stage 1 Screening: Risk Assessment/Case Finding

This stage of screening involves the use of psychometrically sound, typically self-report, questionnaires that cast a fairly wide net to determine the possibility of a particular problem area or mental/addictive disorder and which requires further investigation. In the substance use area, Stage 1 tools may also focus on the level of risk associated with alcohol and drug use per se, the AUDIT perhaps being the best known option for alcohol [6] and the ASSIST for other drugs, excluding tobacco [91]. Having a menu of Stage 1 tools to choose from, ranging from brief one- to three-item instruments to somewhat longer tools that focus on a small number of domains, can facilitate the implementation of systematic screening protocols in emergency rooms, primary care offices, and other service delivery settings where severe time constraints may otherwise preclude a more detailed, systematic screening approach.

Stage 1 tools are characterized by their brevity (typically between 1 and 20 items; completion time less than 5 min) and low-threshold training requirements and scoring algorithms. There have been recent developments toward very brief screeners (one to three items) for alcohol or other drugs in order to facilitate screening in busy settings such as primary care or emergency departments (e.g., [68, 82]) or with high-need populations that cannot tolerate completion of long questionnaires (e.g., people with psychosis: [50]). As noted, the AUDIT [6] is a Stage 1 tool focused on the level of risk of alcohol consumption. The NIDA-Quick Screen focuses on other drug use [66], as do short versions of the ASSIST also developed to facilitate use in high-volume clinical settings [4, 84]. Others are focused on consequences, including substance use/abuse or dependence (e.g., DUDIT, [39]; CAGE, [24]; BASIC, [12]; TWEAK, [77]; and CRAFFT, Knight et al. [46]).

The screening for mental health problems/disorders is also highly relevant for the assessment and treatment of people with identified substance use concerns. With respect to screening for mental health challenges, there is an important distinction between disorder-based tools and those based on a dimensional approach, such as measuring mental distress. Others that are longer such as the Beck Depression Inventory [8], the Beck Anxiety Inventory [9], or screeners for PTSD (SPAN, [15, 60]) and trauma [45] are best considered follow-up Stage 2 tools because of their length and diagnostic specificity. Disorder-based tools that are extremely short, such as those using one to three items for identifying depressive and/or anxiety disorder (e.g., the ADD, [57]), are considered Stage 1 screeners. However, Stage 1 mental health screeners also include brief dimensional measures such as the K6/K10 [44], the five-item mental health component of the SF-36 [11, 89]; the Psychological Screening Inventory (PSI: [48]); and either the Brief Symptom Inventory or the BSRS [23, 49], both being shorter versions of the Symptom Checklist 90-R [10, 22]. For children and adolescents, the Strengths and Difficulties Questionnaire serves as a useful Stage 1 mental health screener [33].

A small number of Stage 1 screening tools focus on *both* mental health and substance use, and these are highly valued because of their broader coverage and, therefore, their applicability in multiple settings involved in a collaborative care arrangement. The GAIN-SS [21] is one such tool rapidly growing in popularity across North America and elsewhere and available in multiple languages.

Biological tests for alcohol and drug use may also be helpful and have the advantage of ease of application in medical settings and their utility as a supplement to self-reported information. Limitations include cost, lack of specificity, and, in some instances, sensitivity to recent substance use. Biological testing includes alcohol breathalyzer testing, measures of tissue damage from chronic substance use such as reflected in the liver enzyme gamma-glutamyl transferase (GGT) or red blood cell mean corpuscular volume (MCV), and hair, saliva, and urine analysis (see [35, 86], for brief reviews).

Time and resources permitting, brief screening across other selected domains is also recommended. Screening for other health problems such as traumatic brain injury, cognitive impairment, fetal alcohol spectrum disorder (FASD), HIV/AIDS, and tobacco use is also of critical importance to treatment and support planning and may be called for in some healthcare settings using additional, brief screeners.

46.4.3.2 Stage 2 Screening: Case Definition

This second step in a staged approach to screening involves the use of psychometrically sound tools that are more specific and longer than those used in Stage 1 and which aim to tentatively identify one or more specific disorders or problem areas. This may include alcohol or other drug use disorders and other mental disorders such as psychotic disorders, major depressive disorder, a variety of anxiety disorders including PTSD, eating disorders, and ADHD. Although more specific and detailed than Stage 1 screeners, the information gathered through the tools in this category of the staged approach is still NOT sufficient on which to base a formal diagnosis, although some of the names of the tools can be misleading in this regard. The administration of a Stage 2 screening tool may involve the same or a different service provider than the one undertaking the Stage 1 screening. In any instances involving a transition to a new partner in a collaborative care process, a motivational approach and transition support to ensure ongoing engagement are critical, especially for people with complex co-occurring conditions.

Screening tools such as the Psychiatric Diagnostic Screening Questionnaire (PDSQ: [94]) and the Modified Mini Screen [3] are particularly helpful as diagnosis-based, Stage 2 screeners. Rush et al. [72] validated the PDSQ, as well as the psychiatric subscale of the widely used Addiction Severity Index for identifying mental disorders among people seeking substance use treatment. Magruder et al. [53] found both the PDSQ and the Conners' Adult ADHD Rating Scale which also performed well in adult substance use treatment settings. For adolescents, the POSIT [20] is more focused on specific problem areas rather than diagnosis (e.g., substance use, health, school, family) and is a well-validated option for Stage 2 screening in several settings. Others for children and youth are the Child Behavior Checklist (CBCL: [1]) and the DISC-R [51] and cover most mental disorders, including substance use disorders. For more discussion on specific screening tools and processes for children and youth, see the narrative review conducted by Rush et al. [69] and synthesized by the Centre for Addiction and Mental Health [17]. As noted earlier, tools such as the Beck Depression Inventory [8] and the Beck Anxiety Inventory [9] are considered to be Stage 2 tools due to their specificity in terms of diagnosis and length. This grouping also includes several mental health screening tools that are dimensional rather than diagnostic in nature such as the longer version of the GHQ-30 and the full SCL-90-R [22].

46.4.4 Assessment

In the staged framework, assessment is also conceptualized as involving two phases. Stage 1 assessment is focused primarily on further information gathering and placement/referral to the most appropriate service setting (i.e., level of care). Upon engagement in the appropriate setting, Stage 2 assessment goes further in examining strengths and needs across several bio-psycho-social-spiritual domains including health and mental health status, family/social situation, environmental risk factors, etc.

One helpful way to conceptualize the distinction between Stage 1 and Stage 2 assessment is that between "placement" and "modality" matching [31, 59]. Placement matching, the aim of Stage 1, refers to initial client assignment to a treatment setting with a certain resource intensity and, therefore, significant cost implications. Modality matching (the aim of Stage 2) refers to client assignment on the basis of the optimal clinical approach and intervention(s), including philosophical and goal orientation such as reduced substance use versus abstinence, based on the full profile of client strengths and needs. The overall assessment process needs to occur within a stepped-care, adaptive treatment strategy that makes ongoing adjustments as new information arises, including the response to treatment, and supported transitions across the various levels of service [63, 64].

46.4.4.1 Stage 1 Assessment: Information Gathering and Service Placement

The essential feature of a Stage 1 assessment, especially in the context of collaborative care across multiple service settings, is the intention to gather enough information on both strengths and needs, including immediate needs for physical and psychosocial stabilization, to formulate an initial placement/referral in an appropriate level of care. This first step involves continued information gathering that is optimally done through the use of valid tools and structured interviews. For substance use services, this would include a determination of the need for withdrawal management which may be initiated in one of the three levels of care: home/mobile, community/medical, or, in the case of complex co-occurring mental and physical problems, a hospital-based service with adequate medical and psychiatric supports. The CWAW-Ar is an assessment tool that supports determination of the need for withdrawal management services [83]. A complementary assessment tool is available for measuring intensity of opiate withdrawal (COWS: [90]). Withdrawal management often needs to be accompanied by a period of stabilization prior to formal engagement in treatment and special care needs to be given to withdrawal management for opioid use disorder given the potential risk of overdose as a result of reduced tolerance and the risk of relapse.

Aside from withdrawal management, a Stage 1 substance use assessment should also determine the need for community or residential treatment at varying levels of duration and intensity. These levels of care are articulated in considerable detail in the ASAM criteria for placement/referral to substance use services [28, 29] and can be tailored for the purposes of need-based planning in specific jurisdictions [75].

It is critical to reemphasize that the initial placement/referral based on the Stage 1 assessment be undertaken in the context of a stepped care, potentially multiservice model – that is, stepping up to a higher level of care if required and stepping down on the basis of progress toward the individual's goals. At moderate-to-high levels of severity and case complexity, this typically requires transition support, including case management and shared e-health information. It also requires monitoring of outcomes, within and posttreatment (see below). The ASAM model specifies the dimensions across which a clinician must explore strengths and needs in order to make the appropriate placement match [29]. These dimensions include

- Acute intoxication and/or withdrawal potential
- Biomedical conditions and complications
- Emotional, behavioral, or cognitive conditions and complications
- Readiness to change
- Relapse, continued use of continued problem potential
- Recovery environment

It is highly recommended that these areas be examined with a semistructured or structured interview approach facilitated by validated instruments that support the initial placement/referral.

Assessment tools and processes for Stage 1 assessment include the GAIN-Q3 Standard MI or the GAIN-I-Lite – these tools being part of the GAIN "family" of substance abuse screening and assessment tools (www.chestnut.org). As with the GAIN-SS, these brief assessment tools are appropriate for use with individuals from age 10 and up. Another instrument for Stage 1 assessment is the Recovery Attitude and Treatment Evaluation (RAATE: [30, 58, 65]).

46.4.4.2 Stage 2 Assessment: Case Conceptualization and Comprehensive Treatment Plan

The next stage of the assessment process involves the creation of a case conceptualization, formulation, and/or diagnosis leading to an individualized and adaptable treatment plan. The language around this overall process changes depending on the discipline and service delivery setting. The central idea, however, is to pull together all the information that has been gathered from validated screening tools, undertake additional information gathering as needed through assessment questionnaires, structured and semistructured interviews, collateral contacts, and case notes from previous service contacts (if available). The resulting case conceptualization or diagnosis informs the treatment plan, including responding to psychosocial and clinical needs and strengths, and facilitating linkage to services. The term "modality matching" summarizes the intention of a Stage 2 assessment, although this may also involve revision of the placement decision made at an earlier stage.

Stage 2 assessment is seen as being grounded in the present context of the person's life situation and problem-focused [42]. This approach, however, should not exclude consideration of critical underlying factors such as trauma, including intergenerational trauma, and neuropsychological mechanisms. A thorough health assessment including a full psychiatric assessment may also be required and is especially indicated for individuals presenting with more complex co-occurring conditions.

It is beyond the scope of this report to delve into all the critical issues involved in the person–clinician interface for purposes of comprehensive assessment and treatment and support planning. There are many excellent reference texts that approach this from various disciplinary perspectives and cited at the outset of this chapter. All such experts acknowledge the role of clinician experience and skills in conducting semistructured or structured interviews that operationalize core principles and practices such as sensitivity to individual differences in culture, diversity, and developmental age, the need for empathy and establishing therapeutic alliance, and the appropriate involvement of family and significant others. In the substance use field, there is a need for such interviews to cover several areas including, but not limited to, substance use history, including age of first use and onset of negative consequences, severity of substance use disorders, level of insight into past and current challenges, social supports and environment risk factors (e.g., for relapse), medical and psychiatric

comorbidity, current phase of use (e.g., intoxicated or in withdrawal), and pressures to seek help and the person's readiness/motivation for change. For many of these areas, the approach is to explore these areas at a deeper level than investigated in Stage 1.

In the substance use field, there have been significant efforts to create integrated assessment packages to support individualized treatment plans and subsequent follow-up determination of outcome. Two well-known comprehensive substance use assessment packages are the Addiction Severity Index [55] and the GAIN-I (www.chestnut.org). The GAIN-I is now used extensively in North America and has the added advantage of being conceptually and instrumentally linked to the GAIN-SS (Stage 1 screener) and the GAIN-Q3 or GAIN-I-Lite (Stage 1 assessment). Another example, with a stronger focus on mental health, is the Psychiatric Research Interview for Substance and Mental Disorders (PRISM) which, although designed primarily as a research tool, provides systematic coverage of alcohol/drugs and mental health experiences and symptoms and functional impairment [37]. There is also the option to administer the full structured interview for DSM-IV disorders (DSM-IV) [25] although this would need to be supplemented with other substance use – specific tools assessing, for example, readiness to change.

46.4.5 Treatment and Support and Outcome Monitoring

Outcome monitoring is a critical component of the staged approach to screening and assessment because of the need to establish baseline status early in the treatment and support process and to inform service delivery on an ongoing basis via measurement-based care and/or engage the client in post-discharge follow-up processes. An important distinction is made between within-treatment and posttreatment outcome monitoring, both of which consider the contact for client and program assessment purposes, as an extension of the treatment and support process itself. This is conceptually quite different than a traditional "research" follow-up and much more likely to engage administrative and clinical staff, as well as clients themselves, in the outcome monitoring process.

46.4.5.1 Stage 1: Within-Treatment Monitoring

Within-treatment outcome monitoring tracks progress on an ongoing basis with very brief but highly relevant clinical tools applied at the front end of periodic therapist–client interactions. Variously referred to as measurement-based care [80], adaptive treatment sequencing [63, 64], routine outcome monitoring [16], or progress monitoring [34], this model evolved largely from the work of Lambert in the mental health area (e.g., [47]) and, in the substance use field [56]. Occurring at the clinical interface of therapist and client, it is critical that the assessment and outcome measures be brief, be implemented within the flow of the clinical encounter, and return feedback immediately in a useful format to further the therapeutic relationship and the client's progress toward goals. Appropriate within-treatment outcome monitoring can be accomplished with repeat application of some screening tools that are sensitive to change over time such as the GAIN-SS [21] and the Brief Addiction Monitor [14]. Others such as Lambert's [47] Outcome Questionnaire (OQ) have been designed specifically to assess psychological processes that cut across many types of mental health problems, including substance use and addictions.

46.4.5.2 Stage 2: Posttreatment Monitoring

Posttreatment outcome monitoring, sometimes referred to as "recovery monitoring" [18], involves the repetition of selected screening/assessment measures at some interval after program admission, such as 3, 6, 12, or 24 months, and determination of changes in these measures [73]. In addition, the follow-up contact is an opportunity to reengage the individual in treatment if indicated, using a guided, motivational return-to-treatment protocol [79]. Posttreatment monitoring is useful as an accountability and program evaluation tool and can also be helpful in identifying clients who may be struggling and need further assistance to recoup gains made in treatment.

Ideally, posttreatment follow-up also involves repeat application of one or more assessment tools or subscales by phone or face-to-face interview. The GAIN-I and GAIN-Q3-standards (www.chestnut.org) on the Addiction Severity Index [55] are useful measures for outcome monitoring. Other measures have been constructed directly from client's reported experience of "recovery" [19]. Locating clients and obtaining good follow-up rates (ideally over 80%) are the Achilles' heel of posttreatment follow-up for substance use programs. There are protocols for achieving substantially higher follow-up rates [78], and these can benefit from collaborative networks working together to locate and engage people in the follow-up process.

46.5 Implementation and Evaluation of Evidence-Based Screening and Assessment

The context in which screening takes place must be carefully considered in both implementation and evaluation of screening and assessment tools and processes. As already mentioned, the role and purpose of screening should be well understood and articulated in the context of the mandate and objectives of the service provider. Organizational policy must also support the implementation of screening and related protocols. Required staff competencies and program design should fit within clear service delivery protocols addressing where, when, and how screening will be administered and how the information gathered will be used. Personnel who are administering the tools must be trained to introduce, administer, score, discuss, and take appropriate action based on the screening results. All of this needs to be clearly conveyed to individuals engaging with the service so that they understand how screening can be helpful and provide fruitful ground for evaluative inquiry.

As noted above, implementing formal screening tools and processes is a logical fit in the specialized substance abuse treatment sector. In these settings, clients have already been identified as needing further screening (e.g., for co-occurring conditions), assessment, or treatment. In other settings where routine screening and assessment of various health concerns are already taking place (i.e., emergency settings, primary care), the rationale for extending screening to identify at-risk substance use and substance-related problems is also clear. Screening in settings such as schools, employment counseling, and justice settings is also important given the evidence that rates of substance use and mental health problems are high and often not identified. While these settings provide important opportunities for early identification and early intervention, there are a number of potential risks that must be considered, including stigma resulting from identification and labeling, social exclusion, limitation of opportunities, and false-positives consuming scarce treatment resources. Risks associated with identification may be greater for some specific groups of people, for example, severe sanctions may be imposed on those identified as being involved in substance using activities by some schools, employment programs, shelter and housing providers, supported housing, long-term care facilities, families, and specific ethno-cultural groups and communities.

With respect to implementation of assessment tools and processes, the issue of staff competencies and qualification is more salient than with respect to screening tools, many of which can be undertaken with much less rigorous training. Importantly, the increasing level of integration of mental health and substance use services [70] is bringing the mental health perspective on "recovery" [81] closer to the substance use field with significant implications for screening and assessment. Among other things, the mental health recovery orientation to service delivery is contributing to the development of what is sometimes referred to as "single-session therapy by walk-in or appointment" that promises brief assessment of the most immediate needs to be addressed largely *from the perspective of the person presenting for assistance* [36]. The focus is very much on rapid linkage which, in many settings, contrasts with a more medical/psychiatric paradigm that requires thorough and, typically, diagnostic assessment.

Models of collaboration within which screening and assessment are core activities provide the field with rich evaluation opportunities, including outcome and process evaluation, and an opportunity to monitor trends and performance. Outcomes can be examined at the individual (i.e., client and clinician), organizational, and community level. For example, at the organizational level, outcome indicators could include changes in staff attitudes, skills, and behavioral engagement in screening and assessment practices and change in referral practices, as well as client perceptions of care. At the community level, indicators could include increased numbers of new clients referred to treatment and reduced number of emergency visits. It is also of interest to evaluate the extent to which the development of collaborative models of screening and assessment contributes to broaden collaborative processes across agencies/service providers – for example, building partnership capital to engage in other joint planning and service delivery. Using a consistent screening tool across a collaborative group of service providers provides an opportunity for decision-makers, funders, and researchers to look at presenting needs across settings and monitor trends over time within the collaborative as well as in comparison to the general population [38].

46.6 Conclusion

There is a very strong rationale for a more proactive concerted effort to screen for mental health problems and at-risk consumption of alcohol and other drugs and related addiction problems given the evidence concerning the level of underdetection in routine practice and the excellent performance of a host of screening tools and processes. Screening in multiple sectors, along with follow-up assessment and intervention, is one strategy to broaden the scope and reach of treatment and support beyond the traditional sector of specialized substance use services. There are many reasons to engage in more proactive screening, and both individual and collaborating partners need to be clear about how the information will be used, including making improvements at the system level. When used for clinical decision making, best practice calls for a staged approach to maximize efficiency of the overall screening and assessment process. The specific tools and processes must be tailored to the setting and target population for which they are being implemented. For example, some tools will work best for screening in primary care and other generic health and social service settings, and others are more appropriate for screening in specialized mental health and substance use settings. That said, whether working in generic settings such as primary care or specialized settings, a collaborative approach, drawing upon multidisciplinary, and potentially multi-provider and multi-sectoral expertise, is needed across the stages of screening and assessment, along with a collaborative response protocol for level-of-care placement/referral for treatment and support.

The evidence is quite strong with respect to the ability of screening tools and processes to identify individuals needing brief intervention or other treatment and support. This evidence underlies the best practice guidelines that call for targeted screening in generic settings such as primary care and universal screening for all clients engaged with specialized mental health and substance use services. However, the effectiveness literature tells us that screening is only one part of the process of engagement and the results are more equivocal in terms of the impact of the screening per se on subsequent case management and health outcomes, the literature on SBIRT in the substance use field being an important exception. Collectively, the literature that cuts across the mental health and substance use area reminds us that screening alone may make little difference without a detailed response plan and follow-up intervention. Further, there is ample evidence that screening for different levels of risk for alcohol and drug use, accompanied by brief intervention or referral to treatment, is effective in engaging people in both these response options and subsequent outcomes [43]. That being said more work is needed on teasing out the most effective ingredients of the overall SBIRT protocol and addressing the challenges implementing SBIRT protocols in healthcare and other settings [41, 92].

References

1. Achenbach TM. Manual for the child behavior checklist/4–18 and 1991 profile. Burlington: Department of Psychology, University of Vermont; 1991.
2. Addiction and Mental Health Collaborative Project Steering Committee. Collaboration for addiction and mental health care: best advice. Ottawa: Canadian Centre on Substance Abuse; 2015.
3. Alexander MJ, Haugland G, Lin SP, Bertollo DN, McCorry FA. Mental health screening in addiction, corrections and social services settings: validating the MMS. Int J Ment Heal Addict. 2008;6:105–9.
4. Ali R, Meena S, Eastwood B, Richards I, Marsden J. Ultra-rapid screening for substance-use disorders: the alcohol, smoking and substance involvement screening test (ASSIST-Lite). Drug Alcohol Depend. 2013;132(1–2):352–61.
5. Babor TF. Treatment systems for population management of substance use disorders: requirements and priorities from a public health perspective. In: el-Guebaly N, Carrà G, Galanter M, editors. Textbook of addiction treatment: international perspectives. Heidelberg/New York/Dordrecht/London: Springer Milan; 2015. p. 1213–29.
6. Babor TF, Higgins-Biddle JC, Saunders JB, Monteiro MG. AUDIT: the alcohol use disorders identification test: guidelines for use in primary care. 2nd ed. Geneva: World Health Organization; 2001.
7. Babor TF, McRee BG, Kassebaum PA, Grimaldi PL, Ahmed K, Bray J. Screening, brief intervention, and referral to treatment (SBIRT) toward a public health approach to the management of substance abuse. Subst Abuse. 2007;28(3):7–30.
8. Beck AT. Beck depression inventory. Philadelphia: Center for Cognitive Therapy; 1961.
9. Beck AT, Epstein N, Brown G, Steer RA. An inventory for measuring clinical anxiety: psychometric properties. J Consult Clin Psychol. 1988;56:893–7.
10. Benjamin AB, Mossman D, Graves NS, Sanders RD. Tests of a symptom checklist to screen for comorbid psychiatric disorders in alcoholism. Compr Psychiatry. 2006;47:227–33.
11. Berwick DM, Murphy JM, Goldman PA, Ware JE, Barsky AJ, Weinstein MC. Performance of a five-item mental health screening test. Med Care. 1991;29:169–76.
12. Bischof G, Reinhardt S, Grothues J, Meyer C, John U, Rumpf HJ. Development and evaluation of a screening instrument for alcohol-use disorders and at-risk drinking: the brief alcohol screening instrument for medical care (BASIC). J Stud Alcohol Drugs. 2007;68(4):607.

13. Blanchette-Martin N, Tremblay J, Ferland F, Rush B, Garceau P, Danielson AM. Co-location of addiction liaison nurses in three Quebec City emergency departments: portrait of services, patients, and treatment trajectories. Can J Addict. 2016;7(3):42–8.

14. Cacciola JS, Alterman AI, DePhilippis D, Drapkin ML, Valadez C Jr, Fala NC, Oslin D, McKay JR. Development and initial evaluation of the brief addiction monitor (BAM). J Subst Abuse Treat. 2013;44(3):256–63.

15. Cameron RP, Gusman D. The primary care PTSD screen (PC-PTSD): development and operating characteristics. Prim Care Psychiatry. 2003;9(1):9–14.

16. Carlier IV, Meuldijk D, Van Vliet IM, Van Fenema E, Van der Wee NJ, Zitman FG. Routine outcome monitoring and feedback on physical or mental health status: evidence and theory. J Eval Clin Pract. 2012;18(1):104–10.

17. Centre for Addiction and Mental Health. Screening for concurrent substance use and mental health problems in youth. Toronto: Centre for Addiction and Mental Health; 2009, http://knowledgex.camh.net/amhspecialists/Screening_assessment/screening/screen_CD_youth/Documents/youth_screening_tools.pdf.

18. Costello MJ, Ropp C, Sousa S, Woo W, Vedelago H, Rush BR. The development and implementation of an outcome monitoring system for an inpatient addiction treatment program in Ontario: lessons learned. Can J Addict. 2016;7(3):15–24.

19. Costello MJ, Sousa S, Ropp C, Rush BR. How to measure addiction recovery? Incorporating perspectives of individuals with lived experience. Int J Ment Heal Addict. 2018;16:1–14.

20. Danseco ER, Marques PR. Development and validation of a POSIT-short form: screening for problem behaviors among adolescents at risk for substance use. J Child Adolesc Subst Abuse. 2002;11(3):17–36.

21. Dennis ML, Chan YF, Funk RR. Development and validation of the GAIN short screener (GSS) for internalizing, externalizing and substance use disorders and crime/violence problems among adolescents and adults. Am J Addict. 2006;15:80–91.

22. Derogatis LR. SCL-90-R administration, scoring, and procedures manual II. Towson: Clinical Psychometric Research; 1983.

23. Derogatis LR, Melisaratos N. The brief symptom inventory: an introductory report. Psychol Med. 1983;13:595–605.

24. Dhalla S, Kopec JA. The CAGE questionnaire for alcohol misuse: a review of reliability and validity studies. Clin Invest Med. 2007;30(1):33–41.

25. First MB, Spitzer RL, Gibbon M, Williams JBW. Structured clinical interview for DSM-IV axis I disorders-patient edition, SCID-I/P, version 2.0. New York: Biometrics Research Department, New York State Psychiatric Institute; 1996.

26. First MB, Tasman A. Clinical guide to the diagnosis and treatment of mental disorders. New York: Wiley; 2010.

27. Flynn PM, Brown BS. Co-occurring disorders in substance abuse treatment: issues and prospects. J Subst Abuse Treat. 2008;34:36–47.

28. Gastfriend DR. Addiction treatment matching: research foundations of the American Society of Addiction Medicine (ASAM) criteria. Binghamton: Haworth Medical Press; 2003.

29. Gastfriend DR, Mee-Lee K. The ASAM patient placement criteria: context, concepts and continuing development. J Addict Dis. 2003;22(Suppl 1):1–8.

30. Gastfriend DR, Filstead WJ, Reif S, Najavits LM, Parrella DP. Validity of assessing treatment readiness in patients with substance use disorders. Am J Addict. 1995;4(3):254–60.

31. Gastfriend DR, Lu S, Sharon E. Placement matching: challenges and technical progress. Subst Use Misuse. 2000;35(12–14):2191–213.

32. Gilbody S, House AO, Sheldon TA. Screening and case finding instruments for depression (review). The Cochrane Collaboration, Wiley; 2007.

33. Goodman A, Goodman R. Strengths and difficulties questionnaire as a dimensional measure of mental health. J Acad Child Adolesc Psychiatry. 2009;48(4):400–3.

34. Goodman JD, McKay JR, DePhilippis D. Progress monitoring in mental health and addiction treatment: a means of improving care. Prof Psychol Res Pract. 2013;44(4):231.

35. Greenfield SF, Hennessy G. Chap. 1: Assessment of the patient. In: Galanter M, Kleber HD, editors. Psychotherapy for the treatment of substance abuse. Arlington: American Psychiatric Publishing Inc; 2011. p. 55–78.

36. Hair HJ, Shortall R, Oldford J. Where's help when we need it? Developing responsive and effective brief counseling services for children, adolescents, and their families. Soc Work Ment Heal. 2013;11(1):16–33.

37. Hasin DS, Trautman KD, Miele GM, Samet S, Smith M, Endicott J. Psychiatric research interview for substance and mental disorders (PRISM): reliability for substance abusers. Am J Psychiatry. 1996;153(9):1195–201.

38. Henderson J, Chaim G. National youth screening project report. Toronto: Centre for Addiction and Mental Health; 2013.

39. Hildebrand M. The psychometric properties of the drug use disorders identification test (DUDIT): a review of recent research. J Subst Abuse Treat. 2015;53:52–9.

40. Hilton T. The promise of PROMIS for addictions. Drug Alcohol Depend. 2011;119:229–34.

41. Johnson M, Jackson R, Guillaume L, Meier P, Goyder E. Barriers and facilitators to implementing screening and brief intervention for alcohol misuse: a systematic review of qualitative evidence. J Publ Heal. 2010;33(3):412–21.

42. Jordan C, Franklin C. Clinical assessment for social workers: quantitative and qualitative methods. 3rd ed. Chicago: Lyceum Books; 2011.

43. Kaner EF, Beyer FR, Muirhead C, Campbell F, Pienaar ED, Bertholet N, Daeppen JB, Saunders JB, Burnand B. Effectiveness of brief alcohol interventions in primary care populations. Cochrane Database Syst Rev. 2018;(2):CD004148.

44. Kessler RC, Andrews G, Colpe LJ, Hiripi E, Mroczek DK, Normand S-LT, Walters EE, Zaslavsky A. Short screening scales to monitor population prevalences and trends in non-specific psychological distress. Psychol Med. 2002;32(6):959–76.

45. Klein S, Alexander DA, Hutchinson JD, Simpson JA, Simpson JM, Bell JS. The Aberdeen trauma screening index: and instrument to predict post-accident psychopathology. Psychol Med. 2002;32:863–71.

46. Knight JR, Shrier LA, Bravender TD, Farrell M, Vander Bilt J, Shaffer HJ. A new brief screen for adolescent substance abuse. Archives of pediatrics & adolescent medicine. 1999;153(6):591–96.

47. Lambert MJ, Burlingame GM, Umphress V, Hansen NB, Vermeersch DA, Clouse GC, Yanchar SC. The reliability and validity of the outcome questionnaire. Clin Psychol Psychother. 1996;3(4):249–58.

48. Lanyon RI. Mental health screening: utility of the psychological screening inventory. Psychol Serv. 2006;3(3):170–80.

49. Lee M, Liao SC, Lee YJ, Wu CH, Tseug MC, Gau SF, Rau CI. Development and verification of validity and reliability of a short screening instrument to identify psychiatric morbidity. J Formos Med Assoc. 2006;102(10):687–94.

50. Ley A, Jeffery D, Shaw S, Weaver T. Development of a brief screen for substance misuse amongst people with severe mental health problems living in the community. J Ment Heal. 2007;16(5):679–90.

51. Lucas CP, Zhang H, Fisher PW, Shaffer D, Regier DA, Narrow WE, Bourdon K, Dulcan MK, Canino G, Rubio-Stipec M, Lahey BB. The DISC predictive scales (DPS): efficiently screening for diagnoses. J Am Acad Child Adolesc Psychiatry. 2001;40:443–9.

52. Lucenko BA, Mancuso D, Felver BEM, Yakup S, Huber A. Co-occurring mental illness among clients in chemical dependency treatment. Olympia: Washington State Department of Social and Health Services Research and Data Analysis Division; 2010. http://publicationsrdadshswagov/1409/ Retrieved 30 June 2010.

53. Magruder KM, Sonne SC, Brady KT, Quello RHM. Screening for co-occurring mental disorders in drug treatment populations. J Drug Issues. 2005;35:593–605.

54. McGovern M, Matzkin AL, Giard J. Assessing the dual diagnosis capability of addiction treatment services: the dual diagnosis capability in addiction treatment (DDCAT) index. J Dual Diagn. 2007;3(2):111–23.

55. McLellan T, Kushner H, Metzger D, Peters R, Smith J, Grissom C, Petinati H, Argeriou M. The fifth edition of the addiction severity index. J Subst Abuse Treat. 1992;9:199–213.

56. McLellan T, Lewis DC, O'Brien CP. Drug dependence, a chronic medical illness: evaluation implica-

tions for treatment, insurance, and outcomes. J Am Med Assoc. 2000;284(13):1689–95.

57. Means-Christensen AJ, Sherbourne CD, Roy-Byrne PP, Craske MG, Stein MB. Using five questions to screen for five common mental disorders in primary care: diagnostic accuracy of the anxiety and depression detector. Gen Hosp Psychiatry. 2006;28(2):108–18.

58. Mee-Lee D. An instrument for treatment progress and matching: the recovery attitude and treatment evaluator (RAATE). J Subst Abuse Treat. 1988;5(3):183–6.

59. Mee-Lee D, Gastfriend DR. Chap. 5: Patient placement criteria. In: Galanter M, Kleber HD, editors. The textbook of substance abuse treatment. Arlington: American Psychiatric Publishing Inc.; 2008.

60. Meltzer-Brody S, Churchill E, Davidson JRT. Derivation of the SPAN, brief diagnostic screening test for post-traumatic stress disorder. Psychiatry Res. 1999;88:63–70.

61. Miller JS, Charles-Jones HD, Barry A, Saunders T. Multidisciplinary primary care mental health teams: a challenge to communication. Prim Care Ment Heal. 2005;3(3):171.

62. Mitchell AJ, Meader N, Bird V, Rizzo M. Clinical recognition and recording of alcohol disorders by clinicians in primary and secondary care: meta-analysis. Br J Psychiatry. 2012;201:93–100.

63. Murphy SA, Collins LM, Rush AJ. Customizing treatment to the patient: adaptive treatment strategies. Drug Alcohol Depend. 2007a;88(Suppl 2):S1.

64. Murphy SA, Oslin DW, Rush AJ, Zhu J. Methodological challenges in constructing effective treatment sequences for chronic psychiatric disorders. Neuropsychopharmacology. 2007b;32(2):257.

65. Najavits LM, Gastfriend DR, Nakayama EY, Barber JP, Blaine J, Frank A, Muenz LR, Thase M. A measure of readiness for substance abuse treatment. Am J Addict. 1997;6(1):74–82.

66. NIDA. Resource guide: Screening for drug use in general medical settings. 2012. https://www.drugabuse.gov/publications/resource-guide-screening-drug-use-in-general-medical-settings/nida-quick-screen. Accessed on 18 June 2019.

67. Parikh S. Screening and treating mental disorders in addiction treatment settings: a stepped care model. Int J Ment Heal Addict. 2008;6:137–40.

68. Ramchand R, Marshall GN, Schell TL, Jaycox LH, Hambarsoomians K, Shetty V, Hinika GS, Cryer HG, Meade P, Belzberg H. Alcohol abuse and illegal drug use among Los Angeles County trauma patients: prevalence and evaluation of single item screener. J Trauma. 2009;66(5):1461–7.

69. Rush BR, Castel S, Somers J, et al. Systematic review and research synthesis of screening tools for mental and substance use disorders appropriate for children and adolescents: technical report (Unpublished manuscript). Toronto: Centre for Addiction and Mental Health; 2009.

70. Rush BR, Castel S. Screening for mental and substance use disorders. In: Cooper D, editor. Care in mental health-substance use (Book 5, chapter 8),

Mental health-substance use book series. Oxford: Radcliffe Publishing Ltd; 2011. p. 89–105.

71. Rush BR, Nadeau L. On the integration of mental health and substance use services and systems. In: Cooper D, editor. Responding in mental health-substance use (Book 3, chapter 13), Mental health-substance use book series. Oxford: Radcliffe Publishing Ltd; 2011. p. 148–75.

72. Rush BR, Castel S, Brands B, Toneatto T, Veldhuizen S. Validation and comparison of diagnostic accuracy of four screening tools for mental disorders in people with substance use disorders. J Subst Abuse Treat. 2013;44(4):375–83.

73. Rush B, Chau N, Rotondi NK, Tan F, Detfurth E. Recovery monitoring for substance use treatment in Ontario: outcome results from a feasibility assessment. Can J Addict. 2016;7(3):5–14.

74. Rush BR, Saini B. Review of coordinated/centralized access mechanisms: evidence, current state and implications. Toronto: Addictions and Mental Health Ontario; 2016.

75. Rush B, Tremblay J, Brown D. Development of a needs-based planning model to estimate required capacity of a substance use treatment system. J Stud Alcohol Drugs Suppl. 2019;27(s18):51–63.

76. Rush B, Urbanoski K. Seven core principles of substance use treatment system design to aid in identifying strengths, gaps, and required enhancements. J Stud Alcohol Drugs Suppl. 2019;27(s18):9–21.

77. Russell M. New assessment tools for risk drinking during pregnancy: T-ACE, TEAK, and others. Alcohol Heal Res World. 1994;18:55–61.

78. Scott CK. A replicable model for achieving over 90% follow-up rates in longitudinal studies of substance abusers. Drug Alcohol Depend. 2004;74:21–36.

79. Scott CK, Dennis ML. Results from two randomized clinical trials evaluating the impact of quarterly recovery management checkups with adult chronic substance users. Addiction. 2009;104:959–71.

80. Scott K, Lewis CC. Using measurement-based care to enhance any treatment. Cogn Behav Pract. 2015;22(1):49–59.

81. Slade M, Longden E. Empirical evidence about recovery and mental health. BMC Psychiatry. 2015;15(1):285.

82. Smith PC, Schmidt SM, Allensworth-Davies D, Saitz R. A single-question screening test for drug use in primary care. Arch Intern Med. 2010;170(13):1155–60.

83. Sullivan JT, Skykora K, Schneiderman J. Assessment of alcohol withdrawal: the revised clinical institute withdrawal assessment for alcohol scale (CIWA-Ar). Br J Addict. 1989;84:1353–7.

84. Tiet QQ, Leyva Y, Moos RH, Smith B. Diagnostic accuracy of a two-item screen for drug use developed from the alcohol, smoking and substance involvement screening test (ASSIST). Drug Alcohol Depend. 2016;164:22–7.

85. Trenoweth S, Moone N, editors. Psychosocial assessment in mental health. Thousand Oaks: Sage; 2017.

86. Tucker J, Murphy JG, Kertesz SG. Chapter 14: Substance use disorders. In: Antony MM, Barlow DH, editors. Handbook of assessment and treatment planning for psychological disorders. New York: Guilford Press; 2011. p. 529–70.

87. Urbanoski K, Rush BR, Wild TC, Bassani D, Castel C. The use of mental health care services by Canadians with co-occurring substance dependence and mental illness. Psychiatr Serv. 2007;58(7):962–9.

88. Urbanoski KA, Cairney J, Bassani D, Rush B. Perceived unmet need for mental health care among Canadians with co-occurring addiction and mental illness. Psychiatr Serv. 2008;59(3):283–9.

89. Ware JE, Sherbourne CD. The MOS 36-item short-form health survey (SF-36). I. Conceptual framework and item selection. Med Care. 1992;30(6):473–83.

90. Wesson DR, Ling W. The clinical opiate withdrawal scale (COWS). J Psychoactive Drugs. 2002;35(2):253–9.

91. WHO Working Group. The alcohol, smoking and substance involvement screening test (ASSIST): development, reliability and feasibility. Addiction. 2002;97(9):1183–94.

92. Williams EC, Johnson ML, Lapham GT, Caldeiro RM, Chew L, Fletcher GS, McCormick KA, Weppner WG, Bradley KA. Strategies to implement alcohol screening and brief intervention in primary care settings: a structured literature review. Psychol Addict Behav. 2011;25(2):206–14.

93. Zimmerman M, Mattia JI. Psychiatric diagnosis in clinical practice: is comorbidity being missed? Compr Psychiatry. 1999;40:182–91.

94. Zimmerman M, Chelminski I. A scale to screen for DSM-IV Axis I disorders in psychiatric out-patients: performance of the psychiatric diagnostic screening questionnaire. Psychol Med. 2006;36(11):1601–11.

Stepped Care Models in Addiction Treatment

47

Ambros Uchtenhagen

Contents

Abstract

Stepped care models aim at matching treatment intensity to defined patient characteristics in a systematic way, thereby avoiding misplacements and making best use of available treatment resources at the same time. In principle, treatment planning for new patients starts with the least intensive care, progressing to more intensive regimes for nonresponders. Such models have been introduced in psychiatry and in other medical fields.

Models of stepwise patient placement in addiction treatment are known from Northern America (Sobell model, model of the American Society of Addiction Medicine, ASAM) for adults and adolescents and special models for dual-diagnosis patients. Another model comes from Europe (the Dutch model for triage and evaluation in addiction treatment MATE; special model for judicial patients). The various elements and procedures of the ASAM and MATE models are described and compared.

An overview on evaluation studies and reviews is presented, concerning feasibility, validity, reliability, effectiveness, and cost-effectiveness of stepped care models. Outcomes are partly positive, but limitations are mentioned, and more research is asked for.

Keywords

Level of care · Needs assessment · Patient placement · Treatment planning

A. Uchtenhagen (✉)
Swiss Research Foundation for Public Health and Addiction, Zurich University, Zurich, Switzerland
e-mail: ambros.uchtenhagen@isgf.uzh.ch

© Springer Nature Switzerland AG 2021
N. el-Guebaly et al. (eds.), *Textbook of Addiction Treatment*,
https://doi.org/10.1007/978-3-030-36391-8_47

47.1   Introduction

47.1.1 A Concept for Patient Placement

It is normal practice to assign a new patient to an appropriate and readily available treatment and to switch a patient not responding to that treatment to another one, be it another intervention type, another medication, or another setting. The therapist makes his or her choice on the basis of guideline recommendations, scientific studies, or personal experience, eventually also on the basis of patient preference.

The concept of stepped care combines a systematized version of such practice with an attempt at matching treatment intensity to patient characteristics. Screening the new patient for specific characteristics provides the basis for treatment indication and placement, starting with the least intensive intervention and stepping up intensity for nonresponders.

Main principle: Patients should be offered the least intensive and intrusive care at first contact, except in case of emergencies and defined complications which ask for an intensive treatment. Otherwise, only nonresponders should receive care along a scale of increased intensity. This principle is aiming to protect patients from intrusive care they do not need and to make best use of available treatment resources by avoiding misplacements. "Stepped care models represent attempts to maximise the effectiveness and efficiency of decisions about allocation of resources in therapy" [11].

47.1.2 Models of Stepped Care

Approaches to stepped care in addiction treatment have been described repeatedly [16]. By now, stepped care models have been introduced in some fields of psychiatry. Guidelines of the National Institute for Clinical Excellence (NICE) provide stepped care models in the UK for the treatment of depression and anxiety [20]. In the USA, such resource allocation issues are mentioned for anxiety disorder, panic disorder, eating disorder, and alcohol dependence [11].

47.1.2.1 From First Line to Intensive Care

In the model proposed by the Sobells [4, 24], the recommended treatment should start with the least restrictive intervention in terms of cost and personal inconvenience for patients. The first step might even involve facilitating "natural recovery" outside of professional services. Stepping up requires a decision about patient progress and depends on the type of disorder and the effectiveness of available treatments. The decisions may be made on the basis of guidelines but should not disregard the risk of inappropriate stepping up and of missed stepping up and should include considerations about costs of treatments at different levels.

47.1.2.2 The ASAM Patient Placement Model

The American Society of Addiction Medicine (ASAM) started to develop the patient placement criteria PPC in 1991, and in 1994 the National Institute of Drug Abuse (NIDA) funded a validity study. Revised versions were published in 1996 (ASAM PPC-2) and in 2001 (ASAM PPC-2R). A further revision will be based on DSM-5 to come.

The follow-up version of the placement criteria is published under the name of ASAM criteria (available in a third edition, referenced under the American Society of Addiction Medicine [2]).

The basis of the model is a concept of individualized treatment: assessment at intake is made in a range of biopsychosocial dimensions (multiaxial DSM diagnoses); assessment dimensions include also readiness to change, continued problem potential, and recovery environment. This is followed by an identification of priority problems, leading to defining the appropriate model and level of service. Progress assessment is used as a basis for eventual reassignment [14, 16, 17].

Placement criteria have been set up for adults and for adolescents. Special attention is also paid to co-occurring mental and substance-related disorders, in patient assessment, as well as in the specifications of services [15]. For dual-diagnosis patient, separate risk dimensions are set up: dangerousness/lethality, interference with addiction recovery efforts, social functioning, ability for self-care, and course of illness. The criteria also advocate for an adequate availability of treatment; by incorporating more use of outpatient care – especially for those in early stages of motivation for change – the criteria help to reduce waiting lists for residential treatment [17].

A supplement was published to delineate specific criteria for the use of pharmacotherapies for alcohol use disorders, for detoxification, and relapse [10].

47.1.2.3 MATE: A Model for Patient Assessment and Referral

The Dutch model for measurement in the addictions for triage and evaluation MATE [21, 22] is a national project, aiming at constructing and testing of a new instrument for the assessment at intake of all problems and needs in relevant domains in substance abuse treatment; the instrument should also be useful as a framework for the application of existing instruments in selected domains for matching, patient allocation, and treatment evaluation in the addictions. The instrument should help to make rational and transparent decisions about providing which and how much treatment to which patients. It was tested for feasibility, reliability, and validity in a population of heavy users, and in a subproject an instrument was developed and tested for judicial clients.

The assessment of substance use disorders at intake is made on the basis of the international classification systems ICD/DSM. Assessment of personal and social functioning is made in order to determine which type of services will be needed; this part of the new instrument is based on the WHO international classification system of functioning, disability, and health ICF. Existing instruments are used for the assessment of comorbidities, new modules for treatment history, motivation, and criminality. Overall, the MATE instrument is composed of ten modules. A manual and a protocol with detailed instructions were published in Dutch.

The MATE was adopted and further developed in Germany. A German version of the instrument was tested and implemented [6–8, 23].

47.1.3 The Main Elements of Stepped Care Models: A Comparative Overview

Stepped care models use three essential elements: patient indicators used for determining the appropriate level of care, treatment typology in regard to intensity of care, assessment, and referral procedures. The following figures summarize the relevant information on these elements in the ASAM and MATE models (Tables 47.1 and 47.2; Figs. 47.1 and 47.2).

MATE criteria were developed for Germany by the German Psychiatric Association and published by the German Ministry of Health.

Detailed criteria listed in the German evaluation protocol for treatment evaluation

Headings:	A 1–12	Seriousness of condition
	B 1–5	Intensity of treatment
	C 1–2	Invasive interventions
	D 1–6	Comorbidities

Source: [8]

Table 47.1 Patient characteristics used for determining appropriate level of care

ASAM assessment dimensions	MATE patient indicators
Acute intoxication and/or withdrawal potential	Addiction severity
Biomedical conditions and complications	Psychiatric impairment
Emotional, behavioral, cognitive conditions/complications	Social stability
Readiness to change	Treatment history 0–1
Relapse/continued use, continued problem potential	Treatment history 2
Recovery environment	Treatment history 3–5
	Treatment history >5

Source for ASAM: Mee-Lee and Shulman [17], Table 27.1. Source for MATE: Schippers and Broekman [21].

Table 47.2 Treatment typology

ASAM levels of care	MATE levels of care
0.5. Early intervention	1. Short outpatient
I. Outpatient treatment	2. Outpatient
II.1. Intensive outpatient	3. Day care/residential
II.5. Partial hospitalization	4. Care (in- and outpatient)
III.1. Low-intensity residential treatment	
III.3. Medium-intensity residential treatment	
III.5. Medium–/high-intensity residential treatment	
III.7. Medically monitored intensive inpatient	
IV. Medically managed intensive inpatient OMT. Opioid maintenance therapy	
Levels of care for adult detoxification	
I-D. ambulatory detoxification without extended on-site monitoring II-D. ambulatory detoxification with extended onsite monitoring	
II 2-D. clinically managed residential detoxification III 7-D. medically monitored inpatient detoxification IV-D. medically managed inpatient detoxification	

Source for ASAM: Mee-Lee and Shulman [17], Table 27.2. Source for MATE: Schippers and Broekman [21].

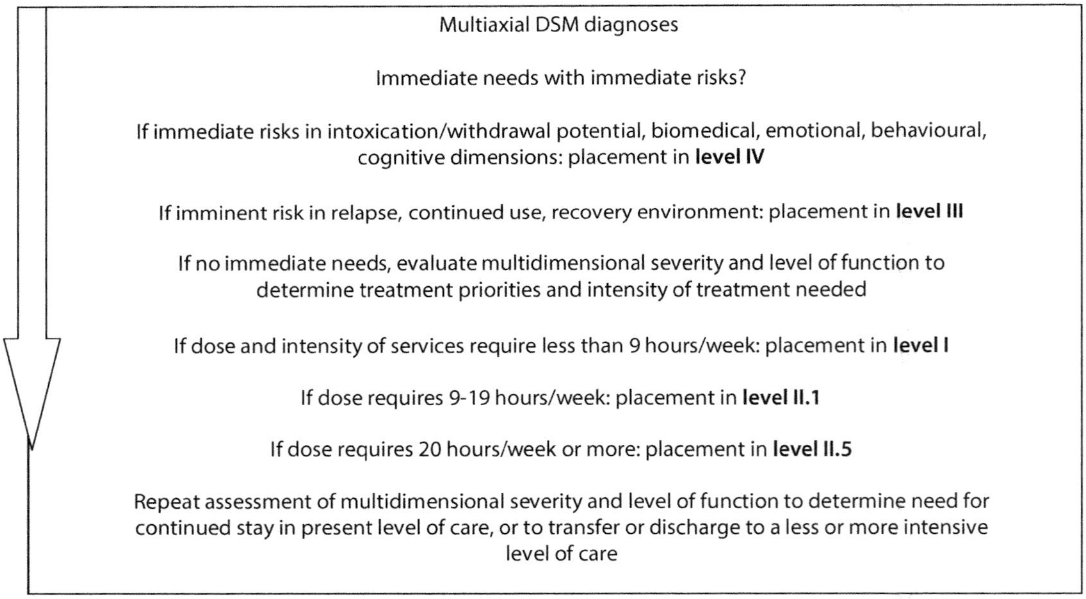

Multiaxial DSM diagnoses

Immediate needs with immediate risks?

If immediate risks in intoxication/withdrawal potential, biomedical, emotional, behavioural, cognitive dimensions: placement in **level IV**

If imminent risk in relapse, continued use, recovery environment: placement in **level III**

If no immediate needs, evaluate multidimensional severity and level of function to determine treatment priorities and intensity of treatment needed

If dose and intensity of services require less than 9 hours/week: placement in **level I**

If dose requires 9-19 hours/week: placement in **level II.1**

If dose requires 20 hours/week or more: placement in **level II.5**

Repeat assessment of multidimensional severity and level of function to determine need for continued stay in present level of care, or to transfer or discharge to a less or more intensive level of care

Fig. 47.1 Assessment and referral procedures in ASAM PPC-2r. (Source: [16], Fig. 6–1)

47.1.4 The NICE Model of Stepped Care

The National Institute for Health and Clinical Excellence (NICE) published recommendations for the psychological treatment of depressions and anxiety disorders in a framework of a stepped care system. The guiding principles are to deliver best possible outcomes while burdening patients as little as possible and to provide scheduled reviews how to step up or down to more or less intensive treatment if appropriate. The system includes three levels of intensity of care (starting with primary care, moving up to self-help interventions, and then to cognitive behavioral therapy) [19].

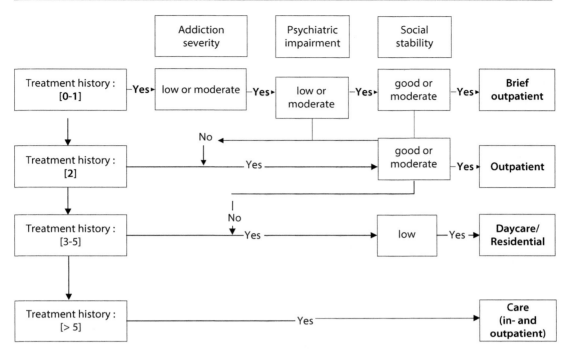

Fig. 47.2 MATE guidance for matching and referral. (Source: [18], Fig. 2)

47.1.5 Evaluation Results and Perspectives

A systematic review was made on the efficacy of stepped care models involving different levels of psychosocial treatment for alcohol use disorders and nicotine dependence, with or without medication [12]. Little evidence was found to suggest that stepping up nonresponders to more intensive therapy improved outcomes. In one study, the application of a stepped care approach was found to reduce treatment costs compared with usual care. There was some evidence that the greater differentiation between the intensity of the interventions offered at each step, the better the outcome. Further research is needed to evaluate the efficacy of stepped care approaches to providing psychosocial treatment.

A summary of research on the ASAM patient placement criteria is presented in the *Textbook of Substance Abuse Treatment*. The authors conclude as follows: "More than a decade of research of the ASAM PPC supports the predictive validity and the cost-effectiveness of the use of

PPC. Based on this research, a variety of computer assisted assessment and placement tools are in development" [16, p. 88]. Another overview is presented in the *Principles of Addiction Medicine*. Nine evaluation studies were performed involving 3641 subjects; controlled studies found that "treatment based on the ASAM PPC are associated with less morbidity, better client functioning, and more efficient service utilization than mismatched treatment" [17, p. 398].

The ASAM placement criteria have been further developed in a guidebook on the treatment of substance abuse issues under the title of ASAM Essentials [1].

Feasibility and field testing of the MATE in a treatment-seeking population were performed in two large treatment settings. Construct validation with related instruments and evaluation of the dimensional structure of modules were performed. Among the results are a satisfactory inter-rater reliability and concurrent validity, indicating the usefulness of the instrument for allocating patients to substance abuse treatment, even in a heterogeneous population [22].

However, there were some problems with clinicians not complying with the guidelines, resulting in mismatched patients usually allocated to outpatient treatment instead of early interventions [18].

A recent manual provides guidance for implementation and comparative research [5]. This manual is now available in English, German, Dutch, Italian, Danish, French, Slovenian, and Portuguese (https://www.mateinfo.eu/german/index).

Another systematic review of stepped care in psychological interventions was made [3]. It identified the underlying assumptions on which the benefits of stepped care depend: equivalence in terms of clinical outcomes, efficiency in terms of resource use and costs, and acceptability of "minimal interventions" to patients and therapists. The review concludes that more research is needed in terms of rigorous evaluations of the underlying assumptions.

A comparison of minimal interventions with a stepped care model for patients with alcohol use disorders in the UK evidenced greater cost savings, greater motivation for change, and greater reduction of alcohol consumption for stepped care 6 months after randomization [9].

47.2   Further Developments

Stepped care models have a considerable potential to improve patient-service matching with improved outcomes and improved use of treatment resources. Stepped care is also considered to be an important element of individualized treatment [13]. A wider implementation of existing or new models however is slow and may meet problems if not politically supported.

References

1. Abigail HJ, Brennan TK, editors. ASAM essentials of Addiction Medicine. 2nd ed. 2015. Retrieved from https://www.asam.org/resources/publications/essentials-of-addiction-med.
2. American Society of Addiction Treatment. ASAM Criteria. Guidelines for placement, continued stay and transfer/discharge of patients with addiction and co-occurring conditions. 3rd ed. 2013. www.asam.org/resources.
3. Bower P, Gilbody S. Stepped care in psychological therapies: access, effectiveness and efficiency. Narrative literature review. Br J Psychiatry. 2005;186:11–7.
4. Breslin F, Sobell M, Sobell L. Problem drinkers: evaluation of stepped care approach. J Subst Abus. 1999;10:217–32.
5. Broekman T, Schippers G. Manual of comparison groups. Composition and use of the comparison scores for the MATE 2–1 and the MATE-Y 2–1. Nijmegen: Bureau Beta; 2018.
6. Buchholz A, Rist F, Küfner H, Kraus L. Die deutsche Version des Measurements in the Addictions for Triage and Evaluation (MATE): Reliabilität, Validität und Anwendbarkeit. Sucht. 2009;55:219–42.
7. Buchholz A, Friedrichs A. ICF in der Suchttherpie. Die Anwendung des MATE-ICN zur Erfassung von Leistungseinschränkungen und Hilfebedarf bei Patienten mit substanzbezogenen Störungen. Konturen Sucht soz Fragen. 2013;27:27–31.
8. Die Drogenbeauftragte der Bundesregierung (Hrsg.). S-3 Leitlinie Methamphetamin-bezogene Störungen. (MATE Kriterien im Anhang). Berlin: Springer; 2016.
9. Drummond C, Coulton S, Darrenn J, Godfrey C, Parrott S, Baxter J, Ford D, Lervy B, Rollnick S, Russell J, Peters T. Effectiveness and cost-effectiveness for a stepped care intervention for alcohol use disorders in primary care: a pilot study. Br J Psychiatry. 2009;195:448–56.
10. Fishman MJ, editor. The ASAM patient placement criteria. Supplement on pharmacotherapies for alcohol use disorders. 1st ed. Philadelphia: Lippincott, Williams and Wilkins; 2010.
11. Haaga DAF. Introduction to the special section on stepped care models in psychotherapy. J Consult Clin Psychol. 2000;68:547–8.
12. Jaehne A, Loessl B, Frick K, Berner M, Hukse G, Balmford J. The efficacy of stepped care models involving psychosocial treatments in alcohol use disorders and nicotine dependence: a systematic review of the literature. Curr Drug Abuse Rev. 2012;5:41–51.
13. Kranzler HR, McKay JR. Personalized treatment of alcohol dependence. Cum Psychiatry Rep. 2012;14:486–93. https://doi.org/10.1007/s11920-012-0296-5.
14. Mee-Lee D, editor. ASAM patient placement criteria for the treatment of substance use disorders. 2nd ed. Revised. American Society of Addiction Medicine. 2001. www.asam/org/publications.patient-placement-criteria/ppc-2r.
15. Mee-Lee D. Development and implementation of patient placement criteria. New developments in addiction treatment. Academic highlights. J Clin Psychiatry. 2006;67(11):1805–7.
16. Mee-Lee D, Gastfriend DR. Patient placement criteria. In: Galanter M, Kleber HD, editors. Textbook

of substance abuse treatment. 4th ed. Arlington: The American Psychiatric Publishing; 2008. p. 79–91.

17. Mee-Lee D, Shulman GD. The ASAM placement criteria and matching patients to treatment. In: Ries RK, Fiellin DA, Miller SC, Saitz R, editors. Principles of addiction medicine. 4th ed. Philadelphia: Kluwer/ Lippincott, Williams & Wilkins; 2009.

18. Merkx MJM, Schippers GM, Koeter MJ, Vujik PJ, Oudejans S, De Vries CCQ, Van den Brink W. Allocation of substance use disorder patients to appropriate levels of care: feasibility of matching guidelines in routine practice in Dutch treatment centres. Addiction. 2007;102:466–74.

19. NHS. n.d. Retrieved from https://www.humber.nhs.uk/advice-health-and-wellbeing/nice_2.htm.

20. Richards DA, Power P, Pagel C, Weaver A, Utley M, Cape J, Pilling S, Lovell K, et al. Delivering stepped care: an analysis of implementation in routine practice. Implement Sci. 2012;7:3.

21. Schippers GM, Broekman TG. MATE, measurements in the addictions for triage and evaluation. Final report. 2007. www.mateinfo.en/pubs/31000068.pdf. Accessed 22 Jan 2013.

22. Schippers GM, Broekman TG, Buchholz A, Koeter MWJ, Van den Brink W. Measurements in the Addictions for Triage and Evaluation (MATE): an instrument based on the World Health Organisation family of international classifications. Addiction. 2010;105:862–71.

23. Schippers GM, Broekman TG, Buchholz A. Handbuch und Leitfaden zur Anwendung des MATE. 2011. http://www.mateinfo.eu/german/index.

24. Sobell MB, Sobell LC. Stepped care as a heuristic approach to the treatment of alcohol problems. J Consult Clin Psychol. 2000;68:573–9.

Therapeutic Communities for Addictions: Essential Elements, Cultural, and Current Issues

48

George De Leon, Fernando B. Perfas,
Aloysius Joseph, and Gregory Bunt

Contents

G. De Leon (✉)
BST at the School of Nursing, NYU,
New York, NY, USA

Department of Psychiatry, NYU School of Medicine,
New York, NY, USA

F. B. Perfas
Daytop International Training Academy,
New York, NY, USA
e-mail: FPerfas@daytop.org

A. Joseph
Daytop International, Inc., New York, NY, USA
e-mail: AJoseph@daytop.org

G. Bunt
Daytop Village, Inc., New York, NY, USA

Department of Psychiatry, NYU Langone
Medical Center,
New York, NY, USA
e-mail: gbunt@daytop.org

© Springer Nature Switzerland AG 2021
N. el-Guebaly et al. (eds.), *Textbook of Addiction Treatment*,
https://doi.org/10.1007/978-3-030-36391-8_48

Abstract

The therapeutic community (TC) is a major treatment modality serving a wide spectrum of substance abuse clients worldwide. The weight of the research evidence developed over some 40 years demonstrates that the TC is an effective and cost-effective treatment particularly for substance abusers with serious social and psychological problems in addition to their drug abuse. This chapter provides an overview of the essential elements of the TC approach: its perspective, method, program model, and adaptation for special populations, settings, and different cultures.

TCs have been successfully modified for special populations of substance users including those with co-occurring disorders, adolescents, women with children, criminal justice clients in prisons, and community-based settings. TC programs have been implemented in Europe, Asia, Africa, Latin America, and the Middle East. And, despite ethnic, social-political, and religious differences, TCs have retained their essential elements and effectiveness across a variety of cultures.

Its evolution over some 50 years has surfaced key issues that challenge the TC to maintain the integrity of its unique social psychological approach – community as method. Several of these are briefly highlighted including funding, workforce, research, treatment fidelity, and the diversity of TC programs. In the current context, the TC is compelled to reassert its place and mission in human services – that of promoting recovery and right living.

Keywords

Therapeutic community · Cultural diversity · Treatment efficacy · International · Treatment perspectives · History

48.1   Introduction

Drug-free residential programs for substance abuse appeared a decade later than did therapeutic communities (TCs) in psychiatric hospitals pioneered by Maxwell Jones and others in the United Kingdom. The term therapeutic community evolved in these hospital settings, although the two models arose independently.

The TC for substance abuse emerged in the late 1950s as a self-help alternative to existing conventional treatments. The originators were recovering alcoholic and drug-addicted individuals [20, 21]. Although its modern antecedents can be traced to Alcoholics Anonymous and Synanon, contemporary TCs for addictions are sophisticated human services institutions. Today, the label therapeutic community is generic, describing a variety of short- and long-term residential and nonresidential programs that serve a wide spectrum of substance abuse clients. Although the TC approach has been adapted for different populations and settings, it is the perspective and method of the traditional long-term residential prototype for adult substance abusers that have documented effectiveness in rehabilitating substance-abusing individuals.

48.2   Essential Elements

48.2.1 The TC Perspective

The TC perspective or theory shapes its program model and its unique approach, community as method. The perspective consists of four interrelated views of the substance use disorder, the individual, recovery process, and healthy living.

48.2.1.1   View of Disorder

Drug abuse is viewed as a disorder of the whole person, affecting some or all areas of functioning. Cognitive and behavioral problems are often present, as are mood disturbances. Thinking may be unrealistic or disorganized; values may be confused, nonexistent, or antisocial. Frequently, the patient exhibits deficits in verbal, reading, writing, or marketable skills. Moral or even spiritual issues, whether expressed in existential or psychological terms, are apparent. Thus, the TC perspective considers the problem to be the individual, not the drug, and addiction is a symptom, not the essence of the disorder.

48.2.1.2 View of the Person

In TCs, individuals are distinguished along dimensions of psychological dysfunction and social deficits rather than according to drug use patterns. Regardless of differences in social background, drug preference, or psychological problems, most individuals admitted to TCs share clinical characteristics (Table 48.1). Whether they are antecedent or consequent to serious involvement with drugs, these characteristics are commonly observed to correlate with chemical dependency. More important, in TCs, a positive change in these characteristics is considered to be essential for stable recovery.

48.2.1.3 View of Recovery

In the TC perspective, recovery extends beyond drug freedom, involving a change in lifestyle and in personal identity. The primary psychological goal is to change the negative patterns of behavior, thinking, and feeling that predispose the individual to drug use; the main social goal is to develop the skills, attitudes, and values of a responsible drug-free lifestyle.

In many TC residents, vocational and educational problems are marked; middle- class, mainstream values are either missing or not sought. Usually these residents emerge from a socially disadvantaged sector. Their recovery in the TC is

Table 48.1 Typical behavioral, cognitive, and emotional characteristics of substance abusers in therapeutic communities

Low tolerance for all forms of discomfort and delay of gratification
Problems with authority
Inability to manage feelings (particularly hostility/anger, guilt, and anxiety)
Poor impulse control (particularly sexual or aggressive impulses)
Poor judgment and reality testing concerning consequences of actions
Unrealistic self-appraisal regarding discrepancies between personal resources and aspirations
Prominence of lying, manipulation, and deception as coping behaviors
Personal and social irresponsibility (e.g., inconsistency or failures in meeting obligations)
Marked deficits in learning and in marketable and communication skills

better termed *habilitation*, the development of a socially productive, conventional lifestyle for the first time. Among individuals from more advantaged backgrounds, the term *rehabilitation* is more suitable, which emphasizes a return to a lifestyle previously lived, known, and perhaps rejected.

48.2.1.4 View of Right Living

TCs adhere to certain precepts and values that constitute a view of healthy personal and social living that guide and reinforce recovery. For example, community sanctions address antisocial behaviors and attitudes; the negative values of the street, jails, or negative peers; and irresponsible or exploitative sexual conduct. Positive values are emphasized as being essential to social learning and personal growth. These values include truth and honesty (in word and deed), a work ethic, self-reliance, earned rewards and achievement, personal accountability, responsible concern (being one's brother's or sister's keeper), social manners, and community involvement. The precepts of right living are constantly reinforced in various formal and informal ways (e.g., signs, seminars, in groups and community meetings).

48.2.2 The TC Approach: Community as Method

The TC approach can be summarized in the phrase "community as method" [2, 3]. A parallel concept – "community as doctor" – in the psychiatric or democratic TC was first coined by Rapoport [16]. Theoretical writings offer a definition of "community as method" as follows: the *purposive* use of the community to teach individuals to *use* the community to change themselves. The fundamental assumption underlying the TC approach is that individuals obtain maximum therapeutic and educational impact when they engage in and learn to use all of the activities, elements of the community as the tools for self-change. Thus, community as method means that the community itself provides a *context* of relationships and activities for social learning. Its membership establishes the *expectations* or standards of participation in community activities; it continually *assesses* how individuals are meeting these expectations and *responds* to them with strategies that promote continued participation.

48.2.3 TC Program Model

The key components of the program model are its social organization (structure), peer and staff roles, groups and individual counseling, community enhancement meetings, community management elements, and program stages. Each component reflects an understanding of the TC perspective, and each is used to transmit community teachings, promote affiliation, and self-change.

48.2.3.1 Social Organization

The TC social organization is stratified with relatively few staff of the TC at the top complemented by resident peers at junior, intermediate, and senior levels. This peer level-to-community structure strengthens the patient's identification with a perceived ordered network of individuals. More important, it arranges relation- ships of mutual responsibility at various levels in the program.

The daily operation of the community itself is the task of the residents, who work together under staff supervision. The broad range of resident job assignments illustrates the extent of the self-help process. Residents perform all house services (e.g., cooking, cleaning, kitchen service, minor repair), serve as apprentices, run all departments, and conduct house meetings, certain seminars, and peer encounter groups.

The TC is managed by the staff, who monitor and evaluate patient status, supervise resident groups, assign and supervise resident jobs, and oversee house operations. The staff members conduct therapeutic groups (other than peer encounter groups), provide individual counseling, and organize social and recreational projects. They make decisions about resident status, e.g., discipline, promotion, transfers, discharges, furloughs, and treatment planning.

48.2.3.2 Peers as Role Models

Peers, serving as role models, and staff members, serving as role models and rational authorities, are the primary mediators of the recovery process. TC members who demonstrate the expected behaviors and reflect the values and teachings of the community are viewed as role models. TCs require multiple resident and staff role models in order to maintain the integrity of the community and ensure the spread of social learning effects.

48.2.3.3 Staff Members as Rational Authorities

Staff members foster the self-help learning process through performance of their managerial and clinical functions described above but also as role models and rational authorities. TC residents often have had difficulties with authorities who have not been trusted or who have been perceived as guides and teachers. There- fore, residents need a positive experience with an authority figure who is viewed as credible, supportive, corrective, and protective so that they may gain authority over themselves (personal autonomy). As rational authorities, staff members provide the reasons for their decisions and explain the meaning of consequences particularly in terms of recovery and personal growth.

48.2.3.4 Therapeutic Educational Activities (Groups and Individual Counseling)

Various forms of group process and individual counseling provide residents with opportunities to express feelings and resolve personal and social issues. They increase communication and interpersonal skills, bring about examination and confrontation of behavior and attitudes, and offer instruction in alternative modes of behavior. The main forms of group activity in the TC are peer-led encounter groups, staff-led therapy, and tutorial groups. Other groups that convene regularly or held as needed supplement the main groups. These vary in focus, format, and composition and include gender, ethnic, age-specific, or health theme groups. Additionally, cognitive-behavioral tutorials using manualized curricula are employed for targeted areas such as relapse prevention, criminal thinking, trauma and PTSD, etc.

One-to-one counseling balances the needs of the individual with those of the community. Peer exchange is ongoing and is the most consistent form of informal counseling in TCs. Staff counseling sessions may be regularly scheduled or conducted as needed. The focus of staff counseling is to address issues that may impede progress and to facilitate the patient's adjustment to and constructive use of the peer community. Counseling is also employed for the purpose of developing an individualized treatment plan.

48.2.3.5 Community Enhancement Activities (Meetings)

Community enhancement activities are the facility-wide meetings that convene daily. These include the morning meeting, the seminar, the house (evening) meeting, and a general meeting. Some of these are held almost daily, while others are called when needed. These gatherings are necessary for building the spirit of community to which members are expected to participate actively. Though different in format, all meetings have the common objective of facilitating the individual's assimilation into the community. The purpose of the morning meeting is to instill a positive attitude in the community at the beginning of the day, motivate residents, create camaraderie, and strengthen unity. Seminars are community-wide teaching sessions led by peers or staff presenting topics that directly or indirectly relate to the TC perspective on recovery and right living. House meetings are coordinated by senior residents to transact community business. General meetings take place only when needed and are usually called so that negative behavior, attitudes, or incidents in the facility can be addressed. While these activities are often facilitated by senior residents, staff are available to oversee them. Community enhancement also occurs in a variety of nonscheduled, informal activities as well. These include activities related to rituals and traditions, celebrations (e.g., birthdays, graduations, phase changes, job changes), ceremonies (e.g., those relating to general and cultural holidays), and memorial observances for deceased residents, family members of residents, and staff members.

48.2.3.6 Community and Clinical Management Elements

Community and clinical management elements maintain the physical and psychological safety of the environment and ensure that resident life is orderly and productive. Thus, they strengthen community as a context for social learning. The main elements that are staff managed, although with some input from the senior resident social hierarchy, are privileges, disciplinary sanctions, surveillance, and urine testing. How- ever, peer confrontation in the form of verbal correctives, affirmations, and feedback (e.g., reactions, advice, information) are ongoing community management activities.

48.2.3.7 Program Stages and Phases

Recovery in the TC is a developmental process that can be understood as a passage through program stages of learning. The learning that occurs at each stage facilitates change at the next, and each change reflects movement toward the goal of recovery. Three major program stages characterize change in long-term residential TCs – *orientation-induction*, *primary treatment*, and *reentry* – and may include additional substages or phases. The original time frame for these stages was grounded in a planned duration of treatment ranging up to 24 months. Current stage and phase durations are shorter commensurate with decreased overall planned durations. Regardless of temporal changes completion of each stage is a celebrated event marking acknowledged programmatic and clinical progress.

Completion marks the end of active program involvement. Graduation itself, however, is an annual event conducted in the facility for individuals who have completed all program stages and have successfully spent some time outside the treatment facility. Thus, the TC experience facilitates a process of change that must continue throughout life; and what is gained in treatment are tools to guide the individual on a path of continued change. Completion, or graduation, therefore, is not an end but a beginning.

48.2.3.8 Aftercare

TCs have always acknowledged the patient's efforts to maintain sobriety and a positive lifestyle beyond graduation. Until recently, long-term TCs addressed key clinical and life adjustment issues of aftercare during the reentry stages of the 2-year program. As noted, funding pressures have resulted in shorter planned durations of residential treatment and the stages and phases therein. This has underscored the necessity for aftercare resources to address both primary treatment and reentry issues. Thus, many contemporary TCs offer post-residential aftercare treatment and social services within their systems, such as intensive day treatment and step-down outpatient ambulatory treatment or through linkages with outside agencies.

48.2.4 The Effectiveness of Therapeutic Communities

Over the past four decades, a considerable scientific knowledge base has developed with follow-up studies on thousands of individuals treated in TCs. The most extensive body of research bearing on the effectiveness of addiction TC programs has amassed from field outcome studies. These all employed similar longitudinal designs that follow admissions to TCs during treatment and 1–5 years (and in one study up to 12 years) after leaving the index treatment.

These studies show that TC admissions have poor profiles in terms of severity of substance use, social deviance, and psychological symptoms. The striking replications across studies leave little doubt as to the reliability of the main conclusion. Namely, there is a consistent relationship between retention in treatment and positive posttreatment outcomes in TCs. Replication studies overseas seem to follow the same trend. This conclusion is supported in the smaller number of controlled and comparative studies involving TC programs (for a recent review of the TC outcome literature in North America, see [4]). Overall, the weight of the research evidence from multiple sources (multi-program field effectiveness studies, single-program controlled studies,

meta-analytic statistical surveys, and cost-benefit studies) is compelling in supporting the hypothesis that the TC is an effective and cost-effective treatment for certain subgroups of substance abusers, particularly those with serious social and psychological problems in addition to their drug abuse.

48.2.5 Adaptations and Modifications of the TC for Special Populations and Settings

The traditional TC model described in this chapter is actually the prototype of a variety of TC-oriented programs. Today, the TC modality consists of a wider range of programs serving a diversity of patients who use a variety of drugs and present with complex social and psychological problems in addition to their substance abuse. Client differences as well as clinical requirements and funding realities have encouraged the development of modified residential TC programs with shorter planned durations of stay (3, 6, and 12 months) as well as TC-oriented day treatment and outpatient ambulatory models. Having become overwhelmed with alcohol and drug abuse problems, correctional facilities, medical and mental hospitals, and community residences and shelters have implemented TC programs within their settings. Additionally, the TC approach has shown to be effective within these specialty settings [4].

Most community-based traditional TCs have expanded their social services or have incorporated new interventions to address the needs of their diverse residents. These changes and additions include family services, primary healthcare specifically geared toward HIV-positive patients and individuals with AIDS, aftercare services particularly for special populations such as substance-abusing inmates leaving prison treatment, relapse prevention training, components of 12-step groups, mental health services, and other evidence-based practices (e.g., cognitive-behavioral therapy, motivational interviewing). Mostly, these modifications and additions enhance but do not substitute for the basic TC approach, community as method. Research literature documents the effectiveness and cost-effectiveness of modified TCs for special populations including homeless mentally ill chemical abusers, those in criminal justice settings, and adolescents (e.g., [2, 6, 9, 17, 19]).

48.2.6 TCs Worldwide

Over some five decades, TC programs have been implemented worldwide. In Europe, the establishment of drug-free therapeutic communities was the main treatment response to the emerging heroin problems in the 1960s and 1970s. The original American TC model was adapted to the European culture, and it integrated the long-standing local traditions and influences. Between 1968 and 1983, the TC approach spread rapidly across virtually all countries in Europe including the United Kingdom and subsequently to Asia, Africa, and Latin America. Globally, it is conservatively estimated that there are over 3000 TCs operating in hospital, prison, juvenile centers, outpatient, and community-based settings.

48.2.7 TC Outcome Research Worldwide

The North American research literature is the most extensive and has been briefly cited above. There is a modest but developing research literature on TCs worldwide particularly of European programs. The main conclusion from recent reviews of the European outcome studies may be briefly summarized.

"Length of stay in treatment and participation in subsequent aftercare were consistent predictors of recovery status. The authors conclude that TCs can promote change regarding various outcome categories. Since recovering addicts often cycle between abstinence and relapse, a continuing care approach is advisable, including assessment of multiple and subjective outcome indicators" [18]. Similar conclusions are obtained in outcome studies of TC programs in Peru and Thailand [10, 11] and Australia [15].

Although treatment process studies are few, emerging research has supported hypotheses concerning the generality of the perspective, model, and method of TC. Utilizing a common assessment instrument (the Survey of Essential Elements Questionnaire SEEQ; [12]), these studies emphasize that differences exist between standard and modified TCs in essential elements within cultures but that the similarities in elements outweigh the differences across cultures [7, 8, 10, 11].

48.2.8 Cultural Adaptations of the TC

Given the complexity of the TC as a social psychological approach, it is understandable that its implementation has been influenced by cultural context. Even within North America, for example, TC programs have adapted to ethnic diversity factors [5]. The adaptation of the TC to cultural diversity or context factors is still greater at the global level.

Beyond the above studies supporting the generality of the essential elements, there has been relatively little empirical research that focuses on cultural influences in the adaptation of the TC. However, a considerable descriptive literature of TCs in different cultures has unfolded over some four decades. Some reports can be found in scientific journals, but most are contained in the published conference proceedings of international and regional TC associations, e.g., the World Federation of Therapeutic Communities (WFTC), the European Federation of Therapeutic Communities (EFTC), the Australasian Therapeutic Communities Association (ATCA), the Latin-American Federation of Therapeutic Communities, and the Asian Federation of Therapeutic Communities.

These writings, along with the few empirical studies and the years of observations by trainers, consultants, and others, have identified various cultural context influences that are embedded in TC programs (see some examples in Table 48.2). It is beyond the purview of this chapter to discuss

Table 48.2 Some examples of cultural elements shaping the unique TC characteristics in different cultures

Gender. In cultures where there are strict norms regarding the mixing of the sexes, there are separate TCs for men and women. The segregation is not driven by clinical rationale intended to better meet the unique needs of a particular gender but more for moral and reasons of propriety.
Religion. In most Eastern TCs, religion and religious practices are integrated into the TC structure. Those who belong to minority religions are encouraged to practice their faith. Major religious holidays are observed, and program activities are tailored around celebrations of such holidays. Even dietary practices are observed.
Social organization. The traditional hierarchical structure of the TC is highly compatible with the formal and often rigid social structure in most conservative cultures. The TC hierarchical structure lends clarity which is consistent with the formal social structures of most of these societies. The delineation and lack of ambiguity of job positions and social status in the community promote social harmony. It also defines the social roles of and expectations from the community members.
Role of the recovering addict as therapist. In most Oriental or Eastern cultures, academic credentials are preferred over experiential training. The contributions of the "recovering" person as therapist are not greatly appreciated, unless the person has a college degree in addition to personal experience. It requires a paradigm shift to consider, for example, a recovering addict or a recovered mentally ill person who become therapists themselves.
Time orientation or temporal perception. Eastern culture has a fluid perception of time in contrast to Western society's highly structured time perception, "on-time" versus "in-time" orientation. Time orientation or how and when activities are implemented has implications in terms of operational efficiency and outcomes. The result-oriented and purpose-driven structure and schedule of the TC compel timeliness in order to comply with the demands and expectations of supporting and maintaining the community. Timeliness is observed across the board out of necessity, transcending cultural temporal perception.
The professional as TC staff. Many TCs outside the United States were founded by professionals who employed the services of TC-recovered ex-addicts as clinical staff along with professional staff. Working as a team, the combination creates a very progressive TC by exploiting the unique contributions of each.
Family. The importance of the family and their role in treatment in various cultures are evident in the popularity of family associations [14]. Some TCs, such as in the case of Indonesia, were conceived by parents who originally sent their children to a Malaysian TC for treatment. In due time, they initiated a TC movement in their own country. Malaysian and Chinese TCs consider family and religion (spirituality) to be central to treatment [1].

these in detail, but several working conclusions are offered concerning the TC's adaptation to cultural influences.

First, the TC perspective (i.e., views of the whole person disorder, recovery, and right living) and its approach (community as method) can be preserved and integrated within diverse cultures. Second, empirical research is needed to abstract a more complete list of cultural influences and to assess their impact on outcomes. Finally, across all cultures, maintaining *fidelity* of practice is necessary to assure the optimal effectiveness of the TC approach, a general issue which is briefly discussed in the last section of this chapter.

48.2.9 Issues and Challenges to the TC

The evolution of the contemporary therapeutic community (TC) for addictions over the past 45 years may be characterized as a movement from the marginal to the mainstream of substance abuse treatment and human services. Currently, TCs serve a wide diversity of clients and problems; they have reshaped staffing composition, reduced the planned duration of residential treatment, reset its treatment goals, and, to a considerable extent, modified the approach itself. These evolutionary changes have surfaced key issues that challenge the TC to maintain the integrity of its unique approach. Several of these are briefly highlighted: funding, workforce, research, treatment fidelity, and the diversity of TCs. Though interrelated, these issues are discussed separately.

Additionally, in the United States, many TC programs have "converted" or begun mergers with physical health clinics with the notion that TC integration with primary healthcare services will produce better outcomes [13]. However, it should be noted this integration may exacerbate the challenges of maintaining treatment fidelity.

48.2.10 Funding and Planned Duration of Treatment

Issue: The success of the TC approach has been demonstrated primarily for residential programs with planned durations of treatment of at least 9–12 months. In recent years, however, fiscal support has been steadily decreasing for long-term treatment in general and for residential treatment in particular. Thus, for the large majority of TCs that depend upon public funding, planned duration of treatment has been reduced often *below the threshold* of time needed to yield positive outcomes. This adjustment to funding pressures potentially undermines the viability of the TC as a cost-effective modality in the healthcare system.

48.2.11 Workforce

Issue: The expansion of the TC to serve special populations in special settings has resulted in a number of problems in the recruitment, retention, and development of experienced staff. General problems include low salaries, limited career goals, and difficult working conditions. However, a specific workforce issue arises from the *diversity of staff* in TCs. The increased number of traditional professional staff from mental health and social services has posed a special challenge to the TC. Based on their education and training, traditional professional staff utilize concepts, vernacular, and methods that often counter or subvert the fundamental mutual self-help features of the TC. Moreover, most professionals and ex-addict paraprofessionals who work in TCs do not undergo rigorous and supervised training on the TC model and its practice.

48.2.12 Research

Issue: Despite decades of therapeutic community (TC) outcome research, some critics have questioned whether the TC is an evidence-based treatment for addictions. Given the relative lack of randomized, double-blind control trials, it is con-cluded that the effectiveness of the TC has not been "proven." Such conclusions contain serious implications for the acceptance and future development of the TC.

A new research agenda should build on the existing knowledge base that documents the contribution of the TC as a major health and human services modality. This agenda should include studies that demonstrate (a) *health and social benefits* (e.g., reduction in drug/alcohol use and social deviancy and increase in employment, education, and overall psychological well-being), (b) *cost-benefits* of both long-term TCs and shorter-term residential programs for specific subgroups of substance abusers, and (c) *collateral benefits* which refers to the *prevention* of trans-genera-tional drug use, HIV, STDs, as well as family breakdown among treatment successes.

48.2.13 Treatment Fidelity

Issue: Understandably, TCs have pursued finan-cial solvency by expanding to serve a wide vari-ety of populations, e.g., mental health, homeless, corrections, juvenile justice, and childcare. Contracts have obligated TCs to meet regulations of community, state, and federal agencies and often to incorporate practices based upon differ-ent professional views of treatment.

This expansion outward of the TC, however, has been at the expense of *inward* refinement of the approach itself. It is one thing to modify and adapt the TC for special populations, settings, and shorter durations of treatment. It is quite another to ignore the development of the TC's unique approach, *community as method*. Thus, if the TC is to retain its unique identity within mainstream human services, it must address the complex issue of treatment *fidelity*.

TC effectiveness and fidelity of treatment are closely related. High-fidelity treatment produces better outcomes [7]. The key strategies needed to assure high-fidelity TCs are staff training based upon critical elements, teaching curricula grounded in a uniform definition of community as method, and appropriate training models that integrate didactic and experiential learning.

Table 48.3 Classification of TC programs

Standard TC programs. These are guided by the TC perspective, retain essential components of the program model, and utilize community as method as the primary approach. They are mainly housed in residential settings, with longer planned durations of treatments, serving the more severe substance abusers (primarily client driven).
Modified TC programs. These are guided by the TC perspective, incorporate essential components of the model, but adapt community as method for special populations (e.g., co-occurring disorders, criminal justice substance abusers, juveniles) and settings (hospitals, shelters, prisons). Key adaptations are more staff directed, greater emphasis on individual differences, moderated intensity of group process, and a more flexible program structure. Additionally, these programs incorporate strategies and services which have proven useful in addressing particular problems and special populations, including pharmacotherapy (e.g., methadone, buprenorphine, psychotropic medications) as well as varieties of counseling and family therapy (client and staff driven).
TC-oriented programs. These *are not* guided by the TC perspective and do not adhere to community as method. Typically, these serve less severe clients in short-term residential or day treatment settings and are eclectic in their approach. They select elements of the TC (e.g., community meetings, peer support group, etc.) but mainly utilize services and practices that are not specific to the TC (primarily staff driven).

48.2.14 Diversity of TC Programs

Issue: The TC approach and model have been successfully adapted and modified for various populations and settings. However, within the wide diversity of programs that represent themselves as TCs, many do not actually implement the TC approach that has proven successful. This often results in variable treatment outcomes and fosters misperceptions of the therapeutic community as an effective evidence-based approach. The credibility of the TC modality in health and human services will require classification of the diversity of programs as well as the development of standards of quality assurance.

48.2.15 Classification of TC Programs

The range of TC programs for substance abuse and related problems can be organized into three broad categories. These are based upon the extent to which a program is guided by the TC perspective (whole person, recovery, and right living), adheres to the approach (community as method), and retains essential components of the program model (see Table 48.3).

Thus, not all programs that label themselves as therapeutic communities are actually TCs. Clarification of differences in programs, the clients they serve, the goals of treatment, and the fidelity of the particular treatment strategies utilized, is necessary to preserve the integrity of the TC approach.

Finally, TCs worldwide are also undergoing many of the evolutionary changes described above, including modifications for special populations and particularly adapting to fiscal pressures to reduce time in residential treatment. A notable development is the rapprochement between the addiction TC and the psychiatric TC pioneered by Maxwell Jones that has been prominent in Europe. Both of these TC approaches share many of the common elements of community as method to treat populations with both substance use and personality disorder. Nevertheless, maintaining uniformity and fidelity of the TC approach in light of these changes remains a challenge.

48.3 Conclusion

Arguably, the therapeutic community for addictions (TC) is the first formal treatment approach that is explicitly *recovery oriented*. Surely, AA and similar mutual self-help approaches facilitate recovery, but these represent themselves as support, not treatment. Pharmacological approaches, notably, methadone maintenance, have as their treatment goal the reduction or elimination of illicit opiate use; and behavioral approaches, such as cognitive-behavioral therapy (CBT), contingency contracting, and motivational enhancement (MET), focus upon reduction, and not necessarily abstinence and recovery, in targeted drug use. In the TC perspective, however, the primary goal of treatment is *recovery* which is broadly defined as changes in lifestyles and identities.

Thus, in the current context of substance abuse policy and issues (e.g., various treatment options, harm reduction strategies, the economic pressures on health care), the overarching challenge of the TC is to reassert its unique place and mission – that of promoting recovery and right living.

References

1. Bunt GC, Kressel D, Stanick V, Au M. Therapeutic community: a three-country comparison. NIDA Int Prog. National Institute on Drug Abuse, Bethesda, MD. 2010.
2. De Leon G, editor. Community as method: therapeutic communities for special populations and special settings. Westport: Greenwood; 1997.
3. De Leon G. The therapeutic community: theory, model, and method. New York: Springer; 2000.
4. De Leon G. Is the therapeutic community an evidence based treatment? What the evidence says. Ther Commun. 2010;31(2):104–75.
5. De Leon G, Melnick G, Schoket D, Jainchill N. Is the therapeutic community culturally relevant? Findings on race/ethnic differences in retention in treatment. J Psychoactive Drugs. 1993;25(1):77–86.
6. De Leon G, Sacks S, Staines G, McKendrick K. Modified therapeutic community for homeless MICAs: treatment outcomes. Am J Drug Alcohol Abuse. 2000;26(3):461–80.
7. Dye M, Ducharme L, Johnson J, Knudsen H, Roman P. Modified therapeutic communities and adherence to traditional elements. J Psychoactive Drugs. 2009;41(3):275–83.
8. Goethels L, Soyez V, De Leon G, Melnick G, Broekert E. Essential elements of treatment: a comparative study of European and American therapeutic communities for addiction. Subst Use Misuse. 2011;46(8):1023a–31a.
9. Jainchill N, Hawke J, Messina M. Post-treatment outcomes among adjudicated adolescent males and females in modified therapeutic community treatment. Subst Use Misuse. 2005;40:975–96.
10. Johnson KW, Young L, Pan T, Zimmerman RS, Vanderhoff KJ. Therapeutic communities (TC) drug treatment success in Thailand: a follow-up study. In: Research monograph. US Department of State's Bureau of International Narcotics and Law Enforcement. Pacific Institute for Research and Evaluation – Louisville Center, Affairs Louisville; 2007.
11. Johnson K, Pan Z, Young L, Vanderhoff J, Shamblen S, Browne T, Linfield K, Suresh G. Therapeutic community drug treatment success in Peru: a follow-up outcome study. Subst Abuse Treat Prev Policy. 2008;3:26.
12. Melnick G, De Leon G. Clarifying the nature of therapeutic community treatment: the survey of essential elements questionnaire (SEEQ). J Subst Abus Treat. 1999;16:307–13.
13. NIDA. (2015, July 23). Therapeutic communities. Retrieved from https://www.drugabuse.gov/publications/research-reports/therapeutic-communities on 2019, March 13.
14. Perfas F. Deconstructing the therapeutic community. New York: Hexagram Publishing; 2012.
15. Pitts J, Yates R. Cost benefits of therapeutic community programming: results of a self- funded survey. Ther Commun. 2010;31(2):129–44.
16. Rapoport R. Community as doctor. London: Tavistock Publications; 1960.
17. Sacks S, Banks S, McKendrick K, Sacks J. Modified therapeutic community for co-occurring disorders: a summary of four studies. J Subst Abus Treat. 2008;34(1):112–22.
18. Vanderplasschen W, Colbert K, Autrique M, Rapp RC, Peace S, Broekaert E, Vandevelde S. Therapeutic communities for addictions: a review of their effectiveness from a recovery-oriented perspective. Sci World J. 2013;2013:1–22.
19. Wexler HK, Prendergast ML. Therapeutic communities in United States' prisons: effectiveness and challenges. Ther commun. 2010;31(2):157, Am J Drug Alcohol Abuse 26(3):461–80.
20. Yablonsky L. The tunnel back. New York: Macmillan; 1965. p. 157–75.
21. Yablonsky L. The therapeutic community: a successful approach for treating substance abusers. New York: Gardner Press; 1989.

Further Reading

Bunt GC, Muehlbach B, Moed CO. The therapeutic community: an international perspective. Subst Abuse. 2008;29(3):81–7.

Spiritual Aspects of the 12-Step Method in Addiction Treatment

49

Marc Galanter

Contents

Abstract

This chapter is directed at defining the nature of spirituality and its relationship to empirical research and clinical practice. An understanding of the spiritual experience can be achieved on the basis of diverse theoretical and empirically grounded sources. Furthermore, the impact of spirituality on addiction in different cultural and clinical settings is explicated by illustrations of its application with regard to Alcoholics Anonymous, Narcotics Anonymous, and Danshukai (Japan).

Keywords

Spirituality · Addiction · Alcoholics anonymous · Treatment · Recovery

49.1 Introduction

49.1.1 AA as a Spiritual Recovery Movement

How does spirituality relate to recovery from addiction? There is a parallel between the way attitudes are transformed in intensely zealous groups and the way the denial of illness and the self-defeating behaviors of people with alcohol and substance use disorders may be reversed through induction into 12-step groups like AA.

Members of the lay public may conclude that certain healthcare issues are inadequately

M. Galanter (✉)
Division of Alcoholism and Drug Abuse, Department of Psychiatry, NYU School of Medicine, New York, NY, USA
e-mail: marcgalanter@nyu.edu

© Springer Nature Switzerland AG 2021
N. el-Guebaly et al. (eds.), *Textbook of Addiction Treatment*,
https://doi.org/10.1007/978-3-030-36391-8_49

addressed by the medical community, particularly when doctors are not sufficiently attentive to the emotional burden that an illness produces. When mutually supportive groups of laymen coalesce to implement a response to this perceived deficit, they may form a spiritual recovery movement [15], one premised on achieving remission based on beliefs independent of evidence- based medicine. Such movements may ascribe their effectiveness to higher metaphysical or nonmaterial forces and claim to offer relief from illness.

AA can be considered as a highly successful example of a spiritual recovery movement, as such movements have three primary characteristics. They (a) claim to provide relief from disease, (b) operate outside the modalities of established empirical medicine, and (c) ascribe their effectiveness to higher metaphysical powers. The appeal of such movements in the contemporary period is due in part to the fact that physicians tend not to attend the spiritual or emotional concerns of their patients [16].

Clearly, the attitudes and behavioral norms that AA espouses are much more in conformity with the values of the larger culture than those of zealous religious sects. The expectation of avoiding drunkenness in AA, normative in our culture, illustrates this. People who are highly distressed over the consequences of their addiction are therefore candidates to respond to the strong ideologic orientation of AA toward recovery and are operantly reinforced by the relief produced by affiliation with the group's ideology and behavioral norms, all related to abstinence and a spiritually grounded lifestyle. Significantly, AA generates distress in its members by pressing them to give up their addictive behaviors, but the distress associated with this conflict is relieved if they sustain affiliation and cleave to the group [20, 21].

49.2   Spiritual Aspects

49.2.1 Spirituality as a Psychological Construct

Two empirically grounded perspectives have played a material role in framing how we conceptualize recovery. One is derived from a model of

psychopathology modeled on the work of Emil Kraepelin [27]. He framed an approach that now characterizes the contemporary medical model for mental disorders, categorizing disease entities diagnosed on the basis of explicit and discrete symptoms. This approach is evident in the development of criteria for substance use disorders employed in recent editions of the symptom-based *Diagnostic and Statistical Manual of Mental Disorders* [2]. From this perspective, a state of remission, colloquially called recovery in rehabilitation circles, can take place with the resolution of the specific symptoms listed as diagnostic criteria. A second perspective on recovery derives from behavioral psychology, whose model of stimulus-response sequences has led to the ordering of experience around discrete phenomena that can be observed by a researcher or clinician. From this perspective, recovery can also be defined in terms of observable, measurable responses to substance use, lending credence to recovery as a process defined in behavioral terms.

Both perspectives are well suited to the study of psychopathology and have lent the addiction field approaches to studying addiction as a disorder, one that is compatible with research approaches employing experimental controls that are used in the physical and biological sciences. Both have therefore had heuristic value in promoting a research field that has yielded many advances in addiction treatment. There is a third perspective, however, that is defined on the basis of addicts' reports of their own subjective experience. These experiences are not directly observable by the clinician but are available only as reported through the prism of the person's own introspection and reflection. This model is more difficult to subject to measurement, but instruments are being developed that can be applied for its study, as will be discussed below. This approach is inherent in the spiritually oriented psychology of Carl Jung [25], who had a direct influence on Bill W's framing of the Alcoholics Anonymous ethos [5]. James [24], often described as the father of American psychology, also discussed mental phenomena in terms of subjectively experienced mystical or spiritual experience. (In fact, he wrote that "the drunken consciousness is one bit of the mystic consciousness" [p. 378].) The need for spiritual redemption was vital in the writings of Viktor Frankl, who wrote *Man's Search for Meaning* [14], and has recently been espoused with regard to psychotherapy by William Miller [31].

This third perspective is related to the model of spiritually grounded recovery we will discuss here, insofar as it emphasizes the achievement of meaningful or positive experiences, rather than a focus on observable, dysfunctional behaviors. Research on this third approach would typically rely on self-report scales, such as those which can be facilitated by development of instruments like the Life Engagement Test [34], the General Well-Being Schedule, or our own Spiritual Self-Rating Scale [17]. We will consider its role in AA, models for how it takes place, and ways it can be measured. In this respect, recovery can be understood as a process whereby an abstinent addicted person is moving toward a positive adaptation in life. This movement can take place with varying degrees of success, depending on the person's own innate capacities and the circumstances in which they find themselves.

49.2.2 Spirituality and Religious Experience

The relative role of spiritual experience in the 12-step recovery process has been investigated from a variety of perspectives, generally in relation to patients' experience in AA. Kelly et al. [26] reviewed studies that applied mediational tests to ascertain how AA achieves beneficial outcomes and found little support for a role of AA's specific spiritual mechanisms. In fact, with regard to religiosity, Tonigan et al. [36] found that, although atheists were less likely to attend AA meetings, those who did join derived equal benefit as did spiritually focused individuals. On the other hand, in one study on persons recovering from cocaine dependence [13], respondents attributed their positive outcomes to religion and spirituality. Additionally, Zemore [39] followed-up a large sample of substance abusers 1 year after inpatient treatment and found that increases in spirituality contributed to the increment in total abstinence associated with 12-step involvement.

Our own experience, as well, is compatible with these findings, as we have found in multiple settings [19] that spirituality is integral to recovery in 12-step groups. This was particularly evident among long-term members.

49.2.3 Spiritually Grounded Recovery in AA

The AA "program of recovery" is mentioned in numerous places in the *Big Book*, Alcoholics Anonymous [1], and is associated there with terms such as "spiritual experience" and "spiritual awakening" and with working AA's 12 steps. Four of the steps include the word God, which is qualified "as we understood Him." Some clarity is lent to this latter phrase in the *Big Book* where it is pointed out that "with few exceptions, our members find that they have tapped an unsuspected inner resource which they presently identify with their own conception of a Power greater than themselves" (p. 569–570). Flexibility on the issue of theistic belief is also made clear in one chapter that addresses any alcoholic person "who feels he is an atheist or agnostic," encouraging their membership as well. The text points out for these members that even "We Agnostics…had to face the fact that we must find a spiritual basis for life" (p. 44) in order to achieve recovery, implying therein the fellowship's distinction between spirituality and theistic religion.

This issue of theistic connotation, however, is as yet resolved relative to the judicial system, where the application of AA is sometimes constrained because of potential church/state conflicts. It is open to question, however, whether the theistic connotations of AA can be modified without vitiating the program's effectiveness. In this relation, it should be noted that in a 5-year follow-up of recovering cocaine-dependent patients, the strength derived from religion and spirituality significantly distinguished between those who had a highly favorable outcome from those who did not [13]. Additionally, attendance at religious services distinguished significantly between criminal justice clients referred for substance abuse treatment who had a positive outcome and those who did not [3].

Spirituality among long-term members is likely instrumental in sustaining the integrity of the fellowship itself. The prominence of spiritually committed long-term members at meetings, and their availability to serve in the sponsorship role, creates readily available models for earnestly held sobriety. They serve as role models for believing commitment to the 12-step spiritual ethos to help newcomers achieve stabilization in membership. Nonetheless, some people attending NA meetings may find it hard to identify with the spiritual orientation of long-term members.

In the clinical context, recovery is based on a person's behavioral and physiologic status, which can be assessed by recourse to criteria employed in the DSM. Some of these criteria are also embodied in the Addiction Severity Index [30], which is employed widely in research to evaluate recovery. These items can be assessed relatively easily, as they are premised on observable behavior or delineated by symptomatology described by patient, family member, or clinician. A spiritually grounded definition of recovery, however, can be useful as well.

Such a concept relates to the importance of non-demographic subject factors, originally proposed as "quality-of-life" issues [4] – among which spirituality can be considered. In this context, a series of suitable criteria for "diagnosing" addiction (a more apt term than "substance dependence") could be developed. They could then be used to assess the spiritual aspect of recovery associated with the 12-step experience. Resolution of these issues could be considered as important to the spiritual aspect of recovery from addiction. A series of criteria could include items such as

- Loss of sense of purpose due to excessive substance use
- A feeling of inadequate social support because of one's addiction
- Continued use of a substance while experiencing moral qualms over its consumption
- Loss of the will to resist temptation when the substance is available

Another aspect of the DSM format can be considered as well. The manual stipulates "course specifiers" of remission such as "on agonist therapy" and "in a controlled environment." These are included because they are explanatory to the clinician. To them could be added "fully engaged in a program of 12-step recovery," which would be equally explanatory to many clinicians.

But are spiritually grounded criteria measurable? In recent years, methodologies have been developed and validated that could be used to assess outcome based on such subjectively experienced criteria. They employ a systematic approach to measurement and can be used to describe spiritually related states:

A. Affective state:
   (i) A sense of well-being, measured by the General Well-Being Schedule [11] (which we employed) or the Subjective Happiness Scale [28]
   (ii) Contentment with one's life circumstances, measured by the Satisfaction with Life Scale [10]
   (iii) Positive affect, assessed with the Positive and Negative Affect Schedule [37], dealing with both variables as separate dimensions, rather than bipolar ends of the same scale
   (iv) Feelings of support, employing a Scale for Perceived Social Support [6]
B. Existential variables: Meaningfulness in one's life: assessed by the Purpose in Life Test [8].
C. Flow: The experience associated with engaging one's highest strengths and talents to meet achievable challenges, as measured by Experience Sampling [9] or the Flow Scale [29].
D. Spirituality: The Spirituality Self-Rating Scale, which we developed and applied to both substance-abusing and non-substance-abusing populations [17], as well as other such scales. By means of our own scale, we were able to distinguish different populations of substance abusers' level of spiritual orientation from the of non-substance populations.

E. Personality assessment: The Classification of Strengths [33], a series of characteristics based on categories of moral excellence drawn from observations across different cultures.

F. AA involvement: Measures of the degree of affiliation and commitment to the AA fellowship [23].

A methodology for defining recovery based on measurements like these may not have the same appeal to biomedically oriented clinicians as does the conventional symptom-based approach, as these measurements are based on self-report of the person's subjective state. Furthermore, the enthusiasm of newfound recovery may yield a Hawthorne effect. The biomedical format currently applied in diagnosis derives from the school of Kraeplin and subsequent investigators like those who developed the Feighner criteria [12] in the 1970s and then in the ensuing DSM system. Spiritual variables, however, have a lineage as well, from William James, Carl Jung, and Bill W.

Spiritual awakening, a key aspect of 12-step recovery, is designated in the twelfth step of Alcoholics Anonymous (AA). Of long-term AA members who reported having had such an awakening, two-thirds reported no craving for alcohol or drugs at the time of the survey. Their responses reflected a major experiential transformation [18], which can be likened to religious conversion, because both involve a major transformation in personal disposition toward a spiritually oriented perspective on life. Pargament [32], who defined *religion* broadly as "the search for significance in ways related to the sacred" (p. 32), wrote of religious conversion as taking place only when a change comes about in both the destinations and pathways of a person's life in connection to the sacred.

49.2.4 Danshukai

The worldwide growth of secular but spiritual mutual aid organizations promoting addiction recovery has led to the option of people achieving addiction recovery outside of professional treatment. One example of the diverse approaches worldwide is Danshukai.

Japan has a history of recovery by mutual support in the Danshukai movement. Danshukai draws on Zen Buddhism and contains elements that parallel AA, such as undercutting denial, a process of amends, and service [38]. Danshukai meetings, however, typically include family members and offer prayers for those who have passed. The meetings are also much more structured than AA meetings, with decreased emphasis on anonymity. Attendees sign in on their entering the meeting, use their full names, and may wear Danshukai pins, indicating their membership.

49.2.5 AA in the Professional Context

The spiritually oriented 12-step approach has been integrated into professional treatment in some settings where it serves as the overriding philosophy of an entire program or, in others, where it is one aspect of a multimodal eclectic approach. The Minnesota Model for treatment, typically located in an isolated institutional setting, is characterized by an intensive inpatient stay during which a primary goal of treatment is to acculturate patients to acceptance of the philosophy of AA and to continue with AA attendance after discharge [7]. Although a variety of exercises are included during the stay, this approach has been criticized as dogmatic because of its sole reliance on the 12-step approach. The outcome of this model, however, has been shown to yield positive results in a survey of patients discharged from one such setting (Hazelden, in Center City, MN) [35], but randomization of patients treated in Minnesota Model facilities with those treated by means of an alternative approach is needed.

A more eclectic option is illustrated in the integration of 12-step groups into a general psychiatric facility for the treatment of patients dually diagnosed for major mental illness and substance abuse. The importance of spirituality in such a highly compromised population was evidenced in our studies [17] in which such patients ranked spiritual issues like belief in God and inner peace higher than tangible benefits like social service support and outpatient treatment. One inherent advantage of this format is that it benefits from the introduction of an inspirational approach to patients who, as Goffman has pointed out [22], have become "degraded" by stigmatization due to their psychiatric disorders.

In summary, spirituality is a matter of personal meaning that is widely accepted. It is also central to the recovery process from addiction for many AA members. The fellowship of AA, in fact, can be considered a movement developed in relation to people's spiritual needs. Although spirituality is subjectively experienced, it can be assessed systematically in given individuals by employing currently available empirical techniques. By such means, an important aspect of addiction recovery can be defined and studied.

References

1. Alcoholics Anonymous World Services. Alcoholics Anonymous: the story of how many thousands of men and women have recovered from alcoholism. New York: Alcoholics Anonymous Publishing; 1955.
2. American Psychiatric Association. Diagnostic and statistical manual of mental disorders, 4th edn, text revision. Washington, D.C.: American Psychiatric Association; 2000.
3. Brown BS, O'Grady K, Battjes RJ, et al. Factors associated with treatment outcomes in an aftercare population. Am J Addict. 2004;13:447–60.
4. Campbell A, Converse PE, Rogers WL. The quality of American life. New York: Russell Sage Foundation; 1976.
5. Cheever S. My name is Bill: Bill Wilson – his life and the creation of Alcoholics Anonymous. New York: Simon & Schuster; 2004.
6. Cohen S, Mermelstein R, Kamarck T, et al. Measuring the functional components of social support. In: Sarason IG, Sarason BR, editors. Social support: theory, research and application. The Hague: Martinus Nijhoff; 1985. p. 73–94.
7. Cook CCH. The Minnesota model in the management of drug and alcohol dependency: miracle, method or myth? Part II: evidence and conclusions. Br J Addict. 1988;83:735–48.
8. Crumbaugh JD, Maholick LT. Manual of instructions for the purpose in life test. Munster: Psychometric Affiliates; 1969.
9. Csikszentmihalyi M, Larson R. Validity and reliability of the experience sampling method. J Nerv Ment Dis. 1987;175:526–36.
10. Diener E, Suh EM, Lucas RE, et al. Subjective well-being: three decades of progress. Psychol Bull. 1999;125:276–302.
11. Dupuy H. The psychological section of the current health and nutrition examination survey. In: Proceedings of the public health conference on records and statistics (1972). DHEW Publication HRA. Rockville: National Center for Health Statistics; 1973. p. 74–1214.
12. Feighner JP, Robins E, Guze SB, et al. Diagnostic criteria for use in psychiatric research. Arch Gen Psychiatry. 1972;26:57–63.
13. Flynn PM, Joe GW, Broome KM, Simpson DD, Brown BS. Looking back on cocaine dependence: reasons for recovery. Am J Addict. 2003;12:398–411.
14. Frankl V. Man's search for meaning. 3rd ed. New York: Touchstone/Simon & Schuster; 1984.
15. Galanter M. Spiritual recovery movements and contemporary medical care. Psychiatry Interpers Biol Proc. 1997;60:236–48.
16. Galanter M. Spirituality and the healthy mind: science, therapy and the need for personal meaning. New York: Oxford University Press; 2005.
17. Galanter M, Dermatis H, Bunt G, et al. Assessment of spirituality and its relevance to addiction treatment. J Subst Abus Treat. 2007;33:257–64.
18. Galanter M, Dermatis H, Sampson C. Spiritual awakening in Alcoholics Anonymous: empirical findings. Alcohol Treat Q. 2014;32:319–34.
19. Galanter M, Dermatis H, Santucci C. Young people in Alcoholics Anonymous: the role of spiritual orientation and AA member affiliation. J Addict Dis. 2012;31:173–82.
20. Galanter M, Dermatis H, Post S, Sampson C. Spirituality-based recovery from drug addiction in the twelve-step fellowship of Narcotics anonymous. J Addict Med. 2013;7(3):189–95.
21. Galanter M, Dermatis H, Stanievich J, Santucci C. Physicians in long-term recovery who are members of Alcoholics Anonymous. Am J Addict. 2013;22(4):323–8.
22. Goffman E. Stigma. New York: Simon & Schuster; 1963.
23. Humphreys K, Kaskutas LA, Weisner C. The Alcoholics Anonymous Affiliation Scale: development, reliability, and norms for diverse treated and untreated populations. Alcohol Clin Exp Res. 1998;22:974–8.
24. James W. The varieties of religious experience. New York: Modern Library; 1929.
25. Jung C. Instinct and unconscious. In: Fordham M, Adler G, McGuire W, Read H, editors. The collected works of C.B. Jung. Princeton: Princeton University Press; 1978.
26. Kelly JF, Magill M, Stout RL. How do people recover from alcohol dependence? A systematic review of the research on mechanisms of behavior change

in Alcoholics Anonymous. Addict Res Theory. 2009;17:236–59.

27. Kraepelin E. Clinical psychiatry: a textbook for students and physicians. New York: Macmillan; 1902.

28. Lyubomirsky S, Lepper HS. A measure of subjective happiness: preliminary reliability and construct validation. Soc Indic Res. 1999;46:137–55.

29. Mayers P. Flow in adolescence and its relation to school experience. PhD thesis, unpublished, University of Chicago. 1978.

30. McLellan AT, Kushner H, Metzger D, et al. The fifth edition of the addiction severity index. J Subst Abus Treat. 1992;9:199–213.

31. Miller WR, editor. Integrating spirituality into treatment. Washington, D.C.: American Psychological Association; 1999.

32. Pargament KI. The psychology of religious coping. New York: Guildford; 1997.

33. Peterson C, Seligman MEP. Character strengths and virtues: a classification and handbook. Washington, D.C.: American Psychological Association; 2004.

34. Scheier MF, Wrosch C, Baum A, et al. The life engagement test: assessing purpose in life. J Behav Med. 2006;29:291–8.

35. Stinchfield R, Owen P. Hazelden's model of treatment and its outcome. Addict Behav. 1998;23:669–83.

36. Tonigan JS, Miller WR, Schermer C. Atheists, agnostics and Alcoholics Anonymous. J Stud Alcohol. 2002;63:534–41.

37. Watson D, Clark LA, Tellegen A. Development and validation of brief measures of positive and negative affect: the PANAS scales. J Pers Soc Psychol. 1988;54:1063–70.

38. White WL. Addiction recovery in Japan. 2016. Accessed at http://www.williamwhitepapers.com/blog/2016/07/additction-recovery-in-japan.html, on 19 March 2019.

39. Zemore SE. A role for spiritual change in the benefits of 12-step involvement. Alcohol Clin Exp Res. 2007;31:76S–9S.

Addiction Recovery in Services and Policy: An International Overview

50

David Best and Rebecca Hamer

Contents

| Abstract |

This chapter provides an overview of the changes occurring in the recovery field in the United States and internationally, with special emphasis on the growing focus on recovery as the guiding vision for drug policy and as a framework for treatment. 'Recovery' goes beyond substance use to encompass improved functioning in all life areas and the realisation of individual aspirations. As substance use disorders are often chronic and relapsing, recovery is conceptualised as a process that unfolds

D. Best (✉)
University of Derby, Derby, UK
e-mail: D.Best@derby.ac.uk

R. Hamer
Sheffield Hallam University, Sheffield, UK

© Springer Nature Switzerland AG 2021
N. el-Guebaly et al. (eds.), *Textbook of Addiction Treatment*,
https://doi.org/10.1007/978-3-030-36391-8_50

over time and requires a continuing care approach. We describe emerging service models, including recovery-oriented systems of care (ROSC) and the centrality of peer-driven recovery supports as part of a social and community emphasis on recovery sustainability. We conclude with some recommendations on strategies that professionals, peers and communities can be used to promote recovery amongst substance-using individuals.

50.1　Introduction

As healthcare evolves, healthcare professionals are grappling with new systems and care models whilst continuing to diagnose and treat human conditions such as substance misuse. However, the way society views addiction has changed over time – from moral failing or crime to chronic brain disease [77], with resulting changes in how addiction is addressed by healthcare services. In this chapter, we describe recent developments in a recovery orientation to substance problems. The chapter examines global research innovations, policy and practice responses and the integration of recovery-oriented approaches into healthcare and social care services.

50.2　Recovery as a Guiding Vision of Substance Use Services and Policy

There are two empirically based elements to the shift in policy and practice: the reconceptualisation of problem drug use as a chronic disorder requiring both treatment and ongoing recovery support and the broadening of what 'recovery' means. First, research in the past 20 years has concluded that addiction is best understood as a chronic disorder equivalent to diabetes, asthma or hypertension [77]. However, unlike these other conditions, treatment for problem drug use (PDU) has historically been delivered using an acute care model: intense episodes of care during which a person, often in crisis, is assessed, treated

and discharged in a relatively short time [27, 56]. Growing evidence for long addiction and treatment 'careers' consisting of multiple cycles of treatment episodes [28, 45] followed by return to active addiction [94] has led to the conclusion that the acute care model is inadequate [44, 56, 78, 79, 87]. Kelly [56] contends that medical intervention alone is insufficient in achieving and maintaining recovery and that it is imperative for ongoing, long-term recovery support to be delivered following stabilisation and treatment phases. A continuum of care model consistent with chronic disease is also aligned with the experience of persons in recovery who overwhelmingly describe recovery as 'a process' versus 'an end point' [60].

The second element of the paradigmatic shift was summarised by McLellan and colleagues as *the immediate goal of reducing alcohol and drug use is necessary but rarely sufficient for the achievement of the longer-term goals of improved personal health and social function and reduced threats to public health and safety – i.e., recovery*' ([79], p. 448). The emerging recovery-oriented model provides a continuum of support designed to promote and sustain improvements in substance use and psychosocial functioning. This reconciles a public health response with a strength- and community-based focus that places the individual at the heart of their own recovery journey and emphasises personal empowerment and individual ownership of recovery. Promoting recovery requires giving individuals the tools and strategies to develop 'capital', a strength-based approach that has gained prominence in both psychology [96] and criminology [92] and is embodied in the addiction field by the construct of 'recovery capital' [35].

Hennessy [40] asserts that the concept of recovery capital provides an exploratory framework with which to identify assets and obstacles to recovery to be built upon or ameliorated in order to support recovery journeys. Amongst the six recovery capital (RC) models included in Hennessy's [40] systematic review, recovery is characterised as ongoing and dynamic, is variable between and within individuals, consists of a broad range of resources from macro, meso- and individual levels, which can interact to further build or deplete RC, and suggests that places, communities and resources can all intersect to generate and embed recovery capital. Finally, recovery is contagious through individuals, groups and society [40].

50.3 What Does 'Recovery' Mean?

The term 'recovery' has been widely used for decades but, until recently, had remained poorly defined. Researchers typically used the term in studies by measuring short-term abstinence (typically a year or less), some from a single substance (e.g., alcohol) and others from all substances (for a discussion, see [60]). In 2005, the Center for Substance Abuse Treatment (CSAT), convened a panel of experts representing a number of key stakeholder groups [20]. The following year, the Betty Ford Center convened a smaller panel of experts and stakeholders that published the first consensus definition of 'recovery' as 'voluntarily maintained lifestyle composed characterised by sobriety, personal health, and citizenship' ([10], p. 221).

The UK Drug Policy Commission [99] echoed these definitions whilst asserting that recovery can be achieved through a diverse range of strategies, including substitution therapy if desired, to provide a holistic continuum of care and support.

White [105] expands upon this, asserting that recovery consists of three elements: sobriety, improvements in global health (referring to the physical, emotional, ontological, life meaning and purpose) and citizenship. The Substance Abuse and Mental Health Services Administration [93] further elaborated a dual conception of recovery for both mental health and problem drug use, delineating ten guiding principles for recovery:

1. Hope: The power of hope is fundamental for individuals, families and communities to feel recovery is possible.
2. Relational: Recovery entails the formation of strong relationships with those who share hope and a vision for recovery, through which new positive identities and roles may be established, providing a sense of belonging, community and agency.
3. Person driven: Recovery is a personal journey, and it is fundamental that each recovery journey is navigated according to individual self-determination.
4. Culture: Recovery pathways are unique according to cultural values and beliefs.
5. Many pathways: The routes to recovery are diverse and comprise a broad spectrum of formal or informal support.
6. Holistic: Recovery is a multi-faceted process entailing improvements across all domains of quality of life and wellbeing.
7. Peer support: Peers are fundamental in providing mutual aid, modelling prosocial behaviour and possibilities to PDU and to communities. Furthermore, peer involvement provides those in recovery with new alternative identities to share their experience to help others and opportunities to reintegrate with and give back to their communities.
8. Strengths/responsibility: Individuals, families and communities all have assets that can be built upon to strengthen recovery.
9. Respect: Discrimination, stigma and ostracisation present significant obstacles to recovery, and so it is crucial that recovery systems recognise the bravery of those pursuing recovery and that their rights are respected.
10. Addresses trauma: Mental health problems and PDU are often preceded and exacerbated by experiences of trauma, whilst trauma similarly presents obstacles to recovery. Therefore, services and systems must be trauma aware and work to ameliorate the destructive effects of posttraumatic stress disorder (PTSD).

Correspondingly, Bassuk et al. [7] attest that 'as a broader definition of recovery gains traction, it is critical that future research expands to mirror the various domains of recovery by including outcomes related to housing, employment, educational status, quality of life, functioning, trauma exposure, mental health status and social support networks'.

50.4 Recovery Prevalence

According to Huskamp and Iglegart [49], 82% of people with substance use disorders do not receive adequate treatment, whilst abstinence rates are complicated by very high mortality rates. Thus, whilst Grella and Lovinger [37] reported an abstinence rate of 80% in the surviving sample, the rate reduced to 30% if the individuals who had died were included in the study. In their review of remission rates, Hser et al. [45] contradicted the idea of 'maturing out' by suggesting that abstinence rates drop to around 30% after 10 years and then remain relatively stable, irrespective of age or chronicity of use. They concluded that opioid addiction is a chronic disorder characterised by frequent relapse, but that 'longer treatment retention is associated with a greater likelihood of cessation, whereas incarceration is negatively linked to subsequent abstinence' (p. 85).

In a review of 415 population and clinical studies between 1868 and 2011, around half of study participants reported remission from substance use disorders at the final study follow-up point. In Fleury et al.'s [31] systematic review and meta-analysis of 21 papers examining remission from substance use disorder, a standard remission rate of 54% and a conservative remission rate of 35% were reported after a mean of 17 years.

In a population-based representative US sample ($n = 39,809$), Kelly et al. [55] found that of respondents answering 'yes' to -'Did you use to have a problem with alcohol or drugs but no longer do?' 9.1% of the sample were in recovery, of whom 46% self-identifying as 'in recovery', whilst 53.9% reported 'assisted' pathway use. Assisted pathways were most common for opioid users and least common for cannabis users.

50.5 What Does Adopting a Recovery Orientation Mean for Addiction Treatment Services?

The paradigm shift discussed above mean that recovery supports need to be expanded in time, in philosophy and in scope. In terms of time, PDUs

have thus far been addressed using intensive, short-term episodes of professionally delivered services. Whilst treatment is generally reported to be effective [101, 102, 103], return to active use following treatment, even amongst those who had achieved abstinence, is high [28, 45, 64, 78, 79]. Kelly [57] notes that in early recovery, people experience higher levels of stress-causing hormones such as cortisol and corticotropin, and thus their ability to learn new skills is hindered whilst their vulnerability to stress-triggered relapse is greater. Consequently, the ongoing recovery support favoured by Kelly [56] factors biological, neurobiological and psychosocial domains within ongoing support, monitoring and intervention to navigate potential or actual relapses along the recovery journey. Kelly [56] identifies four fundamental types of such ongoing recovery support:

- Emotional support
- Tangible support (e.g., links to housing)
- Informational support (advice/learning)
- Social support (sense of belonging)

Recovery support services are increasingly diverse and accessible, and Kelly [56] identifies six types of recovery support services (RSS) in the USA:

- Peer-based recovery support services
- Recovery community centres
- Recover support in education
- Mutual-aid organisations
- Recovery housing
- Clinical models

Most studies exploring the effectiveness of peer recovery support confirm the benefit to participants [7, 29, 98]. Although endorsement of the value of PBRSS is 'tentative', peer support can play a significant role in reducing relapse, building greater trust and relationships between service users and providers, forging prosocial networks and providing greater satisfaction and retention in treatment, so that there is support for integrated peer and professional support [29]. However, the specifics regarding the impact of different levels of peer ability and experience, intervention intensity, duration, frequency and context in addition to the efficacy of peer support for specific populations remains to be explored [7].

Despite the supportive evidence, Greer et al. [36] have identified several barriers and disadvantages peer workers suffer. Stigma from non-peer workers can isolate peers in the workplace and diminishes their achievements. Peer work is also often subject to exploitation, low wages and the expectation of volunteering. As peers often go above and beyond as their motivation is to help their communities, this can be practically, emotionally and financially under-appreciated by employers who do not provide the necessary support, esteem and compensation given the dedication, expertise and passion of most peer workers. Peers may be at heightened risk from vicarious trauma and compassion fatigue which may endanger their own recovery. Further, the interference of peer work with welfare payments can result in individuals being disadvantaged. In Canada, peer work is separated entirely from welfare support and payments, ensuring that their contribution to their communities is suitably facilitated and valued. The BC Centre for Disease Control website features Peer Engagement Best Practice guidance as a result of their 3-year Peer Engagement and Evaluation Project (PEEP).

SAMHSA has begun to develop relevant guidelines ([7], p. 8). Awareness of discrimination, barriers and needs is fundamental if services and systems are to recognise the expertise, value and power that peers bring to recovery services and communities. In addition to asserting PBRSS as an 'evidence-based practice', additional research is required to implement peer support and to foster experiential experts whose knowledge, perspective and empathy inspire recovery [7, 29].

A recovery orientation requires the provision of comprehensive services to address needs in all life areas impaired during active addiction and where improvements are considered an inherent part of recovery, for example, physical and mental health, employment, economic, family and social life. Services addressing these issues have

thus far often been referred to as 'ancillary' in status or 'aftercare' in the timing of delivery in spite of their importance to clients and their role in the transition to stable recovery [65]. Laudet and White [62] examined challenges and life priorities in a sample of 356 community-based persons in abstinent recovery and found that working on one's recovery (e.g., staying sober and 'making recovery a priority') was consistently cited as the top priority (cited by 34–49% across stages). Employment was the second most frequently mentioned priority, cited by the same percentage of persons abstinent over 3 years as working on one's recovery (34.1% each).

As both approaches originate from different models, Galanter [33] contends that treatment and recovery support must be defined as separate but related stages. The implication is that the partnership and streamlining of relationships and referrals between professional treatment and ongoing recovery support services hold great potential for improving service users' recovery chances.

50.6 Recovery-Oriented Systems of Care (ROSC)

In the United States, the shift to a recovery orientation in treatment has been primarily spearheaded by the Substance Abuse and Mental Health Services Administration (SAMHSA), whilst in the United Kingdom, impetus to formalise recovery orientation has come from the English and Scottish Government, as discussed below. The need for this new model was perhaps stated most explicitly by a SAMHSA lead: 'Recovery is more than abstinence from alcohol and drugs; it's about building a full, meaningful, and productive life in the community. Our treatment systems must reflect and help people achieve this broader understanding of recovery' ([23], p. 2). ROSC's goals are to intervene early with individuals, to support sustained recovery and to improve the health and wellness of individuals and families. The ROSC model proposes a multisystem, person-centred continuum of care in which a comprehensive menu of coordinated services and supports is tailored to individuals' recovery stage, needs and chosen pathways [22, 23]. Services and supports are provided in a comprehensive array of domains, including education and job training, housing, childcare, transportation to treatment and work, case management, spiritual support as well as prevention services, for example, relapse prevention, recovery support, education for family members, peer-to-peer services and coaching, self-help and support groups [53, 97].

Services are intended to address the multitude of life areas adversely affected by active substance use and to respond to clients' changing needs across their lifespan. ROSC is responsive to calls for a shift from the acute care model to one more akin to the model used in other chronic conditions [48, 50, 77, 106]. From a systems perspective, this means that the care coordination function of services is conferred a more prominent role in treatment design and delivery. Key principles guiding the recovery orientation include primacy of participation; promoting access and engagement; ensuring continuity of care; employing strength-based assessment; offering individualised recovery planning; functioning as a recovery guide; community mapping, development and inclusion and identifying and addressing barriers to recovery [58, 59].

Implementing ROSC internationally will require transformative changes in agencies and systems, which has implications for the training and evaluation of peer and professional staff and service managers and those responsible for commissioning services.

50.7 What Do Recovery-Oriented Addiction Services Systems Look Like?

In supporting the transition to continuing care approaches, the most common form of aftercare consists of a stepped down course of services typically following intensive inpatient or residential treatment [73, 74, 76]; in spite of its established existence and intuitive appeal, few clients access these resources, and the evidence for

effectiveness remains limited [34, 73]. In the past decade, clinicians have also started to capitalise on health technology such as telephone-based continuing care [75], and several large treatment agencies are developing proprietary web-based online recovery maintenance and support programmes for clients to use after they leave service. Ashford et al. [5] explored digital recovery support services (DRSS), observing that these can take the form of websites, online forums, social networking, smartphone apps and text messaging services. The authors reported that DRSS has not been demonstrated to facilitate and support recovery journeys, due largely to the anecdotal and qualitative nature of accounts. However, its popularity and proliferation support these testimonials. In the USA, 11% of adults in recovery have used one or more DRSS and their digital format can provide more available and accessible recovery support, particularly for especially stigmatised populations [5].

50.8 Individual Recovery Support Services Elements

A range of recovery support services (RSS) have been described in recent articles and monographs that also review the emerging science [53, 61, 97, 104, 105]. Unlike professionally delivered aftercare, peer-based RSS are not only delivered after treatment but can also be provided alongside professional services. This is important as there are often barriers to treatment that include wait lists, finances, stigma and ambivalence about seeking professional help [3, 26, 65, 109]. RSS are often delivered by peers, individuals who have experiential knowledge [17] and work as volunteers or as paid service workers [53] to assist others in initiating and maintaining recovery and enhancing their quality of life [105]. Many individuals in recovery report that being in the company of peers is helpful [35, 63, 71, 86]. In Glasgow, Scotland, one study found that the two strongest predictors of positive quality of life in recovery were spending time with other people in recovery and engagement in meaningful activities, including working, training, volunteering and involvement in community groups [12]. A series of systematic and scoping reviews have surmised the overall promise of peer and self-help group supports in alcohol and drug recovery, albeit this endorsement is tentative due to the lack of methodological rigor and depth of exploration within research [7, 8].

One key aspect of peer involvement is around assertive linkage to prosocial groups. Manning et al. [70] showed significantly greater engagement in mutual aid groups during and after residential treatment when supported by peer assertive linkage (compared to doctor referral or written information). Following up on this, O'Connell et al. [88] used a similar design with patients with co-occurring disorders but added ongoing peer support and found that this condition was associated with lower psychotic symptoms at 9 months and better ongoing treatment engagement.

Andreas et al. [1] reviewed the Peers Reach Out Supporting Peers to Embrace Recovery (PROSPER), a programme involving peer-run groups, coaching, workshops and seminars and extensive training and supervision for peers. Engagement in the programme resulted in increases in self-efficacy, perceived social support, and quality of life. In a Native American context, Kelly et al. [55] found that participation in a peer recovery support service that was community based resulted in reduced recent alcohol and drug use and better rates of employment and stable housing.

Parkman et al. [90] found three factors to determine the efficacy of self-help groups (in this case, for alcohol treatment): attendance, involvement (as a measure of active engagement) and location (proximity to the meeting place and the home of a key worker). Some of the benefits of peer groups are their impact on social networks and sense of identity, as it is the active participation and inclusion in a prosocial group that correlates with positive recovery outcomes.

Perhaps the most well-known and widely available peer self-help model is 12-step mutual aid [54]. In a review article of 12-step facilitation, Kelly [55] reported that eight of the fifteen studies found that the 12-step facilitation produced

superior outcomes on at least one of the outcome indicators. In the same review, Kelly [55] concluded that 'the evidence in this regard is strong. TSF interventions and AA participation is associated with improved substance use outcomes, particularly prolonged abstinence and remission, and is likely to be highly cost-effective' (p. 18). In a 16-year follow-up study of alcohol treatment, [83] reported that, following the initial 6 months of treatment, 12-step involvement was associated with better outcomes than further professional treatment. Humphreys and Moos [47] have argued that whilst an initial episode of specialist treatment may be beneficial, long-term 12-step engagement may be a better predictor of outcomes over time.

There are other models of peer-based recovery support, including the sober residence, a home that offers mutual help-oriented, financially self-sustaining, self-governed, democratic communal-living environments where individuals in recovery can reside for as long as they choose after inpatient treatment or incarceration, during outpatient treatment or as an alternative to treatment [91]. Recovery residences or sober living houses provide stable housing and a structured, prosocial living environment, and such housing comprises a critical component on the continuum of recovery-oriented systems of care [81].

Recovery housing is derived from mutual aid traditions, the most prevalent of which in the States is Oxford Houses Inc., who have established 2287 houses across 44 states [85]. The benefits of the model in terms of substance use and related domains (e.g., employment, criminal involvement) have been documented in peer-reviewed studies across subpopulations [2, 51, 52, 68, 69, 82], as has been its cost-effectiveness [67, 89]. Chavarria et al. [21] conducted a 2-year followup comparing Oxford Houses Inc. and a standard continuing care model and reported that at 2 years, the clients of Oxford Houses Inc. were more than twice as likely to be abstinent, had higher monthly incomes and were less likely to be incarcerated.

There are now national standards governing recovery houses, although there is a lack of empirical findings correlating recovery residences with improved outcomes. Mericle et al. [80] found that the type of recovery house resulted in varying results – houses that were part of a group or a wing of a larger organisation led to increased chances of abstinence, whilst those affiliated with a treatment programme improved employment outcome.

50.9 Therapeutic Communities

Therapeutic Communities (TCs), such as San Patrignano in Italy and River Garden Auchincruive in Scotland, also provide residential, peer designed and led environments in which recovery is facilitated and maintained by the mutually supportive recovery community. Therapeutic Communities (TCs) were developed in the 1960s in the USA in response to the lack of capacity in healthcare and social care services to respond to the treatment needs of problem drug users. These were often privately funded and centred around self-help. Although they filled a certain gap in provision, there were issues of professionalism, the ability to upscale consistently and with leadership powers creating unmoderated, abusive and punitive cultures within communities [100]. Synanon, founded by Charles Dederich, was implicated in intolerance of relapse and aggressive shaming measures such as head shaving, verbal abuse and making residents who failed to adhere to house rules wear signs featuring stigmatising and debasing labels in public [108]. Whilst some such practices persisted until the late 1970s, radicalised communities were increasingly replaced as recognition of variation in recovery, addiction experiences and populations; professional standardisation and progressive policies and procedures permeated the TC field [19].

In a significant departure from the dictatorial early days of Synanon, TCs in various countries across Europe have since developed to meet the needs of specific populations with complex needs such as women and children and individuals with dual (concurrent mental health) diagnoses [100]. TCs are also being established in prisons, and transitioning programmes also assist in reintroducing those who have achieved recovery into

the community [100]. Therapeutic Communities have thus evolved to encompass the current broader vision of recovery, recognising the breadth of need and experience amongst PDU populations and the importance of community reintegration and cohesion. Whilst TCs in Europe were initially inspired by the revised American equivalents, European theories and techniques plus staff comprising of trained professionals and a focus on the family unit marked these communities apart [100].

Vanderplasschen et al. (2014) conducted a literature review of 28 articles set in the USA and 21 undertaken in Europe exploring the efficacy of TCs. The authors note that *'There is some evidence for the effectiveness of TC treatment in terms of reduced substance use and criminal activity, at least in the USA. A small number of studies also showed positive effects on employment, social functioning and general mental health'*. This implies that TCs have been at least tentatively evidenced to provide the multi-faceted improvements in quality of life and social integration now associated with recovery. However, Vanderplasschen et al. [100] also attest that TCs are less effective than other treatments; although, as with other interventions, positive outcomes are strongly correlated with retention and completion. The European evidence base is also methodologically limited; although this similarly suggests TCs offer reductions in problem drug use and criminal justice experiences alongside holistic improvements in quality of life and well-being. With regards to prison-based TCs, evidence provides a strong endorsement with regards to recidivism when compared to other interventions [100].

Recommendations to ensure the future of TCs include demonstrating efficacy and value for money as emphasis on cost-efficacy continues to permeate addiction and recovery landscapes, a focus which holds implications for the training and payment of employees in TCs [100]. Within a social model of recovery, the TC movement has evidenced the importance of peer-based interventions and suggested a recovery pathway independent of 12-step mutual aid, with a fundamentally different conceptualisation of addiction and recovery. The TC approach is entirely consistent with four core tenets of recovery-oriented services: a care coordination across a range of service sectors requiring case management skills and 'outward-looking' specialist treatment services, an increased role for peers, a recognition of the validity of 'expertise by experience' and a continuity of care model that acknowledges the need for integrating acute services with those targeting longer-term changes in wellbeing and social integration.

50.10 What Can Professionals, Peers and Communities Do to Promote Recovery Amongst Problem Drug Users?

For professionals to adapt and embrace the shift to recovery-focused practice, Best et al. [16] emphasise the need for clinicians to transition from 'doing to' to 'working with' service users in order to help them move on. Correspondingly, Humphreys [46] refers to the 'gatekeeper myth' that 'holds that the path to recovery can only be walked with the aid of highly educated specialists in addiction treatment'. The gatekeeper myth and dominance of the professional is, however, being eroded by recovery strategy and practice that places the individual, those with lived and living experience, and communities at the heart of recovery. The individual nature of recovery also means policy; practice and research must pay particular attention to marginalised populations whose cultural and individual needs must be considered.

Whilst women's drug-using careers are shorter and women begin their recovery at an earlier stage than men (Best et al. 2015), they also face a host of issues which complicate and exacerbate their experiences of addiction and recovery.

Women with histories of substance use problems commonly have lifelong experiences of stigmatisation, deprivation, violence and abuse [25, 107]. The symptoms of trauma include disassociation, numbing and avoidance and often aggression/defensiveness which are often both

attempted to be managed by survivors through drug and alcohol abuse and which have often been misinterpreted in services as unwillingness, disobligingness and disinterest in recovery [39].

Herman's [41] pioneering three-stage recovery model advocates for stabilisation in order to provide PTSD survivors with the sense of safety and control essential from which to begin their recovery. The need for all services and systems working with women to be trauma informed continues to gain increasing traction in research findings, strategy and practice recommendations [6, 24, 25, 39, 41].

50.11 The Recovery Landscape in Europe

The final section of the chapter will focus on the gradual emergence of a recovery movement in Europe and the policy and research innovations that have underpinned this transition, starting with the UK, where recovery policies have dominated addiction services since 2008. The origins of a recovery orientation in addiction policy are different in Scotland from England, with Scotland's Road to Recovery [95] building on the success of the Scottish Recovery Network for mental health. In England, the UK Drug Strategy [42] had its origins in the mounting critique of a treatment system predicated on low-intensity treatments [11] and a dissatisfaction with the prevailing treatment system and philosophy [4]. The 2017 English Drug Strategy comprised a continuation of 2010's strategy which marked a discursive and practical shift away from a focus on crime prevention (which relied on maintenance and harm reduction) to a focal inclusion of 'promoting recovery' as one of the main objectives. The English strategy also built upon its predecessor by proposing to:

1. *'Provide stronger governance for delivering the strategy, including a Home Secretary-chaired board and the introduction of a National Recovery Champion.'*
2. *'Expand the data we collect on levels of drug misuse and recovery from dependence and*

develop a set of jointly owned outcome measures to drive action across a broader range of local services.'

3. *Expand on the two overarching aims of the 2010 strategy: to reduce illicit drug use and increase the rate of individuals recovering from their dependence'*

Recent drug strategy in England makes consultation with peers a requirement in treatment providers' decision-making processes and explicitly references the important role peers can have in designing, implementing and reviewing drug and alcohol treatment systems [43]. The UK strategy describes peer support as 'an essential component of successful recovery', emphasising its importance throughout the recovery journey in enhancing treatment engagement and outcomes in addition to reducing stigma. An aspect of PHE's avowed recognition of PBRSS is their intention to explore digital support services in the form of online forums and mandate that community services must develop in line with peer involvement.

Similar to the English endorsement of recovery policy, Scotland's 2008 Road to Recovery and its refresh 'Rights, Respect and Recovery' [95] represented a shift in treatment monitoring in which services were to focus on producing measurable recovery outcomes. In Scotland, the Road to Recovery strategy established the Scottish Recovery Consortium to coordinate services, individuals and communities under a common aim whilst ensuring experiential expertise remains focal in-service design, implementation and in policy and public advocacy and representation. The SRC has an explicit strength-based focus on the benefits recovery brings to society as opposed to the previously dominant narrative of the destructive effects of addiction. Scotland's 2018 Rights, Respect and Recovery was developed in consultation with peers, and acknowledges the nation's flourishing peer recovery groups and communities. Furthermore, the strategy devotes a chapter to 'developing recovery-oriented systems of care', which presents peer

involvement as a human rights-based approach to be implemented through advocacy services promoting participation, equality, empowerment and accountability via peer champions and navigators.

There has been a more recent transition towards recovery-informed policy in Belgium and the Netherlands. In the Netherlands, recovery policies have historically been formulated locally and from the grass roots movements in the absence of national or state policy. Recovery was not explicitly mentioned in national policy until 2010 when a charter was formulated in agreement with 15 professional specialist treatment organisations, wherein it was agreed that quality of life and societal reintegration ought to be the focal principle of recovery interventions [72].

Belgium's recovery strategy comprises a 2016 concept paper which delineates recovery to entail *'strengths-based support, client participation and input, quality of life, social recovery, and attention to different life domains'* [9].

Bellaert et al. [9] contend that this communitarisation is impeding the implementation of parallel mental health and addiction recovery strategies in Belgium due to the division of funding sources, commissioning and implementation bodies, an obstacle the authors suggest may be resolved through bridging between authorities and systems.

The impact of national and policy variations on recovery pathways is currently subject to research investigation in the Recovery Pathways (REC-PATH) study in England, Scotland, the Netherlands and Belgium and is an exploration of recovery pathways by gender [14]. The study has a focus on gender differences in recovery pathways and has used the Life in Recovery method ([30]; Best et al. 2015) to screen for recovery stages and to identify candidate mechanisms for recovery. This builds on work by Kelly [55] on mechanisms for behaviour change in Alcoholics Anonymous (AA). Kelly argues that social-network change (along with cognitive transformations) is critical in male recovery, but that increases in abstinence self-efficacy was the primary mechanism of behaviour change brought about by attendance at the 12-step mutual aid groups for women.

This is crucial in developing a plausible science of recovery in which mechanisms of change can be linked to predictors to increase our understanding of life-course changes. The developing evidence base around recovery capital (summarised by [40]) UK–US research collaborations have been central in developing two key measurement instruments – the Assessment of Recovery Capital [38] and, more recently, the REC-CAP [18]. In both of the underpinning studies, there is evidence supporting a strength-based approach to building resources that are predicated on engaging in prosocial networks and the resulting engagement in meaningful activities.

The UK recovery research model has, consequently, focused on social catalysts for recovery, including the Social Identity Model of Recovery [13] and the Social Identity Model of Cessation Management [32]. In each of these approaches, recovery is seen as resulting from changes in social networks (from using to recovery focused), resulting in shifts in belonging and connected changes in attitudes, values and beliefs.

Much of this work links to a mental health approach to recovery-oriented interventions that is based on a review of the evidence by Leamy et al. [66] that concluded that effective recovery interventions required five change mechanisms – they had to generate positive Connections; they had to inspire Hope; they had to offer positive changes in Identity; they had to support linking people into Meaningful activities; and they had to create Empowerment, summarised in the acronym CHIME. This model has been adapted for the addiction recovery space by Best et al. [15], who has argued that assertive linkage into prosocial groups has the potential to generate the sense of hope that recovery is possible. In this model, hope is seen as the key driver of a dynamic engine in which a virtuous circle of meaningful activity generates a positive sense of identify and growing self-esteem that further perpetuates the cycle of change and recovery growth.

50.12 Conclusion

Whilst there is a growing evidence base around personal recovery pathways and journeys and an increasingly credible evidence base, driven largely by US research, two other key themes are emerging. The first is that recovery models and methods are increasingly influencing policy and practice not only outside of the United States but in the non-English speaking parts of Europe. Secondly, there is a growing awareness that recovery is not a solipsistic activity and that effective recovery models (including policies) require a social and community framing and an improved evidence base around what constitutes an effective and integrated recovery-oriented model of care.

References

1. Alvarez J, Adebanjo AM, Davidson MK, Jason LA, Davis MI. Oxford House: deaf- affirmative support for substance abuse recovery. Am Ann Deaf. 2006;151(4):418–22.
2. Andreas D, Davis Y, Wilson S. Peers Reach Out Supporting Peers to Embrace Recovery (PROSPER): a center for substance abuse treatment recovery community services program, Alcoholism Treatment Quarterly. 2010;28(3):326–38.
3. Appel PW, Ellison AA, Jansky HK, Oldak R. Barriers to enrollment in drug abuse treatment and suggestions for reducing them: opinions of drug injecting street outreach clients and other system stakeholders. Am J Drug Alcohol Abuse. 2004;30(1):129–53.
4. Ashton M. The new abstentionists, druglink, supplement. 2008;1–4.
5. Ashford R, Curtis B, Kelly JF. Systematic review: digital recovery support services used to support substance use disorder recovery. Researchgate. 2019. Accessed May 2019.
6. AVA. Breaking down the barriers: findings of the national commission on domestic and sexual violence and multiple disadvantage. 2019.
7. Bassuk EL, Hanson J, Greene RN, Richard M, Laudet A. Peer-delivered recovery support services for addictions in the United States: a systematic review. J Subst Abus Treat. 2016;63:1–9.
8. Bekkering GE, Mariën D, Parylo O, Hannes K. The effectiveness of self-help groups for adolescent substance misuse: a systematic review. J Child Adolesc Subst Abuse. 2016;25(3):229–44.

9. Bellaert L, Vander Laenen F, Colman C. Belgian policy analysis in ERANID recovery pathways in four European countries- the REC PATH study, Interim Analysis by Best et al. 2019.

10. Belleau C, DuPont R, Erickson C, Flaherty M, Galanter M, Gold M, White W. What is recovery? A working definition from the Betty Ford Institute. J Subst Abus Treat. 2007;33(3):221–8.

11. Best D. Addiction recovery: a movement for social change and personal growth in the UK. Brighton: Pavilion Publishing; 2012.

12. Best D, Gow J, Knox T, Taylor A, Groshkova T, White W. Mapping the recovery stories of drinkers and drug users in Glasgow: quality of life and its associations with measures of recovery capital. Drug Alcohol Rev. 2012;31(3):334–41.

13. Best D, Beckwith M, Haslam C, Haslam SA, Jetten J, Mawson E, Lubman DI. Overcoming alcohol and other drug addiction as a process of social identity transition: The Social Identity Model of Recovery (SIMOR). Addiction Research & Theory. 2016;24(2):1–13.

14. Best D, Vanderplasschen W, Van de Mheen D, De Maeyer J, Colman C, Vanden Laenen F, Irving J, Andersson C, Edwards M, Bellaert L, Martinelli T, Graham S, Hamer R, Nagelhout G. REC-PATH (Recovery Pathways): Overview of a four-country study of pathways to recovery from problematic drug use. Alcoholism Treatment Quarterly. 2018; 36(4):517–29.

15. Best D. Pathways to desistance and recovery: The role of the social contagion of hope. Policy Press: Bristol. 2019.

16. Best D, Bamber S, Battersby A, Gilman M, Groshkova T, Honor S, McCartney D, Yates R, White W. Recovery and straw men: an analysis of the objections raised to the transition to a recovery model in UK addiction services. J Groups Addict Recover. 2010;5(3–4):264–88.

17. Borkman T. Understanding self-help/mutual aid: experiential learning in the commons. New Brunswick: Rutgers University Press; 1999.

18. Cano I, Best D, Edwards M, Lehman J. Recovery capital pathways: modelling the components of recovery wellbeing. Drug Alcohol Depend. 2017;181:11–9.

19. Carroll JF. The evolving American therapeutic community. Alcohol Treat Q. 1993;9(3–4):175–81.

20. Center for Substance Abuse Treatment, editor. National summit on recovery: conference report. Rockville: Substance Abuse and Mental Health Services Administration; 2006.

21. Chavarria J, Stevens EB, Jason LA, Ferrari JR. The effects of self-regulation and self-efficacy on substance use abstinence. Alcohol Treat Q. 2012;30:422–32.

22. Clark W. Recovery-oriented systems of care: SAMHSA/CSAT's public health approach to substance use problems & disorders. Paper presented at the aligning concepts, practice, and contexts to promote long term recovery: an action plan, Philadelphia. 2008. www.ireta.org.

23. Clark W. Recovery as an organizing concept. http://www.nattc.org/learn/topics/rosc/docs/drwestleyclarkinterview.pdf. 2008. 7 Feb 2008.

24. Cohen LR, Hien DA. Treatment outcomes for women with substance abuse and PTSD who have experienced complex trauma. Psychiatric ser. 2006;57(1):100–6. https://doi.org/10.1176/appi.ps.57.1.100.

25. Covington SS. Women and addiction: a trauma-informed approach. J Psycho Drugs. 2008;40(Suppl 5):377–85.

26. Cunningham JA, Sobell LC, Sobell MB, Agrawal S, Toneatto T. Barriers to treatment: why alcohol and drug abusers delay or never seek treatment. Addict Behav. 1993;18(3):347–53.

27. Dennis M, Scott CK. Managing addiction as a chronic condition. NIDA Addict Sci Clin Pract Perspect. 2007;4(1):45–55. addiction recovery in services and policy: an international overview 1079

28. Dennis M, Scott C, Funk R, Foss MA. The duration and correlates of addiction and treatment careers. J Subst Abus Treat. 2005;28(1):S51–62.

29. Eddie D, Hoeppner B, Vilsaint C. Lived experience as clinical assets in new models of care for substance use disorder: a systematic review of recovery coaching and peer recovery support services. Frontiers in Psychology. 2019.

30. Faces and Voices of Recovery. Addiction recovery peer service roles: recovery management in health reform. Faces and Voices of Recovery. Washington: Faces and Voices of Recovery; 2010.

31. Fleury MJ, Djouini A, Huỳnh C, Tremblay J, Ferland F, Ménard JM, Belleville G. Remission from substance use disorders: a systematic review and meta-analysis. Drug Alcohol Depend. 2016;168:293–306.

32. Frings D, Albery IP. The social identity model of cessation maintenance: formulation and initial evidence. Addict Behav. 2015;44:35–42.

33. Galanter M. Combining medically assisted treatment and twelve-step programming: a perspective and review. Am J Drug Alcohol Abuse. 2018;44(2):151–9.

34. Godley MD, Godley SH, Dennis ML, Funk RR, Passetti LL. The effect of assertive continuing care on continuing care linkage, adherence and abstinence following residential treatment for adolescents with substance use disorders. Addiction. 2007;102(1):81–93.

35. Granfield R, Cloud W. Social context and "natural recovery": the role of social capital in the resolution of drug-associated problems. Subst Use Misuse. 2001;36(11):1543–70.

36. Greer AM, Amlani A, Burmeister C, Scott A, Newman C, Lampkin H, Pauly B, Buxton JA. Peer engagement barriers and enablers: insights from people who use drugs in British Columbia, Canada. Can J Public Health. 2019;110(2):227–35.

37. Grella CE, Lovinger K. 30-year trajectories of heroin and other drug use among men and women sampled from methadone treatment in California. Drug Alcohol Depend. 2011;118(2–3):251–8.

38. Groshkova T, Best D, White W. The assessment of recovery capital: properties and psychometrics of a measure of addiction recovery strengths. Drug and Alcohol Review. 2012;32(2):187–94.

39. Hamer R, Best D, Hall L. First year evaluation report: the Stovewood trauma and resilience service. Sheffield, UK: Sheffield Hallam University; 2019.

40. Hennessy E. Recovery capital: a systematic review of the literature. Addict Res Theory. 2017;25:349. https://doi.org/10.1080/16066359.2017.1297990.

41. Herman JL. Trauma and recovery: the aftermath of violence--from domestic abuse to political terror. Hachette; 2015.

42. HM Government. Drug Strategy 2010: Reducing demand, restricting supply, building recovery: Supporting people to live a drug-free life. HM Government: London. 2010.

43. HM Government. 2017 Drug Strategy. HM Government: London. 2017.

44. Hser YI, Anglin MD, Grella C, Longshore D, Prendergast ML. Drug treatment careers. A conceptual framework and existing research findings. J Subst Abus Treat. 1997;14(6):543–58.

45. Hser YI, Evans E, Grella C, Ling W, Anglin D. Long-term course of opioid addiction. Harv Rev Psychiatry. 2015;23(2):76–89.

46. Humphreys K. Addiction Treatment Professionals Are Not the Gatekeepers of Recovery. Subst Use Misuse. [Online]. 2015;50(8–9):1024–7.

47. Humphreys K, Moos R. Can encouraging substance abuse patients to participate in self-help groups reduce demand for health care? A quasi-experimental study. Alcohol Clin Exp Res. 2001;25(5):711–6.

48. Humphreys K, Tucker J. Toward more responsive and effective intervention systems for alcohol-related problems. Addiction. 2002;97(2):126–32.

49. Huskamp HA, Iglehart JK. Mental health and substance-use reforms—milestones reached, challenges ahead. N Engl J Med. 2016;375(7):688–95.

50. Institute of Medicine. Improving the quality of health care for mental and substance use conditions. Washington, DC: National Academy Press; 2005.

51. Jason LA, Davis MI, Ferrari JR, Bishop PD. Oxford house: a review of research and implications for substance abuse recovery and community research. J Drug Educ. 2001;31(1):1–27.

52. Jason LA, Aase DM, Mueller DG, Ferrari JR. Current and previous residents of selfgoverned recovery homes: characteristics of long-term recovery. Alcohol Treat Q. 2009;27(4):442–52.

53. Kaplan L. The role of recovery support services in recovery-oriented systems of care: DHHS publication No. (SMA) 08-4315. Rockville: Center for Substance Abuse Treatment, Substance Abuse and Mental Health Services Administration; 2008.

54. Kelly JF, White WL. Broadening the base of addiction mutual-help organizations. J Groups Addict Recover. 2012;7(2–4):82–101.

55. Kelly J, Bergman B, Hoeppner B, Vilsaint C, White W. Prevalence and pathways of recovery from drug and alcohol problems in the United States population: implications for practice, research, and policy. Drug Alcohol Depend. 2017;181:162–9.

56. Kelly JF. SAMHSA. Report of findings from a systematic review of the scientific literature on recovery support services in the United States. 2018.

57. Kelly JF. E. M. Jellinek's disease concept of alcoholism. Addiction. 2019;114(3):555–9.

58. Kirk T. Creating a recovery-oriented system of care. 2008. http://www.facesandvoicesofrecovery.org/pdf/recovery_symposium/GLATTCInterviewKirk.pdf. Retrieved 7 Feb 2008.

59. Kirk T. Connecticut's journey to a statewide recovery-oriented health-care system: strategies, successes, and challenges. In: Kelly J, White W, editors. Addiction recovery management. New York: Springer Humana Press; 2010. p. 2009–235.

60. Laudet A. What does recovery mean to you? Lessons from the recovery experience for research and practice. J Subst Abus Treat. 2007;33(3):243–56.

61. Laudet A, Humphreys K. Promoting recovery in an evolving context: what do we know and what do we need to know about recovery support services? J Subst Abus Treat. 2013;45(1):126–33.

62. Laudet AB, White W. What are your priorities right now? Identifying service needs across recovery stages to inform service development. J Subst Abus Treat. 2010;38(1):51–9.

63. Laudet AB, Savage R, Mahmood D. Pathways to long-term recovery: a preliminary investigation. J Psychoactive Drugs. 2002;34(3):305–11.

64. Laudet A, Stanick V, Sands B. The effect of onsite 12-step meetings on post-treatment outcomes among polysubstance-dependent outpatient clients. Eval Rev. 2007;31(6):613–46.

65. Laudet AB, Stanick V, Sands B. What could the program have done differently? A qualitative examination of reasons for leaving outpatient treatment. J Subst Abuse Treat. 2009;37(2):182–19066. Addiction Recovery in Services and Policy: An International Overview 1081.

66. Leamy M, Bird V, Le Boutillier C, Williams J, Slade M. Conceptual framework for personal recovery in mental health: systematic review and narrative synthesis. Br J Psychiatry. 2011;199(6):445–52.

67. Lo Sasso AT, Byro E, Jason LA, Ferrari JR, Olson B. Benefits and costs associated with mutual-help community-based recovery homes: the Oxford House model. Eval Program Plann. 2012;35(1):47–53.

68. Majer JM, Jason LA, Ferrari JR, North CS. Comorbidity among Oxford House residents: a preliminary outcome study. Addict Behav. 2002;27(5):837–45.

69. Majer JM, Angulo RS, Aase DM, Jason LA. Gambling behaviors among Oxford House resi-

dents: a preliminary investigation. J Soc Serv Res. 2011;37(4):422–7.

70. Manning V, Best D, Faulkner N, Titherington E, Morinan A, Keaney F, Gossop M, Strang J. Does active referral by a doctor or 12-step peer improve 12-step meeting attendance? Results from a pilot Randomised Control Trial, Drug and Alcohol Dependence. 2012;126(1):131–7.

71. Margolis R, Kilpatrick A, Mooney B. A retrospective look at long-term adolescent recovery: clinicians talk to researchers. J Psychoactive Drugs. 2000;32(1):117–25.

72. Martinelli T, Nagelhout G, Van de Mheen, D. Dutch policy analysis in ERANID recovery pathways in four European countries. The REC PATH study- interim analysis by Best et al. 2019.

73. McKay JR. Effectiveness of continuing care interventions for substance abusers. Implications for the study of long-term treatment effects. Eval Rev. 2001;25(2):211–32.

74. McKay JR. Continuing care research: what we have learned and where we are going. J Subst Abus Treat. 2009;36(2):131–45.

75. McKay JR, Lynch KG, Shepard DS, Morgenstern J, Forman RF, Pettinati HM. Do patient characteristics and initial progress in treatment moderate the effectiveness of telephone-based continuing care for substance use disorders? Addiction. 2005;100(2):216–26.

76. McKay JR, Carise D, Dennis ML, Dupont R, Humphreys K, Kemp J, Schwartzlose J. Extending the benefits of addiction treatment: practical strategies for continuing care and recovery. J Subst Abus Treat. 2009;36(2):127–30.

77. McLellan AT, Lewis DC, O'Brien CP, Kleber HD. Drug dependence, a chronic medical illness: implications for treatment, insurance, and outcomes evaluation. JAMA. 2000;284(13):1689–95.

78. McLellan AT, McKay JR, Forman R, Cacciola J, Kemp J. Reconsidering the evaluation of addiction treatment: from retrospective follow-up to concurrent recovery monitoring. Addiction. 2005;100(4):447–58.

79. McLellan AT, Weinstein RL, Shen Q, Kendig C, Levine M. Improving continuity of care in a public addiction treatment system with clinical case management. Am J Addict. 2005;14(5):426–40.

80. Mericle A, Hemberg J, Stall R, Carrico A. Pathways to recovery: recovery housing models for men who have sex with men (MSM), Addiction Research & Theory. 2019;27(5):373–82.

81. Mericle AA, Polcin DL, Hemberg J, Miles J. Recovery housing: evolving models to address resident needs. Journal of Psychoactive Drugs. 2017;49:352–61.

82. Millar JR, Aase DM, Jason LA, Ferrari JR. Veterans residing in self-governed recovery homes for substance abuse: sociodemographic and psychiatric characteristics. Psychiatr Rehabil J. 2011;35(2):141–4.

83. Moos R, Moos B. Rates and predictors of relapse after natural and treated remission from alcohol use disorders, Addiction. 2006:101(2);212–22.

84. Murphy MK, Bijur PE, Rosenbloom D, Bernstein SL, Gallagher EJ. Feasibility of a - computer-assisted alcohol SBIRT program in an urban emergency department: patient and research staff perspectives. Addict Sci Clin Pract. 2013;8(1):2. https://doi.org/10.1186/1940-0640-8-2, 1940- 0640-8-2 [pii].

85. NARR. A Primer on recovery residences: FAQs from the National Association of Recovery Residences, Atlanta, GA: NARR; 2012.

86. Nealon-Woods MA, Ferrari JR, Jason LA. Twelve- step program use among Oxford House residents: spirituality or social support in sobriety? J Subst Abus. 1995;7(3):311–8.

87. O'Brien C, McLellan A. Myths about the treatment of addiction. Lancet. 1996;347(8996):237–40.

88. O'Connell MJ, Flanagan EH, Delphin-Rittmon ME, Davidson L. Enhancing outcomes for persons with co-occurring disorders through skills training and peer recovery support. J Ment Health. 2017;29(1):1–6.

89. Olson BD, Viola J, Jason LA, Davis MI, Ferrari JR, Rabin-Belyaev O. Economic costs of Oxford House inpatient treatment and incarceration: a preliminary report. J Prev Interv Community. 2006;31(1–2):63–72.

90. Parkman TJ, Lloyd C, Splisbury K. Self-help groups for alcohol dependency: a scoping review. J Groups Addict Recover. 2015;10(2):102–24.

91. Polcin DL. A model for sober housing during outpatient treatment. J Psychoactive Drugs. 2009;41(2):153–61.

92. Ronel N, Elisha E. A different perspective: introducing positive criminology. Int J Offender Ther Comp Criminol. 2011;55(2):305–25. https://doi.org/10.1177/0306624X09357772.

93. SAMHSA. What's recovery? SAMHSA's working definition. 2012.

94. Scott CK, Foss MA, Dennis ML. Pathways in the relapse–treatment–recovery cycle over 3 years. J Subst Abus Treat. 2005;28(1):S63–72.

95. Scottish Government. The road to recovery: a new approach to Scotland's drug problem. Edinburgh: Scottish Government; 2008.

96. Seligman M. Authentic happiness. Boston: Nicholas Brealey Publishing; 2003.

97. Sheedy CK, Whitter M, editors. Guiding principles and elements of recovery-oriented systems of care: what do we know from the research? HHS publication No. (SMA) 09-4439. Rockville: Center for Substance Abuse Treatment, Substance Abuse and Mental Health Services Administration; 2009.

98. Tonigan JS. Alcoholics anonymous outcomes and benefits. Recent Dev Alcohol. 2008;18:357–72.

99. UK Drug Policy Commission Consensus Group. A vision for recovery. London: UKDPC; 2008.

100. Vanderplasschen W, Vandevelde S, Broekaert E. Therapeutic communities for treating addictions in Europe. Evidence, current practices and future

challenges. Ghent, Belgium: University of Ghent; 2014.

101. Waldron HB, Turner CW. Evidence-based psychosocial treatments for adolescent substance abuse. J Clin Child Adolesc Psychol. 2008;37(1):238–61.

102. Weisner C, Delucchi K, Matzger H, Schmidt L. The role of community services and informal support on five-year drinking trajectories of alcohol dependent and problem drinkers. J Stud Alcohol. 2003;64(6):862–73.

103. Weisner C, Matzger H, Kaskutas LA. How important is treatment? One-year outcomes of treated and untreated alcohol-dependent individuals. Addiction. 2003;98(7):901–11.

104. White W, editor. Recovery management and recovery-oriented systems of care: scientific rationale and promising practices. Pittsburgh: Northeast Addiction Technology Transfer Center, Great Lakes Addiction Technology Transfer Center, Philadelphia Department of Behavioral Health & Mental Retardation Services; 2008.

105. White W, editor. Peer-based addiction recovery support: history, theory, practice and scientific evaluation. Philadelphia: Great Lakes Addiction Technology Transfer Center, Philadelphia Department of Behavioral Health & Mental Retardation Services; 2009.

106. White W, Boyle M, Loveland D, Corrington P. What is behavioral health recovery management? A brief primer. 2005. www.addictionmanagement.org/recovery%20management.pdf. Retrieved 13 Feb 2008.

107. Wincup E. Gender, recovery and contemporary UK drug policy. Drugs and Alcohol Today. 2016;16(1):39–48.

108. Yablonsky L. The anticriminal society: Synanon. Fed. Probation. 1962;26:50.

109. Zemore SE, Mulia N, Ye Y, Borges G, Greenfield TK. Gender, acculturation, and other barriers to alcohol treatment utilization among Latinos in three National Alcohol Surveys. J Subst Abus Treat. 2009;36(4):446–56.

Strategies of Drug Prevention in the Workplace: An International Perspective of Drug Testing and Employee Assistance Programs

51

David E. Smith, Lisa Marzilli,
and Leigh Dickerson Davidson

Contents

Abstract

Drug testing in the workplace is not universal and is regulated by various governmental agencies at the federal, state, and municipal levels, as well as by select industries. Safety-sensitive occupations are typically targeted and various industries and agencies have specific drug testing protocols. In the United States, drug testing is highly structured and much of it falls under the purview of a Presidential Executive Order issued in 1986, with subsequent legislation calling for a drug-free workplace. An assigned Medical Review Officer (MRO) resolves any questionable results, be it a false-negative or false-positive drug test report.

In the European Union and other countries, drug testing is much less uniform, as attitudes to workplace alcohol and drug use are quite variable with no "standard approach." While the use of illicit drugs spurred widespread drug testing in the United States, prescribed medications that may impact workplace safety

D. E. Smith (✉) · L. D. Davidson
David E. Smith, MD & Associates,
San Francisco, CA, USA
e-mail: DrSmith@DrDave.org

L. Marzilli
Dominion Diagnostics Lab, Narragansett, RI, USA

© Springer Nature Switzerland AG 2021
N. el-Guebaly et al. (eds.), *Textbook of Addiction Treatment*,
https://doi.org/10.1007/978-3-030-36391-8_51

have become a controversial issue and have not been fully addressed. Many companies establish Employee Assistance Programs (EAPs) that are designed to help employees deal with life issues, including work–life stressors, family issues, financial concerns, relationship challenges, productivity issues, and concerns of substance use and abuse. Various services are provided to the employee, largely free of charge, relating to substance misuse and its effect on job performance. While the effectiveness of US programs is easier to assess due to consistency in approach, the variability of European programs makes them more difficult to evaluate.

Keywords

Addiction · Drug testing · Employee Assistance Programs · Medical Review Officer · Substance abuse · Workplace safety

51.1 Introduction

The majority of people using alcohol and other drugs, both legal, such as prescription medications, and illicit, are employed.

Substance misuse in the workplace is a major public health and economic issue, as the majority of substance misusers are employed. Substance use disorder (SUD), including alcohol use, is associated with increased accidents, absenteeism, and health costs. Therefore, modern concepts of drug use prevention, including drug testing, apply to the workplace and, when effected, produce benefits for both the employee and the employer.

As defined by DuPont [10], drug use prevention can be divided into three levels:

1. The primary strategy is aimed at preventing any illegal drug use. Drug use laws vary from country to country, so a broader concept relates to preventing use that produces impairment and threatens safety. Experts such as DuPont stress that any drug use by youth when the brain is still developing can be problematic, and a drug-free workplace can be a motivating factor for youth to avoid drug use.
2. Secondary prevention focuses on reducing the consequences of illicit drug use, such as workplace accidents and health costs for chronic diseases, for example, hepatitis and heart disease.
3. Tertiary prevention focuses on the individual who has a defined addictive disorder that requires treatment. With the passage of the Affordable Care Act in the United States, substance abuse is viewed as a medical issue that requires treatment before the individual can return to duty. If cleared, these individuals are protected by the Americans with Disabilities Act of 1990 (ADA) as long as they maintain their recovery in an appropriate monitoring system.

The secondary and tertiary levels of prevention are applicable to the workplace to reduce injury, accidents, and medical complications; all of which are costly to the employer and damaging to the worker. Different reduction strategies are used for each level, with drug testing and Employee Assistance Programs considered essential.

Most substance misuse in the workplace falls into one of the following areas: desired improvement in performance/productivity, relief of boredom, alleviation of physical and/or psychological pain/discomfort, addiction, or self-medication to relieve the side effects (e.g., hangovers, anxiety, etc.) of alcohol and other drugs. Substances ranging from opioids to stimulants may be used, depending on the user's objectives and preferences [25].

Drug-facilitated work impairment may not be noticeable or significant in ordinary situations. Emergencies, however, or unexpected demands on the worker, may precipitate unfortunate consequences. In addition, preoccupation with issues resulting from the worker's substance misuse, such as family arguments or contemplation of procuring more drugs, may reduce the worker's attentiveness to the requirements of the job. The employer may also be impacted by the worker's theft or misuse of company resources to obtain additional drugs, absenteeism, turnover, violation of governmental guidelines for a drug-free workplace, or adverse publicity [25].

Cannabis use, particularly its principal psychoactive ingredient delta-9-tetrahydrocannabinol (THC), has been associated with negative health outcomes, including cannabinoid-induced hyperemesis and cannabis-induced psychosis. Cannabis use is associated with drugged driving and increased risk of accidents. This is relevant to the workplace as a majority of workers drive as part of their employment [14].

Cognitive risks have also been associated with chronic cannabis use, including impaired learning and executive function. High potency THC compounds have been associated with greater psychiatric and neurological risks, including diminution of gray matter, particularly in adolescent early onset users whose brains are still maturing.

51.2 Drug Prevention in the Workplace

In the United States, drug testing to promote workplace safety and deter drug use is regulated by various governmental agencies at the federal, state, and municipal levels. And some employers' insurance carriers require specific drug testing programs. Different protocols exist for various industries and agencies; however, certain elements are consistent. Some companies require testing of every employee, others require preemployment testing only, and still others require periodic testing for employees holding safety-sensitive positions. Particularly after an accident, most employers require testing for potential drug or alcohol use. With the legalization of medical and recreational marijuana in many states, this has created another layer of complexity. The consequences of verifiable illicit drug/alcohol use in the workplace range from disciplinary action, referral to treatment, suspension, or employment termination.

The era of drug use prevention (other than alcohol) in the workplace began in the United States in the 1980s with the establishment of the Drug-Free Workplace Program, Executive Order #12564 [12]. This paralleled the drug epidemic permeating industrial settings and contributed to several highly publicized fatal accidents in which several employees tested positive for marijuana. As a result, in 1986 the US Federal Government issued Executive Order #12564:

> The Federal Government, as the largest employer in the nation, can and should show the way towards achieving drug-free workplaces through a program designed to offer drug users a helping hand and, at the same time, demonstrating to drug users and potential drug users that drugs will not be tolerated in the Federal workplace....

The Executive Order mandated that most Federal agencies, under the purview of the Executive Department, required the following: employees must refrain from illicit drug use, agencies implement and develop Employee Assistance Programs (EAPs), and they establish standard drug testing policies and procedures. The focus of the drug-free workplace was to eliminate illicit drug use of heroin, cocaine, amphetamines, marijuana, and 1, 1-phenylcyclohexyl (PCP). This panel became known as the National Institute on Drug Abuse-5 (NIDA-5). However, because alcohol was and is the primary drug problem in the industrial setting, both in the United States and worldwide, the Omnibus Transportation Employee Testing Act of 1991 included alcohol. According to the Division of Workplace Programs of the Substance Abuse and Mental Health Services Administration (SAMHSA) in the United States, the majority of active illicit drug/alcohol users are employed full-time and constitute two-thirds or more of the adult population [15]. The 2013 SAMHSA National Survey on Drug Use and Health reported that 68.9% of the estimated 22.4 million illicit drug users, age 18 or older, were employed full or part-time, while upward of 75% of adult binge and heavy alcohol drinkers were employed [24]. And in 2018, the number of users that were employed full-time rose to nearly 75% [7, 14].

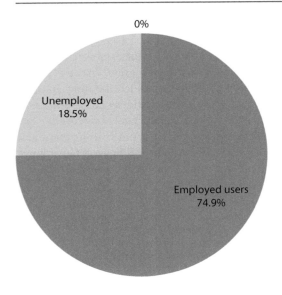

The majority of current drug users are employed (current users of illicit drugs, ages 18 and over). (Source: National Survey on Drug Use and Health: National Findings)

While illicit drugs were the main impetus for establishing the drug-free workplace regulation in the 1980s in the United States, prescribed medications, especially opioids, became a growing issue, ravaging all regions of the United States. The resulting restrictions on prescribed opioids beginning in 2016 and becoming even more stringent in 2018 have created a shift to the utilization of heroin, illicit fentanyl, and other synthetic opioids (Centers for Disease Control). In 2017, the Centers for Disease Control (CDC) reported that over 70,200 drug overdose deaths involved opioids, and the primary driver was attributed to synthetic opioids (illicit fentanyl and analogues). Unintentional overdoses in the US workplace due to nonmedical use of drugs and alcohol increased over 25% each year from 2012 to 2017. The challenges employers face in this climate have resulted in far-reaching consequences beyond the scope of this chapter. It is worth noting that on January 1, 2018, the Federal Department of Transportation (DOT) added four additional drugs for screening: hydrocodone, hydromorphone, oxycodone, and oxymorphone.

US legislation established the designation of "Medical Review Officer" (MRO) [3, 20] in the 1980s specifically for the evaluation of "questionable" drug test results. A limited number of professional organizations offer courses to provide clinical training in the review and analysis of drug test results and a formal certification of MRO. The Medical Review Officer Certification Council (MROCC) promotes and preserves the highest quality of standards among MROs and their team members by setting standards, defining MRO competencies, promoting a Code of Ethics, offering certification examinations, and providing publications and educational activities. The role of the MRO in assessing safety in the workplace with prescribed medications, specifically opioids, continues to be extremely challenging.

Many companies that operate internationally have established EAPs designed to help them address safety and productivity issues by providing various services to behaviorally effected employees in order to alleviate and resolve issues interfering with their job performance. The Employee Assistance Professionals Association lists several national and regional EAP associations and organizations at www. EAPASSN.org.

51.3 Drug Testing in the United States Workplace

Workplace drug testing in the United States is highly structured and is intended to foster workplace safety standards and creates a healthy work environment [2, 6]. Tests are generally administered in a nonmedical setting, where body fluids, most commonly urine, are collected and analyzed. The sample passes through a rigorous and well-documented "chain of custody" process. The frequency, type, and drugs tested for typically depend on the industry and various government regulatory agencies involved. Companies and organizations with US government contracts must be compliant with regulations regarding drug use in the workplace.

Drug testing is most common in settings where employees perform hazardous or safety-related tasks: such as operation of heavy equipment; transportation of passengers, medical, and surgical procedures; operation of nuclear power plants, public safety, and law enforcement. Every branch of the military has a specific program for drug testing of its service members.

There are several instances that will initiate an order for a drug test. Some of these include preemployment, after an accident/incident, impaired performance on the job, observed use of drugs or alcohol, random assignment, voluntary, follow-up to treatment, and return to work. Continued monitoring and random drug testing may be instituted as part of an employee's recovery plan and often in conjunction with a medical professional.

Interpreting drug test results is more nuanced than a simple "positive" or "negative" if a valid result is to be obtained. Individuals may test positive if they are prescribed an opioid pain medication, for example. If a specimen is compromised or adulterated, either intentionally or inadvertently, an erroneous result report is likely to occur. For this reason, it is advisable that a qualified MRO be available to certify the results obtained. It must be noted that while MRO protocols are quite rigorous to assess sample adulteration, Internet search engines and individual initiative offer an ever-growing abundance of information on specimen tampering. Laboratories provide testing for validity markers (i.e., temperature, pH, and specific gravity) in order to assess for adulteration.

Medically prescribed drugs do not necessarily result in impairment or risk of accident on the job. Therefore, the focus in the United States as it relates to drug testing has been on substance use prevention and education. New synthetic drugs (e.g., synthetic cannabinoids, synthetic stimulants, etc.) that are continually emerging are not included on a standard drug test and pose a challenge to employers.

Random drug testing is mandated by many regulatory agencies in order to accurately assess whether or not an employee is using alcohol or illicit drugs. Employee identifications are typically generated in a random fashion, and the employee must report for a drug test within 24–48 hours at a location determined by the employer. After the specimen is collected, it may be analyzed on site immediately or may be shipped via overnight express to a centralized laboratory. Samples are usually "split" in the event there is a need to repeat and further analyze the specimen. For example, an employee may dispute the result at which time the MRO would intervene and review the results report or potentially request a retest in order to validate the findings.

Though specimen testing is largely via urine sample, other testing matrices may be utilized, such as blood, saliva, and hair. Regardless of the specimen collected, all must follow a rigorous protocol in order to balance the following: the employee's right to privacy, monitoring for specimen tampering, adherence to the process in the "chain of custody," and ensuring a valid and secure results report.

Components of specimen collection

- Employee's right to privacy
- Chain of custody
- Federal custody and control form (CCF)
- Integrity, security, and identification
- Temperature recording
- Tamper-evident bottle seal

Employees testing "positive" with an unexpected result are sometimes suspended from work until the results are reviewed and verified by the MRO. The specimen integrity, chain of command, potential shipping delay, or ambiguous result may require further investigation. Assessing the employee's use of over-the-counter (OTC) medications is also critical, as some of these products interfere with the laboratory testing, causing a false-positive result. In this case, the MRO must carefully review, assess, and interpret the results report for further clarification. Depending on the sensitivity and specificity of the drug testing methodology, foodstuffs like poppy seeds may also generate a false-positive result for opiates. For this reason, workplace testing in the United States has established cutoff levels for opiates above the levels generally triggered by poppy seed ingestion.

Similarly, a policy to raise the marijuana cutoff level has been instituted to address the issue of second-hand smoke or "passive inhalation" when in the presence of an individual smoking marijuana. However, with the legalization of medical and recreational marijuana in many states across the United States, many challenges continue to manifest. State laws and employer policies are highly variable, and the issue of impairment on the job must be addressed. That said, the DOT has not waivered or modified their drug testing program, even though the Department of Justice (DOJ) has issued guidelines for prosecutors in states that have enacted laws authorizing the use of medical or recreational marijuana. Currently, MROs are prohibited from verifying a DOT drug test as "negative" based upon a physician recommending an employee use of "medical marijuana." For more detailed information on this topic, visit the US Department of Transportation website for the full manuscript and current ruling posted 2019 (USDOT/documents/medical-marijuana.pdf).

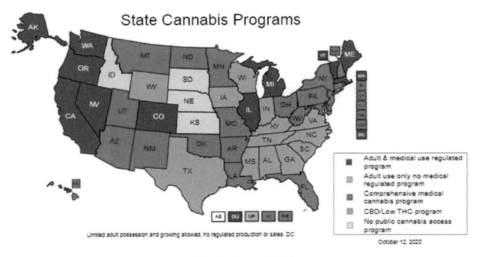

Current state. Approved Marijuana status, August 2018. (Source: DEA)

While federal mandates for safety-sensitive jobs are clearly defined, the decision-making for private employers is extremely challenging as it relates to marijuana use. And according to the National Safety Council Report (February 2019 [19]), roughly 15 million employed individuals are struggling with some degree of substance misuse disorder. The top two substances are alcohol and cannabis, followed by opioid pain medications, benzodiazepines, and many other illicit drugs.

With the October 2018 legalization of cannabis in Canada, the Occupational and Environmental Medical Association of Canada (OEMAC) issued a position statement in September 2018 stating that "current evidence indicates cannabis is the most commonly encountered agent in workplace drug testing in Canada and, second to alcohol, the most prevalent substance implicated in driving under the influence." The document concludes that use of cannabis can lead to impairment, that motor vehicle or equipment operation is not advisable, that workplace drug and alcohol policies be updated, and that additional research and education are needed [21].

Some US states, including California, Massachusetts, and Nevada, have seen double-digit increases in the number of employees who test positive for marijuana. The complexity of this changing landscape has forced several private companies (in several states that have legalized medical and recreational cannabis use) to drop marijuana from their drug testing profile [13, 23].

Another significant challenge that is not captured by the NIDA-5 testing panel is the ever-growing issue of "designer drugs," now globally referred to as novel psychoactive substances (NPS). In 2008, synthetic cannabinoids (e.g., K2, spice, etc.) and synthetic stimulants were just emerging in the United States. Continued modification of these substances and creations of new products (e.g., illicit fentanyl and other synthetic opioids) have made it nearly impossible for a basic drug test to detect use [18]. Impairment on the job without the objective evidence from a drug test has created yet another dilemma for MRO recommendations and employer risks.

Over the last 5 years beginning in 2014, illicit fentanyl and fentanyl analogues have created severe risks in health-hazard exposure. The National Institute for Occupational Safety and Health's (NIOSH) 2018 guidance is available for reference, providing an in-depth review on preventing occupational exposure to these potentially lethal products [13].

Nonetheless, drug testing remains crucial for effective identification, intervention, and monitoring in the workplace. This medical test produces a results report that provides objective data that may be used for nullification purposes and also provides a platform to monitor effectiveness of treatment after an SUD has been diagnosed in the individual. The MRO designation was partly established so employees would not be denied necessary prescribed medications in overzealous attempts to extinguish illicit drug use.

The following graphic illustrates the MRO decision tree and laboratory analysis:

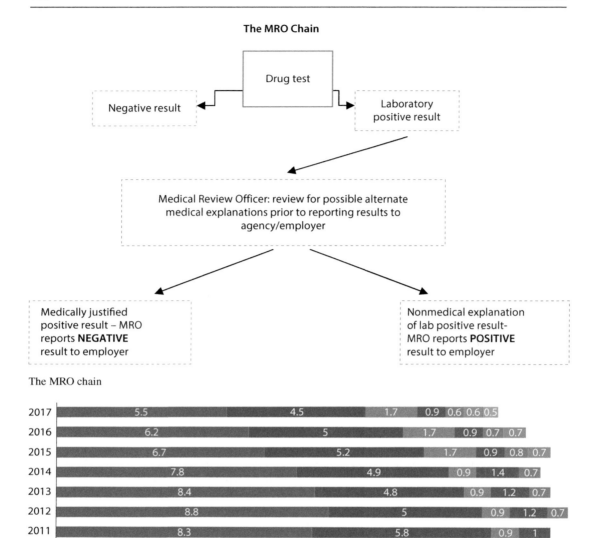

Top controlled prescription drugs sold to domestic retail level purchasers in billions of dosage units, 2009–2017. (Source: Automation of Reports and Consolidated Orders Systems, DEA)

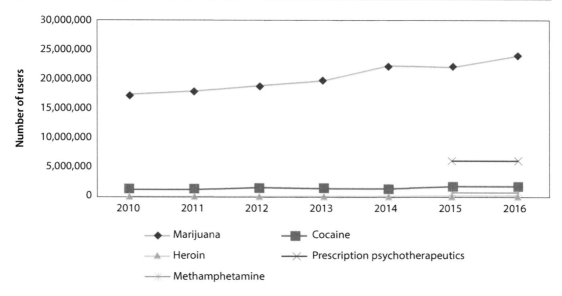

Number of past month, nonmedical users of psychotherapeutic drugs compared to other select drugs of abuse, 2010–2016. (Source: Substance Abuse and Mental Health Services Administration, National Survey on Drug Use and Health)

Though opioid-prescribing regulations and restrictions continue to tighten in the United States, they remain an issue for employees that use pain medications appropriately (with a valid physician prescription). Differentiating between appropriate use, misuse, abuse, addiction, and drug diversion in the workplace is crucial so that legitimate pain management is not confused with inappropriate use that results in negative health consequences and/or safety risks in the workplace. In these circumstances, when an employee's drug test indicates a "positive" opioid detection, the MRO must notify the employee and request a copy of the physician's prescription, to include a clinical diagnosis for treatment. Typically, the MRO will instruct the employee to cease work and immediately report to the supervisor. If the employee supplies the information to support medication use, the MRO will review the documents and notify the employer that the individual is medically cleared to return to work as long as no documented issues with performance or behavior have been observed.

Opioids, even when used for appropriate pain management, may potentially lead to workplace accidents, performance problems, and other medical, psychological, and behavioral problems. Side effects associated with opioid treatment include drowsiness, inattentiveness, impaired judgment, poor hand/eye coordination, tolerance and dose escalation, physical dependence, loss of function, perception of emotional pain as physical pain, and hyperalgesia (continual increases in dosage resulting in escalation of pain and the perception of pain).

To date, there continues to be an issue of establishing set protocols for appropriate use of prescription medications as it relates to proper assessment of workplace performance. An individual's right to privacy is a significant factor. In the United States, the Americans with Disabilities Act (ADA) became law in 1990 to prohibit discrimination against individuals suffering from a disability in the workplace, schools, transportation, and all public and private areas that are open to the general public [17]. Several amendments to the civil rights law have been made over the years to guarantee civil rights protection for both public and private employers (more than 15 employees). Two recent settlements serve as a reminder that employers must be prudent when assessing cases that involve employees prescribed medication use and their ability to perform job duties.

MRO courses such as those presented by the Medical Review Officer Certification Council

(MROCC) provide clinical training on opioid medications and the potential of negative consequences such as intoxication, addiction, and overdose, as well as information on several other medications and substances of abuse, including stimulants like amphetamine, methamphetamine, and cocaine that are widely used and misused in the workplace. The latest Federal DEA data published in 2018 reports a significant escalation of coca production, cocaine trafficking, and imports have reached an all-time high in the United States [26]. As supply rises and prices fall, access and use increase [18].

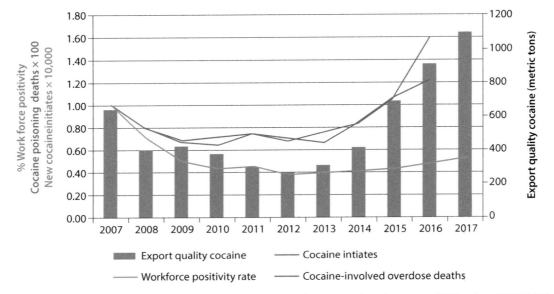

U.S. cocaine indicators and Colombia export quality cocaine production, based on 2007 value, 2007–2017. (Source: DEA National Forensic Laboratory Information System, August 2017)

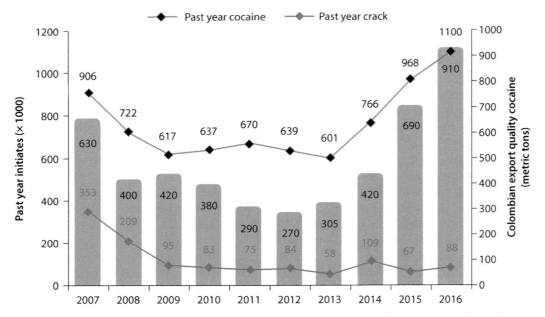

Past year cocaine initiates and export quality cocaine production. (Source: National Survey on Drug Use and Health and United States Government)

By definition in the Diagnostic and Statistical Manual of Mental Disorder's fifth Edition (DSM-V), SUD can affect workplace functioning due to dependence, abuse, intoxication, delirium, withdrawal, induction of psychotic disorder with hallucination or delusions, induced mood disorder, and many other negative consequences. And there are many adverse events that may require immediate medical attention whether or not the substance is legal (such as alcohol), prescribed by a physician, or obtained illegally. This potential for an adverse drug reaction is further heightened when multiple drugs/substances are ingested.

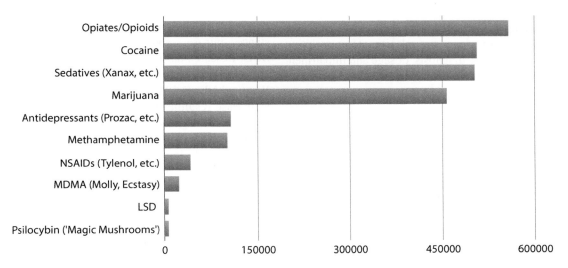

Emergency Department Admissions (2011). (Source: DEA.org)

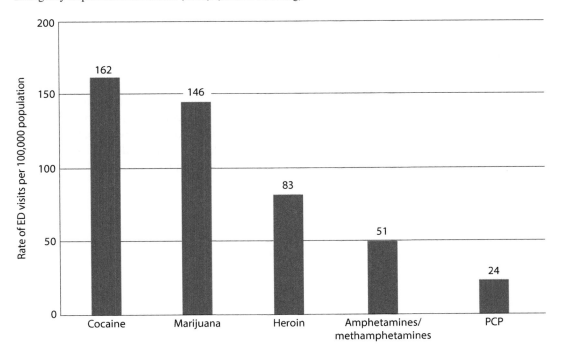

Source: DAWN data, 2011

51.4 Alcohol Testing

The relationship between blood alcohol concentration (BAC) and accident risk is well established. The US National Transportation Safety Board (NTSB) is currently campaigning to reduce the BAC limits for all drivers.

For other substances like opioids and amphetamines, discerning impairment and accident risk is not well defined and can be extremely challenging for an MRO to assess. Even in cases where an employee has a legitimate prescription and qualifying diagnosis, dosage and impairment are not linear and clearly defined, as is the case with alcohol consumption.

Levels of alcohol intoxication

Blood alcohol concentration (BAC)	Percent of drivers too intoxicated to drive	Increased risk of accident
0.02% Restraint/awareness	5%	^1
0.04% Comprehension	15%	1×
0.06% Judgment	35%	2×
0.08% Muscle control	65%	4×
0.10% Coordination	100%	8×
0.20% Equilibrium/sleep		65×
0.30% Stupor		600×
0.40% Coma		
0.50% Death		

Because alcohol is rapidly metabolized, it is detectable only for approximately 6–8 hours when utilizing urine as the medium for drug testing. However, alcohol metabolites are present in the urine for up to 72 hours as ethyl glucuronide (EtG) and ethyl sulfate (EtS). The standard NIDA-5 does not include tests for these metabolites. In the event the MRO deems necessary, tests for EtG and EtS are available.

Identification of SUD in the workplace requires appropriate training and professional evaluation. As emphasized by Dr. Wesley H. Clark, former Director of the Center for Substance Abuse Treatment (CSAT) and faculty member of the now-discontinued ASAM MRO course, a positive toxicology report or an adverse drug reaction does not necessarily indicate substance misuse, abuse, or a diagnosis of SUD. Research has indicated there is a spectrum of substance use ranging from "I Like....I Want....I NEED." The DSM-V defines addiction as disease resulting in a pathological state with characteristic signs and symptoms.

Over time, morphological changes in the brain progress and impair rational thinking and decision-making. Predictable and often catastrophic consequences result when SUD is left untreated. It is characterized by the compulsive desire for the substance (or behavior known as *process* addiction), a loss of control when exposed, and continued use despite negative consequences. Though many individuals use alcohol and other substances and engage in unhealthy behaviors in the workplace, it is worth stating that only approximately 10% of those exposed actually progress to a diagnosis of SUD and require intensive treatment before returning to work.

Drug testing in the workplace is an essential component of a comprehensive workplace program. It provides objective evidence to accurately assess alcohol and drug consumption. Unfortunately, implementation in US industry is quite variable.

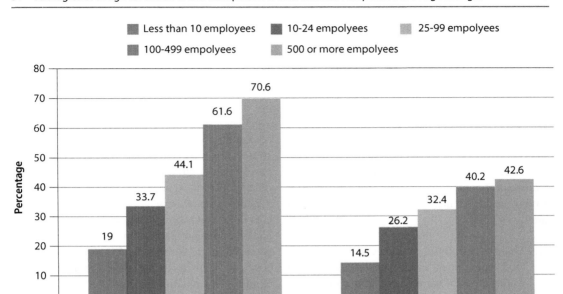

Type of drug and alcohol testing program, age 18–64. (Source: Worker Substance Use and Workplace Policies and Programs, 2007 NSDUH)

Treatment for SUD will assist those afflicted personally and professionally and foster a healthy workplace environment. Studies prepared by the Division of Workplace Programs of SAMHSA have shown that individuals' physical and mental health improve significantly during and after treatment, resulting in a major reduction in health care utilization. Recognizing that SUD is a disease has benefits for the employer when the employee is referred to treatment and is willing to accept and engage the process. If the employee successfully completes initial treatment, the employer is able to retain a trained, experienced employee and eliminate the cost of recruiting and training a new employee. And with continued treatment and monitoring, the employee provides a positive example for other fellow employees who may be suffering in silence.

51.5 Drug Testing in the European Workplace

In Europe and other countries, drug testing in the workplace is far less standardized and much more controversial than the United States. Varied social norms and cultural trends must be balanced with the need for safety in the workplace. National legislation varies widely in terms of the following: the employees' rights and obligations for being subject to testing, the conditions under which testing takes place, whether specimen collection is "observed," processed, and transported. Many other challenges exist when legislation and protocols are not clearly defined, for example, the need and availability of a qualified individual to interpret drug test results and the process of how these results are communicated to employer and employee. Further complicating the matter is that amounts of allowable intake of alcohol and other substances in the workplace setting vary widely.

Without consistent regulations and policies, it is difficult to create a standardized drug use prevention in the workplace program in Europe (and other countries), although efforts are underway to address this gap. Some countries have no specialized programs, while others have limited programs, but attitudes are beginning to change. In fact, the UK and several Scandinavian countries have developed comprehensive workplace drug testing policies and programs. Corral, Duran, and Isusi [9] examined the types of regulations in place across a wide swath of the European countries in their report, "Use of Alcohol and Drugs at the Workplace," for the European Foundation for the Improvement of Living and Working Conditions (Eurofound). As in the United States, drug testing is mandated by a variety of governmental regulatory agencies and industries, but in many of these countries, employees have a much "louder voice" than is acceptable in the United States.

A sampling of study results cited in the European Foundation for the Improvement of Living and Working Conditions [11] document are listed below:

(a) There is a cultural tolerance of alcohol use (and sometimes other substances) in the workplace that varies from country to country. This approach is diametrically opposed to the United States where the model is a zero-tolerance policy.

(b) A majority of employers and employees do not agree with the use of alcohol and drugs in the workplace; however, cultural views on alcohol consumption and various substances are less rigid than the United States, so protocols for implementing policies are quite difficult to enforce and are highly variable.

(c) The cultural stance on alcohol and drug use in the workplace has grown more conservative over the years and has been addressed in a variety of studies. The Swedish Construction Federation reported that it was no longer socially acceptable to consume drugs in the workplace, a stark contrast to attitudes in the construction industry 40 years prior.

(d) In Portugal, there has been a growing awareness of the consequences of alcohol and drug use in the workplace. In early 2010, 90% of Portuguese enterprises had concerns related to employees' general health problems, increased incidence of sick leave and short-term absenteeism, reduced performance levels, labor conflicts, and an unsettled work environment.

(e) One Italian study reported that employees addicted to drugs/alcohol had more than double the rate of absenteeism compared to employees that did not use these substances [16].

(f) In Austria, alcohol-dependent employees took sick leave 16 times more frequently and reported "feeling sick" 2.5 times more often than those employees who were not alcohol dependent.

Other European studies investigating the use of alcohol and drugs in the workplace demonstrated that their use negatively impacted work performance, attitude, and morale and contributed to workplace accidents resulting in harm to a fellow employee. A 2008 Latvian report indicated that there were substantial economic losses and a damaged public image when accidents occurred in the workplace. As community members continued to discuss these incidences, the employer's reputation declined.

Other studies and reports have documented significant economic costs of substance misuse in the workplace. In Norway, alcohol-related illness accounted for substantial financial losses in millions of euros. And in the early 2010 period, Austrian alcohol use accounted for 1.5–2.5% of total payroll costs. The Austrian Federal Economic Chamber (*Wirtschaftskammer Osterreich*, www.wko.at) stated in this same era that a worker with alcohol and drug problems performed at roughly 75% of potential. Considering this information and more gathered since that time, European employers are closely examining the need for a new approach to strictly limit the use of alcohol and other substances in the workplace.

Unfortunately, there is often a delayed recognition of an employees' excessive consumption of alcohol/other drugs in the workplace. A German study indicated the delayed response time was nearly 10 years for men and 2–5 years for women. And more often than not, at this point, the employee was terminated. In contrast, the approach in the United States for first-time offenders is a strategy of intervention, treatment, continued monitoring, and reintegration into the workplace.

The European Workplace Drug Testing Society (www.EWDTS.org) works to examine issues relating to workplace drug testing and organizes annual conferences, providing an opportunity for all stakeholders to share ideas and discuss best-practice approaches. EWDTS' mission statement is in part "....to ensure that drug testing in Europe is performed in a standard and legal manner...." The website provides brief summaries of workplace drug testing in various countries [27].

Though there is no centralized statistical information source in Europe and surrounding countries, the European Monitoring Centre for Drugs and Drug Addiction [4] reported that cocaine consumption was second to cannabis. A slightly different conclusion on drug prevalence in the UK workplace by drug testing provider Concateno [8] reported cannabis was the most frequently consumed, closely followed by opioids. The report also discussed the fact that patterns of drug use change with age. For instance, cannabis use appears to decrease with age, while the use of opioids increases. Amphetamines, methamphetamine, and the stimulant class as a whole have been and continue to be a growing problem.

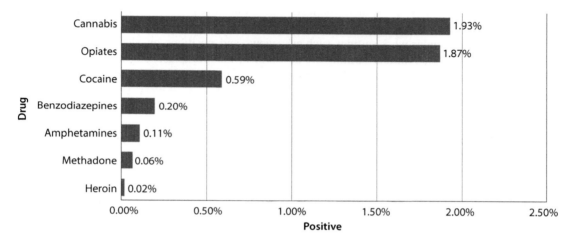

UK drug prevalence within the workplace 2007–2011

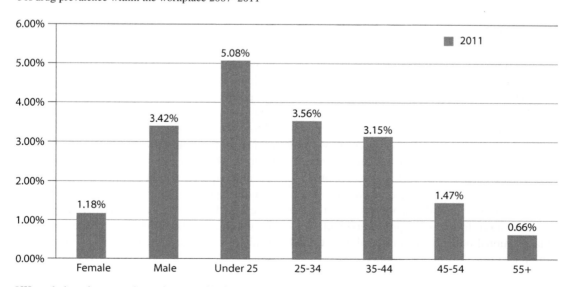

UK workplace drug prevalence demographic for 2011

In France, the National Research and Safety Institute for the Prevention of Occupational Accidents and Diseases in the workplace has a program to train employers and supervisors to identify employees of concern and assist them in actionable plan forward. The German Centre for Addiction Issues commissioned an expert report on the practice of company-based drug prevention, and in 2006, it was debuted by policy makers, health insurers, and other social partners.

Several European nations have recognized that alcohol and drug use represents a severe problem for a significant percentage of the working population. National estimates indicate that 5–20% of workers are impaired by substance use, and particular work settings such as construction, transportation, and farming are at greater risk. Alcohol and drug consumption in the workplace often results in negative consequences such as a higher incidence of sick leave, reduced productivity, impaired performance, and avoidable accidents. Because the United States has more consistent national polices in workplace testing, comprehensive data is available to assess interventions, rehabilitation, and workplace reentry. Unfortunately, this type of information is lacking in the European countries.

Most European countries have some general legislation and agreements in place to prohibit or regulate the consumption of alcohol and other substances in the workplace, but there is considerable diversity regarding implementation and legal enforcement. In Germany, Belgium, and Denmark, "collective social agreements" are implemented in lieu of pure coercive measures. Until national labor codes and statutes are collectively agreed upon, many interventions are loosely labeled as "disciplinary," and corrective actions are taken to merely limit the use of alcohol and drugs in the workplace. However, companies that operate in multiple nations are forced to institute more formal drug-prevention and drug-interventional policies. International airlines and shipping firms illustrate this example.

European studies appear to place more emphasis on work-related reasons for alcohol and substance use, including strenuous physical work, poor working conditions, low job satisfaction, personal issues, relationship challenges, and lack of recognition of employees' rights. The intention appears to focus on what leads to substance use rather than flatly banning use and consumption in the workplace. Additionally, European cultures generally have a more tolerant view of alcohol use during the workday. Until the 1970s, this sentiment was more pervasive in the United States, and it was not unusual for a businessmen of the time to engage in a "three-martini lunch." But for the past several decades, the emphasis in the United States is for a drug-free workplace and zero-tolerance policy. Several recent reports indicate that European nations are changing their views and positions on alcohol/drug consumption in the workplace. As the economy globalizes, further study is needed to determine the most effective workplace programs to mitigate accidents and provide healthy and safe working environments. There is certainly a vested interest on behalf of employer groups to ensure productivity and safety.

51.6 Employee Assistance Programs

The key to an effective workplace program is a comprehensive Employee Assistance Program (EAP) [22]. Identification of the behaviorally impaired employee due to alcohol or substance misuse and/or abuse provides an opportunity for evaluation and referral to appropriate treatment, as opposed to a sudden disciplinary termination. The American Society of Addiction Medicine (ASAM) assessment and patient placement criteria [1] are most effective for such evaluation and referral. Although companies in the United States are not required to have workplace EAPs and treatment programs, many do because of insurance and liability risks. SAMHSA studies and reports have established that these programs result in excellent benefits, both economic and social. It has been shown that treatment averts many negative outcomes, saves money in overall health care costs, and reduces accident risk in the workplace.

EAPs for alcohol-use disorder gained prominence after World War II, largely due to the influence of Alcoholics Anonymous (AA), which was established in the 1930s. Individuals influential in the AA movement, such as Marty Mann, who helped found the National Committee for Education on Alcoholism (now known as the National Council on Alcoholism and Drug Dependence (NCADD)), and Dr. Ruth Fox, who helped form the New York Society of Alcoholism, were among the guiding forces behind the formation of the American Society of Addiction Medicine (ASAM).

ASAM [5] has developed a very clear clinical definition of the disease of addiction:

> Addiction is a primary, chronic disease of the brain reward, motivation, memory, and related circuitry. Dysfunction in these circuits leads to characteristic biological, psychological, social, and spiritual manifestations. This is reflected in an individual pathologically pursuing reward and/or relief by substance use and other behaviors.
>
> Addiction is characterized by an inability to consistently abstain, impairment in behavioral control, continual craving, diminished recognition of significant problems with one's behaviors and interpersonal relationships, and a dysfunctional emotional response. Like other chronic diseases, addiction often involves cycles of relapse and remission. Without treatment or engagement in recovery activities, addiction is progressive and can result in disability or premature death.

The 4 Cs of Addiction:

- Craving
- Loss of Control
- Compulsive Use
- Continued Use Despite Harm

That said, some employees use narcotic pain medication under the care of a physician with a valid prescription. Differentiating appropriate use and potential misuse, abuse, addiction, or diversion in the workplace is crucial so that legitimate pain management is not confused with misuse. Evaluation and selection of an appropriate laboratory for drug testing are essential. In addition, it is necessary to engage a highly qualified MRO to interpret the drug test results in order to clarify false positives or negatives and to

ensure that appropriate reporting and assessment take place.

EAPs may be funded by employers, employee benefit organizations, or unions and are often provided at no cost to the employee. They are designed to provide short-term counseling for a variety of personal issues, including legal, financial, relationship challenges, life events, and substance use disorders (SUD) – all of which may affect workplace performance. For issues that cannot be resolved quickly, referrals and other resources are provided. One might compare the services provided by an EAP to that of an ambulance – get to the patient quickly, stabilize the condition, and transfer to a facility for further evaluation and care if necessary. Confidentiality of an employee's visit with a counselor is required, as the session content cannot ethically be reported to the employer for any reason.

EAPs are available internationally. The Employee Assistance Professionals Association is a worldwide association (www.EAPASSN. org), and there are other national organizations focused in Europe, Canada, Australia, the UK, Ireland, and the Asia Pacific Region.

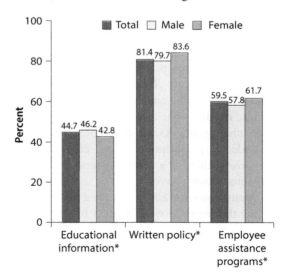

Workplace provides educational information, written policy, or employee assistance program concerning drug or alcohol use among full-time workers aged 18–64, by gender: annual averages, 2008–2012. *Difference between male and females is significant at the .05 level. (Source: SAMHSA, Center for Behavioral Health Statistics and quality, National Surveys on Drug Use and Health (NSDUHs), 2008–2010 (revised March 2012), and 2011–2012)

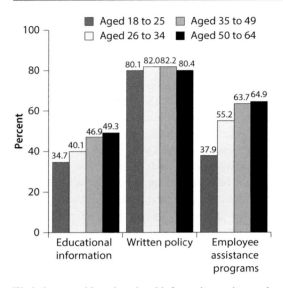

Workplace provides educational information, written policy, or employee assistance program concerning drug or alcohol use among full-time workers aged 18–64, by gender: annual averages, 2008–2012. (Source: SAMHSA, Center for Behavioral Health Statistics and quality, National Surveys on Drug Use and Health (NSDUHs), 2008–2010 (revised March 2012), and 2011–2012)

EAPs typically have a strong component of the recognition, referral, and treatment of substance misuse and abuse. Some large programs may engage Substance Abuse Professionals (SAPs) who have specialized training to identify potential drug problems and provide referral to treatment. They may also identify practitioners who enable employees to abuse drugs, misuse their medications, or divert for sale and profit. As many employer benefits include a prescription drug plan for the employee, there is a vested interest in containing unnecessary costs.

Many times, the EAP will play a role in monitoring the return to work process for employees suffering from SUD. This outcome is "best-case scenario" and benefits both the employer and employee. Monitoring with objective markers such as random drug testing, assuring the employee is attending psychotherapy sessions, and encouraging utilization of a 12-Step program are some of the ways the employee can be supported toward successful outcomes.

51.7 Summary

In reviewing the topic of alcohol and substance use in the workplace, drug testing, and management, it is clear there is no uniform approach. When considering the topic from an international prospective, cultural norms and views further vary the landscape of management approaches.

The United States has a well-defined and structured approach, including strict discipline, mandates, treatment, rehabilitation, and drug test monitoring prior to reentry into the workplace. In the European countries, the approach is less rigid and focuses more on the reasons why employees ingest alcohol/substances in the workplace, which appears to engage an approach of prevention and rehabilitation without placing the employee immediately at risk of consequence and potential job loss.

EAPs offer benefits to both employers and employees. For the employer, they provide an avenue for maintaining productivity, reducing absenteeism and workplace accidents, and retaining experienced and seasoned employees. For the employee, an EAP provides a lifeline in the event of serious life challenges and, in the event of a developing substance use disorder, a structured path with a compassionate and medically proven venue for treatment and continued monitoring.

Glossary

AA Alcoholics Anonymous
ASAM American Society of Addiction Medicine
CSAT Center for Substance Abuse Treatment, SAMHSA (USA)
DAWN Drug Abuse Warning Network (USA)
DOJ Department of Justice (USA)
DOT Department of Transportation (USA)
EAPA Employee Assistance Professionals Association
EMCDDA European Monitoring Centre for Drugs and Drug Addiction
EAP Employee Assistance Program
MRO Medical Review Officer
MROCC Medical Review Officer Certification Council

NCADD National Council on Alcoholism and Drug Dependence (USA)

NIDA National Institute on Drug Abuse (USA)

NIOSH National Institute for Occupational Safety and Health (USA)

NSDUH National Survey on Drug Use and Health (USA)

OTC Over-the-counter, that is, medications available without a prescription

SAMHSA Substance Abuse and Mental Health Services Administration (USA)

SAP Substance Abuse Professional

Appendix: Additional Graphics (U.S.) and Other Data

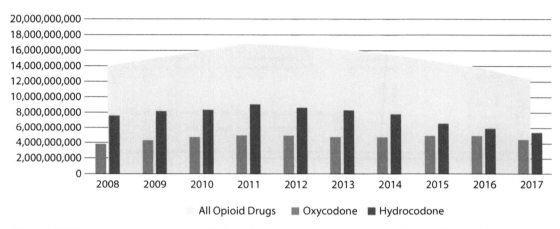

All opioid CPDs compared to the number of hydrocodone and oxycodone prescription drugs sold to retail level purchasers in billions of dosage units, 2008–2017. (Source: DEA)

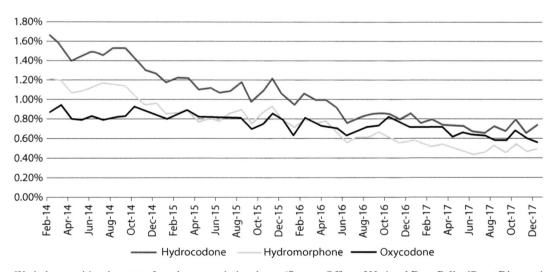

Workplace positive drug tests for select prescription drugs. (Source: Office of National Drug Policy/Quest Diagnostics Drug Testing Index)

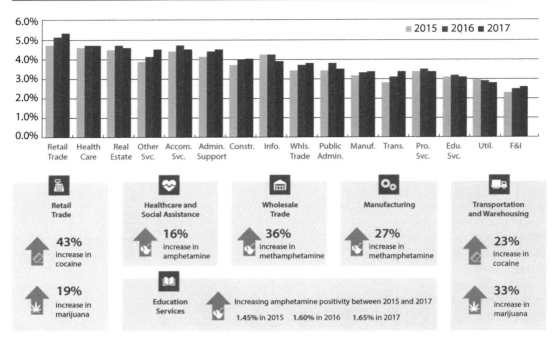

Drug positivity rates by industry sector. (Source: Quest Diagnostics Drug Testing Index™, 2018)

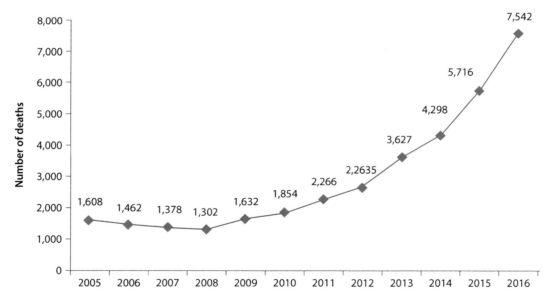

Psychostimulant-involved drug poisoning deaths, 2005–2016. (Source: National Center for Health Statistics/Centers for Disease Control and Prevention)

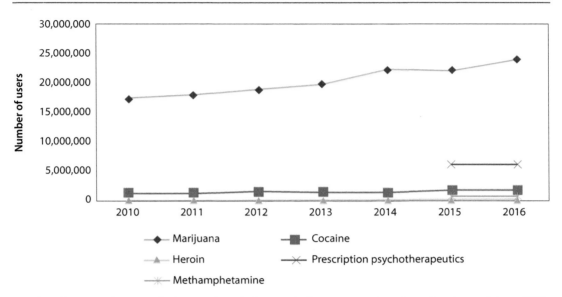

Number of past month, nonmedical users of psychotherapeutic drugs compared to other select drugs of abuse, 2010–2016. (Source: Substance Abuse and Mental Health Services Administration, National Survey on Drug Use and Health)

Supplemental Table 2D

Estimated numbers[a,b] and age-adjusted rates per 100,000 population of drug poisoning-related emergency department visits by selected substances — United States, January 1–September 30, 2016

Socio-demographic characteristics	All drug poisonings[c]		All opioid poisonings[d]		Heroin poisonings[e]		Methadone poisonings[f]		Poisonings by other opioids[g]		Cocaine poisonings[h]		Methamphetamine poisonings[i]	
	Rate[j]	SE	Rate	SE	Rate	SE	Rate	SE	Rate	SE	Rate	SE	Rate	SE
All visits	174.4	266	41.9	1.51	25.0	1.27	1.2	0.07	16.1	0.34	3.2	0.11	5.3	0.15
Sex														
Male	166.0	3.10	51.6	2.02	34.7	1.74	1.3	0.08	16.1	0.42	4.1	0.17	6.2	0.22
Female	182.8	2.52	32.1	1.07	15.2	0.85	1.1	0.08	16.1	0.36	2.3	0.11	4.3	0.15
Age Groups														
0–14	136.2	5.89	3.9	0.27	k	k	k	k	3.8	0.26	1.0	0.12	4.2	0.30
15–19	311.0	9.85	25.9	1.49	11.1	1.05	k	k	14.8	0.83	2.2	0.27	8.4	0.59
20–24	279.5	12.13	96.7	7.44	71.9	6.50	1.1	0.20	24.4	1.42	5.1	0.45	12.0	0.83
25–34	259.0	12.86	107.3	8.90	79.5	7.64	2.3	0.31	26.6	1.56	6.5	0.46	10.4	0.63
35–44	179.7	7.23	55.9	4.12	33.8	3.33	2.0	0.21	20.7	1.04	4.9	0.37	6.1	0.40
45–54	145.4	5.22	38.8	2.46	17.6	1.79	1.6	0.19	20.1	0.92	4.0	0.38	3.0	0.29
55–64	106.0	3.36	26.0	1.37	7.4	0.74	1.6	0.23	17.3	0.80	2.1	0.23	1.3	0.17
≥65	87.7	2.44	13.0	0.60	1.0	0.15	0.5	0.09	11.6	0.56	0.5	0.08	0.4	0.07
US. census region of residence														
Northeast	205.0	9.26	76.3	6.41	57.6	5.49	1.7	0.22	17.7	1.07	4.0	0.33	2.4	0.20
Midwest	198.0	6.42	52.6	3.68	35.1	3.05	1.0	0.13	17.0	0.81	3.7	0.30	6.1	0.38
South	159.6	3.83	30.6	1.77	14.6	1.48	0.9	0.08	15.5	0.49	3.5	0.18	5.1	0.22
West	155.8	3.36	26.1	1.06	9.5	0.70	1.4	0.15	15.5	0.52	1.5	0.14	6.9	0.35

Source: Annual Surveillance Report of Drug-Related Risks and Outcomes. U.S. CDC National Center for Injury Prevention and Control (2018)

References

1. ASAM. The ASAM criteria. Rockville: American Society of Addiction Medicine; n.d. Retrieved 6/17/2019 from https://www.asam.org/resources/the-asam-criteria/about.
2. ASAM. Drug testing in workplace settings. Chevy Chase: American Society of Addiction Medicine; 2002. Retrieved 6/18/2019 from http://www.asam.org/advocacy/find-a-policy-statement/view-policy-statement/public-policy-statements/2011/12/15/drug-testing-in-workplace-settings.
3. ASAM. The role of medical review officers. Chevy Chase: American Society of Addiction Medicine; 1991, rev. 1992. Retrieved 6/18/2019 from https://www.asam.org/advocacy/find-a-policy-statement/view-policy-statement/public-policy-statements/2011/12/16/the-role-of-medical-review-officers.
4. EMCDDA. European drug report 2013: trends and developments. Lisbon: European Monitoring Centre for Drugs and Drug Addiction; 2013. 80p. Retrieved 6/10/2013 from http://www.emcdda.europa.eu/attachements.cfm/att_212374_EN_TDAT13001ENN.pdf.
5. ASAM. Public policy statement: definition of addiction. Rockville: American Society of Addiction Medicine; 2011. Retrieved 6/13/2019 from http://www.asam.org/for-the-public/definition-of-addiction.
6. ASAM. Drug testing: a white paper of the American Society of Addiction Medicine (ASAM). Rockville: American Society of Addiction Medicine; 2013. Retrieved 6/17/2019 from https://www.asam.org/docs/default-source/public-policy-statements/drug-testing-a-white-paper-by-asam.pdf.
7. Centers for Disease Control and Prevention. 2018 Annual Surveillance Report of Drug-Related Risks and Outcomes — United States. Surveillance Special Report. Centers for Disease Control and Prevention, U.S. Department of Health and Human Services. 2018. Retrieved 6/17/2019 from https://www.cdc.gov/drugoverdose/pdf/pubs/2018-cdc-drug-surveillance-report.pdf.
8. Concateno. High society: drug prevalence in the UK workplace. 1st ed. Abingdon: Concateno Global Drug Testing Services; 2012. Retrieved 7/3/2013 from http://www.scribd.com/doc/98867797/High-Society-drug-prevalence-in-the-UK-workplace-Concateno.
9. Corral A, Durán J, Isusi I. Use of alcohol and drugs at the workplace. Dublin & Brussels: European Foundation for the Improvement of Living and Working Conditions (Eurofound). 2012. Retrieved 6/10/2013 from http://www.eurofound.europa.eu/publications/htmlfiles/ef12231.htm.
10. DuPont RL. Chemical slavery: understanding addiction and stopping the drug epidemic. Rockville: Institute for Behavior and Health; 2018.
11. European Foundation for the Improvement of Living and Working Conditions. Use of alcohol and drugs in the workplace. 2012. Retrieved 6/13/2019 from https://www.eurofound.europa.eu/publications/report/2012/use-of-alcohol-and-drugs-at-the-workplace.
12. Executive Order 12564. Drug-Free Federal Workplace. Federal Register 51 FR 32889, 3 CFR, 1986 Comp. 1986. p. 224. Retrieved from 6/13/2013 http://www.archives.gov/federal-register/codification/executive-order/12564.html.
13. Howard J, Hornsby-Myers J. Fentanyls and the safety of first responders: science and recommendations. [web log post]. NIOSH science blog, National Institute for Occupational Safety and Health. 2018, June 26. Retrieved 6/17/2019 from https://blogs-origin.cdc.gov/niosh-science-blog/2018/06/26/fentanyls-and-first-responders/.
14. Kosnett MJ. Presentation on how to assess the impact of Cannabis on driving and workplace performance. San Francisco: American College of Medical Toxicology; 2019.
15. Larson SL, Eyerman J, Foster MS, Gfroerer JC. Worker substance use and workplace policies and programs (DHHS publication no. SMA 07-4273, analytic series A-29). Rockville: Substance Abuse and Mental Health Services Administration, Office of Applied Studies; 2007. Retrieved 6/13/2013 from http://samhsa.gov/data/work2k7/Work.htm.
16. Mariotti O. Droghe e lavoro. G Ital Med Lav Ergon. 2004;26(3):1–21.
17. Mora J. EEOC scrutinizes employer policies regarding prescription drug use. [web log post]. Absence Management and Reasonable Accommodation, ADA, EEOC, Workplace Policies and Processes. Seyfarth Shaw, LLP, Chicago. 2018, June. Retrieved 6/17/2019 from https://www.laborandemploymentlawcounsel.com/category/absence-management-reasonable-accommodation/page/2/.
18. National Drug Early Warning System (NDEWS). Emerging Drug Threats Reports, 2017–2019. Center for Substance Abuse Research, University of Maryland. 2019. Retrieved 6/17/2019 from https://ndews.umd.edu/resources/dea-emerging-threat-reports/.
19. National Safety Council. Implications of drug use for employers: who's affected? 2019. Retrieved 6/13/2019 from https://www.nsc.org/work-safety/safety-topics/drugs-at-work/whos-affected.
20. Nationwide Medical Review. n.d. About the Medical Review Officer. Retrieved 6/18/2019 from http://drugfreeworkplace.com/mro-resources/medical-review-officer/.
21. Occupational and Environmental Medical Association of Canada (OEMAC). Position Statement on the Implications of Cannabis Use for Safety-Sensitive Work. 2018. Retrieved 6/17/2019 from https://oemac.org/wp-content/uploads/2018/09/Position-Statement-on-the-Implications-of-cannabis-use.pdf.
22. Office of Disability Employment Policy. Employee assistance programs for a new generation of employees. Washington, D.C.: U.S. Department of Labor;

2009. Retrieved 6/17/2019 from http://www.askearn. org/wp-content/uploads/2019/01/employeeassis- tance.pdf.

23. Roosevelt M. In the age of legal marijuana, many employers drop 'zero tolerance' drug tests. Los Angeles Times. 2019, April 12. Retrieved 6/17/2019 from https://www.latimes.com/busi- ness/la-fi-marijuana-drug-test-hiring-20190412- story.html.

24. Substance Abuse and Mental Health Services Administration (SAMHSA), Office of Applied Studies. Drug Abuse Warning Network, 2005: selected tables of national estimates of Drug-Related Emergency Department Visits. Rockville. 2009. Retrieved 6/18/2019 from https://www.datafiles.sam- hsa.gov/study-series/drug-abuse-warning-network- dawn-nid13516 (includes years 2004–2011).

25. Smith DE, Wesson DR, Zerkin EL, Novey JH, editors. Substance abuse in the workplace. San Francisco: Haight Ashbury Publications; 1984.

26. U.S. Dept. of Justice. Drug Enforcement Administration. 2018. National Drug Threat Assessment, 2018. Retrieved 6/17/2019 from https:// www.dea.gov/sites/default/files/2018-11/DIR- 032-18%202018%20NDTA%20%5Bfinal%5D%20 low%20resolution11-20.pdf.

27. Verstraete AG, Pierce A. Workplace drug testing in Europe. Forensic Sci Int. 2001;121(1-2):2–6. Retrieved 6/18/2019 from https://www.ncbi.nlm.nih. gov/pubmed/11516880.

Harm-Reduction Interventions

52

Dagmar Hedrich and Richard Lionel Hartnoll

Contents

Abstract

The goal of harm reduction is to reduce both the individual and societal harms of drug use through knowledge-based interventions that change risks, risk behaviours and risk settings. This chapter describes the main harm-reduction interventions implemented in many countries around the world, synthesises evidence on their effectiveness and risks and summarises key lessons learned. The focus is on illegal drugs, especially opioids and the central nervous system stimulants. The interventions covered are opioid substitution treatment; needle and syringe programmes; supervised drug consumption facilities; drug overdose prevention; outreach, peer education and health promotion; testing, vaccination and treatment of drug-related infectious diseases; and interventions for stimulant users. Key themes stressed include the following: that harm reduction does not replace the need for treatment but adds to the capacity to respond effectively to the wide range of health and social challenges raised by drug use; that the scientific evidence shows that harm-reduction interventions are effective in terms of their stated goals, as long as they are implemented appropriately within their contextual settings,

D. Hedrich (✉) · R. L. Hartnoll
European Monitoring Centre for Drugs and Drug Addiction, Lisbon, Portugal
e-mail: dagmar.hedrich@emcdda.europa.eu

© Springer Nature Switzerland AG 2021
N. el-Guebaly et al. (eds.), *Textbook of Addiction Treatment*,
https://doi.org/10.1007/978-3-030-36391-8_52

and that single interventions are far more effective when implemented together as part of a broader public health policy, including steps to facilitate healthier living and safer social environments.

Keywords

Risk behaviour · Harm reduction · Needle syringe programme · Overdose prevention Naloxone · Supervised drug consumption Outreach · Peer education · HIV · Hepatitis C Combination intervention

52.1   Introduction

The goal of harm reduction is to reduce individual and societal harms of drug use through policies and interventions that change risks, risk behaviours and risk settings. Harm reduction is based on the concept of harmful drug use and does not assume that drug use per se is harmful. It is a pragmatic approach that aims to reduce harmful correlates and consequences of drug use through a package of evidence-based, targeted interventions tailored to local settings and needs.

Drug-related harm refers both to individual consequences, such as dependence, overdoses or infectious diseases, as well as to social, economic and public health harms to the community (crime, healthcare costs and high HIV prevalence). The underlying public health paradigm is broader than individual-centred treatment and involves balancing individual and societal needs.

Harm reduction as a policy started to gain acceptance in Europe with the emergence of HIV/AIDS amongst drug injectors in the mid-1980s and is now a major pillar of drug policy in all EU member states [38]. Globally it is supported by at least 87 countries [90] and promoted by the WHO, United Nations and European Union as a key element of a comprehensive approach.

Harm reduction entails a coordinated response from a range of actors, including treatment, prevention, public health, law enforcement, community groups and local authorities [21, 74, 79, 100]. It goes beyond interventions for individuals by stressing enabling environments to enhance protective factors, reduce harms and promote public health.

Harm reduction incorporates an important ethical dimension concerning human rights, equality of access to services, respect for privacy and confidentiality and efforts to counteract social exclusion and stigma [79].

Much drug-related harm is linked to heavy consumption of opioids, the central nervous system (CNS) stimulants or multiple drug combinations, including alcohol and other CNS depressants. There is a strong relationship between drug injecting and more severe levels of harm, though problems can arise with other routes of administration. Heavy drug use is often strongly correlated with unsafe sexual practices, including unprotected sex, multiple partners and sometimes selling sex for money or drugs.

Risk behaviours occur within a wider social context. Structural factors such as the policy and legislative framework can generate risk environments that increase social exclusion, deter help seeking for fear of arrest or exacerbate the spread of infectious diseases [17, 75, 80]. The diversity of settings implies diversity of risks and responses [34].

This chapter describes the major harm-reduction interventions, syntheses evidence on their effectiveness and summarises key lessons learned. It draws on a wide range of sources from research and practice, including scientific reviews, evidence-based guidelines and practical manuals. The interventions covered are the following:

- Opioid substitution treatment
- Needle and syringe programmes
- Supervised drug consumption facilities
- Overdose prevention interventions
- Outreach, peer education and health promotion
- Testing, vaccination and treatment of infectious diseases
- Interventions for stimulant use

The focus is on illegal drugs, especially opioids and the central nervous system stimulants. Harm-reduction approaches have been applied to other drugs including alcohol, cannabis and tobacco and to other user groups such as young recreational drug users [79, 83].

52.2 Interventions

52.2.1 Opioid Substitution Treatment

Other chapters in this textbook cover opioid substitution treatment (OST) as treatment for opioid dependence. In this section, the emphasis is on OST for reducing individual and social harms associated with illicit opioid use. Methadone is the main drug employed, though buprenorphine has become more common following the 1990s. In some European countries and Canada, heroin-assisted treatment is provided to long-term heroin dependent individuals who have not responded well on methadone [64, 91]. Whilst naltrexone, an opioid receptor antagonist, has also been researched as treatment for relapse prevention, its effectiveness is limited by poor adherence, and maintenance with methadone or buprenorphine remains the preferred treatment [18]. OST is usually combined with psychosocial treatment, counselling and other health and social services.

Within a harm-reduction paradigm, OST consists of the (usually long term) prescription of opioid agonists to prevent withdrawal symptoms and craving, enabling users to lead more stable lives and reduce illicit heroin use, risk behaviour and criminal activity. Apart from reduced illicit heroin use, which has been demonstrated in numerous studies (see Chap. 10 in this textbook), specific harm-reduction outcomes that are sought include reductions in prevalence and frequency of drug injecting, prevalence and frequency of sharing drug using paraphernalia, incidence and prevalence of infectious diseases (especially HIV and hepatitis C), rates of drug-related mortality (especially overdoses) [70] and rates of drug-related crime. Reductions in high-risk sexual behaviours, as well as improvements in health and social functioning, are also the objectives.

Reviews of multiple studies with robust designs all found strong evidence that OST is effective in reducing self-reported prevalence and frequency of injecting, sharing of injecting equipment and injecting risk behaviour scores [30, 44, 49, 50, 53]. The same reviews found clear, consistent evidence that OST in community settings is effective in reducing HIV transmission, especially amongst those in continuous treatment and when dosages are adequate [26]; for example, MacArthur [49] estimated that OST is associated with a 54% reduction in risk of HIV infection amongst people who inject drugs.

The effectiveness of OST in reducing HCV transmission has been harder to determine. This is probably because HCV is more easily transmitted through injecting risk behaviours and because baseline prevalence levels of HCV in drug-injecting populations are often high. However, a recent systematic review [73] found that OST is associated with a reduced risk of HCV acquisition, which is strengthened in studies assessing OST and needle and syringe programme (NSP) in combination. There is accumulating evidence on the impact of combining these prevention interventions on hepatitis elimination (e.g., [63, 67, 97]), and a recent global mathematical model [39] underlines the importance of bringing harm-reduction services up to scale, highlighting their key role in prevention.

There is long-standing, strong evidence that OST reduces substantially the risk of overdose mortality, as long as doses are sufficient and continuity of treatment is maintained [16, 43, 52].

There is clear and consistent evidence from many studies that criminal activity, arrest and incarceration rates decline markedly after patients enter OST and that this effect is stronger the longer they remain in treatment [62]. This is particularly true of drug-related criminal activity such as drug-dealing and acquisitive crime. Where sufficient coverage of the opioid-using population is achieved, decreases in drug-related crime at the individual level are reflected in reduced levels of crime at community level [62].

A systematic review of 21 studies conducted in prison settings concluded that the benefits of OST provided in prison are similar to those obtained in community settings [36]. OST was significantly associated with reduced heroin use, injecting and syringe-sharing in prison if doses were adequate. Prerelease OST was significantly associated with increased treatment entry and retention after release if arrangements existed to continue treatment. For other outcomes, associations with prerelease OST were weaker. Whilst some post-release reductions in heroin use were observed, evidence regarding crime and re-incarceration was equivocal. Due to lack of studies, there was insufficient evidence concerning HIV/HCV incidence, either in prison or post release. Disruption of OST continuity, especially due to brief periods of imprisonment, was associated with very significant increases in HCV incidence [19]. In a national prospective, observational study in England prison-based opioid substitution therapy was associated with a 75% reduction in all-cause mortality and an 85% reduction in fatal drug-related poisoning in the first month after release [51]. In a meta-analysis and systematic review by Moore et al. [59], opioid substitution treatment with methadone provided during incarceration was found to be effective in reducing post-incarceration illicit opioid use and injecting.

Benefits of OST that have been clearly established include reduced illicit heroin use, injecting and risk behaviours, reduced overdose mortality and criminal activity and reduced HIV and HCV incidence – especially in combination with high-scale NSP. There is also evidence that OST facilitates improved adherence to HIV treatment [65] and leads to reductions in high-risk sexual behaviours [30].

In prison settings, OST presents an opportunity to recruit problem opioid users into treatment, to reduce illicit opioid use and risk behaviours in prison, and potentially to minimise overdose risks on release [22]. If liaison with community-based programmes exists, prison OST facilitates continuity of treatment and longer-term benefits can be achieved. For prison-ers in OST before imprisonment, prison OST provides treatment continuity, especially important for drug users who are incarcerated for short periods. A population-based retrospective cohort study amongst Canadian convicted offenders documents that the adherence to OST had a positive impact not only on overdose deaths but also on other causes of mortality after release [84].

There are also limitations. OST is suitable neither for users of non-opioid drugs nor for drug users who have only recently started to use opioids, even though during the early stages of use they may be at particular risk of becoming infected (especially with HCV) through using another person's paraphernalia. Even in countries with high levels of OST provision, coverage of the total opioid-dependent population rarely exceeds 60% [24, 25]. Whilst other treatment modalities meet some of the shortfall, there remain important populations of problematic drug users who do not come for treatment or who do not fare well in treatment. As described above, other approaches need to be pursued alongside or in combination with OST to optimise its effects.

Specific risks of OST include increased mortality risk during induction into treatment and immediately after leaving treatment, which should be dealt with by both public health and clinical mitigation strategies [89]. Methadone overdoses can occur in association with careless overprescribing or use of illicit methadone from diversion or thefts. A different challenge arises from the accumulation of ageing, long-term patients on OST, many with multiple comorbidities. A harm-reduction approach not only includes encouraging OST clients to become drug free when they can but also accepts that for some this is not possible.

Several important lessons learned should be stressed. Adequate doses are essential. Whilst individual dosage levels vary, positive outcomes are mostly achieved when average programmed methadone dosages are in the 60–120 mg range [26, 102]. Continuity too is vital, accompanied by appropriate socio-psychological support and health education input.

52.2.2 Needle and Syringe Programmes

A needle and syringe programme (NSP) is a specialised service, offered by low-threshold drugs- and health agencies including through outreach, and that consists of distributing syringes, needles and other sterile injecting equipment to people who inject drugs. These agencies are usually located close to areas where drug injecting is prevalent and form part of a wider network of local services. Their primary objective is to facilitate more hygienic injecting practices and reduce sharing or reuse of needles, syringes and other items in order to prevent drug-use-related complications, especially the transmission of HIV and HCV. Most needle and syringe service providers also offer equipment for safer non-injecting use of drugs.

NSPs often serve as important contact points for drug users who have little contact with treatment or other health services. Thus, a supplementary objective is to deliver health promotion and facilitate access to healthcare, including entry to OST or other treatment. They routinely distribute condoms and offer advice on safer sex. They may also provide counselling and testing for infectious diseases and sexually transmitted infections (STIs), as well as vaccination for hepatitis B and basic healthcare. In some countries, NSPs are mainly implemented through national networks of pharmacies. In other settings pharmacy-based programmes and vending machines supplement specialised NSPs. In some countries, NSPs have been established in prisons.

A broad body of evidence indicates that NSPs are effective, as part of a multicomponent set of responses, in limiting the transmission of blood-borne infections, without increasing the prevalence or frequency of injecting [2, 13, 66, 95]. There are methodological difficulties in separating the impact of NSPs from the influence of other interventions and local contextual factors, which means that rigorous scientific studies of the effectiveness of NSPs as a single intervention are limited. Evidence from systematic reviews of NSPs across a range of settings and countries indicates that they are effective in reducing self-reported risk behaviours associated with inject-ing [50] and in reducing the transmission of HIV amongst people who inject drugs [2]. A recent systematic review [73] found greater heterogeneity between studies and weaker evidence for impact of NSP on HCV acquisition. High NSP coverage (defined as regular attendance at an NSP or all injections being covered by a new needle/syringe) was associated with a reduction in the risk of HCV acquisition in studies in Europe, whilst the effect was not clear for studies conducted in North America. The lack of evidence from US studies can be attributed to a mixture of confounding, differences in injecting patterns, potential selection bias and misclassification of exposure [73]. There is also evidence that NSPs and other harm-reduction interventions are cost-effective [101].

Benefits of NSPs, when implemented appropriately and at sufficient scale, include important reductions in injecting risk behaviours and HIV transmission. In combination with opioid substitution treatment, they make a significant contribution to reducing not only HIV but also HCV transmission. There is no evidence that the establishment of NSPs encourages non-injectors to start injecting or that injection frequency increases amongst attenders [79]. There were no reports of adverse events involving syringes in studies of prison-based NSPs.

Important lessons have been learned over the past three decades. It is essential to aim for full coverage of clients' injecting needs. Restrictions on the number of needles and syringes distributed, or insistence on returning used equipment, can be counter-productive, especially for high-frequency injectors such as cocaine users, since this can facilitate reuse and sharing. The underlying principle should be at least 100% coverage of each injection and distribution according to need rather than one-for-one exchange. It is also important to achieve wide coverage of local populations of drug injectors. Many NSPs allow secondary distribution, where clients distribute clean needles and syringes to partners or peers. Mobile units and outreach are valuable to further extend coverage.

Injecting equipment should take account of local context and the type and preparation of drugs injected. Injectors in different settings often have preferences for certain types or sizes of equipment. Apart from needles and syringes, NSPs should provide other injecting-related items, including alcohol swabs, sterile water, filters, mixing vessels (e.g., spoons or "cookers") and acidifiers to assist with dissolving the substance to be injected [21].

Health promotion activities among people who use drugs should address viral infections such as HIV and hepatitis B and C, that is, how they are transmitted and how they can be avoided, practical advice on hygiene and safer injecting, as well as information on STIs and reducing sexual risks. They should also include provision of condoms, information on health and social services and, when appropriate, referral to drug treatment. Whilst staff can encourage clients to consider entering treatment or changing to safer routes of administration, this should not be linked to pressure such as implied withdrawal of services. Since NSPs come in contact with out-of-treatment drug injectors, it is valuable if they can carry out on-site counselling, testing and monitoring of HIV, viral hepatitis, STIs and TB, as well as vaccination for hepatitis B. Some NSPs also provide basic healthcare (e.g., wound dressing) or train clients in overdose prevention and management, including giving out naloxone. Testing and behaviour change counselling are essential not only for those who are seropositive but also for those who test negative since it is important to avoid complacency (see Sect. 52.2.6 in this chapter).

Reuse of injection equipment for administering injections to more than one person or introducing the syringe in a shared repository of drugs, reuse of syringe barrels or of the whole syringe and informal cleaning have been identified by WHO [105] as high-risk practices. To increase one-time use of injection equipment in medical settings, WHO issue a recommendation for the use of syringes with a reuse prevention feature. Research on low dead space syringes (LDSS) suggests that they reduce the amount of blood remaining in the syringe after completely pushing down the plunger – and subsequently, after rinsing with water, HIV viral burden may be reduced by a factor of 1000 compared to high

dead space syringes [106]. A model described LDSS as a potential powerful HIV prevention strategy, and recent real-life data from the UK show an association between exclusive LDSS use with lower prevalence of HCV amongst people who had started injecting recently, suggesting LDSS use may be protective against HCV [96]. However, there is a risk that promoting LDSS may appear to accept sharing, in contradiction to the clear message that syringes should never be reused or shared.

Safe disposal of used equipment is important. NSPs can facilitate safe disposal by receiving used syringes or by providing puncture-resistant disposal containers to clients. However, if carrying used needles and syringes is a criminal offence or may be used as evidence of drug use, clients may be reluctant to bring used equipment back.

Accessibility and acceptability to target populations are important. This means setting up NSPs in locations with easy access and a minimum of bureaucratic entry requirements. Opening hours should include evenings and weekends. Staff should be positive and sympathetic.

NSPs are mostly implemented in urban settings with a higher prevalence of injecting. In smaller towns and rural settings, a pharmacy-based model may be more appropriate. Apart from (free) distribution through NSPs, needles and syringes can be purchased at pharmacies in many countries, though various formal or informal restrictions can discourage people from using this option, and even a low price may be a disincentive for low-income populations.

The distribution of non-injecting paraphernalia such as safer smoking kits is among the main harm-reduction measures suggested for people who smoke heroin, crack cocaine or methamphetamine (crystal) [82]. A pilot study by Pizzey and Hunt [72] suggested that distributing foil and smoking materials from needle and syringe programmes helps to promote transitions from heroin injecting to chasing. An online survey amongst managers of 80 NSPs in Canada showed that efforts to reduce harm of non-injecting routes of administration are increasing. A majority of programmes educated clients on reducing risks associated with sharing crack cocaine smoking equipment and most of them also distributed equipment (crack pipes). The most common reasons for not distributing safer smoking equipment were not enough funding and lack of client demand [93].

Despite clear evidence on the benefits of NSPs, opposition from local policymakers, professionals and community groups can limit the possibilities of establishing an effective network of NSPs. Thus, a process of consultation with relevant local bodies is essential. Careful planning and co-ordination with local health and treatment services are important to establish clear procedures for referral links. Agreement needs to be reached with justice and police officials to avoid counter-productive interventions.

52.2.3 Supervised Drug Consumption Facilities

Drug consumption rooms (DCRs) are professionally supervised healthcare facilities where drug users can use drugs in safer and more hygienic conditions [37]. DCRs seek to attract hard-to-reach populations of drug users, especially marginalised groups and those who use drugs on the streets or in other risky and unhygienic conditions. They aim to reduce morbidity and mortality by providing a safe environment for more hygienic drug use and by training clients in safer drug use. At the same time, they seek to reduce public drug use and to improve public amenity in areas surrounding urban drug markets. A further aim is to promote access to social, health and drug treatment facilities [42]. Since 1986, more than 150 DCRs have been set up in 10 European countries as well as in Canada, Australia and Mexico [24, 25]. They are highly targeted services addressing specific local problems within a wider network of services, and access is typically restricted to registered service users. They usually operate as an integrated part of low-threshold facilities for drug users or the homeless, though some are stand-alone units. Most target drug injectors, though increasingly also cover users who inhale or smoke drugs. At times, their estab-

lishment has been controversial due to concerns that they may encourage drug use, delay treatment entry or aggravate problems of local drug markets, and initiatives to establish DCRs have been prevented by political intervention.

Evidence shows that DCRs succeed in reaching their target populations and achieve immediate improvements in terms of better hygiene and safer use for clients who use the services. There is consistent evidence that DCR use is associated with self-reported reductions in injecting risk behaviour such as syringe sharing as well as reductions in improperly discarded syringes, so DCRs are also likely to be beneficial in reducing drug use in public and related problems of public disorder. Studies on overdose-related morbidity and mortality suggest a protective effect of DCRs [37, 42]. Regarding transmission of HIV and HCV, due to a lack of robust studies and methodological problems such as isolating the effect of DCRs from other interventions or low coverage of the risk population, there is insufficient evidence either to support or discount the effectiveness of DCRs [3, 50].

Benefits of DCRs include improvements in safe, hygienic drug use, especially amongst regular clients, increased access to health and social services and reduced public drug use and associated nuisance. The availability of safer injecting facilities does not increase drug use or frequency of injecting; it facilitates rather than delays treatment entry, and does not result in higher rates of local drug-related crime.

DCRs have mostly been established in specific urban settings with problems of public drug use and overdose or where there are subpopulations of drug users with limited possibilities of hygienic injection (e.g., homeless, living in insecure accommodation or shelters). As with NSPs, consultation with local key actors is essential to minimise community resistance or counter-productive police responses.

52.2.4 Overdose Prevention

Large increases in opioid overdose deaths in the USA and Canada over the last decade raised alarm about the overprescribing of strong opioids and the significantly increased presence of fentanyl (a highly potent opioid) in the illicit heroin market [54, 85], trends not observed in Europe. However, although rising overdose deaths often trigger concern, efforts to develop interventions specifically targeted at reducing overdose deaths have historically emerged more slowly than responses to other drug-related problems like dependence, crime or HIV/AIDS.

As noted above, effective drug treatment, in particular OST, significantly reduces overdose mortality, and DCRs can contribute at local level if capacity is sufficient. A more specific and promising approach to reducing opioid overdose deaths is offered by community-based overdose prevention programmes that include peer naloxone distribution.

Naloxone is an opioid-antagonist used in medical emergencies to reverse respiratory depression caused by opioid overdose. It has no effect on non-opioid drug overdoses and has a high safety margin. It is available in injectable form and also as an intranasal spray since 2015.

The aim of naloxone distribution programmes is to increase the availability of effective medication in places where overdoses are more likely to occur. Overdose is common amongst opioid users, and most overdoses happen in the presence of a witness, often in the users' home. Many people who die from opioid overdose fail to receive proper medical attention because witnesses (often other drug users) do not recognise the seriousness of the situation, delay, or do not call emergency services for fear of police involvement.

Peer naloxone distribution programmes work by training drug users and other likely first responders (e.g., peers, families), as well as front-line services such as healthcare providers, staff in homeless shelters and, in some cases, police officers, on how to recognise and respond to an overdose, including administration of naloxone, until emergency medical help is obtained. Naloxone is distributed to trained participants, to be at hand if they witness an overdose.

While local naloxone projects started in the USA and Europe in the 1990s [92], they have only recently been scaled up in some locations. Given the dramatic rates of fatal opioid overdoses in the USA and Canada, federal, state and local governments have prioritised increased access to naloxone and overdose education, and naloxone distribution programmes are implemented as a harm-reduction strategy. Nationwide take-home naloxone programmes exist in European countries with high rates of drug-related deaths (including the UK, Norway and Denmark).

A study covering the first 8 years of naloxone provision by community-based organisations across the USA documented that over 150,000 laypersons had been trained and 26,463 overdoses reversed [99]. A systematic review of 21 studies reporting outcomes of take-home naloxone programmes found evidence that educational and training interventions, complemented by naloxone distribution, may decrease overdose-related mortality and that opioid-dependent patients and their peers involved in such programmes improve their knowledge on the correct use of naloxone and management of witnessed overdoses [57]. A meta-analysis of pooled data from four studies on bystander naloxone administration and from five studies on overdose education programmes [29] confirmed an association of naloxone programmes with increased odds of recovery and improved knowledge of overdose recognition and management in nonclinical settings. Furthermore, naloxone distribution was found to be cost-effective [12]. In a pre-post evaluation of a national naloxone programme (Scotland), brief training and standardised naloxone supply for individuals at risk of opioid overdose in prison were effective in reducing by 36% the proportion of opioid-related deaths occurring in the 4 weeks following release from prison [5]. A recent study in the USA analysed whether different laws affecting the accessibility of naloxone correlated with the number of overdoses and deaths [1]. The researchers found that only laws allowing widest access via direct dispensing by pharmacists appeared to be useful in reducing opioid-related fatalities, but noted an increase in non-fatal overdoses in communities where access to naloxone is improved.

Benefits include substantial reductions in opioid overdose deaths, if sufficient coverage of risk populations can be achieved. Giving people, who are likely to witness an overdose, access to naloxone is recommended by WHO in guidelines on community management of overdose and as a component of a comprehensive package of services for people who use drugs. The introduction of naloxone nasal sprays promises to ease the administration of naloxone and improves safety through avoidance of needlestick injuries when treating a population at high risk of blood-borne infections.

Raising overdose risk awareness and increasing response skills amongst professionals in contact with drug users, and disseminating overdose risk information to users, their peers and families constitute an other important part of a comprehensive programme to reduce overdose mortality. Counselling on overdose risk should be a key component of prison release or treatment discharge protocols. Crisis intervention and counselling at hospital emergency rooms following admission for overdose have been tried in some countries.

Since in the USA a significant proportion of drug overdose deaths are associated with prescription opioids and sedatives, prescription monitoring and co-prescribing of naloxone to long-term pain patients have been suggested among various responses to curb the epidemic of overdose deaths [11].

52.2.5 Outreach, Peer Education and Health Promotion

Community-based outreach aims to facilitate improvements in health and reductions in risks and harms for individuals and groups who are not effectively reached by fixed-site services or through traditional health education channels [76]. It seeks to achieve this through identifying and contacting target groups of drug users in different community settings in order to deliver in situ interventions to hard-to-reach populations as well as to provide a contact point for increasing access to a range of other services. Depending on circumstances, interventions may include dissemination of information on drug- and sex-related harms and risk behaviours; provision of advice and counselling on individual behaviour change; distribution of prevention and safer use materials such as sterile injecting equipment, condoms and lubricants; overdose prevention training, including take-home naloxone distribution; and measures to facilitate access to healthcare, social services and drug treatment. The focus may be on individual risk reduction, or it may also include attempts to change social norms concerning risk behaviours amongst the target populations concerned.

Outreach projects may operate from a stand-alone base, but they are often attached to other community health and social services such as NSPs, street-level low-threshold services, treatment centres, etc. Target groups may include homeless, migrant or minority group users with limited access to services, street users, sex workers, chaotic stimulant and multiple drug users or more private, closed groups.

Different models of outreach have been described [60, 76, 77, 78]. Some are based on professional youth or community health workers, others originated from ethnographic research involving indigenous leaders to target risk networks and individuals, others have focussed on promoting peer-driven outreach, whilst others have developed out of advocacy or self-help organisations. Some concentrate more on the individual level (e.g., information and awareness raising, referral or support for change), whilst others give greater emphasis to a network approach involving peer education and modification of peer norms or empowerment of vulnerable groups.

Reviews of studies of outreach interventions to prevent HIV infection conclude that outreach is an effective strategy for reaching hard-to-reach, hidden populations of people who inject drugs, enabling them to reduce their risk behaviours and increase protective behaviours [50, 60, 88].

Studies of network approaches suggest that, given guidance and nominal incentives, injecting drug users can play a more extensive role in community outreach efforts than the traditional model allows. New models of care, developed in the context of viral hepatitis elimination, show that referrals made by peer outreach teams or using specialised liaison nurses help to engage with homeless individuals with multiple comorbidities and help undiagnosed people who inject drugs to access voluntary testing [33, 46].

Outreach is a flexible and effective component of local harm-reduction strategies. It is essential that outreach workers can establish rapport with target populations and gain acceptance as trusted and knowledgeable sources of information and advice. It is vital to ensure confidentiality and to communicate messages clearly. Outreach workers need adequate training, support and protection, especially in peer-driven interventions. This is helped by clear guidelines covering objectives, services offered, responsibilities and limits (personal, professional, legal, etc.). Concrete procedures with other local agencies are important to maximise the uptake of referrals. Drug users and user organisations should be actively involved as partners in planning and conducting outreach.

52.2.6 Testing, Vaccination and Treatment of Infectious Diseases

Public health guidelines recommend a comprehensive and integrated approach to preventing and treating infectious diseases amongst high-risk populations with focus on the individual's overall health and social conditions. This section highlights key points for practitioners and managers involved in harm-reduction interventions for people who use drugs. Innovative technologies are influencing algorithms for diagnosing infections, and new highly effective treatments have led to rapid changes regarding hepatitis C. Extensive, up-to-date information on public health policy, scientific evidence and clinical practice can be found in reviews and guidelines by public health institutions (e.g., ECDC, CDC and WHO) [8, 20, 21, 22, 104].

Recommended core measures include provider-initiated offer of voluntary, confidential screening for HIV, hepatitis B and C, common STDs and TB; vaccination for hepatitis A and B, and where clinically indicated for tetanus, influenza and pneumococcus (HIV positive) and antiviral treatment for HIV and hepatitis C; as well as treatment for STDs and TB [21]. Care should be taken about potential medication interactions, including methadone, especially in the treatment of people with co-infections.

Many people who inject drugs may be unaware that they are infected. Accessible testing in settings where people who use drugs are reached offers an opportunity to provide information and health education and to identify cases for vaccination or treatment. Knowledge of sero-status provides an informed basis for discussing changes in drug use and sexual behaviour with clients and has been found to be associated with positive behaviour changes [20].

Access to and uptake of testing and treatment of infectious diseases and STIs can be increased through on-site screening at services for drug users (drug treatment centres, NSPs or DCRs). Rapid testing techniques now allow this in diverse contexts, including low-threshold services and outreach. Where possible, treatment should take place at the same sites to improve uptake. If not possible, then active referral pathways to public health facilities should be established.

Screening programmes for infectious diseases need to be tailored to clients' life situations and be highly accessible and quick. Thus, the use of point-of-care rapid tests is common. For HIV antibodies, inexpensive enzyme immunoassays using unprocessed blood (finger stick) or oral fluid specimens provide results within 20 minutes. HIV self-testing (HIVST) is recommended by WHO for reaching as-yet undiagnosed populations. Rapid HIV testing kits for home use are approved in the USA and other countries and are available from major pharmacies; some harm-reduction agencies include HIVST kits amongst a range of prevention materials.

When positive, rapid tests require laboratory confirmation with serum or plasma. Delays between first test and confirmation (and treatment start) often cause loss to follow-up. New technical devices (platforms) allow detection and quantification of HIV nucleic acid and HCV viral load at the point of care using unprocessed whole blood specimens. Mechanisms linking those infected to treatment need to be established; as infections can be asymptomatic, starting treatment may not be a priority from the client's perspective. Whilst testing has already moved towards point of care, a new approach to prevent loss to follow-up is to combine diagnosis and start of antiviral treatment in the same visit.

Testing can also provide opportunities to encourage partners to be tested and to participate in changes needed to reduce risks. Periodic health checks and monitoring of seronegative individuals, as well as those successfully treated, help to reinforce protective behaviours and identify reinfection. It also contributes to monitoring programme effectiveness.

52.2.6.1 Agenda 2030 for Sustainable Development

Target 3 of the agenda for global development (SDG 2030) aims at ending the epidemics of AIDS, tuberculosis, malaria and neglected tropical diseases and combat hepatitis, water-borne diseases and other communicable diseases by 2030. Recent advances in the treatment of hepatitis C led WHO to add the elimination of viral hepatitis as a public health threat by 2030 as an additional goal.

Antiretroviral treatment (ART) is a highly effective treatment for HIV and reduces viral load amongst those who adhere to it to undetectable levels. A policy of universal test and treat – making ART available to all HIV-infected persons regardless of CD4 count – is recommended by WHO since 2014. Earliest ART initiation results in successful treatment outcomes amongst PWID with no increase in self-reported risk behaviour. Early diagnosis and engagement in OST should be promoted whilst enhancing care for those with advanced HIV disease and history of imprisonment [61].

New hepatitis C treatments with combinations of drugs called direct-acting antivirals (DAAs) achieve high cure rates even amongst active PWID – in terms of a sustained virologic response (SVR) – with few side effects and after treatment periods of 12 weeks or less. Treating HIV and HCV in those infected not only benefits individuals but has an important preventive effect since it reduces infectivity and thus the risk of transmission to others [100].

Recommendations by the European Association for the Study of the Liver (EASL) on treatment of hepatitis C [68] recommend prioritising groups with high risk of transmission – including active PWID and people in prison, for viral hepatitis treatment as a way to significantly decrease incidence. As reinfection can occur amongst those who remain involved in high-risk practices, maintaining an offer of high-scale harm-reduction measures alongside treatment of infection is essential. This includes education and support to reduce risks, access to clean injecting equipment, effective treatment of drug dependence and reducing stigma related to drug use and infection. For populations exposed to high-risk drug use environments, DCRs can complement other measures. Active PWID are not eligible for direct-acting antiviral treatment in some health systems, and research on how to overcome further client- or provider-related barriers to treatment initiation is needed [98].

For those uninfected, taking ART as preventive measure (pre-exposure prophylaxis PrEP) has been shown to be effective in men who have sex with men (MSM) and heterosexually active men and women [8, 41]. A randomised controlled trial of tenofovir covering over 2400 PWID in Bangkok showed a 49% reduction in HIV incidence related to PrEP over placebo. Based on these findings, the US Centers for Disease Control and Prevention (CDC) recommend PrEP be considered 'as one of several prevention options for persons at very high risk for HIV acquisition through the injection of illicit drugs' [7]. PWID may still be largely unaware of PrEP, but recent studies show that they are interested in taking it [4, 86].

Universal vaccination of children for hepatitis B and vaccination campaigns targeting high-risk groups mean that hepatitis B should become increasingly rare. Meanwhile, it is valuable to continue screening for HBV and, where appropriate, offer vaccination using the Accelerated Schedule [103].

STIs increase the risk of sexual transmission of HIV [9]. Thus, identification and treatment of common STIs is one of the principles of HIV prevention strategies amongst sexually active individuals, especially in high-risk populations.

Investment in prevention, scaling up harm-reduction interventions for PWID, remains a crucial priority for halting the HIV and HCV epidemics [39, 47].

52.2.7 Interventions for Stimulant Use

After alcohol and tobacco, amphetamine-type substances and cocaine are the most prevalent substances used worldwide. It is estimated that one in five to seven recent stimulant users develop a problematic consumption pattern [15, 69]. Apart from dependence, harms especially associated with chronic stimulant use include cardiovascular and cerebrovascular diseases; pulmonary damage; mental health problems such as acute psychotic episodes, depression and anxiety; chaotic behaviour, including higher rates of needle sharing associated with intensive, high-frequency injection; and sexual behaviours that increase transmission risks of HIV and STIs. In high cocaine prevalence areas, significant numbers of acute cocaine episodes ('overamping'[1]) are seen by medical emergency services, and deaths involving cocaine (injected or smoked) and psy-

chostimulants have increased in the USA in recent years [40].

The likelihood of harm varies according to context. For example, crack cocaine is more common amongst highly marginalised groups and is associated with elevated levels of HIV transmission risk, especially for women who trade sex for money or drugs [23, 56]. Crack is sometimes injected as well as smoked, adding a further risk dimension [81]. Transmission of HCV may occur through sharing crack pipes via oral sores and cracked lips [27, 55]. Methamphetamine use, especially by men who have sex with men (MSM), is associated with high levels of sexual risk behaviour [87]. 'Chemsex', the intentional combination of sex with the use of certain psychoactive drugs amongst MSM can bear high risks of infection transmission, and concerns small subgroups of MSM who typically present further risk factors [94]. High levels of cocaine use may also be found amongst socially integrated users who sniff rather than inject or smoke the drug. Whilst health risks are lower, they still remain, especially through sexual risk behaviour and sharing straws (HCV). The social networks and economic resources of socially integrated cocaine users may enable them to resolve problems without contacting services [14]. For the most part, problem stimulant use is associated with lower socioeconomic status and a range of social and legal problems, in addition to a variety of psychiatric comorbidities [31].

Harm-reduction interventions for stimulant users include safer smoking equipment (pipes and foil), outreach and peer-driven programmes, sexual risk reduction education, information campaigns including web-based dissemination, assertive community treatment, environments to reduce anxiety and increase control over use in a non-rushed environment, such as supervised consumption facilities, as well as various innovative approaches based on alternative medicine [71].

There are few high-quality scientific studies of interventions to reduce specifically the harms of CNS stimulants. Systematic reviews on treatment for psychostimulants indicate that the addition of

---

[1]The term 'overamping' is used to describe the variety of negative of uncomfortable physical and psychological effects; can include paranoia, increased heart rate, discomfort, violence, anxiety, sweating and other experiences – See: https://harmreduction.org/issues/overdose-prevention/overview/stimulant-overamping-basics/what-is-overamping/

psychosocial treatment such as contingency management, cognitive behavioural therapy, motivational interviewing and others may offer modest improvements compared to treatment as usual (usually characterised by group counselling or case management), probably reducing the dropout rate and increasing the longest period of abstinence [58]. Retention rates in treatment tend to be low, reducing the potential for systematic efforts to reduce risk behaviours.

A systematic review addressing pharmacotherapy for cocaine use [10] found no evidence of effectiveness of any class of drug in increasing abstinence, reducing use or improving treatment retention rates. There were some indications that particular drugs may be beneficial, such as sertraline to maintain abstinence, antipsychotics to improve treatment retention and psychostimulants and anti-depressants to increase abstinence in comorbid opioid users. Work on a cocaine vaccine progresses slowly and is still in early stages of optimising vaccine formulations to improve efficacy [45].

A review of whether substitution with medications that have psychostimulant effect is effective for treating patients with cocaine dependence [6] assessed nine CNS stimulants (bupropion, dexamphetamine, lisdexamfetamine, methylphenidate, modafinil, mazindol, methamphetamine, mixed amphetamine salts and selegiline) and found mixed results, suggesting research to further evaluate the approach in combination with behavioural and psychosocial input to stabilise drug use and lifestyle.

NSPs are an effective intervention to reduce injecting-related risks for injecting stimulant users as well as opioid users. However, as noted earlier, people who inject stimulants inject frequently and need a plentiful supply of sterile syringes and needles. Given the chaotic lifestyle, frenetic drug-using behaviours and disturbed sleep patterns often seen in compulsive stimulant injectors, providing adequate coverage of injecting needs, potentially for up to 24 hours per day, is a challenge for any service. Mobile units and syringe dispensing machines can help extend coverage in terms of times and places.

Most DCRs were initially established for heroin injectors and often did not admit cocaine injectors or smokers but have increasingly adapted to client needs by setting up separate rooms for those who smoke or inhale drugs. This has proved to be feasible, attracting important subgroups such as crack-using sex workers, and appears to provide benefits similar to those that obtain for heroin users [35, 82].

It has been suggested that traditional harm-reduction services fail to reach problem stimulant users due to opiate-centred services and social barriers to young or female users [31]. Thus, greater emphasis needs to be placed on outreach and peer education approaches (see Sect. 52.2.5), especially for younger users. In response to the risks associated with smoking crack, some programmes in the USA, Brazil, Canada and France have developed 'crack kits' [82]. These include a Pyrex Tube, rubber mouthpieces, filters, lip balm, sterile compresses, chewing gum for salivation and condoms. Initial results suggest that sharing of crack pipes decreased dramatically, whilst crack users reduced injecting and more often smoked cocaine [48]. However, crack kits are controversial and rarely funded.

Regarding crack, there is some evidence that the severity of mental health harms associated with cocaine is related more to the intensity and context of use than to the specific form of cocaine used [32]. Harm-reduction measures aimed at safer, more controlled, less intensive use of cocaine together with steps to stabilise the social situation may help to decrease mental health problems.

Other approaches include acupuncture as an adjunct to treatment to reduce craving, though a systematic review of controlled trials found no evidence of effectiveness [28], or providing accessible and flexible walk-in calming environments to reduce agitation and anxiety levels. Advice, counselling and treatment services for socially integrated users may be more attractive if separated from services for opioid users and drug injectors and if they operate at appropriate hours, for example, evenings.

Interventions for less intensive users include information dissemination on managing mental health risks or on stimulant use via flyers, websites, personal messaging via mobile phones or "pill testing" in nightlife settings [31, 82].

Patterns of stimulant use and risks can vary greatly from one setting to another. For example, in some former Soviet Union republics, home production of stimulants is associated with specific and highly risky patterns of drug consumption [31], and in the UK, groin injection of crack cocaine raises special challenges [81]. In some settings, women are particularly at risk. This means that interventions need to be thoughtfully planned to take account of local circumstances and vulnerable groups. This should include critical reflection on whether any unintended negative effects might arise. Whilst there is much room for innovative development of harm-reduction responses, it should be stressed that all interventions for stimulant users need to give high priority to sexual risks as well as to drug-related risks.

52.3 Conclusion

This chapter has provided an overview of interventions that contribute to reducing drug-related harms. Above and beyond any particular intervention, it must be emphasised that single interventions are far more effective when implemented together as part of a broader package, including policies to facilitate enabling environments that foster healthier and safer living.

Harm reduction does not replace the need for treatment but adds to our capacity to respond effectively to the wide range of health and social challenges raised by drug use. Apart from skills in dealing with individual clients, practitioners need an understanding of the social, community and public health settings within which drug use and drug-related harms arise, as well as an awareness of how social responses can have unintended consequences. Willingness and abil-

ity to co-operate within a local network of agencies and listen to the concerns of drug users themselves is essential. This involves a broad vision of drug use, harms and responses and willingness to think outside of traditional individual psychiatric and social casework paradigms.

References

1. Abouk R, Pacula RL, Powell D. Association between state laws facilitating pharmacy distribution of naloxone and risk of fatal overdose. JAMA Intern Med. 2019;07410:1–7. https://doi.org/10.1001/jamainternmed.2019.0272.
2. Aspinall EJ, Nambiar D, Goldberg DJ, Hickman M, Weir A, Van Velzen E, et al. Are needle and syringe programmes associated with a reduction in hiv transmission among people who inject drugs: a systematic review and meta-analysis. Int J Epidemiol. 2014;43(1):235–48. https://doi.org/10.1093/ije/dyt243.
3. Belackova V, Salmon AM. Overview of international literature - supervised injecting facilities & drug consumption rooms - Issue 1. (1st ed.) (Vol. 1). Sydney: Uniting MSIC; 2017. Retrieved from https://www.researchgate.net/publication/323445212_Overview_of_international_literature_-_supervised_injecting_facilities_drug_consumption_rooms_-_Issue_1.
4. Biello KB, Edeza A, Salhaney P, Biancarelli DL, Mimiaga MJ, Drainoni ML, et al. A missing perspective: injectable pre-exposure prophylaxis for people who inject drugs. AIDS Care. 2019;31:1214–20. https://doi.org/10.1080/09540121.2019.1587356.
5. Bird SM, Mcauley A, Perry S, Hunter C. Effectiveness of Scotland's National Naloxone Programme for reducing opioid-related deaths: a before (2006-10) versus after (2011-13) comparison. Addiction. 2016;111(5):883–91. https://doi.org/10.1111/add.13265.
6. Castells X, Cunill R, Vidal X, Capellà D. Psychostimulant drugs for cocaine dependence (review) summary of findings for the main comparison. Cochrane Database Syst Rev. 2016;(9):CD007380. https://doi.org/10.1002/14651858.CD007380.pub4. www.cochranelibrary.com.
7. Centers for Disease Control and Prevention (CDC). Update to Interim Guidance for Preexposure Prophylaxis (PrEP) for the Prevention of HIV Infection: PrEP for injecting drug users. MMWR Morb Mortal Wkly Rep. 2013;62(23):463–5.
8. Centers for Disease Control and Prevention (CDC). Preexposure prophylaxis for the prevention of HIV

infection in the United States—2017 update: a clinical practice guideline. Atlanta: US Department of Health and Human Services, CDC; 2018. https://www.cdc.gov/hiv/pdf/risk/prep/cdc-hiv-prep-guidelines-2017.pdf, https://doi.org/10.1016/S0040-4039(01)91800-3.

9. Centers for Disease Control and Prevention (CDC). STDs and HIV – CDC Fact Sheet. cdc.gov. (no year) Availabe online: https://www.cdc.gov/std/hiv/stdfact-std-hiv-detailed.htm.

10. Chan B, Kondo K, Ayers C, Freeman M, Montgomery J, Paynter R, Kansagara D. Pharmacotherapy for stimulant use disorders: a systematic review of the evidence. Washington, D.C.: Department of Veterans Affairs (US); 2018. Retrieved from https://www.ncbi.nlm.nih.gov/books/NBK536789/pdf/Bookshelf_NBK536789.pdf.

11. Christie C, Baker C, Cooper R, Kennedy PJ, Madras BJ, Bondi P. Recommendations by the President's Commission on combating drug addiction and the opioid crisis. Washington, D.C.: The White House; 2017. Retrieved from https://www.whitehouse.gov/sites/whitehouse.gov/files/images/Final_Report_Draft_11-15-2017.pdf.

12. Coffin PO, Sullivan SD. Cost-effectiveness of distributing naloxone to heroin users for lay overdose reversal. Ann Intern Med. 2013;158(1):1–9. https://doi.org/10.7326/0003-4819-158-1-201301010-00003.

13. Committee on the Prevention of HIV Infection among Injecting Drug Users in High-Risk Countries. Preventing HIV infection among injecting drug users in high risk countries: an assessment of the evidence. Washington, D.C.: The National Academies Press; 2006. Retrieved from http://www.nap.edu/catalog.php?record_id=11731.

14. Decorte T. The taming of cocaine: cocaine use in European and American cities. Brussels: VUB University Press; 2001.

15. Degenhardt L, Baxter AJ, Lee YY, Hall W, Sara GE, Johns N, et al. The global epidemiology and burden of psychostimulant dependence: findings from the global burden of disease study 2010. Drug Alcohol Depend. 2014;137:36–47. https://doi.org/10.1016/j.drugalcdep.2013.12.025.

16. Degenhardt L, Bucello C, Mathers B, Briegleb C, Ali H, Hickman M, McLaren J. Mortality among regular or dependent users of heroin and other opioids: a systematic review and meta-analysis of cohort studies. Addiction. 2011;106(1):32–51. https://doi.org/10.1111/j.1360-0443.2010.03140.x.

17. Degenhardt L, Mathers B, Vickerman P, Rhodes T, Latkin C, Hickman M. Prevention of HIV infection for people who inject drugs: why individual, structural, and combination approaches are needed. Lancet. 2010;376(9737):285–301. https://doi.org/10.1016/S0140-6736(10)60742-8.

18. Degenhardt L, Stockings E, Strang J, Marsden J, Hall WD. Illicit drug dependence. In: Patel V, Chisholm D, Parikh R, Charlson FJ, Degenhardt L, editors. Disease control priorities - mental, neurological, and substance use disorders, third edition (volume

4). Washington, D.C.: The International Bank for Reconstruction and Development/The World Bank; 2016. p. 109–26. Retrieved from https://www.ncbi.nlm.nih.gov/books/NBK361945/.

19. Dolan KA, Shearer J, White B, Zhou J, Kaldor J, Wodak AD. Four-year follow-up of imprisoned male heroin users and methadone treatment: mortality, re-incarceration and hepatitis C infection. Addiction. 2005;100(6):820–8. https://doi.org/10.1111/j.1360-0443.2005.01050.x.

20. European Centre for Disease Prevention and Control. Public health guidance on HIV, hepatitis B and C testing in the EU/EEA – an integrated approach. Stockholm: European Center for Disease Prevention and Control; 2018. https://doi.org/10.2900/424242.

21. European Centre for Disease Prevention and Control (ECDC), European Monitoring Centre for Drugs and Drug Addiction (EMCDDA). ECDC and EMCDDA guidance: prevention and control of infectious diseases among people who inject drugs. Stockholm/Lisbon: ECDC & EMCDDA; 2011. https://doi.org/10.1186/1471-2334-14-S6-S11.

22. European Centre for Disease Prevention and Control (ECDC), European Monitoring Centre for Drugs and Drug Addiction (EMCDDA). Public health guidance on prevention and control of blood-borne viruses in prison settings. Stockholm/Lisbon: ECDC & EMCDDA; 2018. https://doi.org/10.2900/042079.

23. European Monitoring Centre for Drugs and Drug Addiction. Health and social responses to drug problems: a European guide. Luxembourg: Publications Office of the European Union; 2017. https://doi.org/10.2810/244934.

24. European Monitoring Centre for Drugs and Drug Addiction. Drug consumption rooms: an overview of provisions and evidence. 2018. Retrieved from emcdda.europa.eu/topics/pods/drug-consumption-rooms.

25. European Monitoring Centre for Drugs and Drug Addiction. European drugs report 2019: trends and developments. Luxembourg: Office for Official Publications of the European Union; 2018. https://doi.org/10.2810/191370.

26. Faggiano F, Vigna-Taglianti F, Versino E, Lemma P. Methadone maintenance at different dosages for opioid dependence (review). Cochrane Libr. 2008;(3):3–5. https://doi.org/10.1002/14651858.CD002208. Copyright.

27. Fischer B, Powis J, Firestone Cruz M, Rudzinski K, Rehm J. Hepatitis C virus transmission among oral crack users: viral detection on crack paraphernalia. Eur J Gastroenterol Hepatol. 2008;20(1):29–32. https://doi.org/10.1097/MEG.0b013e3282f16a8c.

28. Gates S, Smith LA, Foxcroft DR. Auricular acupuncture for cocaine dependence. Cochrane Database Syst Rev. 2006;(1):CD005192. https://doi.org/10.1002/14651858.CD005192.pub2.

29. Giglio RE, Li G, DiMaggio CJ. Effectiveness of bystander naloxone administration and over-

dose education programs: a meta-analysis. Inj Epidemiol. 2015;2(1):10. https://doi.org/10.1186/s40621-015-0041-8.

30. Gowing L, Farrell MF, Bornemann R, Sullivan LE, Ali R. Oral substitution treatment of injecting opioid users for prevention of HIV infection. Cochrane Database Syst Rev. 2011;(8):CD004145. https://doi.org/10.1002/14651858.CD004145.pub4.

31. Grund J, Coffin P, Jauffret-Roustide M, Dijkstra M, de Bruin D. The fast and furious — cocaine, amphetamines and harm reduction. In: Rhodes T, Hedrich D, editors. Harm reduction: evidence, impacts and challenges. Luxembourg: Publications Office of the European Union; 2010. p. 191–232.

32. Haasen C, Prinzleve M, Gossop M, Fischer G, Casas M. Relationship between cocaine use and mental health problems in a sample of European cocaine powder or crack users. World Psychiatry. 2005;4(3):173–6. Retrieved from http://www.pubmedcentral.nih.gov/articlerender.fcgi?artid=1414771&tool=pmcentrez&rendertype=abstract.

33. Harris M, Bonnington O, Harrison G, Hickman M, Irving W, Roberts K, et al. Understanding hepatitis C intervention success—qualitative findings from the HepCATT study. J Viral Hepat. 2018;25(7):762–70. https://doi.org/10.1111/jvh.12869.

34. Hartnoll R, Gyarmathy A, Zabransky T. Variations in problem drug use patterns and their implications for harm reduction. In: Rhodes T, Hedrich D, editors. Harm Reduction: evidence, impacts and challenges. Luxembourg: Publications Office of the European Union; 2010. p. 405–32. Retrieved from http://www.emcdda.europa.eu/attachements.cfm/att_101261_EN_emcdda-harmred-mon-ch15-web.pdf.

35. Hedrich D. European report on drug consumption rooms. EMCDDA technical papers. Luxembourg: Office for Official Publications of the European Union; 2004. Retrieved from http://www.emcdda.europa.eu/system/files/publications/339/Consumption_rooms_101741.pdf.

36. Hedrich D, Alves P, Farrell M, Stöver H, Møller L, Mayet S. The effectiveness of opioid maintenance treatment in prison settings: a systematic review. Addiction. 2012;107(3):501–17. https://doi.org/10.1111/j.1360-0443.2011.03676.x.

37. Hedrich D, Kerr T, Dubois-Arber F. Drug consumption facilities in Europe and beyond. In: Rhodes T, Hedrich D, editors. Harm reduction: evidence, impacts and challenges. Luxembourg: Publications Office of the European Union; 2010. p. 305–31. https://doi.org/10.2810/29497.

38. Hedrich D, Pirona A, Wiessing L. From margin to mainstream: the evolution of harm reduction responses to problem drug use in Europe. Drugs Educ Prev Policy. 2008;15(6):503–17. https://doi.org/10.1080/09687630802227673.

39. Heffernan A, Cooke GS, Nayagam S, Thursz M, Hallett TB. Scaling up prevention and treatment towards the elimination of hepatitis C: a global mathematical model. Lancet. 2019;393(10178):1319–29. https://doi.org/10.1016/S0140-6736(18)32277-3.

40. Kariisa M, Scholl L, Wilson N, Seth P, Hoots B. Drug overdose deaths involving cocaine and psychostimulants with abuse potential — United States, 2003–2017. MMWR Morb Mortal Wkly Rep. 2019;68(17):388–95. https://doi.org/10.15585/mmwr.mm6817a3.

41. Kennedy C, Fonner V. Pre-exposure prophylaxis for people who inject drugs: a systematic review (WHO Guidel). Geneva: WHO; 2014. p. 1–24.

42. Kennedy MC, Karamouzian M, Kerr T. Public health and public order outcomes associated with supervised drug consumption facilities: a systematic review. Curr HIV/AIDS Rep. 2017;14(5):161–83. https://doi.org/10.1007/s11904-017-0363-y.

43. Kimber J, Copeland L, Hickman M, Macleod J, McKenzie J, De Angelis D, Robertson JR. Survival and cessation in injecting drug users: prospective observational study of outcomes and effect of opiate substitution treatment. BMJ. 2010;341:c3172. Retrieved from http://www.pubmedcentral.nih.gov/articlerender.fcgi?artid=2895695&tool=pmcentrez&rendertype=abstract.

44. Kimber J, Palmateer N, Hutchinson S, Hickman M, Goldberg D, Rhodes T. Harm reduction among injecting drug users — evidence of effectiveness. In: Rhodes T, Hedrich D, editors. Harm Reduction: evidence, impacts and challenges. Luxembourg: Publications Office of the European Union; 2010. p. 115–64. Retrieved from http://www.emcdda.europa.eu/attachements.cfm/att_101268_EN_emcdda-harmred-mon-ch5-web.pdf.

45. Kimishima A, Olson ME, Janda KD. Investigations into the efficacy of multi-component cocaine vaccines. Bioorg Med Chem Lett. 2018;28(16):2779–83. https://doi.org/10.1016/j.bmcl.2017.12.043.

46. Lambert JS, Murtagh R, Menezes D, O'Carroll A, Murphy C, Cullen W, et al. "HepCheck Dublin": an intensified hepatitis C screening programme in a homeless population demonstrates the need for alternative models of care. BMC Infect Dis. 2019;19(1):1–9. https://doi.org/10.1186/s12879-019-3748-2.

47. Larney S, Peacock A, Leung J, Colledge S, Hickman MM, Vickerman P, et al. Global, regional, and country-level coverage of interventions to prevent and manage HIV and hepatitis C among people who inject drugs: a systematic review. Lancet Glob Health. 2017;5(12):e1208–20. https://doi.org/10.1016/S2214-109X(17)30373-X.

48. Leonard L, DeRubeis E, Pelude L, Medd E, Birkett N, Seto J. "I inject less as I have easier access to pipes". Injecting, and sharing of crack-smoking materials, decline as safer crack-smoking resources are distributed. Int J Drug Policy. 2008;19(3):255–64. https://doi.org/10.1016/j.drugpo.2007.02.008.

49. MacArthur GJ, Minozzi S, Martin N, Vickerman P, Deren S, Bruneau J, et al. Opiate substitution treat-

ment and HIV transmission in people who inject drugs: systematic review and meta-analysis. BMJ. 2012;345:e5945. https://doi.org/10.1136/bmj.e5945.

50. MacArthur GJ, van Velzen E, Palmateer N, Kimber J, Pharris A, Hope V, et al. Interventions to prevent HIV and hepatitis C in people who inject drugs: a review of reviews to assess evidence of effectiveness. Int J Drug Policy. 2014;25(1):34–52. https://doi.org/10.1016/j.drugpo.2013.07.001.

51. Marsden J, Stillwell G, Jones H, Cooper A, Eastwood B, Farrell M, et al. Does exposure to opioid substitution treatment in prison reduce the risk of death after release? A national prospective observational study in England. Addiction. 2017;112(8):1408–18. https://doi.org/10.1111/add.13779.

52. Mathers BM, Degenhardt L, Bucello C, Lemon J, Wiessing L, Hickman M. Mortality among people who inject drugs: a systematic review and meta-analysis. Bull World Health Organ. 2013;91(2):102–23. https://doi.org/10.2471/blt.12.108282.

53. Mattick RP, Breen C, Kimber J, Davoli M. Methadone maintenance therapy versus no opioid replacement therapy for opioid dependence. Cochrane Database Syst Rev. 2009;(3):CD002209. https://doi.org/10.1002/14651858.CD002209.pub2.

54. Mattson CL, O'Donnell J, Kariisa M, Seth P, Scholl L, Gladden RM. Opportunities to prevent overdose deaths involving prescription and illicit opioids, 11 states, July 2016–June 2017. MMWR Morb Mortal Wkly Rep. 2018;67(34):945–51. https://doi.org/10.15585/mmwr.mm6734a2.

55. McMahon JM, Simm M, Milano D, Clatts M. Detection of hepatitis C virus in the nasal secretions of an intranasal drug-user. Ann Clin Microbiol Antimicrob. 2004;3:4–7. https://doi.org/10.1186/1476-0711-3-6.

56. Medina-Perucha L, Family H, Scott J, Chapman S, Dack C. Factors associated with sexual risks and risk of STIs, HIV and other blood-borne viruses among women using heroin and other Drugs: a systematic literature review. AIDS Behav. 2019;23(1):222–51. https://doi.org/10.1007/s10461-018-2238-7.

57. Minozzi S, Amato L, Davoli M. Preventing fatal overdoses: a systematic review of the effectiveness of take-home naloxone. EMCDDA Papers. Lisbon: EMCDDA; 2015. Retrieved from http://www.emcdda.europa.eu/system/files/publications/932/TDAU14009ENN.web_.pdf.

58. Minozzi S, Saulle R, Franco DC, Amato L. Psychosocial interventions for psychostimulant misuse (review) summary of findings for the main comparison. Cochrane Database Syst Rev. 2016;(9):CD011866. https://doi.org/10.1002/14651858.CD011866.pub2. www.cochranelibrary.com.

59. Moore KE, Roberts W, Reid HH, Smith KMZ, Oberleitner LMS, McKee SA. Effectiveness of medication assisted treatment for opioid use in prison and jail settings: a meta-analysis and systematic review. J Subst Abuse Treat. 2019;99:32–43. https://doi.org/10.1016/j.jsat.2018.12.003.

60. Needle RH, Burrows D, Friedman SR, Dorabjee J, Touzé G, Badrieva L, et al. Effectiveness of community-based outreach in preventing HIV/AIDS among injecting drug users. Int J Drug Policy. 2005;16(Supplement 1):45–57. https://doi.org/10.1016/j.drugpo.2005.02.009.

61. Nguyen HH, Bui DD, Dinh TTT, Pham LQ, Nguyen VTT, Tran TH, et al. A prospective "test-and-treat" demonstration project among people who inject drugs in Vietnam. J Int AIDS Soc. 2018;21(7):1–9. https://doi.org/10.1002/jia2.25151.

62. NIDA International Program. Part B: 20 questions and answers regarding methadone maintenance treatment research. Does methadone maintenance treatment reduce criminal activity? 2006. Retrieved 21 Mar 2013, from https://www.drugabuse.gov/sites/default/files/pdf/partb.pdf.

63. Nolan S, Dias Lima V, Fairbairn N, Kerr T, Montaner J, Grebely J, Wood E. The impact of methadone maintenance therapy on hepatitis C incidence among illicit drug users. Addiction. 2014;109(12):2053–9. https://doi.org/10.1111/add.12682.

64. Oviedo-Joekes E, Guh D, Brissette S, Marchand K, MacDonald S, Lock K, et al. Hydromorphone compared with diacetylmorphine for long-term opioid dependence: a randomized clinical trial. JAMA Psychiatry. 2016;73(5):447–55. https://doi.org/10.1001/jamapsychiatry.2016.0109.

65. Palepu A, Tyndall MW, Joy R, Kerr T, Wood E, Press N, et al. Antiretroviral adherence and HIV treatment outcomes among HIV/HCV co-infected injection drug users: the role of methadone maintenance therapy. Drug Alcohol Depend. 2006;84(2):188–94. https://doi.org/10.1016/j.drugalcdep.2006.02.003.

66. Palmateer N, Kimber J, Hickman M, Hutchinson S, Rhodes T, Goldberg D. Evidence for the effectiveness of sterile injecting equipment provision in preventing hepatitis C and human immunodeficiency virus transmission among injecting drug users: a review of reviews. Addiction. 2010;105(5):844–59. https://doi.org/10.1111/j.1360-0443.2009.02888.x.

67. Palmateer NE, Taylor A, Goldberg DJ, Munro A, Aitken C, Shepherd SJ, et al. Rapid decline in HCV incidence among people who inject drugs associated with national scale-up in coverage of a combination of harm reduction interventions. PLoS One. 2014;9(8):e104515. https://doi.org/10.1371/journal.pone.0104515.

68. Pawlotsky J-M, Negro F, Aghemo A, Berenguer M, Dalgard O, Dusheiko G, et al. EASL recommendations on treatment of hepatitis C 2018. J Hepatol. 2018;69(2):461–511. https://doi.org/10.1016/j.jhep.2018.03.026.

69. Peacock A, Leung J, Larney S, Colledge S, Hickman M, Rehm J, et al. Global statistics on alcohol, tobacco and illicit drug use: 2017 status report. Addiction. 2018;113(10):1905–26. https://doi.org/10.1111/add.14234.

70. Pierce M, Bird SM, Hickman M, Marsden J, Dunn G, Jones A, Millar T. Impact of treatment for opioid dependence on fatal drug-related poisoning: a national cohort study in England. Addiction. 2016;111(2):298–308. https://doi.org/10.1111/add.13193.

71. Pinkham S, Stone C. A global review of the harm reduction response to amphetamines. 2015. https://doi.org/ISBN 978-0-9927609-6-0.

72. Pizzey R, Hunt N. Distributing foil from needle and syringe programmes (NSPs) to promote transitions from heroin injecting to chasing: an evaluation. Harm Reduct J. 2008;5:24. https://doi.org/10.1186/1477-7517-5-24.

73. Platt L, Minozzi S, Reed J, Vickerman P, Hagan H, French C, et al. Needle syringe programmes and opioid substitution therapy for preventing HCV transmission among people who inject drugs: findings from a cochrane review and meta-analysis. Addiction. 2017;113:545. https://doi.org/10.1111/add.14012.

74. Rhodes T. The 'risk environment': a framework for understanding and reducing drug-related harm. Int J Drug Policy. 2002;13(2):85–94. Retrieved from http://www.ijdp.org/article/S0955-3959(02)00007-5/abstract.

75. Rhodes T. Risk environments and drug harms: a social science for harm reduction approach. Int J Drug Policy. 2009;20(3):193–201. https://doi.org/10.1016/j.drugpo.2008.10.003.

76. Rhodes T, Hartnoll R. Reaching the hard to reach: models of HIV outreach health education. In: Aggleton P, Hart G, Davies P, editors. AIDS: responses, interventions and care. London: The Falmer Press; 1991. p. 233–48.

77. Rhodes T, Hartnoll R. AIDS, drugs and prevention: perspectives on individual and community action. London/New York: Routledge; 1996.

78. Rhodes T, Hartnoll R, Johnson A. Out of the agency and on to the streets: a review of HIV outreach health education in Europe and in the United States. London: University of London Birkbeck College; 1991.

79. Rhodes T, Hedrich D, editors. Harm reduction: evidence, impacts and challenges. Luxembourg: Publications Office of the European Union; 2010. https://doi.org/10.2810/29497.

80. Rhodes T, Hedrich D. Harm reduction and the mainstream. In: Rhodes T, Hedrich D, editors. Harm reduction: evidence, impacts and challenges. Luxembourg: Publications Office of the European Union; 2010. p. 19–33.

81. Rhodes T, Stoneman A, Hope V, Hunt N, Martin A, Judd A. Groin injecting in the context of crack cocaine and homelessness: from "risk boundary" to "acceptable risk"? Int J Drug Policy. 2006;17(3):164–70. https://doi.org/10.1016/j.drugpo.2006.02.011.

82. Rigoni R, Breeksema J, Woods S. In: Mainline & GIZ, Eds, editor. Speed Limits: harm reduction for people who use stimulants. Amsterdam: Mainline Foundation; 2018. Retrieved from http://fileserver.idpc.net/library/Mainline_REPORT_complete.pdf.

83. Ritter A, Cameron J. A review of the efficacy and effectiveness of harm reduction strategies for alcohol, tobacco and illicit drugs. Drug Alcohol Rev. 2006;25(6):611–24. https://doi.org/10.1080/09595230600944529.

84. Russolillo A, Moniruzzaman A, Somers JM. Methadone maintenance treatment and mortality in people with criminal convictions: a population-based retrospective cohort study from Canada. PLoS Med. 2018;15(7):1–19. https://doi.org/10.1371/journal.pmed.1002625.

85. Scholl L, Seth P, Wilson N, Baldwin G, Kariisa M, Wilson N, Baldwin G. Drug and opioid-involved overdose deaths — United States, 2013–2017. MMWR Morb Mortal Wkly Rep. 2018;67(5152):1419. https://doi.org/10.15585/mmwr.mm6751521e1.

86. Sherman SG, Schneider KE, Nyeong Park J, Allen ST, Hunt D, Chaulk P, Weir WB. PrEP awareness, eligibility, and interest among people who inject drugs in Baltimore, Maryland. Drug Alcohol Depend. 2019;195(Feb):148–55. https://doi.org/10.1038/nm.2451.A.

87. Shoptaw S, Reback CJ. Associations between methamphetamine use and HIV among men who have sex with men: a model for guiding public policy. J Urban Health. 2006;83(6):1151–7. https://doi.org/10.1007/s11524-006-9119-5.

88. Simoni JM, Nelson KM, Franks JC, Yard SS, Lehavot K. Are peer interventions for HIV efficacious? A systematic review. AIDS Behav. 2011;15(8):1589–95. https://doi.org/10.1007/s10461-011-9963-5.

89. Sordo L, Barrio G, Bravo MJ, Indave BI, Degenhardt L, Wiessing L, et al. Mortality risk during and after opioid substitution treatment: systematic review and meta-analysis of cohort studies. BMJ. 2017;357:j1550. https://doi.org/10.1136/bmj.j1550.

90. Stone K, Shirley-Beavan S. The global state of harm reduction 2018. London: Harm Reduction International; 2018.

91. Strang J, Groshkova T, Metrebian N. New heroin-assisted treatment. Lux: Office for Official Publications of the European Union; 2012. Retrieved from http://www.emcdda.europa.eu/system/files/publications/690/Heroin_Insight_335259.pdf.

92. Strang J, McDonald R. Preventing opioid overdose deaths with take-home naloxone. EMCDDA insights (Vol. 20). Luxembourg: Publications Office of the European Union; 2016. Retrieved from http://www.emcdda.europa.eu/system/files/publications/2089/TDXD15020ENN.pdf.

93. Strike C, Watson TM. Education and equipment for people who smoke crack cocaine in Canada:

progress and limits. Harm Reduct J. 2017;14(1):94. https://doi.org/10.1186/s12954-017-0144-3.

94. Stuart D. A chemsex crucible: the context and the controversy. J Fam Plann Reprod Health Care. 2016;42(4):295–6. https://doi.org/10.1136/jfprhc-2016-101603.

95. Sweeney S, Ward Z, Platt L, Guinness L, Hickman M, Hope V, et al. Evaluating the cost-effectiveness of existing needle and syringe programmes in preventing hepatitis C transmission in people who inject drugs. Addiction. 2019;114:560–70. https://doi.org/10.1111/add.14519.

96. Trickey A, May MT, Hope V, Ward Z, Desai M, Heinsbroek E, et al. Usage of low dead space syringes and association with hepatitis C prevalence amongst people who inject drugs in the UK. Drug Alcohol Depend. 2018;192:118–24. https://doi.org/10.1016/j.drugalcdep.2018.07.041.

97. Vickerman P, Martin N, Turner K, Hickman M. Can needle and syringe programmes and opiate substitution therapy achieve substantial reductions in hepatitis C virus prevalence? Model projections for different epidemic settings. Addiction. 2012;107(11):1984–95. https://doi.org/10.1111/j.1360-0443.2012.03932.x.

98. Ward KM, Falade-Nwulia O, Moon J, Sutcliffe CG, Brinkley S, Haselhuhn T, et al. A randomized controlled trial of cash incentives or peer support to increase HCV treatment for persons with HIV who use drugs: the CHAMPS study. Open Forum Infect Dis. 2019;6:1–9. https://doi.org/10.1093/ofid/ofz166.

99. Wheeler E, Jones TS, Gilbert MK, Davidson PJ. Opioid overdose prevention programs providing naloxone to laypersons - United States, 2014. MMWR Morb Mortal Wkly Rep. 2015;64(23):631–5. https://doi.org/mm6423a2 [pii].

100. WHO, UNODC, UNAIDS. Technical guide for countries to set targets for universal access to HIV prevention, treatment and care for injecting drug users, 2012 revision. Geneva: World Health Organization; 2013. Retrieved from http://www.who.int/hiv/pub/idu/targets_universal_access/en/index.html.

101. Wilson DP, Donald B, Shattock AJ, Wilson D, Fraser-Hurt N. The cost-effectiveness of harm reduction. Int J Drug Policy. 2015;26:S5. https://doi.org/10.1016/j.drugpo.2014.11.007.

102. World Health Organization. Guidelines for the psychosocially assisted pharmacological treatment of opioid dependence. Guidelines for the psychosocially assisted pharmacological treatment of opioid dependence. Geneva: World Health Organization; 2009, Distribution and Sales Geneva 27 CH-1211 Switzerland. Retrieved from http://www.who.int/substance_abuse/publications/opioid_dependence_guidelines.pdf.

103. World Health Organization. Guidance on prevention of viral hepatitis B and C among people who inject drugs. Geneva: World Health Organization; 2012.

104. World Health Organization. Guidelines for the screening care and treatment of persons with chronic hepatitis C infection. Geneva: World Health Organization; 2016. https://doi.org/ISBN 978 92 4 154961 5.

105. World Health Organization. WHO guideline on the use of safety-engineered syringes for intramuscular, intradermal and subcutaneous injections in health-care settings, vol. 26. Geneva: WHO; 2016. https://doi.org/10.1016/j.neuron.2013.04.023.

106. Zule WA, Cross HE, Stover J, Pretorius C. Are major reductions in new HIV infections possible with people who inject drugs? The case for low dead-space syringes in highly affected countries. Int J Drug Policy. 2013;24(1):1–7. https://doi.org/10.1016/j.drugpo.2012.07.002.

.

Part V

Policies and Training in Addiction

Alexander Baldacchino and Barbara Broers

Policy and Training in Addiction: An Introduction

Alexander M. Baldacchino and Barbara Broers

Content

Worldwide, around 271 million people (5.5% of the global population) aged 15–64 years, used illegal drugs at least once during 2017 [1]. These drugs predominantly include cannabinoids, opioids, cocaine and/or amphetamine-type stimulant (ATS) groups. Some 31 million people who use drugs suffer from drug use disorders (DUDs), meaning that their drug use is harmful to the point where they may need advice or treatment. Some 585,000 people are estimated to have died as a result of drug use in 2017. Opioids take a large share, accounting for 76% of deaths amongst people using drugs. About 11.3 million persons in 2017 have a recent history of intravenous drug use. This subgroup endures the great-

A. M. Baldacchino (✉)
Population and Behavioural Science Division (Psychiatry and Addictions), University of St Andrews and NHS Fife, St Andrews, UK
e-mail: amb30@st-andrews.ac.uk

B. Broers
Unit for Dependencies, Division for Primary Care, Department for Community Medicine, Primary Care and Emergencies, Geneva University Hospitals, Geneva, Switzerland
e-mail: barbara.broers@unige.ch

est health risks with almost half of them living with Hepatitis C, 1.4 million living with HIV and one million living with both of these preventable conditions. The disability-adjusted life year (DALY) in 2017 attributable to illicit drug use was estimated to be 27.8 million. This was compared with tobacco use and alcohol use, accounting for 170.9 million and 85 million in the DALY [2].

Surveys on drug use amongst the general population show that the extent of drug use amongst young people remains higher than that amongst older people, although there are some exceptions associated with the traditional use of drugs, such as opium or khat. Most research suggests that adolescence (12 to 17 years old) is a critical risk period for the initiation of substance use and that substance use may peak amongst young people aged 18–25 years [1].

There have been steps taken at a global level to set strategies for response to the world drug problem. The Joint UN Ministerial Political Declaration and Plan of Action in 2014 [3] explicitly reaffirmed that DUD is a health problem with a need to further strengthen public health systems that are responsive to current and emerging drug-related problems. The adoption of target 3.5 of the Sustainable Development Goals [4] also reaffirms this vision of strengthening the prevention and treatment of substance abuse, including narcotic drug abuse and harmful use of alcohol.

The outcome document of the special session of the United Nations General Assembly on the World Drug Problem held in 2016 [5] contains more than 100 recommendations on promoting evidence-based prevention, care and other measures to address both supply and demand. Additionally, World Health Organization (WHO) and United Nation Office for Drug Control (UNODC) have developed close collaborations to support the implementation of development of comprehensive, integrated health-based approaches to drug policies that can reduce demand for illicit substances, relieve suffering and decrease drug- and alcohol-related harm to individuals, families, communities and societies [6].

In order to benefit optimally from the international covenants and policy environment, a series of consultations with the WHO technical focal points from all member states was conducted. With close collaboration with sister UN and other international drug policy agencies, a framework to strengthen public health responses to drug and alcohol problems was agreed. The underpinning principles behind this framework include interventions that are evidence based, adopt a life-course approach, promote multi-sectorial action and observe standard of care across a continuum which is gender and culture sensitive. The drivers behind this framework include an active engagement of civil society that has the voices of both service users and care providers that value the protection and promotion of equity and universal rights to access optimal treatment and harm reduction interventions.

The framework incorporates five overarching strategic domains:

1. *Governance:* This includes the adoption of evidence-based and cost-effective interventions as part of the universal health coverage benefit package; develop and update evidence-informed national substance use policies and associated legislation with a strong public health component in consultation with stakeholders from public, private, as well as civil society sectors; set up an inter-sectoral coordination mechanism to facilitate implementation and monitoring of evidence-based substance use policies and legislation and allocate specific budget allocations within the health and welfare sectors to address prevention, management, rehabilitation, recovery and monitoring and evaluation of drug- and alcohol-use problems; develop programmes offering alternatives to incarcerate illicit drug offenders.

2. *Health Sector Responses:* Integrate screening and brief interventions for substance-use disorders and management of overdose in primary health care and emergency rooms; develop and strengthen specialised services for holistic and integrated management of substance use disorders, including pharmacological and psychosocial interventions; introduce and/or rapidly scale up the comprehensive package of services for harm reduction; ensure availability of essential medicines in management of substance-use disorders; facilitate and promote establishment of self- help and mutual aid groups and develop/strengthen capacity to conduct and utilise implementation research.

3. *Promotion and Prevention:* Embed universal substance-use prevention programmes in the broader health policies and strategies based on rigorous local needs and resource assessments and design and implement age-specific substance use prevention programmes in community, education and work place settings.

4. *Monitoring and Surveillance:* Identify a standard set of comparable core indicators to monitor the substance use situation including for inclusion in the existing surveys and develop a system for national substance use monitoring and surveillance system to collect and report core set of indicators using standardised data collection tools and methodologies.

5. *International and Regional Cooperation:* Promote active sharing of information and evidence between professionals and civil society organisations from countries of the region at national and international policy forums on substance use.

The second edition of this ISAM Textbook reflects the increasing importance of the interplay amongst policy, legal, quality and other governance-led standards within the field of addiction medicine as summarised by the above framework. The quality standards will be discussed by Marica Ferri et al. from the EMCDDA with ethical and legal aspects addressed by Ambros Uchtenhagen. Evidence-based policy can only be delivered if the appropriate methodologies are established. This will be addressed separately by Robin Room and Ambros Uchtenhagen.

However, one aspect that as yet has not been fully developed in the above framework is the global recognition to increase and improve our addiction medicine workforce. The framework recognises the need to develop capacity of personnel in health and social welfare sector for substance-use prevention, treatment, care and rehabilitation through integrating the component in preservice and in-service teaching/ training and as a part of continuing professional education/recertification processes. This is the International Society of Addiction Medicine's core mission and involves the long-term commitment from relevant stakeholders to improve undergraduate addiction medicine training and postgraduate specialisation in addiction medicine. This is most relevant to the future medical workforce who will increasingly be treating complex cases with multi-morbidities (mental and physical) directly or indirectly related to polydrug misuse and/or multiple dependencies (pharmacological and behavioural). Additionally, this is as equally relevant to other clinicians working in the field of addiction medicine who, with the medical workforce, are increasingly encouraged to work within an environment that encourages shared decision and multidisciplinary teamwork.

Training in addiction medicine needs to be both knowledge and competence based, especially when one reaches postgraduate/specialisation stage of the professional career [7]. This has been shown to influence positively the clinical, educational, information and research governance requirements to complex interventions. The result will be a competent and confident workforce that enables and sustains delivery of efficacious and effective health sector and culturally sensitive and non-stigmatising responses. Further challenges faced with establishing such a competitive-based informed learning environment are discussed by Nady el-Guebaly et al., Steve Gust et al., Christine Goodair et al. and Cor de Jong et al. separately addressing some of the solutions.

References

1. World Drug Report 2019 (United Nations Publication, Sales No. E.19.XI.9).
2. Peacock, et al. Global statistics on alcohol, tobacco and illicit drug use: 2017 status report. Addiction. 2018;113(10):1905–26.
3. Commission on Narcotic Drugs, UNODC, Vienna, March 2014.
4. United Nations General Assembly Resolution 70/1, transforming our world: the 2030 Agenda for Sustainable Development.
5. United Nations General Assembly Special Session, 2016, on the world drug problem outcome document (A/S-30/L.1) "Our joint commitment to effectively addressing and countering the world drug problem"; United Nations, New York.
6. UNODC–WHO International Standards for the Treatment of Drug Use Disorders. World Health Organization and United Nations Office on Drugs and Crime, 2018.
7. Fleury G, Milin R, Crockford D, Buckley L, Charney D, George TP, el-Guebaly N. Training in substance related and addictive disorders. Parts 1 and 2. Position Papers. Canadian Psychiatric Association. 2015

Good Practice and Quality Standards

54

Marica Ferri and Paul Griffiths

Contents

Abstract

The present chapter is aimed at enabling the readers to understand the methods and the available tools to ascertain whether an evidence-based recommendation is appropriate for real-world patients in specific contexts. In times of a wide availability of real-time information on potentially anything, it is crucial to develop an individual capacity for critical assessment of scientific literature including strategies to search for updated and reliable sources of evidence. The methods, the processes, and the practical meaning of the most popular tools for the promotion of quality are presented with links to current projects and free-of-cost resources for professionals. The ultimate goal of evidence-based medicine is to provide patients with the best possible interventions. To reach this goal, knowledge has to be translated into practice. Guidelines and standards are popular instruments to disseminate and implement evidence-based recommendations. Nevertheless, to implement them into specific contexts, some decisions are needed. The chapter includes a description of the main approaches used to adapt or adopt guidelines and standards.

Quality is never an accident. It is always the result of intelligent effort. There must be the will to produce a superior thing. —John Ruskin

M. Ferri (✉) · P. Griffiths
EMCDDA, Lisbon, Portugal
e-mail: marica.ferri@emcdda.europa.eu

© Springer Nature Switzerland AG 2021
N. el-Guebaly et al. (eds.), *Textbook of Addiction Treatment*,
https://doi.org/10.1007/978-3-030-36391-8_54

54.1   Introduction

The promotion of quality of health and social interventions and the exchange of good practices are recognized as an important strategy both to improve the effectiveness of drug-related interventions and to ensure the efficient use of limited resources. Guidelines and standards, in particular, are among the most frequently used tools for the promotion of quality through the translation of knowledge into the daily practice of treatment of drug addiction. But publishing new guidelines and standards is not always needed; often the existing good-quality guidance documents can be adapted to suit a specific national or local context.

New disciplines focusing on methods for successful knowledge transfer to action, such as implementation science, translational science, and knowledge mobilization, have emerged. A common recommendation to successful implementation is the promotion of participation among all the stakeholders, starting with medical doctors and health professionals and including decision makers, patients and their families, and the public in general. It is therefore important that the professionals in the treatment of drug addiction are familiar with the terminology and the methods of quality promotion, as these are increasingly part of their daily activity.

The contents of the evidence base change rapidly, as new studies contribute to new results. This is why it is important to master the methods to ascertain whether a recommendation is appropriate for real-world patients in specific contexts. It becomes crucial to develop an individual capacity for critical assessment and to know where to search for updated and reliable sources of evidence. This chapter seeks to address these concerns. It describes the evolution from evidence base to implementation and provides details on the terminology and references for further reading. The methods, processes, and the practical meaning of the most popular tools for the promotion of quality are also presented here with links to current projects and free-of-cost resources for professionals, researchers, and patients. In particular, it details how time and resources can be saved by *adapting* or *adopting* already published evidence-based guidelines to specific needs and contexts. The current initiatives for the development of quality standards in drug addiction treatment at international and at the national level are described and compared, and for each of them, the links for free downloading of documents are included. To complement the information on implementation, the chapter includes also a description and references to some recent initiatives in the medical field, in which the participation of drug addiction treatment professionals is crucial but still not sufficient. All these initiatives are studying strategies to effectively communicate with decision makers and patients. In addition, two examples of the use of standards are compared more in-depth: one case as part of an accreditation system, and the other as support for implementation and the measuring of quality criteria.

54.2   From Knowledge to Implementation

54.2.1   Knowledge Translation into Practice: From Evidence to Change

The overall aim of good practice sharing and standards development is the achievement of improvement in the quality of treatment. Quality is not an abstract concept but rather an umbrella definition for a series of measurable achievements in the health and well-being of the treated patients.

"Primum non nocere" – first of all, do not harm –, the phrase attributed to the Hippocratic Oath, reminds us that the first aim of a health intervention is to avoid harm. And it is exactly with this intention that the pioneers of the evidence-based medicine called the attention on the discrepancies between research results and medical practice, which would have cost human lives [11]. According to their claims, the timely application to the practice of the results from clinical research would have saved many lives and reduced subsequent costs to society [16]. For example, randomized controlled trials proving the effectiveness of systemic glucocorticosteroids administered to pregnant women at risk of preterm delivery to reduce respiratory distress syndrome in newborn

babies were available already in the 1970s, but it took almost 20 years before this intervention became common practice [39].

The possible effect of the delay in the adoption of this practice was that a significant number of premature babies probably suffered and possibly died and needed more expensive treatment than was necessary [38].

The movement for the systematic collection of scientific results for dissemination outside the restricted circles of researchers and academics became known worldwide at the beginning of the 1990s [41] and was boosted by the foundation of the Cochrane Collaboration, an international organization aimed at helping "healthcare providers, policy-makers, patients, their advocates and carers, make well-informed decisions about health care, by preparing, updating, and promoting the accessibility of Cochrane Reviews" [10].

In 1998, an editorial group specifically devoted to the study of interventions for drugs and alcohol-related problems was founded with its base in Rome [13], and since then around 70 reviews on prevention, treatment, and harm reduction have been published and systematically updated.

The availability of good quality research on the effectiveness of treatment for drug problems has dramatically increased over the last years, even though important gaps remain to be bridged with evidence [47]. The availability of studies and systematic reviews nurtured the production of clinical guidelines as a major tool for the dissemination and application of evidence in practice.

For example, a survey for the identification of treatment guidelines in Europe identified more than 140 sets of guidelines for the treatment of drug addiction [18]. Nevertheless, the practical effects of such a massive effort to produce clinical guidelines were not clear. When measured, the impact on the quality of treatment seemed not impressive. Some surveys performed in the medical field, not specifically in the drug addiction one, showed that clinical guidelines are applied to practice in only 50–70% of day-to-day decisions, and the main reason given for not applying them is that they are of limited relevance to patients and healthcare staff [36]. Moreover, in a debate promoted by the British Medical Journal about the effectiveness of guidelines [23], it was

pointed out that to ensure clinical guidelines have an impact on actual care and practice, activities beyond the mere production and dissemination should be instigated [21].

This type of considerations along with the need to reduce cost and improve quality and outcomes must be at the base of the evolution toward the *knowledge translation into practice* approach [5]. Moving from the concept of evidence to that of knowledge expands an idea already present in the definition of evidence-based medicine. The practice of evidence-based medicine integrates clinical expertise with the best available evidence from systematic research, explained David Sackett [41]. "Without clinical expertise, practice risks becoming tyrannized by evidence, for even excellent external evidence may be inapplicable to or inappropriate for an individual patient" reinforced. Probably "knowledge" is a better term to put together evidence with expertise. *Knowledge translation* has been defined as a "dynamic and iterative process that includes the synthesis, dissemination, exchange and ethically sound application of knowledge to improve health, provide more effective health services and products, and strengthen the health care system" [9]. Knowledge translation is not the only term that has been used to name this tendency toward the practical use of knowledge to improve practice. According to Straus et al. [45], more than 90 terms were identified in the literature. According to them, in Europe, preferences are for "implementation science" or "research utilization," whereas the terms "dissemination and diffusion," "research use," and "knowledge transfer and uptake" are more frequently preferred in the United States. The Canadian "knowledge translation" has been adapted by others, including the United States National Center for Dissemination of Disability Research and the World Health Organization (WHO).

The lowest common denominator among the above-described different terms is a move beyond the dissemination of knowledge into the actual use of it to transform practice. "Knowledge creation (i.e., primary research), knowledge distillation (i.e., the creation of systematic reviews and guidelines) and knowledge dissemination (i.e., appearances in journals and presentations) are not enough on their own to ensure the use of knowledge in decision-making" [45].

A definition of the "best-practice" concept was recently developed by a group of European experts convened by the European Monitoring Centre for Drugs and Drug Addiction (EMCDDA). In brief, best practice is the best application of the available evidence to current activities in the drug field. Several factors were identified as contributing to making an intervention qualify as "best practice." In summary, a best-practice intervention is based on the most robust scientific evidence available regarding what is known to be effective in producing successful outcomes, and it is tailored to the needs of those it addresses. Methods used will be transparent, reliable, and transferable and can be updated as the knowledge base develops. Concerning implementation, local contextual factors will be taken into account, and the intervention will be harmonized with other actions as a part of a comprehensive approach to drug problems. A best practice is closely linked to the concept of "evidence-based practice," and it requires the careful integration of both scientific knowledge and implementation expertise to appropriately adapt the intervention to the single individual and/or to a specific context. A best-practice intervention should provide better outcomes than other interventions and therefore also allow a rational allocation of resources [21].

There remain challenges associated with the promotion of best practice through guidelines, standards, and other similar tools. The first is to make sure that they are based on reliable scientific evidence and that they are regularly updated when new systematic reviews are published. The second is to make the best use of the currently existing guidelines. Finally, it is important to ensure that guidelines and standards are appropriately implemented.

54.2.2 Quality of Interventions: The Main Tools and Their Life Cycle

Clinical guidelines are the main instrument to disseminate evidence-based interventions via

recommendations for practice that are based on a clear methodology for the appraisal, synthesis, and grading of the available evidence [12]. Evidence-based guidelines are produced by convening multidisciplinary groups of experts who systematically assess the quality of the available evidence and classify the recommendations according to the level of supporting evidence. The level of evidence is determined by a synthesis of relevant studies' design (systematic reviews), the number of participants studied, and the number of studies sharing the same results along with the overall measure of effect found by pooling the results of the studies. Each recommendation should be accompanied by an indication of its strength, which clarifies how and when this applies to the patients. Although the level of evidence influences the strength of a recommendation, there are conditions under which, even where there is a lack of evidence from studies, the appointed group of experts may attribute a high strength to some recommendations. This is the case for some interventions, such as hydration for hospital patients or blankets to prevent heat loss in trauma patients, that are supported by practical experience and do not need to be based on experimental evidence. Guidelines may, therefore, include a statement such as "we recommend that this intervention is offered to most patients, even though there are no studies which prove or refute the effects, and this recommendation is based only on expert opinion." In some milestone manuals for guidelines development, these are indicated as *good practice points* [44].

Another example is where patients cannot be directly studied for ethical reasons (such as exposing newborn babies to different drug therapies). In such cases, the recommendations can be based on the results of studies on other types of patients, by analogy. In practical terms, this system, which separates the level of evidence from strength of recommendations, produces two separate – but not completely independent – scores. In general, evidence-based guidelines are published by independent organizations that can assemble experts who are free from conflicts of interest and who represent different fields and professions. These groups generally involve as many stakeholders as necessary to ensure they appropriately address all the different aspects of a question, including patients' preferences and practical concerns arising from the experience of the carers [18].

In 2000, a collaboration was established of people interested in addressing the shortcomings of the grading systems used in guideline development, "the grading of recommendations assessment, development, and evaluation" (GRADE) working group [26]. Over the years, this group has developed and continuously updated a common, sensible, and transparent approach to grading the quality of evidence and the strength of recommendations. This system has been adopted by several international organizations among which are the EMCDDA (the Best Practice Portal); the World Health Organization (WHO); Agency for Healthcare Research and Quality (AHRQ), United States; and the National Institute for Clinical Excellence (NICE) in the United Kingdom. The complete list of the organizations that have adopted GRADE can be found in its website (http://www.gradeworkinggroup.org/).

The evidence-based clinical guidelines are meant to facilitate the application of updated evidence to practice, and therefore, they are supposed to be timely revised. An indication of a specific date for revision should be stated clearly, and the choice of this date should be based on an assessment of the time in which new evidence is likely to be available.

This anticipation of a date for the availability of new evidence is in general possible because evidence-based clinical guidelines are based on systematic reviews of studies. These reviews are identified through structured "search strategies" based on a list of "clinical questions" that the guidelines should address. Based on those questions – which should be relevant to the patients and detailed enough to allow the appropriate search for the available evidence [42] – the methodologists search, identify, and select some systematic reviews of evidence. The latter are based on published and unpublished studies and should also identify – in ad hoc created registries [51] – the ongoing studies. Those registries collect information from the very beginning of the clinical studies and follow up each step until the publication. The

entity (or the individual researcher) registering a clinical trial is requested to include a date of completion. Although these dates can be changed during the study period, they provide an idea when new results can be available.

Several tools have been developed to assess the quality dimensions in guidelines, one of them being the "appraisal of guidelines for research and evaluation" [1], which was created to address the issue of variability in guideline quality by assessing methodological rigor and transparency. The updated version, "AGREE II" (AGREE Next Steps Consortium [2]), is composed of six domains aimed at assessing whether or not the scope and purpose of the guidelines is clearly indicated; the stakeholders' involvement is sufficient to represent the views of the intended users; the process of development is rigorous; the presentation and text are clear; and the guidelines are fit for purpose and free from conflicts of interest.

Worldwide, there are currently several international inventories of guidelines that can be consulted to find relevant documents. Among those, the more important are the inventory maintained by the Guidelines International Network (http://www.g-i-n.net/library) containing over 6000 sets of guidelines for evidence-based healthcare (in multiple languages) and the National Guidelines Clearinghouse (http://www.guideline.gov/), an initiative of the Agency for Healthcare Research and Quality (AHRQ) in the United States, which publishes guidelines from any countries provided they are in English. The website of the National Guidelines Clearinghouse offers an automated function to compare different guidelines and obtain the synthesis of guidelines. The main aim of the inventories of guidelines is to avoid duplication of efforts making good quality guidelines available for adoption or adaptation in different contexts.

54.2.2.1 Adaptation of Guidelines to Everyday Practice Under Local Circumstances

Clinical guidelines can be elaborated and published at several levels: international, national, or local level. The World Health Organization, for example, published guidelines and principles on the treatment of drug addiction [50].

Being a very resource-intensive activity, guidelines are in general commissioned to specialized national agencies that have the capacity for convening many stakeholders from all the involved parts and reduce the risks of conflicts of interest. Examples of agencies to develop clinical guidelines are the National Institute for Clinical Excellence in the United Kingdom; the Scottish Intercollegiate Guidelines Network; the Finnish STAKES, National Research and Development Centre for Welfare and Health; the French National Health Authority (HAS); the New Zealand Guideline Group (went in voluntary liquidation in 2012); the Canadian Task Force on Preventive Health Care; and many others. An indicative list of organizations that develop and publish guidelines is available on the website of the Guidelines International Network [25].

Guidelines that are published at a general level may require some further elaboration before they can be effectively applied to everyday practice.

The translation of evidence-based recommendations into practice is the so-called implementation process.

Implementation activities can follow two general approaches mainly depending on the "distance" between the context where the guidelines were issued and that where they have to be implemented. In some cases, it is sufficient to *adopt* the guidelines through the development of protocols at the service level in which the guidelines' recommendations are broken down into actions and responsibilities, agreed by the healthcare personnel. This type of protocols (which can be also called *clinical pathways*) supplements clinical recommendations with hospital (or service)-specific details and, in some cases, can emend those recommendations which are considered not fitting with the local context [24]. These protocols can be disseminated in the realm of some peer-led educational activities, and they can include reminders and other initiatives aimed at reinforcing the application of recommendations in practice [7] (Table 54.1).

Table 54.1 Quality standards in the treatment of drug addiction

Title and year of publication	Supporting organization	Target groups	Structure of the standards	Web address
European Minimum Quality Standards (EQUS), 2012	European Commission	Professionals performing interventions; service directors and managers responsible for the functioning of their institutions and staff; and health authorities, planners, and policymakers who are mainly concerned with the drug demand reduction activities at the system and network levels	Structural standards of services Process standards at the service level Process standards of interventions Outcome standards at the system level	www.isgf.ch
Proposed continental minimum quality standards for the treatment of drug dependence, 2012	African Union [3]	Unspecified	14 principles of effective drug dependence treatment 15 standards for the treatment of drug dependence and 3 standards for evaluation and assessment	http://www.au.int/en/

Table 54.1 (continued)

Title and year of publication	Supporting organization	Target groups	Structure of the standards	Web address
Principles of drug dependence treatment, 2008	UNODC WHO [49]	https://www.unodc.org/docs/treatment/UNODC-WHO_2016_treatment_standards_E.pdf	9 principles: description and justification components Actions to promote each principle	http://www.who.int/substance_abuse/publications/principles_drug_dependence_treatment.pdf
National standards Service delivery for people with coexisting mental health and addiction, 2010	New Zealand Ministry of Health	This guidance document is aimed at all those who have an interest and responsibility for planning, funding, and providing mental health and addiction services including District Health Boards, non-governmental organizations and the Ministry of Health. The content will be of interest to staff working in services, consumers, and service users, carers, and others who have contact with these services	General principles Tips for mental health and addiction planners and funders Tips for mental health and addiction service managers and clinical leaders Suggested actions for local planning	http://www.health.govt.nz/publication/service-delivery-people-co-existing- mental-health-and-addiction-problems- integrated-solutions-2010
Principles of drug addiction treatment, 2012	National Institute for Drug Addiction (NIDA), USA	Unspecified	13 principles of effective treatment 22 frequently asked questions	http://www.drugabuse.gov/publications/term/33/Guidelines%20and%20Manuals
Alcohol dependence and harmful alcohol use quality standard, 2011	National Institute for Clinical Excellence (UK)	The public, health and social care professionals, commissioners, and service providers	13 statements and 13 quality measures for: structure process outcome	http://publications.nice.org.uk/alcohol-dependence-and-harmful-alcohol-use- quality-standard-qs11/list-of-statements
Quality standard for drug use disorders, 2012	National Institute for Clinical Excellence (UK)	The public, health and social care professionals, commissioners, and service providers	10 statements and quality measures for: structure process outcome	http://publications.nice.org.uk/quality-standard-for-drug-use-disorders-qs23
Quality framework for mental health services in Ireland, 2005	Mental Health Commission Ireland	Service users as well as the different nature and scale of organizations involved in service delivery	8 themes 24 standards 163 criteria	http://www.mhcirl.ie/Standards_Quality_Assurance/ Quality_Framework.pdf
Standards for integrated care pathways for mental health December 2007	NHS Quality Improvement Scotland	Local management, health staff at the service level	9 process standards 21 care assessment, planning, delivery, and outcome standards 16 condition-specific standards (only one relevant to drug addiction) 2 service improvement standards	http://www.healthcareimprovementscotland.org/programmes/mental_health/icps_for_mental_health/standards_for_integrated_care.aspx

In other cases, an *adaptation* process is put in place, where the source guidelines are further analyzed by a group of local experts who draft new contextual-wise recommendations. Customizing clinical practice guidelines to a particular context and involving local stakeholders and the end-users of the guideline in this process have been identified as ways to improve acceptance and adherence [27]. In general, but not necessarily, the *adaptation* occurs when (inter) national guidelines are to be applied at the local level. In this case, the adaptation process can consider more than one set of guidelines and imply a process similar to the one needed for drafting a new guideline. The major difference lies in the search for source documents that, in the case of an *adaptation*, focus on guidelines rather than on systematic reviews of evidence (and or primary studies) as in the case of development of a new guideline.

ADAPTE (www.Adapte.org) is an international organization of methodologists, researchers, guideline developers, and guideline implementers who aim to promote the development and use of clinical practice guidelines through the adaptation of existing guidelines. The organization created a resource toolkit that can be freely downloaded in the Guidelines International Network website (www.g-i-n.net).

Quality standards are becoming an increasingly popular tool for ensuring the quality of interventions in healthcare. In general terms, standards are principles and sets of rules about what to do and what to have [6] presented as voluntary to many potential adopters. According to one of the most known organizations for standards development, a standard is a document, established by consensus and approved by a recognized body, that provides, for common and repeated use, rules, guidelines, or characteristics for activities or their results, aimed at the achievement of the optimum degree of order in a given context [28]. Typically, the standards proposed in the health field refer to content issues, processes, or structural (formal) aspects of quality assurance, such as environment and staffing composition.

Quality standards can be developed by private sector organizations as it is the case for the International Standards Organization [29]; national private, nonprofit organizations like the American National Standards Institute (ANSI); the Association Franc¸aise de Normalisations (AFNOR); and the British Standards Institute (BSI). The great majority of these organizations have been founded at the beginning of the twentieth century and some after the Second World War. Standards can also be developed by international governmental organizations like the United Nations, the Organization for Economic Co-operation and Development, and the European Union. Standards are a good way to propose harmonization, especially by those organizations whose members are sovereign states that cannot be obliged to follow some rules [6]. Nevertheless, there are also several national organizations, especially in the health field, which develop quality standards. In the case of these organizations, quality standards are intended as sets of rules based on evidence and used to implement the interventions recommended in clinical guidelines. The standards which are developed by the National Institute of Clinical Evidence in the United Kingdom, for example, are typically composed of a general statement and a measure that can be used to assess the quality of care or service provider specified in the statement. "The quality statements are clear, measurable and concise and describe high-priority areas for quality improvement. They are aspirational (they describe high-quality care or service provision) but achievable" [34].

Several international organizations are undertaking standards development for health interventions in drug demand reduction.

The European Commission financed a study on the Development of a European Union Framework for minimum quality standards and benchmarks in drug demand reduction (EQUS) [43], proposing a set of 22 quality standards for treatment (the study included also 33 standards for prevention and 16 for harm reduction).

According to the background paper of this project, in the medical sciences, quality standards are determined by different stakeholders: health authorities, insurance companies, service providers, professionals, and patients. Each of these professional categories brings different goals, interests, and priorities that need to be reflected in the standards in the light of the underlying scientific evidence. The project, whose lead investigator was Ambros Uchtenaghen [48], divided the quality standards into three dimensions:

1. *Structural quality*, for example, standards relating to the physical environment, staff, training, etc.
2. *Process quality*, for example, standards relating to the process of an intervention, diagnostic assessment
3. *Outcome quality and economic quality*, for example, standards to measure the cost-benefit ratio

The *structural standards for services* cover areas like the physical accessibility of treatment services (which need to be located in places easily reached by public transport) or the environment where the treatment takes place, which should be adequate (to allow privacy during consultations) and safe. Another important aspect is the need for a documented diagnosis as a basis for treatment choice. Staff education and composition are also mentioned in terms of ensuring the presence of medical and nursing staff along with psychologists or social workers and multidisciplinarity with at least three professions represented.

The *process standards at the service level* included the assessment of substance use history, diagnosis, and treatment history along with the somatic and the social status for each patient including an assessment of the psychiatric conditions.

Each patient should be provided with information on the treatment options available and should be provided with a treatment plan tailored to his/her individual needs.

Treatment plans, assessments, changes, unexpected events, and any relevant information should be recorded and kept confidential. Each treatment service should promote cooperation with other agencies and services to ensure an appropriate response to the needs of their patients (whenever a service is not equipped to deal with all needs of a given patient, another appropriate service is at hand for referral) and should ensure continuous education for the staff members.

The *outcome standards proposed at the system level* included the goals of health and social stabilization of patients and the reduction of illegal or non-prescribed psychotropic substances. Monitoring included the level of utilization (each service should provide information on the number of slots or bed utilized) and the ratio of discharges occurred as planned or for different reasons.

Internal and external evaluation of services was also proposed as a standard.

Beyond the list of proposed standards, the project-added value lies in the process adopted to consult the stakeholders and to identify several levels of standards. Namely, the stakeholders were interviewed by rounds of Internet-based consultations about the level of implementation status and acceptability of the proposed standards in their respective countries. Through this strategy, it was possible to identify a long list of standards and grade them by priority of implementation. The European Minimum Quality Standards (EQUS) study also included a review of existing quality standards already implemented at the national level, involving experts from 24 European countries. Concerning drug treatment processes, the standards most frequently reported as already implemented were in the areas of client data confidentiality and assessment of clients' drug use history, whereas the standards concerned with routine cooperation with other services, and those focusing on continuous staff training, were less often implemented. In the area of treatment outcomes, the two types of the standard most frequently reported as implemented were those with goals linked to health improvement and reduced substance use. Among the standards less likely to be applied were those focusing on external evaluation and monitoring client discharge; problems related to the implementation of these standards were reported.

This approach may allow the participating countries to set their own goals and to pace their achievement according to their own capacity and priorities. This process would also be greatly facilitated by the existence of the European Monitoring Centre for Drugs and Drug Addiction (EMCDDA), a decentralized agency whose aim is to provide sound and comparable information on drugs in Europe. Thanks to its impartiality and comprehensiveness of information, EMCDDA can support the countries volunteering for the adoption of the quality standards in setting their goals and measuring their successes.

In September 2015, the Council of the European Union adopted Council conclusions on the implementation of minimum quality standards in drug demand reduction in the EU. The list of 16 standards was the result of an initiative of the Italian Presidency that, taking over the priority of defining quality standards based on the project EQUS, set by the Greek Presidency, convened a group of European experts. The expert group cross-analyzed different sets of international standards, comparing them against the principles of the European Drugs Strategy.

These standards represent a minimum benchmark of quality for interventions in: drug use prevention, risk and harm reduction, treatment, social integration, and rehabilitation. Although non-binding for national governments, the document represents the political will of EU countries to address demand reduction interventions with an evidence-based approach. These guidelines have been drawn up in the context of Action 9 of the EU Action Plan on Drugs (2013–2016) (Table 54.2).

In general terms, it can be observed that the existing standards (at their different level of implementation) seem to be triggered by several reasons: the harmonization of the existing services, the translation in practice of the evidence-based guidelines, the consistency between policy decisions and service provision, and the need to measure the results of interventions. These reasons are diversely reflected in the initiatives mentioned mainly about the level, where the standards are proposed. The life cycle of quality standards depends on the supporting evidence, but not completely. When it comes to human rights or general safety measures, the relevant principles are imperishable.

Clinical pathways are structured, multidisciplinary plans of care designed to support the implementation of clinical guidelines and protocols. In the recent past, it was considered that this definition was variedly interpreted by different stakeholders until a recent systematic review [31] clarified the concept.

The clinical pathways are essential to the translation of evidence-based guidelines at the service level. They are meant to "detail essential steps in care of patients with a specific clinical problem" and sequence "the actions of a multidisciplinary team" [14]. In clarifying which actions should be undertaken to practice evidence-based recommendations, clinical pathways "facilitate translation of national guidelines into local protocols" [8] and allow continuous improvement by monitoring and evaluating variances.

Clinical pathways are commonly adopted in the United States, where, in 2003, it was reported that almost 80% of the hospitals used this tool [31]. Evidence supports the adoption of clinical pathways at the hospital level for the reduction of

Table 54.2 Processes for the adaptation of guidelines at the local level

Document	Process	Professionals' involvement	Output	Definition
Guidelines (national or international)	Adoption	Service personnel	Service protocol/ clinical pathway	A comprehensive set of rigid criteria outlining the management steps for a single clinical condition or aspects of the organization (http://www. openclinical.org/guidelines.html#gandp)
Guidelines	Adaptation	Stakeholders	Locally adapted guidelines	The local adaptation of national guidelines has been proposed as a way of increasing the benefit of local ownership while maintaining scientific validity [30]

in-hospital complications (such as infections, bleeding, and pneumonia), improved documentation, and possibly a reduction in the length of stay [40]. An experience of integrated clinical pathways in mental health has been reported in Scotland, where the National Health Service (NHS) Scotland is taking a national approach to improving the quality and safety of mental health services. The program started with the publication of national standards by NHS Quality Improvement Scotland (NHS QIS), setting out the framework for development at the local level.

The emphasis of development and implementation of the ICPs lies with local NHS boards to ensure they are developed with local ownership and to meet the needs of the local population. However, to ensure accreditation by NHS QIS, the local ICPs must incorporate the national standards and evidence improvement to the quality of care provided [17]. In Belgium, there is the European Association for the development of clinical pathways (http://www.e-p-a.org/about-epa/index.html). Among the objectives of this organization, there is the setup of an international network for pooling know-how on clinical pathways and the promotion and fostering of international cooperation between healthcare researchers, managers, and healthcare providers from European countries and the wider international community. The association has a journal that publishes research results on the development of clinical pathways.

54.2.3 Participation: A Key for Successful Implementation

Two core elements underlie all the instruments for quality improvement mentioned above (evidence-based clinical guidelines, quality standards, and clinical pathways): (i) the evidence base and (ii) stakeholders' consensus. The last three decades have been devoted to define and share a valid methodology for the identification assessment and synthesis of the available evidence. This activity successfully brought to a general understanding of the terminology and the sources of correct information. Nowadays the

role of evidence to base decisions is widely recognized, and the access to good quality sources of evidence is increasingly available.

The new challenge seems to lie on the promotion of an authentic participatory implementation of evidence-based interventions.

The same pioneers of the evidence-based medicine are now exploring strategies to communicating and involving two crucial stakeholders: the decision makers and the patients (this latter category includes also family members, civil society organizations, community representatives [15]). Projects like SUPPORT, financed by the European Commission's 6th Framework Programme [32], and the most recent DECIDE [46], co-funded by the European Commission under the Seventh Framework Programme, are both aimed at supporting decision makers in the use of evidence.

SUPPORT targets policymakers as a diverse group that includes cabinet members (e.g., Ministers of Health or Finance), elected officials (e.g., chairs of legislative committees), senior civil servants (e.g., directors of primary healthcare programs), and high-level political appointees (e.g., heads of government agencies). In spite of being aware of the differences that can exist among the countries due to the different political systems, the leading project managers of SUPPORT state that what all the decision makers have in common is the authority to make or influence decisions directly. The project encompasses several tools for boosting evidence-based decision making in various settings including low- and middle-income countries and high-income countries. As the other mentioned project, DECIDE, also SUPPORT, sought strategies for the involvement of the public in evidence-based decision making [35]. In particular, DECIDE, whose target is Europe, is composed of eight work packages, three of which are devoted to identifying best strategies to communicate with specific target groups such as health professionals, policymakers and managers, and patients and public.

The two projects have similar objectives though following different approaches: DECIDE focuses on guidelines and recommendations, while SUPPORT aims to support policy-relevant reviews and trials. DECIDE on the other hand is developing tools that will help policymakers to decide about, say, whether to pay for particular healthcare innovation in their region. Additionally, it is developing tools to make understanding the research information that forms the basis for guideline recommendations easier for a wide audience, including policymakers and the public. To some extent, DECIDE builds on the work of SUPPORT.

Even though these projects are important, quite often the exercise of knowledge translation brings to the appreciation of huge gaps in knowledge, gaps that are difficult to fill with methods for gathering consensus and taking decisions in the lack of evidence. The only possible way forward to fill those gaps is to propose new studies to find answers. These new studies should rely on mixed methods to get sound evidence from several sources and, of course, to be based on the priorities of the end-users of the answers they should provide, such as the patients [33]. In the United Kingdom, Sir Iain Chalmers, one of the founders of the Cochrane Collaboration, has undertaken a new initiative for the proactive involvement of patients in the setting of research priorities through the James Lind Alliance initiative (Petit-Zeman S FAU – Cowan and Cowan [2]). The James Lind Alliance brings together patients, carers, and clinicians to identify and prioritize the uncertainties, or "unanswered questions," about the effects of treatments, which they agree are most important, and makes the list of research questions public and available for researchers and research funders. Not always is the area of addiction represented in these initiatives. The main linkages are granted by the Cochrane Group on Drugs and Alcohol and by the European Monitoring Centre for Drugs and Drug Addiction which is working in partnership to bring the typical problems of this field in the broader perspective of knowledge translation.

Some of the characteristics of the drug addiction field can be shared by other medical conditions. For example, the behavioral component calls for research that cannot be only based on experimental studies. An important aspect of

knowledge can be found in long-term observational studies, and in some cases, they require qualitative analysis which is more difficult to be systematically retrieved with the typical search strategies adopted in systematic reviews and even more difficult to be assessed for quality and included in the meta-analysis [22]. Nevertheless, there are some added values in the drug addiction field which compensate for those extra efforts. The impact of interventions on public health and security makes drug addiction an important point on every political agenda and needs to be based on the best available evidence.

54.2.3.1 Implementation Strategies

In recent years, it became clear that implementation is key to effective evidence-based interventions. Particular attention has been paid to the identification of strategies to implement interventions in specific contexts and for specific targets. The implementation of evidence-based interventions can be particularly challenging in the case of drug-related interventions for a number of reasons: (i) these interventions involve not only health but also social and policy elements; (ii) some drug-related interventions are highly controversial, as is the case with drug consumption rooms, for example, and (iii) they involve all relevant communities.

For these reasons, it is helpful to consider the lessons learnt in other fields, that is, not only in health but also in education, social work, and so on [20]. For example, Powell et al. (2015) consulted experts through a DELPHI consultation and identified 73 strategies for implementing interventions in education [4]. The list of actions and strategies proposed by the experts included:

- Obtaining funding
- Using train-the-trainer strategies
- Creating new teams
- Obtaining formal commitments
- Changing physical structure and equipment
- Developing tools and processes for the monitoring of quality
- Promoting ongoing consultation
- Using data experts
- Working with educational institutions

A prerequisite for implementation is the setting of objectives and measurable outcomes; tools such as Support and DECIDE, mentioned above, support this exercise. Another important aspect to consider is that the process of implementation can be also assessed through dimensions such as the implementation climate in an organization; the degree to which an evidence-based practice is adopted over time; the level of fidelity with which an intervention is implemented by staff; or the costs of an implementation process [4].

The deeper reflection on the importance of implementation resulted in the establishment of several initiatives and collaborations around the world. Examples include the Society for implementation research collaboration (SIRC http://societyforimplementationresearchcollaboration.org) and the European Implementation Collaborative (https://implementation.eu/). These initiatives are devoted to improve the implementation of evidence-based interventions by facilitating communication and collaboration between implementation research teams, researchers, and community providers. They hold conferences and develop tools and materials to facilitate implementation. A large number of aspects are covered in these resources, some of which are developed by other researchers and made available on institutional websites. Topics covered span from measuring the fidelity of implementation to dimensions needed for effective changes, decision-making tools, and evaluation tools.

54.2.3.2 Training Initiatives

The training of professionals is a central element for the implementation of good quality interventions. Training sessions can address behavior change as well as skills to deliver specific interventions. A recent example of training for professionals is the Universal Prevention Curriculum, which was adapted to the European context through a European-funded project (UPC-ADAPT).

Many European countries offer training programs for intervention providers. These range from specialist university programs, as it is the case in Germany and Czechia, to specific courses offered in many countries as part of the university curricula for health or social welfare degrees.

54.2.4 Examples of Frameworks for Quality Standards

Several evidence-based guidelines, issued at the international and national levels, are currently available for the treatment of drug addiction, in particular for the combined pharmacological and psychological approaches to opioid dependence. Quality standards are also becoming widely available, and combined also with training initiatives for professionals. As the majority of quality standards have been developed in the context of prevention, the first training initiatives target prevention professionals [19].

Two examples of national quality standards for drug addiction treatment in Europe can be drawn from Czechia and the United Kingdom.

In Czechia, the implementation of quality standards for the treatment of drug addiction dates back to 1995 for an initiative of the Interdepartmental National Drug Commission (now Government Council for Drug Policy Coordination). Called minimal standards, these were adopted by the Association of Non-Governmental Organizations (ANO) for Addiction Prevention and Treatment for evaluating the quality of member organizations and newly established facilities. After further elaboration occurred in the subsequent 4 years, those standards became the basis for a certification process, which recognizes that a specific service provider is in line with predefined quality standards. Since 2004, the adherence to quality standards has been assessed by specifically trained external evaluators. The current process for the certification of treatment providers was kicked off in 2005, and it included a transition period to allow the treatment provider services to start the certification process. After that period, certification became a prerequisite for applying for state grant programs. The overall aim of the certification process was the improvement of the quality of the network of services including a cost-effective administration of public funds. With the certification process came the integration of drug addiction services into the medical and social national system.

The underlying principles are as follows: (i) voluntariness – certification is not required to provide drug services but only to apply for public funds; (ii) transparency – the evaluation process is carried out according to published criteria; and (iii) objectivity – the actual evaluation of quality is performed by an independent agency who appoints trained evaluators, and the facility providers can point out any possible conflict of interest.

The standards are at the base of the certification and accreditation process. The core activity of the certification process includes that a group of trained assessors visit the service providers to collect relevant information. Active participants in this process are the facilities requesting the certificate of quality (those wishing to apply for public funds); the certification agency (an independent institution that arranges on-site examinations, communication between the parties of the certification processes, and training of certificators); the certification team carrying out on-site examinations (composed by at least three trained certificators); the Certification Board of the Government Council for Drug Policy Coordination (deciding about certification request results and validity of certification ranging from 1 to 4 years); and the Executive Board of the Government Council for Drug Policy Coordination – to which the facilities can address their complaints about, for example, the composition of the certification team. Before the certification can start, the agency and the requesting facility have to agree on the date and the composition of the team of assessors. Subsequently, several previously identified employees and clients are interviewed with semi-structured questionnaires. The on-site examination, in general, lasts 1 day, at the end of which the team of assessors drafts a report with a proposal for certification or suggestions for improvement. The report is shared with the interested facility, which is allowed to comment in writing.

The report is therefore completed and forwarded by the certification agency to the Certification Board of the Government Council for Drug Policy for the final decision.

Overall the process takes around 2 months, and the facilities requesting certification have 15 days to contest the results.

In the United Kingdom, the National Institute for Clinical Excellence (NICE) publishes evidence-based clinical guidelines for many different medical disciplines including drug addiction. Sets of quality standards are derived from the best available evidence such as NICE guidance and other evidence sources accredited. They are developed in collaboration with NHS and social care professionals, their partners, and service users. The standards consider issues like evidence of effectiveness and cost-effectiveness, people's experience, safety, equality, and cost impact. The quality standards are considered central to supporting the government's vision for an NHS and social care system focused on delivering the best possible outcomes for people who use services [37]. This act clarifies that the Secretary of State "must have regard to the quality standards prepared by NICE." The care system should consider those standards in planning and delivering services to secure continuous improvement in quality. NICE quality standards do not provide service specifications but rather define priority areas for quality improvement. Nevertheless, those standards are the basis to ensure that the providers of health and adult social care in England meet the standards of quality and safety required by the Care Quality Commission.

The standards developed by NICE are typically composed of a general statement complemented by a measure. These quality measures are drafted only after the quality statement wording has been agreed and addresses the structure of care or services, process of care or service provision, and, if appropriate, outcome of care or service provision. The majority of measures refer to process and are expressed as a numerator and denominator to define a proportion, in which the numerator is a subset of the denominator population. For example, for the standard "People who inject drugs have access to needle and syringe programmes in accordance with NICE guidance," there is a measure at the structure level, which is "Evidence of local arrangements to ensure people who inject drugs have access to needle and syringe programmes in accordance with NICE guidance," complemented by a measure of outcome: (i) proportion of people who inject drugs who access needle and syringe programs, wherein the numerator is the number of people who access needle and syringe programs and the denominator is the estimated prevalence of injecting drug users and (ii) incidence of blood-borne viruses among people who inject drugs.

To clarify the implications of the standard, a breakdown of meanings of the standard for each stakeholder is included: service providers ensure systems are in place for people who inject drugs to have access to needle and syringe programs in accordance with NICE guidance; needle and syringe program staff ensure people who inject drugs have access to needle and syringe programs in accordance with NICE guidance; commissioners ensure they commission services for people who inject drugs to have access to needle and syringe programs in accordance with NICE guidance; and people who inject drugs have access to needle and syringe programs that are nearby, have suitable opening hours, and provide injecting equipment and advice on reducing the risk of harm. The standards include also that the sources of data be considered in the measurement. Furthermore, at NICE, there is an implementation team to support key audiences and organizations to maximize the uptake of guidance and quality standards. The team assesses the aids and barriers to implementation and provides practical support tools for commissioning, service improvement and audit, education, and learning. The team prepares reports on the uptake of guidance that are used to inform the development of the quality standard. The implementation team collaborates with national bodies and local organizations, through local implementation consultants, to support the use of quality standards and to facilitate shared learning.

Overall, the process to produce standards at the National Institute for Clinical Excellence lasts indicatively for 42 weeks.

These two examples suggest the possibility of different approaches to the use of quality standards. In the Czech experience, the development of the standards represents an initial effort, whereas the actual focus seems to lie on the certification and accreditation process including several levels of training and a "learning by experience" process. Furthermore, the entire experience initiated around 20 years ago has been conceived and developed specifically in the treatment of drug addiction.

On the other hand, the National Institute for Clinical Evidence has created, along with the Department of Health and other key partners, a core library of topics for quality standard development in health-related topics, among which alcohol dependence and drug use were included. In this case, the focus seems to be on the development itself of the standards which *translate the evidence-based guidelines* into general statements and measures of outcomes at the system level including the indication of the sources of data to be used for the assessment of the implementation. Furthermore, NICE offers the support of an implementation team to enhance local adoption initiatives.

54.3 Conclusion

Quality of intervention is entrenched to the evidence base, and in the last 20 years, important progress has been made in the availability of good quality systematic reviews of effectiveness in the field of drug addiction treatment. Nevertheless, important gaps in knowledge still exist and need to be addressed by further investment in research. To ensure that research answers concrete problems arising from the daily experience of those affected by the drug problems at several levels, it is crucial that the end-users of research results – such as practitioners, patients, and decision makers – are involved in the selection of priority for investigation.

Currently, the attention seems to be focused on how to better communicate evidence to policymakers, patients, and the general public. The achievement and maintenance of quality in the treatment of drug addiction need the participation of all the stakeholders. The agencies providing data to assess the current situation and set the future goals, the decision-makers at the system level, and those managing the local, regional, and national services, have to collaborate with the practitioners to offer the best possible treatment to the drug users. The drug users, the families, and the public have to proactively be involved in any decision and should be able to speak out their needs and problems.

The tools to translate evidence into the quality of treatment have to be understandable by all the relevant stakeholders to empower them in a reiterative process of testing and learning lessons.

Quality is a continuous process where each new achievement has to be seen as a step toward new goals.

Glossary

Accreditation is the process by which an institution delivering a service is independently assessed for quality against some predefined criteria. Accreditation requires a set of minimum standards, which are set by the accrediting body.

Benchmarking is the process of comparing service processes and performance metrics to best practices from other services. Dimensions typically measured are quality, time, and cost.

Clinical pathways are structured, multidisciplinary plans of care designed to support the implementation of clinical guidelines and protocols.

Guidance is a general term that covers documents such as guidelines and quality standards.

Guidelines are "statements that include recommendations intended to optimise patient care that is informed by a systematic review of evidence and an assessment of the benefits and harms of alternative care options" (Institute of Medicine 2011). They are designed to assist

carers' and clients' decisions about appropriate interventions in specific circumstances.

Protocols in general, are documents that specify the procedures to follow to perform some tasks, typically those used to conduct a study or to implement some guidelines at the individual service level.

Standards and quality standards are principles and sets of rules based on evidence [6], which are used to implement the interventions recommended in guidelines. They can refer to content issues, processes, or structural (formal) aspects of quality assurance, such as environment and staffing composition. In some cases, standards are legally binding.

References

1. AGREE Collaboration. Development and validation of an international appraisal instrument for assessing the quality of clinical practice guidelines: the AGREE project. Qual Saf Health Care. 2003;12:18–23.
2. Brouwers M, Kho ME, Browman GP, Cluzeau F, feder G, Fervers B, Hanna S, Makarski J on behalf of the AGREE Next Steps Consortium. AGREE II: Advancing guideline development, reporting and evaluation in healthcare. Can Med Assoc J. Dec 2010; 182:E839–842; doi: 10.1503/cmaj.090449
3. African Union. Proposed continental minimum quality standards for the treatment of drug dependence. 2012. http://www.au.int/ar/sites/default/files/02%20 Concept%20Note.pdf.
4. Albers B, Pattuwage L. Implementation in education: findings from a scoping review. Melbourne: Evidence for Learning; 2017.
5. Brownson RC, Colditz GA, Proctor EK. Dissemination and implementation research in health. New York: Oxford University Press; 2012.
6. Brunsson N, Jacobsson B, editors. A world of standards. New York: Oxford University Press; 2000.
7. Burgers JS, Grol R, Klazinga NS, Mäkelä M, Zaat J, AGREE Collaboration. Towards evidence-based clinical practice: an international survey of 18 clinical guidelines programs. Int J Qual Health Care. 2003;15(1):31–45, http://intqhc.oxfordjournals.org/ content/15/1/31. Abstract.
8. Campbell H, Hotchkiss R, Bradshaw N, Porteous M. Integrated care pathways. BMJ. 1998;316(7125):133–7, PM: 9462322.
9. Canadian Institutes of Health Research. About knowledge translation. 2012.
10. Chalmers I, Glasziou P. Avoidable waste in the production and reporting of research evidence. Lancet.

2004;374(9683):86–9, http://www.sciencedirect.com/science/article/ pii/S0140673609603299.

11. Cochrane AL. Effectiveness and efficiency: random reflections on health services. London: Royal Society of Medicine Press; 1999.

12. Connis RT, Nickinovich DG, Caplan RA, Arens JF. The development of evidence-based clinical practice guidelines. Integrating medical science and practice. Int J Technol Assess Health Care. 2000;16(4):1003–12, PM:11155824.

13. Davoli M, Ferri M. The Cochrane Review Group on drugs and alcohol. Addiction. 2000;95(10):1473–4, PM:11070523.

14. De Bleser L, Depreitere R, De WK, Vanhaecht K, Vlayen J, Sermeus W. Defining pathways. J Nurs Manag. 2006;14(7):553–63, PM:17004966.

15. Deber RB, Kraetschmer N, Urowitz S, Sharpe N. Patient, consumer, client, or customer: what do people want to be called? Health Expect. 2005;8(4):345–51, PM:16266422.

16. Egger M, Smith GD. Meta-analysis. Potentials and promise. Br Med J. 1997;315(7119):1371–4, PM:9432250.

17. El-Ghorr A, et al. Scotland's national approach to improving mental health services: integrated care pathways as tools for redesign and continuous quality improvement. Int J Care Pathways. 2010;14(2):57–64.

18. EMCDDA. Guidelines for the treatment of drug dependence: a European perspective. Luxembourg: Publications Office of the European Union; 2011.

19. EMCDDA. European drug prevention quality standards. A manual for prevention professionals. Lisbon: Publications Office of the European Union; 2012.

20. EMCDDA. Health and social responses to drug problems: a European guide. Lisbon: Publications Office of the European Union; 2017. October 2017.

21. Ferri M, Bo A. Drug demand reduction: global evidence for local action, drugs in focus briefings from the European Monitoring Centre for Drugs and Drug Addiction 1. Lisbon: Publications Office of the European Union # European Monitoring Centre for Drugs and Drug Addiction; 2012.

22. Gough B, Madill A. Subjectivity in psychological science: from problem to prospect. Psychol Methods. 2012;17(3):374–84.

23. Grol R, Wensing M. What drives change? Barriers to and incentives for achieving evidence-based practice. Med J Aust. 2004;180(Suppl):S57–60.

24. Groot P, Hommersom A, Lucas P. Adaptation of clinical practice guidelines. Stud Health Technol Inf. 2008;139:121–39, PM:18806324.

25. Guidelines International Network. Annual report 2012. Ref Type: Online Source. 2012.

26. Guyatt GH, et al. GRADE guidelines: 4. Rating the quality of evidence-study limitations (risk of bias). J Clin Epidemiol. 2011;64(4):407–15.

27. Harrison MB, Legare F, Graham ID, Fervers B. Adapting clinical practice guidelines to local context and assessing barriers to their use. CMAJ. 2010;182(2):E78–84, PM:19969563.

28. ISO. ISO/TMB policy and principles statement global relevance of ISO technical work and publications. 2004. http://www.iso.org/iso/global_relevance.pdf.

29. ISO. Structure and governance. Geneva: International Standards Organization; 2013. Ref Type: Online Source.

30. Khunti K, Lakhani M. Barriers to the implementation of guidelines in general practice. Asthma Gen Pract. 1998;6(1):7–8.

31. Kinsman L, Rotter T, James E, Snow P, Willis J. What is a clinical pathway? Development of a definition to inform the debate. BMC Med. 2010;8:31, PM:20507550.

32. Lavis JN, et al. SUPPORT tools for evidence-informed health policymaking (STP). Health Res Policy Syst. 2009;7(Suppl 1):I1.

33. Liberati A. Need to realign patient-oriented and commercial and academic research. Lancet. 2011;378(9805):1777–8, http://linkinghub.elsevier.com/retrieve/pii/S0140673611617728.

34. NICE. Health and social care directorate quality standards process guide. Manchester: National Institute for Health and Clinical Excellence; 2012.

35. Oxman AD, Lewin S, Lavis JN, Fretheim A. SUPPORT tools for evidence-informed health policy making (STP) 15: engaging the public in evidence-informed policymaking. Health Res Policy Syst. 2009;7(Suppl 1):S15, PM:20018105.

36. Parchman ML, Scoglio CM, Schumm P. Understanding the implementation of evidence-based care: a structural network approach. Implement Sci. 2011;6:14.

37. Parliament of the United Kingdom, Health and Social Care Act. Ref Type: Online Source Petit-Zeman S, FAU - Cowan K, Cowan K Patients/carers and clinicians can set joint priorities for research in cleft lip and palate. (1872–8464 (Electronic)). 2012.

38. Rennick GJ. Use of systemic glucocorticosteroids in pregnancy: be alert but not alarmed. Australas J Dermatol. 2006;47(1):34–6, PM:16405480.

39. Roberts D, Dalziel S. Antenatal corticosteroids for accelerating fetal lung maturation for women at risk of preterm birth. Cochrane Database Syst Rev. 2006;(3):CD004454. Available at: PM:16856047.

40. Rotter T, Kinsman L, James E, Machotta A, Gothe H, Willis J, et al. Clinical pathways: effects on professional practice, patient outcomes, length of stay and hospital costs. Cochrane Database Syst Rev. 2010;17(3):CD006632. https://doi.org/10.1002/14651858.CD006632.pub2. Review.

41. Sackett DL, Rosenberg WM, Gray JA, Haynes RB, Richardson WS. Evidence based medicine: what it is and what it isn't. BMJ. 1996;312(7023):71–2, PM:8555924.

42. Schardt C, Adams MB, Owens T, Keitz S, Fontelo P. Utilization of the PICO framework to improve

searching PubMed for clinical questions. BMC Med Inform Decis Mak. 2007;7:16, PM:17573961.

43. Schaub MP, Uchtenhagen A, EQUS Expert Group. Building a European consensus on minimum quality standards for drug treatment, rehabilitation and harm reduction. Eur Addict Res. 2013;19(6):314–24. https://doi.org/10.1159/000350740. Epub 2013 Jun 14.

44. SIGN. SIGN 50: a guideline developer's handbook. Scotland: Scottish Intercollegiate Guidelines Network; 2011.

45. Straus SE, Tetroe J, Graham I. Defining knowledge translation. Can Med Assoc J. 2009;181(3–4):165–8, http://www.cmaj.ca/content/181/3-4/165.short.

46. Treweek S, Oxman AD, Alderson P, Bossuyt PM, Brandt L, Brozek J, et al. Developing and evaluating communication strategies to support informed deci-sions and practice based on evidence (DECIDE): protocol and preliminary results. Implement Sci. 2013;8:6.

47. Turner BJ, McLellan AT. Methodological challenges and limitations of research on alcohol consumption and effect on common clinical conditions: evidence from six systematic reviews. J Gen Intern Med. 2009;24(10):1156–60, PM:19672662.

48. Uchtenhagen A, Schaub M. Minimum quality standards in drug demand reduction EQUS. 2011.

49. UNODC. International standards on drug use prevention. Ref Type: Online Source. 2013

50. WHO. Guidelines for the psychosocially assisted pharmacological treatment of opioid dependence. Geneva: World Health Organisation; 2009.

51. WHO. International clinical trials registry platform (ICTRP). 2013. http://www.who.int/ictrp/en/.

The United Nations Drug Conventions: Evidence on Effects and Impact

55

Robin Room

Contents

Abstract

The three international drug treaties cover many psychoactive substances ("drugs"), although not tobacco (now under a separate treaty) or alcohol. They include a penal regime to enforce the limitation of use to medical or scientific purposes, a trade regime concerning drugs for medical use, and a planning scheme to ensure adequate supplies of medical opiates. The system, initiated in

R. Room (✉)
Centre for Alcohol Policy Research, La Trobe University, Bundoora, VIC, Australia

Centre for Social Research on Alcohol & Drugs, Department of Public Health Sciences, Stockholm University, Stockholm, Sweden
e-mail: r.room@latrobe.edu.au

1912, had shifted its main focus by the time of the 1988 treaty to combating the illicit markets, which accompany a prohibitory system. The place of the drug treaties in the United Nations system and the bodies which make up the system are briefly characterised. Nearly every country has signed each treaty, though often with reservations. The option this opens up of denouncing and re-acceding with reservations has also been successfully used by Bolivia concerning coca leaves. The system has assured access to pain medication in most high-income countries, but not in much of the world, where the system's emphasis on law enforcement has often indirectly but effectively cut off supplies. In terms of controlling legal medical markets, the system has had mixed success. But the

© Springer Nature Switzerland AG 2021
N. el-Guebaly et al. (eds.), *Textbook of Addiction Treatment*,
https://doi.org/10.1007/978-3-030-36391-8_55

system has mostly failed in cutting off the illicit drug trade. In a system that has been committed to a prohibitory approach, there are recent signs of change, particularly in the Americas; the legalisation of cannabis in Canada and much of the USA poses a new challenge to the status quo in the international system.

Keywords

Drug treaties · Cannabis · Opioids
Medication supply · Legalisation
Prohibition effects

55.1   Introduction

The United Nations drug control system is organised around three international treaties: the Single Convention on Narcotic Drugs of 1961, as amended by a Protocol of 1972; the Convention on Psychotropic Substances of 1971; and the UN Convention against Trafficking in Narcotic Drugs and Psychotropic Substances of 1988. Their texts, and the official commentaries on them, are conveniently available online: https://www. unodc.org/unodc/treaties/index.html

The treaties, of course, do not cover the whole range of psychoactive substances. There is a separate treaty on tobacco, the Framework Convention on Tobacco Control of 2003, negotiated under the auspices of the World Health Organization (WHO), and an International Convention against Doping in Sport (many of the substances covered by it are psychoactive), which was adopted in 2005 under the auspices of UNESCO. Notably absent from the list of substances under international control is alcohol, although it was actually the subject of the first international drug treaty, controlling "trade spirits" in colonial Africa, negotiated in 1889 but now in abeyance [8]. The 2012 WHO Expert Committee on Drug Dependence briefly discussed whether alcohol would qualify for listing under the UN drug conventions, but though this was referred for consideration at a future Expert Committee meeting [30:16], as of 2019 this has not occurred.

From the perspective of the inherent harmfulness of different psychoactive substances (e.g. [19]), what is included and excluded in the three "drug treaties" is not easily defensible, except as reflecting the vagaries of history. But despite the ongoing convergence in scientific thinking about psychoactive substances [10], it is still true that discussions of international drug control which take account of the whole range of drugs and their regulation are rare (for an exception, see [7]).

In this chapter, however, attention remains focused on the three UN drug treaties. We consider the intended functions of the treaties, the institutional arrangements for their implementation, and what evidence is available on effects and impact of the system. A brief discussion of potential future developments is also included.

55.2   Intended Functions of the Treaties

The treaties have three main functions: as a penal regime to enforce limitation of use of scheduled substances to medical or scientific purposes; as a specialised trade treaty, controlling international trade in psychoactive substances for medical use; and as a central planning scheme to ensure adequate supplies, particularly of opiates for medical use.

55.2.1 A Penal Regime to Enforce Drug Prohibition

The Single Convention, as its name conveys, replaced an array of treaties and protocols, which had accumulated since the first opium treaty, the Hague Convention of 1912. But the Single Convention went well beyond what was in the previous treaties, signalling a change in the system's orientation [9]. Whereas the prime concern of the previous treaties had been with regulating international trade in plant-derived drugs (opiates, cocaine and cannabis), the 1961 Convention introduced requirements that possession and delivery, along with a wide variety of market-related actions concerning the drugs covered, be criminalised under a country's domestic laws [4]. What had been a system concerned primarily with controlling international movement of drugs became a system committed to enforcing prohibitions on nonmedical use of the drugs, with each country's criminal laws as means of enforcement. The international prohibition system, as it now exists, can thus be said to have begun with the 1961 treaty.

The 1971 treaty greatly expanded the scope of the system by including a wide range of synthetic substances, many of them with pharmaceutical uses. The market controls in the 1971 treaty are weaker than those in the 1961 treaty, reflecting the powerful influence of the pharmaceutical industry on the treaty negotiations [18]. The requirement concerning criminalisation under domestic law is more simply stated than in the 1961 treaty, requiring penalisation of "any action contrary to a law or regulation adopted in pursuance of its obligations under this Convention". Since the Convention requires a medical prescription to authorise use of a covered drug, any possession or use without a prescription should thus be criminalised.

The 1988 treaty, as its name reveals, represented a further shift in the system's focus, with more attention focused on combatting the illicit markets which had emerged as a by-product of the prohibition system, including, for the first time, controls on precursor chemicals used in the preparation of controlled drugs. But, in an effort to eliminate any remaining ambiguity, it also included a further provision on criminalisation at the level of the individual drug user: that a signatory country should "establish as a criminal offence under its domestic law, when committed intentionally, the possession, purchase or cultivation of narcotic drugs or psychotropic substances for personal consumption".

The system of treaties inaugurated by the 1961 Convention, then, has as a main goal the elimination or at least suppression of any nonmedical use of drugs, aiming to eliminate illicit markets in drugs by a five-pronged approach: (1) particularly for drugs covered by the 1961 treaty,

by restriction of the supply of the drugs, limiting production to the estimated medical need for the drugs; (2) by a system of export and import permits, restricting legitimate trade in the drugs in accordance with a receiving country's wishes; (3) by requiring that most substances covered by the treaties be in a prescription system, as a way of confining availability to medical control and use; (4) by criminalising production, sale, and other market activities outside those permitted for drugs for medical use; and (5) by criminalising users for purchase or possession of drugs other than for medical purposes.

55.2.2 A Trading and Marketing Control Regime

The treaties also set up a trading and marketing regime, a special kind of trade treaty which aims more to structure and direct international trade, rather than the more usual main aim of trade treaties – to facilitate trade. Requiring that an import permit be issued by the receiving country before drugs can be shipped to it means that a country can control and indeed cut off the legal supply of a drug to its residents.

Although the drug treaty system was established before the formation of the current system of international trade treaties, it has served an informal function of protecting the substances under its jurisdiction from any trade disputes seeking to open up markets for controlled drugs. This contrasts with the situation for alcohol and tobacco [3, 21, 26].

55.2.3 A Central Planning Scheme to Supply Medical Needs

Particularly through the 1961 treaty and its predecessors, and particularly for opiates, the international system is intended to ensure that supplies of opium-derived drugs for medical use are available globally. Each signatory country is supposed to send to the International Narcotics Control Board (INCB) annual data on medical use of opioids and estimates of requirements for the next year. There is a system of permits for countries to grow opium to meet the demands of the medicinal market (in the mid-2010s, around half the legal supply was grown in Tasmania – [14]). Particularly with respect to opium, the aim is to create a globally controlled system of cultivation, manufacture, and supply, which will ensure that medical needs, everywhere, for opioid medications are met.

55.3 Institutional Arrangements for Implementation of the Treaties

In the United Nations system, the drug treaties come under the jurisdiction of the UN's Economic and Social Council (ECOSOC), which serves as the final deciding body for issues, such as the scheduling of drugs under the treaties, and determines whether a conference should be called to consider amendments to the treaties. The political body governing the drug system is the Commission on Narcotic Drugs (CND), with 53 member states elected by ECOSOC, but with proceedings open to attendance by other UN member states. The CND meets annually for several days in March in Vienna, in proceedings including plenary sessions, a Committee of the Whole for the discussion of proposed resolutions, and committee meetings. Each year, the CND adopts resolutions following discussions which are often lengthy, since its decisions are customarily made by consensus.

The administrative body for the system is the UN Office on Drugs and Crime (UNODC), which has responsibility also for the two UN crime treaties (on transnational organised crime and against corruption). UNODC has a limited "regular budget" as part of the UN system, and relies, for 90% of its funding, on "voluntary contributions", mainly from governments. Since these contributions are usually earmarked for specific projects, donor countries have a large say in determining the directions of the UNODC's work. In 2012, UNODC had about 500 employees, spread around the world – a smaller number than the US Drug Enforcement Agency had posted outside the USA [25].

The International Narcotics Control Board (INCB) is a board consisting of 13 individual members elected by ECOSOC, 3 of them from a list of 5 nominated by the World Health Organization. They are supposed to serve as independent experts, not as representatives of any state; a unit within the UNODC serves as the INCB's secretariat. In addition to technical duties such as running the international market for opiate medications, the INCB has regarded itself as the "guardian of the treaties", issuing an annual detailed global report on the state of compliance as the INCB defines it [5].

The World Health Organization also has responsibilities, under the 1961 and 1971 treaties, for providing scientific and medical expertise, particularly concerning the classification and scheduling of psychoactive substances under the Conventions. According to the 1971 Convention, its assessments "shall be determinative as to medical and scientific matters". These responsibilities are primarily assigned to the Expert Committee on Drug Dependence, which is supposed to be constituted every 2 years for a process involving first pre-review and then 2 years later a detailed review concerning classification of particular substances. However, the meetings were less frequent in the decade of the 2000s, due to WHO's limited resources, but have become annual since 2014, with two meetings in 2018. Recognising that the present scheduling of many substances had not been re-examined in the light of scientific and other developments for many years, an Expert Committee meeting proposed that each scheduled substance be re-reviewed every 20 years; the first ECDD review ever on cannabis was conducted in late 2018 [17], recommending that cannabis be rescheduled under the treaties to legitimate medical use. The ECDD is also charged with tackling classification of the diverse category of new psychoactive substances, of which 750 have been reported to the system since 2009. Despite the increased frequency of meetings, resources remain inadequate for the tasks the ECDD system is assigned. An ECDD meeting has also pointed out that the language of the Conventions does not map easily onto current scientific language concerning drugs [30:16, 23–35].

Over a number of years, the drug treaty system and the WHO drifted apart. A signal of this has been the divergence between the CND and WHO's Expert Committee on scheduling of specific substances [1:213–214, 2:232]. Another signal of the division had been over the place of harm reduction in the treatment of drug problems. In public health in general, the reduction of harm is a central commitment and strategy, and as the global public health agency, WHO was necessarily committed to its promotion. However, prior to 2009 the USA had insisted that the concept and term "harm reduction" not be used in the work of the international treaty agencies. After 2009, relationships between UNODC and WHO improved again, including joint work on treatment guidelines [25]. But in general, the UNDCP has operated in substantial isolation from other UN bodies [2:237].

55.4   What Can Be Said About the Effects and Impact of the System?

One measure of the success of the system is its near-universality, in terms of formal adherence to the treaties. Each year's INCB report notes with some pride the tally of countries which are signed up to each treaty. The desire for universality triumphed in the case of Bolivia's denunciation and reaccession to the 1961 treaty, despite disapproval by the INCB and other guardians of the system. Bolivia took this route to add a reservation to the treaty, which would then allow Bolivians to chew coca leaves without contravening Bolivia's treaty commitments. Thwarted in an attempt to make this change by international consensus, Bolivia denounced (announced its withdrawal from) the treaty, proposing to reaccede with a reservation concerning coca-chewing if the reservation was accepted [23]. If one-third of countries acceding to the treaty had objected, Bolivia's reaccession would not have gone into effect. It is a mark of the system's commitment to universality that there were only a few objections, despite considerable displeasure expressed by the INCB and others about Bolivia's reservation.

A second measure is in terms of its success in ensuring access to pain medication. For developed countries, this is not generally a problem. But the WHO has estimated that 80% of the world's population lacks adequate access to effective pain medication [29]. Part of the problem, of course, is a lack of resources to procure or supply the medication. But another part is the indirect result of the treaty system. In consequence of the system's emphasis on law enforcement, decisions on importation of controlled drugs are often in the hands of police, who may choose to restrict or stop imports in order to impede diversion of the medicine to illicit markets. Reflecting concern about this, the WHO Expert Committee decided that ketamine, a cheap and relatively safe anaesthetic widely used in poor countries, should not be brought under the treaties. "Concerns were raised that if ketamine were placed under international control, this would adversely impact its availability and accessibility. This in turn would limit access to essential and emergency surgery, which would constitute a public-health crisis in countries where no affordable alternative anaesthetic is available. On this basis, the Expert Committee decided that bringing ketamine under international control is not appropriate" [30:9]. Reflecting a greater priority still being placed on the prohibition of nonmedical use than on the availability of needed medications, many national delegations and three regional groupings expressed concerns or regret about the WHO's decision at the May 2013 meeting of the CND [13:11], and China pressed again on this issue for two further years [2:232].

A third measure is in terms of success in controlling legal markets. Here the system can show some success, among mixed results. The pre-Single Convention system succeeded (aided by the Depression) in substantially reducing world consumption of opium in the years prior to World War II. The current system, however, has not impeded the substantial rise, in recent years, in prescribed use of opioids in North America, which accounts for the lion's share of global use of prescribed opioids. In general, the conclusion of Bruun et al. [8] remains true: the system's successes tend to occur where "it has been the conduct of professions and private enterprise which has been influenced". Large firms and state-licensed professionals have something to gain from cooperation with a control system, and with such levers of influence drug control systems have had some successes, for instance, in getting chemical industries to control chemical precursors, and in changing doctors' prescribing patterns when drugs, such as the barbiturates, prove to be more dangerous than was thought. Nevertheless, the sharp rise in opioid use and deaths in the early twenty-first century, particularly in North America [11, 12], was to a substantial degree fuelled by prescribed medications; pharmaceutical firms and professionals involved were not sufficiently persuaded or deterred from profit-seeking by the control system. The lack of any trade disputes about drugs under the system's control, in an era when free-market ideology has been dominant, might also be regarded as an unheralded success for the system.

A fourth measure, of course, is the system's degree of success in eliminating or at least reducing illicit trade, markets, and use. Here the overall result must be viewed as a failure. In 1998, the UN system set a 10-year goal of "eliminating or significantly reducing the illicit cultivation of coca bush, the cannabis plant, and the opium poppy by the year 2008". The UNODC's 2014 Annual Report concluded "that overall the global situation … is generally stable" [27]. Twenty years after it was set, the goal of reducing illicit markets remained a vain hope.

55.5 Signs and Directions of Change

The failure of the international drug prohibition system in terms of its most public goal, of eliminating or minimising illicit markets, has been apparent for some decades. At national and subnational levels, there have been initiatives and experiments since the 1960s in moving in other directions, although these initiatives have been greatly hampered by the perceived necessity of operating within the constraints of the international system. Thus even the Dutch "coffee shop" system for quasi-legal retail sale of cannabis, the most far-reaching attempt prior to 2010 to move from an illicit to a regulated market, was handicapped by the "back door" problem – that cannabis which was sold under license at the front door had come in the back door illegally, since no way could be found to reconcile a legal wholesale supply with national obligations under the treaty [16].

But there have been signs of change in the 2010s, particularly in the Americas. A diverse array of Latin American countries have shown a growing impatience with the status quo and have been willing to push against the longstanding "Washington consensus" for the status quo on drug policies. First, several retired Latin American presidents, and then some sitting presidents, have expressed the need for new directions. The motivations have been diverse. In Mexico and Central America, the primary issue has been the carnage in their populations from a "war on drugs" aimed at cutting off the supply to the insatiable demand from northern neighbours. In Bolivia, as mentioned, legalisation of the folk custom of coca-leaf chewing has been a main concern. In countries like Uruguay, efforts to create a regulated legal cannabis market are aimed primarily at removing a main source of criminalisation of young people. With a report from the Organization of American States (OAS) exploring alternative scenarios for the future [20], these impulses at national levels took on a collective form in the region's intergovernmental agency.

At least as important have been the changes in North America, particularly concerning cannabis. In November 2012, votes on popular initiatives for regulated cannabis markets in Colorado and Washington began concrete processes of change likely to have lasting effects, no matter how the US federal government may position itself. At about the same time, trends in opinion polls among US adults for the first time showed a popular majority for legalising cannabis [28]. By the end of 2018, 9 US states had legalised commercial sales of cannabis for recreational use and 14 more had decriminalised possession [31]. Cannabis became legal throughout Canada on 17 October 2018, sold in some provinces in government stores [6]. Changes in the legal status of cannabis do not, of course, deal with the drug problem as a whole. But, since three-quarters of the illicit drug users in the world use only cannabis, in numeric terms, such changes in the status of cannabis will have a large effect.

The direction and extent of any changes in the international drug treaties and control system are still unclear. The OAS report lays out some alternative scenarios for the future. Other recent reports have laid out options for change in the treaties and have discussed more and less likely scenarios [24], including a potential Framework Convention on Cannabis, which might supersede the handling of cannabis in the Single Convention [22]. But, at least in the short run, it is more likely that changes will be piecemeal and country-specific, rather than at the system level – whether involving changes made within the rules of the system, as in the case of Bolivia, or beyond the rules, as with cannabis buyers' clubs in Spain and other parts of Europe [15] and with the North American shifts on cannabis.

national levels. The system has also been overwhelmed by the large number of "new psychoactive substances" for potential control. But there is, as yet, little appetite within the system for reform.

Clinical Relevance

In considering both patient drug use patterns and whether and what psychoactive medications to prescribe, a clinician needs to take into account the legal status of a substance. However, in terms of the drug's actions and utility, the clinician should look beyond the legal divisions between medications, illicit drugs, and legal substances like nicotine and alcohol.

There has been substantial overpromotion, in affluent societies, of psychoactive medications, particularly medicinal opioids, and clinicians need to exercise care in their prescription.

Key Points

- The international drug control system is nearly universal, but somewhat ossified and resistant to change.
- It classifies psychoactive drugs in terms of their potency and potential harm but provides for potential medical use of most controlled drugs. It does not deal with some drugs in wide use in Western societies, notably alcohol.
- It has not succeeded in its goal of eliminating illicit supply of drugs for non-medical use. It succeeds in ensuring supplies for medical use in wealthy countries, but not in much of the world, where actions against the illicit market also cut off medical supplies. Particularly in North America, there has been an oversupply and overuse of medicinal opioids.
- The system's prohibition of nonmedical cannabis and restrictions on medicinal cannabis are under siege and increasingly ignored at national and sub-

Acknowledgement Dave Bewley-Taylor and Ambros Uchtenhagen are thanked for suggestions and prompts on the first version of this article, but are not of course responsible for the results.

References

1. Babor T, Caulkins J, Edwards G, Fischer B, Foxcroft D, Humphreys K, Obot I, Rehm J, Reuter P, Room R, Rossow I, Strang J. Drug policy and the public good. 1st ed. Oxford: Oxford University Press; 2010.
2. Babor T, Caulkins J, Fischer B, Foxcroft D, Humphreys K, Medina-Mora ME, Obot I, Rehm J, Reuter P, Room R, Rossow I, Strang J. Drug policy and the public good. 2nd ed. Oxford: Oxford University Press; 2018.
3. Baumberg B, Anderson P. Trade and health: how World Trade Organization (WTO) law affects alcohol and public health. Addiction. 2008;103:1952–8.
4. Bewley-Taylor D, Jelsma M. Regime change: revisiting the 1961 single convention on narcotic drugs. Int J Drug Policy. 2012;23:72–81.
5. Bewley-Taylor D, Trace M. The INCB: watchdog or Guardian of the UN drug control conventions? Beckley Park, Oxford, UK: Beckley Foundation; 2006. http://www.beckleyfoundation.org/pdf/Report_07.pdf.

6. Bilefsky D. Legalizing recreational marijuana, Canada begins a national experiment New York Times, 17 October 2018. https://www.nytimes.com/2018/10/17/world/canada/marijuana-pot-cannabis-legalization.html.

7. Braithwaite J, Drahos P. Drugs. In: Global business regulation. Cambridge: Cambridge University Press; 2000. p. 360–98.

8. Bruun K, Pan L, Rexed I. The Gentlemen's Club: international control of drugs and alcohol. Chicago and London: University of Chicago Press; 1975.

9. Carstairs C. The stages of the international drug control system. Drug Alcohol Rev. 2005;24:57–65.

10. Courtwright DT. Mr. ATOD's wild ride: what do alcohol, tobacco, and other drugs have in common? Soc Hist Alcohol Drugs. 2005;20:105–24.

11. Fischer B, Keates A, Bühringer G, Reimer J, Rehm J. Non-medical use of prescription opioids and prescription opioid-related harms: why so markedly higher in North America compared to the rest of the world? Addiction. 2014;109(2):177–81.

12. Helmerhorst GTT, Teunis T, Janssen SJ, Ring D. An epidemic of the use, misuse and overdose of opioids and deaths due to overdose, in the United States and Canada: is Europe next? Bone Joint J. 2017;99(7):856–64.

13. IDPC. The 2013 commission on narcotic drugs: report of proceedings. London: International Drug Policy Consortium; 2013. http://idpc.net/publications/2013/05/idpc-report-of-proceedings-the-2013-commission-on-narcotic-drugs.

14. INCB. Part 3. Supply of opiate raw materials and demand for opiates for medical and scientific purposes. In: Narcotic Drugs: Estimated World Requirements for 2018; Statistics for 2016 (E/INCB/2017/2). New York: International Narcotics Control Bureau; 2017. http://www.incb.org/incb/en/narcotic-drugs/Technical_Reports/2017/narcotic-drugs-technical-report-2017.html.

15. Jelsma M. The development of international drug control: lessons learned and strategic challenges for the future. Working paper prepared for the first meeting of the global commission on drug policies, Geneva, 24–25 January 2011. http://www.canadianharmreduction.com/sites/default/files/Dvlpt%20of%20Intnl%20Drug%20Control%20-%20Lessons%20%26%20Challenges%20-%202011_0.pdf.

16. Korf D. An open front door: The coffee shop phenomenon in the Netherlands. In: Rødner Sznitman S, Olsson B, Room R, editors. A cannabis reader: global issues and local experiences – perspectives on cannabis controversies, treatment and regulation in Europe, EMCCDA monograph no, vol. 8. Luxembourg: Office for Official Publications of the European Communities; 2008. p. 140–54. http://www.emcdda.europa.eu/attachements.cfm/att_53355_EN_emcdda-cannabis-mon-full-2vols-web.pdf.

17. Mayor S. WHO proposes rescheduling cannabis to allow medical applications. BMJ. 2019;364:I574.

18. McAllister WB. Conflict of interest in the international drug control system. J Policy History. 1991;3:143–66.

19. Nutt DJ, King LA, Phillips LD. Drug harms in the UK: a multicriteria decision analysis. Lancet. 2010;376:1588–65.

20. OAS. The drug problem in the Americas. Washington, D.C.: Organization of American States; 2013. http://www.oas.org/en/media_center/press_release.asp?sCodigo=E-194/13.

21. O'Brien P. Australia's double standard on Thailand's alcohol warning labels. Drug Alcohol Rev. 2013;32:5–10.

22. Room R, Fischer B, Hall W, Lenton S, Reuter P. Cannabis policy: moving beyond stalemate. Oxford: Oxford University Press; 2010.

23. Room R. Reform by subtraction: the path of denunciation of international drug treaties and reaccession with reservations. Int J Drug Policy. 2012;23:401–6.

24. Room R, editor. Roadmaps to reforming the UN drug conventions. Beckley Park, Oxford, UK: Beckley Foundation; 2012. http://www.beckleyfoundation.org/wp-content/uploads/2012/12/Roadmaps_to_Reform.pdf.

25. Room R, Reuter P. How well do international drug conventions protect public health? Lancet. 2012;379:84–91.

26. Shaffer ER, Brenner JE, Houston TP. International trade agreements: a threat to tobacco control policy. Tobacco Control. 2005;14(Suppl II):ii19–25. http://www.ncbi.nlm.nih.gov/pmc/articles/PMC1766197/pdf/v014p0ii19.pdf.

27. UNODC. UNODC Annual Report. Vienna: united nations office on drugs and crime, 2014. https://www.unodc.org/documents/AnnualReport2014/Annual_Report_2014_WEB.pdf.

28. Walsh J. Q&A: legal marijuana in Colorado and Washington. Washington, D.C.: Brookings Institution; 2013. http://www.brookings.edu/research/papers/2013/05/21-legal-marijuana-colorado-washington.

29. WHO. Access to controlled medications programme. In: Briefing note. Geneva: World Health Organization; 2007. http://www.who.int/medicines/areas/quality_safety/ACMP_BrNoteGenrl_EN_Feb09.pdf.

30. WHO. WHO expert committee on drug dependence: thirty-fifth report. Geneva: World Health Organization; 2012. http://apps.who.int/iris/bitstream/10665/77747/1/WHO_trs_973_eng.pdf

31. Wikipedia. Legality of cannabis by U.S. jurisdiction. 2018. Accessed 27 Dec. https://en.wikipedia.org/wiki/Legality_of_cannabis_by_U.S._jurisdiction.

Ethical and Legal Aspects of Interventions in Addiction Treatment

56

Ambros Uchtenhagen

Contents

Abstract

The United Nations (UN) conventions present the international legal framework; they urge member states to provide treatment and rehabilitation but prohibit consumption and possession of scheduled drugs. This creates problems for providing treatment and harm reduction programs to patients who are not or not yet ready to stop illicit drug use. Other international documents, notably from the World Health Organization and the United Nations Office on Drugs and Crime, are strongly in favor of agonist substitution treatment and harm reduction measures. Within this framework, national legislation has much room for diverse preferences; the International Narcotic Control Board regularly comments the national practices, as well as the European Monitoring Centre for Drugs and Drug Addiction for the EU member states. An international trend gradually prefers therapeutic measures over criminal sanctions for drug users.

The international ethical framework is set by the universal declaration and European convention on human rights, striking a balance between individual rights and societal interests. Less ambiguous guidance comes from medical ethics claiming the full range of patient's rights for addicted persons.

Note: Some of the material is based on earlier work of the author about ethical aspects of treatment and care in addiction [50–53].

A. Uchtenhagen (✉)
Swiss Research Foundation for Public Health and Addiction, Zurich University, Zurich, Switzerland
e-mail: ambros.uchtenhagen@isgf.uzh.ch

The respective conduct codes for medical professions are regional or national and include procedures how to deal with ethical conflicts. Conflicting situations frequently occur, for example, around the principles of autonomy or of confidentiality.

An essential ethical element of treatment is its effectiveness and avoidance of harm, asking for scientific evaluation of therapeutic approaches, services, and systems. The ethical acceptability of agonist substitution treatment and of harm reduction measures is based on rigorous evidence of their effectiveness. Other aspects concern the limits of social acceptability of addictive behavior and the limits of what can be attained for an individual patient by therapeutic interventions; avoidance of harm often is the more immediate objective than full recovery. In a public health perspective, effects at population level rather than at individual level are a priority, aiming at good coverage of treatment needs by good accessibility and affordability of services.

56.1 Introduction

Addiction treatment is historically, and until present, guided by the basic understanding of addictive behavior. Interventions are shaped accordingly to prevailing paradigms explaining substance use and substance dependence. Legislation is a preferred instrument to limit consumption and addictive behavior, through preventive interventions as well as sanctions. The development of liberal societies caring for individual freedom and responsibility, less interference with lifestyles and personal choices, and the need for ethical standards in human behavior came to the forefront and resulted in various rules guiding interventions and therapist's conduct. This process in the area of addiction treatment has been taken at hand, but with persisting differences in orientation and a need for conflict management.

56.2 International Frameworks and National Diversities

56.2.1 Legal Aspects

56.2.1.1 The International Framework: The United Nations Conventions

The UN conventions of 1961, 1971, and 1988 have some implications for delivering addiction treatment.

The Single Convention urges "to take all practicable measures for the prevention of abuse of drugs and for the early identification, treatment, education, after-care, rehabilitation, and social reintegration of the persons involved." While this Article 38 does not indicate how treatment should be delivered, Resolution II declares that "one of the most effective methods of treatment for addiction is treatment in a hospital institution having a drug free atmosphere," and urges the provision of such facilities [56].

The Convention on Psychotropic Substances of 1971 [57] restricts the "use and possession of, substances in Schedules II, III and IV to medical and scientific purposes," thereby criminalizing patients in treatment who continue, sporadically or regularly, to use illicit drugs (schedules II, III, and IV include drugs such as barbiturates, benzodiazepines, and buprenorphine). Art. 7 states, for schedule I drugs, to "prohibit all use except for scientific and very limited medical purposes by duly authorized persons." What the limitations are is open to interpretation. Art. 9 requires "that substances in Schedules II, III and IV be supplied or dispensed for use by individuals pursuant to medical prescription only, except when individuals may lawfully obtain, use, dispense or administer such substances in the duly authorized exercise of therapeutic or scientific functions." Licensed pharmacists, however, may "supply, at their discretion and without prescription, for use for medical purposes by individuals in exceptional cases, small quantities, within limits to be defined by the Parties, of substances in Schedules III and IV." Art. 20 urges to "take all practicable measures for the prevention of abuse of psychotropic substances and for the early identification, treatment, education, after-care, rehabilitation and social reintegration of the persons involved." Also, treatment may be provided either as an alternative to conviction or punishment or, in addition to punishment, if abusers of psychotropic substances have committed such offences (Art. 22).

According to the 1988 Convention [58], preparatory acts for personal use of scheduled substances are criminal offences (Art. 3,2):

> Subject to its constitutional principles and the basic concepts of its legal system, each Party shall adopt such measures as may be necessary to establish as a criminal offence under its domestic law, when committed intentionally, the possession, purchase or cultivation of narcotic drugs or psychotropic substances for personal consumption contrary to the provisions of the 1961 Convention, the 1961 Convention as amended or the 1971 Convention.

Implicitly, this includes criminalization of use (no use without preparatory acts). The International Narcotic Control Board (INCB) was set up in 1968, with the main task to control and facilitate the implementation of the Single Convention at national level. The following conventions have revised and restated the functions of the Board.

In summary, the UN conventions urge the treatment and rehabilitation of drug abusers but prohibit the consumption of narcotics and psychotropic substances (including tranquilizers and sedatives), which creates problems for patients in treatment (continued use is often a reason to exclude patients from treatment) and even more problems for harm reduction approaches designed to diminish the medical risks of substance use (for persons in addiction treatment and outside of treatment). Agonist maintenance treatment is viewed critically by INCB as a potential source of diversion of narcotics to the illegal market [29]. However, the conventions allow diversion to treatment as an alternative to punishment.

56.2.1.2 Other International Frameworks

Some international documents are mentioned here with relevance to addiction treatment and specifically in regard to agonist maintenance treatment and harm reduction interventions. These evidence-based documents present strong recommendations which are not legally binding.

The World Health Organization (WHO) and the United Nations Office on Crime and Drugs (UNODC) published Principles of Drug Dependence Treatment in 2008. This chapter is in strong support of agonist maintenance treatment for opioid dependence: "Opioid agonist pharmacotherapy is one of the most effective treatment options for opioid dependence when methadone or buprenorphine are administered at an individualized dosage for a period of several months to years." The chapter also urges to implement legal frameworks, which guarantee protection from potential sanctions for those seeking treatment [69].

The UNODC, WHO, and United Nations Programme on HIV/AIDS (UNAIDS) "Technical Guide for countries to set targets for universal access to HIV prevention, treatment and care for injecting drug users," published in 2009, has a range of preventive measures (e.g., needle and syringe exchange programs) among its recommendations, thereby complementing the treatment recommendations [59].

In Europe, the EU Action Plan 2005–2008 [16] foresaw harm reduction measures as a specific action for the implementation of Objective 14 (prevention of health risks related to drug use) and Objective 15 (availability and access to harm reduction services). The implementation process and the available evidence on outcomes are presented in a monograph [41].

56.2.1.3 Diversity of National Legislation

At the national level, narcotic laws and policy guidelines mirror a diversity of principles, priorities, and preferences, even when countries have ratified the UN conventions. Treatment of substance abuse is one of the essential elements, but how it is defined, for whom it is available, under which circumstances, and which approaches are officially accepted are all subject to major differences. One example is the national guidelines for substitution treatments of opiate dependence; an analysis of 28 national guidelines found a large variety of indication criteria and practices [53].

At present, the diversity of legislations and regulations is best documented in regard to Cannabis. The alternatives to prohibition, in the sense of the UN conventions, range from decriminalization of use and preparatory acts for personal use to a replacement of illicit markets by tolerated controlled markets without legalization, to partial or full legalization in analogy to alcohol and tobacco. *Decriminalization* means or preferring administrative instead of criminal sanctions, or no sanctions within age limits and allowed quantities. A *tolerated controlled market* is based on issuing licenses for production, marketing, and sale of cannabis products under specified conditions. Compliance with the conditions is controlled and licenses are withdrawn in case of non-compliance. License holders pay taxes for their profits. *Legalization* may be restricted for defined target groups (e.g., residents only, medical cannabis prescribed to patients suffering from specified conditions, adult members of cannabis social clubs). Legal availability of cannabis may be restricted with age limits, quantities allowed per time period, and Tetrahydrocannabinol (THC) content in order to prevent negative effects of use. Maximum prices apply in certain jurisdictions, in order to avoid a competitive illegal market with lower prices (overview in Uchtenhagen 2016).

An official source of information on problems with the implementation of the UN conventions is presented in the annual reports of the International Narcotic Control Board (INCB). The 2011 report includes, for example, information on unacceptable treatment problems, such as diversion of prescribed pain medications or allowing safe injection rooms ([29], p. 38). The setting up of the lack of aftercare is admonished (p. 59). On the other hand, large compulsory treatment centers are mentioned (p. 78), as well

as detoxification, rehabilitation, and counseling services (p. 83); opiate substitution treatment (p. 51, 78); and needle/syringe exchange programs (p. 51), without indicating their acceptability and outcomes.

The 2018 report provides, in Chap. 1, recent developments in the use and regulation of the medical use of Cannabinoids and Cannabis, as well as recent changes in national legislation in regard of non-medical cannabis use (legalizing production, sale, possession, and consumption). Concerns are expressed about diversion of medical cannabis for non-medical use, weakening public awareness of risks resulting in facilitating legalization of non-medical cannabis. Chap. 2 provides information about the compliance with the treaties by national authorities in member states. Chap. 3 gives a detailed overview on the worldwide situation in the production and use of scheduled drugs worldwide, followed by Chap. 4 with recommendations (not legally binding) to governments and involved organizations.

A complete and updated collection of national drug laws and drug policies is presented by the European Monitoring Centre on Drugs and Drug Abuse (EMCDDA); it includes not only the EU member states but also acceding and candidate countries as well as neighboring and Central Asian countries [15]. The same source provides systematic information on treatment approaches and harm reduction approaches in these countries.

56.2.1.4 Sanctions

Use and possession of illegal drugs for personal use are prohibited in a range of countries. For Europe, an analysis of national practices is presented [14]. Only rarely, prison sentences are handed out in case of infraction. In other regions, imprisonment and compulsory treatment are more common, for example, in labor camps [67].

In some countries, drug possession is an offence, which may entail imprisonment or even capital punishment. A systematic overview is not available. In Islamic law, use of any drugs including alcohol is prohibited and sanctioned, but it also provides care for those suffering from medical conditions.

A high-level organization, the Global Commission for Drug Policy, strongly recommends to avoid criminal sanctions for the use of all scheduled drugs and the stigmatization of all substance users [21].

Agonist maintenance therapy is prohibited in Russia [37], while a growing number of countries support and expand this approach, replacing criminal sanctions.

56.2.2 Ethical Aspects

56.2.2.1 Ethical Basis of Interventions: Human Rights

The Universal Declaration of Human Rights [54] contains a number of relevant conditions, such as no discrimination (Art. 2), no degrading or inhuman treatment (Art. 5), and right of equal access to medical care and social services (Art. 25/1), but also that everyone has duties to the community (Art. 29/1) and that limitations of rights and freedom are admissible on the basis of "just requirements of morality, public order and the general welfare" (Art. 29/2).

In view of conflicts this may create, a recent initiative proposes the formulation of meta-rules, providing guidance on how to resolve conflicts in human rights [4].

The European Convention on Human Rights [7] further stipulates that a person's liberty may be deprived in case of lawful detention of alcoholics or drug addicts (Art. 5/1/e), with a right to appeal to a court (Art. 5/4).

In summary, these statements try to establish a balance between protecting the individual rights of the person and respecting the needs of society for public order, general welfare, and even morality. There is large room for interpretation, so that every society can decide on the compatibility of addictive behavior with the nature and extent of the above-mentioned requirements. Compulsory measures against persons with substance dependence may be admissible on the basis of national laws.

A step further is made in the EU, where the Commission has issued guidelines on the regulation of patient rights. A growing number of member states have adopted laws or regulations, granting patients the right to self-determination (no interventions without informed consent) and confidentiality [17]. Only exceptionally, involuntary interventions are allowed, for example in cases of criminal behavior or deficient power of judgment. This creates a new ethical dilemma in case of serious destructive behavior as a symptom of the patient's condition. It is argued that treating physicians in such a case have a responsibility to protect the patient from the negative consequences of behavior, even through involuntary intervention.

Again a new situation has been created with the UN Convention on the Rights of disabled persons (CRPD), in force since May 2008, ratified by 177 member states [55]. This convention grants all human rights to persons with any kind of disability, including psychiatric conditions and therefore also with substance use disorders. Some of the specific rights cover the freedom of accommodation, of mobility, of social participation, not easy to be reconciled with addictive behaviors. All signatories are obliged to send annually a report to the Secretary General on how these rights are implemented at the national level.

56.2.2.2 Ethical Basis of Interventions: Medical Ethics

Medical ethics apply only if and inasmuch as substance dependence is understood as a medical condition. This has been the official position of the leading medical organizations since decades (and brain research has identified it as a "brain disease," thereby giving it a biological basis) [33]. The substance-dependent person is a patient and should enjoy the status and all the rights of patients.

The current medical science defines substance dependence as a condition with diagnostic criteria, described in the generally acknowledged diagnostic systems, such as International Classification of Diseases ICD-10 of World Health Organization [68] and Diagnostic-Statistical Manual of Mental Disorders DSM-IV TR of the American Psychiatric Association [2]. The criteria include biological symptoms (tolerance, withdrawal symptoms in case of discontinued use), psychological symptoms (craving, desire to reduce consumption), and behavioral symptoms (loss of control over consumption, consuming in spite of perceived negative consequences).

ICD-10 includes a diagnosis of harmful use (with negative health consequences of use), while DSM-IV includes a diagnosis of abuse. These conditions are also considered to be a medical condition inviting therapeutic interventions.

What are the consequences for the treatment of addiction? Examples of the general conduct codes are the Standards of Conduct of the American Medical Association [1] and the Good Medical Practice of the British General Medical Council [22]. Main issues are the patient's autonomy of decision, informed consent, dignity and confidentiality, nondiscriminatory beneficence, and non-maleficence, but also keeping up professional standards by continued education and networking with other services and colleagues in order to provide the best possible care. In addition, the American recommendations include a responsibility to seek change in official or legal requirements, which are contrary to the best interests of the patient. These codes usually acknowledge the occurrence of ethical conflicts and provide links for support in such cases.

In the absence of specific rules for the treatment of substance dependence, the general ethical rules for good medical practice apply. The four major principles are as follows: do no harm, improve the well-being, respect the autonomy, and apply justice. It is obvious that even these few principles cannot be followed without creating conflict [43].

Involuntary intervention to prevent harm is in conflict with the autonomy of an unwilling patient. Treating all patients as being equal (principle of justice) is impossible where the resources are limited. Also confidentiality and data protection often are in conflict with administrative and law enforcement interests in case of illicit drug use. All such conflicts must be carefully examined, in the best interest of all concerned. When the patient's interests collide with those of relatives or other third parties, a common solution

must be found to the extent possible. It is advisable to recur to an ethical consilium if major consequences are expected from the decision. The principle of respecting the autonomy of the patient must never be overruled in the name of some abstract societal value without the presence of concrete harm implications for others.

56.2.2.3 Ethical Justification of Interventions

Human rights as well as medical ethics mention the interests of society, which may be in conflict with the interests of the individual. In fact, the ethical justification to interfere with a person's substance use or dependence resides in negative societal consequences. In the case of substance dependence, treatment is justified in order to avoid such negative consequences. Among the appropriate measures are all treatments which help to bring a majority of people with addictive behavior or dependence into treatment, without disregarding their autonomy, and to optimize accessibility of treatment services. In the case of hazardous and harmful use, treatment by early and short interventions (e.g., motivational interviewing) can have positive effects.

As in other medical fields, therapeutic interventions are justifiable if efficient and effective. This principle is part of what is named "consequential ethics," in contrast to dogmatic ethics which call for complying with a given norm whatever the consequences may be. A good example of consequential ethics is the acceptance of harm reduction measures for persons using drugs. On the one hand, a growing number of research findings on positive effects of harm reduction measures justify their integration into the range of interventions for substance users and substance dependence. On the other hand, a dogmatic position is exemplified with the refusal of all interventions except detoxification and abstinence-oriented treatment.

Substance use is a factor in many social and cultural events, as a facilitator of social contact and a source of emotional well-being but also of destructive or aggressive behavior. The acceptable limits of intoxication and behavior, of substances used, and of opportunities for consumption, are culture specific and are to be respected when dealing with substance dependence [11]. For instance, a major difference between Western and Asian cultures is the place of the individual within the family system; while the individual's interests and autonomy are a core concept of most Western psychotherapies, the integrity and the interests of the family are the higher value in many Asian societies.

In a paternalistic attitude, substance-dependent persons must be protected against wasting their personal resources and potential achievements. However, such an attitude collides with the present position that interference is only justified on the basis of negative consequences of a person's behavior for others. Also, many people have lived or live a productive life in spite of their substance dependence, and to interfere with their lifestyle would cause more ethical concerns than to respect their autonomy.

Developing one's own resources and shaping one's own life is to be facilitated by education and by societal organization, but it is ultimately in the responsibility of the person itself. Conditional are the freedom of choice and the freedom of the will. Is addiction leaving any room for choices, is it a negation of free will and therefore the basis for involuntary intervention? This has been debated extensively. At present and on the basis of research evidence, we have a more differentiated view. The decision of many to change their lifestyle and go to treatment [5, 12] or to stop the dependence without professional support (the so-called self-healers) [31] demonstrates the ability of many persons with substance dependence or addictive behavior to make a choice and stick to it.

This notion is reinforced by observations of regaining consumption control by former addicts [30], and that not the substance alone but also the personality and the social environment had a role in the development of dependence, and that many users keep their consumption under control or regain control under more favorable conditions [42, 71].

A basic ambivalence – substance dependence as a medical condition or a moral weakness – is reflected in the opposition of medical and moral treatment. Moral treatment is understood to be educational and admonishing. The medical approach is to help the addict in getting motivated for change by appropriate empathy and information, while confrontation and reproaches risk reinforcing the resistance against any change. It is important to give the patient the feeling that they are taking the decisions and doing the necessary steps forward themselves. Special methods have been developed for enhancing the motivation for change, and they have become an important element in today's treatment of alcohol and other drug problems [25, 39].

In summary, treatment of substance dependence is expected to help the individual to make his own choices and to regain self-responsibility, rather than to make the decisions for him.

56.2.2.4 The Goals of Treatment: A Hierarchy of Objectives

The goals to be reached through treatments of substance dependence (and which therefore are the criteria for measuring outcome in treatment evaluation research) have changed over the last decades. While the goal of abstinence was traditionally on top of the list, the present situation can be summarized as follows: the primary goal is the patient's survival, moving to health improvements (or at least prevention of deterioration), to improvements in social integration, to reductions in substance use (moving away from addictive behavior), to improvements in quality of life (as defined subjectively by the patient), and ultimately resulting in a responsible and satisfactory lifestyle. Abstinence is not always needed for reaching these objectives, nor does abstinence guarantee to reach them.

A national example of listing the objectives is given in the report on Models of Care by the UK Department of Health [8]:

- Reduction of psychological, social, and other problems directly related to drug use
- Reduction of psychological, social, or other problems not directly attributable to drug use
- Reduction of harmful or risky behaviors associated with the use of drugs (e.g., sharing injecting equipment)

- Attainment of controlled, nondependent, or non-problematic drug use
- Abstinence from main problem drugs
- Abstinence from all drugs

This document fully endorses the principle of consequential ethics in prioritizing the reduction of the various forms of drug-related harm, including social, medical, legal, and financial problems, until the drug-dependent patient is ready and able to come off drugs.

56.2.2.5 Cure or Care?

Treatment is often identified with cure (in the sense of healing an illness), while care means serving a chronic patient without chances for healing. As such, care is an equivalent to harm reduction, meaning all interventions designed to improve the health and social status of a chronic addict who continues a dependent behavior (harm reduction is more than HIV prevention). The present debate on treatment and harm reduction is often a debate on opposing principles of action which cannot be reconciled. In this debate, harm reduction has been disqualified as an approach to prolong dependence, to make substance use acceptable for young people, and to undermine the readiness of addicts for treatment. A recent movement to promote recovery as a complete resocialization without drugs disqualifies agonist maintenance treatment, which is only accepted as "maintenance to abstinence."

Today, in the light of the updated treatment objectives, harm reduction is considered an ally rather than an opponent of treatment. Accordingly, the treatment system must be an integrated system that enables abstinence and harm reduction services to work together, in order to provide a continuum of care, including:

- Easily accessible low threshold services that meet the immediate needs of continuing drug users
- Clear processes for motivating users to move away from drug-dependent lifestyles
- Clear processes for referring users into structured treatment programs that promote stabilization or abstinence (quoted from Ref. [46], p. 6)

56.2.2.6 Tailoring Treatment to Individual Needs

Bearing in mind the diversity of etiology, symptoms, and stages of substance dependence, it becomes obvious that treatment cannot be uniform for all dependent persons. In addition, treatment needs in different age groups and other target groups (gender, ethnicity, comorbidity, etc.) may differ considerably as well. Treatment must respond to the specific needs of an individual patient, on the basis of a comprehensive needs assessment and a treatment planning process where patient and therapist work together on a shared understanding of what is needed and what should be done.

This concept of a needs-based treatment has been intensively researched. I mention two large studies from USA: the National Treatment Improvement Evaluation Study (NTIES) documented the results of needs-based treatment planning and found a significant correlation between 1-year outcomes (measured as drug-free urines) and the number of needs included in the treatment plan [24]. A comparison of basic, average, and enhanced services for heroin dependence evidenced better retention and outcomes in services, where psychiatric and social care was available to patients [35]. In both studies, covering the needs for psychiatric care and living conditions (housing, jobs) was found to be especially important. This again has consequences for the hierarchy of objectives: a reduction of substance use is facilitated by improved living conditions and not necessarily their precondition. "Matching treatment settings, interventions, and services to an individual's particular problems and needs is critical to his or her ultimate success in returning to productive functioning in the family, workplace, and society" is therefore one of the principles of addiction treatment [40].

56.2.2.7 Public Health Interventions Versus Individual Care

Coverage of Treatment Needs Reaching the majority of drug injectors became a primary objective in order to slow down the HIV epidemic. The public health priority is to offer treatment to all persons in need of treatment.

Individual care is optimized by high-quality treatment, but public health cannot accept high-quality standards for a few as long as the many are not reached adequately. This principle includes monitoring of the treatment needs in a given population and, accordingly, careful planning of the treatment system as a whole. The responsibilities – ethically and professionally – are well distributed: medical practitioners are responsible for good individual care, service directors are responsible for good practice in their services, and health authorities are responsible for good coverage of treatment needs.

Cost Effectiveness of Interventions When caring for the treatment system as a whole, the next step is to take the responsibility for making best use of the available human and financial resources for treatment. This means to look at how much effective treatment is provided at what costs. It does not suffice to give a priority to treatments with good evidence for effectiveness but to treatments which provide effectiveness at the lowest costs in terms of staff and budget. A recent approach was efforts which intend to make best use of resources through models of stepped care, matching patients to specific treatments, on the basis of their characteristics and needs (see Chap. 82 "Stepped Care Models in Addiction" in this section).

Harm Reduction An efficient protection of public health goes beyond providing treatment for substance-dependent persons. It includes all measures which are effective in protecting the health and social status of active users, in the interest of users as well as of the population at large.

Accessibility and Affordability of Treatment Neglect of patients in need of treatment can take many forms. For instance, an analysis of national guidelines for substitution treatments of opiate dependence showed a range of restrictive access criteria, such as minimal age, minimal duration of dependence, polydrug use, and lack of confidentiality, and likewise restrictive criteria for a continuation of treatment, such as persistent illicit substance use or bureaucratic limitation of treatment duration [53]. Other examples are the denial of social support and/or medical care to active alcohol or drug users or smokers. Examples are the denial of liver transplants to persons with alcohol problems, in spite of research evidence that survival rates in those who continue to drink are not lower than in other patients [19], and the denial of Hepatitis C treatment with Interferon to active drug injectors on the basis of wrongly presumed lack of compliance [10]. Excluding addiction treatment from health insurance and reserving treatment to those who can pay for it are other examples.

In summary, the ethical implications are obvious: without appropriate accessibility and affordability of treatment, there is no way to reach the "health for all" goal of good coverage and of treating all patients as equal.

Quasi-Compulsory and Compulsory Treatment Is it advisable to force individuals with addictive behavior or dependence into treatment, when they are not motivated to engage in it by themselves, in view of an objective of optimal coverage? It is a common understanding that those individuals do not opt for treatment unless there is some external or internal force behind such a decision. The forces are quite different, ranging from health concerns to social pressure by family or employer to legal pressure in order to avoid losing the driver's license or going to prison. This is called the "continuum of coercion" [61]. The scientific evidence on the effectiveness of such "coercion" is contradictory [23, 70]. A recent multi-country study on quasi-compulsory treatment (QCT, treatment on court order as an alternative to imprisonment, with the consent of the patient) documented that perceived pressure does not translate into higher motivation; no significant differences in outcome were found between QCT patients and control groups of voluntary patients [46].

Coercion through mutually agreed consequences of substance use during treatment (contingency management) is recognized to be helpful, but more so when using positive rein-forcers than sanctions [38, 44]. From an ethical standpoint, it is reluctantly accepted under the term of "Ulysses coercion" (Odysseus wanted to be bound to the mast of his ship in order to resist the temptations of the sirens, [48]).

In summary, the findings indicate that coercion may have a role in supporting patient motivation for change, on the basis of informed consent, but it cannot replace motivation by compulsory measures without consent.

56.2.2.8 The Case of Agonist Maintenance Treatment

Rationale and Origins At first view, prescribing agonists with dependence liability to persons suffering from substance dependence seems to be paradox. One of the main arguments against agonist prescribing refers to a prolongation of dependence, which is considered to be unethical. How can we understand the rise and successes of this therapeutic approach (also known under the terms substitution or replacement treatment)? The main objective is to replace uncontrolled use of an addictive substance, by the controlled provision of a medication acting on the same receptors, as the original substance. The secondary objectives to be reached are reduction of the uncontrolled substance use, reduction of adverse health and social effects of uncontrolled use (including a reduction in drug-related delinquency), and normalization of lifestyle (including drug-free social contacts, improved housing, and employment conditions). These objectives are in line with the hierarchy outlined above. The primary objective is reached by prescribing and controlled intake of an agonist, the secondary objectives by eliminating the need to purchase the original substance of dependence and by ancillary care.

The introduction of agonist maintenance treatment is closely linked to the experience of unsuccessful detoxification and abstinence-based treatment. Maintenance without substitution of the problem drug was practiced in Roman times (the emperor Marc Aurel was maintained on opium by Galenus, the eminent physician), and daily dosages of opium were provided to

dependent persons in Southeast Asia in the nine-teenth century [62]; ironically, after the ban of opium, these persons switched to heroin [63]. First attempts at substitution were to replace opium by alcohol in the sixteenth century [13], morphine by heroin [32], and morphine by cocaine [20] in the nineteenth century. These attempts were far from being successful. A first well-designed and scientifically based model was developed by Dole and Nyswander: the methadone maintenance scheme [9]. They used oral methadone, a full opiate agonist with a longer half-life than injected heroin (controlled intake of one dose per day can block the heroin craving effectively). The model included ancillary care for medical and social conditions of enrolled patients.

Apart from opiate replacement, only nicotine replacement has been introduced into present medical practice, while former alcohol maintenance for alcoholics is discontinued.

Result Methadone maintenance is one of the most frequently and best researched therapeutic approaches. Extensive reviews of the pharmacological aspects, of service delivery, and of therapeutic outcomes, have been published [3, 18, 27, 49, 60]. In addition to methadone, buprenorphine and retarded morphine have been introduced and researched as replacement medicines in the treatment of opioid dependence, with similar outcomes. For chronic opiate individuals who failed to profit from those agonist maintenance treatments, pharmaceutical heroin was tested and introduced as a "last resort" therapeutic approach with equally good results [47]. The positive findings in terms of health and social improvements, including a massive reduction of delinquency, were complemented by the fact that agonist maintenance treatment has the greatest potential to bring heroin-dependent persons into contact with therapy and care. It therefore became one of the most welcome instruments for limiting the spread of blood-borne diseases – HIV/Aids and hepatitis – among drug injectors. The reduction of risky injecting behavior and of seroconversion rates in methadone patients became evidenced for community-based programs [36] and for prison-based programs [45]. Economic evaluation documented the cost-effectiveness of methadone and buprenorphine maintenance treatment [6].

Based on the evidence, methadone and buprenorphine have been scheduled by the World Health Organization as essential medicines [64, 65]. Also, international evidence-based scientific guidelines for agonist maintenance treatments have been published [66].

Concerns A major concern was a weakening of the motivation to change and therefore a prolongation of addictive behavior through agonist maintenance treatment. There is no evidence for this claim. A multisite major cohort study showed a relapse rate of methadone maintenance patients to daily opiate use of only 27% at 12-year follow-up [34]. The Drug Abuse Treatment Outcome Study (DATOS) study from USA and the National Treatment Outcome Research Study (NTORS) study of the UK, both multisite prospective cohort studies, found comparable outcomes at 5-year follow-up in patients who were enrolled in residential drug-free and in methadone maintenance treatment [26, 28].

In summary, the ethical justification of agonist maintenance treatment in the modern form was to provide otherwise treatment-resistant heroin addicts with an effective approach to improve their health and social situation without asking for total abstinence from narcotic substances.

56.2.2.9 Conflicts in Ethical and Legal Orientation

In numerous concrete situations, human rights and medical ethics are difficult or impossible to respect as well as national or local legal conditions. A number of such situations has have been indicated throughout this text. Sometimes, an appropriate conflict management may help, especially if the application of an opportunity principle is permitted. In other situations, there is no such solution. The way out is indicated by the ethical code of AMA: to engage in an effort to change laws which prove to be incompatible with responsible care for the addicts [1].

56.3 Conclusion

The essential ethical message is well summarized in the WHO international guidelines for the psychosocially assisted pharmacological treatment of opioid dependence [66]:

> **Clinical Relevance**
> When making clinical decisions for the treatment of people with opioid dependence, ethical principles should be considered, together with evidence from clinical trials; the human rights of opioid dependent individuals should always be respected. Treatment decisions should be based on standard principles of medical care ethics – providing equitable access to treatment and psychosocial support that best meets the needs of the individual patient. Treatment should respect and validate the autonomy of the individual, with patients being fully informed about the risks and benefits of treatment choices. Furthermore, programs should create supportive environments and relationships to facilitate treatment, provide coordinated treatment of comorbid mental and physical disorders, and address relevant psychosocial factors.
>
> There is not much to be added. The statement applies fully as the main recommendation for all treatments of substance dependence. It is a perpetual agenda for future generations. The task is to update the key elements of this chapter: the legal framework for the treatment of addictive behavior and dependence, at international, national, and local levels; to reflect the ethical positions, their consequences, and limitations in the best interest of patients and all other concerned population segments; the changing societal norms as well as the changing background and needs of the individual patients.

Key Points

Clinicians engaged in the treatment and
care of addicted persons find, in this chapter, the necessary information needed to
keep their interventions within legal and
ethical guidelines and to shape institutional
care concepts accordingly, in the interest of
acceptability and adequacy to societal and
patient expectations.

References

1. AMA. Principles of medical ethics. In: Code of medical ethics. Chicago: American Medical Association;
   2001.
2. APA. Diagnostic and statistical manual of mental disorders DSM IV TR. Arlington: American Psychiatric
   Association; 2000.
3. Arif A, Westermeyer J. Methadone maintenance in the
   management of opioid dependence: an international
   review. New York: Praeger; 1990.
4. Arosemena G. Conflicts of rights in international
   human rights: a meta-rule analysis. Glob Const.
   2013;2:6–36.
5. Bergmark A. Specific and contextual treatment mechanisms. Nordic Stud Alcohol Drugs.
   2008;25:277–85.
6. Connock M, Juarez-Garcia A, Jowett S, Frew E, Liu Z,
   Taylor RJ, Fry-Smith A, Day E, Lintzeris N, Roberts
   T, Burls A, Taylor RS. Methadone and buprenorphine
   for the management of opioid dependence: a systematic review and economic evaluation. Health Technol
   Assess. 2007;11:1–171.
7. Council of Europe. Convention for the protection of
   human rights and dignity of the human being with
   regard to the application of biology and medicine:
   convention on human rights and biomedicine. Rome:
   Council of Europe; 1950.
8. Department of Health. Models of care for substance
   misuse treatment. Promoting quality, efficiency and
   effectiveness in drug misuse treatment services.
   London: Department of Health; 2002.
9. Dole VP, Nyswander ME. A medical treatment
   for diacetyl-morphine (heroin) addiction. JAMA.
   1965;193:646–50.
10. Edlin BR, Keal KH, Lorwock J, Kral AH, Ciccarone
    DH, Moore LD, Lo B. Is it justifiable to withhold
    treatment for hepatitis C from illicit drug users? New
    Engl J Med. 2001;345:211–5.
11. Edwards G, Arif A. Dug problems in a socio-cultural
    context. A basis for policy and programme plan-
    ning. Public health papers No. 73. World Health
    Organisation, Geneva. 1980.
12. Ekendahl M. Will and skill – an exploratory study
    of substance abuser's attitudes towards life-style
    changes. Eur Addict Res. 2007;13:148–55.
13. Elliot HM. Memoirs of Jahangir. Lahore: Islamic
    Book Service; 1920.
14. EMCDDA. Special issue 2009. Drug offences; sen-
    tencing and other outcomes. European Monitoring
    Centre on Drugs and Drug Addiction, Lisbon. http://
    www.emcdda.europa.eu/publications/selected-issues/
    sentencing-statistics. 2009. Accessed 14 Feb 2013.
15. EMCDDA. http://www.emcdda.europa.eu/publica-
    tions/country-overviews. 2012.
16. EU. EU drug action plan. Brussels, Amtsblatt der
    Europäischen Union 2005/C168/01. 2005.
17. European Commission. Patients rights in the European
    Union. Report on a mapping exercise. Publication
    Office of the European Union, Luxembourg. 2016.
18. Farrell M, Ward J, Mattick R, Hall W, Stimson GV,
    des Jarlais D, Gossop M, Strang J. Methadone main-
    tenance treatment in opiate dependence: a review. Brit
    Med J. 2004;309:997–1001.
19. Fireman M, Rabkin JM. Outcome of liver transplan-
    tation in patients with alcohol and other chemical
    dependence. Psychosomatics. 2001;42:172–3.
20. Freud S. Über coca. Centralblatt für die gesamte
    Therapie. 1884;2:289–314.
21. GCDPR. The global commission on drug policy
    report. www.globalcommissionondrugs.org/wp-con-
    tent/uploads/2017/10/GCDP_War on drugs. 2011.
22. General Medical Council. Good medical practice.
    Regulating doctors. Ensuring good medical practice.
    London: General Medical Council; 2006.
23. Gerdner A. Patient and programme factors with
    impact on outcome in Swedish compulsory care
    of addicts: a systematic review. Lund University,
    Sweden. 1998.
24. Gerstein DR, Datta AR, Ingels JS, Johnson RA,
    Rasinski KA, Schildhaus S, Talley K. NTIES. The
    National Treatment Improvement Evaluation Study.
    Final report. Chicago: National Opin- ion Research
    Center; 1997.
25. Gossop M. Treating drug misuse problems: evidence
    of effectiveness. London: National Treatment Agency
    for Substance Misuse; 2006.
26. Gossop M, Marsden J, Stewart D, Kidd T. The National
    Treatment Outcome Research Study (NTORS): 4–5
    year follow-up results. Addiction. 2003;98:291–303.
27. Health Canada. Literature review – methadone
    maintenance treatment. Ottawa: Public Works and
    Government Services Canada; 2008.
28. Hubbard RL, Craddock SG, Anderson J. Overview
    of 5-year follow-up outcomes in the drug abuse treat-
    ment outcome studies (DATOS). J Subst Abus Treat.
    2003;25:126–34.
29. INCB. Report of the international narcotic control
    board for 2011. http://www.incb.org/incb/en/publica-
    tions/annual-reports/annual-report-2011.html. 2011.
30. Kaya CY, Tugai Y, Filar JA, Agrawal MR, Ali RL,
    Gowing LR, Cooke R. Heroin users in Australia: pop-
    ulation trends. Drug Alcohol Rev. 2004;23:107–16.

31. Klingemann H, Sobell LC. Promoting self-change from addictive behaviors. Practical implications for policy, prevention and treatment. New York: Springer; 2007.

32. Kramer JC. Heroin in the treatment of morphine addiction. J Psychedelic Drugs. 1977;197:193–7.

33. Leshner A. Addiction is a brain disease, and it matters. Science. 1997;278:45–7.

34. Marsh KL, Joe GW, Simpson DD, Lehmann WEK. Treatment history. In: Simpson DD, Sells SB, editors. Opioid addiction and treatment: a 12-year follow-up. Malabar: Krieger; 1990. p. 137–56.

35. McLellan AT, Grissom GR, Zanis D, Randall M, Brill P, O'Brien CP. Problem-service 'matching' in addiction treatment. A prospective study in 4 programs. Arch Gen Psychiat. 1997;54:730–5.

36. Metzger DS, Woody GE, McLellan AT. Human immunodeficiency virus seroconversion among intravenous drug users in- and out-of-treatment: an 18-month prospective follow-up. J Acquir Immune Defic Syndr. 1993;6:1049–56.

37. MHR. Order from the Ministry of Health of Russia dated 14 August 1995 #239, titled About additional measures on control of narcotic drugs, dangerous substances and poisons. 1995.

38. Miller N, Flaherty JA. Effectiveness of coerced addiction treatment (alternative conse- quences) a review of the clinical research. J Subst Abus Treat. 2000;18:9–16.

39. Moyer A, Finney JW, Swearingen CE, Vergun P. Brief interventions for alcohol problems: a meta-analytic review of controlled investigations into treatment-seeking and non-treatment- seeking populations. Addiction. 2002;97:279–92.

40. NIDA. Principles of drug addiction treatment. A research-based guide. Bethesda: National Institute of Drug Abuse; 2012.

41. Rhodes T, Hedrich D, editors. Harm reduction: evidence, impact and challenges. Lisbon: EMCDDA Monograph. European Monitoring Centre for Drugs and Drug Addiction; 2010.

42. Robins LN. Vietnam veterans rapid recovery from heroin addiction – a fluke or normal expectation. Addiction. 1993;88:1041–54.

43. Rust A. Ethische aspekte. In: Uchtenhagen A, Zieglgänsberger W, editors. Suchtmedizin. konzepte, strategien und therapeutisches management. Munich: Urban & Fischer; 2000. p. 573–84.

44. Schumacher JE, Milby JB, Wallace D, Meehan DC, Kertesz S, Vuchinich R, Dunning J, Usdan S. Meta-analysis of day treatment and contingency-management dismantling research: Birmingham homeless cocaine studies (1990–2006). J Consult Clin Psychol. 2007;75:823–8.

45. Stallwitz A, Stoever H. The impact of substitution treatment in prisons – a literature review. Int J Drug Policy, 18. 2007:464–74.

46. Stevens A, Hallam C, Trace M. Treatment for dependent drug use. A guide for policymakers. London: Beckley Foundation; 2006.

47. Strang J, Groshkova T, Metrebian N. New heroin-assisted treatment: recent evidence and current practices of supervised injectable heroin treatment in Europe and beyond. European Monitoring Centre for Drugs and Drug Addiction. 2012; Publications Office of the European Union.

48. Tännsjö T. Coercive care. The ethics of choice in health and medicine. London: Routledge; 1999.

49. Uchtenhagen A. Substitution management in opioid dependence. In: Fleischhacker WW, Brooks DJ, editors. Addictions, mechanisms, phenomenology and treatment; 2003. p. 33–60.

50. Uchtenhagen A. Treatment of substance dependence: ethical aspects. In: Helmchen H, Sartorius N, editors. Ethics in psychiatry – European contributions. Amsterdam: Springer; 2010a. p. 381–400.

51. Uchtenhagen A. Ethical perspectives in caring for people living with addictions: the European experience. Int Rev Psychiatry. 2010b;22:274–80.

52. Uchtenhagen A, Guggenbühl L. Adequacy in drug abuse treatment and Care in Europe (ADAT). Commissioned by World Health Organisation, Regional Office for Europe. Zurich: Research Institute for Public Health and Addiction; 2000.

53. Uchtenhagen A, Ladjevic T, Rehm J. Guidelines for psychosocially assisted pharmacological treatment of persons dependent on opioids. Working paper for World Health Organisation. Zurich: Research Institute for Public Health and Addiction; 2005.

54. UN. Universal declaration of human rights. New York: United Nations; 1948.

55. UN. Convention the rights of persons with disabilities. 2008. Retrieved from https://www.un.org/development/desa/disabilities/convention-on-the-r%20%20ights-of-persons-w%20ith-disabilities.html.

56. UN. Single convention on narcotic drugs. New York: United Nations; 1961.

57. UN. Convention on psychotropic substances. New York: United Nations; 1971.

58. UN. United Nations convention against illicit traffic in narcotic drugs and psychotropic substances. New York: United Nations; 1988.

59. UNODC/WHO/UNAIDS. Technical guide for countries to set targets for universal access to HIV prevention, treatment and care for injecting drug users. Vienna: United Nations Office on Drugs and Crime; 2009.

60. Ward J, Mattick R, Hall W. Methadone maintenance treatment and other opioid replacement therapies. Amsterdam: Harwood; 1998.

61. Weisner C. Coercion in alcohol treatment. In: Institute of Medicine, editor. Broadening the base for the treatment of alcohol problems. Washington, DC: The National Academic Press; 1990. p. 579–610.

62. Westermeyer J. Poppies, pipes and people: opium and its use in Laos. Berkeley: University of California Press; 1982.

63. Westermeyer J. The switch from opium to heroin smoking. Addiction. 2006;92:686–7.

64. WHO. Proposal for the inclusion of Methadone in the WHO model list of essential medicines. Geneva: World Health Organisation; 2004a.

65. WHO. Proposal for the inclusion of buprenorphine in the WHO model list of essential medicines. Geneva: World Health Organisation; 2004b.

66. WHO. Guidelines for psychosocially assisted pharmacological treatments of opioid dependence. Geneva: World Health Organisation; 2008.

67. WHO. Assessment of compulsory treatment of people who use drugs in Cambodia, China, Malaysia and Viet Nam: an application of selected human rights principles. Manila: World Health Organisation; 2009.

68. WHO. International classification of diseases (10th ed) version for 2010. World Health Organisation. 2010.

69. WHO/UNODC. Principles of drug dependence treatment. A discussion paper. Geneva: World Health Organisation; 2008.

70. Wild DC, Cunningham JA, Ryan RM. Social pressure, coercion, and client engagement at treatment entry: a self-determination theory perspective. Addict Behav. 2006;31:1858–72.

71. Zinberg NE. Drug, set and setting. New Haven: Yale University Press; 1984.

Monitoring and Evaluation of Addiction Treatment

57

Ambros Uchtenhagen

Contents

Abstract

Monitoring and evaluation (M & E) are research activities dedicated to document and analyze the processes and outcomes of addiction treatment. Before starting M & E, some conceptual issues apply, such as considering the objectives of a given treatment or treatment system, the outcome indicators to be used, the characteristics of the target population, and the basic understanding of the nature of addiction.

A range of different goals can be envisaged in M & E projects, from measuring treatment implementation and the use of the available resources to measuring efficacy and effectiveness. The overall goal, in general, is the improvement of services and treatment systems. The main steps in developing M & E projects are determining the research questions, the appropriate type and design of evaluation, and the resources and partners needed. Also, it is helpful to identify expected problems and obstacles.

Lists of evidence-based guidelines and instruments for evaluation are attached, as well as lists of high-quality publications reviewing the outcomes of evaluation studies.

Keywords

Monitoring · Evaluation · Tretament Workbooks · Outcome

A. Uchtenhagen (✉)
Swiss Research Foundation for Public Health and
Addiction, Zurich University, Zurich, Switzerland
e-mail: ambros.uchtenhagen@isgf.uzh.ch

© Springer Nature Switzerland AG 2021
N. el-Guebaly et al. (eds.), *Textbook of Addiction Treatment*,
https://doi.org/10.1007/978-3-030-36391-8_57

57.1   Introduction

Monitoring and evaluation (M & E) are essential instruments for an optimal drug demand reduction through treatment and prevention. They serve the commitment to effective interventions, which are based on scientific evidence. Only a good knowledge on the effects of interventions can provide the evidence base for an adequate substance abuse policy.

The main objective of M & E is to assess the available intervention system at country, regional, or local level, to determine its adequacy for covering the treatment needs in the respective population, and to measure its intermediate, short-term, and long-term outcomes. This is instrumental for a targeted improvement of available intervention systems, as well as for an adaptation to new challenges from changes in substance-using populations, and the health and social consequences of use. Monitoring trends in substance-using populations out of treatment is helpful in order to observe such changes, for example, the arrival of new drugs.

M & E also covers structural and procedural properties of services and systems, as major instrumental elements for outcomes.

M & E can also serve other purposes, such as providing arguments for legitimizing the treatment or prevention approach against repressive approaches.

57.2   Main Aspects of Monitoring and Evaluation

57.2.1 Definitions and Rationale

There are no universally accepted definitions. Monitoring and evaluation are performed in many fields of activities, such as health and education, and the aims and definitions are adjusted to the respective field. For this chapter, the following definitions and rationale apply.

57.2.1.1   Monitoring Treatment
Monitoring is an activity to continuously document defined indicators of treatment implementation and outcomes.

Rationale: To determine the level of service performance and treatment results, as a starting point for improvements and for measuring change as a result of improvements.

57.2.1.2   Process Evaluation of Treatment
Process evaluation is a one-time or repetitive activity to document how therapeutic interventions are implemented, in terms of coping with predetermined rules and criteria.

Rationale: To determine the level of service responsiveness to needs and compliance with expected performance, in order to facilitate the expected results.

57.2.1.3   Outcome Evaluation of Treatment
Outcome evaluation is a one-time or repetitive activity to document the consequences of therapeutic interventions for the target population and/or any other sector of the population, in terms of predetermined goals and indicators.

Rationale: To measure the intended and unintended effects of therapeutic interventions, in order to determine the value of a given intervention, a service, or treatment system to serve the expected treatment objectives.

57.2.1.4   Economic Evaluation of Treatment
Economic evaluations are a specific type of outcome evaluation. They measure the proportions of costs and benefits of an intervention, a service, or a treatment system. Costs and benefits are measured at the individual or at society level. In cost-effectiveness evaluation, effectiveness is expressed in terms of costs per unit of outcome. Cost-utility evaluation determines the gains in years and quality of life in relation to costs.

Rationale: To explore satisfaction with the results of investments made.

57.2.1.5   Meta-Evaluation
The growing number of evaluation studies and their unequal quality invited an effort to review evaluation studies, on the basis of rigorous method-

ological analysis, resulting in reliable information about "what works" and "what works for whom."

57.2.1.6 Comparable Terms

Other terms for process and outcome evaluation, especially in the educational field, are formative and summative evaluations. Formative evaluation is typically conducted during the development or improvement of a program or course. Summative evaluation involves making judgments about the efficacy of a program or course at its conclusion.

For other and partly overlapping definitions of terms, see the referenced evaluation guidelines of the World Health Organization [5] and the European Monitoring Centre for Drugs and Drug Addiction [7, 9].

57.2.2 Preparing for Monitoring and Evaluation

A detailed M & E project is the key to the feasibility of data collection, to the validity of data, and to the usefulness of results. The following issues and steps must be considered before starting a project. It is recommendable to set up an M & E project in collaboration with an expert.

57.2.2.1 Conceptual Issues

Treatment Objectives

The specific objectives of a given therapeutic method or of a given program determine the type of outcome data to be collected, in order to know how far outcome responds to the objectives. Objectives may be reduction of main substance use or any substance use, abstinence from main substance use or any substance use, health improvements, reduction or abstinence of illegal activities, social integration such as gainful employment or participating in a social network, or complete recovery [8].

Outcome Criteria

If no specific treatment objectives are in place, any M & E project has to determine which type of outcomes are to be measured. This may be those mentioned earlier, but also others such as the quality of life of patients/clients or the reduc-

Table 57.1 Outcome indicators

Retention rate	Measuring time in treatment
Status at discharge	Regular versus irregular discharge (drop-out, exclusion)
Addictive behavior	Consumption patterns of legal and illegal addictive substances
Risk-taking behavior	Injecting drugs, needle sharing, and unsafe sex
Health status	Changes in somatic and psychological health
Social reintegration	Changes in living arrangements, employment, social networking, and criminal activities
Quality of life	Subjective Well-being

tion of negative consequences of addiction at population level in terms of substance-related crime and nuisance or blood-borne infectious disease. The following is a catalog of the most frequently used outcome indicators (adapted from [9], Table 2) (Table 57.1):

The choice of outcome criteria should meet the interests of all stakeholders, including the mandating and/or funding bodies for the project.

Characteristics of the Target Population

Intermediate, short-term, and long-term outcomes of therapeutic interventions are diverse for different target populations. Age, gender, level of education, level of social integration and social support, religious affiliation, health factors such as comorbidity, etc. have a potential to influence how well a person responds to a therapeutic intervention or program. Data collection therefore must be tailored to the specificities of the target groups an intervention or service is meant to serve.

Understanding Addiction

Also, the kind of data to be collected for M & E depends on how addictive behavior is interpreted. Various paradigms apply here: the use of psychotropic substances can be understood as self-medication for symptom relief [18], as a special variation of self-manipulation, tailoring use to a desired state of mind, or as instrumental for self-enhancement, optimizing function and output [15]. Or else, substance use is understood as a lifestyle phenomenon, in the sense of "consumerism" or of an expression of subcultural identity.

On the other side, addiction is understood as a brain disease, following repetitive substance use, resulting in structural changes [20] or on a vulnerability-stress model focusing on the impact of genetic and environmental factors on the brain changes [34]. For each of these paradigms, specific contextual data and patient/client characteristics are of interest in order to explain the value of intervention outcomes.

Also, understanding addiction as a chronic relapsing disorder has consequences for the design and methodology of evaluation studies [22]. Or else, addiction is conceived in a synthetic theory as a pathology of the motivational system, resulting in a deficit of other satisfactory/pleasurable experience, restricting such experience to repetitive substance use [36].

57.2.2.2 Goals of Monitoring and Evaluation Projects

M & E projects are made for a variety of purposes (see also Ref. [9], Chap. 1). The purpose is relevant for the research questions to be answered by the project; the research questions are relevant for the design and methodology to be used as well as for the data which are necessary for answering the questions.

Measuring Program Implementation

A comparison is made between the intended standards of a therapeutic program or protocol and the de facto characteristics of its implementation. It includes structural and procedural aspects. Among the many issues of interest are the indication criteria, staff composition and qualifications, infrastructure and location of service, links with other services, etc. It may also include an estimation of how well the treatment needs in the regional/local population are covered.

Such projects are mainly of the process evaluation type. A recent example is part of the WHO collaborative study on substitution therapy of opioid dependence and human immunodeficiency virus/acquired immunodeficiency syndrome (HIV/AIDS) [19]. Continuous monitoring of the process has the advantage to document changes made over time in terms of program implementation.

Measuring Use of Resources

In an overall purpose to make best use of available human and financial resources, M & E projects can measure the overall utilization of the treatment capacity or the utilization by the intended target population. They can compare outcomes between services receiving similar investments and serving similar populations. More difficult and demanding are economic evaluations as mentioned earlier.

Measuring Efficacy and Effectiveness

Efficacy of therapeutic interventions is, as a rule, determined by clinical trials, using a randomized controlled design. These trials provide us with data showing the relative efficacy of a given intervention or medication in comparison to another intervention or medication, if the treatment is allocated at random and the sample characteristics are comparable.

In contrast, the effectiveness of an intervention or a treatment service is defined by how well an intervention or a service works in practice and produces the desired results. It is usually measured by cohort studies, including outcome evaluation with or without elements of process evaluation.

Efficacy and effectiveness studies contribute to a better knowledge on what treatment is best suitable, have the best chances for which patients/clients under which conditions, and thereby improve the indication criteria for patient/client placement.

Legitimation of Treatment

A frequent purpose of evaluation projects is demonstrating the value of a given intervention or service, in terms of desired outcomes, patient/client satisfaction, and positive economic balance of input and outcome. This can be done through a single-service follow-up study or a nonrandomized comparative study. The main issues why it is important to assure the legitimacy must be considered in the research questions and the study design.

Improvement of Services and Treatment Systems

M & E studies can provide data which allow to identify weaknesses, to initiate changes, and—in a repetitive effort—to document the intended and unintended effects of such changes. Process evaluation and qualitative data are most helpful for improvement purposes [27].

57.2.2.3 Determining the Research Questions

The questions to be answered by an M & E project depend on the aims and must be made explicit, for an agreement between all stakeholders. The questions determine what kind of samples is needed, which data must be collected, and which study design is most appropriate.

Additional research questions may be included in order to address special interests by staff, funding agency, or other stakeholders. The inclusion of such questions has a potential to enhance cooperation and compliance with the main study.

The following types of research questions can be considered (see also WHO 2000, workbook 1 step 5, and [9], Chap. 3):

- *Descriptive questions* for precise information about observations made.
- *Normative questions* aiming at a comparison between observations and expectations (e.g., standards).
- *Impact questions* exploring the role of interventions or elements thereof for the observed outcomes.

57.2.2.4 Typology of Treatment Evaluation

There is no universally accepted typology. The following is mainly based on the types presented in the EMCDDA Guidelines [9] and in the WHO/ United Nations Office on Drugs and Crime. (UNODC)/EMCDDA Evaluation workbooks [39].

Needs Assessment Evaluation

Needs assessment studies are used to determine and improve the coverage of treatment needs in a given population, in order to tailor treatment capacity, mix of services, and networking among services accordingly (WHO evaluation workbook 3).

Structure Evaluation

Evaluation of the appropriateness of infrastructure and other structural elements to facilitate the desired outcomes of treatment. This includes location, safety provisions, financial resources, staff composition and qualification, governance, and organization.

Process Evaluation

Process evaluation documents and analyzes how treatment is delivered. Assessment procedures, indication criteria, treatment planning, programming, qualification and attitudes of staff, continued training of staff, house rules, sanctions, etc. are some of the elements to be considered (WHO workbook 4, extensive list of available instruments for process evaluation on the EMCDDA instrument bank EIB).

Outcome Evaluation

The focus is on the consequences of treatment for patients/clients, their families, and the community. It provides information on which treatment modality has which consequences for which target groups under which conditions. It may consider the impact on other treatment approaches. It may become relevant for treatment motivation in the target population.

Outcome is measured against predefined behavior norms (normative evaluation), baseline pretreatment status (evaluation of change during treatment), or predefined treatment goals (goal-attainment evaluation). Outcome evaluation mainly uses quantitative methods (by randomized controlled trials (RCTs) or cohort studies), eventually a combination of quantitative and qualitative methods (WHO workbook 7, instruments on EIB of EMCDDA).

Patient/Client Satisfaction Evaluation

Patient/client satisfaction studies measure to what extent treatment provision and treatment results meet the expectations of patients/clients. They are a major source for service improvement, together with retention rates and drop-out rates (WHO workbook 6, instruments on EIB of EMCDDA).

Economic Evaluations

Various designs are used to describe and analyze economic factors in addiction treatment. Cost analysis measures the cost factors and overall costs of treatment (e.g., per patient day, per treatment episode, per treatment modality, etc.). Cost-benefit evaluation determines the relation between costs and financial benefits (e.g., in terms of reduced health and social costs in a defined posttreatment period as compared to pretreatment values). Cost-effectiveness evaluation measures costs in relation to a specific unit of outcome (e.g., significant health improvement or significant reduction in addictive behavior). Cost-utility evaluation measures the utility of treatment for patients/clients, for example, in terms of disability-adjusted life years—DALYs [2] or as quality-adjusted life years—QALYs [25, 37]. For cost evaluations, see also WHO workbook 5; for economic evaluations, WHO workbook 8; and for instruments, see EIB of EMCDDA.

Formal Evaluation
This is an assessment of service compliance with professional, ethical, and legal standards.

Meta-Evaluation
Meta-evaluation is made on the basis of recognized procedures to combine quantitative results from several studies about the same or similar interventions, in order to establish composite outcome scores. This allows assessing the effectiveness of a given intervention with greater confidence than on the basis of a single study.

57.2.2.5 Evaluation by Whom?
External Evaluation
Outcome or/and process evaluation of treatment services or interventions by research professionals who are independent from the evaluated agency. This is the preferred modality because eventual bias in collecting client data is avoided, and the credibility of the study is enhanced. Disadvantages in comparison to internal evaluation may be the higher costs and resistance or noncompliance of treatment staff.

Internal Evaluation (Self-Evaluation)
This can be used as an internal learning process about the treatment program or in case of restricted funds for evaluation studies. However, internal evaluation is not recommended for out-come studies because credibility is lower in comparison to external evaluation. Collaboration with an external evaluation specialist is an advantage.

57.2.2.6 Evaluation Level and Timing
Evaluation Level
The target of M & E projects can be a specific type of intervention or therapeutic method. It can also be a specific service or setting for delivering treatment. In contrast to single intervention and service follow-up studies, a comparative evaluation focuses on the functioning and outcomes of a local, regional, or national treatment network of services or of the overall treatment system. Choosing the target implies the choice of an adequate type and design of the project.

One-Time and Repetitive Evaluation
One-time evaluation studies are frequently made for all purposes. More relevant are repeated studies or a continuous monitoring system, allowing for a documentation of specific changes in implementation and outcomes over time. However, such an approach has important cost implications. A possible compromise is the combination of a relatively simple monitoring of routine data with a more extensive evaluation study if indicated by changes in the monitoring data or after important program changes.

57.2.2.7 Resources
Estimations must be made on the amount of funds and type of manpower in order to conduct the planned M & E project, and the availability of these resources must be checked in advance, in order to avoid delays or restrictions during implementation. Also, the infrastructure for data storage and analysis must be made available.

In view of the difference in available resources between high-income and low−/middle-income countries, priority-oriented monitoring and evaluation research, as well as transnational collaboration, is recommendable.

Financial Resources
If an M & E study is mandated by an external agency (governmental or nongovernmental), the

budget available for the study must be identified, in order to design the study accordingly. Or else, the research group planning the study has to present a budget proposal and apply to a funding agency (Research council, Foundation, Health Authority, etc.).

If there are doubts about the feasibility of the study (e.g., access to services and patients/clients), a stepwise procedure may be preferred. In this case, a separate budget for the feasibility study is needed, and the results will determine the budget of the ensuing evaluation study.

Human Resources

Which staff is needed for carrying out a planned project? Various functions must be considered: expert support for setting up the research questions and protocol, for determining the appropriate methods and instruments, for training of interviewers, etc. Staff responsible for data collection, interviewers, staff for data control and entering into a master file, statistician for data analysis, etc. are needed. It is helpful to identify staff in advance, in order to avoid delays in implementation and in order to establish a realistic budget.

Infrastructure

Access to the necessary equipment for staff and for safe storage of data is to be ensured, as well as the disposition of the appropriate software for data handling and analysis.

57.2.2.8   Partners

Most M & E projects are a collaborative effort between various partners, especially in case of external evaluation of services and networks. Clear agreements on functions, responsibilities, temporal availability, and costs are recommended, eventually with written contracts.

Funding Partners

Agreements on the overall budget, bookkeeping, financial controls, timing of payments, and financial reports help to prevent misunderstandings and litigations. Such agreements should be made to protect the interests of all parties.

Therapeutic Partners

All projects on external evaluation are based on collaboration between researchers and treatment providers. Agreements are needed on the access to patient/client data and service data, access to patients/clients for external interviewers, responsible person in a given service for organizing and facilitating the research process, ownership of data, and arrangements for publishing the study results. Procedures in case of upcoming problems during project implementation should also be agreed upon in advance.

A special situation is created in case of a systematic evaluation at the system level, involving all or selected treatment providers.

Research Partners

In case multiple researchers or research groups are involved, a clear working arrangement should identify the functions, tasks, and responsibilities of the individual persons. If a service provider hires a researcher or research group for an internal or external evaluation, or monitoring system, there is also a need to identify the various functions, tasks, and responsibilities.

57.2.2.9   Expected Obstacles

Most problems occurring during project implementation are due to missing or incomplete preparation. However, even a carefully prepared project may meet some obstacles. Some of the frequent ones are mentioned here.

Compliance with Protocol

Staff involved in project implementation may disregard details of the research protocol and thereby weaken data reliability, even if well instructed. This may also happen in case of changes of staff. Tutoring staff activities over the entire duration of the project helps to avoid such failures. Also, efforts to make a strong evaluation culture at the system level acceptable will contribute essentially to overcome this type of obstacle.

Resistance from Patients/Clients

One of the most common problems is the refusal to participate in a randomized study, resulting in an unacceptable degree of sample selectivity. This is especially to be expected if a control group with placebos or other forms of low therapeutic value are used or patients/clients are not confident that their data will be well protected against external parties, for example, in studies involving illicit substance use and/or drug-related criminal activities. Informed consent should cover not only aims and design of the study but also measures taken to guarantee data protection.

External Interference

It may so happen that family members of patients/client or other third parties raise opposition against an M & E project, on the basis of ethical concerns. It is advisable to have an explicit permission from an ethical committee, if not already prescribed by law.

57.2.3 Implementation of Monitoring and Evaluation

57.2.3.1 Available Guidelines and Instruments for Treatment Evaluation

International Guidelines for Treatment Evaluation

From the number of evaluation guidelines, a few are mentioned here, on the basis of their wide international applicability. It is highly recommendable to consult one or more guidelines before starting an M & E project.

WHO/UNODC/EMCDDA Evaluation of Psychoactive Substance Use Disorder Treatment Workbook Series (WHO 2000)

This publication consists of a series of workbooks intended to educate program planners, managers, staff, and other decision-makers about the evaluation of services and systems for the treatment of psychoactive substance use disorders. The objective of this series is to enhance their capacity for carrying out evaluation activities. The broader goal of the workbooks is to enhance treatment efficacy and cost-effectiveness, using the information that comes from these evaluation activities.

EMCDDA Guidelines for the Evaluation of Treatment in the Field of Problem Drug Use. A Manual for Researchers and Professionals [29, 9]

This publication provides basic information on the options, elements, and procedures of drug-related treatment evaluation. It also contains an overview of European and international evaluation and research networks.

Instruments for Treatment Evaluation

The EMCDDA evaluation instrument bank (EIB) covers a range of available instruments ready for data collection, including information on the target group specificity, the available languages (mostly English), copyrights, and eventual restrictions for use. Instruments are available for needs assessment and planning, for mediating and risk factors, for process and outcome evaluation, for patient/client satisfaction, and for staff knowledge and satisfaction.

The WHO/UNODC/EMCDDA evaluation workbooks present many instruments in the context of the various steps and approaches of treatment evaluation (WHO 2000).

A recent instrument for assessing and improving addiction treatment at the system level is the WHO Substance Abuse Instrument for Mapping Services (SAIMS) in high-income and middle−/low-income countries and disadvantaged regions [40].

57.2.3.2 Adaptation of Guidelines to Special Situations

Recommendations

The recommendations made in guidelines do not always respond to the specificity of a given project. However, major deviations from recommendations should be highlighted and reasons should be given. Special situation may arise from restricted resources or ethical restrictions. While there is some research on how to adapt treatment guidelines to clinical practice [13], no such systematic effort is known for evaluation guidelines.

An innovative attempt is to be expected from the WHO SAIMS project [40].

57.2.3.3 Meta-Analysis and Reviews of Evaluation Studies

Two organizations have been established in order to review and analyze evaluation studies selected for their rigorous methodology: the Cochrane Collaboration and the Campbell Collaboration.

The Cochrane Collaboration (www.cochrane.org) has its focus on evaluation of medical treatments, while the Campbell collaboration (www.campbellcollaboration.org) has its focus on social interventions.

Both organizations make their reviews available in their respective online libraries (www.thecochranelibrary.com, www.campbellcollaboration.org/library.php). A growing number of reviews cover pharmacological and psychosocial treatments in addiction and their outcomes.

57.2.3.4 Study Designs and Protocols

The choice of the appropriate study design depends on the research questions and on the available resources. The most frequently used designs are presented in Table 57.2 (see also Ref. [9], Chap. 3, Table 1).

Cross-Sectional Studies

Cross-sectional studies are one-time studies to compare treatment services, treatment populations, and treatment outcomes at a given moment in time (e.g., intermediate outcomes during treatment or after terminating treatment). Cross-

Table 57.2 Main types of study designs

Cross-sectional studies	Comparing interventions/services at a given point in time
Cohort studies	Comparing measurements of single interventions/services or several interventions/services at multiple points in time (baseline data, intermediate outcomes, outcomes at follow-up). Cohort studies are made prospectively or retrospectively (on the basis of past data files)
Randomized controlled studies RCT	
Quasi-experimental studies	
Comparing outcomes if interventions are assigned to patients/clients at random, not as in clinical practice (observational studies)	
RCT with special randomization procedures	

sectional studies cannot describe processes of change over time.

Cohort Studies

Cohort studies describe the course and outcomes of treatment populations, which receive their treatment as usual in practice, not allocated by randomization (observational or "naturalistic" studies). Cohort studies use retrospective or prospective data.

Longitudinal Retrospective Studies

Anamnestic data on pretreatment characteristics and outcomes of treatment populations are used to describe the therapeutic results of a given intervention/service alone or in comparison with other interventions/services. This type of study is more economic in comparison to prospective studies, which need multiple, at least two, measurement points in time; its usefulness, however, depends on the availability and quality of anamnestic data.

Longitudinal Prospective Studies

Collecting pretreatment, during-treatment, and posttreatment data at different time points allows a focused and detailed description of the treatment process and results. It avoids biased or missing baseline data and therefore provides for more reliable results of effectiveness. Prominent national studies comparing cohorts from different treatment settings are the DATOS study in the USA [28] and the National Treatment Outcome Research Study (NTORS) study in the UK [11].

Randomized Controlled Studies

Randomized controlled studies (RCT) are the "gold standard" for evaluating specific therapeutic modalities and medications in clinical research. Patients are allocated "at random" to an experimental group or to a control group, thereby minimizing selection factors between the two groups. As not all patients are willing to accept randomization, especially if not allocated to their preferred intervention, this design may suffer from refusal to participate or from elevated dropout rates. Randomized studies allow to identify the effectiveness of a modality or medication but do not provide results of effectiveness due to their selectivity. An updated collection of RCTs on addiction treatment can be found in the Cochrane library.

Double-Blind Randomized

If assignment to the experimental or the control group is not revealed to patients and therapists, their preferences are better (although not completely) ruled out, and the study gets more reliable results about comparative treatment efficacy. This design is mainly used for a comparison of medications; psychosocial interventions cannot be "blinded."

Quasi-Experimental Designs

Instead of comparing two or more modalities, the effects of an experimental modality can be compared to the course while waiting to be accepted for that modality. In this case, the control group receives treatment as usual or no treatment while waiting.

In the Zelen design, informed consent is only asked after randomization and only from patients assigned to the experimental group, while those who are randomized to treatment as usual need not consent to participation in the study [31]. This design makes it easier for patients to participate because they do not have to consent to be randomized. Of course, blinding is not possible in this design.

Another design uses different sequences of treatment modalities, for example, A-B-A compared with B-A-B or B-B-A.

Role of Methodology for the Quality of Results

Grading of Evidence

Treatment evaluation searches for scientific evidence that can be used as a basis for therapeutic recommendations. However, there are grades of evidence, depending on the type of study design (see also Ref. [12]). The following is an adapted version (Table 57.3).

Standards for Consensus Building

Where evidence from quantitative studies is not available or feasible, recommendations

Table 57.3 Grading of evidence grade definition

A	Highest degree of evidence: Review from multiple randomized controlled studies (RCT) with convergent results
B	High degree of evidence; results from single RCT and controlled clinical studies
C	Moderate degree of evidence: Prospective comparative longitudinal studies (observational studies without control design)
D	Low degree of evidence: Single intervention/ service follow-up studies, case studies E very low degree of evidence: Nonsystematic observations
Z	Not known

for good practice are mainly based on expert opinion. In order to optimize the consensus-building process, rigorous rules have been established [1].

57.2.3.5 Quantitative and Qualitative Methods

Quantitative Methods

Quantitative methods are used for outcome evaluation. They consist in collecting empirical data via standardized instruments (surveys, questionnaires, pre- and post-tests) for statistical analysis and mathematical modeling and in producing numerical results (statistics, percentages), which answer specific research questions. Data may come from existing databases (secondary data) or are collected directly from treatment samples (face to face, per telephone, or electronic media). Questionnaires may be self-administered or administered by trained interviewers. Sample size and homogeneity, reliability and validity of data, and appropriate statistical methods and models are essential for representative results.

Not all patients/clients who participate in a randomized evaluation study are compliant with the study protocol and available for follow-up data collection. Two concepts are therefore used for statistical analysis: the intention-to-treat (ITT) concept includes all participants who have been randomized, ignoring noncompliance and withdrawal, while the per-protocol concept includes only participants without any major protocol violations [14].

Qualitative Methods

Qualitative methods are mainly used for process evaluation. When indicating problem areas in the provision of treatments, they can also be useful for improvements and for generating new research questions. They provide information for the construction of questionnaires in process and outcome evaluation, and they can be used for the interpretation of quantitative findings [23].

The main methods are participant observation, semi-structured interviews, focus groups, and narrative research (see Ref. [9]). A standardized method for the selection of interview and focus group partners is the theoretical sampling model, allowing for the broadest possible spectrum of views and perspectives [10, 30].

57.2.3.6 Use of Results

It is advisable to determine at an early stage of an M & E project how the results will be communicated, by whom and how. This includes issues like data ownership and authorship in publications. In order to avoid later litigations, all agreements should be documented in written.

A first start to communicate evaluation results are intermediate and comprehensive final reports; for recommended components see [39] (workbook 2, step 4) and the EMCDDA Guidelines for treatment evaluation ([9], Chap. 6). Reports must at least be accessible to all stakeholders of an evaluation project. On the basis of the final results, a publication plan can help to make the best use of those. The scientific community is best reached by publications in peer-reviewed journals, and a wider audience eventually by open access journals, books, good practice documents (e.g., Ref. [33]), pamphlets, mass media articles, etc.

Once the results are known, what they mean and to whom they might be communicated should also be discussed in order to optimize their potential impact on treatments, on service planning and improvement, on treatment policy, etc.

57.2.3.7 Checklists for Assuring the Evaluation Process

All those involved in planning and implementation of a given project can profit from checklists which help to keep all elements of the project under control. The EMCDDA Guidelines for treatment evaluation present useful checklists for the preparation and implementation, as well as for the evaluation process ([9], Chap. 5).

57.2.4 Treatment Outcomes: Selected Evidence-Based Guidelines and Systematic Reviews

- Effectiveness of Therapeutic Communities: a systematic review [21].
- Principles of Drug Dependence Treatment. A Research Based Guide (NIDA [24]).
- Guidelines for the Psychosocially Assisted Pharmacological Treatment of Opioid Dependence [38].
- Contemporary Drug Abuse Treatment. A Review of the Evidence Base (UNODC [32]).
- Reviews for specific interventions:
- Calabria et al. [4]
- Humphreys and McLellan [17]
- Malivert et al. [21]
- Hertzler et al. [16]
- O'Donnell et al. [26]
- Werb et al. [35]
- Bomparis [3]

57.2.4.1 Cochrane Library (Selected Reviews)

- Psychological therapies for pathological and problem gambling (2011)
- Methadone for non-cancer pain in adults (2012)
- Psychosocial interventions to reduce alcohol consumption in concurrent problem alcohol and illicit drug users (2012)

- Nicotine replacement therapy for smoking cessation (2012)
- Mobile phone–based interventions for smoking cessation (2012)
- Combined pharmacotherapy and behavioral interventions for smoking cessation (2012)
- Psychosocial interventions for benzodiazepine harmful use, abuse, and dependence (2012)
- Effects of psychostimulant drugs on cocaine dependence (2010)
- Acamprosate for alcohol dependence (2010)
- Opioid antagonists for alcohol dependence (2010)
- Psychosocial interventions for reducing injection and sexual risk behavior for preventing HIV in drug users (2010)
- Psychosocial interventions for people with both mental illness and substance abuse (2010)
- Buprenorphine maintenance versus placebo or methadone maintenance for opioid dependence (2008)
- Psychosocial interventions for cocaine and psychostimulant amphetamines related disorders (2007)
- Alcoholics Anonymous and other 12-step programs for alcohol dependence (2006)
- Methadone maintenance at different dosages for opioid dependence (2003)

57.2.4.2 Campbell Library (Selected Reviews)

- Effects of early, brief, computerized interventions on Risky Alcohol and Cannabis Use Among Young People: A Systematic Review (2013)
- The Effectiveness of Incarceration-Based Drug Treatment on Criminal Behavior: A Systematic Review (2012)
- Brief Strategic Family Therapy for Young People in Treatment for Non-Opioid Drug Use (2012)
- Effects of drug substitution programs on offending among drug addicts (2009)
- Case management for persons with substance use disorders (2009)
- Motivational interviewing for substance abuse (2009)

Key Points

This chapter focuses on how treatment services and networks can be analyzed in regard to their functioning and usefulness, in a systematic long-term process, or in time-limited research projects. Essential elements are conceptual preparation of what should be learned (type of evidence), which patients and professional partners should be involved, what resources are needed and available, advantages and limitations of methods to be applied, and use of results in the interest of patients and all concerned.

Clinical Relevance

Treatment is about improving the symptoms of medical conditions, to learn about which interventions are effective for whom in the short and long term, and how to improve the patient's quality of life in caring for incurable conditions. This chapter helps clinicians to assess the patient situation beyond a formal diagnosis in all relevant aspects to develop and follow up an individual treatment plan and to learn about the effectiveness and side effects of their interventions.

References

1. AGREE II. Appraisal of guidelines for research and evaluation II. The AGREE Next Steps Consortium. 2009. www.agreetrust.org.
2. Anand S, Hanson K. Disability adjusted life years: a critical review. J Health Econ. 1997;16:658–702.
3. Bomparis N. Internet interventions for adult illicit substance users: a meta-analysis. Addiction. 2017;112:1521–32.
4. Calabria B, et al. Systematic review of prospective studies, investigating remission from amphetamine, cannabis, cocaine, or opioid dependence. Addict Behav. 2010;35:731–9.
5. Campbell collaboration. www.campbellcollaboration. org, Campbell library www.campbellcollaboration. org/library.

6. Cochrane collaboration. www.cochrane.org, Cochrane library www.thecochranelibrary.com.

7. EIB: Evaluation instrument bank of the european monitoring centre for drugs and drug addiction, Lisbon. www.emcdda.europa.eu/eib.

8. El-Guebaly N. The meanings of recovery from addiction: evolution and promises. J Addict Med. 2012:6–19.

9. EMCDDA. Guidelines for the evaluation of treatment in the field of problem drug use. A manual for researchers and professionals. Lisbon: European Monitoring Centre for Drugs and Drug Addiction; 2007.

10. Glaser BG, Straus AI. The discovery of grounded theory: strategies for qualitative research. Chicago: Aldine Publishing Company; 1967.

11. Gossop M, Marsden J, Stewart D, Kidd T. The National Treatment Outcome Research Study (NTORS): 4–5 year follow-up results. Addiction. 2003;98:291–303.

12. GRADE working group. Grading quality of evidence and strength of recommendations. BMJ. 2004;328:1490.

13. Graham ID, Harrison MB. Evaluation and adaptation of clinical practice guidelines. Evid Based Nurs. 2005;8:68–72.

14. Gupta SK. Intention-to-treat concept: a review. Perspect Clin Res. 2011;2:109–12.

15. Harris J. Enhancing evolution. The ethical case for making better people. Oxford: Princeton University Press; 2007.

16. Hertzler B, et al. Contingency management in substance abuse treatment: a structured review of the evidence for its transportability. Drug Alcohol Dependence. 2013;122:1–10.

17. Humphreys K, McLellan AT. A policy oriented review of strategies for improving the outcomes of services for substance abuse disorder patients. Addiction. 2011;106:2058–66.

18. Khantzian EJ. The self-medication hypothesis of substance use disorders: a reconsideration and recent applications. Harv Rev Psychiatry. 1997;4:231–44.

19. Lawrinson P, Ali R, Uchtenhagen A, et al. Key findings from WHO collaborative study on substitution therapy of opioid dependence and HIV/AIDS. Addiction. 2008;103:1484–92.

20. Leshner I. Addiction is a brain disease, and it matters. Science. 1997;278:45–7.

21. Malivert M, Fatséas M, Denis C, et al. Effectiveness of therapeutic communities: a systematic review. Eur Addict Res. 2012;18:1–11.

22. McLellan AT, Lewis DC, O'Brien CP, Kleber HD. Drug dependence, a chronic medical illness. Implications for treatment, insurance and outcomes evaluation. JAMA. 2000;284:1689–96.

23. Neale J, Allen D, Coombes L. Qualitative research methods within the addictions. Addiction. 2005;100:1584.

24. NIDA. Principles of drug addiction treatment. A research-based guide. 3rd ed. Bethesda: National Institute of Drug Abuse; 2012.

25. Nord E. Methods for quality adjustment of life years. Soc Sci Med. 1992;34:559–69.

26. O'Donnell A, et al. The impact of brief alcohol interventions in primary healthcare. A systematic review of reviews. Alcohol Alcoholism. 2013;49:66–78.

27. Rush B, Krywonis M. Evaluation and continuous quality improvement of substance abuse services and systems. Toronto: Addiction Research Foundation; 1996.

28. Simpson DD, editor. Special section: 5-year follow-up treatment outcome studies from DATOS. J Subst Abus Treat. 2003;25:123–86.

29. Steven A, Hallam C, Trace M. Treatment for dependent drug use. A guide for policymakers. The Beckley Foundation. 2006. http://beckleyfoundation.org/.

30. Strübing J. Grounded theory. Wiesbaden: Verlag für Sozialwissenschaften; 2004.

31. Torgerson DJ, Roland M. What is Zelen design? BMJ. 1998;316:606.

32. UNODC. Contemporary drug abuse treatment. A review of the evidence base. New York: United Nations; 2002.

33. UNODC. International network of drug dependence, treatment and rehabilitation resource centers. Good practice documents. 2008. www.unodc.org/treatment/

34. Volkow ND, Fowler JS, Wang G-J. The addicted human brain viewed in the light of imaging studies: brain circuits and treatment strategies. Neuropharmacology. 2004;47:3–13.

35. Werb D, et al. The effectiveness of compulsory drug treatment: a systematic review. Internat J Drug Policy. 2016;28:1–9.

36. West R, Brown J. Theory of addiction. Hoboken: Wiley Blackwell, The Addiction Press; 2013.

37. Whitehead SJ, Ali S. Health outcomes in economic evaluation; the QALY and utilities. Br Med Bull. 2010;96:5–21.

38. WHO. Guidelines for the psychosocially assisted pharmacological treatment of opioid dependence. Geneva: World Health Organization; 2009.

39. WHO/UNODC/EMCDDA. Evaluation of psychoactive substance use disorder treatment, workbook series. Geneva: World Health Organisation; 2000.

40. WHO. Assessment of treatment Systems for Substance use Disorders using the WHO-SAIMS (substance-abuse instrument for mapping services). Interim report. Geneva: World Health Organisation; 2010.

Pathways to the Specialty Recognition of Addiction Medicine

58

Cornelis A. J. De Jong, David Crockford,
Gabrielle Welle-Strand, Shelly Iskandar,
Siddharth Sarkar, Paul S. Haber,
and Michael Miller

Contents

C. A. J. De Jong (✉)
Radboud University, Nijmegen, The Netherlands

D. Crockford
Department of Psychiatry, University of Calgary,
Calgary, AB, Canada
e-mail: david.crockford@albertahealthservices.ca

G. Welle-Strand
Norwegian Center of Addiction Research/Oslo
University Hospital, Oslo, Norway
e-mail: gabwel@online.no

S. Iskandar
Psychiatric Department, Hasan Sadikin Hospital,
Padjajaran University, Bandung, Indonesia

S. Sarkar
Department of Psychiatry and National Drug
Dependence Treatment Center, All India Institute of
Medical Sciences, New Delhi, India

P. S. Haber
Drug Health Services, Sydney Local Health District,
The University of Sydney Central Clinical School,
Sydney, NSW, Australia
e-mail: paul.haber@sydney.edu.au

M. Miller
Department of Psychiatry, University of Wisconsin,
Madison, WI, USA
e-mail: michael.miller@uwmf.wisc.edu

© Springer Nature Switzerland AG 2021
N. el-Guebaly et al. (eds.), *Textbook of Addiction Treatment*,
https://doi.org/10.1007/978-3-030-36391-8_58

Abstract

In the first edition of the International Society of Addicted Medicine (ISAM) textbook, specialized ways of training from The Netherlands, Canada, Norway and Indonesia were presented. In this chapter, an update of the training in these countries is presented. Contributions from India, Australia and the United States are new.

Although there are, of course, differences based on local settings and prevalence of substance-related disorders, there is a more or less consensus on the content of the educational courses. All contributions illustrate that it is not that difficult to reach consensus on a national level. What makes them all different is the adaptation to local educational and licensing requirements that govern the national practice of medicine.

A preliminary conclusion is that the process towards an Addiction Medicine (AM) specialty is universally incremental and currently in transition, creating unique challenges in implementation but also opportunities for international group support and collaboration.

Keywords

Addiction Medicine (AM) · Addiction Psychiatry · Educational courses · SWOT analysis · Medical speciality development International survey · Undergraduate curricula in AM · Postgraduate addiction-oriented courses

58.1 Introduction

Substance use disorders (SUD) affect every medical practice. It is a recent development that medical doctors specialize in the field of Addiction Medicine (AM). In the section on Education and Training in the first edition of the ISAM textbook, specialized ways of training in The Netherlands [6], Canada [5], Norway [19] and Indonesia [4] were presented. At the end of the introduction of the section, it was concluded that the initiatives described were uniformly recent ones and are at various stages of development [8]. It was hoped for that the section could promote more international collaboration and support. Concerning the training in different countries, it was also concluded that there is no 'one size model fitting all'.

A review paper summarized scientific publications that outlined the content of Addiction Medicine curricula and evaluated the evidence for efficacy for training in Addiction Medicine. One of the conclusions was that Addiction Medicine should get the same priority as other chronic diseases do and that it must be integrated into the core of medical curricula of under- and postgraduate training of medical doctors.

An international consultation on training in Addiction Medicine led to a global core set of knowledge, skills and attitudes and recommendations for the under- and postgraduate training of medical doctors. The need to tailor a curriculum to national settings and different specialities was recognized [2]. The journey towards specialty recognition must also adapt to local educational and licensing requirements that govern the national practice of medicine.

In this chapter, we will present an update of the training in Norway, The Netherlands, Canada and Indonesia. Initiatives from India, Australia and the United States are new in the chapter.

Some countries have adopted a focus on primary care; others have a focus on specialties, including psychiatry, internal medicine and community health, and most are adopting a multiple approach. In most paragraphs, the strengths, weaknesses, opportunities and threats are described, sometimes as a special subparagraph. A preliminary conclusion is that the process towards an AM specialty is universally incremental and currently in transition, creating unique challenges in implementation but also opportunities for international group support and collaboration.

58.2 The Netherlands

Between 2000 and 2005, it became clear for the medical directors in the Addiction Treatment facilities in the Netherlands that the quality of Addiction Medicine (AM) was problematic. This was due to shortage of medical doctors interested in AM, medical doctors in the field without proper training, low perspective for career and being faced with the fact that the best doctors leave to specialize as psychiatrists, internists, neurologists or general physicians (GPs). In just two years, we managed to start a full-time, two-year professional training in AM in the Netherlands. In 2012, AM was approved as a medical subspecialty by the Royal Dutch Society of Medicine. The development of the Dutch Master in Addiction Medicine (MiAM) was described in detail in 2013(7).

The aim of this section is to describe the present status of the Dutch MiAM, to present an evaluation of the seven groups of medical doctors that graduated and to describe the process of re-registration of the doctors who were enrolled in the register from the start. First, some words will be spent on addiction psychiatry.

Addiction is not a special area of attention in the training for psychiatrists, and addiction psychiatry is not yet a super-specialty in the Netherlands. There are two structured ways to learn more on addiction as a graduated psychiatrist. The Radboud Center of Social Sciences of the Radboud University offers a 10-day course on addiction psychiatry for psychiatrists, focusing on the increase of knowledge and skills in individual psychiatrists. Multidisciplinary In-Company courses in addiction psychiatry for psychiatrists, psychologists and nursing specialists, focusing on increasing the quality of the integral care of the mental health institute for psychiatric patients with a co-occurring substance-related disorder, are developed and implemented by the first author (CDJ).

In the competency-based MiAM, theoretical courses are integrated with learning in clinical practice under guidance of an experienced clinical teacher: a dual education paradigm. The theoretical courses consist of evidence-based medicine, communication and basic psychotherapeutic skills, neurobiology of addiction, Addiction Medicine, addiction and psychiatry, clinical leadership and public health. The seven main competencies are concretized in 31 Entrustable Professional Activities (EPAs). EPAs are the units of a professional practice that constitute what clinicians do as daily work (8). They are integrated in a personal education plan (PEP) and are evaluated by different ways of

examining and with a focus on stimulating self-reflection.

From the start of the MiAM in 2007 till 2019, a total of 139 medical doctors in 7 batches started the course, 65 women (47%) and 74 men (53%) with a mean age of 41.7 (SD 8.8) in a range of 26–59. Not all were native Dutch medical doctors, 39 (28%) came to the Netherlands and integrated as medical professionals after graduating as doctors again in the Netherlands. Many of them were refugees. Overall, 104 did graduate (75%) and 35 terminated the course prematurely (25%). The reasons for ending the course prematurely vary: severe physical illnesses, psychiatric or personality disorders, burnout, conflicts with management or a supervisor, inappropriate learning attitude or a combination of these.

In recent years, addiction doctors have gained a place within the medical community. Since the start of MiAM, the addiction doctor has become more professional and can therefore be designated as a treatment coordinator within the institutions for mental healthcare and addiction care. The programme is highly condensed, and 2 years is not enough to fully cover all aspects of AM. Although most graduates continue working in the addiction treatment centres, some of them wanted more and started psychiatry training to combine their clinical work as a PhD candidate.

Until the start of the MiAM in 2007, most doctors only worked in the specialized field of care for patients with SUD. In 2019, they also worked in general psychiatry, and there are opportunities for primary care, emergency care, liaison psychiatry, pain clinics and so on.

One of the challenges is to reassess the competences listed with the updated Canadian Medical Education Directives for Specialists (CanMEDS) competencies (9) and, above all, to integrate the educational milestones into clinical practice to illustrate how the competence of an addiction doctor progresses during his career—the journey from beginner to master.

In 2019, almost 200 medical doctors were included in the register of the Dutch Medical Society. In 2016–2017, there were almost 100 job offers. With an output of graduated doctors of 20 per 2 years from the MiAM, these job offers will never be fulfilled. The situation for the future is even worse because it is expected that almost 40% of the registered will end their career within 10 years.

Postgraduates are registered as addiction specialists and have to re-register every 5 years. In order to keep the registration, one needs to meet certain criteria, for instance, for at least 16 h a week for the duration of 5 years, they need to have worked in patient care, attended training workshops and symposia, and participated in peer training meetings. The Dutch Society of Addiction Medicine developed the content and process of the individual evaluation programme that starts in 2020. Every Addiction Medicine Specialist will have to present a personal education plan, which will be evaluated every 5 years by a review committee. For former students of the MiAM, this will merely be a continuation of personalized learning. The older and mostly the self-taught group of experienced doctors face a new approach of lifelong learning.

58.3 Canada

Canadian medical practice, particularly in acute care settings, has needed to rapidly evolve to the opioid crisis, growing stimulant problems and the legalization of cannabis nationally. Substance use problems are cited as the third most important in order of competence for newly practising primary care physicians, ahead of ischaemic heart disease and diabetes [13]. Relatively small numbers of clinicians skilled in AM have been previously tied to a lack of available training in Canada, but that appears to be changing [13]. A number of initiatives nationally are underway to promote best practices and validate the special knowledge, skills and practices required for the practice of AM.

Initially, Canadian physicians sought specialty recognition through Certification and Board Diplomas of the American and International Societies of Addiction Medicine, which would be subsequently recognized by the Canadian Society of Addiction Medicine [7]. The strength of this was that it was accessible through a practice-eligible route, requiring less investment by prac-

tising physicians. But, while certification could ensure a certain knowledge base in AM, it may not ensure competence to practice AM or meaningfully structure training.

As medical training in Canada has shifted to being competency-based training [9], AM training initiatives have followed suit. The two primary licensing Colleges in Canada, the College of Family Physicians of Canada (CFPC) for primary care physicians and the Royal College of Physicians and Surgeons of Canada (RCPSC) for specialists, each approved added competencies for AM in 2016. The CFPC awards a Certificate of Added Competence (CAC), and the RCPSC awards a diploma in an Area of Focused Competence (AFC). They have slightly different but complementary approaches.

The CAC in AM approved by the CFPC in 2018 aims to determine competence at the advanced skills level for primary care providers. The CFPC has developed 13 priority topics specific to AM with key features to each. The priority topics were developed by a nominal group using an individual survey, followed by group discussion and consensus, as well as from a larger national survey of family practitioners. The priority topics include: (1) clinical boundaries; (2) AM screening, assessment and triage; (3) treatment planning and continuing care; (4) management of intoxication and withdrawal; (5) harm reduction within the continuum of care; (6) pharmacology; (7) psychotherapeutic techniques; (8) concurrent mental health disorders; (9) medical comorbidities; (10) pain and addiction; (11) special populations; (12) advocacy; and (13) provider health resilience. Each priority topic has key features to further specify and define them. Competence is indicated by consistent demonstration of most of the key features across a good sample of priority topics. Initial CACs will be awarded to family physicians who have previously acquired competence deemed worthy of recognition through practice experience, successful completion of a residency training programme and/or continuing professional development, and demonstrated leadership in the domain of the CAC. Thereafter, CACs are to be awarded based on the credentials and documented evidence as judged by a peer review committee process. It has led to the development of 1-year fellowships for primary care physicians in AM across Canada at multiple training sites. The strength of the CAC process is in its flexibility and accessibility to current primary care practitioners, as well as new graduates, so it is expected that there will be significant uptake of CACs and extend the specialty recognition of AM for those in primary care.

The AFC in AM approved by the RCPSC in 2019 applies to all medical specialties, so the development of the training requirements has been more complicated than that for the CAC. For residency training programmes to have an AFC programme in AM, they have to be accredited by the RSPSC, which can take 1–2 years to meet their requirements. To receive an AFC diploma in AM, trainees must be certified in their entry route discipline, in order to be eligible to submit a Royal College competency portfolio in AM to the AFC Program Committee at the accredited programme. Competencies are described in the CanMEDS roles [10] where diplomats are expected to function as a competent specialist in AM capable of enhanced practice within the scope of their discipline. The competency portfolio addresses eight goals, each having multiple milestones with standards of assessment and specific supporting documents that are required to be signed off upon by their supervisor. The eight goals include the responsibility for: (1) evaluation of patients for substance use or addiction(s) in urgent and elective settings; (2) acute stabilization and management of patients with addiction; (3) comprehensive ongoing management for patients with addiction; (4) health promotion practices for patients with addiction; (5) engaging and supporting individuals within a patient's social network; (6) acting as a resource for other health providers; (7) advocacy for patients with addiction, for addiction treatment or for addiction prevention and (8) advancement of the discipline of AM through teaching and scholarly activity. The AFC requirements are quite stringent, so it may be challenging for specialty residency training programmes beyond those in very large urban centres to be able to establish AFC accredited programmes and attract residents or fellows who are willing to commit further training time beyond the 5 years they already require for their specialty. Those who do the training, however, will be highly skilled and potentially greater advocates for the future of AM. By the standards being applicable to all specialties, it may also facilitate greater cross-pollenization in AM across specialties.

Specialty recognition of AM in Canada continues to expand through practice-eligible routes and formal residency training programmes, with there now being CACs and AFC diplomas for primary care and specialists, respectively. If the AFC diplomas are embraced by medical specialists, this may set the stage for the development of formal sub-specialties in AM in the future.

58.4 Norway

The development of the specialty in Norway was described in detail in 2015 [19]. The specialty and interim regulations were approved by the Ministry of Health in 2014, and the first AM Specialist was approved in 2015.

58.4.1 The Specialty Regulations and Other Requirements to Become a Specialist in Addiction Medicine

The specialty regulations are as follows: 5 years of internship in accredited institutions is required of which 42 months of internship in AM, including 12 months in a detoxification department, 6 months in inpatient/residential treatment, 12 months in outpatient treatment and, for the last 12 months, a range of services can be chosen. Twelve months of internship should be in psychiatry and a minimum of 6 months of these in an acute ward. The last 6 months of internship can be in other relevant areas of medicine, including somatic wards, pharmacology, psychiatry or general practice.

In addition, the candidate must have 270 h of national coursework during the 5 years and at least 70 h of hospital coursework a year. The candidate must receive individual clinical supervision of at least 1 h per week throughout the clinical training and also group-based supervision. Further, the candidate must receive at least 30 h of specialized supervision in a specific therapeutic method.

58.4.2　The Status in June 2019

Overall, 129 doctors have been accredited full specialists in AM after interim regulations. Additionally, more than 100 medical doctors are in training across the country to become full specialists in AM. It is expected that approximately 20 of these candidates will be accredited full specialists in AM after the Specialty regulations in 2019.

Teaching hospitals have been established in all regions and at all larger hospitals in Norway. A total of 20 hospitals/institutions have been accredited as teaching hospitals.

A national coursework has been established. All candidates entering the structured education in AM will take part in a 4-week compulsory coursework over 2 years, covering a wide range of essential knowledge needed to be a specialist in AM. The third group of candidates in this compulsory coursework will finish the 4 weeks in the autumn of 2019, and a fourth group will be started the same autumn. Other coursework that have been established are courses of cognitive therapy, psychodynamic therapy and group therapy; pharmacology; treatment of attention deficit hyperactivity disorder (ADHD) for substance-dependent patients; as well as clinical toxicology. The candidate is also expected to use an online self-study portal and can, in this way, achieve competence in specific teaching goals.

58.4.3　National Conference in Addiction Medicine

Each year, a national conference for AM specialists, candidates and other medical doctors with interest in AM is arranged by the Norwegian Association of Addiction Medicine in order to further develop the new specialty and focus on new development and research in the addiction field. This conference is also an important meeting place for the new specialty.

58.4.4　Strengths, Weaknesses, Opportunities and Threats Analysis

The strengths of the full specialty in AM in Norway are several. We have successfully established the full specialty with accredited specialists and teaching hospitals in all regions of the country. The new specialty means that patients with substance use problems will receive specialist evaluation and treatment from well-qualified doctors in AM. The requirements for AM specialists are the same as for any other specialty in medicine, giving AM specialists a similar status as other medical specialists. The recruitment to the new specialty is very good because the medical doctors now have a possibility to make a career in AM. This means that the medical doctors will stay in the addiction field to a far greater extent than previously.

A weakness regarding the AM specialty is that not all the hospitals have enough specialists yet. However, as long as the recruitment into the specialty is very good, this is a situation which will improve with more medical doctors being accredited as specialists. Another possible weakness is that there is too little emphasis on somatic diseases in the specialist requirements.

Addiction research in Norway has developed a lot during the last 10–15 years and many PhD diplomas have been acquired both by medical doctors, psychologists and other professionals. Doctors in AM have good possibilities to finish a PhD as part of their specialist education or in addition to their specialty. Another opportunity is that having an AM specialty makes it easier to cooperate with regard to both treatment and research with somatic and psychiatric specialists, regarding acknowledging the many patients with co-occurring substance use problems and somatic and psychiatric diseases.

The establishment of the AM specialty has been viewed as a threat by some of the other professionals in the addiction field. The treatment of substance use disorders in Norway is a multi-professional area, where social workers, psychologist, nurses, medical doctors and other professions work. It will be up to the AM specialists to prove that better educated medical doctors will be an asset, not only for the patients but also for the other professionals in the addiction field.

58.4.5 Conclusion

The full medical specialty in AM is well established in Norway. So far, 129 specialists in AM have been accredited. More than 100 specialist candidates are in structured training all over Norway to become full specialists in AM. There are enough medical doctors who want to start the structured training in AM. More than 20 teaching hospitals/institutions in AM across the country have been accredited. The national coursework for the candidates has been established and is well functioning. A yearly conference for AM has been established as an important meeting place for the thriving and developing specialty. A lot of work over a long time by many pioneering medical doctors in the addiction field has led to the successful establishment of a full specialty in AM in Norway. The Norwegian Medical Association views the establishment of the AM specialty as a success, in terms of how fast the specialty has developed and how well the AM specialists and training of the new candidates is spread around the hospitals in Norway during such a limited time period.

58.5 Indonesia

The development of a National Training Program on AM in Indonesia was described earlier [4]. Here, we describe the progress for the under- and postgraduate training. First, we like to globally describe the undergraduate AM Training (AMT). In 2019, the Atma Jaya Catholic University is the only medical school that provides AMT in a 5-week elective block for fourth-year medical students at the final semester of the pre-clinical level. After following the block, the participant is expected to have (1) increased knowledge and understanding of the basics of substance use and addiction (epidemiology, neurobiology, psychology, clinical, socio-cultural and medicolegal aspects) skills; (2) developed clinical skills (screening, diagnosis, early treatment), addiction counselling and public education; and (3) expressed positive attitudes towards patients with substance use and addiction.

The academic staff (Astri Parawita Ayu, Isadora Gracia and Kevin Kristian) that contributes to the AM block is mainly from the department of psychiatry. Atma Jaya has been organizing the AM block since 2009, and several evaluations have been performed. The AMT block improved students' attitude towards patients with addiction and changed their perceptions of addiction. Further development is threatened by the fact that human resources in the school of medicine are scarce. In 2019, the dean had requested the AMT team to propose topics that can be embedded in the medical curriculum and distributed throughout the pre-clinical and clinical training. Such a request is an opportunity to develop AMT in Atma Jaya further. To answer the dean, the academic staff and five students are running a training need assessment [15] among medical doctors who work in all primary healthcare facilities in Jakarta. Hopefully, other universities can collaborate, and replication of such an assessment by other universities will make the results eligible at the national level.

The Indonesian Standard Competency for Medical Doctors states that a general practitioner (GP) has to be competent in making a clinical diagnosis for a substance use disorder and providing initial treatment and referring a patient. However, there is no national curriculum for medical doctors in Indonesia yet. Each university has to develop its own excellency in one to three topics. Atma Jaya University is one of the universities that has a focus on addiction in the form of an elective block.

In Universitas Padjadjaran (UNPAD), another academic university, the focus is more on postgraduate programmes [4], and the Indonesian Short Course on Addiction Medicine (ISCAN) was developed in 2010 [14]. After 2012, two batches of this 6-month course were conducted on the weekends for postgraduate medical doctors from all over Indonesia.

The first batch consists of 25 participants, most of them were recommended by municipal health departments in West Java as the requirements to be funded by UNPAD. The second batch were 30 participants, all of them were recommended and supported by national narcotics boards. We had evaluation on satisfaction to the topics and lecturers (Likert scale from 1–10). The average was an 8 for topics and lecturers in the first and second batch. We also have pre- and post-test for every module. It showed good improvement on knowledge. In general, the participants stated that the programme has been done well. They enjoyed the programme, although they had to spend their weekend to attend. The training would improve if behavioural addictions could also be tackled during the course, and if more workshops were integrated to improve their skills.

In 2017, the Department of Psychiatry of Medical Faculty-Universitas Indonesia/Cipto Mangunkusumo Hospital had started a training programme of subspecialty in addiction psychiatry in collaboration with the Kurihama Medical and Addiction Center, Japan, and Flinders University, Australia. Psychiatrists who want to become a consultant in addiction can enrol in this 2-year programme. By the end of the training, participants are expected to achieve academic and professional competence related to addiction psychiatry. In 2019, four addiction psychiatrists have graduated from such training. The training programme consists of a range of topics concerning drugs and behavioural addictions and characteristic psychiatric comorbidities. Participants are obliged to follow clinical rotation at hospitals, community services, prisons and the national rehabilitation centre. The academic activities include webinar lectures, case presentations, and, by the end of the training, participants should submit a research report.

A standard curriculum is needed for medical doctors, nurses, psychologists and pharmacists to develop interprofessional education modules.

Specific training programmes for each professional to gain knowledge and develop special skills in providing addiction services from a positive attitude towards patients with substance-related disorders. For residents in psychiatry, a 3-month stage in the addiction division is obligatory. The continuity and development of those programmes face a lot of obstacles due to the willingness and leadership of the stakeholders, including lecturers, resources and budget.

The problem with the development of addiction curriculum in Indonesia is because there is no strong intention from stakeholders to provide standard services [3]. Several focus group discussions with stakeholders showed that addiction problems are increasing, and it was regarded as very important to provide standard competence for healthcare providers' work in the addiction field. However, there are no collaborating efforts to make AM curricula in Indonesia a priority yet.

Small and separate programmes have been developed in collaboration with the International Consortium of Universities for Drug Demand Reduction (ICUDDR), the Colombo Plan and the U.S. Bureau of International Narcotics and Law Enforcement Affairs (INL). Indonesian universities can use the whole or a part of the curriculum developed by ICUDDR.

Universities also work together with the national and provincial narcotic board and local governments to provide a 2-day addiction training for primary healthcare doctors. The problem is that they only offer little knowledge, and the training does not really improve the doctors' skills. Furthermore, there is no continuation of the training, and the rapid changes in the role of the primary health doctor limit the effects of the training. In this respect, national addiction curricula and standard competencies are needed.

The development of AMT in Indonesia has several strengths. The foundation of AM has been made, starting from a previous project Integrated Management of Prevention and Control & Treatment of hiv/aids (IMPACT). There are some psychiatrists and lecturers who are interested in AM, and collaboration with addiction experts in Indonesia and abroad has been established. However, there is not yet a strong leader to bring together all AMT programmes, there is lack of support and budget from stakeholders such as faculty and government, and there is too limited time allocated for the development of an addiction curriculum due to overburden of the academic staff.

Although it is quite hard to develop AMT properly, there are opportunities for the future that are hopeful. Professional organizations acknowledge the need to improve skills of healthcare providers working in the addition field. There are new leaders and governmental regulations supporting addiction treatment, including training of professionals working in AM. Several non-governmental organizations are funding the development of AM curricula.

In our opinion, strong leadership and willingness to collaborate nationally and internationally are the keys to develop sustainable national addiction curricula.

58.6 India

In India, training in addiction has been ingrained in the 3-year postgraduate psychiatry course. Selection for the course is held generally through nationally competitive entrance examinations for medical graduates. The means and mechanisms for implementation of addiction training vary from institution to institution. Typically, case-based teaching is carried out as a part of the general psychiatric evaluations and mentoring from faculty members. Some of the institutions have dedicated clinics or centres where the postgraduate trainees are posted during their rotations, which last from weeks to up to 6 months. Seminars, case conferences and didactic lectures are the methods through which theoretical aspects of addiction psychiatry are discussed during the postgraduate general psychiatry training. The emphases on the addiction-related topics vary, but they form a part of the overall teaching curricula for the psychiatric trainees. Assessment is generally case-based and through written summative assessments, wherein addiction psychiatry may be an overall part of the psychiatric syllabus. There is heterogeneity and substantial variation in the manner in which teaching-learning of addiction psychiatry is carried out in different centres.

Overseeing the training programmes, a need has been felt for development of super-specialty courses in addiction psychiatry, on similar lines as super-specialty training in cardiology and neurosurgery after broad-based postgraduate training in medicine or surgery, respectively. Thus, the Doctorate in Medicine Addiction Psychiatry course has been launched, the first of such courses being instituted about 5 years back. Currently, at least four centres in India are running this course: All India Institute of Medical Sciences, New Delhi; Postgraduate Institute of Medical Education and Research, Chandigarh; National Institute of Mental Health and Neurosciences, Bengaluru; and All India Institute of Medical Sciences, Rishikesh. This 3-year super-specialty course is open to medical graduates who have completed a 3-year postgraduate degree in psychiatry, and selection is done through nationally open competitive examinations. The aim is to develop addiction psychiatry specialists who have wide clinical and research experience, deep theoretical knowledge and who are attuned to national realities in healthcare. They would be expected to provide better care for patients suffering from addictions and provide input for policy matters when required, apart from advancing the science related to AM.

Currently, the curricula vary across the centres offering the super-specialty course. The institutes have their own curricular structure, posting schedules, teaching-learning methods and assessment strategies. The variability enables utilization of the strengths and resources of each of the centre (e.g. research focus, clinical focus or public health engagement). The trainees have to engage in research or complete a dissertation under the guidance of a faculty member. Graduates from the super-specialty course in addiction psychiatry have been recruited in different teaching and clinical institutions.

The All India Institute of Medical Sciences, New Delhi, started the course in 2016 January. There are about five positions per year (highest in the country till date). Trainees have exposure to inpatient and outpatient clinical care, including outreach methadone and buprenorphine dispensing and engagement in community services. They are trained in laboratory services and psychotherapy for patients with addictions. Consultation liaison addiction psychiatry services help them see referrals from other departments and the interface of addiction and multiple medical illnesses. The institute has a system of structured formative assessments as well, through written examination and case discussion. The trainees partake in teaching of other postgraduate students and indulge in peer-teaching as well. Many of them have undertaken additional research pursuits and have volunteered their time for organizing Continuing Medical Education (CME) and conferences in addiction psychiatry.

The strengths of a super-specialty in addiction psychiatry include deep focus on the various aspects of addiction, the availability of dedicated and experienced professionals and presence of a comparable accreditation framework as other super-specialty disciplines. The weaknesses include lack of wider and specific demand from patients and prospective employers, variations in the conduct and emphasis of the course across centres and the lack of an association dedicated specifically towards addiction psychiatry. The opportunities presented are the cross-institution dialogue for exchange of curricula and students, regularization into annual meeting and conferences, utilization of the super-specialty trainees to impart supervision and teaching to medical students and interns, changes in summative and formative assessment methods to reduce subjectivity, and greater exposure from humanistic and legal perspectives of addiction. The threats include failure to develop proper referral mechanisms so that the patients are able to reach the super-specialists, and inability to expand the number of centres offering the course due to dynamically changing healthcare priorities.

The number of positions for such super-specialty doctors have been limited (less than 20 psychiatry specialists who have completed the course), which is paltry compared to the large population of India (over a billion and counting). The overall number of medical health professionals and psychiatrists are limited in the country, and such super-specialty courses are nascent and niche. Yet, the keen interest shown by trainees has been encouraging. We hope that with time, the graduates of this super-specialty course would be able to provide leadership in the field of addiction psychiatry, by expanding clinical care, training other medical graduates, conducting relevant and ethical research, providing policy directions and advocating for the cause of those who have been suffering from addictive disorders.

58.7 Australia

The training in AM in Australia was described in detail in 2011 [11] and 2013 [12]. The Australian Medical and Professional Society on Alcohol and other Drugs (AMPSAD) began in 1981 and developed a short training course, but this was undertaken by very few medical practitioners.

The Chapter of AM (AChAM) formed in December 2001 within the Royal Australasian College of Physicians (RACP) [16], and the Australian government recognized AM as a medical specialty in November 2009. RACP is the largest specialist college in Australasia mainly comprising specialists in the various branches of internal medicine. AChAM has adopted a well-established and widely accepted training scheme. Specialist reimbursement item numbers commenced operating in November 2010 and were upgraded to match those of other RACP specialists in 2016. The number of trainees has been slowly growing, but there is still a significant shortage of AM specialists.

The Royal Australian and New Zealand College of Psychiatry (RANZCP) [17] established the Section of Addiction Psychiatry, initially, as a special interest group without formal training. Addiction psychiatry is now a recognized subspecialty of psychiatry with about 150 members and requires 2 years of clinical training (RANZCP). It leads to the Certificate of Advanced Training in Addiction Psychiatry and includes a formal education programme, case history and clinical skills development described as Entrustable Professional Activities (EPAs). This training is well structured and requires assessment of written assignments but without examination. There is healthy interest in this programme from trainees and a growing clinical workforce.

There is a special-interest network for general practitioners (GPs) interested in drugs and alcohol. This is one of the 29 of networks with a specific interest. As a part of GP training, candidates can do extended skills posts for 6–12 months, and AM is one of the options. There are no specific training requirements beyond this. A number of GPs have proceeded to AM specialist training as described in the next section.

58.7.1 Addiction Medicine Training Programme

Advanced training in AM follows a modification of the general Postgraduate Physician Training, which comprises 3 years of basic training in internal medicine post internship, followed by 3 years of advanced training in the chosen field. There is a written examination early during the third year of training, and successful candidates proceed to a difficult clinical examination in general internal medicine later that year. Once the clinical examination is passed, trainees may enter advanced training in AM or another field. Assessment is by assignments and supervisor reports on clinical work, but there is no examination. A key difference for AM is that the RACP clinical examination is not required for AM training. However, the title Fellow of RACP (FRACP) is not awarded unless the clinical examination is passed. Specialist physicians with FRACP have broader internal medicine training and clinical privileges compared to AM specialists (FAChAM). Remuneration is now the same.

Basic physician training is one pathway for entry, but it is only adopted by a minority of current AM trainees. Entry via other clinical training is accepted and provides flexibility (RACP).

Advanced training extends for 3 years of supervised clinical postings and structured learning activities (RACP). Core training requires at least 18 months in a clinical AM position. Of the total, at least 12 months must be spent in an ambulatory (community) assessment and/or detoxification service, in opioid agonist prescribing. Six months is required in a consultation-liaison term in a general hospital, in an in-patient

unit and in a pain clinic. These attachments may be part-time and undertaken concurrently. Experience in Psychiatry is also required as part of AM rotation and/or as a separate rotation.

The curriculum for AM covers the broad themes of clinical assessment and management of alcohol and other substance use disorders in a broad range of settings, including consultation liaison in hospitals and other health services; public health and prevention of alcohol and other drug use–related harms; regulatory issues; and medicolegal and forensic aspects of the practice. The curriculum is supported by a number of online training modules accessible to accredited trainees via the RACP website. There is a weekly national training symposium that can be accessed face to face or by webinar.

Trainees work in accredited clinical sites for clinical training. Site accreditation for the AM training programme is the responsibility of Chapter Education Committee (ChEC) to ensure:

- An appropriate level of supervision by Fellows of the Chapter with Supervisor training.
- Exposure to a wide range of clinical presentations.
- Opportunities and support for continuing education and research.
- Suitable infrastructure for training–equipment, clinical and educational resources, quarantined training time.

Trainees are encouraged to nominate a mentor separate from their supervisor.

58.7.2 Outcomes to Date

Informal feedback has highlighted several strengths of the programme. Trainees appreciate rotation through different treatment services with exposure to diverse models of care and supervisors. In particular, the breadth of AM practice incorporating behavioural medicine, physical health and mental health is appealing to trainees. The focus on self-directed adult learning has been welcomed. The online training modules are popular, with standardized teaching that is accessible at any time. The public health workbook and the research project were considered valuable learning activities.

The number of trainees has been slowly growing and while there were 30 trainees active in 2019, the number remains insufficient to meet workforce demands. In particular, most trainees are in the most populous state (New South Wales) with very few in other states.

58.8   United States

Health professions' academicians, under the leadership of David Lewis, MD, now the Donald G. Millar Emeritus Professor of Alcohol and Addiction Studies at Brown University, created the Association for Medical Education and Research in Substance Abuse (AMERSA) in 1976, an interdisciplinary professional society of faculty members in professional schools of medicine, nursing, psychology, social work and other disciplines. AMERSA (www.amersa.org) has been the most consistent driver of improvement in the curricula of professional schools so that all graduates are more knowledgeable about addiction, addiction treatment and the health impacts of unhealthy substance use. Sadly, the goals of AMERSA in this regard remain unfulfilled, as the incorporation of content about addiction and recovery into the curricula of professional schools remains spotty.

The American Society of AM (ASAM), the largest professional association of physicians (and, since 2013, other professionals) devoted to improving addiction treatment quality and access (www.asam.org), has long had a committee on medical education, but ASAM's most prominent success has been in offering continuing education courses to persons already in practice. The ASAM Annual Conference and State of the Art Conference attract attendees from dozens of nations worldwide. ASAM also had a fellowship committee in the 1990s, which collected information about AM fellowship programmes in existence at academic medical centres and located in treatment programmes; none of these were accredited at that time by the Accreditation Council on Graduate Medical Education (ACGME) [1].

In 1993, the field of psychiatry took the lead in developing ACGME accredited training for physicians [18]. These fellowship programmes in addiction psychiatry were open to psychiatrists who had completed general psychiatry training. There are currently 49 accredited fellowships in addiction psychiatry. Most of these programmes would admit a non-psychiatrist into training, but such graduates would not be eligible for certification in the field. Completion of a fellowship by a psychiatrist could lead to certification by the American Board of Medical Specialties (ABMS) and its member board, the American Board of Psychiatry and Neurology, in addiction psychiatry; physicians from internal medicine, family medicine or other disciplines completing an addiction psychiatry fellowship were not able to secure any certification recognized by the ABMS.

In 2007, ASAM decided that a necessary step in securing ABMS recognition of AM would be to have physician certification conferred not by a membership society such as ASAM, but by a free-standing certification board. Thus, ASAM assisted in the creation of the American Board of Addiction Medicine (ABAM), which began offering the national certification examination in 2010. ABAM created a sister organization named The ABAM Foundation renamed The Addiction Medicine Foundation, or TAMF, and on January 1, 2019, renamed the American College of Academic Addiction Medicine, ACAAM, www. acaam.org. The mission of ABAM was to certify individual physicians, via an examination, in the specialty of AM, while the mission of TAMF was to accredit fellowship training programmes in AM. The ABAM Foundation developed educational objectives for training programmes and accreditation guidelines for training programmes, and it did its best to have its processes mirror those of the ACGME in establishing educational objectives and a core curriculum for graduate medical education (GME) programmes. By 2018, ACAAM oversaw the development of 52 fellowship programmes which met the rigorous accreditation standards it had set. Around the time that the American Board of Preventive Medicine (ABPM), one of the 24 member boards of the ABMS, developed an application to the ABMS Board of Directors (with the assistance of ABAM

Directors and staff), TAMF approached the ACGME about taking over the accreditation of AM Fellowships. The ABMS approved the application of the ABPM in 2015, and a certification programme for physicians in the subspecialty of AM was established by ABPM under the auspices of the ABMS. The first examination offered by the ABPM was in 2017. The first training programmes accredited by the ACGME in 2018 were sponsored by various primary residency programmes and 1 year in duration. The ACGME will have accredited 54 AM Fellowships by June 2019 (ACGME). These are sponsored largely by academic departments in academic medical centres: 13 in Department of Internal Medicine, 25 in Department of Family Medicine, 27 in Department of Psychiatry, 1 in Department of Paediatrics and none in Department of Obstetrics and Gynaecology. Thus, graduate medical education at the fellowship level in the subspecialty of AM is now on a par with fellowship training in other medical disciplines. Of the total 74 ACGME and ACAAM accredited fellowships, 2 are in Puerto Rico and 3 are in Canada.

Undergraduate Medical Education (medical school training) in addiction continues to be far less robust than the scope of the public health problem of addiction and unhealthy substance use. The existence of ACGME accredited training programmes has gotten the attention of Deans of Schools of Medicine, and there is growing advocacy to expand and improve the education of all physicians in this area. ASAM continues to be interested in improvement in medical school curricula in addiction. A separate group, the Coalition on Physician Education (COPE) in Substance Use Disorders (https://www.copenow.org/), was created in the wake of a Leadership Conference on Medical Education in Substance Abuse co-sponsored by the ABAM Foundation and the White House Office on National Drug Control Policy in 2008. COPE continues to advocate for curriculum development in medical schools in addiction.

Parallel to medical education in allopathic medicine leading to a Doctor of Medicine (MD) degree is the education of physicians in osteopathic medicine. The American Osteopathic Association (AOA) accredits osteopathic medical schools akin to the way the American Association of Medical Colleges accredits allopathic medical schools, and the AOA also accredits osteopathic residency programmes akin to the way the ACGME accredits residencies. The AOA also offers certification programmes for individuals holding a Doctor of Osteopathy (DO) degree, and there is a subspecialty society for osteopathic physicians, the American Academy of Osteopathic Addiction Medicine (AAOAM). The AOA does not accredit any fellowships in Addiction Medicine, but physicians with DO degrees may enrol in ACGME accredited fellowship programmes in AM.

58.9 Conclusion

In this chapter, examples of the development of Addiction Medicine as a (sub)specialty are described. If we compare the situation in the countries that were described in 2015 with the current state of affairs, it appears that considerable progress has been made. Furthermore, we have the impression that the content of the training courses is not very different between the seven countries. All over the world, professionals in AM seem to share the same ideas about addiction and patients with substance-related disorders. Of course, the training courses are adapted, for instance, to prevalence of the use of certain psychoactive substances and their related disorders. To teach AM, they all adopted a framework of competencies similar to CanMEDS, but we are aware of different educational methods.

In general, it is encouraging that in a few countries, there is an AM specialty. In others, individual professionals or professional communities in the field are working on the establishment of AM as a specialty. In some countries, the focus is more on increasing the quality and quantity of training programmes in Addiction Psychiatry. We can confirm the statement that there is not 'one size that fits all' [8].

If we look in more detail to the line of development in the seven countries described, we notice, however, significant differences. Concerning the development and implementation of Addiction Medicine, the strengths, weak-

Table 58.1 Strengths, weaknesses, opportunities and threats during the development and implementation of Addiction Medicine as a specialty in seven countries

	Strengths	Weaknesses	Opportunities	Threats
The Netherlands	Recognized as specialty by the medical community. Dual educational system. Gained a place in medical community	Short (2 years) educational course and therefore different from other specialties. Still a small group of specialists.	Re-registration process guarantees quality. Emphasizes the existence of a specific group of specialists Destigmatization of patients with SUD	A lot of job offers and 40% leaving AM within 10 years Discussions and conflicts with other medical specialists on whose territory patients should be treated
Canada	The initiatives to improve the quality of Addiction Medicine are widely supported by the medical community	AM still part of other specialties	Growing interest in AM in several other specialties and acknowledgement of the importance by licensing authorities	Few AM specialists outside of major urban centres
Norway	Better educated doctors mean better treatment for patients. Recognized as specialty by the medical community. The requirements for AM specialists are the same as for any other specialty in medicine	Too little emphasis on somatic diseases in the specialist requirements	Chances for scientific research in the field of AM	It is up to the AM specialists to prove that better educated medical doctors will be an asset to the addiction field
Indonesia	In universities, there is a growing interest in and implementation of undergraduate education in AM and postgraduate Addiction Psychiatry. Well-appreciated short training in AM	No progress in establishing AM as a specialty	Professional organizations acknowledge the need to improve skills of healthcare providers working in the addition field International collaboration on AM	No strong leadership yet to convince the government of the importance of AM for public health. Limited resources and budget
India	Training in addiction has been ingrained in the three-year postgraduate psychiatry course.	No initiatives for an AM specialty, heterogeneity and substantial variation in teaching–learning of addiction psychiatry.	Development of super-specialty courses in addiction psychiatry	Failure to develop proper referral mechanisms for patients to reach the super-specialists, and inability to expand the number of centres offering the course
Australia	Addiction psychiatry is a recognized subspecialty of psychiatry, including a formal education programme. Dual-education system for advanced training in AM	There is still a significant shortage of AM specialists	Well-evaluated advanced training in AM and healthy interest in the Addiction Psychiatry programme from trainees	Too few specialists in less populated areas
United States	Accredited fellowships in Addiction Psychiatry. Fellowship level in the subspecialty of AM is now on a par with fellowship training in other medical disciplines	Addiction and recovery into the curricula of professional schools remains spotty	Formal agreement on AM as subspecialty by the medical communities	Undergraduate Medical Education in addiction continues to be far less robust than the scope of the public health problem of addiction

nesses, opportunities and threats are summarized in Table 58.1.

Working on the development of AM and setting up an AM specialty can certainly lead to AM being recognized as a successful specialty, as is clear in the Netherlands and Norway. However, the journey is not always that simple or successful. In the United States, it took a long time to get approval to establish AM as a specialty, and in Australia, it is quite difficult to attract enough trainees to meet the need for sufficient AM specialists. However, there is a stimulating message for the AM field: it is possible to set up an AM specialty. Even if it is not possible, the endeavour will still help the medical community to realize and to recognize that addiction is a chronic disease and thereby contributes to the destigmatization of patients.

Nevertheless, there is still a lot of work to do. The connection between the undergraduate curricula in AM and the postgraduate development or addiction-oriented courses in the training of other specialists is still lacunar in most countries. This also means that young doctors are usually unaware that it can be very interesting and beneficial to work with this group of patients. In case of a well-established AM speciality, the duration of the training is sometimes too short, and the content is not always properly attuned to, for example, the comorbidity of patients with a substance-related disorder. In large countries such as Canada, Indonesia, India and Australia, in particular, it is difficult to establish sufficient AM specialists outside of major urban centres or to create good training places there.

Although professional organizations acknowledge the need to improve knowledge and skills of healthcare providers working in the addiction field, inspiring leadership from the AM community is needed to make efforts in the development of training and teaching that matter. We have the impression that in our era social media stimulates international group support and that this should be encouraged in every possible way.

The increased interest in addiction and training in Addiction Medicine also stimulates scientific research in that field. After the recognition of AM as a specialty, it forces professional organizations to develop standards for the re-registration of AM specialists.

Finally, the recent progress in the development in AM should be stimulating for professionals in countries that are working in the field of AM and are struggling to take further steps; there is hope!

Acknowledgements The Netherlands
Michel Wolters,
Tactus Addiction Treatment, Enschede, The Netherlands/Dutch Society of Addiction Medicine
Norway
Rune Tore Strøm,
Norwegian Association of Addiction Medicine/Oslo University
Hospital, Guri Spilhaug,
Norwegian Association of Addiction Medicine/Oslo University Hospital
Indonesia
Kristiana Siste,
Department of Psychiatry, Medical Faculty, Universitas Indonesia/CiptoMangunkusumo Hospital
Astri P. Ayu,
Addiction Medicine Study Group | Department of Psychiatry and Behavioural Sciences | School of Medicine and Health Sciences Atma Jaya Catholic University of Indonesia, Jakarta, Indonesia
India
Anju Dhawan,
Department of Psychiatry and National Drug Dependence Treatment Center, All India Institute of Medical Sciences, New Delhi, India
Australia
Dan Lubman,
Eastern Health Clinical School, Monash Addiction Research Centre, Monash University, Richmond Victoria, Australia
United States
Randall Brown,
Department of Family Medicine & Community Health, University of Wisconsin, United States

References

1. ACGME. Medpage Today, from https://www.medpagetoday.com/meetingcoverage/asam/72392. 2018. Accessed 18 Aug, 2019.
2. Ayu AP, El-Guebaly N, Schellekens A, De Jong C, Welle-Strand G, Small W, et al. Core addiction medicine competencies for doctors: an international consultation on training. Subst Abus. 2017;38(4):483–7. https://doi.org/10.1080/08897077.2017.1355868.
3. Ayu AP, Iskandar S, Siste K, De Jong C, Schellekens A. Addiction training for health professionals as an

antidote to the addiction health burden in Indonesia. Addiction. 2016;111(8):1498–9. https://doi.org/10.1111/add.13407.

4. Ayu AP, Schellekens AFA, Iskandar S, Pinxten L, De Jong CAJ. The development of a National Training Program on Addiction Medicine in Indonesia. In: el-Guebaly N, Carrà G, Galanter M, editors. Textbook of addiction treatment: international perspectives, vol. XII. Milan Heidelberg New York Dordrecht London: Springer; 2015. p. 2424–30.

5. Crockford D, el-Guebaly N. Medical education in addiction and related disorders: the Canadian experience. In: el-Guebaly N, Carrà G, Galanter M, editors. Textbook of addiction treatment: international perspectives, vol. XII. Milan Heidelberg New York Dordrecht London: Springer; 2015. p. 2395–409.

6. DeJong CAJ, Luycks L. Addiction medicine training in The Netherlands. In: el-Guebaly N, Carrà G, Galanter M, editors. Textbook of addiction treatment: international perspectives, vol. XII. Milan Heidelberg New York Dordrecht London: Springer; 2015. p. 2381–95.

7. el-Guebaly N. Educational opportunities and a call for synergy. Can J Addict. 2014;5(3):3–4.

8. el-Guebaly N, De Jong CAJ. Education and training: an introduction. In: el-Guebaly N, Carrà G, Galanter M, editors. Textbook of addiction treatment: international perspectives, vol. XII. Milan Heidelberg New York Dordrecht London: Springer; 2015. p. 2377–9.

9. Frank JR, Snell LS, Cate OT, Holmboe ES, Carraccio C, Swing SR, et al. Competency-based medical education: theory to practice. Med Teach. 2010;32(8):638–45. https://doi.org/10.3109/0142159X.2010.501190.

10. Frank JR, Snell L, Sherbino J. CanMEDS 2015 physician competency framework. Ottawa: Royal College of Physicians and Surgeons of Canada; 2015.

11. Haber PS, Murnion BP. Training in Addiction Medicine in Australia. Subst Abus. 2011;32(2):115–9. https://doi.org/10.1080/08897077.2011.555718. 933123228 [pii]

12. Haber PS, Murnion BP. Training in addiction medicine in Australia. In: Haber PS, editor. International perspectives on training in addiction medicine. London and New York: Routledge, Taylor & Francis Group; 2013.

13. Hering RD, Lefebvre LG, Stewart PA, Selby PL. Increasing addiction medicine capacity in Canada: the case for collaboration in education and research. Can J Addict. 2014;5(3):10–4.

14. Pinxten WJ, De Jong C, Hidayat T, Istiqomah AN, Achmad YM, Raya RP, et al. Developing a competence-based addiction medicine curriculum in Indonesia: the training needs assessment. Subst Abus. 2011;32(2):101–7. https://doi.org/10.1080/08897077.2011.555710. 933149398 [pii]

15. Pinxten WJL, Fitriana E, De Jong C, Klimas J, Tobin H, Barry T, et al. Excellent reliability and validity of the Addiction Medicine Training Need Assessment Scale across four countries. J Subst Abus Treat. 2019;99:61–6. https://doi.org/10.1016/j.jsat.2019.01.009.

16. RACP. from https://www.racp.edu.au/trainees/advanced-training/advanced-training-programs/addiction-medicine.

17. RANZCP. from https://www.ranzcp.org/pre-fellowship/about-the-training-program/certificates-of-advanced-training/addiction-psychiatry.

18. Tontchev GV, Housel TR, Callahan JF, Kunz KB, Miller MM, Blondell RD. Specialized training on addictions for physicians in the United States. Subst Abus. 2011;32(2):84–92. https://doi.org/10.1080/08897077.2011.555702.

19. Welle-Strand GK. Development of a full medical speciality in addiction medicine: the Norwegian experience. In: el-Guebaly N, Carrà G, Galanter M, editors. Textbook of addiction treatment: international perspectives, vol. XII. Milan Heidelberg New York Dordrecht London: Springer; 2015. p. 2409–23.

International Society of Addiction Medicine's International Certification of Addiction Medicine: The First 15 Years

59

Nady el-Guebaly and Claudio Violato

Contents

Abstract

This chapter reviews 15 years of effort by the International Society of Addiction Medicine to develop a multiple-choice test of knowledge and clinical judgment in the field. The process of establishing a pool of questions as well as criteria for eligibility to challenge such an examination is described.

Lessons derived from the repeated administration of the exam are reviewed. An international examination is possible, involving questions with good psychometric properties. The challenges of striving for an "a-cultural examination" as well as the necessities of cost accessibility, security, and sensitivity are reported.

Keywords

Certification · Multiple choice · Performance levels · Core competencies

59.1 Introduction

In 1999, the International Society of Addiction Medicine (ISAM) came into being. Its mission was to promote an international agenda, including advancing the knowledge about addiction seen as a treatable disease, advocating for the major role physicians play in its management as well as enhancing the credibility of their role, and, last, developing educational kits accessible to an international audience.

N. el-Guebaly (✉)
Division of Addiction, Department of Psychiatry, University of Calgary, Calgary, AB, Canada
e-mail: nady.el-Guebaly@ahs.ca

C. Violato
University of Minnesota Medical School, Minneapolis, MN, USA
e-mail: cviolato@umn.edu

© Springer Nature Switzerland AG 2021
N. el-Guebaly et al. (eds.), *Textbook of Addiction Treatment*,
https://doi.org/10.1007/978-3-030-36391-8_59

The need for improved medical education in the field is well recognized in both developed and developing countries and is detailed in other chapters of this textbook's section. The call for educating all physicians in playing their respective roles in the care of patients affected with the disorders of addiction has been made repeatedly [2, 3, 13]. An increasing number of generalists and specialist physicians are dedicating a major portion, if not all of their practice, to this significant public health issue. Enhancing their credibility and validating their practice through a formal process of certification became a goal of ISAM.

There is a growing international consensus about the core competencies required of every physician in treating abusing or addicted patients. They are screening, brief intervention, including motivational interviewing, and awareness of referral for treatment options, including mutual help. In the USA, these competencies are known by their acronym Screening, Brief Intervention, Referral to Treatment (SBIRT) [8]. By comparison, the boundaries of individual specialty competencies are understandably less defined. Based on core concepts from the basic sciences, evidence-based practices include, but are not limited to, prevention strategies; diagnosis, assessment, and early interventions; detoxification and craving; relapse prevention; psychotherapy, Cognitive Behavioral Therapy (CBT), 12-step, motivational enhancement, contingency management, and cue exposure; psychopharmacology, general and specific, including maintenance and medication interaction; physical and psychiatric concurrent disorders, primary or secondary disorders; ethical and legal issues around the workplace, including a physician's own impairment; chronic pain; forensic issues; cultural factors; age and gender issues; and behavioral addictions.

In the USA, the first medical association's certification examination in the field was held in 1983 by the California Society of Addiction Medicine, followed by the first national examination in 1986 under the auspices of the American Society of Addiction Medicine (ASAM). The American Academy of Addiction Psychiatry established the first subspecialty examination under the auspices of the American Boards in

1993. In 2009, the American Society of Addiction Medicine created an independent American Board of Addiction Medicine (ABAM), followed, in 2016, by admission to the American Boards as part of the American Board of Preventive Medicine (ABPN). Currently, those board certifications or diplomas are valid for 10 years. A commitment to maintenance of certification through documented lifelong learning and assessment of practice-based performance is also required. The criteria of eligibility for challenging these examinations limit the access to candidates mostly from within North America. Examples of other national efforts to validate the training of Addiction Medicine specialists are described in Chap. 59, Education: International Pathways.

59.2 The Certification Process

59.2.1 Chronological Development of an International Certification

Based on the US experience, in September 2003, in Amsterdam, the Board of the International Society of Addiction Medicine (ISAM) accepted to set up a valid and affordable international certification. An Editorial Board was formed composed of 10 senior clinician members of ISAM from 7 countries. An expert in medical education research, including examination psychometrics (C.V.), joined that Board.

ISAM initially recognized three English language multiauthored textbooks as a repository of current knowledge in the field through their successive editions [6, 11, 12]. The most current editions are Galanter, Kleber, and Brady 2015 [7] and Miller et al. 2018 [9]. These texts are backed by some 150 peer-reviewed journals in the field, ranging from basic science to clinical practice. An increasing number of research institutes are disseminating information across the world, including leading institutions such as, in the USA, the National Institute of Drug Abuse and the National Institute on Alcohol Abuse and Alcoholism.

To meet the criterion of affordability as well as reducing the differential access to the literature in different parts of the world, the knowledge basis of the examination was originally based on a primary reliance on the Principles of Addiction Medicine [11]. Since then, further changes have occurred: the nomenclatures of Diagnostic and Statistical Manual of Mental Disorders (fifth ed.; DSM-5; [1]) and International Statistical Classification of Diseases and Related Health Problems, 11th Revision (ICD 11) [16]. Since 2015, the main reference for the ISAM Certification has become the Textbook of Addiction Treatment: International Perspectives [4].

From the onset as part of the drafting of multiple-choice questions, a concerted effort was made to select as many "culture-neutral" questions as possible. Half of the Editorial Board were holders of ASAM certificates and aware of the preponderance of research data based on US populations in the textbooks that would be of lesser significance in other continents. This meant that the epidemiological database had to shift to the data collected by international bodies such as the World Health Organization (WHO) and the United Nations Office on Drugs and Crime (UNODC). Another implication was the exclusion of questions about national legislation replaced by questions about the International Conventions. At the end, from an initial pool of 450 questions, 200 multiple choice questions (MCQs) were selected at a 2-day meeting in September 2004 in Calgary. It was recommended that four options for each MCQ were sufficient (25% chance per option instead of five with 20% chance). From the very onset, it was clearly stated that the certification would be a test of knowledge with some vignettes assessing clinical judgment. The number of questions allocated to each content area was debated at length. It was eventually agreed that the proportion of content questions would reflect the extent of coverage of the topic in the selected textbooks. A subsequent update of the exam questions in 2015, using the Textbook of Addiction Treatment: International Perspectives, similarly reflects the major content areas (see Table 59.1).

Table 59.1 List of certification examination content areas and questions (2016)

Content area	Number of questions
I. Basic sciences and clinical foundations	20
II. Screening and early interventions	30
III. Drugs of abuse and pharmacotherapies for substance use disorders	35
IV. Behavioral approaches	20
V. Social therapies, treatment settings and systems approach to addiction treatment	20
VI. Behavioral addictions and management applications	20
VII. Medical disorders, complications of alcohol and drugs, pain and addiction	28
VIII. Psychiatric comorbidity complications of alcohol and other drugs	27
IX. Children, adolescents, young adults, and special populations	25
Total	225

59.2.2 The Minimum Performance Level Method

To fulfill their mandate of protecting the public, licensure and certification boards in the health professions need to determine which candidates are qualified to attain certification (pass the examinations) or not (fail). Many of these organizations use criterion-referenced testing with predetermined cutoff scores for pass/fail on licensing or certification examinations. There are many ways to set such cutoff scores, but most rely on expert judgment, employing empirical approaches such as the Nedelsky [10] procedure, based on the principle of minimum performance levels (MPLs). Accordingly, we employed a modified Nedelsky procedure for setting cutoff scores using MPLs.

In this criterion-referenced testing procedure, the total test score MPL is the sum of each item MPL [15]. The item writer, therefore, sets an MPL for each item. The MPL is the value ranging between 0.25 and 1.0, which reflects the probability that even a minimally competent candidate can answer this item correctly. An MPL of

0.25 indicates a very difficult item with an MPL of 1.0 reflecting an easy one.

59.2.2.1 Example Item from an ISAM Examination

An added formulation of buprenorphine designed to discourage intravenous use contains? (stem)

(a) Gabapentin (distracter)
(b) Nalmefene (distracter)
(c) Acetylcysteine (distracter)
(d) *Naloxone (keyed response)

A = 1.0 b = 0.75 c = 0.75 d*

MPL = 1/(4 − sum of p) = 1/(4−2:50) = 0:67

Each question having undergone a thorough and rigorous editing process receives an MPL. The construction and psychometric analysis of the exam is under the auspices of faculty from the Cumming School of Medicine at the University of Calgary as well as the University of Minnesota Medical School.

To renew the pool from September 2006, 25 "dummy" or experimental questions were added for psychometric testing and formed the basis of new yearly questions. This is a common practice in the testing industry to identify questions performing well enough to be retained for future test takers. More recently, feedback from the examination applicants also inform the need to upgrade specific questions for the next exam sitting.

The current exam is in two parts with an allowed duration of 2 h and 15 min each.

59.2.3 Psychometric Analysis

59.2.3.1 Item Analysis

A complete analysis of the test requires an item analysis. There are three essential features that constitute an item analysis: (1) difficulty of the item, (2) item discrimination, and (3) distracter effectiveness [5].

The difficulty of the item is the percentage or proportion of people who got the item correct. Item discrimination has to do with the extent to which an item distinguishes or "discriminates" between high test scorers and low test scorers.

Distracter effectiveness refers to the ability of distracters in attracting responses. A distracter that attracts no response is not effective; it begins to become effective when it attracts some responses.

59.2.3.2 Reliability and Validity

The reliability of scores is assessed using the coefficient α. Coefficient α estimates the amount of variability in applicants' scores that is due to the difference in ability rather than random influences such as guessing. In the initial series of applicants, the reliabilities of all subtests ranged from adequate to good. In an 8-year study (2011–2018) of the overall test and subtests, alpha has ranged from 0.68 to 0.87, adequate to good. Validity of a test has to do with extent to which it measures whatever it is supposed to measure. As very careful attention is given to the development of the appropriate sampling of the subject matter and content (i.e., addiction medicine) of the ISAM test, it has adequate content validity. Empirical evidence of validity is sought by evaluating the correlations between the subscales of the test. Over the 8-year study period, subscale correlations have ranged from 0.25 to 0.78, providing evidence of both discriminant and convergent validity [14].

59.2.4 Criteria of Eligibility and Applicants' Countries of Practice

To enhance access to the examination by an international audience, the following eligibility criteria were recommended:

• Graduation from a medical school recognized by the WHO
• Valid license to practice medicine from a licensing jurisdiction (national, regional)
• Good standing in medical community, evidenced by at least three letters of recommendation, from physicians knowing the applicant for at least 2 years, including, if possible, one current ISAM member

- Completion of a formal university-based 1-year fellowship or equivalent in the addiction field
- Documented substantial portion of medical practice including evidence of continuing education (conferences, workshops, courses, etc.) over a 3-year period in the addiction field

The above criteria seem to be within the reach of all applicants, and no noticeable impediment to access of the required information has been recorded.

Fee

An international money order payable to the International Society of Addiction Medicine for US$800 (non-ISAM members), US$700 (ISAM members), and US$725 US (Affiliate Societies' members) is forwarded, along with the application.

From 2005 to 2018 inclusive, the examination has been held 23 times. Practitioners from Canada, Egypt, and Saudi Arabia have formed the bulk of the applicants so far. Candidates from Antigua, Hong Kong, Iceland, India, Iran, Jordan, Kuwait, Oman, Sudan, Turkey, UAE, the UK, Ukraine, the USA, and Vietnam have also challenged the examination. The overall pass rate has been a steady 78% so far.

59.2.5 Lessons Learned

In North America, the Canadian Society of Addiction Medicine recognizes both ASAM and ISAM certificates as equivalent. These qualifications are readily recognized to designate experts in courts and with independent medical examinations (IMEs) for a host of insurance and other agencies.

In Egypt, the ISAM certification is recognized by the Ministry of Health as a professional qualifier. The universities have agreed to use the examination as an end of training knowledge qualifier followed by a clinical skills examination.

A dialogue is ongoing, in several countries in Europe, to use the certification as adjunct to local diplomas. Setting a valid and reliable examina-

tion is a time- and resource-intensive exercise, and from our experience, the process of testing core knowledge does not need to be duplicated in every country. Potential addition of questions of national interest to the core questions is a possibility.

As the ISAM certification enters its 15th year, a review of the experience leads to the following conclusions:

1. An international certification examination is possible! While the experience so far focuses on Canada and the Middle East, the process is slowly gaining credibility, judging from the inquiries from other regions. The examination is also available to international fellows training in North America's leading institutions. Local leadership support to disseminate information and promote the value of a clinical knowledge qualifier is critical.

2. The questions show good discriminatory performance. Following the first exam set of 200, 9 questions were dropped and new ones added from the pool, and 36 others had their MPL readjusted, "raising the bar." To renew the pool, 25 "dummy" questions were added to be tested in each examination. The first major editorial update was conducted in 2010, resulting in the replacement of one-third of the questions by new ones and another third being modified. Only the references of the remaining third were updated. A second update occurred in 2015–2016, with the inclusion of the new reference source, The Textbook of Addiction Treatment: International Perspectives. The third cycle of editorial update will begin in 2020, coinciding with the publication of the second edition of the Textbook of Addiction Treatment: International Perspectives.

3. The careful development of the ISAM test has resulted in evidence for both validity (content, empirical) and reliability (internal consistency), and items that are carefully reviewed and evaluated for difficulty, discrimination, and distracter effectiveness.

4. The recommended curriculum should inform examination and vice versa. Topics where

the candidates are the weakest included pain and addiction; behavioral addictions; and diagnosis, assessment, and early intervention. In several countries, the field of addiction is limited to the management of substance misuse. Addition of "local" questions to the core examination has been proposed to accommodate the local legislative and possible cultural needs.

5. An "a-cultural" examination may be only a goal to strive for. Biological or laboratory tests may be largely culture-free, although epigenetic findings are showing a number of ethnic differences. Epidemiological data, psychological treatments, mutual help resources, and workplace guidelines are more influenced by the local culture. Many countries forbid the use of methadone maintenance, for example. Can a core examination be fair globally when the medical practices are subject to different cultural and economic constraints? Candidates appreciate the need to be aware of evidence-based treatment options available in other parts of the world and may promote their culturally sensitive adaptation in their own country.

6. The cost, integrity, and sensitivity of the examination are critical in all areas of the world but particularly in developing countries. Requests have been made to create a network of examination centers where the certification could be disseminated electronically. While this remains under consideration, there remains concerns about test security as well as a sustainable critical mass of applicants.

7. We have moved from a reliance on national textbooks to an internationally collaborated textbook, which is available in electronic version.

8. Each successful candidate receives a numbered certificate to avoid forgery. Displays of association membership certificates in practitioners' offices as evidence of competence have been reported. This increases the need for a recognized certificate, testing clinical knowledge through MCQs, and clinical vignettes.

9. The repeated experience of the examination in developing countries is that the pool of often university-based candidates readily achieves pass and higher scores. This pool is however finite. This observation calls for enhanced national efforts to increase the pool of justified candidates practicing evidence-based medicine across the nation.

10. Presenting standardized review courses and complementing the test of clinical knowledge with a standardized objective structural clinical exam (OSCE), administered locally, is the next frontier.

There is no doubt that language proficiency can be a barrier. Discussions have been underway to translate the examination into Spanish and Italian. Settings where a computerized version of the examination can be administered are being contemplated. The security of this process may be improving. The cost remains significant. The search for funding support is ongoing. Several examination sets are being administered by different academic institutions worldwide; must we reinvent the wheel time and time again?

Key Points

- An international examination is possible, involving questions with good psychometric properties.
- The eligibility criteria appear to be within reach of many countries with some English proficiency.
- The examination sections address a broad-based addiction medicine practice.
- The certification is a test of knowledge with some vignettes addressing clinical judgment.
- The ISAM Certification can be a useful adjunct to local diplomas.
- Cultural adaptation can be facilitated through evidence-based treatment options in the examination.

Acknowledgment to the ISAM Editorial Board of Examiners (2004–2011) Dr. Maria Delgado (Argentina); Dr. Paul Haber (Australia); Dr. Bill Campbell, Dr. Sam Chang, Dr. Raju Hajela, Dr. Ron Lim (Canada); Dr. Salwa Erfan and Dr. Tarek Gawad (Egypt); Dr. Hannu Alho (Finland); Dr. Char-Nie Chen (Hong Kong); Dr. Thor Tyrfingsson (Iceland); Dr. Flavio Poldrugo (Italy); Dr. Doug Talbott and Dr. Greg Bunt (USA); Dr. Nady el-Guebaly (Chair), Dr. Claudio Violato (Consultant), Marilyn Dorozio and Cheryl Noonan (Administrative Assistance).

(2016) Dr. Oscar D'Agnone (UK), Dr. Cor de Jong (Netherlands), Dr. Tarek Gawad (UAE), Dr. Laura Evans (Canada), Marta Torrens (Spain)

References

1. American Psychiatric Association. Diagnostic and statistical manual of mental disorders. 5th ed. Arlington: Author; 2013.

2. Ayu AP, De Jong C. Addiction training in medical education. In: el-Guebaly N, Carrà G, Galanter. Eds. The textbook of addiction treatment: international perspectives. Springer Milan Heidelberg, New York, Dordrecht. London. 2015.

3. Crockford D, el-Guebaly N. Addiction treatment in medical education: the Canadian experience. In: el-Guebaly N, Carrà G, Galanter. Eds. The textbook of addiction treatment: international perspectives. Springer Milan Heidelberg, New York, Dordrecht. London. 2015.

4. el-Guebaly N, Carrà G, Galanter M, editors. Textbook of addiction treatment: international perspectives, vol. 1–4. Italia: Springer Verlag; 2015.

5. el-Guebaly N, Violato C. The international certification of addiction medicine: validating clinical knowledge across borders. Subst Abus. 2011;32(2):77–83.

6. Galanter M, Kleber HD, editors. Textbook of substance abuse treatment. 4th ed. Arlington: American Psychiatric Publishing; 2008.

7. Galanter M, Kleber HD, Brady K, editors. Textbook of substance abuse treatment. 5th ed. Arlington: American Psychiatric Publishing; 2015.

8. Madras BK, Compton WM, Avula D, et al. Screening, brief interventions, referral to treatment (SBIRT) for illicit drug and alcohol use at multiple health care sites: comparison at intake and 6 months later. Drug Alcohol Depend. 2009;99:280–95.

9. Miller SC, Fiellin DA, Rosenthal RN, Saitz R. Principles of addiction medicine. 6th ed. Philadelphia: Wolters Kluwer; 2019.

10. Nedelsky L. Absolute grading standards for objective tests. Educ Psychol Meas. 1954;14:3–19.

11. Ries R, Fiellin DA, Miller SC, Saitz R. Principles of addiction medicine. 4th ed. Philadelphia: Lippincott Williams & Wilkins; 2009.

12. Ruiz P, Strain E. Substance abuse. A comprehensive textbook. 5th ed. Philadelphia: Lippincott Williams & Wilkins; 2011.

13. Soyka M, Gorelick DA. Why should addiction medicine be an attractive field for young physicians? Addiction. 2009;104:169–72.

14. Violato C. Assessing competence in medicine and other health professions. New York: Taylor & Francis; 2019.

15. Violato C, Marini A, Lee C. A validity study of expert judgment procedures for setting cutoff scores on high-stakes credentialing examinations using cluster analysis. Eval Health Prof. 2003;26:59–72.

16. World Health Organization. International statistical classification of diseases and related health problems (11th Revision). 2018. Retrieved from https://icd.who.int/browse11/l-m/en.

National Institute on Drug Abuse International Fellowships: Research Training for Addiction Specialists

60

Steven W. Gust

Contents

Abstract

Despite the widespread prevalence and increasing risk of disability or death associated with drug use disorders, access to evidence-based treatment is rare. The United Nations estimates that only one in six people who need drug treatment receive it, and cites the lack of research and training as barriers to expanding evidence-based treatment. Professional associations in the United States and the United Kingdom call for mentored research training to help health care professionals learn how to conduct research and understand and implement research findings in practice. Recent evaluations of research training programs found that physicians, service planners, and policymakers benefitted from mentored research training. Effective mentoring programs helped trainees conduct research, analyze data, publish findings, present at scientific meetings, collaborate with senior researchers, meet government officials, and continue networking after the conclusion of the fellowship. These components of effective research training programs are available through fellowships offered by the National Institute on Drug Abuse (NIDA) International Program. The NIDA fellowships for postdoctoral, mid-career, and senior addiction specialists are reviewed, including credential and citizenship requirements for applicants, and professional advantages are described. Former fellows head academic research centers and

S. W. Gust (✉)
International Program, National Institute on Drug Abuse, National Institutes of Health, US Department of Health and Human Services,
Washington, DC, USA
e-mail: ipdirector@nida.nih.gov

© Springer Nature Switzerland AG 2021
N. el-Guebaly et al. (eds.), *Textbook of Addiction Treatment*,
https://doi.org/10.1007/978-3-030-36391-8_60

nongovernmental organizations, provide addiction treatment, serve as government officials, and play key roles in international drug policy. NIDA fellows collaborate with international partners, receive grants from NIDA and other funders, publish articles, and present at conferences. They form a global network of drug abuse scientists working collaboratively to develop, validate, and implement evidence-based treatment and prevention programs around the world.

Keywords

NIDA International · Addiction Research · Drug Abuse Fellowships

60.1　Introduction

Training an international cohort of health care professionals to research and treat drug use disorders is an increasingly urgent priority. The United Nations Office on Drugs and Crime (UNODC) estimated that 275 million people aged 16–64 used drugs in 2016 [1]. Of those individuals, 31 million were diagnosed with a substance use disorder. In 2015, drug use was associated with 450,000 deaths, an increase of 60% since 2000 [1]. The Global Burden of Disease research team reported that 31.8 million disability-adjusted life years (DALYs) in 2016 were attributable to drug use as a risk factor [2]. In 2017, drug use disorders were ranked 21 among the top sources of DALYs for men, an increase of 26.6% since 2007 [3]. Foreman and colleagues predict that by 2040, drug use disorders will be among the top 10 causes of years of life lost in Australasia, Eastern Europe, and high-income North America [4].

Despite the widespread prevalence and growing risk of disability or death associated with drug use disorders, access to evidence-based treatment remains limited. UNODC reports that only one in six individuals who need drug treatment have access to treatment services [1]. Barriers to evidence-based drug treatment include a lack of research, particularly in real-world

health care settings, and a shortage of health care professionals trained in public health and medical models of drug treatment [5].

In the United States, the American Board of Medical Specialties formally recognized Addiction Medicine as a subspecialty in March 2016. Decades earlier, National Consensus Standards on postgraduate medical fellowship training in alcoholism and drug abuse called for a "meaningful, supervised research experience" ([6], p., 6). The Consensus Standard priorities included learning about research methods and how to design and interpret research studies. Conducting an independent research project was "desirable" ([6], p., 10). In 2018, the Association for Multidisciplinary Education and Research in Substance Use and Addiction (AMERSA) revised its standards for health care professional training. AMERSA recommends that physicians, nurses, pharmacists, social workers, and physician assistants who assess and treat patients who use alcohol and drugs should learn how to understand and implement research findings in treatment and participate in interdisciplinary activities, including research [7]. The United Kingdom General Medical Council essential capabilities for postgraduate medical curricula include "Research and Scholarship" among nine domains. The 2017 document describes requirements that doctors-in-training understand research methods and principles, learn to interpret public health epidemiology findings, and know how to translate research into practice [8].

Medical students who participate in mentored research programs develop positive opinions about both clinical care and academic research in substance abuse [9, 10]. Recent evaluations of research training programs conducted in both low- and high-income countries found that mentored research programs influenced fellows' research careers and success. This was especially true of programs that helped trainees develop and publish their own research and provided long-term networking after the conclusion of the fellowship [11–17]. For fellowships that focused on trainees from low-income countries, mentored research that prepared individuals for independent careers was enhanced by international collaboration with senior researchers, participation in workshops and scientific meetings, guidance in data analysis and scientific writing, and visits to the US National Institutes of Health (NIH) [18–20]. Treatment providers, service planners, and policymakers from low- and middle-income countries also benefitted from research training programs [14, 21].

60.2 Fellowships Supported by the National Institute on Drug Abuse International Program

Since 1990, the NIDA International Program has developed drug abuse research fellowships to facilitate an international network of scientists trained to investigate the causes, prevention, treatment, and consequences of drug use and addiction. NIDA's global network now includes scientists and drug abuse professionals from more than 110 countries who have completed more than 500 fellowships. Fellows work with NIDA grantees at US institutions and have conducted research in every aspect of the NIDA portfolio, including preclinical research and studies in epidemiology, prevention, treatment, and clinical trials.

NIDA currently supports four postdoctoral fellowship programs, a fellowship for mid-career drug abuse professionals from eligible low- and middle-income countries, and two professional development programs for senior scientists. NIDA International fellowship programs train substance use researchers from other countries in US research methods, help fellows enhance their understanding of the scientific basis of drug use and addiction, and promote research collaboration by introducing NIDA grantees to talented drug use researchers from other countries. The seven fellowship and scientific exchange programs expand the Institute's ability to build networks, mentor junior investigators, conduct needs assessments, and transfer knowledge. Table 60.1 summarizes the fellowship career levels, activities, eligibility requirements, and application deadlines. Additional details are available

on the NIDA International Program website: https://www.drugabuse.gov/international/fellowships-landing.

The four INVEST fellowships combine postdoctoral research training in the United States with professional development activities such as preparing publications, poster or oral presentations at scientific meetings, and grant-writing guidance. The program is designed to enhance the ability of junior drug use scientists from other countries to conduct independent research upon return to their home country. Three fellowships are open to applicants from any other country—the INVEST Drug Abuse Research Fellowships, INVEST/Clinical Trials Network (CTN) Drug Abuse Research Fellowships, and the INVEST Drug Abuse Prevention Research Fellowship. The INVEST NIDA–Inserm Postdoctoral Drug Abuse Research Fellowship is restricted to US and French scientists, with US researchers working at Inserm laboratories in France and French researchers working with NIDA grantees in the United States. All fellows are invited to present their research at an appropriate scientific meeting, such as the NIDA International Forum satellite to the College on Problems of Drug Dependence, and meetings sponsored by the Society for Prevention Research or the Society for Neuroscience.

The NIDA Hubert H. Humphrey Drug Abuse Research Fellowships bring fellows from eligible low- and middle-income countries to study and work with colleagues in the United States. NIDA Humphrey Fellowships are part of a larger program coordinated by the US Department of State that provides mid-career experts with advanced leadership training that includes academic, practical, and cultural activities in the United States. NIDA Humphrey Fellows also receive training in addiction science and public health through specialized coursework, professional affiliations with US substance abuse experts, visits to NIH, and participation in the NIDA International Forum. The fellowships are particularly appropriate for treatment providers and policymakers who need to understand the science of addiction in order to adopt evidence-based treatment practice guidelines and government policies.

Table 60.1 NIDA International Program training opportunities for US and international scientists

Career level	Program name	Eligible audience	What fellowship includes	Application deadline
Postdoctoral training	INVEST Drug Abuse Research Fellowship	Non-US citizens, any topic	12-month training and professional development with a NIDA grantee at a US institution. May apply to renew once.	October 1
	INVEST/Clinical Trials Network (CTN) Drug Abuse Research Fellowship	Non-US citizens, topic of interest to CTN	12-month training and professional development with a NIDA grantee affiliated with a CTN Node at a US institution. May apply to renew once.	October 1
	INVEST Prevention Drug Abuse Research Fellowship	Non-US citizens or permanent residents conducting prevention research	12-month training and professional development with a NIDA-supported prevention researcher at a US institution. May apply to renew once.	October 1
	INVEST NIDA–Inserm Postdoctoral Drug Abuse Research Fellowship	French citizens work with a NIDA grantee at a US institution US citizens work at an Inserm lab in France	6- to 12-month training and professional development. May apply to renew once.	Applications may be submitted at any time
Mid-career training	NIDA Hubert H. Humphrey Drug Abuse Research Fellowship	US State Department identifies eligible countries and reviews applications	10-month academic study and professional development activities	Deadlines vary Apply through US Embassy or Fulbright Commission in eligible countries
Senior researcher exchanges	Distinguished International Scientist Collaboration Award (DISCA) and USDISCA	DISCA: Non-US citizens visit NIDA grantees in US USDISCA: US citizens and permanent residents visit research partners in other countries	Research exchange visits of at least 1 month to finalize a specific task that could not be completed without face-to-face consultation	December 1

The competitive Distinguished International Scientist Collaboration Awards (DISCA) and the companion Distinguished International Scientist Collaboration Awards for US Citizens and Permanent Residents (USDISCA) programs support brief research exchange visits between senior researchers from other countries and NIDA grantees. The research team must propose a specific task that could not be completed without face-to-face consultation.

60.3 Professional Advantages of the National Institute on Drug Abuse International Program Fellowships

Former NIDA International Program Fellows advance scientific knowledge on drug use and addiction through their research and professional careers. Former fellows head academic research centers and nongovernmental organizations, provide addiction treatment, serve as government officials, and play key roles in international drug policy through international organizations such as the Colombo Plan Drug Advisory Programme, European Union, Inter-American Drug Abuse Control Commission (CICAD) at the Organization of American States, United Nations, and the World Health Organization (WHO). For example, former NIDA International Program fellows played key roles in developing WHO and UNODC guidelines for substance use treatment and prevention, pharmacological and psychosocial approaches to treating opioid dependence, community efforts to address opioid overdose, treating substance use disorders in pregnant women and people involved in the criminal justice system, and the effects of nonmedical cannabis use. Former NIDA Fellows also contributed to the joint European Monitoring Centre for Drugs and Drug Addiction/Organization of American States handbook on building a national drug observatory, and have led the Drug Advisory Programme at the Colombo Plan.

Fellows conduct and publish peer-reviewed research. An analysis of fellows' publications during 2016 and 2017 identified 561 unique articles published in peer-reviewed publications indexed by the NIH PubMed database. More than half (52.4%) of former NIDA International Program postdoctoral fellows and more than one-fourth (25.8%) of all former fellows published articles during that time frame [22].

An evaluation of the Virginia Commonwealth University host campus for the NIDA Humphrey Fellowship program found that former fellows reported collaborating with international partners, receiving grants, publishing articles, presenting at conferences, and obtaining new credentials since completing their fellowships. Of the 108 former fellows from 52 countries, 34.7% had collaborated with a US partner, 24.3% had collaborated with other former fellows, and 19% had received grant support. Nearly one-third (30%) had published a manuscript, 49% had presented at a conference, and 46% had conducted research. About one-fourth had received a license or certification (26%), and 21% had enrolled in an academic program since completing their fellowship [23].

The NIDA International Program helps fellows build on their research training through the annual NIDA International Forum. About 200 researchers participate, nearly half from the United States and other high-income countries. Former fellows and other participants make oral or poster presentations, network with former mentors and other fellows, and establish new research partnerships. Between 2012 and 2017, more than 30 NIDA grants were associated with the Forum; the foreign principal investigator on 23 of those grants was a former NIDA International Program fellow [22].

60.4   The Way Forward

Although the NIDA International Program fellowships are unique, a few other NIH research training programs are available for addiction specialists who are not US citizens or permanent residents. The Visiting Program supports NIDA Intramural Research Program (IRP) fellowships for non-US postdoctoral researchers and temporary full-time research positions for international scientists. NIDA IRP also offers limited predoctoral research opportunities for international students. The NIDA IRP training opportunities are online at https://irp. drugabuse.gov/training/. Information about other NIH Institutes that participate in the NIH Visiting Program is available at https://www.ors.od.nih. gov/pes/dis/VisitingScientists/Pages/default.aspx. The NIH Fogarty International Center (https://fic. nih.gov) supports a number of training programs for scientists and clinicians from low- and middle-income countries, and NIDA participates in the Fogarty D43 institutional training grant for Chronic, Non-Communicable Diseases and Disorders Across the Lifespan.

NIDA promotes international collaborative research through a dedicated funding opportunity (PA-18-773, International Collaborative Research on Drug Abuse and Addiction Research) that requires a partnership between a US scientist and their partners in another country. Many other NIH funding opportunities are open to participation by non-US researchers. Each funding opportunity announcement includes an eligibility section that will specify what types of foreign participation are permitted for that announcement. Currently, about 8% of the NIDA research portfolio is allocated for international research, primarily through grants to US domestic organizations with foreign partners. All international research must meet special requirements, such as providing access to unusual talent, resources, populations, or environmental conditions not available domestically, demonstrating how the international research will significantly advance US health sciences, and documenting relevance to the NIDA mission.

NIDA works closely with international organizations devoted to improving drug addiction research and treatment, such as CICAD, Colombo Plan, European Monitoring Centre for Drugs and Drug Addiction, International Consortium of Universities for Drug Demand Reduction (ICUDDR), International Society of Substance Use Professionals, UNODC, and WHO. Most of these training programs are designed for the global health care workforce, but few offer mentored research training. ICUDDR members are developing undergraduate, graduate, and postdoctoral training programs within their own universities, and international research training opportunities will expand as these programs mature.

60.5   Conclusions

The need for evidence-based drug use and addiction treatment is increasing, along with the need for addiction specialists who understand the principles of research and know how to implement findings into practice. Organizations such as AMERSA and the UK General Medical Council call research training essential for qualified addiction specialists. Practitioners who participate in effective research training programs report improved job satisfaction and professional success in both clinical and research careers. Effective research training programs include components such as conducting research, analyzing data, publishing findings, presenting at scientific meetings, collaborating with senior

researchers, meeting government officials, and networking after the conclusion of the fellowship. Since their creation in 1990, the NIDA International Program drug abuse research fellowships have provided effective mentoring and networking for addiction specialists from other countries. The NIDA fellows' successful clinical and research careers document the professional advantages mentored research training can offer.

NIDA will continue to support its international drug abuse research fellowships, adapting and expanding the program as funding permits to meet the growing demand for mentored addiction research opportunities. The current NIDA–Inserm fellowship provides a model for addiction research training partnerships with similar institutions in other countries: NIDA supports French researchers who train in the United States, and Inserm supports US researchers who train in France. We invite current and new partners interested in addiction research training to join NIDA in meeting this critical need.

Key Points

– Professional associations such as the American Board of Medical Specialties and credentialing bodies such as the UK General Medical Council recommend research training to help addiction specialists evaluate and implement research findings in practice.

– Since 1990, NIDA has supported more than 500 research training fellowships for postdoctoral researchers, mid-career professionals, and senior scientists from 110 countries.

– These NIDA International Fellowships include components proven to be effective, such as conducting research, analyzing data, publishing findings, presenting at scientific meetings, collaborating with senior researchers, meeting government officials, and networking after the conclusion of the fellowship.

- – NIDA International Fellowships contribute to former Fellows' successful careers and advance scientific knowledge about drug abuse:
  - – Former fellows head academic research centers and nongovernmental organizations, provide addiction treatment, serve as government officials, and play key roles in international drug policy through roles at international organizations.
  - – Between 2012 and 2017, more than 30 NIDA grants were associated with the NIDA International Forum; the foreign principal investigator on 23 of those grants was a former NIDA International Program fellow.
  - – In 2016–2017, former NIDA fellows published 521 unique research articles indexed by PubMed.

Clinical Relevance

Clinicians are better prepared to adopt evidence-based treatments if they have research experience and can integrate published research findings into practice.

References

1. United Nations Office on Drugs and Crime (UNODC). World Drug Report 2018 (United Nations publication, Sales No. E.18.XL.9). Vienna: UNODC. 2018. Retrieved from https://www.unodc.org/wdr2018/. Accessed 9 Mar 2019.
2. GBD 2016 Alcohol and Drug Use Collaborators. The global burden of disease attributable to alcohol and drug use in 195 countries and territories, 1990–2016: a systematic analysis for the Global Burden of Disease Study 2016. Lancet Psychiatry. 2018;5(12):987–1012. https://doi.org/10.1016/S2215-0366(18)30337-7.
3. GBD 2017 DALYs and HALE Collaborators. Global, regional, and national disability-adjusted life-years (DALYs) for 359 diseases and injuries and healthy life expectancy (HALE) for 195 countries and territories,1990–2017: a systematic analysis for the Global Burden of Disease Study 2017. Lancet. 2018;392(10159):1859–922. https://doi.org/10.1016/S0140-6736(18)32335-3.
4. Foreman KJ, Marquez N, Dolgert A, Fukutaki K, Fullman N, McGaughey M, Pletcher MA, Smith AE, Tang K, Yuan CW, Brown JC, Friedman J, He J, Heuton KR, Holmberg M, Patel DJ, Reidy P, Carter A, Cercy K, Chapin A, Douwes-Schultz D, Frank T, Goettsch F, Liu PY, Nandakumar V, Reitsma MB, Reuter V, Sadat N, Sorensen RJD, Srinivasan V, Updike RL, York H, Lopez AD, Lozano R, Lim SS, Mokdad AH, Vollset SE, Murray CJL. Forecasting life expectancy, years of life lost, and all-cause and cause-specific mortality for 250 causes of death: reference and alternative scenarios for 2016-2040 for 195 countries and territories. Lancet. 2018;392(10159):2052–90. https://doi.org/10.1016/S0140-6736(18)31694-5.
5. United Nations Office on Drugs and Crime (UNODC). UNODC treatment of stimulant use disorders: current practices and promising perspectives. Discussion Paper. Vienna: UNODC. 2019. Retrieved from https://www.unodc.org/documents/drug-prevention-and-treatment/Treatment_of_PSUD_for_print_1X_09.03.19.pdf. Accessed 9 Mar 2019.
6. Galanter M, Kaufman E, Schnoll S, Burns J. Postgraduate medical fellowship training in alcoholism and drug abuse: National Consensus Standards. Am J Drug Alcohol Abuse. 1991;17(1):1–12.
7. Association for Multidisciplinary Education and Research in Substance Use and Addiction (AMERSA). Specific disciplines addressing substance use: AMERSA in the 21st Century – 2018 Update. Cranston, RI. 2018. Retrieved from https://amersa.org/wp-content/uploads/AMERSA-Competencies-Final-31119.pdf. Accessed 24 Apr 2014.
8. General Medical Council. Generic professional capabilities framework. Manchester. 2017. Retrieved from https://www.gmc-uk.org/-/media/documents/generic-professional-capabilities-framework%2D%2D0817_pdf-70417127.pdf. Accessed 24 Apr 2019.
9. Solomon SS, Tom SC, Pichert J, Wasserman D, Powers AC. Impact of medical student research in the development of physician-scientists. J Investig Med. 2003;51(3):149–56. https://doi.org/10.1136/jim-51-03-17. https://jim.bmj.com/content/51/3/149.long. Accessed 24 Apr 2019.
10. Truncali A, Kalet AL, Gillespie C, More F, Naegle M, Lee JD, Huben L, Kerr D, Gourevitch MN. Engaging health professional students in substance abuse research: development and early evaluation of the SARET program. J Addict Med. 2012;6(3):196–204. https://doi.org/10.1097/ADM.0b013e31825f77db.
11. Brown AM, Chipps TM, Gebretsadik T, Ware LB, Islam JY, Finck LR, Barnett J, Hartert TV. Training the next generation of physician researchers - Vanderbilt Medical Scholars Program. BMC Med Educ. 2018;18(1):5. https://doi.org/10.1186/s12909-017-1103-0.
12. Campbell ANC, Back SE, Ostroff JS, Hien DA, Gourevitch MN, Sheffer CE, Brady KT, Hanley K, Bereket S, Book S. Addiction research training pro-

grams: four case studies and recommendations for evaluation. J Addict Med. 2018;11(5):333–8. https://doi.org/10.1097/ADM.0000000000000328.

13. Hanley K, Bereket S, Tuchman E, More FG, Naegle MA, Kalet A, Goldfeld K, Gourevitch MN. Evaluation of the Substance Abuse Research and Education Training (SARET) program: stimulating health professional students to pursue careers in substance use research. Subst Abus. 2018;39(4):476–83. https://doi.org/10.1080/08897077.2018.1449167.

14. Semrau M, Alem A, Abdulmalik J, Docrat S, Evans-Lacko S, Gureje O, Kigozi F, Lempp H, Lund C, Petersen I, Shidhaye R, Thornicroft G, Hanlon C. Developing capacity-building activities for mental health system strengthening in low- and middle-income countries for service users and caregivers, service planners, and researchers. Epidemiol Psychiatr Sci. 2018;27:11–21. https://doi.org/10.1017/S2045796017000452.

15. Krupat E, Camargo CA Jr, Strewler GJ, Espinola JA, Fleenor TJ Jr, Dienstag JL. Factors associated with physicians' choice of a career in research: a retrospective report 15 years after medical school graduation. Adv Health Sci Educ Theory Pract. 2017;22(1):5–15. https://doi.org/10.1007/s10459-016-9678-5.

16. Ognibene FP, Gallin JI, Baum BJ, Wyatt RG, Gottesman MM. Outcomes from the NIH Clinical Research Training Program: a mentored research experience to enhance career development of clinician-scientists. Acad Med. 2016;91(12):1684–90. https://doi.org/10.1097/ACM.0000000000001245.

17. Pfund C, Byars-Winston A, Branchaw J, Hurtado S, Eagan K. Defining attributes and metrics of effective research mentoring relationships. AIDS and Behavior. 2016;2:238–48. https://doi.org/10.1007/s10461-016-1384-z.

18. Magidson JF, Stevenson A, Ng LC, Hock RS, Borba CP, Namey LB, Carney J, Joska JA, Kagee A, Fekadu A, Bangsberg DR, Safren SA, Fricchione GL, Henderson DC. Massachusetts General Hospital global psychiatric clinical research training program: a new fellowship in global mental health. Acad Psychiatry. 2016;40(4):695–7. https://doi.org/10.1007/s40596-015-0388-8.

19. Bloomfield GS, Xavier D, Belis D, Alam D, Davis P, Dorairaj P, Ghannem H, Gilman RH, Kamath D, Kimaiyo S, Levitt N, Martinez H, Mejicano G, Miranda JJ, Koehlmoos TP, Rabadán-Diehl C, Ramirez-Zea M, Rubinstein A, Sacksteder KA, Steyn K, Tandon N, Vedanthan R, Wolbach T, Wu Y, Yan LL. Training and capacity building in LMIC for research in heart and lung diseases: the NHLBI-UnitedHealth Global Health Centers of Excellence Program. Glob Heart. 2016;11(1):17–25. https://doi.org/10.1016/j.gheart.2016.01.004.

20. ESSENCE on Health Research. Seven principles for strengthening research capacity in low- and middle-income countries: Simple ideas in a complex world. Essence Good practice document series. World Health Organization reference number: TDR/ESSENCE/2.14 Geneva. 2014. https://www.who.int/tdr/publications/Essence_report2014_OK.pdf?ua=1. Accessed 24 Apr 2019.

21. Rawson RA, Woody G, Kresina TF, Gust S. The globalization of addiction research: capacity-building mechanisms and selected examples. Harv Rev Psychiatry. 2015;23(2):147–56. https://doi.org/10.1097/HRP.0000000000000067.

22. Gust SW, McCormally J. NIDA International Program: leveraging international research to improve treatment for opioid use disorders. Curr Opin Psychiatry. 2018;31(4):287–93. https://doi.org/10.1097/YCO.0000000000000426.

23. Leonchuk L, Koch JR, Breland A, Balster R, Kliewer W. Evaluation of the VCU humphrey fellowship program: a mixed-method approach. Oral presentation at the NIDA International Forum, June 8, 2019. San Diego. 2018. Available by email request to ip@nida.nih.gov.

Undergraduate Medical Training in Substance Misuse

61

Ilana B. Crome and Christine M. Goodair

Contents

Abstract

Whilst addiction psychiatry is a recognised subspecialty in the UK, research into UK medical schools during the 1990s showed very low levels of exposure of future doctors to teaching on drug and alcohol misuse issues. Substance misuse is prevalent in almost all branches of medicine. As a result, there are extensive opportunities to teach and learn about it. However, this also leads to the risk that the topic may be fragmented, poorly coordinated and spread too thinly, so that it is often ultimately barely visible to students. In the UK, a 'Substance Misuse in the Undergraduate Medical Curriculum Project' was funded with the aim of improving the teaching of substance misuse to medical undergraduates so as to enhance medical education in addictions and improve treatment services in the future.

I. B. Crome
Keele University, Staffordshire, UK

St George's, University of London, London, UK

C. M. Goodair (✉)
Population Health Research Institute, St George's,
University of London, London, UK
e-mail: cgoodair@sgul.ac.uk

© Springer Nature Switzerland AG 2021
N. el-Guebaly et al. (eds.), *Textbook of Addiction Treatment*,
https://doi.org/10.1007/978-3-030-36391-8_61

Keywords

Medical education · Undergraduate ·
Addiction · Curriculum Substance Misuse

61.1 Introduction

This chapter focuses on the need for training and education on substance-related disorders for undergraduate medical students and describes initiatives undertaken in the UK. It provides a brief historical and contextual introduction, describes work undertaken and explores issues of sustainability within a constant changing health landscape.

61.2 Historical and Contextual

Substance misuse has been a national and international public health challenge for many years. The use and misuse of alcohol, drugs (licit and illicit), prescribed and over-the-counter medications, and tobacco impacts individual patients, their families and communities. Doctors and other health professionals across all medical specialities are highly likely to encounter individuals with substance-related health problems, given the extent of these problems. All health professionals have a key role in improving not only the health of their individual patients but also the nation's public health. This was recognised by both the World Health Organization [25] and the United Nations [18, 19] who have recommended to governments that substance misuse should be included in medical teaching.

UK statistics show that, in 2016, there were estimated to be 77,900 deaths attributable to smoking amongst adults aged 35 and over based on the original cause of death. Hospital admissions estimated to be attributable to

smoking indicates that 22% of all admissions were for respiratory diseases, 15% for circulatory diseases and 9% for cancers. Of the admissions for cancers, 47% were caused by smoking,

with 40% of admissions for respiratory diseases that can be caused by smoking, were estimated to be attributable to smoking [20, 21]. The total cost to society (in England) is approximately £12.9 billion a year and includes the cost to the NHS of treating diseases caused by smoking and lost productivity due to premature deaths, smoking breaks and absenteeism [1].

In 2017–2018, there were 338,000 estimated admissions to hospitals that were attributable to alcohol, and, in England, in 2017, there were 5,843 alcohol-specific deaths with alcoholic liver disease accounting for 80% of the deaths, and 9% were from mental and behavioural disorders due to the use of alcohol [23]. Alcohol is estimated to cost the NHS around £3.5 billion per year [14].

About 3 million adults aged 16–59 in England and Wales in 2017–2018 had used illicit drugs, with Class A drug use (typically opioids and cocaine) increasing since 2011–2012. In 2017–2018, there were 7258 hospital admissions for drug-related mental and behavioural disorders, and 2503 deaths were related to poisoning by drug misuse. In the same period, 268,390 individuals were in contact with drug and alcohol services during 2017–2018 with those in treatment for opiate dependence making up the largest proportion of the total numbers in treatment (53% or 141,189) [20–22].

In 2014, the National Treatment Agency estimated that the overall annual cost of drug misuse was around £15.4 billion. A total of £13.9 billion was due to drug-related crime, while around £0.5 billion was NHS costs for treating drug misuse [2].

Research, including surveys into the undergraduate medical UK curricula between the late 1980s and 2004, found that substance misuse was generally very poorly represented in the training of future doctors, and the number of hours allocated to formal teaching about substance misuse was small. It was taught mainly within the disciplines of psychiatry and pharmacology, thus reinforcing the false notion that substance misuse is a niche specialty topic [3, 4, 7, 12]. Whilst it was found that there were numerous initiatives in North America, some establishing a core curriculum and others developing teaching and learning innovations, very little innovation was taking place in the UK. The lessons were clear: substance misuse has to be integrated into the curriculum of medical students, and it has to be a topic introduced from the very beginning of the course—not least for students' own health and professional behaviour.

Previous initiatives undertaken by St George's, University of London, and the World Health Organization (WHO) on substance misuse education for doctors, pharmacists and nurses resulted in the WHO recommending to governments that substance misuse should be included in the medical curricula [6, 11, 25].

Proposals were submitted to the Department of Health to develop a consensus approach to the enhancement of substance misuse training in medical and nursing schools in the UK. Funding was awarded in 2005 to improve the education of doctors in substance misuse and to develop a consensus approach to substance misuse training in medical schools, and a national project, 'Substance Misuse in the Undergraduate Curriculum', was established and led by Professor Hamid Ghodse, Director of the then International Centre for Drug Policy at St George's Medical School.

61.3 Description of the Project

This project has comprised three phases. In Phase 1, during 2005–2007, a UK corporate guidance document was developed that set out core aims and learning outcomes for substance misuse teaching and learning in the undergraduate medical curricula. Phase 2, during 2008–2011, focused on implementing the guidance through the appointment of curriculum coordinators in English medical schools to identify what substance misuse teaching was being undertaken, and to recommend changes to ensure that substance misuse issues were fully covered. Phase 3, from 2012 onwards, concentrated on developing and extensively revising a set of factsheets, initially written in Phase 2, and which covered substance misuse relevant to a range of clinical conditions, groups of patients, specialities and settings.

61.3.1 Phase 1

Building on the research done in the late 1980s and 1990s, during Phase 1, the project further reviewed the ways in which substance misuse problems was being taught in all UK medical schools [3, 6, 7, 12, 13]. It sought to establish the reasons for ineffectiveness and to make proposals for improvement in medical schools throughout the country. The project aimed to understand the reasons why medical education was not preparing doctors appropriately in this respect; to identify initiatives that different medical schools could take to improve matters; and make recommendations for further action.

A survey was undertaken in 2005 which provided an overview of the state of substance misuse education in all UK medical schools. The aim of the survey was to gather information about substance misuse teaching and learning, including strategies medical schools used for embedding the topic in the curriculum, and to collect examples of good quality learning materials. Responses were obtained from each of the 32 UK medical schools.

The survey findings included the following:

- There was no commonality of approach in what was taught about substance misuse: learning outcomes differed hugely in style, level of detail and emphasis.
- Many schools covered a lot about alcohol, but relatively few covered teaching about drugs—with this aspect frequently being left to psychiatrists only.
- Only two schools planned and coordinated their substance misuse curriculum as a whole. Mostly, the teaching was concentrated in the specialty niches.
- Assessment of substance misuse within curricula was rarely planned. As 'blueprinting' against curriculum outcomes was being increasingly introduced, more formal planning in this area was expected.
- About half the schools had some provision of optional learning about substance misuse through 'student-selected components' (SSCs).

The main outcome of Phase 1 of the project was the production of a UK-wide consensus guidance document on substance misuse in the undergraduate medical curriculum and agreed by all medical schools. The document, 'Substance misuse in the undergraduate medical curriculum' set out core aims and learning outcomes for undergraduate curricula [15].

This guidance document, endorsed by the Chief Medical Officer (England) and the General Medical Council, was a milestone in medical education on substance misuse, setting out three core aims for undergraduate medical education in substance misuse that are still relevant today.

1. Students should be able to recognise, assess and understand the management of substance misuse and associated health and social problems, and contribute to the prevention of addiction.
2. Students should be aware of the effects of substance misuse on their own behaviour and health and on their professional practice and conduct.
3. Students' education and training should challenge the stigma and discrimination that are often experienced by people with addiction problems.

61.4 Substance Misuse Core Curriculum Aims and Learning Outcomes

It is acknowledged that one of the difficulties in mapping and tracking the teaching of substance misuse is that topics associated with substance misuse permeate the whole curriculum and are not simply confined to certain clinical specialties or basic science subject disciplines. In order to aid curriculum planning and integration of substance misuse topics into appropriate course areas, the outcomes have been grouped under six key areas:

1. Bio-psychosocial models of addiction
2. Professionalism and self-care
3. Clinical assessment of patients
4. Treatment interventions
5. Epidemiology, public health and society
6. Specific disease and specialty topics

The outcomes are presented as high-level outcomes, so as to make them as flexible as possible in comparing them with and applying them to the diversity of UK curricula. Each area is mapped on to the outcomes prescribed by the General Medical Council (GMC) in Tomorrow's Doctors 2003 (paragraphs 4–10), the relevant sections of which are summarised under each of the areas. Keywords are highlighted in italics within each of the learning outcomes so as to help curriculum mapping.

61.4.1 Core Topics and Learning Outcomes

1. Bio-psychosocial Models of Addiction
On graduation, students should be able to:

- Define *substance misuse*, mechanisms of dependence (both physical and psychological), tolerance, withdrawal and addictive behaviour
- Demonstrate awareness of the range of substances that can be misused; the different *types and classes of licit, illicit and over-the-counter (OTC) substances*; and other colloquial names and their effects
- Demonstrate awareness of the psychological, social and biological aspects of *dependence*; the interactions between such factors in the individual; and the different *models* used to describe addiction
- Describe the *mechanisms of tolerance, dependence and withdrawal* of different drugs and the involvement of different neurotransmitter systems

Meets GMC outcome:

- *4b – Know about, understand and be able to apply and integrate the clinical, basic, behavioural and social sciences on which medical practice is based*

2. Professionalism, Fitness to Practise and Students' Own Health

On graduation, students should be able to:

- Describe the *principles of rational prescribing* and the use of psychoactive medication
- Demonstrate *professional behaviour* towards individuals with problems of addiction, which incorporates a non-judgemental compassionate approach and respect for a patient's autonomy
- Describe the *ethical and legal issues* associated with dealing with cases of substance misuse
- Explain and outline the problems of *iatrogenic addiction*
- Describe the *risk factors* for substance misuse in medical students and in health professionals
- Describe how substance misuse problems may affect a *health professional's* judgement, performance and care of their patients
- Describe the need to balance due concern for the health of a colleague with responsibilities for the *safety and welfare of patients*
- Outline the role of the medical schools and the GMC in ensuring students and doctors' *fitness to practise*
- Describe the *sources of help* for students and doctors with drug and alcohol-related problems

Meets GMC outcomes:

- *4a (i) – Know and understand our guidance on the principles of good medical*

practice and the standards of competence, care and conduct expected of doctors in the UK.
- *4d – Recognise personal and professional limits and be willing to ask for help where necessary and recognise the duty to protect patients and others by taking action if a colleague's health, performance or conduct is putting patients at risk.*
- *5c – Be willing to respond constructively to the outcome of appraisal, performance review and assessment.*
- *10 – Graduates must be aware of the health hazards of medical practice, the importance of their own health and the effect that their health has on their ability to practise safely and effectively as a doctor.*

3. Clinical Assessment of Patients

On graduation, students should be able to:

- Describe the major *clinical features* of alcohol abuse, drug dependence and tobacco use
- Describe the possible *outcomes of different treatment regimens for substance misuse* and discuss the prognosis and management
- Take a focused drug and alcohol *history*
- Elicit signs of misuse of alcohol, tobacco and illicit or over-the-counter (OTC) drugs through *physical and mental state examinations* and identify and prioritise medical and psychosocial problems associated with substance misuse
- Demonstrate appropriate skills for communicating sensitively with patients about substance misuse issues and know how to *deal with challenging, aggressive or intoxicated patients*, balancing

assessment need with their own safety and that of others

- Appropriately order and interpret *urine, blood and other appropriate tests* for drugs of addiction; use standardised *screening and assessment instruments* to detect alcohol and drug levels; and describe other special investigations and how to interpret results
- Carry out a *psychological assessment* of a patient's readiness to implement change

Meets GMC outcomes:

- 4a(iii) – *Know about and understand how errors can happen in practice and the principles of managing risks*
- 4c – *Be able to perform clinical and practical skills safely*
- 6b – *Be able to communicate effectively with individuals and groups*
- 6c – *Understand the principles of audit and the importance of using the results of audit to improve practice*

4. Treatment Interventions
On graduation, students should be able to:

- Describe the *common treatment regimens* for various types of addictions and withdrawal states
- Describe the basis of *commonly used therapies* for addiction
- Describe the variety of UK agencies to which patients with addiction problems can be referred, and how and where to make appropriate *referrals for treatment*
- Demonstrate awareness of risk related to *needle use and disposal* for health-care workers and patients and risk prevention
- Advise a patient appropriately on *reducing or abstaining from drinking and*

smoking and list appropriate agencies or individuals to which patients can be referred to create a treatment plan

- Advise women on the effect of substance use and the impact on *foetal and maternal health*
- Demonstrate awareness of the need to assess patients' *capacity to consent* to treatment
- Describe the impact of substance misuse on *drug interactions* and a patient's compliance with treatment

Meets GMC outcomes:

- 4b – *Know about, understand and be able to apply and integrate the clinical, basic, behavioural and social sciences on which medical practice is based*
- 7a – *Know about, understand and respect the roles and expertise of other health and social care professionals*

5. Epidemiology, Public Health and Society
On graduation, students should be able to:

- Outline *UK policies* on misuse of drugs, drug prescribing and dispensing, and on alcohol and smoking
- Outline *UK legislation* controlling drugs, alcohol and tobacco, including the legal alcohol limits for driving
- Explain *hazardous and harmful levels of alcohol consumption*, and the *recommended limits for alcohol consumption*
- Outline UK *strategies for the prevention and treatment of drug misuse*
- Outline *international policies and strategies* to limit drug supply and demand
- Describe the *epidemiology* of alcohol consumption, smoking, drug misuse in the general population, vulnerable groups and specifically in doctors and other health care professionals

- Describe the problems associated with *self-medication*
- Demonstrate awareness of the risks in different *work environments* and the need for employers to have *drug and alcohol policies*
- Describe the *effects of addiction* on individuals, their families, friends and colleagues in a range of age-groups; from children and adolescents to older people
- Describe the long-term *physical, psychological and social consequences* of various types of addiction and substance misuse, including the economic consequences and the links between crime and substance misuse
- Describe the risks to the children of addicted parents, including *child protection policies* and a doctor's duty to implement these

Meets GMC outcomes:

- *4a(ii) – Know about and understand the environment in which medicine is practised in the UK*
- *4a(iii) – Know about and understand how errors can happen in practice and the principles of managing risks*
- *4b – Know about, understand and be able to apply and integrate the clinical, basic, behavioural and social sciences on which medical practice is based*
- *6c – Understand the principles of audit and the importance of using the results of audit to improve practice*

6. Specific Disease and Speciality Topics
On graduation, students should be able to:

- Recognise *life-threatening complications* of substance misuse, including septicaemia, pulmonary emboli and overdose and be able to carry out appropriate interventions
- Describe and explain the links between substance misuse and:
  - Accidents and violence (including sexual assault and sexually transmitted diseases—STDs)
  - Lung disease, specifically tobacco, 'crack' cocaine and cannabis
  - Anxiety, depression, dementia, schizophrenia
  - Acute psychotic episodes
  - Self-harm and suicide
  - Heart disease, hypertension and myocardial infarct and cocaine use
  - Liver disease, pancreatitis and gastritis
  - Infectious diseases, including human immunodeficiency virus (HIV) and hepatitis B and C virus infections

From International Centre for Drug Policy [17] *Substance Misuse in the Undergraduate Curriculum Project Report, Appendix 1.*

61.4.2 Phase 2

The second phase (2008–2011) provided a time-limited period of intensive support for the development and implementation of the new curriculum guidance into the teaching and learning opportunities of the medical schools at a local level, and into their local curriculum planning processes; promoted a self-sustaining network of all English medical schools involved in changing their curricula; and developed and validated a toolkit [16] of guidance for the effective implementation/development of substance misuse training in the undergraduate medical curriculum. A series of fact sheets, written by clinicians with in-depth knowledge of substance misuse, were produced to provide concise, relevant and up-to-date information on specific areas of substance misuse teaching. They were found to be very valuable resource since they provided a framework for developing current teaching material as well as being used as stand-alone teaching resources.

Each medical school was required to identify a local academic champion whose role was to motivate change and to supervise the work of the appointed local curriculum coordinator to implement the integration of substance misuse teaching and assessment in the undergraduate curriculum. Specifically, the role of the local curriculum development coordinators was to manage the implementation of the substance misuse Toolkit across the medical school for undergraduate education; to map and review the current curriculum compared to the guidance recommendations; and to make recommendations for implementation. These roles were supported by a national coordinator whose key task was to oversee the management of the implementation phase and work with the participating schools.

In the UK, medical education is regulated by the General Medical Council, with all school curricula being bound by the structures and demands of the key policy documents 'Tomorrow's Doctors' [8, 9]. Undergraduate medical training in the UK was comprehensively reformed, following the recommendations of 'Tomorrow's Doctors' [8, 9] and the subsequent Outcomes for Graduates [10]. Although curricula are structured differently across the participating medical schools, they all share the aims of providing high-quality medical education for students and of producing well trained and competent doctors [24].

Within the participating medical schools, a range of teaching and learning methods and corresponding range of assessment methods are used. Curricula set around a pre-clinical phase of learning (typically for 2 years), followed by a clinical phase, moving away from purely academic and theoretical studies towards more applied work. Intensive patient contact and clinical experience are used by some of the schools, whilst others use the approach of learning through a problem/case-based learning (PBL/CBL). This approach typically uses patient 'cases' or particular medical 'problems' to exemplify the learning

required of students throughout the course. These cases are likely to link to a spiral curriculum, where layers of learning, for example, around physiology, anatomy or basic science, are revisited repeatedly in increasing detail. PBL or CBL course structures are more likely to include clinical placements right from the start of the course.

In each participating medical school, the current teaching and learning of substance misuse within the undergraduate medical curriculum was identified. Coordinators undertook a mapping exercise that enabled them to construct a comprehensive overview of substance misuse teaching within their respective school, and for their findings to be aligned to the substance misuse learning outcomes from the core curriculum guidance. This process identified what was covered, not covered and what could be added to within substance misuse teaching, including areas of commonality across the schools.

Broad areas that were identified as needing more development through this process included professionalism (e.g. attitudes, values, judgement, coping with substance misuse on placements); iatrogenic addiction; fitness to practise issues; self-care; child-related issues (e.g. parenting, potential neglect, foetal and maternal health); drug policies and work environment; strategies and policies on drug use; treatments for addicts (e.g. engagement, motivation, referrals, risk-reduction strategies); sources of help for students/doctors who misuse substances; specific clinical issues (e.g. needle use, outcomes of addiction, prescribing, neurological issues, complications, drug use/types); and communication issues (including capacity to consent). It was encouraging to note that such a key topic for future public health as 'advising a patient appropriately on reducing or abstaining from drinking and smoking and implementing a treatment plan with the patient' was one of the most widely covered topics. Concurrently, student views and experiences of substance misuse teaching were gathered through surveys and focus groups in some of the participating schools. The findings from each survey were compiled, and in summary, the views of students were that they perceived substance misuse to be an important aspect of undergraduate medical education, with the teaching being comprehensive and sufficient. Overall, the bio-psychosocial aspects of addiction were covered well in teaching sessions, but more could be done regarding the clinical assessment of patients. Most of the teaching and learning was perceived to occur through independent study or via formal sessions, such as lectures or intercalation degrees.

Students perceived the teaching of alcohol, smoking and illicit drug use to be well covered; however, they felt that they could be taught more about over-the-counter drugs and prescription drug misuse. Students also recommended more teaching on how to manage addicts and about the effects of different substances when used on their own or combined. Students varied in their confidence of performing different skills with patients who misuse substances and did not feel particularly confident in taking an illicit drug history, discussing options for patients to cut down to stop alcohol or illicit drug use, and in recommending appropriate organisations which could help patients stop misusing substances.

The work during this phase enabled the changes to their curricula made by the coordinators to be delivered over a rapid timescale, and brought about important changes to the teaching and learning opportunities for future doctors. These changes addressed key recommendations that were made to improve substance misuse learning. In addition to modifying the learning outcomes, the coordinators, supported by the academic champions, introduced a range of initiatives, including new lectures and special study module components, and provided additional substance misuse resources for students to use, which supported the taught sessions. Initiatives were undertaken to raise awareness of substance misuse issues, including workshops, quizzes and working with external organisations. The toolkit and fast fact sheets that were developed across the two phases of the project were also important in providing useful materials for use in a wide variety of settings, disciplines and learning opportunities, and for integration across all years of training. These fact sheets have continued to be updated and the number of titles expanded to reflect changes such as the development of e-cigarettes, and emerging issues like gambling, and novel psychoactive substances. (https://www.addiction-ssa.org/hot-topic/factsheets/).

61.5 Opportunities and Threats

Major changes or re-structuring of curricula poses both opportunities and pitfalls for substance misuse teaching. New recommendations made during a re-structuring may build on developments to date, potentially with additional substance misuse learning opportunities, but positive changes can also fall by the wayside, especially if local enthusiasm and championing of the issue falter.

Taking new opportunities as they arise may enable sustainability. Making use of those areas of teaching which are currently 'hot topics' could be helpful, such as the question of professionalism, substance misuse by older people, teaching about emerging drugs such as novel psychoactive drugs, e-cigarettes and training in prescribing for medical cannabis. Similarly, a focus on issues of public concern, such as addiction to prescribed drugs, drug deaths, from both illicit and licit substances, might help maintain and highlight the need for substance misuse teaching to be clearly evident in the curriculum.

61.6 Evaluation

Although there was no formal evaluation of the project as it was not part of the funding, the National Steering Group for the Project decided to incorporate it within the timescale of the project as it was felt that this is an integral part of any training programme or initiative. In 2010, a small working group was established to evaluate the development, implementation and short-term outcome of the substance misuse undergraduate medical curriculum project. The views of both curriculum coordinators and academic champions were collected through interviews, questionnaires and a focus group.

The evaluation component of the project produced several recommendations concerning resources, training and sustainability:

- A core expert group/advisory panel should continue to meet on a biannual or annual basis for 2–3 years to ensure that substance misuse teaching objectives remain embedded within undergraduate curricula so that the following recommendations are actioned
- To develop a generic 1-day curriculum mapping/review training course that could be accessed online or rolled out as a package for others working on similar projects. This would be delivered on commencement of the curriculum development post
- To develop a database/resource of all SSCs and SSMs currently offered by medical schools in the area of substance misuse
- To develop a resource-sharing portal where all project resources can be collated and accessed for teaching purposes, including a core list of recommended addiction teaching and learning resources.
- To maintain and update the fact sheets
- To develop guidance on topics and questions for assessment and to provide questions for the Medical Schools Council Assessment Alliance (MSCAA) common assessment ban of questions
- To identify a 'link person' for substance misuse teaching should be identified in each participating school
- To develop specifically designed tools, such as Google desktop or Google box to assist the process of curriculum mapping. Such software might potentially be used to create a database with ability to rate content
- To ensure continuity of undergraduate substance misuse–related learning outcomes through to postgraduate education and with appropriate professional postgraduate medical education initiatives
- Relationships with Third Sector providers and other partners should be built to ensure that teaching via placements continues.
- In the light of ongoing changes to drug and alcohol service provision, medical schools should actively seek recognition of time and resources for teaching undergraduate medical students to be included within commissioning tender documents and service specifications [17].

We are well aware that the changes in the treatment policy landscape in the UK has also resulted in a reduction in addiction psychiatry services over the past decade. This has very serious implications for training since the number of specialist addiction psychiatrists, who often contribute to teaching medical students as described earlier and also provide clinical placements, has been halved [5].

A key question now, some years on from the conclusion of the major phases of the project, is how best to sustain the positive changes implemented in the teaching of substance misuse to future doctors, so that future graduating medical students continue to be better equipped to deal with substance misuse? This undoubtedly requires a group of passionate and compassionate addiction specialists who can act as lecturers, trainers, mentors, supervisors and advisors for medical students, as well as for generalist or specialist doctors and their teams. The range of medical specialties to which substance misusers present.

How will different models of learning be implemented and compared? How can substance misuse education be 'normalised' within curricula so this is not perceived as an optional extra, rather than an essential component? Who will ensure that the new emerging issues described earlier, for example, the training needed for prescription of medical cannabis, the recognition of substance use in older people, the rising numbers of alcohol- and drug-related admissions and deaths, are highlighted in the undergraduate and postgraduate medical curricula. How will post-qualification postgraduate training and continuing professional development be organised? And what about other professional groups who play a major role in the detection and treatment of addiction problems?

61.7 Conclusions

This model comprising national guidance on core curriculum content, a toolkit to aid the implementation process and which is supported with teaching resources, has the potential to be adapted and implemented in many different settings and professional disciplines such as nursing, pharmacy and psychology. It can be extended to provide in-depth specialist professional training as well as continuing professional development for general practitioners, psychiatrists and medical specialists such as physicians, obstetricians and surgeons, as well as dentists. It is eminently suitable for undergraduate, postgraduate and continuing professional training for those professional groups allied to the medical profession, including nurses, occupational therapists, social workers, psychologists and pharmacists. This model and the curriculum content provide a core learning resource for any organisation that is considering the development and implementation of a programme on substance misuse. While some components are universally applicable, some may need to be developed with the particular programme in mind. However, this gives the opportunity for some initiatives to take account of their own special circumstances and expand the resources in line with their needs.

It still seems paradoxical that given the nature and extent of addiction problems in almost every branch of medicine, it is not accepted, and therefore acceptable, that addiction training is considered a 'must have' like cancer, heart disease and diabetes rather than a possible optional extra for which a case still has to be made.

A national strategy which has direction and funding from government and coordinated support from diverse stakeholders is a valuable start. Educators with the range of clinical skills and up-to-date knowledge base are an essential element for the introduction and continuation of integration of substance misuse education into the undergraduate medical school curriculum, specialist programmes and continuing development.

61.7.1 Clinical Relevance

As substances are ubiquitous, substance problems resonate throughout virtually every medical speciality. Patients will be misusing combinations of tobacco, alcohol, prescribed and over-the-counter medications, as well as illicit drugs. Thus, they will present with overt and covert clinical symptoms and syndromes related to substance use, misuse and dependence. Without a detailed understanding of the complex interrelationships, patient care will be compromised. Hence, it is essential that medical students have a systematic knowledge of the effects, side effects, consequences and causes of substance misuse, in order that they can undertake a thorough assessment. Training in detailed history taking will lead to more accurate diagnosis, which can inform better targeted treatment. Since there are a range of effective psychological and pharmacological treatments available for the management of substance-related conditions, students need to have the opportunity to develop the skills to administer these interventions. Doctors also need to understand how the medical profession interacts with other colleagues, for example, nurses, psychologists, pharmacists, in the provision of comprehensive services for patients. Furthermore, exposure of students to collaborative working and integration of medical, social and psychological approaches within a multidisciplinary team structure can demonstrate how patients can be adequately supported to achieve the best possible outcomes. Finally, there are exciting new developments in neuroscience, and it is important that tomorrow's doctors gain a deeper appreciation of the biological basis of addiction, while not detracting from the contribution of psychosocial treatment and the role of a public health approach.

In conclusion, it is important to bring out some key points that should be taken into account:

- The use and misuse of alcohol, illicit drugs, tobacco, prescribed and over-the-counter medications are a major public health challenge facing society today. It impacts not only patients but also their families and their communities in general.

- Those who suffer physical, psychological and social harms as a result of misuse of substances will almost certainly be seen by doctors and their teams at some stage. Therefore, the medical profession has a vital role to play in the recognition, assessment and management of problems associated with substance misuse.

- However, the changes in commissioning addiction treatment services to organisations which are not part of the National Health Service, as well as the significant reduction in funding for treatment facilities, have implications far beyond the implementation of interventions. It threatens the provision of appropriate high-quality teaching and training for future medical students and trainee doctors in the numerous specialties to which patients with substance problems present.

- If health professionals are to succeed in dealing with the problem of substance abuse, they require a systematic training so that they have better understanding of the nature and complexity of the problems associated with substance misuse as well as the interventions which are available.

- They need to be continually updated as new scientific developments emerge and debate some controversial issues, which have recently surfaced, such as the use of medical cannabis, vaping cigarettes and other substances, and the misuse of prescribed medication, for example, gabapentinoids.

- Thus, a sustainable strategy, which sees as its core aim for medical education that medical students have the skills and knowledge to effectively manage substance misuse when they meet it, needs to be outlined and realised.

- Ensuring financial assistance for qualified staff to support implementation of the new curriculum at a local level has contributed to improvements in the extent and quality of teaching on substance misuse issues. This depends on high-level support within medical schools and at governmental level so that the programme can be initiated, maintained and evaluated so it becomes a salient component of the undergraduate medical course.

References

1. ASH Tobacco Economics Factsheet. 2017. Retrieved from http://ash.org.uk/category/information-and-resources/fact-sheets/.
2. Barber S, Harker R, Pratt A. Human and financial costs of drug addiction, House of Commons Library Debate Pack Number CDP-0230, 21 November 2017.
3. Crome I. The trouble with training; substance misuse in British Medical Schools revisited. What are the issues? Drug-Educ Prev Policy. 1999;6(1):111–23. https://doi.org/10.1080/09687639997331.
4. Crome IB, Sheikh N. Undergraduate medical school education in substance misuse in Britain iii: can medical students drive change? Drugs Educ Prev Policy. 2004;11(6):483–503. https://doi.org/10.1080/0968763041000170132.
5. Drummond. Cuts to addiction services are a false economy. BMJ. 2017;357:j2704. https://doi.org/10.1136/bmj.j2704.
6. Falkowski J, Ghodse AH. An international survey of the educational activities of schools nursing on psychoactive drugs. Bull World Health Organ. 1990;68(4):479–82.
7. Falkowski J, Ghodse AH. Undergraduate Medical School Training in Psychoactive drugs and Rational Prescribing in the United Kingdom. Br J Addict. 1989;84:1539–42. https://doi.org/10.1111/j.1360-0443.1989.tb03937.x.
8. General Medical Council. Tomorrow's doctors: recommendations on undergraduate medical education. 2003. Retrieved from https://www.educaionmedica.net/pdf/documentos/modelos/tomorrowdoc.pdf.
9. General Medical Council. Tomorrow's doctors: outcomes and standards for undergraduate medical education. 2009. Retrieved from http://www.ub.edu/medicina_unitateducaciomedica/documentos/TomorrowsDoctors_2009.pdf.
10. General Medical Council. Outcomes for graduates. 2015. Retrieved from https://www.gmc-uk.org/education/undergraduate/undergrad_outcomes.asp.
11. Ghodse AH. Report of the WHO meeting on Nursing Midwifery. Education in the rational use of psychoactive drugs, Islamabad 7–11 Aug 1989.
12. Glass IB. Undergraduate training in substance abuse in the United Kingdom. Br J Addict. 1989;84(2):197–202. https://doi.org/10.1111/j.1360-0443.1989.tb00569.x.

13. Goodair C, Crome I. Improving the landscape of substance misuse teaching in undergraduate medical education in english medical schools from concept to implementation. Can J. Addict. 2014;5(3):5–10. Special Education Issue.

14. The Guardian. Alcohol and the NHS - five key questions. 2016. Retrieved from https://www.theguardian.com/news/datablog/2016/jan/22/alcohol-and-the-nhs-five-key-questions.

15. International Centre for Drug Policy. Substance misuse in the undergraduate curriculum. 2007. Retrieved from https://www.sgul.ac.uk/research/population-health/our-projects/substance-misuse-in-the-undergraduate-medical-curriculum.

16. International Centre for Drug Policy. Substance misuse in the undergraduate curriculum: a toolkit for teaching and learning. 2011. Retrieved from https://www.sgul.ac.uk/images/docs/idcp%20pdfs/Substance%20misuse%20in%20the%20undergrad%20medical%20curiculum/ToolkitFinalVersion14Aug12CG.pdf.

17. International Centre for Drug Policy. Substance misuse in the undergraduate curriculum project report. 2012. Retrieved from https://www.sgul.ac.uk/research/population-health/our-projects/substance-misuse-in-the-undergraduate-medical-curriculum.

18. International Narcotics Control Board. Annex IV Letter from the President of the International Narcotics control Board to all countries. Report of the International Narcotics Control Board on the Availability of Internationally Controlled Drugs: Ensuring Adequate Access for Medical and Scientific Purposes. New York: United Nations, p. 73–4. 2010. Retrieved from http://www.incb.org/incb/en/publications/annual-reports/annual-report-2001-2010.html.

19. International Narcotics Control Board. Europe National legislation, policy and action paragraph 699. Report of the International Narcotics Control Board 2009. New York: United Nations, p. 109. 2010. Retrieved from http://www.incb.org/incb/en/publications/annual-reports/annual-report-2009.htm.

20. NHS Digital. Statistics on smoking - England, 2018. Retrieved from https://digital.nhs.uk/data-and-information/publications/statistical/statistics-on-smoking/statistics-on-smoking-england-2018/part-1-smoking-related-ill-health-and-mortality.

21. NHS Digital. Statistics on drug misuse, England, 2018 (November update). Retrieved from https://digital.nhs.uk/data-and-information/publications/statistical/statistics-on-drug-misuse/november-2018-update.

22. National Statistics. Drug misuse: findings from the 2017 to 2018 CSEW. 2018. Retrieved from https://www.gov.uk/government/statistics/drug-misuse-findings-from-the-2017-to-2018-csew.

23. NHS Digital. Statistics on alcohol, England 2019. Retrieved from https://digital.nhs.uk/data-and-information/publications/statistical/statistics-on-alcohol/2019/part-2.

24. Royal College of Psychiatrists (2018). CR211: Our Invisible Addicts. Royal College of Psychiatrists, London.

25. World Health Organization, United Nations Fund for Drug Abuse Control. Role of schools of pharmacy in the rational use of psychoactive drugs: report from a national seminar in Chengdu, People's Republic of China, in December, 1988.